Diversified Health Occupations

Diversified Health Occupations

Sixth Edition

Louise Simmers, M.Ed., R.N.

THOMSON

DELMAR LEARNING™

Australia   Canada   Mexico   Singapore   Spain   United   Kingdom   United States

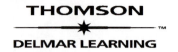

Diversified Health Occupations, Sixth Edition
Louise Simmers

Executive Director:
William Brottmiller

Executive Editor:
Cathy L. Esperti

Acquisitions Editor:
Sherry Gomoll

Developmental Editor:
Marah Bellegarde

Executive Marketing Manager:
Dawn F. Gerrain

Channel Manager:
Jennifer McAvey

Editorial Assistant:
Jennifer Conklin

Art/Design Coordinator:
Connie Lundberg-Watkins

Project Editor:
Bryan Viggiani

Production Editor:
Anne Sherman

Technology Production Coordinator:
Sherry Conners

Library of Congress Cataloging-in-Publication Data
Simmers, Louise.
    Diversified health occupations / Louise Simmers. -- 6th ed.
        p. cm.
Includes bibliographical references and index.
ISBN-13: 978-1-4018-1456-4
ISBN-10: 1-4018-1456-5
    1. Allied health personnel -- Vocational guidance.
I. Title.
        R697.A4S5 2003
        610.69--dc21
                                                2002041716

International Divisions List

Asia (Including India):
Thomson Learning
60 Albert Street, #15-01
Albert Complex
Singapore 189969
Tel 65 336-6411
Fax 65 336-7411

Australia/New Zealand:
Nelson
102 Dodds Street
South Melbourne
Victoria 3205
Australia
Tel 61 (0)3 9685-4111
Fax 61 (0)3 9685-4199

Latin America:
Thomson Learning
Seneca 53
Colonia Polanco
11560 Mexico, D.F. Mexico
Tel (525) 281-2906
Fax (525) 281-2656

Canada:
Nelson
1120 Birchmount Road
Toronto, Ontario
Canada M1K 5G4
Tel (416) 752-9100
Fax (416) 752-8102

UK/Europe/Middle East/Africa:
Thomson Learning
Berkshire House
1680-173 High Holborn
London WC1V 7AA
United Kingdom
Tel 44 (0)20 497-1422
Fax 44 (0)20 497-1426

Spain (includes Portugal):
Paraninfo
Calle Magallanes 25
28015 Madrid
España
Tel 34 (0)91 446-3350
Fax 34 (0)91 445-6218

NOTICE TO THE READER

Contents

Preface xii

How to Use Text xvi

Acknowledgments xviii

PART 1

Basic Health Care Concepts and Skills **xx**

UNIT 1
Health Care Systems **2**

Objectives	2
Key Terms	3
1:1 History of Health Care	3
1:2 Private Health Care Facilities	8
1:3 Government Agencies	11
1:4 Voluntary or Nonprofit Agencies	11
1:5 Health Insurance Plans	12
1:6 Organizational Structure	13
1:7 Trends in Health Care	15
Summary	22
Internet Searches	22
Review Questions	23
Suggested References	23

UNIT 2
Careers in Health Care **25**

Objectives	25
Key Terms	26
2:1 Introduction to Health Careers	27
2:2 Dental Careers	30
2:3 Diagnostic Services	32
2:4 Emergency Medical Services	36
2:5 Health Information and Communication Services	38
2:6 Hospital/Health Care Facility Services	40
2:7 Medical Careers	41
2:8 Mental and Social Services	43
2:9 Mortuary Careers	45
2:10 Nursing Careers	46
2:11 Nutrition and Dietary Services	48
2:12 Therapeutic Services	49
2:13 Veterinary Careers	55
2:14 Vision Services	56
Summary	57
Internet Searches	58
Review Questions	58
Suggested References	58

UNIT 3
Personal Qualities of a Health Care Worker **60**

Objectives	60
Key Terms	61
3:1 Personal Appearance	61
3:2 Personal Characteristics	63
3:3 Teamwork	65
3:4 Professional Leadership	66
3:5 Stress	67
3:6 Time Management	69
Summary	71
Internet Searches	72
Review Questions	72
Suggested References	72

UNIT 4
Legal and Ethical Responsibilities   74

Objectives	74
Key Terms	75
4:1 Legal Responsibilities	75
4:2 Ethics	79
4:3 Patients' Rights	80
4:4 Advance Directives for Health Care	81
4:5 Professional Standards	83
Summary	85
Internet Searches	85
Review Questions	86
Suggested References	86

UNIT 5
Medical Terminology   87

Objectives	87
Key Terms	88
5:1 Using Medical Abbreviations	88
5:2 Interpreting Word Parts	95
Summary	100
Internet Searches	101
Review Questions	101
Suggested References	101

UNIT 6
Anatomy and Physiology   102

Objectives	102
6:1 Basic Structure of the Human Body	103
6:2 Body Planes, Directions, and Cavities	110
6:3 Integumentary System	113
6:4 Skeletal System	117
6:5 Muscular System	124
6:6 Nervous System	128
6:7 Special Senses	135
6:8 Circulatory System	141
6:9 Lymphatic System	152
6:10 Respiratory System	155
6:11 Digestive System	161
6:12 Urinary System	167
6:13 Endocrine System	172
6:14 Reproductive System	177
Summary	186
Internet Searches	186
Review Questions	186
Suggested References	187

UNIT 7
Human Growth and Development   188

Objectives	188
Key Terms	189
7:1 Life Stages	189
7:2 Death and Dying	199
7:3 Human Needs	201
7:4 Effective Communications	206
Summary	212
Internet Searches	213
Review Questions	213
Suggested References	214

UNIT 8
Cultural Diversity   215

Objectives	215
Key Terms	216
8:1 Culture, Ethnicity, and Race	216
8:2 Bias, Prejudice, and Stereotyping	218
8:3 Understanding Cultural Diversity	219
8:4 Respecting Cultural Diversity	230
Summary	230
Internet Searches	231
Review Questions	231
Suggested References	232

UNIT 9
Geriatric Care   233

Objectives	234
Key Terms	234
9:1 Myths on Aging	234
9:2 Physical Changes of Aging	236
9:3 Psychosocial Changes of Aging	242
9:4 Confusion and Disorientation in the Elderly	245
9:5 Meeting the Needs of the Elderly	248
Summary	250
Internet Searches	250
Review Questions	250
Suggested References	251

UNIT 10
Nutrition and Diets — 252

Objectives	252
Key Terms	253
10:1 Fundamentals of Nutrition	253
10:2 Essential Nutrients	254
10:3 Utilization of Nutrients	258
10:4 Maintenance of Good Nutrition	259
10:5 Therapeutic Diets	261
Summary	265
Internet Searches	265
Review Questions	265
Suggested References	266

UNIT 11
Computers in Health Care — 267

Objectives	267
Key Terms	268
11:1 Introduction	268
11:2 What is a Computer System?	269
11:3 Computer Applications	271
11:4 Using the Internet	278
Summary	280
Internet Searches	280
Review Questions	280
Suggested References	281

UNIT 12
Promotion of Safety — 282

Objectives	282
Key Terms	283
12:1 Using Body Mechanics	283
12:2 Preventing Accidents and Injuries	285
12:3 Observing Fire Safety	291
Summary	295
Internet Searches	295
Review Questions	296
Suggested References	296

UNIT 13
Infection Control — 297

Objectives	297
Key Terms	298
13:1 Understanding the Principles of Infection Control	298
13:2 Washing Hands	303
13:3 Observing Standard Precautions	306
13:4 Sterilizing with an Autoclave	314
A: Wrapping Items for Autoclaving	316
B: Loading and Operating an Autoclave	319
13:5 Using Chemicals for Disinfection	321
13:6 Cleaning with an Ultrasonic Unit	323
13:7 Using Sterile Techniques	326
A: Opening Sterile Packages	328
B: Preparing a Sterile Dressing Tray	330
C: Donning and Removing Sterile Gloves	332
D: Changing a Sterile Dressing	334
13:8 Maintaining Transmission-Based Isolation Precautions	336
A: Donning and Removing Transmission-Based Isolation Garments	341
B: Working in a Hospital Transmission-Based Isolation Unit	344
Summary	346
Internet Searches	346
Review Questions	347
Suggested References	347

UNIT 14
Vital Signs — 348

Objectives	348
Key Terms	349
14:1 Measuring and Recording Vital Signs	349
14:2 Measuring and Recording Temperature	351
A: Cleaning a Clinical Thermometer	355
B: Measuring and Recording Oral Temperature	356
C: Measuring and Recording Rectal Temperature	358
D: Measuring and Recording Axillary Temperature	359
E: Measuring and Recording Tympanic (Aural) Temperature	360
F: Measuring Temperature with an Electronic Thermometer	362
14:3 Measuring and Recording Pulse	363
14:4 Measuring and Recording Respirations	365
14:5 Graphing TPR	367
14:6 Measuring and Recording Apical Pulse	369
14:7 Measuring and Recording Blood Pressure	372
Summary	376
Internet Searches	377
Review Questions	377
Suggested References	377

UNIT 15
First Aid   378

Objectives   378
Key Terms   379
15:1   Providing First Aid   379
15:2   Performing Cardiopulmonary
      Resuscitation   382
      A: Performing CPR—One-Person
         Rescue   387
      B: Performing CPR—Two-Person
         Rescue   390
      C and D: Performing CPR on Infants
         and Children   392
      E: Performing CPR—Obstructed
         Airway on Conscious, Adult Victim   394
      F: Performing CPR—Obstructed
         Airway on Unconscious Victim   395
15:3   Providing First Aid for Bleeding
      and Wounds   398
15:4   Providing First Aid for Shock   403
15:5   Providing First Aid for Poisoning   406
15:6   Providing First Aid for Burns   410
15:7   Providing First Aid for Heat Exposure   415
15:8   Providing First Aid for Cold Exposure   417
15:9   Providing First Aid for Bone
      and Joint Injuries   419
15:10 Providing First Aid for Specific Injuries   425
15:11 Providing First Aid for Sudden Illness   432
15:12 Applying Dressings and Bandages   437
Summary   443
Internet Searches   443
Review Questions   443
Suggested References   443

UNIT 16
Preparing for the World of Work   445

Objectives   445
Key Terms   446
16:1   Developing Job-Keeping Skills   446
16:2   Writing a Letter of Application
      and Preparing a Resumé   448
16:3   Completing Job Application Forms   454
16:4   Participating in a Job Interview   456
16:5   Determining Net Income   460
16:6   Calculating a Budge   462
Summary   464
Internet Searches   464
Review Questions   464
Suggested References   465

PART 2:
Special Health Care Skills   466

UNIT 17
Dental Assistant Skills   468

Objectives   468
Key Terms   469
Career Highlight   470
17:1   Identifying the Structures
      and Tissues of a Tooth   470
17:2   Identifying the Teeth   474
17:3   Identifying Teeth by Using the Universal
      Numbering System and the Federation
      Dentaire International System   476
      A: Identifying Teeth Using the
         Universal Numbering System   479
      B: Identifying Teeth Using the
         Federation Dentaire International
         System   480
17:4   Identifying the Surfaces of the Teeth   481
17:5   Charting Conditions of the Teeth   483
17:6   Operating and Maintaining Dental
      Equipment   489
17:7   Identifying Dental Instruments
      and Preparing Dental Trays   498
17:8   Positioning a Patient in the Dental Chair   505
17:9   Demonstrating Brushing and Flossing
      Techniques   507
      A: Demonstrating Brushing Technique   508
      B: Demonstrating Flossing Technique   509
17:10 Taking Impressions and Pouring Models   510
      A: Preparing Alginate   513
      B: Preparing Rubber Base (Polysulfide)   515
      C: Pouring a Plaster Model   517
      D: Pouring a Stone Model   520
      E: Trimming a Model   521
17:11 Making Custom Trays   522
17:12 Maintaining and Loading an Anesthetic
      Aspirating Syringe   524
      A: Maintaining an Anesthetic Aspirating
         Syringe   527
      B: Loading an Anesthetic Aspirating
         Syringe   528
17:13 Mixing Dental Cements and Bases   529
      A: Preparing Varnish   530
      B: Preparing Calcium Hydroxide   532
      C: Preparing Carboxylate   533
      D: Preparing Zinc Oxide Eugenol (ZOE)   534

17:14 Preparing Restorative Materials—
Amalgam and Composite 535
A: Preparing Amalgam 538
B: Preparing Composite 539
17:15 Developing and Mounting
Dental X-Rays 541
A: Developing Dental X-Rays 544
B: Mounting Dental X-Rays 546
Summary 547
Internet Searches 547
Review Questions 547
Suggested References 548

UNIT 18
Laboratory Assistant Skills 550

Objectives 550
Key Terms 551
Career Highlight 551
18:1 Operating the Microscope 553
18:2 Obtaining and Handling Cultures 557
A: Obtaining a Culture Specimen 559
B: Preparing a Direct Smear 561
C: Streaking an Agar Plate 562
D: Transferring Culture from Agar
Plate to Slide 564
E: Staining with Gram's Stain 565
18:3 Puncturing the Skin to Obtain
Capillary Blood 567
18:4 Performing a Microhematocrit 570
18:5 Measuring Hemoglobin 574
A: Measuring Hemoglobin with a
Hemoglobinometer 575
B: Measuring Hemoglobin with
a Photometer 577
18:6 Counting Blood Cells 579
A: Counting Erythrocytes 582
B: Counting Leukocytes 585
18:7 Preparing and Staining a Blood Film
or Smear 587
A: Preparing a Blood Film or Smear 588
B: Staining a Blood Film or Smear 590
18:8 Testing for Blood Types 591
18:9 Performing an Erythrocyte
Sedimentation Rate 595
18:10 Measuring Blood-Sugar (Glucose) Level 598
18:11 Testing Urine 602
18:12 Using Reagent Strips to Test Urine 602
18:13 Measuring Specific Gravity 607
18:14 Preparing Urine for Microscopic
Examination 610

Summary 613
Internet Searches 614
Review Questions 614
Suggested References 614

UNIT 19
Medical Assistant Skills 616

Objectives 616
Key Terms 617
Career Highlight 617
19:1 Measuring/Recording Height
and Weight 618
A: Measuring/Recording Height
and Weight 621
B: Measuring/Recording Height
and Weight of an Infant 623
19:2 Positioning a Patient 625
19:3 Screening for Vision Problems 630
19:4 Assisting with Physical Examinations 634
A: Eye, Ear, Nose, and Throat
Examination 637
B: Assisting with a Gynecological
Examination 638
C: Assisting with a General Physical
Examination 640
19:5 Assisting with Minor Surgery and Suture
Removal 642
A: Assisting with Minor Surgery 644
B: Assisting with Suture Removal 646
19:6 Recording and Mounting an
Electrocardiogram 647
19:7 Using the *Physicians' Desk
Reference* (PDR) 658
19:8 Working with Math and Medications 660
A: Using Roman Numerals 663
B: Converting Metric Measurements 663
C: Converting Household (English)
Measurements 665
Summary 666
Internet Searches 666
Review Questions 667
Suggested References 667

UNIT 20
Nurse Assistant Skills 669

Objectives 669
Key Terms 670
Career Highlight 670

20:1 Admitting, Transferring, and Discharging
      Patients   672
      A: Admitting the Patient   674
      B: Transferring the Patient   676
      C: Discharging the Patient   677
20:2 Positioning, Turning, Moving,
      and Transferring Patients   679
      A: Aligning the Patient   682
      B: Moving the Patient Up in Bed   684
      C: Turning the Patient Away to Change
         Position   686
      D: Turning the Patient Inward to Change
         Position   687
      E: Sitting Up to Dangle   689
      F: Transferring a Patient to a Chair or
         Wheelchair   690
      G: Transferring a Patient to a Stretcher   693
      H: Using a Mechanical Lift to Transfer
         a Patient   695
20:3 Bedmaking   698
      A: Making a Closed Bed   699
      B: Making an Occupied Bed   702
      C: Opening a Closed Bed   705
      D: Placing a Bed Cradle   706
20:4 Administering Personal Hygiene   707
      A: Providing Routine Oral Hygiene   710
      B: Cleaning Dentures   712
      C: Giving Special Mouth Care   713
      D: Administering Daily Hair Care   715
      E: Providing Nail Care   716
      F: Giving a Backrub   717
      G: Shaving a Patient   719
      H: Changing a Patient's Gown or Pajamas   721
      I: Giving a Complete Bed Bath / 723
      J: Helping a Patient Take a Tub Bath
         or Shower   727
20:5 Measuring and Recording Intake
      and Output   728
20:6 Feeding a Patient   734
20:7 Assisting with a Bedpan/Urinal   737
      A: Assisting with a Bedpan   739
      B: Assisting with a Urinal   741
20:8 Providing Catheter and
      Urinary-Drainage-Unit Care   742
      A: Providing Catheter Care   745
      B: Emptying a Urinary-Drainage Unit   747
20:9 Providing Ostomy Care   748
20:10 Collecting Stool/Urine Specimens   752
      A: Collecting a Routine Urine Specimen   756
      B: Collecting a Midstream Urine Specimen   757
      C: Collecting a 24-Hour Urine Specimen   759

      D: Collecting a Stool Specimen   760
      E: Preparing and Testing a
         Hemoccult Slide   761
20:11 Enemas and Rectal Treatments   763
      A: Giving a Tap-Water or Soap-Solution
         Enema   764
      B: Giving a Disposable Enema   767
      C: Giving an Oil Retention Enema   769
      D: Inserting a Rectal Tube   770
20:12 Applying Restraints   772
      A: Applying Limb Restraints   774
      B: Applying a Jacket Restraint   775
20:13 Administering Pre- and Postoperative Care 777
      A: Shaving the Operative Area   781
      B: Administering Preoperative Care   783
      C: Preparing a Postoperative Unit   784
      D: Applying Surgical Hose   785
20:14 Applying Binders   787
20:15 Administering Oxygen   789
20:16 Giving Postmortem Care   794
Summary   796
Internet Searches   797
Review Questions   797
Suggested References   797

UNIT 21
Physical Therapy Skills   **799**

Objectives   799
Key Terms   800
Career Highlight   800
21:1 Performing Range-of-Motion (ROM)
      Exercises   801
21:2 Ambulating Patients Who Use
      Transfer (Gait) Belts, Crutches,
      Canes, or Walkers   808
      A: Ambulating a Patient with a
         Transfer (Gait) Belt   813
      B: Ambulating a Patient Who Uses
         Crutches   815
      C: Ambulating a Patient Who Uses
         a Cane   818
      D: Ambulating a Patient Who Uses
         a Walker   819
21:3 Administering Heat/Cold Applications   821
      A: Applying an Ice Bag or Ice Collar   823
      B: Applying a Warm-Water Bag   825
      C: Applying an Aquamatic Pad   827
      D: Applying a Moist Compress   828
      E: Administering a Sitz Bath   830

Summary   832
Internet Searches   832
Review Questions   832
Suggested References   833

UNIT 22
Business and
Accounting Skills   834

Objectives   834
Key Terms   835
22:1   Filing Records   835
22:2   Using the Telephone   842
22:3   Scheduling Appointments   847
22:4   Completing Medical Records
       and Forms   850
22:5   Composing Business Letters   856
22:6   Completing Insurance Forms   862
22:7   Maintaining a Bookkeeping System   868

22:8   Writing Checks, Deposit Slips,
       and Receipts   873
       A: Writing Checks   876
       B: Writing Deposit Slips   878
       C: Writing Receipts   879
Summary   880
Internet Searches   880
Review Questions   881
Suggested References   881

Appendix A: Career and Technology
             Student Organizations   883

Appendix B: Metric Conversion Charts   887

Appendix C: 24-Hour Clock (Military
             Time) Conversion Chart   889

Glossary   890

Index   911

Preface

Diversified Health Occupations, 6th edition was written to provide the beginning student in health occupations with the basic entry-level knowledge and skills required for a variety of health occupations. Although each specific health occupation requires specialized knowledge and skills, some knowledge and skills are applicable to many different health occupations. In short, this book was developed to provide some of the core knowledge and skills that can be used in several different fields.

ORGANIZATION OF TEXT

Diversified Health Occupations is divided into two main parts. Part 1 provides the student with the basic knowledge and skills required for many different health occupations. Part 2 introduces the student to basic entry-level skills required for some specific health occupations. Each part is subdivided into units.

Unit Organization

Each unit has a list of objectives, key terms (with pronunciations for more difficult words), and a list of suggested references and resources from which the student can obtain additional information. For each skill included in the text, both the knowledge necessary for the skill and the procedure to perform the skill are provided. By understanding the principles and the procedure, the student will develop a deeper understanding of why certain things are done and will be able to perform more competently. Procedures may vary slightly depending on the type of agency and on the kind of equipment and supplies used. By understanding the underlying principles, however, the student can adapt the procedure as necessary and still observe correct technique.

Information Sections (Textbook): The information sections provide the basic knowledge the student must acquire. These sections explain why the knowledge is important, the basic facts regarding the particular topic, and how this information is applied in various health careers. Most information sections refer the student to the assignment sheets found in the student workbook.

Assignment Sheets (Workbook): After students have read an information section, they are instructed to go to the corresponding assignment sheet. The assignment sheets allow them to test their comprehension and to return to the information section to check their answers. This enables them to reinforce their understanding prior to moving on to another information section.

Procedure Sections (Textbook): The procedure sections provide step-by-step instructions on how to perform specific procedures. The student follows the steps while practicing the procedures. Each procedure begins with a list of the necessary equipment and supplies. *Note, Caution,* and *Checkpoint* may appear within the procedure. **Note** urges careful reading of the comments that follow. These comments usually stress points of knowledge or explain why certain techniques are used. **Caution** indicates that a safety factor is involved and that students should proceed carefully while doing the step in order to avoid injuring themselves or a patient. **Checkpoint** alerts students to ask the instructor to check their work at that point in the procedure. Checkpoints are usually located at a critical stage. Each procedure section refers the student to a specific evaluation sheet in the workbook.

Evaluation Sheets (Workbook): Each evaluation sheet contains a list of criteria on which the students will be tested after they have mastered a particular procedure. When a student feels he or she has mastered a particular procedure, he or she signs the evaluation sheet and gives it to the instructor. The instructor can grade the student by using the listed criteria and checking each step against actual performance.

 Because regulations vary from state to state regarding which procedures can be performed by a student in health occupations, it is important to check the specific regulations for your state. A health occupation worker should never perform any procedure without checking legal responsibilities. In addition, a student should perform no procedure unless the student has been properly taught the procedure and has been authorized to perform it.

Added Features:

◆ More than 100 new photos and illustrations have been added to enhance learning and clarify technical content.

◆ The text material covers the *National Health Care Skill Standards,* helping instructors implement the curriculum elements of this important document.

◆ Internet search topics have been added at the end of each unit to encourage the student to explore the Internet to obtain current information on the many aspects of health care.

◆ Review questions have been added to the end of each unit to enable the student to test his or her knowledge of information provided in the unit.

◆ Career information has been updated and is stressed throughout the textbook to provide current information on a wide variety of health care careers.

◆ Additional emphasis has been placed on dealing with cultural diversity, technological advances, legal responsibilities, new federal legislation pertaining to health care providers, infection control standards, and safety.

◆ Various icons have been included throughout the textbook. These icons denote the integration of academics, such as math, science, and communication; occupational safety issues, such as standard precautions, and OBRA requirements; and workplace readiness issues such as career, legal, and technology information. An icon key similar to the one below can be found on the opening page of every unit. The icons and their meaning are as follows:

 Observe Standard Precautions

 Safety—Proceed with Caution

 Math Skill

 Science Skill

 Communications Skill

 Instructors Check—Call Instructor at This Point

 OBRA Requirement—Based on Federal Law

 Legal Responsibility

 Career Information

 Technology

Enhanced Content:

◆ Vital, updated information on standard precautions, OBRA requirements, and transmission-based isolation techniques have been included.

◆ A new section on teamwork describes the basic principles of a health care team, benefits of teamwork, personal qualities needed by each team member, and ways to solve conflicts that may occur.

◆ A new section on professional leadership describes the qualities of a leader, the three main types of leaders, and how to be an effective leader.

◆ A new section on stress describes the body's response to stress, how to recognize and deal with stressors, how to use problem-solving techniques, and ways to decrease or prevent stress.

◆ A new section on time management discusses why it is important, how to set both short- and long-term goals, ways to effectively manage time, and how to establish a time management system.

◆ A new section on Internet searches explains how search engines work, discusses many of the current search engines in use, and describes effective ways to conduct searches.

EXTENSIVE TEACHING AND LEARNING PACKAGE

Diversified Health Occupations, 6th Edition, has a complete and specially designed supplement package to enhance student learning and workplace preparation. It is also designed to assist instructors in planning and implementing their instructional programs for the most efficient use of time and resources. The package contains:

Diversified Health Occupations, 6e Electronic Book

Order # 140181462X

The entire *Diversified Health Occupations,* 6e is now offered in electronic format. Available on-line in PDF form for easy download.

Diversified Health Occupations Teacher's Resource Kit

Order # 1401814603

A complete guide to implementing a *Diversified Health Occupations* course. The kit explains how to apply content to applied academics and the *National Health Care Skill Standards.* It also provides

◆ Classroom management activities

◆ Lesson Plans

◆ Various Testing Materials

◆ Classroom Activities

◆ Internet Activities

◆ Leadership-Development Activities

◆ A computerized testbank on CD containing over 1,800 modifiable questions and answers.

◆ Delmar Learning's Medical Terminology Image Library, 2nd edition – Over 500 images, including full-color photographs, anatomic art, and line illustrations, that can be viewed directly off the CD-ROM, pasted into a presentation software program, or used to create color transparencies.

◆ Anatomy and Physiology Transparency Masters to reinforce learning in a visual format.

Diversified Health Occupations Electronic Teacher's Resource Kit

Order # 1401814654

An electronic version of the printed Teacher's Resource Kit is now available on-line. Same great content, just in electronic form.

Diversified Health Occupations, 6th edition, Computerized Testbank

Order # 140181459X

A computerized testbank on CD now with over *1,800 modifiable test questions.* The user can also add his/her own questions. This software allows the user to create tests in less than 5 minutes with the ability to print them out in a variety of layouts. Has electronic "take-home testing" (put test on disk) and Internet-based testing capabilities. Additionally, the software allows the user to include multimedia into the electronic tests (video, audio).

Diversified Health Occupations, 6th edition, Student Workbook

Order # 1401814573

This workbook, updated to reflect the *Diversified Health Occupations,* 6th edition text, contains perforated, performance-based assignment and evaluation sheets. The assignment sheets help students review what they have learned. The evaluation sheets provide criteria or standards for judging student performance for each procedure in the text.

WebTutor to Accompany Diversified Health Occupations, 6e

Web CT version: Order # 1401814638
Blackboard version: Order # 1401814646

WebTutor is an Internet-based course management and delivery system designed to accompany the text. Its content is available for use in either WebCT or Blackboard. Available to supplement on-site delivery or as the course management platform for an on-line course, WebTutor contains:

◆ Threaded discussion topics

◆ Weblinks which offer links to other sites that contain additional information pertinent to topics being discussed

◆ Learning Links which offer students a short assignment using the Internet

◆ Flashcards for review of key terms

◆ On-line quizzes for each chapter

◆ Plus a host of other great features.

Visit **e.thomsonlearning.com** to find out more.

Diversified Health Occupations, 6th edition, Activity Software

Order # 1401814611

This game software allows students to assess their health occupations knowledge in a self-paced, non-competitive environment, against the clock, or in a team setting. It features over 800 questions in the following formats: multiple choice, labeling, fill-in-the-blank, crossword puzzles, concentration, and hangman. This activity software can be used in the classroom, in a computer lab, or at home.

Diversified Health Occupations, 6th edition, Instructor's Manual

Order # 1401814581

Provides easy-to-find answers to questions found in the *student workbook*.

Diversified Health Occupations Video Series

A set of four videos that correlate to the text. The videos present career- and workplace-readiness issues.

Complete Video Package

Order # 082737982X

Video 1: Is a Career in Health Care for You? **Order # 0827382766;** Video 2: A Day in the Life of Health Care Services, **Order # 0827382774;** Video 3: Professional and Personal Standards for Health Care Careers, **Order # 0827382782;** Video 4: How to Succeed in Your Health Care Career, **Order # 0827382790.**

Electronic Versions

Want to go paperless? Delmar Learning has the solution for you. The following products are now available in an electronic format.

Diversified Health Occupations, 6th edition E-Book
Order # 140181462X

Diversified Health Occupations, 6th edition Electronic Teachers Resource Kit
Order # 1401814654

Computerized Testbank to Accompany Diversified Health Occupations, 6th edition
Order # 140181459X

WebTutor to Accompany Diversified Health Occupations, 6e
Web CT version: Order # 1401814638
Blackboard version: Order # 1410814646

Activity Software to Accompany Diversified Health Occupations, 6e
Order # 1401814611

About the Author

Louise Simmers received a B.S. in nursing from the University of Maryland and an M.Ed. in Vocational Education from Kent State University. She has worked as a public health nurse, medical-surgical nurse, charge nurse in a coronary-intensive care unit, instructor of practical nursing, and health occupations teacher and school-to-work coordinator at the Madison Comprehensive High School in Mansfield, OH. She is a member of the University of Maryland Nursing Alumni Association, Sigma Theta Tau, Phi Kappa Phi, National Education Association, and American Vocational Association, and is a volunteer worker for the Richland County Red Cross. As an active member of the Health Occupations Division of the Ohio Vocational Association, Ms. Simmers has served on numerous committees and was elected to serve as president of this organization for 1982–1983. In 1980, she received the Vocational Educator of the Year Award for Health Occupations in the State of Ohio and in 1990, she received the Diversified Health Occupations Instructor of the Year Award for the State of Ohio.

How to Use

Objectives

Objectives. Review this series of goals before you begin reading a chapter to help you focus your study. Then, when you have completed the chapter, go back and review these goals to see if you have grasped the key points of the chapter.

Icons

Icons are used throughout the text to highlight specific pieces of information. This **icon key** is presented to reinforce the meaning of the icons so when you see the icons used in text you will "understand what they stand for.

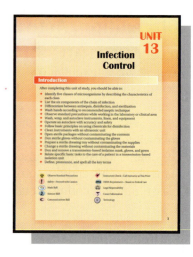

Key Terms

Key Terms highlight the critical vocabulary words you will need to learn. Pronunciations are also included for the harder-to-pronounce words. These terms are highlighted within the text where they are defined. You will also find these terms listed in the glossary section. Use this listing as part of your study and review of critical terms.

Career Highlights

Career Highlights appear in Special Health Care Skills units. By reading and understanding the material presented in these boxes, you will learn the educational requirements of each profession, potential places of employment, and additional tasks you may have to perform that are not specifically discussed within the unit.

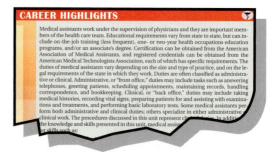

Related Health Careers

RELATED HEALTH CAREERS

- Athletic Trainer
- Chiropractor
- Orthopedist
- Osteopathic physician
- Physiatrist
- Physical Therapist
- Podiatrist
- Prosthetist
- Radiologic Technologist
- Sports Medicine

Related Health Careers appear in Unit 6, *Anatomy and Physiology.* By reviewing the information presented in these boxes, you will relate specific health careers to specific body systems.

Procedures Sections

Procedures Sections provide step-by-step instructions on how to perform the procedure outlined in the Information section. Practice these procedures until you perform them correctly and proficiently.

PROCEDURE 13:2
Washing Hands

Equipment and Supplies

Paper towels, running water, waste container, hand brush or orange/cuticle stick, soap

Procedure

1. Assemble all equipment. Stand back slightly from the sink so you do not contaminate your uniform or clothing. Avoid touching the inside of the sink with your hands since it is considered contaminated.
2. Turn the faucet on by holding a paper towel in your hand and the faucet (see fig... ...the temperature of the ...ter your hands.
4. Use soap to get a lather on your hands.
5. Put the palms of your hands together and rub them using friction and a circular motion for approximately 10 to 15 seconds.
6. Put the palm of one hand on the back of the other hand. Rub together several times. Repeat this after reversing position of hands (see figure 13-8B).
7. Interlace the fingers on both hands and rub them back and forth (see figure 13-8C).
8. Clean the nails with an orange/cuticle stick and/or hand brush (see figures 13-8D and E).

⚠ **CAUTION:** Use the blunt end of orange/cuticle stick to avoid injury.

13:2 INFORMATION
Washing Hands

OBRA Handwashing is a basic task required in any health occupation. The method described in this unit has been developed to ensure that a thorough cleansing occurs. An aseptic technique is a method followed to prevent the spread of germs or pathogens. *Handwashing is the most important method used to practice aseptic technique.* Handwashing is also the most effective way to prevent the spread of infection.

The hands are a perfect medium for the spread of pathogens. Thoroughly washing the ...prevent and control the spread of ...one person to another. It also ...ealth worker f...

♦ After picking up any item off the floor
♦ After personal use of the bathroom
♦ After you cough, sneeze, or use a tissue
♦ Before and after any contact with your mouth or mucous membrane, such as eating, drinking, smoking, applying lip balm, or inserting or removing contact lenses

The recommended method for handwashing is based on the following principles; they should be observed whenever hands are washed:

♦ Soap is used as a cleansing agent because it aids in the removal of germs through its sudsy action and alkali content. Pathogens are trapped in the soapsuds and rinsed away. Use liquid soap from a dispenser whenever possible because bar soap can contain microorganisms.
♦ Warm water should be used. This is less d...

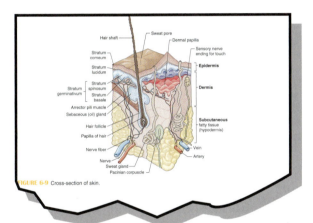

Hair shaft
Sweat pore
Dermal papilla
Sensory nerve ending for touch
Epidermis
Stratum corneum
Stratum lucidum
Stratum germinativum
Stratum spinosum
Stratum basale
Dermis
Arrector pili muscle
Sebaceous (oil) gland
Hair follicle
Subcutaneous fatty tissue (hypodermis)
Papilla of hair
Nerve fiber
Vein
Artery
Nerve
Sweat gland
Pacinian corpuscle

FIGURE 6-9 Cross-section of skin.

Full-color photos are used throughout the text to illustrate important techniques you will be required to know and demonstrate when working within a health care field.

Full-Color Photos and Illustrations

Information Sections explain the basic facts of the topic, why you would need this information, and how the information is applied to various health care fields.

Illustrations are presented in full color that demonstrate important health care concepts, including the inner workings of the body. Use these illustrations for review while studying.

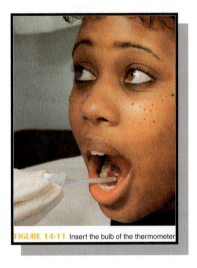

FIGURE 14-11 Insert the bulb of the thermometer

INTERNET SEARCHES

Use the suggested search engines in Unit 11:4 of this textbook to search the Internet for additional information on the following topics:

1. *Cultural diversity:* search words such as culture, ethnicity, and race to obtain additional information on characteristics and examples for each.
2. *Ethnic groups:* search countries of origin for information on different ethnic groups or on your own ethnic group; for example, if you are ...an-I... ...rch for information on both

Internet Searches

Internet Searches can enhance your comprehension of the chapter information by offering you the chance to read information on the chapter topics.

REVIEW QUESTIONS

1. Differentiate between culture, ethnicity, and race.
2. Name five (5) common ethnic groups and at least two (2) countries of origin for each group.
3. Create examples of how a bias, prejudice, and stereotype may interfere with providing quality health care.
4. Describe your family structure. Is it a nuclear or extended family? Is it patriarchal or ...atriarchal or neither? Why?
...al acculturation occur... ...the United...

Review Questions

Review Questions have been added to enhance your comprehension of chapter content. After you have completed the chapter reading, try to answer the review questions at the end of the chapter. If you find yourself unable to answer the questions go back and review the chapter again.

Acknowledgments

This 6th edition of *Diversified Health Occupations* is dedicated to my grandchildren, Kaleigh Ann Nartker and Hayden Michael Kobelak, who have brought so much joy and pleasure into my life.

The author would like to thank everyone who participated in the development of this text, including

Nancy L. Raynor, Chief Consultant, Health Occupations Education, State of North Carolina, who served as a consultant

Dr. Charles Nichols, Department Head, and Ray Jacobs, Teacher Educator, Kent State University

Nancy Webber, R.N., Diversified Health Occupations Instructor

Each person who consented to be a subject in the photographs

Administrative staff at Madison Comprehensive High School

Carolynn Townsend, Lisa Shearer Cooper, Donna Story, and Dorothy Fishman, who contributed unit information

Kathryn G. Cutlip, Health and Safety Services Director at Richland County Red Cross, who reviewed and contributed information for the First Aid Unit

Sharon Logan, a true friend and health care professional, who never hesitates to review new material, research information, critique the manuscript, and offer encouragement.

The author and Delmar Learning would like to thank those individuals who reviewed the manuscript and offered suggestions, feedback, and assistance. The text has been improved as a result of the reviewers' helpful, insightful, and creative suggestions. Their work is greatly appreciated.

Susan Berridge, BSN, MA
Health Occupations Instructor

Jackson Area Career Center
Jackson, MI

Tom Chartier, BAE/EMT-I
Vocational Health Instructor
Woodburg Central High School
Moville, IA

Marilyn Cloutier
Health Careers Instructor
South Vigo High School
Terre Haute, IN

Joan Wolf, RN, MS
Health Occupations Instructor
Indian Valley S.D.
Gnadenhutten, OH

Lois Thomson, MED MT(ASCP)
Health Occupations Instructor
Cypress Creek High School
Houston, TX

Joy Steele, RN
Health Occupations Instructor
Howard School of Academics and Technology
Chattanooga, TN

The author also wishes to thank the following companies, associations, and individuals for information and/or illustrations.

A-dec, Inc.
American Cancer Society
American Optometric Association
Becton Dickinson
Boehringer Mannheim
Brevis Corporation
Briggs Corporation
Centers for Disease Control and Prevention
Choice in Dying
CIBA Pharmaceutical Company
The Clorox Company
Control-o-fax Office Systems

Deborah Funk, M.D.
G.E. Medical Systems
Health Occupations Students of America
HemoCue®
Hollister Incorporated
J.T. Posey Company
Kerr Corporation
Medline Industries
Miltex Instrument Company
Omron Healthcare
Phoenix Society of Burn Survivors, Inc.
Photodisc

Physician's Record Company
Patrick Reineck, D.D.S.
Sage Products, Inc.
Skills USA-VICA
Robert A. Silverman
Smead Manufacturing
Spacelabs Medical, Inc.
Ron Stram, M.D.
Sunrise Medical
3M Company
W.A. Foote Memorial Hospital
US Army

Part 1

Basic Health Care Concepts & Skills

A Letter to the Student

Welcome to the world of health occupations. You have chosen a career in a field that offers endless opportunities. If you learn and master the knowledge and skills required, you can find employment in any number of rewarding occupations.

There will always be a need for workers in health occupations because such workers provide services that cannot be performed by automation or a machine. Thus, although the future will bring changes, you will always be an important part of providing care or services needed.

The material that follows will provide you with a good start toward your career goal. As you learn to use the information presented in the pages that follow, I encourage you to always continue to learn and to grow. All material is presented in a manner to make learning as easy as possible. However, you must still make the effort to achieve the standards set and to perform to the best of your ability.

I expect that you will find this book different from previous books that you have used. If you read the pages that begin each part, you will understand how to use this book. I think you will enjoy working with it, because it will allow you to constantly see how much progress you are making. In addition, it is probably the only book you will have used that allows you to practice tests or evaluations before you actually take them.

One final word. You are entering a field that provides one of the greatest rewards: that of working to assist others. Although the work is hard at times, you will always have the satisfaction of knowing that you are helping other people. So, be proud of yourself. When you learn the concepts and skills well, you will provide services that are appreciated by all.

Introduction

This part is divided into 16 units. Each unit covers several topics. The topics presented are designed to provide you with the basic knowledge and skills required for many different health careers. Before starting a unit, read the unit objectives so you will know exactly what is expected of you. The objectives identify the competencies you should have mastered upon completing the unit.

Diversified Health Occupations, 6th edition, has a textbook and a workbook. Each unit in the textbook is subdivided into Information sections. At the end of most of these sections you will find a statement telling you to go to the workbook to complete an assignment sheet on the information covered. Some units also include Procedure sections, each of which refers you to an evaluation sheet in the workbook. Following are brief explanations of these main components.

1. *Information Sections (Textbook):* The Information sections are designed to provide the basic knowledge you must acquire. These sections explain why the knowledge is important, the basic facts regarding the particular topic, and how this information is applied in various health careers. Most Information sections refer you to specific assignment sheets in the workbook.

   Some Information sections are designed to provide the basic knowledge you must have to perform a given procedure. These sections explain why things are done, give necessary facts, stress key points that should be observed, and, again, refer you to specific assignment sheets in the workbook.

2. *Assignment Sheets (Workbook):* The assignment sheets provide review of the main facts and information presented in the textbook. After you have read an Information section in the text, try to answer the questions on the assignment sheet. Refer back to the Information section to see whether your answers are correct. Let your instructor grade your completed assignment sheets. Note and learn from any changes or corrections. Be sure you understand the information before going on to another Information section or performing the corresponding procedure.

3. *Procedure Sections (Textbook):* The Procedure sections provide step-by-step instructions on how to perform the procedures. Follow the steps while you practice the procedures. Each procedure begins with a list of the necessary equipment and supplies. On occasion, you will see any or all of three words within the procedure sections: **Note, Caution,** and **Checkpoint. Note** means to carefully read the comments following. These comments usually stress points of knowledge or explain why certain techniques are used. **Caution** means that a safety factor is involved and that you should proceed carefully while doing the step in order to avoid injuring yourself or the patient. **Checkpoint** means to ask your instructor to check you at that point in the procedure. Checkpoints are usually located at critical points in the procedures. Each procedure section refers you to a specific evaluation sheet in the workbook.

4. *Evaluation Sheets (Workbook):* Each evaluation sheet contains a list of criteria on which you will be tested when you have mastered a particular procedure. Make sure that your performance meets the standards set. When you feel you have mastered a particular procedure, sign the evaluation sheet and give it to your instructor. Your instructor will grade you by using the listed criteria and checking each step against your performance.

In addition to these components, you will also find a list of Suggested References at the end of each unit in the textbook. If you want additional information about the topics discussed, refer to these references.

Finally, you will notice various icons throughout the textbook. The purpose of these icons is to accentuate particular factors or denote specific types of knowledge. The icons and their meanings are as follows:

 Observe Standard Precautions   Instructors Check—Call Instructor at This Point

 Safety—Proceed with Caution   OBRA Requirement— Based on Federal Law

 Math Skill   Legal Responsibility

 Science Skill   Career Information

 Communications Skill   Technology

UNIT 1

Health Care Systems

Unit Objectives

After completing this unit of study, you should be able to:

- Differentiate between early beliefs about the cause of disease and treatment and current beliefs about disease and treatment

- Identify at least 10 major events in the history of health care

- Describe at least eight types of private health care facilities

- Analyze at least three government agencies and the services offered by each

- Describe at least three services offered by voluntary or nonprofit agencies

- Compare the basic principles of at least four different health insurance plans

- Explain the purpose of organizational structures in health care facilities

- Identify at least five current trends or changes in health care

- Define, pronounce, and spell all the key terms

 Observe Standard Precautions

 Safety—Proceed with Caution

 Math Skill

 Science Skill

 C Communications Skill

 Instructors Check—Call Instructor at This Point

 **OBRA** OBRA Requirement— Based on Federal Law

 Legal Responsibility

 Career Information

 Technology

KEY TERMS

Agency for Health Care Policy
   and Research (AHCPR)
alternative therapies
assisted living facilities
Centers for Disease Control
   and Prevention (CDC)
clinics
complementary therapies
cost containment
dental offices
diagnostic related groups
   (DRGs)
emergency care services
Food and Drug Administration
   (FDA)
genetic counseling centers
geriatric care
health departments
health insurance plans

health maintenance
   organizations (HMOs)
holistic health care
home health care
hospice
hospitals
independent living facilities
industrial health care centers
laboratories
long-term care facilities (LTCs
   or LTCFs)
managed care
Medicaid
medical offices
Medicare
mental health
National Institutes of Health
   (NIH)
nonprofit agencies

Occupational Safety and
   Health Administration
   (OSHA)
Omnibus Budget
   Reconciliation Act (OBRA)
optical centers
organizational structure
preferred provider
   organizations (PPOs)
rehabilitation
school health services
U.S. Department of Health and
   Human Services (USDHHS)
voluntary agencies
wellness
Workers' Compensation
World Health Organization
   (WHO)

NOTE: *To further emphasize the Key Terms, they appear in color in the unit copy. You will notice beginning in Unit 2 on page 26 that pronunciations have been provided for the more difficult key terms. The single accent mark, _'_, shows where the main stress is placed when saying the word. The double accent, _"_, shows secondary stress (if present in the word).*

1:1 INFORMATION
History of Health Care

A summary of the major events in the history of health care is shown in table 1-1. In ancient times, the belief that disease and illness were caused by demons and evil spirits resulted in treatment being directed toward eliminating the evil spirits. As knowledge evolved through the centuries, and disease-producing organisms were discovered, treatment was directed toward eliminating the organisms. The most rapid advances in health care occurred during the 20th century. The potential for even greater advances exists for the 21st century.

TABLE 1-1 History of Health Care

TIME PERIOD	HISTORICAL EVENTS IN HEALTH CARE
4000 BC–3000 BC Primitive Times	Believed that illness and disease caused by supernatural spirits and demons Tribal witch doctors treated illness with ceremonies to drive out evil spirits Herbs and plants used as medicines and some, such as morphine for pain and digitalis for the heart, are still used today Trepanation or trephining, boring a hole in the skull, was used to treat insanity, epilepsy, and headache Average life span was 20 years

(continued)

TABLE 1-1 History of Health Care *(Continued)*

TIME PERIOD	HISTORICAL EVENTS IN HEALTH CARE
3000 BC–300 BC **Ancient Egyptians**	Earliest people known to maintain accurate health records Called upon the gods to heal them when disease occurred Physicians were priests who studied medicine and surgery in temple medical schools Imhotep (2725? BC) may have been the first physician Believed body was a system of channels for air, tears, blood, urine, sperm, and feces If channels became "clogged," bloodletting or leeches were used to "open" them Used magic and medicinal plants to treat disease Average life span was 20 to 30 years
1700 BC–220 AD **Ancient Chinese**	Religious prohibitions against dissection resulted in inadequate knowledge of body structure Carefully monitored the pulse to determine the condition of the body Believed in the need to treat the whole body by curing the spirit and nourishing the body Recorded a pharmacopoeia of medications based mainly on the use of herbs Used acupuncture, or puncture of the skin by needles, to relieve pain and congestion Also used moxibustion (a powdered substance was placed on the skin and then burned to cause a blister) to treat disease Began the search for medical reasons for illness Average life span was 20 to 30 years

1200 BC –200 BC
Ancient Greeks
	Began modern medical science by observing human body and effects of disease
	Biochemist Alcmaeon in 6th century BC identified the brain as the physiological site of the senses
	Hippocrates (460–377 BC) called the Father of Medicine:
	    Developed an organized method to observe the human body
	    Recorded signs and symptoms of many diseases
	    Created a high standard of ethics, the Oath of Hippocrates, used by physicians today
	Aristotle (384–322 BC) dissected animals and is called founder of comparative anatomy
	Believed illness is a result of natural causes
	Used therapies such as massage, art therapy, and herbal treatment which are still used today
	Stressed diet and cleanliness as ways to prevent disease
	Average life span was 25 to 35 years

753 BC–410 AD
Ancient Romans
	First to organize medical care by providing care for injured soldiers
	Early hospitals developed when physicians cared for ill people in rooms in their homes
	Later hospitals were religious and charitable institutions housed in monasteries and convents
	Began public health and sanitation systems:
	    Created aqueducts to carry clean water to the cities
	    Built sewers to carry waste materials away from the cities
	    Used filtering systems in public baths to prevent disease
	    Drained marshes to reduce the incidence of malaria
	Claudius Galen (129–199? AD), a physician, established many medical beliefs:
	    Body regulated by four fluids or humors: blood, phlegm, black bile, and yellow bile
	    An imbalance in the humors resulted in illness
	    Described symptoms of inflammation and studied infectious diseases
	    Dissected animals and determined function of muscles, kidney, and bladder
	Diet, exercise, and medications were used to treat disease
	Average life span was 25 to 35 years

(continued)

TABLE 1-1 History of Health Care *(Continued)*

TIME PERIOD	HISTORICAL EVENTS IN HEALTH CARE
400–800 AD **Dark Ages**	Emphasis was placed on saving the soul and the study of medicine was prohibited Prayer and divine intervention were used to treat illness and disease Monks and priests provided custodial care for sick people Medications were mainly herbal mixtures Average life span was 20 to 30 years

800–1400 AD
Middle Ages
	Renewed interest in the medical practice of Greeks and Romans
	Physicians began to obtain knowledge at medical universities in the 9th century
	A pandemic (worldwide epidemic) of the bubonic plague (black death) killed ¾ of the population of Europe and Asia
	Major diseases were smallpox, diphtheria, tuberculosis, typhoid, the plague, and malaria
	Arab physicians used their knowledge of chemistry to advance pharmacology
	Rhazes (al-Razi), an Arab physician, became known as the Arab Hippocrates:
	    Based diagnoses on observations of the signs and symptoms of disease
	    Developed criteria for distinguishing between smallpox and measles in 910 AD
	    Suggested blood was the cause of many infectious diseases
	    Began the use of animal gut for suture material
	Arabs began requiring that physicians pass examinations and obtain licenses
	Avenzoar, a physician, described the parasite causing scabies in 12th century
	Average life span was 20 to 35 years

1350–1650 AD
Renaissance
	Rebirth of the science of medicine
	Dissection of the body began to allow a better understanding of anatomy and physiology
	Artists Michelangelo (1475–1564) and Leonardo da Vinci (1452–1519) used dissection in order to draw the human body more realistically
	First chairs (positions of authority) of medicine created at Oxford and Cambridge in England in 1440
	Development of the printing press allowed knowledge to be spread to others
	First anatomy book was published by Andreas Vesalius (1514–1564)
	First book on dietetics written by Isaac Judaeus
	Michael Servetus (1511–1553):
	    Described the circulatory system in the lungs
	    Explained how digestion is a source of heat for the body
	Roger Bacon (1214?–1294):
	    Promoted chemical remedies to treat disease
	    Researched optics and refraction (bending of light rays)
	Average life span was 30 to 40 years

16th and 17th
Centuries
	Causes of disease were still not known and many people died from infections and puerperal (childbirth) fever
	Ambroise Pare (1510–1590), a French Surgeon, known as Father of Modern Surgery:
	    Established use of ligatures to bind arteries and stop bleeding
	    Eliminated use of boiling oil to cauterize wounds
	    Improved treatment of fractures and promoted use of artificial limbs
	Gabriel Fallopius (1523–1562):
	    Identified the fallopian tubes in the female
	    Described the tympanic membrane in the ear
	William Harvey (1578–1657) described the circulation of blood to and from the heart in 1628
	Anton van Leeuwenhoek (1632–1723) invented the microscope in 1666
	Bartolomeo Eustachio identified the eustachian tube leading from the ear to the throat
	Scientific societies, such as the Royal Society of London, were established
	Apothecaries (early pharmacists) made, prescribed, and sold medications
	Average life span was 35 to 45 years

(continued)

TABLE 1-1 History of Health Care *(Continued)*

TIME PERIOD	HISTORICAL EVENTS IN HEALTH CARE

18th Century	Gabriel Fahrenheit (1686–1736) created the first mercury thermometer in 1714
	Joseph Priestley (1733–1804) discovered the element oxygen in 1774
	John Hunter (1728–1793), an English surgeon:
	    Established scientific surgical procedures
	    Introduced tube feeding in 1778
	Benjamin Franklin (1706–1790) invented bifocals for glasses
	James Lind prescribed lime juice containing vitamin C to prevent scurvy in 1795
	Edward Jenner (1749–1823) developed a vaccination for smallpox in 1796
	Average life span was 40 to 50 years

19th Century	Royal College of Surgeons (medical school) founded in London in 1800
	French barbers acted as surgeons by extracting teeth, using leeches for treatment, and giving enemas
	First successful blood transfusion was performed on humans in 1818 by James Blundell
	Rene Laennec (1781–1826) invented the stethoscope in 1819
	Dr. Philippe Pinel (1755–1826) began humane treatment for mental illness
	Theodor Fliedner started one of the first training programs for nurses in Germany in 1836; provided Florence Nightingale with her formal training
	In the 1840s, Ignaz Semmelweis (1818–1865) encouraged physicians to wash hands with lime after performing autopsies and before delivering babies to prevent puerperal (childbirth) fever, but the idea was resisted by hospital and medical personnel
	Dr. William Morton (1819–1868), American dentist, began using ether as an anesthetic in 1846
	Dr. James Simpson (1811–1870) began using chloroform as an anesthetic in 1847
	Elizabeth Blackwell (1821–1910) became the first female physician in the United States in 1849
	Florence Nightingale (1820–1910) was the founder of modern nursing:
	    Established efficient and sanitary nursing units during Crimean War in 1854
	    Opened Nightingale School and Home for Nurses at St. Thomas' Hospital in London in 1860
	    Began the professional education of nurses
	Dorothea Dix (1802–1887) appointed Superintendent of Female Nurses of the Army in 1861
	International Red Cross was founded in 1863
	Joseph Lister (1827–1912) started using disinfectants and antiseptics during surgery to prevent infection in 1865
	Elizabeth Garrett Anderson (1836–1917) became the first female physician in Britain in 1870 and the first woman member of the British Medical Association in 1873
	Paul Ehrlich (1854–1915), a German bacteriologist, developed methods of detecting and differentiating between various diseases, developed the foundation for modern theories of immunity, and used chemicals to eliminate microorganisms
	Clara Barton (1821–1912) founded the American Red Cross in 1881
	Louis Pasteur (1822–1895) contributed many discoveries to the practice of medicine including:
	    Proving that microorganisms cause disease
	    Pasteurizing milk to kill bacteria
	    Creating a vaccine for rabies in 1885
	Gregory Mendel (1822–1884) established principles of heredity and dominant/recessive patterns
	Robert Koch (1843–1910), called the Father of Microbiology, developed the culture plate method to identify pathogens and isolated the bacteria causing tuberculosis
	Dimitri Ivanofski discovered viruses in 1892
	Lillian Wald (1867–1940) established the Henry Street Settlement in New York City in 1893 (the start of public health nursing)
	Wilhelm Roentgen (1845–1923) discovered Roentgenograms (X-rays) in 1895
	Almroth Wright developed vaccine for typhoid fever in 1897
	Bacteria causing gonorrhea and leprosy were discovered and identified
	Average life span was 40 to 60 years

(continued)

TABLE 1-1 History of Health Care *(Continued)*

TIME PERIOD	HISTORICAL EVENTS IN HEALTH CARE
20th Century	Walter Reed demonstrated that mosquitoes carry yellow fever in 1900 Carl Landsteiner classified the ABO blood groups in 1901 Dr. Elie Metchnikoff (1845–1916) identified how white blood cells protect against disease Marie Curie (1867–1934) isolated radium in 1910 Sigmund Freud's (1856–1939) studies formed the basis for psychology and psychiatry Frederick Banting and Charles Best discovered and used insulin to treat diabetes in 1922 Health insurance plans and social reforms developed in the 1920s Mary Breckinridge (1881–1965) founded Frontier Nursing Service in 1925 to deliver health care to rural Kentuckians John Enders and Frederick Robbins developed methods to grow viruses in cultures in 1930s Sir Alexander Fleming (1881–1955) discovered penicillin in 1928 Gerhard Domagk (1895–1964) developed sulfa drugs to fight infections Dr. George Papanicolaou developed the Pap test to detect cervical cancer in females The first kidney dialysis machine was developed in 1944 Jonas Salk (1914–1995) developed the polio vaccine using dead polio virus in 1952 Francis Crick and James Watson described the structure of DNA and how it carries genetic information in 1953 The first heart-lung machine was used for open-heart surgery in 1953 The first successful kidney transplant in humans was performed by Joseph Murray in 1954 Albert Sabin (1906–1993) developed an oral live-virus polio vaccine in the mid 1950s Birth control pills approved by FDA in 1960 An arm severed at the shoulder was successfully reattached to body in 1962 The first liver transplant was performed by Thomas Starzl in 1963 The first lung transplant was performed by James Hardy in 1964 Medicare and Medicaid 1965 Amendment to Social Security Act marked the entry of the federal government into the health care arena as a major purchaser of health services The first successful heart transplant was performed by Christian Barnard in 1968 The first hospice was founded in England in 1967 Hargobind Khorana synthesized a gene in 1970 Health Maintenance Organization Act of 1973 established standards for HMOs and provided an alternative to private health insurance Physicians used amniocentesis to diagnose inherited diseases before birth in 1975 Computerized axial tomography (CAT) scan was developed in 1975 New Jersey Supreme Court ruled that parents of a comatose woman had the power to remove life support systems in 1975 The first "test tube" baby, Louise Brown, was born in England in 1978 Genetic engineering led to development of vaccines against hepatitis, herpes simplex, and chicken pox in 1980s Acquired Immune Deficiency Syndrome (AIDS) was identified as a disease in 1981 Dr. William DeVries implanted the first artificial heart, the Jarvik-7, in 1982 Cyclosporine, a drug to suppress the immune system after organ transplants, approved in 1983 The Human Immunodeficiency virus (HIV) causing AIDS was identified in 1984 The Omnibus Budget Reconciliation Act (OBRA) of 1987 established regulations for the education and certification of nursing assistants The Omnibus Budget Reconciliation Act of 1989 created an agency for health care policy and research to develop outcome measures of health care quality The first gene therapy to treat disease occurred in 1990 Identification of genes causing diseases increased rapidly in the 1990s A sheep was cloned in 1997 Average life span was 60 to 70 years

TABLE 1-1 History of Health Care, *(Continued)*

TIME PERIOD	HISTORICAL EVENTS IN HEALTH CARE
Potential for the 21st Century	Cures for AIDS, cancer, and heart disease are found
	Genetic manipulation to prevent inherited diseases is a common practice
	Development of methods to slow the aging process or stop aging are created
	Nerves in the brain and spinal cord are regenerated to eliminate paralysis
	Transplants of every organ in the body, including the brain, are possible
	Antibiotics are developed that do not allow pathogens to develop resistance
	Average life span is increased to 90 to 100 years and beyond

1:2 INFORMATION
Private Health Care Facilities

Today, health care systems include the many agencies, facilities, and personnel involved in the delivery of health care. According to U.S. government statistics, health care is one of the largest and fastest-growing industries in the United States. This industry employs over 10 million workers in over 200 different health careers. It attracts people with a wide range of educational backgrounds because it offers multiple career options. By the year 2008, employment is expected to increase to over 14 million workers. Health care has become a 2-billion-dollar-per-day business.

Many different health care facilities provide services that are a part of the industry called *health care,* figure 1-1. Most private health care facilities require a fee for services. In some cases, grants and contributions help provide financial support for these facilities. A basic description of the various facilities will help provide an understanding of the many different types of services included under the umbrella of the health care industry.

Hospitals are one of the major types of health care facilities. They vary in size and types of service provided. Some hospitals are small and serve the basic needs of a community; others are large, complex centers offering a wide range of services including diagnosis, treatment, education, and research. Hospitals are also classified as private or proprietary (operated for profit), religious, nonprofit or voluntary, and government, depending on the sources of income received by the hospital. Some hospitals are general hospitals treating a wide range of conditions, but others are speciality hospitals caring for only special conditions or age groups. Examples of speciality hospitals include burn hospitals, oncology (cancer) hospitals, pediatric (or children's) hospitals, psychiatric hospitals (dealing with mental diseases and disorders), orthopedic hospitals (dealing with bone, joint, or muscle disease), and rehabilitative hospitals (offering services such as physical and occupational therapy). Government hospitals are operated by federal, state, and local government agencies. They include the many facilities located throughout the world that provide care for government service personnel and their dependents. Other examples of government hospitals include Veterans Administration hospitals (which provide care for veterans), state psychiatric hospitals, and state rehabilitation centers. University or college medical centers provide hospital services along with research and education. They can be funded by private and/or governmental sources. In any type of hospital facility, a wide range of trained health workers is needed at all levels.

Long-term care facilities (LTCs or LTCFs) mainly provide assistance and care for elderly patients, usually called *residents.* However, they also provide care for individuals with disabilities or handicaps and individuals with chronic or long-term illness. Some facilities are called *nursing homes* or *geriatric homes.* These are designed to provide basic physical and emotional care to individuals who can no longer care for themselves. The facilities help individuals with activities of daily living (ADLs), provide a safe and secure environment, and promote opportunities for social interactions. Other long-term care facilities are called *extended care facilities* or *skilled care facilities.* These are designed to provide skilled nursing care and rehabilitative care to prepare patients* or residents for

*In some health care facilities, patients are referred to as clients. For the purposes of this text, patient will be used.

return to home environments or other long-term care facilities. Some skilled care facilities have *subacute units* designed to provide services to patients who need rehabilitation to recover from a major illness or surgery, treatment for cancer, or treatments such as dialysis for kidney disease or heart monitoring. **Independent living** and **assisted living** facilities allow individuals who can care for themselves to rent or purchase an apartment in the facility. Services such as meals, housekeeping, laundry, transportation, social events, and basic medical care (such as assisting with medications) are provided. Most assisted or independent living facilities are associated with nursing homes, extended care facilities, and/or skilled care facilities. This allows an individual to move readily from one level of care to the next when health needs change. Many long-term care facilities also offer special services such as the delivery of meals to the homes of the elderly, chronically ill, or people with disabilities. Some facilities offer senior citizen or adult day care centers, which provide social activities and other services for the elderly. The need for long-term care facilities has increased dramatically because of the large increase in the number of elderly people. Therefore, many health career opportunities are available in these facilities.

Medical offices vary from offices that are privately owned by one doctor to large complexes that operate as corporations and employ many doctors and other health care professionals. Medical services obtained in these facilities can include diagnosis (determining the nature of an illness), treatment, examination, basic laboratory testing, minor surgery, and other similar care. Some medical doctors treat a wide variety of illnesses and age groups, but others specialize in and handle only certain age groups or conditions. Examples of specialities include pediatrics (infants and children), cardiology (diseases and disorders of the heart), and obstetrics (care of the pregnant female).

Dental offices vary in size from offices that are privately owned by one or more dentists to dental clinics that employ a number of dentists. In some areas, major retail or department stores operate dental clinics. Dental services can include general care provided to all age groups or specialized care offered to certain age groups or for certain dental conditions.

Clinics, also called satellite clinics or satellite centers, are health care facilities found in many types of health care. Some clinics are composed of a group of medical or dental doctors who share

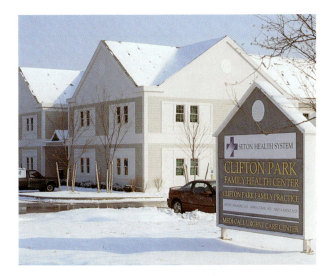
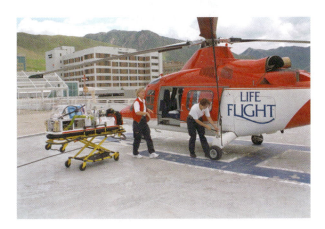
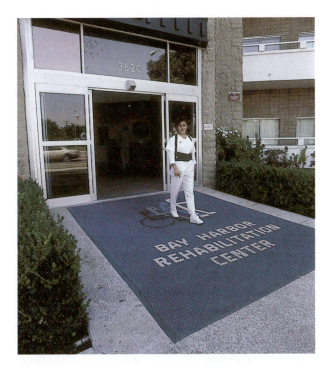

FIGURE 1-1 Different health care facilities.

a facility and other personnel. Other clinics are operated by private groups who provide special care. Examples include surgical clinics or surgicenters that perform minor surgical procedures; urgent or emergency care clinics; rehabilitation clinics that offer physical, occupational, speech, and other similar therapies; and specialty clinics such as diabetic or oncology (cancer) clinics. Many hospitals operate clinics for outpatients (patients who are not admitted to the hospital). Health departments offer clinics for pediatric health care, treatment of sexually transmitted diseases and respiratory disease, immunizations, and other special services. Medical centers at colleges or universities offer clinics for various health conditions. These clinics often offer free care and treatment to provide learning experiences for medical students.

Optical centers can be individually owned by an ophthalmologist or optometrist or they can be part of a large chain of stores. They provide vision examinations, prescribe eyeglasses or contact lenses, and check for the presence of eye diseases.

Emergency care services provide special care for victims of accidents or sudden illness. Facilities providing these services include ambulance services, both private and governmental; rescue squads, frequently operated by fire departments; emergency care clinics and centers; emergency rooms operated by hospitals; and helicopter or airplane emergency services that rapidly transport patients to medical facilities for special care.

Laboratories are often a part of other facilities but can operate as separate health care services. Medical laboratories can perform special diagnostic tests such as blood or urine tests. Dental laboratories can prepare dentures (false teeth) and many other devices used to repair or replace teeth. Medical and dental offices, small hospitals, clinics, and many other health care facilities frequently use the services provided by laboratories.

Home health care agencies are designed to provide care in a patient's home, figure 1-2. The services of these agencies are frequently used by the elderly and disabled. Examples of such services include nursing care, personal care, therapy (physical, occupational, speech, respiratory, etc.), and homemaking (food preparation, cleaning, etc.). Health departments, hospitals, private agencies, government agencies, and nonprofit or volunteer groups can offer home care services.

Hospice agencies provide care for terminally ill persons with life expectancies of 6 months or less. Care can be provided in the person's home or

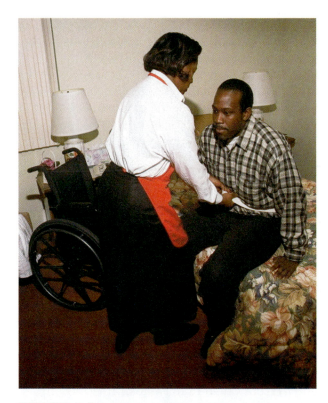

FIGURE 1-2 Many types of health care can be provided in a patient's home.

in a hospice facility. Care is directed toward allowing the person to die with dignity and in comfort. Psychological, social, spiritual, and financial counseling are provided for both the patient and the family.

Mental health facilities treat patients with mental disorders and diseases. Examples of these facilities include guidance and counseling centers, psychiatric clinics and hospitals, chemical abuse treatment centers (dealing with alcohol and drug abuse), and physical abuse treatment centers (dealing with child abuse, spousal abuse, etc.).

Genetic counseling centers can be an independent facility or located in another facility such as a hospital, clinic, or physician's office. Genetic counselors work with couples or individuals who are pregnant or considering a pregnancy. They perform prenatal screening tests, check for genetic abnormalities and birth defects, explain the results of the tests, identify medical options when a birth defect is present, and help the individuals cope with the psychological issues caused by a genetic disorder. Counselors frequently consult with couples prior to a pregnancy if the woman is in her late childbearing years, has a family history of genetic disease, or is of a specific race or nationality with a prevalence of genetic disease.

Rehabilitation facilities are located in hospitals, clinics, and/or private centers. They provide care to help patients with physical or mental disabilities obtain maximum self-care and function. Services may include physical, occupational, recreational, speech, and hearing therapy.

Health maintenance organizations (HMOs) provide total health care directed toward preventive health care. Services include examinations, basic medical services, health education, and hospitalization or rehabilitation services as needed. Some HMOs are operated by large industries or corporations; others are operated by private agencies. They often use the services of other health care facilities including medical and dental offices, hospitals, rehabilitative centers, home health care agencies, clinics, and laboratories.

Industrial health care centers or *occupational health clinics* are found in large companies or industries. Such centers provide health care for employees of the industry or business by performing basic examinations; teaching accident prevention and safety; and providing emergency care.

School health services are found in schools and colleges. These services provide emergency care for victims of accidents and sudden illness; perform tests to check for health conditions such as speech, vision, and hearing problems; promote health education; and maintain a safe and sanitary school environment. Many school health services also provide counseling.

1:3 INFORMATION Government Agencies

In addition to the government health care facilities mentioned previously, other health services are offered at international, national, state, and local levels. Government services are tax supported.

The **World Health Organization (WHO)** is an international agency sponsored by the United Nations. It compiles statistics and information on disease, publishes health information, and investigates and addresses serious health problems throughout the world.

The **U.S. Department of Health and Human Services (USDHHS)** is a national agency that deals with the health problems in the United States. One division of the USDHHS is the **National Institutes of Health (NIH),** which is involved in research on disease. Another division is the **Centers for Disease Control and Prevention (CDC),** which is concerned with causes, spread, and control of diseases in populations. The **Food and Drug Administration (FDA)** is a federal agency responsible for regulating food and drug products sold to the public. The **Agency for Health Care Policy and Research (AHCPR)** is a federal agency established in 1990 to research the quality of health care delivery and identify the standards of treatment that should be provided by health care facilities. Another important federal agency is the **Occupational Safety and Health Administration (OSHA).** It establishes and enforces standards that protect workers from job-related injuries and illnesses.

State and local (county and city) **health departments** provide health services as directed by the Department of Health and Human Services (USDHHS) and also provide specific services needed by the state or local community. Examples of services include immunization for disease control; inspections for environmental health and sanitation; communicable disease control; collection of statistics and records related to health; health education; clinics for health care and prevention; and other services needed in a community.

1:4 INFORMATION Voluntary or Nonprofit Agencies

Voluntary agencies, frequently called **nonprofit agencies,** are supported by donations, membership fees, fundraisers, and federal or state grants. They provide health services at national, state, and local levels.

Examples of nonprofit agencies include the American Cancer Society, the American Heart Association, the American Respiratory Disease Association, the American Diabetes Association, the National Association of Mental Health, the National Foundation of the March of Dimes, and the American Red Cross. Many of these organizations have national offices as well as branch offices in states and/or local communities.

As indicated by their names, many such organizations focus on one specific disease or group of diseases. Each organization typically studies the disease, provides funding to encourage research directed at curing or treating the disease, and promotes public education regarding information obtained through research. These organizations also provide special services to victims of disease, such as purchasing medical equipment and supplies, providing treatment centers, and supplying information regarding other community agencies that offer assistance.

Nonprofit agencies employ many health care workers in addition to using volunteer workers to provide services.

1:5 INFORMATION Health Insurance Plans

The cost of health care is a major concern of everyone who needs health services. Statistics show that the cost of health care is over 12 percent of the gross national product (the total amount of money spent on all goods and services). Also, health care costs are increasing much faster than other costs of living. In order to pay for the costs of health care, most people rely on **health insurance plans.** Without insurance, the cost of an illness can mean financial disaster for an individual or family.

Health insurance plans are offered by several thousand insurance agencies. A common example is Blue Cross–Blue Shield, figure 1-3. In this type of plan, a premium (or payment) is made to the insurance company. When the insured individual incurs health care expenses covered by the insurance plan, the insurance company pays for

the services. The amount of payment and the type of services covered vary from plan to plan. Most insurance plans have limits on payments and deductibles. *Deductibles* are amounts that must be paid by the patient for medical services before the policy begins to pay. *Co-insurance* requires that specific percentages of expenses are shared by the patient and insurance company. For example, in an 80%–20% co-insurance, the company pays 80% of covered expenses, and the patient pays the remaining 20%. Some policies require a *co-payment*, a specific amount of money a patient pays for a particular service, for example, $10 for each physician visit regardless of the total cost of the visit. Many individuals have insurance coverage through their places of employment (called employer-sponsored health insurance or group insurance), where the premiums are paid by the employer. In most cases, the individual also pays a percentage of the premium. Private policies are also available for purchase by individuals.

A health maintenance organization (HMO) is another type of health insurance plan. A monthly fee or premium is paid for membership, and the fee stays the same regardless of the amount of health care used. The premium can be paid by an employer and/or an individual. Total care provided is directed toward preventive type health care. An individual insured under this type of plan has ready access to health examinations and early treatment and detection of disease. Because most other types of insurance plans do not cover routine examinations and preventive care, the individual insured by an HMO can therefore theoretically maintain a better state of health. The disadvantage of an HMO is that the insured is required to use only HMO-affiliated health care providers (doctors, labs, hospitals) for health care. If a nonaffiliated health care provider is used instead, the insured usually must pay for the care.

A **preferred provider organization (PPO)** is another type of health insurance plan usually provided by large industries or companies to their employees. The industry or company forms a contract with certain health care agencies, such as a large hospital and/or specific doctors and dentists, to provide certain types of health care at reduced rates. Employees are restricted to using the specific hospital and/or doctors, but the industry or company can provide health care at lower rates.

The government also provides health insurance plans for certain groups of people. Two of the main plans are Medicare and Medicaid.

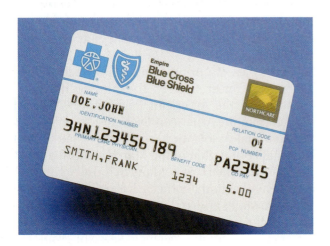

FIGURE 1-3 Health insurance plans help pay for the costs of health care.

Medicare is a federal government program that provides health care for almost all individuals over the age of 65 and for any person with a disability who has received Social Security benefits for at least 2 years. Medicare consists of two kinds of coverage: type A for hospital insurance, and type B for medical insurance. Type A covers hospital services and care provided by an extended care facility or home-health care agency after hospitalization. Type B offers additional coverage for doctor's services, outpatient treatments, therapy, and other health care. The individual does pay a premium for type B coverage and also must pay an initial deductible for services. In addition, Medicare pays for only 80% of the services; the individual must either pay the balance or have another insurance policy to cover the expenses.

Medicaid is a medical assistance program operated by individual states. Benefits and individuals covered under this program vary slightly from state to state. This health insurance plan usually pays for the health care of individuals with low incomes, children who qualify for public assistance, and individuals who are physically disabled or blind.

The *State Children's Health Insurance Program (SCHIP)* was established in 1997 to provide health care to uninsured children of working families who earn too little to afford private insurance but too much to be eligible for Medicaid. It provides inpatient and outpatient hospital services, physician's surgical and medical care, laboratory and X-ray tests, and well-baby and well-child care, including immunizations.

Workers' Compensation is a health insurance plan providing treatment for workers injured on the job. It is administered by the state, and payments are made by employers and the state. In addition to providing payment for needed health care, this plan also reimburses the worker for wages lost because of on-the-job injury.

The United States government provides health care for all military personnel. A health insurance plan called TRICARE, formerly called CHAMPUS (the Civilian Health and Medical Programs for the Uniform Services), provides care for all active duty members and their families, survivors of military personnel, and retired members of the Armed Forces. The Veterans Administration provides for military veterans.

Managed care is an approach that has developed in response to rising health care costs. Employers as well as insurance companies who pay large medical bills want to ensure that such money is spent efficiently rather than wastefully. The principle behind managed care is that all health care provided to a patient must have a purpose. A second opinion or verification of need is frequently required before care can be provided. Every effort is made to provide preventive care and early diagnosis of disease to avoid the high cost of treating disease. For example, routine physical examinations, well-baby care, immunizations, and wellness education to promote good nutrition, exercise, weight control, and healthy living practices are usually provided under managed care. Employers and insurance companies create a network of doctors, specialists, therapists, and health care facilities that provide care at the most reasonable cost. Health maintenance organizations and preferred provider organizations are the main providers of managed care, but many private insurance companies are establishing health care networks to provide care to their subscribers. As these health care networks compete for the consumer dollar, they are required to provide quality care at the lowest possible cost. The health care consumer who is enrolled in a managed care plan receives quality care at the most reasonable cost, but is restricted in choice of health care providers.

Health insurance plans do not solve all the problems of health care costs, but they do help many people by paying for all or part of the cost of health services.

1:6 INFORMATION Organizational Structure

All health care facilities must have some type of **organizational structure.** The structure may be complex, as in larger facilities, or simple, as in smaller facilities. Organizational structure always, however, encompasses a line of authority or chain of command. The organizational structure should indicate areas of responsibility and lead to the most efficient operation of the facility.

A sample organizational chart for a large general hospital is shown in figure 1-4. This chart shows organization by department. Each department, in turn, can have an organizational chart similar to the one shown for the nursing department in figure 1-4. A sample organizational chart for a small medical office is shown in figure 1-5. The organizational structure will vary with the size of the office and the number of people employed.

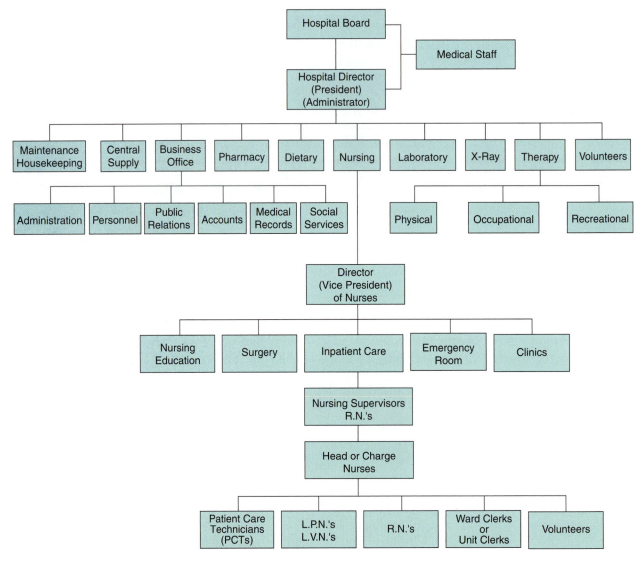

FIGURE 1-4 A sample hospital organizational chart.

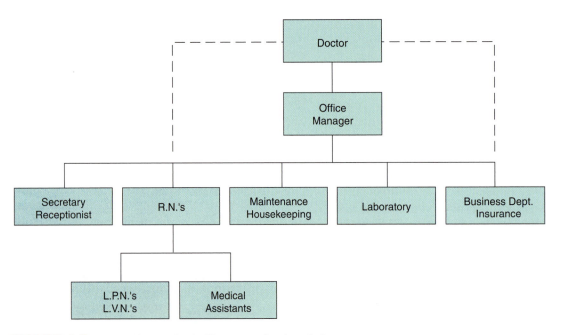

FIGURE 1-5 A sample medical office organizational chart.

In both organizational charts illustrated, the lines of authority are clearly indicated. It is important for health care workers to identify and understand their respective positions in a given facility's organizational structure. By doing this, they will know their lines of authority and understand who are the immediate supervisors in charge of their work. Health care workers must always take questions, reports, and problems to their immediate supervisors, who are responsible for providing necessary assistance. If immediate supervisors cannot answer the question or solve the problem, it is their responsibility to take the situation to the next level in the organizational chart. It is also important for health care workers to understand the functions and goals of the organization.

1:7 INFORMATION Trends in Health Care

Health care has seen many changes during the past several decades, and many additional changes will occur in the years to come. An awareness of such changes and trends is important for any health care worker.

COST CONTAINMENT

Cost containment, a term heard frequently in health care circles, means trying to control the rising cost of health care and achieving the maximum benefit for every dollar spent. One reason for high health care costs is technological advances. Highly technical procedures such as heart, lung, liver, or kidney transplants can cost hundreds of thousands of dollars. Even so, many of these procedures are performed daily throughout the United States. Artificial hearts are another new technology being used. Computers that can be used to examine internal body parts are valuable diagnostic tools, but these devices can cost millions of dollars. Advanced technology does allow people to survive illnesses that used to be fatal, but these individuals may require expensive and lifelong care. A second reason for high health care costs is the aging population. This group of individuals increases the use of pharmaceutical products (medications), has more chronic diseases, and often needs frequent health care services.

An increase in health related lawsuits also contributes to an increase in health care costs. Health care providers are forced to obtain expensive malpractice insurance, order diagnostic tests even though they might not be necessary, and make every effort to avoid lawsuits by practicing defensive health care. Since these expenses must be paid, health care costs could rise to levels that could prohibit providing services to all individuals. However, everyone should have equal access to care regardless of the ability to pay. All aspects of health care are therefore directed toward cost containment. Although there is no firm answer to controlling health costs, most agencies that deliver health care are trying to provide quality care at the lowest possible price. Some methods of cost containment that are used include:

◆ *Diagnostic related groups (DRGs):* one way Congress is trying to control costs for government insurance plans such as Medicare and Medicaid. Under this plan, patients with certain diagnoses who are admitted to hospitals are classified in one payment group. A limit is placed on the cost of care, and the agency providing care receives this set amount. This encourages the agency to make every effort to provide care within the expense limit allowed. If the cost of care is less than the amount paid, the agency keeps the extra money. If the cost of care is more than the amount paid, the agency must accept the loss.

◆ *Combination of services:* done to eliminate duplication of services. Clinics, laboratories shared by different agencies, health maintenance organizations (HMOs), preferred provider organizations (PPOs), and other similar agencies all represent attempts to control the rising cost of health care. When health care agencies join together or share specific services, care can be provided to a larger number of people at a decreased cost per person. For example, a large medical laboratory with expensive computerized equipment performing thousands of tests per day can provide quality service at a much lower price than smaller laboratories with less expensive equipment capable of performing only a limited numbers of tests per day.

◆ *Outpatient services:* patients receive care without being admitted to hospitals or other care facilities. Hospital care is expensive. Reducing the length of hospital stays or decreasing the need for hospital admissions lowers the cost of health care. For example, patients who had open-heart surgery used to spend several weeks in a hospital. Today the average length of stay is 5 to 7 days. Less expensive home care or transfer to a skilled-care facility can be used for individuals who require additional assistance. Surgery, X-rays, diagnostic tests, and many other procedures that once required admission to a hospital are now done on an outpatient basis.

◆ *Mass or bulk purchasing:* buying equipment and supplies in larger quantities at reduced prices. This can be done by combining the purchases of different departments in a single agency, or by combining the purchases of several different agencies. A major health care system purchasing medical supplies for hundreds or thousands of health care agencies can obtain much lower prices than an individual agency. Computerized inventory can be used to determine when supplies are needed and to prevent overstocks and waste.

◆ *Early intervention and preventive services:* providing care before acute or chronic disease occurs. Preventing illness is always more cost effective than treating illness. Methods used to prevent illness include patient education, immunizations, regular physical examinations to detect problems early, incentives for individuals to participate in preventive activities, and easy access for all individuals to preventive health care services. Studies have shown that individuals with limited access to health services and restricted finances use expensive emergency rooms and acute care facilities much more frequently. Providing early intervention and care to these individuals is much more cost-efficient.

◆ *Energy conservation:* monitoring the use of energy to control costs and conserve resources. Major expenses for every health care industry/ agency are electricity, water, and/or gas. Most large health care facilities perform energy audits to determine how resources are being used and to calculate ways to conserve energy. Methods that can be used for energy conservation include designing and building new energy-efficient facilities; constantly monitoring and maintaining heating/cooling systems; using insulation and thermopane windows to prevent hot/cool air loss; repairing plumbing fixtures immediately to stop water loss; replacing energy-consuming light bulbs with fluorescent or energy-efficient bulbs; installing infrared sensors to turn water faucets on and off; and using alternative forms of energy such as solar power. Recycling is also a form of energy conservation, and most health care facilities recycle many different materials.

The preceding are just a few examples of cost containment. Many other methods will undoubtedly be applied in the years ahead. It is important to note that the quality of health care should not be lowered simply to control costs. To prevent this from happening, the Agency for Health Care Policy and Research (AHCPR) researches the quality of health care delivery and identifies the standards of treatment that should be provided. In addition, every health care worker must make every effort to provide quality care while doing everything possible to avoid waste and keep expenditures down. Health care consumers must assume more responsibility for their own care, become better informed of all options for health care services, and follow preventive measures to avoid or limit illness and disease. Everyone working together can help control the rising cost of health care.

HOME HEALTH CARE

Home health care is a rapidly growing field. Diagnostic related groups and shorter hospital stays have created a need for providing care in the home. Years ago, home care was the usual method of treatment. Doctors made house calls, private duty nurses cared for patients in the patients' homes, babies were delivered at home, and patients died at home. Current trends show a return to some of these practices. Home care is also another form of cost containment because it is usually less expensive to provide this type of care. All aspects of health care can be involved. Nursing care; physical and occupational therapy; respiratory therapy; social services; nutritional and food services; and other types of care can be provided in the home environment.

GERIATRIC CARE

Geriatric care, or care for the elderly, is another field that will continue to experience rapid growth in the future (figure 1-6). This is caused in part by the large number of individuals

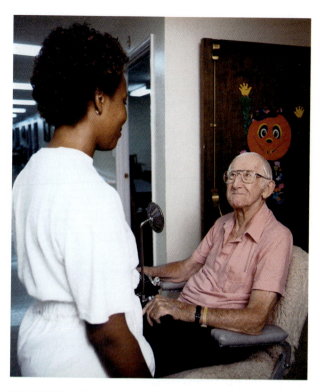

FIGURE 1-6 Geriatric care is a field that will continue to experience rapid growth.

continuing education, periodic evaluation of performance, and retraining and/or testing if a nursing assistant does not work in a health care facility for more than two years. Each state then maintains a registry of qualified individuals. The Omnibus Budget Reconciliation Act also requires compliance with patients'/residents' rights, and forces states to establish guidelines to ensure that such rights are observed and enforced. These regulations serve to ensure certain standards of care. As the need for geriatric care increases, additional regulations may be created. It is important that every health care worker be informed about all OBRA regulations in order to comply with these regulations.

TELEMEDICINE

Telemedicine involves the use of video, audio, and computer systems to provide medical and/or health care services. New technology now allows interactive services between health care providers even though they are in different locations. For example, emergency medical technicians (EMTs), at the scene of an accident or illness, can use technology to transmit medical data such as an electrocardiogram to an emergency room physician. The physician can then monitor the data and direct the care of the patient. Surgeons using a computer can guide a remote controlled arm (robotic) to perform surgery on a patient many miles away. In other instances, a surgeon can direct the work of another surgeon by watching the procedure on video beamed by a satellite system.

As consumers become computer literate, more health care services will be provided electronically. Telemedicine machines, operating over telephone lines, are "user-friendly," compact, and less expensive than when they were developed. They are already allowing individuals with chronic illnesses or disabilities to receive care in the comfort of their homes. This decreases the need for trips to medical care facilities. Patients can test blood sugar levels, oxygen levels, blood pressure measurements, and other vital signs, and send the results to a physician/nurse; monitor pacemakers; use on-line courses to learn how to manage their condition; schedule an "appointment" to talk with a health care provider "face to face" through video monitors; receive

who are experiencing longer life spans thanks to advances in health care. Many people now enjoy life spans of eighty years or more. Years ago, very few people lived to be 100 years old. This is becoming more and more common. Also, the "baby boom" generation—the large number of people born after World War II—will reach the geriatric age classification in the near future. Many different facilities will be involved in providing care and resources for this age group. Adult day care centers, retirement communities, assisted/independent living facilities, long-term care facilities, and other organizations will all see increased demand for the services they provide.

OBRA The **Omnibus Budget Reconciliation Act (OBRA)** of 1987 has led to the development of many regulations regarding long-term care and home health care. This act requires states to establish training and competency evaluation programs for nursing and geriatric assistants. Each assistant working in a long-term care facility or home health care is now required under federal law to complete a mandatory, state-approved training program and pass a written and/or competency examination to obtain certification or registration. OBRA also requires

electronic reminders to take medications or perform diagnostic tests; and receive answers to specific health questions. In rural areas, where specialty care is often limited, telemedicine can provide a patient with access to specialists thousands of miles away. Telemedicine will become a very important way of delivering health care in future years.

WELLNESS

Wellness, or the state of being in optimum health with a balanced relationship between physical, mental, and social health, is another major trend in health care. People are more aware of the need to maintain health and prevent disease because disease prevention improves the quality of life and saves costs. More individuals are recognizing the importance of exercise, good nutrition, weight control, and healthy living habits, figure 1-7. This has led to the establishment of wellness centers, weight control facilities, health food stores, nutrition services, stress reduction counseling, and habit cessation management.

Wellness is determined by the lifestyle choices made by an individual and involves many factors. Some of the factors and ways to promote wellness include:

◆ *Physical wellness:* promoted by a well-balanced diet; regular exercise; routine physical examinations and immunizations; regular dental and vision examinations; and avoidance of alcohol, tobacco, caffeine, drugs, environmental contaminants, and risky sexual behavior

◆ *Emotional wellness:* promoted by understanding personal feelings and expressing them appropriately, accepting one's limitations, adjusting to change, coping with stress, enjoying life, and maintaining an optimistic outlook

◆ *Social wellness:* promoted by showing concern, fairness, affection, tolerance, and respect for others; communicating and interacting well with others; sharing ideas and thoughts; and practicing honesty and loyalty

◆ *Mental and intellectual wellness:* promoted by being creative, logical, curious, and open-minded; using common sense; obtaining

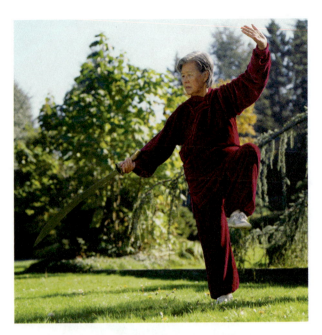

FIGURE 1-7 Individuals are recognizing the importance of exercise and healthy living habits. *(Courtesy of Photodisc)*

continual learning; questioning and evaluating information and situations; learning from life experiences; and using flexibility and creativity to solve problems

◆ *Spiritual wellness:* promoted by using values, ethics, and morals to find meaning, direction, and purpose to life; often includes believing in a higher authority and observing religious practices

The trend toward wellness has led to **holistic health care,** or care that promotes physical, emotional, social, intellectual, and spiritual well-being by treating the whole body, mind, and spirit. Each patient is recognized as a unique person with different needs. Holistic health care uses many methods of diagnosis and treatment in addition to traditional Western medical practice. Treatment is directed towards protection and restoration. It is based on the body's natural healing powers, the various ways different tissues and systems in the body influence each other, and the effect of the external environment. It is essential to remember that the patient is responsible for choosing his or her own care. Health care workers must respect the patient's choices and provide care that promotes the well-being of the whole person.

ALTERNATIVE AND COMPLEMENTARY METHODS OF HEALTH CARE

The most common health care system in the United States is the biomedical or "Western" system. It is based on evaluating the physical signs and symptoms of a patient, determining the cause of disease, and treating the cause. A major trend, however, is an increase in the use of alternative or complementary health care therapies. **Alternative therapies** can be defined as methods of treatment that are used in place of biomedical therapies. **Complementary therapies** are methods of treatment that are used in conjunction with conventional medical therapies. Even though the two terms are different, the term "alternative" is usually applied whether or not the therapy is used in place of, or in conjunction with, conventional medical therapies.

The interest in holistic health care has increased the use of alternative/complementary therapies. Common threads in these therapies are that they consider the whole individual and recognize that the health of each part has an effect on the person's total health status; that each person has a life force or special type of energy that can be used in the healing process; and that skilled practitioners, rituals, and specialized practices are a part of the therapy. Many of these therapies are based on cultural values and beliefs. A few examples of alternative/complementary practitioners include:

◆ *Ayurvedic practitioners:* use an ancient philosophy, ayurveda, developed in India to determine a person's predominant dosha (body type) and prescribe diet, herbal treatment, exercise, yoga, massage, minerals, and living practices to restore and maintain harmony in the body.

◆ *Chinese medicine practitioners:* use an ancient holistic-based healing practice based on the belief that a life energy (Chi) flows through every living person in an invisible system of meridians (pathways) to link the organs together and connect them to the external environment or universe; use acupuncture, acupressure, tai chi, and herbal remedies to maintain the proper flow of energy and promote health.

◆ *Chiropractors:* believe that the brain sends vital energy to all body parts through nerves in the spinal cord; when there is a misalignment of the vertebrae (bones), pressure is placed on spinal nerves which results in disease and pain; use spinal manipulation, massage, and exercise to adjust the position of the vertebrae and restore the flow of energy.

◆ *Homeopaths:* believe in the ability of the body to heal itself through the actions of the immune system; use minute diluted doses of drugs made from plant, animal, and mineral substances to cause symptoms similar to the disease and activate the immune system.

◆ *Hypnotists:* help an individual obtain a trance-like state with the belief that the person will be receptive to verbal suggestions and able to make a desired behavior change.

◆ *Naturopaths:* use only natural therapies such as fasting, special diets, lifestyle-changes, and supportive approaches to promote healing; avoid the use of surgery or medicinal agents to treat disease.

Many different therapies are used in alternative/complementary medicine. Some of these therapies are discussed in table 1-2. Most of the therapies are noninvasive and holistic. In many instances, they are less expensive than other traditional treatments.

Because of the increased use of alternative and complementary therapies, the federal government established the Office of Alternative Medicine (OAM) at the National Institutes of Health in 1992. Its purpose is to research the various therapies and determine standards of quality care. In addition, many states have passed laws to govern the use of various therapies. Some states have established standards for some therapies, forbidden the use of others, labeled specific therapies experimental, and require a license or certain educational requirements before a practitioner can administer a particular therapy. It is essential for health care workers to learn the legal requirements of their states regarding the different alternative/complementary therapies. Health care workers must also remember that patients have the right to choose their own type of care. A nonjudgmental attitude is essential.

TABLE 1-2 Alternative and Complementary Therapies

THERAPY	BASIC DESCRIPTION
Acupressure (Shiatsu)	Pressure is applied with fingers, palms, thumbs, or elbows to specific pressure points of the body to stimulate and regulate the flow of energy; based on the belief that Qi (life energy) flows through meridians (pathways) in the body, and illness and pain occur when the flow is blocked; used to treat muscular–joint pain, depression, digestive problems, and respiratory disorders; *Shiatsu* is the Japanese form of acupressure
Acupuncture	Ancient Chinese therapy that involves the insertion of very thin needles into specific points along the meridians (pathways) in the body to stimulate and balance the flow of energy; at times, heat (moxibustion) or electrical stimulation is applied to the needles; based on the belief that Chi (life energy) flows through the meridians and illness and pain occur when the flow is blocked; used to relieve pain, especially headache and back pain, reduce stress-related illnesses, and treat drug dependency and obesity
Antioxidants (Free Radicals)	Nutritional therapy that encourages the use of substances called antioxidants to prevent or inhibit oxidation (chemical process in which a substance is joined to oxygen) and neutralize free radicals (molecules that can damage body cells by altering the genetic code); examples of antioxidants are vitamins A, C, and E, and selenium; may prevent heart disease, cataracts, and some types of cancer
Aromatherapy	Therapeutic use of selected fragrances (concentrated essences or essential oils that have been extracted from roots, bark, plants, and/or flowers) to alter mood and restore the body, mind, and spirit; fragrances may be diluted in oils for massages or placed in warm water or candles for inhalation; used to relieve tense muscles and tension headaches or backaches, lower blood pressure, and cause a stimulating, uplifting, relaxing, or soothing effect
Biofeedback	Relaxation therapy that uses monitoring devices to provide a patient with information about his/her reaction to stress by showing the effect of stress on heart rate, respirations, blood pressure, muscle tension, and skin temperature; patient is then taught relaxation methods to gain "mind" or voluntary control over the physical responses; used to treat hypertension (high blood pressure), migraine headaches, and stress-related illnesses, and to enhance relaxation
Healing Touch (Reiki)	Ancient Japanese/Tibetan healing art based on the idea that disease causes an imbalance in the body's energy field; begins with centering (inward focus of total serenity) before gentle hand pressure is applied to the body's chakras (energy centers) to harness and balance the life energy force, help clear blockages, and stimulate healing; at times, hands are positioned slightly above the energy centers; used to promote relaxation, reduce pain, and promote wound healing
Herbal or Botanical Medicine	Uses herbal medicines that have been used in almost all cultures since primitive times; based on the belief that herbs and plant extracts, from roots, stems, seeds, flowers, and leaves, contain compounds that alter blood chemistry, remove impurities, strengthen the immune system, and protect against disease
Homeopathy	Uses very minute, dilute, doses of drugs made from natural substances to produce symptoms of the disease being treated; based on the belief that these substances stimulate the immune system to remove toxins and heal the body; very controversial form of treatment
Hydrotherapy	Uses water in any form, internally and externally, for healing purposes; common external examples include water aerobics and exercises, massage in or under water, soaking in hot springs or tubs, and steam vapors; a common internal example is a diet that encourages drinking large amounts of water to help cleanse the body and stimulate the digestive tract
Hypnotherapy (Hypnosis)	Technique used to induce a trance-like state so a person is more receptive to suggestion; enhances a person's ability to form images; used to encourage desired behavior changes
Imagery	Technique of using imagination and as many senses as possible to visualize a pleasant and soothing image; used to decrease tension, anxiety, and adverse effects of chemotherapy
Ionization Therapy	Special machines called air ionizers are used to produce negatively charged air particles or ions; used to treat common respiratory disorders

(continued)

TABLE 1-2 Alternative and Complementary Therapies *(Continued)*

THERAPY	BASIC DESCRIPTION
Macrobiotic Diet	Macrobiotic (meaning "long life") is a nutrition therapy based on the Taoist concept of the balance between yin (cold, death, and darkness) and yang (heat, life, and light) and the belief that different foods represent yin (sweet foods) and yang (meat and eggs); diet encourages balanced foods such as brown rice, whole grains, nuts, vegetables, fruits, and fish; discourages overindulgence of yin or yang foods; processed and treated foods, red meat, sugar, dairy products, eggs, and caffeine should be avoided; similar to the American Dietary Association's low-fat, low-cholesterol, and high-fiber diet
Meditation	Therapy that teaches breathing and muscle relaxation techniques to quiet the mind by focusing attention on obtaining a sense of oneness within oneself; used to reduce stress and pain, slow heart rate, lower blood pressure, and stimulate relaxation
Pet Therapy	Uses pets, such as dogs, cats, and birds, to enhance health and stimulate an interest in life; helps individuals overcome physical limitations, decrease depression, increase self-esteem, socialize, and lower stress levels and blood pressure
Phytochemicals	Nutritional therapy that recommends foods containing phytochemicals (nonnutritive plant chemicals that store nutrients and provide aroma and color in plants) with the belief that the chemicals help prevent disease; found mainly in a wide variety of fruits and vegetables, so these are recommended for daily consumption; used to prevent heart disease, stroke, cancer, and cataracts
Play Therapy	Uses toys to allow children to learn about situations, share experiences, and express their emotions; important aspect of psychotherapy for children with limited language ability
Positive Thought	Therapy that involves developing self-awareness, self-esteem, and love for oneself to allow the body to heal itself and eliminate disease; based on the belief that disease is a negative process that can be reversed by an individual's mental processes
Reflexology	Ancient healing art based on the concept that the body is divided into ten equal zones that run from the head to the toes; illness or disease of a body part causes deposits of calcium or acids in the corresponding part of the foot; therapy involves applying pressure on specific points on the foot so energy movement is directed toward the affected body part; used to promote healing and relaxation, reduce stress, improve circulation, and treat asthma, sinus infections, irritable bowel syndrome, kidney stones, and constipation
Spiritual Therapies	Based on the belief that a state of wholeness or health depends not only on physical health, but the spiritual aspects of an individual; uses prayer, meditation, self-evaluation, and spiritual guidance to allow an individual to use the powers within to increase the sense of well-being and promote healing
Tai Chi	Based on the ancient theory that health is harmony with nature and the universe and a balanced state of yin (cold) and yang (heat); uses a series of sequential, slow, graceful, and precise body movements combined with breathing techniques to improve energy flow (Qi) within the body; improves stamina, balance, and coordination and leads to a sense of well-being; used to treat digestive disorders, stress, depression, and arthritis
Therapeutic (Swedish) Massage	Uses kneeling, gliding, friction, tapping, and vibration motions by the hands to increase circulation of the blood and lymph, relieve musculoskeletal stiffness, pain, and spasm, increase range-of-motion, and induce relaxation
Therapeutic Touch	Based on an ancient healing practice with the belief that illness is an imbalance in an individual's energy field; the practitioner assesses alterations or changes in a patient's energy fields, places his/her hands on or slightly above the patient's body, and balances the energy flow to stimulate self-healing; used to encourage relaxation, stimulate wound healing, increase the energy level, and decrease anxiety
Yoga	Hindu discipline that uses concentration, specific positions, and ancient ritual movements to maintain the balance and flow of life energy; encourages the use of both the body and mind to achieve a state of perfect spiritual insight and tranquility; used to increase spiritual enlightenment and well-being, develop an awareness of the body to improve coordination, relieve stress and anxiety, and increase muscle tone

NATIONAL HEALTH CARE PLAN

The high cost of health care and large number of uninsured individuals have created a demand for a national health care plan. Many different types of plans have been proposed. One plan involves nationalized medicine, where the federal government would pay for all health services and levy taxes to pay for those services. Another plan involves the creation of health care cooperatives, which would allow consumers to purchase health care at lower costs. A third plan is based on managed care and requires employers to provide coverage and the federal government to subsidize insurance for the poor. Still another plan would allow each state to establish its own health care plan paid for by employers, individuals, and/or government subsidies.

The main goal in health care reform is to ensure that all Americans can get health coverage. Related problems include the cost of creating such a system, the fact that those with insurance may pay more to cover uninsured individuals, the lack of freedom in choosing health care providers, and the regulations that will have to be created to establish a national health care system.

Although the preceding are just several of the trends in health care, they do illustrate how health care has changed and how it will continue to change. Every health care worker must stay abreast of such changes and make every attempt to learn about them.

STUDENT: *Go to the workbook and complete the assignment sheet for Unit 1, Health Care Systems.*

UNIT 1 SUMMARY

Health care, one of the largest and fastest growing industries in the United States, encompasses many different types of facilities that provide health-related services. These include hospitals; long-term care facilities; medical and dental offices; clinics; laboratories; industrial and school health services; and many others. Government and nonprofit or voluntary agencies also provide health care services. All health care facilities require different health care workers at all levels of training.

Many types of health insurance plans are available to help pay the costs of health care. Insurance does not usually cover the entire cost of care, however. It is important for consumers to be aware of the types of coverage provided by their respective insurance plans.

Organizational structure is important in all health care facilities. The structure can be complex or simple, but it should show a line of authority or chain of command within the facility and indicate areas of responsibility.

As health care continues to grow as an industry, changes and trends will occur. Issues of primary importance are cost containment to control the high cost of health care, home health care, care for the elderly, telemedicine, wellness to prevent disease, alternative and complementary methods of health care, and a national health care plan.

INTERNET SEARCHES

Use the suggested search engines in Unit 11:4 of this textbook to search the Internet for additional information on the following topics:

1. *Private health care facilities:* search for information on each of the specific types of facilities; for example, hospitals, hospice care, or emergency care services.

2. *Government agencies:* search for more detailed information about the activities of the World Health Organization, U.S. Department of Health and Human Services, National Institutes of Health, Centers for Disease Control and Prevention, Food and Drug Administration, and Occupational Safety and Health Administration.

3. *Voluntary or nonprofit agencies:* search for information on the purposes and activities of organizations such as the American Cancer Society, American Heart Association, American Respiratory Disease Association, American Diabetes Association, National Association of

Mental Health, National Foundation of the March of Dimes, and the American Red Cross.

4. *Health insurance:* search the Internet to find specific names of companies that are health maintenance organizations or preferred provider organizations. Check to see how their coverage for individuals is the same or how it is different.

5. *Government health care insurance:* search the Internet to learn about benefits provided under Medicare, Medicaid, and the State Children's Health Insurance Program.

6. *History of health care:* research individual names or discoveries such as the polio vaccine to gain more insight into how major developments in health care occurred.

7. *Trends in health care:* research topics such as home health care, Omnibus Budget Reconciliation Act of 1987, telemedicine, holistic health care, cost containment, geriatric care, and wellness to obtain additional information on the present effect on health care.

8. *Alternative/complementary methods of health care:* search the Internet for additional information on specific therapies such as acupuncture. Refer to table 1-2 for a list of many different therapies.

REVIEW QUESTIONS

1. Differentiate between a private or proprietary, religious, nonprofit or voluntary, and government type of hospital.

2. Identify at least six (6) different types of private health care facilities by stating the functions of the facility or the type of health care provided.

3. Name each of the following federal agencies and briefly describe its function:
   a. CDC   d. OSHA
   b. FDA   e. USDHHS
   c. NIH   f. WHO

4. What does the term "deductible" mean on health insurance policies? co-insurance? co-payment?

5. Why is it important for every health care worker to know the organizational structure for his/her place of employment?

6. Create a time line for the history of health care showing the twenty (20) events you feel had the most impact on modern day care.

7. List six (6) specific ways to control the rising cost of health care.

8. Review all the alternative/complementary therapies shown in table 1-2. Identify two therapies that you feel would be beneficial. Explain why you think the therapies might be effective.

UNIT 1
SUGGESTED REFERENCES

Alternative Link Systems, Inc. *The State Legal Guide to Complementary and Alternative Medicine and Nursing.* Clifton Park, NY: Delmar Learning, 2001.

American Medical Association. *Alternative Health Methods.* Chicago, IL: American Medical Association, 1995.

Deem, Saitofi, and Joseph Deem. *Health Care Exploration.* Clifton Park, NY: Delmar Learning, 2000

Fugh-Berman, Adriane. *Alternative Medicine— What Works.* Philadelphia, PA: Lippincott, Williams, & Wilkins, 1998.

Hegner, Barbara, Esther Caldwell, and Joan Needham. *Nursing Assistant: A Nursing Process Approach.* 8th ed. Clifton Park, NY: Delmar Learning, 1999.

Heshmet, Shabram. *Health Care Economics: Understanding an Integrated Health Care Delivery System.* Clifton Park, NY: Delmar Learning, 2001.

Hover-Kramer, Dorothea. *Healing Touch: A Resource for Health Professionals.* Clifton Park, NY: Delmar Learning, 2002.

Jonas, Wayne, and Jeffrey Levin. *Essentials of Complementary and Alternative Medicine.* Philadelphia, PA: Lippincott, Williams, & Wilkins, 1999.

Keegan, Lynn. *Healing and Complementary and Alternative Therapies.* Clifton Park, NY: Delmar Learning, 1999.

Keegan, Lynn. *Healing Nutrition.* 2nd ed. Clifton Park, NY: Delmar Learning, 2002.

Mitchell, Joyce, and Lee Haroun. *Introduction to Health Care.* Clifton Park, NY: Delmar Learning, 2002.

Nielsen, Ronald. *OSHA Regulations and Guidelines: A Guide for Health Care Providers.* Clifton Park, NY: Delmar Learning, 2000.

Raffel, Marshall W., and Camille K. Barsukiewicz. *The US Health System Origins and Functions:* 5th ed. Clifton Park, NY: Delmar Learning, 2002.

Segen, Joseph. *Dictionary of Alternative Medicine.* Norwalk, CT: Appleton–Lange, 1998.

Umlauf, Mary. *Healing Meditation.* Clifton Park, NY: Delmar Learning, 1997.

U.S. Department of Labor. *Occupational Outlook Handbook.* Washington, D.C.: U.S. Government Printing Office, updated annually.

Williams, Stephen. *Essentials of Health Services.* 2nd ed. Clifton Park, NY: Delmar Learning, 2001.

Williams, Stephen, and Paul Torrens. *Introduction to Health Services.* 6th ed. Clifton Park, NY: Delmar Learning, 2002.

UNIT 2

Careers in Health Care

Unit Objectives

After completing this unit of study, you should be able to:

- ◆ Compare the educational requirements for associate's, bachelor's, and master's degrees
- ◆ Contrast certification, registration, and licensure
- ◆ Describe at least 10 different health careers by including a definition of the career, three duties, educational requirements, and employment opportunities
- ◆ Investigate at least one health career by writing to listed sources or using the Internet to request additional information on the career
- ◆ Interpret at least 10 abbreviations used to identify health occupations workers
- ◆ Define, pronounce, and spell all the key terms (see page 3 for explanation of accent mark use)

 Observe Standard Precautions

 Safety—Proceed with Caution

 Math Skill

 Science Skill

 C Communications Skill

 Instructors Check—Call Instructor at This Point

 **OBRA** OBRA Requirement— Based on Federal Law

 Legal Responsibility

 Career Information

 Technology

KEY TERMS

admitting officers/clerks

art, music, dance therapists

associate's degree

athletic trainers (ATs)

audiologists

bachelor's degree

biomedical equipment
  technicians (BETs)

cardiovascular technologist

central/sterile supply workers

certification

continuing education units
  (CEUs)

dental assistants (DAs)

dental hygienists
  (den'-tall hi-geen'-ists)

dental laboratory technicians

dentists (DMDs or DDSs)

dialysis technicians
  (die-ahl'-ih-sis tek-nish'ins)

dietetic assistants

dietetic technicians (DTs)

dietitians (RDs)

Doctor of Chiropractic (DC)
  (Ky-row-prak'-tik)

Doctor of Medicine (MD)

Doctor of Osteopathic
  Medicine (DO)
  (Oss-tee-ohp'-ath-ik)

Doctor of Podiatric Medicine
  (DPM)
  (Poh"-dee'-ah-trik)

doctorate/doctor's degree

electrocardiograph (ECG)
  technicians
  *(ee-lek"-trow-car'-dee-oh-graf
  tek-nish'-ins)*

electroencephalographic (EEG)
  technologist
  *(ee-lek"-troh-en-sef-ahl-oh-
  graf'-ik tek-nahl'-oh-jist)*

electroneurodiagnostic
  technologist
  *(ee-lek"-troh-new-roh-die-ag-
  nah'-stik)*

embalmers
  (em-bahl'-mers)

emergency medical technician
  (EMT)

endodontics
  (en'-doe-don'-tiks)

entrepreneur
  (on"trah-peh-nor')

funeral directors

geriatric aides/assistants
  (jerry-at'-rik)

health care administrators

health occupations education
  (HOE)

home health care assistants

housekeeping workers/
  sanitary managers

licensed practical/vocational
  nurses (LPNs/LVNs)

licensure
  (ly'-sehn-shur)

massage therapists

master's degree

medical assistants (MAs)

medical illustrators

medical laboratory assistants

medical laboratory technicians
  (MLTs)

medical laboratory
  technologists (MTs)

medical librarians

medical records administrators
  (RAs)

medical records technicians

medical transcriptionists

mortuary assistants

multicompetent/multiskilled
  worker

nurse assistants

occupational therapists (OTs)

occupational therapy
  assistants (OTAs)

ophthalmic assistants (OAs)

ophthalmic laboratory
  technicians

ophthalmic medical
  technologists (OMTs)

ophthalmic technicians (OTs)

ophthalmologists

opticians
  (ahp-tish'-ins)

optometrists (ODs)
  (ah'-tom'-eh-trists)

oral surgery

orthodontics
  (or"-thow-don'-tiks)

paramedic (EMT-P)

patient care technicians (PCTs)

pedodontics
  (peh"-doe-don'-tiks)

perfusionists
  (purr-few'-shun-ists)

periodontics
  (peh"-ree-oh-don'-tiks)

pharmacists (PharmDs)
  (far'-mah-sists)

pharmacy technicians

phlebotomists

physical therapists (PTs)

physical therapist assistants
  (PTAs)

physicians

physician assistants (PAs)

prosthodontics
  (pross"-thow-don'-tiks)

psychiatric/mental health
  technicians

psychiatrists

psychologists
  (sy-koll"-oh-jists)

radiologic technologists (RTs)
  *(ray"-dee-oh-loge'-ik tek-
  nahl'-oh-jists)*

recreational therapists (TRs)

recreational therapy assistants

registered nurses (RNs)

registration

respiratory therapists (RTs)

respiratory therapy
  technicians (RTTs)

social workers (SWs)

speech–language therapists

surgical technologists/
  technicians (STs)

unit secretaries/ward
  clerks/unit coordinators

veterinarians (DVMs or VMDs)
  (vet"-eh-ran-air'-e-ans)

veterinary assistants

veterinary technicians (VTs)

2:1 INFORMATION Introduction to Health Careers

There are over 200 different health care careers, so it would be impossible to discuss all of them in this unit. A broad overview of a variety of careers is presented, however.

Educational requirements for health careers depend on many factors and can vary from state to state. Basic preparation begins in high school (secondary education) and should include the sciences, social studies, English, and mathematics. General typing and accounting skills are also utilized in many health occupations. Secondary vocational **health occupations education (HOE)** programs can prepare a student for immediate employment in many health careers or for additional education after graduation. Post-secondary education (after high school) can include training in a vocational–technical school, community college, or university. Some careers require an **associate's degree,** which is awarded by a vocational-technical school or a community college after completion of a prescribed two-year course of study. Other careers require a **bachelor's degree**, which is awarded by a college or university after a prescribed course of study that usually lasts for four or more years. In some cases, a **master's degree** is required. This is awarded by a college or university after completion of one or more years of work beyond a bachelor's degree. Other careers require a **doctorate**, or **doctor's degree**, which is awarded by a college or university after completion of two or more years of work beyond a bachelor's or master's degree. Some doctorates can require four to six years of additional study.

CERTIFICATION, REGISTRATION, AND LICENSURE

Three other terms associated with health careers are *certification, registration,* and *licensure.* These are methods used to ensure the skill and competency of health care personnel and to protect the consumer or patient.

Certification means that a person has fulfilled requirements of education and performance and meets the standards and qualifications established by the professional association or government agency that regulates a particular career. A certificate or statement is issued by the association. Examples of certified positions include certified dental assistant, certified laboratory technician, and certified medical assistant.

Registration is required in some health occupations. This is performed by a regulatory body (professional association or state board) that administers examinations and maintains a current list ("registry") of qualified personnel in a given health care area. Examples of registered positions include registered dietitian, registered respiratory therapist, and registered radiologic technologist.

Licensure is a process whereby a government agency authorizes individuals to work in a given occupation. Health occupations requiring licensure can vary from state to state. Obtaining and retaining licensure usually requires that a person complete an approved educational program, pass a state board test, and maintain certain standards. Examples of licensed positions include physician, dentist, physical therapist, registered nurse, and licensed practical/vocational nurse.

For most health careers, graduation from an accredited program is required before certification, registration, and/or licensure will be granted. Accreditation ensures that the program of study meets the established quality competency standards and prepares students for employment in the health career. It is important for a student to make sure that a technical school, college, or university offers accredited programs of study before enrolling. Two major accrediting agencies for health care programs are the Commission on Accreditation of Allied Health Education Programs (CAAHEP) and the Accrediting Bureau of Health Education Schools (ABHES). A student can contact these agencies to determine whether a health occupations program at a specific school is accredited.

Continuing education units (CEUs) are required to renew licenses or maintain certification or registration in many states, figure 2-1. An individual must obtain additional hours of education in the specific health career area during a specified period of time. For example, many states require registered nurses to obtain 24 to 48 CEUs every one to two years in order to renew

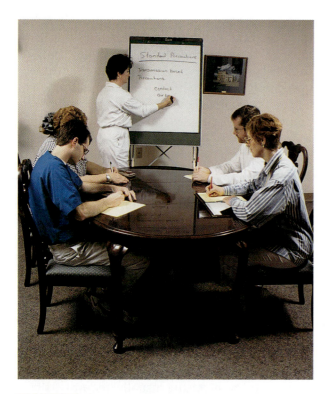

FIGURE 2-1 Continuing education units (CEUs) are required to renew licenses or maintain certification or registration in many states.

licenses. Health care workers should be aware of the state requirements regarding CEUs for their given careers.

EDUCATION LEVELS, TRENDS, AND OPPORTUNITIES

Generally speaking, training for most health occupations can be categorized into four levels, table 2-1.

A new trend in health occupations is that of the **multicompetent or multiskilled worker**. Because of high health care costs, smaller facilities and rural areas often cannot afford to hire a specialist for every aspect of care. Therefore, workers are hired who can perform a variety of health care skills. For example, a health care worker may be hired to perform the skills of both an electrocardiograph (ECG or EKG) technician (who records electrical activity of the heart) and an electroencephalographic (EEG) technologist (who records electrical activity of the brain). Another example might involve combining the basic skills of radiology, medical laboratory, and respiratory therapy. At times, workers trained in one field or occupation receive additional education to work in a second and even third occupation. In other cases, educational programs have been established to prepare multicompetent workers.

Another opportunity available in many health occupations is that of entrepreneur. An **entrepreneur** is an individual who organizes, manages, and assumes the risk of a business. Some health care careers allow an individual to work as an independent entrepreneur, while others encourage the use of groups of cooperating individuals. Many entrepreneurs must work under the direction or guidance of physicians or dentists. Because the opportunity to be self-employed and to be involved in the business area of health care exists, educational programs are including business skills with career objectives. A common example is combining a bachelor's degree in a specific health care career with a master's degree in business. Some health care providers who may be entrepreneurial include dental laboratory technicians, dental hygienists, nurse practitioners, physical therapists, physician assistants, respiratory therapists, recreational therapists, physicians, dentists, chiropractors, and optometrists. While entrepreneurship involves many risks and requires a certain level of education and ability, it can be an extremely satisfying choice for the individual who is well motivated, self-confident, responsible, creative, and independent.

NATIONAL HEALTH CARE SKILL STANDARDS

The National Health Care Skill Standards (NHCSS) were developed to indicate the knowledge and skills that are expected of health care workers primarily at the entry and technical levels. The six groups of standards include the following:

◆ Health Care Core Standards: specify the knowledge and skills that the vast majority of health care workers should have; discusses an academic foundation, communication skills, employability skills, legal responsibilities, ethics, safety practices, teamwork, and knowledge about the systems in the health care environment.

◆ Therapeutic/Diagnostic Core Standards: specify the knowledge and skills required to focus

TABLE 2-1 Education and Levels of Training

CAREER LEVEL	EDUCATIONAL REQUIREMENT	EXAMPLES
Professional	Four or more years of college with bachelor's, master's, or doctoral degree	Medical doctor Dentist
Technologist or Therapist	Three to four years of college plus work experience, usually bachelor's degree and at times, master's degree	Medical laboratory technologist Physical therapist Speech therapist Respiratory therapist
Technician	Two-year associate's degree, special health occupations education, or three to four years of on-the-job training	Dental laboratory technician Medical laboratory technician Surgical technician
Aide or Assistant	One or more years of training combining classroom and/or on-the-job training	Dental assistant Medical assistant Nurse assistant

on direct client care in both the therapeutic and diagnostic occupations; includes health maintenance practices, client interaction, intrateam communication, monitoring client status, and client movement.

◆ Therapeutic Cluster Standards: specify the knowledge and skills required of workers in health occupations that are involved in changing the health status of the client over time; includes data collection, treatment planning, implementing procedures, and client status evaluation.

◆ Diagnostic Cluster Standards: specify the knowledge and skills required of workers in health occupations that are involved in creating a picture of the health status of the client at a single point in time; includes planning, preparation, procedure, evaluation, and reporting.

◆ Information Services Cluster Standards: specify the knowledge and skills required of workers in health occupations that are involved with the documentation of client care; includes analysis, abstracting and coding, information systems, documentation, and operations to enter, retrieve, and maintain information.

◆ Environmental Services Cluster Standards: specify the knowledge and skills required of workers in health occupations that are involved with creating a therapeutic environment to provide direct or indirect client care; includes environmental operations, aseptic procedures, resource management, and aesthetics.

Examples of some of the health careers included in the NHCSS Clusters are shown on table 2-2. The careers listed are discussed in detail in this unit.

INTRODUCTION TO HEALTH CAREERS

In the following discussion of health careers, a basic description of the job duties for each career is provided. The various levels in each health occupation are also given. In addition, tables for each career group show educational requirements, job outlook, and average yearly earnings. In order to simplify the information presented in these tables, the highest level of education for each career group is listed. The designations used are as follows:

◆ on-the-job training: "on-the-job"

◆ health occupations education program: "HOE program"

◆ two-year associate's degree: "associate's degree"

◆ four-year bachelor's degree: "bachelor's degree"

◆ master's degree with one or more years beyond a bachelor's degree: "master's degree"

◆ doctorate with four or more years beyond a bachelor's degree: "doctoral degree"

It is important to note that although many health careers begin with vocational HOE programs, obtaining additional education after

TABLE 2-2 Examples of Health Careers in the NHCSS Clusters

THERAPEUTIC CLUSTER	DIAGNOSTIC CLUSTER	INFORMATION SERVICES CLUSTER	ENVIRONMENTAL SERVICES CLUSTER
Art/Music/Dance Therapist	Electrocardiographic Technician	Admitting Officer/Clerk	Biomedical Engineer
Athletic Trainer	Electroencephalographic Technician	Biomedical Writer	Biomedical Equipment Technician
Audiologist	Diagnostic Imaging Technician	Health Care Administrator	Central/Sterile Supply Worker
Chiropractor	Genetic Counselor	Health Educator	Environmental Health Scientist
Dental Careers	Medical Laboratory Careers	Health Sciences Librarian	Housekeeping Worker
Dialysis Technician	Phlebotomist	Insurance Processor	Sanitary Manager
Dietetic Technician	Radiologic Technologist	Medical Billing Officer	
Dietitian	Sonographer	Medical Illustrator	
Emergency Medical Careers		Medical Photographer	
Massage Therapist		Medical Records Administrator	
Medical Assistant		Medical Records Technician	
Mental Health Technician		Unit Secretary/ Coordinator	
Nursing Careers			
Occupational Therapist			
Ophthalmologist			
Optometrist			
Perfusionist			
Pharmacy Careers			
Physical Therapist			
Physician Assistant			
Physician			
Psychiatrist			
Psychologist			
Radiation Therapist			
Recreational Therapist			
Respiratory Therapist			
Social Worker/Sociologist			
Speech–Language Therapist			
Veterinarian			
Veterinary Technician			

graduation from HOE programs allows health care workers to progress in career level to higher-paying positions. The job outlook or expected job growth through the year 2010 is stated in the tables as "below average," "average," or "above average." Average yearly earning is presented as a range of income, because earnings will vary according to geographical location, specialty area, level of education, and work experience.

All career information presented includes a basic introduction. *Because requirements for various health occupations can vary from state to state, it is important for students to obtain information pertinent to their respective states.* More detailed information on any given occupation discussed can be obtained from the sources listed for that occupation's career cluster or from the references listed at the end of this unit.

2:2 INFORMATION Dental Careers

Dental workers focus on the health of the teeth and the soft tissues of the mouth. Care is directed toward preventing dental disease; repairing or replacing diseased or damaged teeth; and treating the gingiva (gums) and other supporting structures of the teeth.

Places of employment include private dental offices, laboratories, and clinics; or dental departments in hospitals, schools, health departments, or government agencies.

Most dental professionals work in general dentistry practices where all types of dental conditions are treated in people of all ages. Some, however, work in specialty areas such as the following:

◆ **Endodontics**—treatment of diseases of the pulp, nerves, blood vessels, and roots of the teeth; often called root canal treatment

◆ **Orthodontics**—alignment or straightening of the teeth

◆ **Oral Surgery**—surgery on the teeth, mouth, and jaw

◆ **Pedodontics**—dental treatment of children and adolescents

◆ **Periodontics**—treatment and prevention of diseases of the gums, bone, and structures supporting the teeth

◆ **Prosthodontics**—replacement of natural teeth with artificial teeth or dentures

Levels of workers in dentistry include dentist, dental hygienist, dental laboratory technician, and dental assistant (see table 2-3).

Dentists (DMD or DDS) are doctors who examine teeth and mouth tissues to diagnose and treat disease and abnormalities; perform surgery on the teeth, gums, and tissues; and work to prevent dental disease. They also supervise the work of other dental workers. Most are entrepreneurs.

Dental hygienists work under the supervision of dentists. They perform preliminary examinations of the teeth and mouth, remove stains and deposits from teeth, expose and develop X-rays, and perform other preventive or therapeutic (treatment) services to help the patient develop and maintain good dental health. In some states, dental hygienists are authorized to place and carve restorative materials, polish restorations, remove sutures, and/or administer anesthesia. Dental hygienists can be entrepreneurs.

Dental laboratory technicians make and repair a variety of dental prostheses (artificial devices) such as dentures, crowns, bridges, and orthodontic appliances according to the specifications of dentists. Specialities include dental ceramist and orthodontic technician. Some dental laboratory technicians are entrepreneurs.

TABLE 2-3 Dental Careers

OCCUPATION	EDUCATION REQUIRED	JOB OUTLOOK TO YEAR 2010	AVERAGE YEARLY EARNINGS
Dentist (DMD or DDS)	Doctor of Dental Medicine (DMD) or Doctor of Dental Surgery (DDS); 2 or more years additional education for specialization; licensure in state of practice	Below average growth	$84,000–$200,000
Dental Hygienist (DH) Licensed Dental Hygienist (LDH)	Associate's, bachelor's, or master's degree; licensure in state of practice	Above average growth	$33,700–$69,000
Dental Laboratory Technician (DLT)	3–4 years on-the-job or 1–2 years HOE program or associate's degree; certification can be obtained from National Board for Certification in Dental Technology	Average growth	$19,400–$52,600
Dental Assistant (DA) and Certified Dental Assistant (CDA)	1–3 years on-the-job or 1–2 years in HOE program or associate's degree; licensure or registration required in some states; certification can be obtained from Dental Assisting National Board	Above average growth	$15,600–$31,200

Dental assistants (DA), working under the supervision of dentists, prepare patients for examinations; pass instruments; prepare dental materials; take and develop X-rays; teach preventive dental care; sterilize instruments; and/or perform dental receptionist duties such as scheduling appointments and handling accounts. Their duties may be limited by the dental practice laws of the state in which they work.

ADDITIONAL SOURCES OF INFORMATION

◆ American Dental Education Association
1625 Massachusetts Avenue, NW
Washington, DC 20036
Internet address: *www.adea.org*

◆ American Dental Assistants Association
203 N. LaSalle Street
Chicago, IL 60601
Internet address: *www.dentalassistant.org*

◆ American Dental Association
211 E. Chicago Avenue
Chicago, IL 60611
Internet address: *www.ada.org*

◆ American Dental Hygienists' Association
444 N. Michigan Avenue, Suite 3400
Chicago, IL 60611
Internet address: *www.adha.org*

◆ Dental Assisting National Board, Inc.
676 North Saint Clair, Suite 1880
Chicago, IL 60611
Internet address: *www.dentalassisting.com*

◆ National Association of Dental Laboratories
1530 Metropolitan Boulevard
Tallahassee, FL 32308
Internet address: *www.nadl.org*

◆ National Association of Advisors for the Health Professions, Inc.
P.O. Box 1518
Champaign, IL 61824-1518
Internet address: *www.naahp.org*

◆ For information about specific tasks of a dental assistant, ask your instructor for the Guideline for Clinical Rotations in the *Diversified Health Occupations Teacher's Resource Kit*. Additional career information is provided in the Career Highlight Section of Unit 17 in this textbook.

2:3 INFORMATION
Diagnostic Services

Health workers in the diagnostic services perform tests or evaluations that aid in the detection, diagnosis, and treatment of disease, injury, or other physical conditions.

Many workers are employed in hospital laboratories, but others work in private laboratories, doctors' offices, clinics, public health agencies, pharmaceutical (drug) firms, and research or government agencies. In some occupations, individuals are entrepreneurs, owning and operating their own businesses.

Many careers fall under the designation of diagnostic services. Some of the more common ones are discussed in this unit. There are various levels of workers in most fields (see table 2-4). **Electrocardiograph (ECG) technicians** operate electrocardiograph machines, which record electrical impulses that originate in the heart. Physicians (especially cardiologists) use the electrocardiogram (ECG/EKG) to help diagnose heart disease and to note changes in the condition of a patient's heart. ECG or cardiac technicians having more advanced training also perform stress tests (which record the action of the heart during physical activity), Holter monitorings (ECGs lasting 24–48 hours, see figure 2-2), thallium scans (a nuclear scan after thallium is injected), and other specialized cardiac tests that frequently involve the use of computers. An associate's or bachelor's degree leads to a position as a **cardiovascular technologist**. These individuals assist with cardiac catheterization procedures and angioplasty (a procedure to remove blockages in blood vessels), monitor patients during open-heart surgery and the implantation of pacemakers, and perform tests to check circulation in blood vessels. Some specialize in using ultrasound (high frequency sound waves) to diagnose heart conditions and are called *echocardiographers*.

An **electroencephalographic (EEG) technologist** operates an instrument called an electroencephalograph, which records the electrical activity of the brain. The record produced, called an electroencephalogram, is used by a variety of physicians, especially neurologists (doctors specializing in nerve and brain diseases), to diagnose

TABLE 2-4 Diagnostic Services

OCCUPATION	EDUCATION REQUIRED	JOB OUTLOOK TO YEAR 2010	AVERAGE YEARLY EARNINGS
Cardiovascular Technologist **Registered Diagnostic Vascular Technician (RDVT)**	Associate's or bachelor's degree; registration can be obtained from Cardiovascular Credentialing International	Average growth	$27,500–$53,200
Electrocardiograph (ECG Technician)	1–12 months on-the-job or 6–12-month-HOE program; credentials can be obtained from National Board of Cardiovascular Testing	Below average growth	$17,300–$32,800
Electroencephalographic (EEG) Technologist and Electroneurodiagnostic Technologist	Few have 1–2 years on-the-job; most have 1–2-year HOE certification program or associate's degree; registration can be obtained from American Board of Registration of EEG Technologists	Below average growth	$25,300–$46,200
Medical (Clinical) Laboratory Technologist (MT) **Certified Medical (Clinical) Laboratory Technologist (CMT)** **Registered Medical (Clinical) Laboratory Technologist (RMT)**	Bachelor's or master's degree; licensure or registration required in some states; certification can be obtained from International Society for Clinical Laboratory Technology or American Medical Technologists Association National Certification Agency for Medical Laboratory Personnel	Average growth	$33,600–$55,200
Medical (Clinical) Laboratory Technician (MLT) **Certified Laboratory Technician (CLT)**	2-year HOE certification program or associate's degree; licensure or registration required in some states; certification can be obtained from International Society for Clinical Laboratory Technology or American Medical Technologists Association National Certification Agency for Medical Laboratory Personnel	Average growth	$25,700–$33,500
Medical (Clinical) Laboratory Assistant	1–2-year HOE program or on-the-job training; certification can be obtained from the Board of Certified Laboratory Assistants	Below average growth	$12,800–$26,300
Phlebotomist	1–2 years on-the-job or HOE program or 10–20 hour certification program	Average growth	$12,800–$26,300
Radiologic Technologist ARRT (Registered)	Associate's degree or bachelor's degree; licensure required in most states; registration can be obtained from American Registry of Radiologic Technologies (ARRT)	Above average growth	$28,900–$51,400
Biomedical Equipment Technician CBET (certified)	Associate's degree or bachelor's degree; certification can be obtained from International Certification Commission for Clinical Engineering and Biomedical Technology of the Association for the Advancement of Medical Instrumentation	Above average growth	$22,500–$52,400

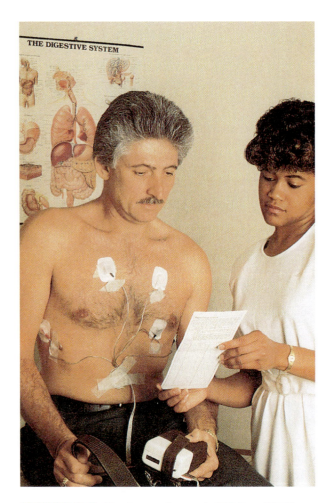

FIGURE 2-2 Electrocardiograph (ECG or EKG) technicians assist with Holter monitorings of the heart.

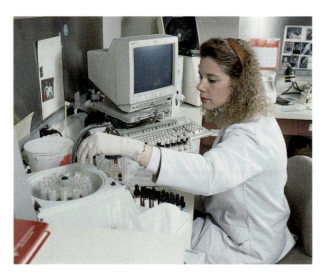

FIGURE 2-3 Medical laboratory technologists perform computerized blood analysis tests. *(Photo by Marcia Butterfield, courtesy of W. A. Foote Memorial Hospital, Jackson, MI)*

and evaluate diseases and disorders of the brain, such as brain tumors, strokes, toxic/metabolic disorders, epilepsy, and sleep disorders. Advanced training leads to a position as an **electroneurodiagnostic technologist**. In addition to performing EEGs, these individuals perform nerve conduction tests, measure sensory and physical responses to specific stimuli, and operate other monitoring devices. Technologists who specialize in administering sleep disorder evaluations are called *polysomnographic technologists*.

Medical laboratory technologists (MTs), also called clinical laboratory technologists, work under the supervision of doctors called pathologists. They study tissues, fluids, and cells of the human body to help determine the presence and/or cause of disease. They perform complicated chemical, microscopic, and automated analyzer/computer tests (see figure 2-3). In small

laboratories, technologists perform many types of tests. In larger laboratories, they may specialize. Examples of specialization include: biochemistry (chemical analysis of body fluids), blood bank technology (collection and preparation of blood and blood products for transfusions), cytotechnology (study of human body cells and cellular abnormalities), hematology (study of blood cells), histology (study of human body tissue), and microbiology (study of bacteria and other microorganisms).

Medical laboratory technicians (MLTs), working under the supervision of medical technologists or pathologists, perform many of the routine tests that do not require the advanced knowledge held by a medical technologist. Like the technologist, the technician can specialize in a particular field or perform a variety of tests.

Medical laboratory assistants, working under the supervision of medical technologists, technicians, or pathologists, perform basic laboratory tests; prepare specimens for examination or testing; and perform other laboratory duties such as cleaning and helping to maintain equipment.

Phlebotomists (see figure 2-4), or venipuncture technicians, collect blood and prepare it for testing. In some states, they perform blood tests under the supervision of medical technologists or pathologists.

Radiologic technologists (RTs), working under the supervision of doctors called radiologists, use X-rays, radiation, nuclear medicine,

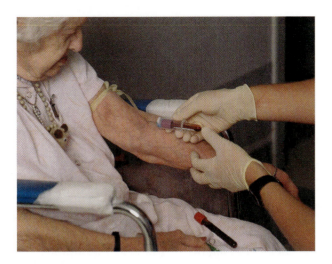

FIGURE 2-4 Phlebotomists collect blood and prepare it for testing.

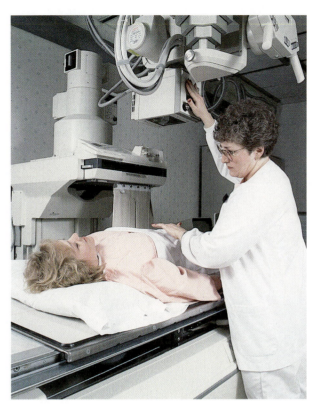

FIGURE 2-5 Radiologic technologists take X-rays used in the diagnosis of disease. *(Photo by Marcia Butterfield, courtesy of W. A. Foote Memorial Hospital, Jackson, MI)*

ultrasound, and magnetic resonance to diagnose and treat disease. Most techniques are noninvasive, which means examining or treating the internal organs of patients without entering the body. In many cases, recent advances in this field have eliminated the need for surgery and, therefore, offer less risk to patients. Radiologic technologists use different types of scanners to produce images of body parts. Examples include X-ray machines, fluoroscopes, ultrasonic scanners, computerized tomography (CT) scanners (formerly known as computerized axial tomography [CAT] scanners), magnetic resonance imagers (MRI), and positron emission tomography (PET) scanners. Many radiologic technologists also provide radiation treatment. Specific job titles exist for technologists who specialize. *Radiographers* (see figure 2-5) take X-rays of the body for diagnosis purposes. *Radiation therapists* administer prescribed doses of radiation to treat disease (usually cancer). *Nuclear medicine technologists* prepare radioactive substances for administration to patients. Once administered, these professionals use films, images on a screen, or body specimens such as blood or urine to determine how the radioactive substances pass through or localize in different parts of the body. This information is used by physicians to detect abnormalities or diagnose disease. *Ultrasound technologists,* or *sonographers,* use equipment that sends high frequency sound waves into the body. As the sound waves bounce back from the part being examined, an image of the part is viewed on a screen. This can be recorded on a printout strip or be photographed. Ultrasound is frequently used to examine the fetus (developing infant) in a pregnant woman and can reveal the sex of the unborn child. Ultrasound is also used for neurosonography (the brain), vascular (blood vessels and blood flow), and echocardiography (the heart) examinations. Magnetic resonance imaging (MRI) uses superconductive magnets and radio waves to produce detailed images of internal anatomy. The information is processed by a computer and displayed on a videoscreen. Examples of MRI use include identifying multiple sclerosis and detecting hemorrhaging (bleeding) in the brain. A positron emission scanner (PET), another diagnostic device, uses electrons to scan the body for disease processes.

Biomedical equipment technicians (BETs) work with the many different machines used to diagnose, treat, and monitor patients. They install, test, service, and repair equipment such as patient monitors, kidney hemodialysis units, diagnostic imaging scanners, incubators, electrocardiographs, X-ray units, pacemakers, sterilizers, blood-gas analyzers, heart-lung machines, respirators, and other similar devices.

Lives depend on the accuracy and proper operation of many of these machines, so constant maintenance and testing for defects is critical. Some biomedical equipment technicians also teach other staff members how to use biomedical equipment.

ADDITIONAL SOURCES OF INFORMATION

◆ Alliance of Cardiovascular Professionals
910 Charles Street
Fredericksburg, VA 22401

◆ American College of Radiology
1891 Preston White Drive
Reston, VA 22091
Internet address: *www.acr.org*

◆ American Medical Technologists
710 Higgins Road
Park Ridge, IL 60068
Internet address: *www.amt1.com*

◆ American Registry of Radiologic Technologists
1255 Northland Drive
St. Paul, MN 55120
Internet address: *www.arrt.org*

◆ American Society for Clinical Laboratory Science
7910 Woodmont Avenue, Suite 530
Bethesda, MD 20814
Internet address: *www.ascls.org*

◆ American Society of Electroneurodiagnostic Technologists
204 W. 7th Street
Carroll, IA 51401
Internet address: *www.aset.org*

◆ American Society of Radiologic Technologists
15000 Central Avenue SE
Albuquerque, NM 87123
Internet address: *www.asrt.org*

◆ Association for the Advancement of Medical Instrumentation
1110 North Globe Road, Suite 220
Arlington, VA 22201-4795
Internet address: *www.aami.org*

◆ Cardiovascular Credentialing International (CCI)
4456 Corporation Lane
Virginia Beach, VA 23462
Internet address: *www.cci-online.org*

◆ International Society for Clinical Laboratory Technology
917 Locust Street, Suite 1100
St. Louis, MO 63101

◆ National Accrediting Agency for Clinical Laboratory Sciences
8410 West Bryn Mawr Avenue, Suite 670
Chicago, IL 60631-3415
Internet address: *www.nca-info.org*

◆ National Association of Health Career Schools
750 First Street NE, Suite 940
Washington, DC 20002
Internet address: *www.NAHCS.org*

◆ Society of Diagnostic Medical Sonography
12770 Coit Road, Suite 708
Dallas, TX 75251
Internet address: *www.sdms.org*

◆ For information about specific tasks of a medical laboratory assistant/technician and a radiology assistant/technician, ask your instructor for the Guideline for Clinical Rotations in the *Diversified Health Occupations Teacher's Resource Kit*. Additional career information for medical laboratory assistants/technicians is provided in the Career Highlight Section of Unit 18 in this textbook.

2:4 INFORMATION Emergency Medical Services

Emergency medical services personnel (see figure 2-6) provide emergency, prehospital care to victims of accidents, injuries, or sudden illnesses. Although individuals with only basic training in first aid do sometimes work in this field, **emergency medical technician (EMT)** training is required for most jobs. Formal EMT training is available in all states and is offered by fire, police, and health departments, hospitals, vocational schools, and as a nondegree course in technical/community colleges and universities.

Places of employment include fire and police departments; rescue squads; ambulance services; hospital or private emergency rooms; urgent care centers; industry; emergency helicopter services; and the military. Some EMTs are entrepreneurs. Emergency medical technicians sometimes serve as volunteers in fire and rescue departments.

Levels of EMT include the EMT ambulance/ basic, EMT intermediate, and EMT paramedic (see table 2-5). Another emergency medical person is a first responder.

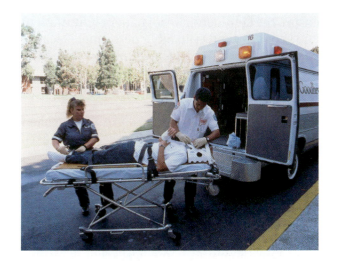

FIGURE 2-6 Emergency medical technicians (EMTs) provide emergency, prehospital care to victims of accidents, injuries, or sudden illness.

A first responder is the first person to arrive at the scene of an illness or injury. Common examples include police officers, security guards, fire department personnel, and immediate family members. The first responder frequently must provide basic emergency medical care. A certified first responder (CFR) course prepares individuals by teaching airway management, oxygen administration, bleeding control, and cardiopulmonary resuscitation (CPR).

Emergency medical technicians ambulance/ basic (EMT-B) provide care for a wide range of illnesses and injuries including medical emergencies, bleeding, fractures, airway obstruction, basic life support (BLS), oxygen administration, emergency childbirth, rescue of trapped persons, and transporting of victims.

Emergency medical technician defibrillator (EMT-D) is a new level of EMT-B. It allows EMT-Bs with additional training and competency in basic life support to administer electrical defibrillation to certain heart attack victims.

Emergency medical technicians intermediate (EMT-I) perform the same tasks as do EMT-Bs

TABLE 2-5 Emergency Medical Services

OCCUPATION	EDUCATION REQUIRED	JOB OUTLOOK TO YEAR 2010	AVERAGE YEARLY EARNINGS
Emergency Medical Technician Paramedic (EMT-P) (EMT-4)	EMT-Intermediate plus additional 6–9 months to 2 years (over 1000 hours) approved paramedic training or associate's degree; 6 months experience as paramedic; state certification; registration or licensure required in most states; other states identify as EMT-1, EMT-2, EMT-3, and EMT-4 and administer their own certification examination	Above average growth	$24,700–$48,500
Emergency Medical Technician Intermediate (EMT-I) (EMT-2 and EMT-3)	EMT-Basic plus additional approved training of at least 35–55 hours with clinical experience; state certification; registration required in some states; other states identify as EMT-1, EMT-2, EMT-3, and EMT-4 and administer their own certification examination	Above average growth	$21,200–$40,100
Emergency Medical Technician Ambulance/ Basic (EMT-B) (EMT-1)	Usually minimum 110 hours approved EMT program with 10 hours of internship in emergency room; state certification; registration by National Registry of EMTs (NREMT) required in some states; other states identify as EMT-1, EMT-2, EMT-3, and EMT-4 and administer their own certification examination	Above average growth	$19,200–$32,300

along with assessing patients, managing shock, using intravenous equipment, and inserting esophageal airways.

Emergency medical technicians **paramedic (EMT-P)** perform all the basic EMT duties plus in-depth patient assessment, provision of advanced cardiac life support (ACLS), ECG interpretation, endotracheal intubation, drug administration, and operation of complex equipment.

ADDITIONAL SOURCES OF INFORMATION

- National Association of Emergency Medical Technicians
  408 Monroe Street
  Clinton, MS 39056
  Internet address: *www.naemt.org*

- National Highway Transportation Safety Administration (NHTSA)
  EMS Division
  400 7th Street SW, NTS-14
  Washington, DC 20002
  Internet address:
  www.nhtsa.dot.gov/people/injury/ems

- National Registry of Emergency Medical Technicians
  6610 Bush Boulevard
  P. O. Box 29233
  Columbus, OH 43229
  Internet address: *www.nremt.org*

2:5 INFORMATION
Health Information and Communication Services

Health information and communication services employ many different types of health workers at all levels. Careers include medical records workers (who maintain complete accurate patient records), medical illustrators, photographers, writers, and librarians (see table 2-6). Computers are used in almost all the careers.

Places of employment include hospitals, clinics, research centers, health departments, long-term care facilities, colleges, law firms, health maintenance organizations (HMOs), and insurance companies.

Medical records administrators (RAs) plan the systems for storing and obtaining information from records; prepare information for legal actions and insurance claims; compile statistics for organizations and government agencies; manage medical records departments; ensure the confidentiality of patient information; and supervise and train other personnel. Because computers are used in almost all aspects of the job, it is essential for the medical records administrator to be able to operate and use a variety of computer programs.

Medical records technicians, also called health information technicians (see figure 2-7), organize and code patient records; gather statistical or research data; and record information. Computers have simplified many of the duties and are used to organize records; compile and report statistical data; and perform similar tasks. Computer operation is an important part of the education program for medical records technicians. Medical records departments also employ clerks, who organize records. Clerks typically complete a one- or two-year vocational program, or are trained on the job.

Medical transcriptionists use a word processor to enter data that has been dictated on an audiotape recorder by physicians or other health care professionals. Examples of data include physical examination reports, surgical reports, consultation findings, progress notes, and radiology reports.

Unit secretaries, ward clerks, or **unit coordinators** are employed in hospitals, extended care facilities, clinics, and other health facilities to record information on records; schedule procedures or tests; answer telephones; order supplies; and work with computers to record or obtain information.

Medical illustrators use their artistic and creative talents to produce illustrations, charts, graphs, and diagrams for health textbooks, journals, magazines, and exhibits. Another related field is a medical photographer who takes photographs or records videotapes of surgical procedures, health education information, documentation of conditions before and after reconstructive surgery, and legal information such as injuries received in an accident.

Medical librarians, also called health sciences librarians, organize books, journals, and other print materials to provide health information to other health care professionals. They use the computer to create information centers for large health care facilities or to provide information

TABLE 2-6 Health Information and Communication Services

OCCUPATION	EDUCATION REQUIRED	JOB OUTLOOK TO YEAR 2010	AVERAGE YEARLY EARNINGS
Medical Records (Health Information) Administrator Registered (RRA)	Bachelor's degree; registration can be obtained from American Health Information Management Association (AHIMA)	Average growth	$32,600–$70,400
Medical Records (Health Information) Technician Accredited (ART)	Independent Study Program in Health Information Technology with 30 semester hours of academic credit in medical records in an accredited program or associate's degree; Pass written examination of American Health Information Management Association (AHIMA); certification can be obtained from American Medical Records Association	Above average growth	$19,500–$40,500
Medical Transcriptionist American Medical Transcriptionist (AMT)	1 or more years vocational or technical education program, on-the-job training, or correspondence course; certification can be obtained from American Medical Transcriptionists	Average growth	$14,500–$29,900
Unit Secretary Ward Clerk Unit Coordinator Medical Records Clerk	1 or more years vocational or technical education program; some have on-the-job training	Average growth	$14,200–$34,300
Medical Illustrator	Bachelor's or master's degree; certification can be obtained from Association of Medical Illustrators	Average growth	$35,000–$65,200
Medical Librarian	Master's degree in library science	Average growth	$35,400–$136,300

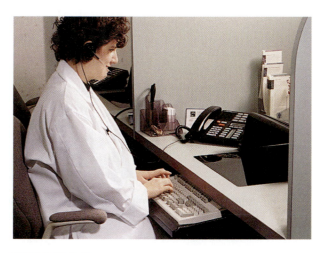

FIGURE 2-7 Medical records technicians organize and code patients' records.

to health care providers. Some librarians specialize in researching information for large pharmaceutical companies, insurance agencies, lawyers, industry, and/or government agencies.

ADDITIONAL SOURCES OF INFORMATION

◆ American Association for Medical Transcription
100 Sycamore Avenue
Modesto, CA 95354
Internet address: *www.aamt.org*

◆ American Health Information Management Association
233 N. Michigan Avenue, Suite 2150
Chicago, IL 60601
Internet address: *www.ahima.org*

◆ American Medical Association
Commission on Accreditation of Allied Health Education Programs
515 N. State Street
Chicago, IL 60610
Internet address: *www.ama-assn.org*

◆ Association of Medical Illustrators
2965 Flowers Road South, Suite 105
Atlanta, GA 30341
Internet address:
www.medical-illustrators.org

◆ Medical Library Association
65 East Wacker Plaza, Suite 1900
Chicago, IL 60602
Internet address: *www.mlanet.org*

2:6 INFORMATION Hospital/Health Care Facility Services

Any hospital or large health care facility requires workers to operate the support departments such as administration, the business office, the admissions office, central/sterile supply, and housekeeping. Each department has workers at all levels and with varying levels of education (see table 2-7).

Places of employment include hospitals, clinics, long-term care facilities, health maintenance organizations (HMOs), and public health or governmental agencies.

Health care administrators or health services managers plan, direct, coordinate, and supervise delivery of health care and manage the operation of health care facilities. They are frequently called chief executive officers (CEOs). A health care administrator may be responsible for personnel; supervise department heads; determine budget and finance; establish policies and procedures; perform public relations duties; and coordinate all activities in the facility. Duties depend on the size of the facility.

Admitting officers/clerks work in the admissions department of a health care facility. They are responsible for obtaining all necessary information when a patient is admitted to the facility; assigning rooms; maintaining records; and processing information when the patient is discharged. An admitting department manager is a higher level of worker in this field, usually having an associate's or bachelor's degree.

Central/sterile supply workers (see figure 2-8), are involved in ordering, maintaining, and supplying all the equipment and supplies used by other departments in a health care facility. They sterilize instruments or supplies, maintain equipment, inventory materials, and fill requisitions from other departments.

Housekeeping workers/sanitary managers, also called environmental service workers, help maintain the cleanliness of the health care facility in order to provide a pleasant, sanitary environment.

TABLE 2-7 Hospital/Health Care Facility Services

OCCUPATION	EDUCATION REQUIRED	JOB OUTLOOK TO YEAR 2010	AVERAGE YEARLY EARNINGS
Health Care Administrator Health Services Manager	Usually master's or doctorate, but smaller facilities may accept a bachelor's degree; licensure required for long-term care facilities; certification can be obtained from American College of Health Care Executives	Above average growth	$48,500–$196,000
Admitting Officer or Clerk	1–2-year HOE or business/office vocational/technical education; admitting officer may require bachelor's degree; few have on-the-job training	Average growth	$12,200–$26,600
Central/Sterile Supply Technician	On-the-job training or 1–2-year HOE program	Average growth	$12,200–$23,500
Housekeeping Worker Sanitary Manager	On-the-job training or 1-year vocational program	Above average growth	$12,200–$24,700

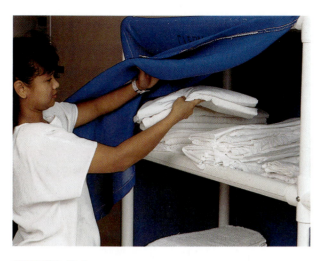

FIGURE 2-8 Central/sterile supply workers prepare all the equipment and supplies used by other departments in a health care facility.

ADDITIONAL SOURCES OF INFORMATION

◆ American College of Health Care Administrators
1800 Diagonal Road, Suite 355
Alexandria, VA 22314
Internet address: *www.achca.org*

◆ American College of Healthcare Executives
One North Franklin Street, Suite 1700
Chicago, IL 60606
Internet address: *www.ache.org*

◆ American Health Care Association
1201 L Street NW
Washington, DC 20005
Internet address: *www.ahca.org*

◆ American Hospital Association
1 North Franklin Street
Chicago, IL 60606
Internet address: *www.aha.org*

2:7 INFORMATION *Medical Careers*

Medical careers is a broad category encompassing physicians (doctors) and other individuals who work in any of the varied careers under the supervision of physicians. All such careers focus on diagnosing, treating, or preventing diseases and disorders of the human body.

Places of employment include private practices, clinics, hospitals, public health agencies, research facilities, health maintenance organizations (HMOs), government agencies, and colleges or universities.

Levels include physician, physician assistant, and medical assistant (see table 2-8).

Physicians examine patients, obtain medical histories, order tests, make diagnoses, perform surgery, treat diseases/disorders, and teach preventive health. Several classifications are as follows:

◆ **Doctor of Medicine (MD)**—Diagnoses, treats, and prevents diseases or disorders; may specialize as noted in table 2-9.

◆ **Doctor of Osteopathic Medicine (DO)**—Treats diseases/disorders, placing special emphasis on the nervous, muscular, and skeletal systems, and the relationship between the body, mind, and emotions; may also specialize.

◆ **Doctor of Podiatric Medicine (DPM)**—Examines, diagnoses, and treats diseases/disorders of the feet or of the leg below the knee.

◆ **Doctor of Chiropractic (DC)**—Focuses on ensuring proper alignment of the spine and optimal operation of the nervous system to maintain health.

Physician assistants (PAs), working under the supervision of physicians, take medical histories; perform routine physical examinations and basic diagnostic tests; make preliminary diagnoses; treat minor injuries; and prescribe and administer appropriate treatments.

Medical assistants (MAs), working under the supervision of physicians, prepare patients for examinations; take vital signs and medical histories; assist with procedures and treatments; perform basic laboratory tests; prepare and maintain equipment and supplies; and/or perform secretarial–receptionist duties (see figure 2-9). The type of facility and physician determines the kinds of duties. The range of duties is determined by state law. Assistants working for physicians who specialize are called specialty assistants. For example, an assistant working for a pediatrician is called a pediatric assistant.

TABLE 2-8 Medical Careers

OCCUPATION	EDUCATION REQUIRED	JOB OUTLOOK TO YEAR 2010	AVERAGE YEARLY EARNINGS
Physician	Doctor's degree; 3–8 years additional postgraduate training of internship and residency depending on specialty selected; state licensure; board certification in specialty area	Above average growth	$120,000–$305,000
Physician Assistant (PA) **PAC (certified)**	2 or more years of college and usually a bachelor's degree; 2 or more years accredited physician assistant program with certificate, associate's, or bachelor's degree; registration, certification, or licensure required in most states; certification from National Commission on Certification of Physician's Assistants	Above average growth	$38,600–$83,200
Medical Assistant (MA) **CMA (certified)** **RMA (registered)**	1–2-year HOE program or associate's degree; certification can be obtained from American Association of Medical Assistants (AAMA); after graduation from CAAHEP or ABHES accredited medical assistant program registered credentials can be obtained from American Medical Technologists (AMT)	Above average growth	$15,200–$33,400

ADDITIONAL SOURCES OF INFORMATION

◆ American Academy of Physician Assistants
950 N. Washington Street
Alexandria, VA 22314
Internet address: *www.aapa.org*

◆ American Association of Medical Assistants
20 N. Wacker Drive, Suite 1575
Chicago, IL 60606-2963
Internet address: *www.aama-ntl.org*

◆ American Chiropractic Association
1701 Clarendon Boulevard
Arlington, VA 22209
Internet address: *www.amerchiro.org*

◆ American Medical Association
515 North State Street
Chicago, IL 60610
Internet address: *www.ama-assn.org*

◆ American Osteopathic Association
142 East Ontario Street
Chicago, IL 60611
Internet address: *www.aoa-net.org*

◆ American Podiatric Medical Association
9312 Old Georgetown Road
Bethesda, MD 20814
Internet address: *www.apma.org*

◆ American Society of Podiatric Medical Assistants
2124 S. Austin Boulevard
Cicero, IL 60804
Internet address: *www.aspma.org*

◆ Registered Medical Assistants of the American Medical Technologists
710 Higgins Road
Park Ridge, IL 60068

◆ For information about specific tasks of a medical assistant, ask your instructor for the Guideline for Clinical Rotations in the *Diversified Health Occupations Teacher's Resource Kit.* Additional career information is provided in the Career Highlight Section of Unit 19 in this textbook.

TABLE 2-9 Medical Specialties

PHYSICIAN'S TITLE	SPECIALTY
Anesthesiologist	Administration of medications to cause loss of sensation or feeling during surgery
Cardiologist	Diseases of the heart and blood vessels
Dermatologist	Diseases of the skin
Emergency Physician	Acute illness or injury
Endocrinologist	Diseases of the endocrine glands
Family Physician/Practice	Promote wellness, treat illness or injury in all age groups
Gastroenterologist	Diseases and disorders of the stomach and intestine
Gerontologist	Diseases of elderly individuals
Gynecologist	Diseases of the female reproductive organs
Internist	Diseases of the internal organs (lungs, heart, glands, intestines, kidneys)
Neurologist	Disorders of the brain and nervous system
Obstetrician	Pregnancy and childbirth
Oncologist	Diagnosis and treatment of tumors (cancer)
Ophthalmologist	Diseases and disorders of the eye
Orthopedist	Diseases and disorders of muscles and bones
Otolaryngologist	Disease of the ear, nose, and throat
Pathologist	Diagnose disease by studying changes in organs, tissues, and cells
Pediatrician	Diseases and disorders of children
Physiatrist	Physical medicine and rehabilitation
Plastic Surgeon	Corrective surgery to repair injured or malformed body parts
Proctologist	Diseases of the lower part of the large intestine
Psychiatrist	Diseases and disorders of the mind
Radiologist	Use of X-rays and radiation to diagnose and treat disease
Sports Medicine	Prevention and treatment of injuries sustained in athletic events
Surgeon	Surgery to correct deformities or treat injuries or disease
Thoracic Surgeon	Surgery of the lungs, heart, or chest cavity
Urologist	Diseases of the kidney, bladder, or urinary system

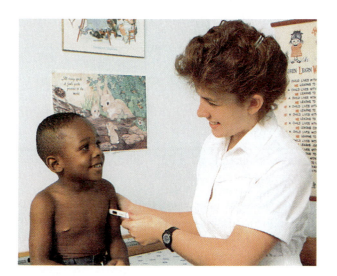

FIGURE 2-9 Medical assistants take vital signs and prepare patients for examinations.

2:8 INFORMATION Mental and Social Services

Mental services professionals focus on helping people with mental or emotional disorders or those who are developmentally delayed or mentally impaired. Social workers help people deal with illnesses, employment, or community problems. Workers in both fields try to help individuals function to their maximum capacities.

Places of employment include hospitals; psychiatric hospitals or clinics; home health care agencies; public health departments; government agencies; crisis or counseling centers; drug and alcohol treatment facilities; prisons; educational institutions; and long-term care facilities.

Levels of employment range from psychiatrist (a physician), who diagnoses and treats mental illness, to psychologist and psychiatric technician. There are also various levels (including assistant) employed in the field of social work (see table 2-10).

Psychiatrists are physicians who specialize in diagnosing and treating mental illness. Specialties include child or adolescent psychiatry, geriatric psychiatry, and drug/chemical abuse.

Psychologists study human behavior and use this knowledge to help individuals deal with problems of everyday living. Many specialize in specific aspects of psychology, which include child psychology, adolescent psychology, geriatric psychology, behavior modification, drug/chemical abuse, and physical/sexual abuse.

Psychiatric/mental health technicians, working under the supervision of psychiatrists or psychologists, help patients and their families follow treatment and rehabilitation plans. They provide understanding and encouragement; assist with physical care; observe and report behavior; and help teach patients constructive social behavior. Assistants or aides who have completed one or more years in an HOE program are also employed in this field.

Social workers, also called sociologists, case managers, or counselors (see figure 2-10), aid people who have difficulty coping with various problems by helping them make adjustments in their lives and/or by referring them to community resources for assistance. Specialties include child welfare, geriatrics, family, correctional (jail), and occupational social work. Many areas employ assistants or technicians who have one or more years of an HOE program.

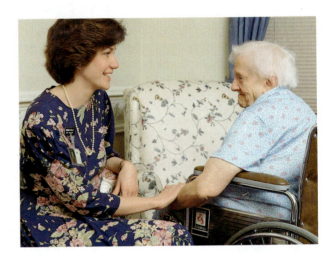

FIGURE 2-10 Social workers help people make life adjustments and refer patients to community resources for assistance.

TABLE 2-10 Mental and Social Services

OCCUPATION	EDUCATION REQUIRED	JOB OUTLOOK TO YEAR 2010	AVERAGE YEARLY EARNINGS
Psychiatrist	Doctor's degree; 2–7 years postgraduate specialty training; state licensure; certification in psychiatry	Above average growth	$95,500–$245,000
Psychologist PsyD (Doctor of Psychology)	Bachelor's or master's degree; doctor of psychology required for many positions; licensure or certification required in all states; certification for specialty areas available from American Board of Professional Psychology	Average growth	$24,900–$71,800 or $38,900–$92,500 with doctorate
Psychiatric/Mental Health Technicians	Associate's degree; licensure required in some states; a few states require a nursing degree	Above average growth	$18,600–$31,300
Social Workers/ Sociologists	Bachelor's or master's degree or Doctor of Philosophy or Social Work (DSW); licensure, certification, or registration required in all states; credentials available from National Association of Social Workers	Above average growth	$28,600–$56,800

ADDITIONAL SOURCES OF INFORMATION

◆ American Psychiatric Association
1400 K Street NW
Washington, DC 20005
Internet address: *www.psych.org*

◆ American Psychological Association
750 1st Street NE
Washington, DC 20002-4242
Internet address: *www.apa.org*

◆ American Sociological Association
1307 New York Avenue NW, Suite 700
Washington, DC 20005
Internet address: *www.asanet.org*

◆ Center for Mental Health Services
Internet address: *www.mentalhealth.org*

◆ National Association of Social Workers
750 First Street NE, Suite 700
Washington, DC 20002-4241
Internet address: *www.naswdc.org*

◆ National Mental Health Association
1021 Prince Street
Alexandria, VA 22314
Internet address: *www.nmha.org*

2:9 INFORMATION Mortuary Careers

Workers in mortuary careers provide a service that is needed by everyone. Even though funeral practices and rites vary because of cultural diversity and religion, most services involve preparation of the body, performance of a ceremony that honors the deceased and meets the spiritual needs of the living, and cremation or burial of the remains.

Places of employment are funeral homes or mortuaries, crematoriums, or cemetery associations.

Levels include funeral director, embalmer, and mortuary assistant (see table 2-11).

Funeral directors, also called morticians or undertakers, provide support to the survivors; interview the family of the deceased to establish details of the funeral ceremonies or review arrangements the deceased person requested prior to death; prepare the body following legal requirements; secure information for legal documents; file death certificates; arrange and direct all the details of the wake and services; make arrangements for burial or cremation; and direct all business activities of the funeral home. Frequently, funeral directors help surviving individuals adapt to the death by providing post-death counseling and support group activities. Most funeral directors are also licensed embalmers.

Embalmers prepare the body for interment by washing the body with germicidal soap, replacing the blood with embalming fluid to preserve the body, reshaping and restructuring disfigured bodies, applying cosmetics to create a natural appearance, dressing the body, and placing it in a casket. They are also responsible for maintaining embalming reports and itemized lists of clothing or valuables.

Mortuary assistants work under the supervision of the funeral director and/or embalmer. They may assist with preparation of the body, drive the hearse to pick up the body after death or to take it to the burial site, arrange flowers for the viewing, assist with preparations for the funeral service, help with filing and maintenance of records, clean the funeral home, and other similar duties.

TABLE 2-11 Mortuary Careers

OCCUPATION	EDUCATION REQUIRED	JOB OUTLOOK TO YEAR 2010	AVERAGE YEARLY EARNINGS
Funeral Director (Mortician)	2–4 years in a mortuary science college or associate's or bachelor's degree; licensure required in all states except Colorado	Above average	$25,500–$86,500
Embalmer	2–4 years in a mortuary science college or associate's or bachelor's degree; licensure required in all states	Above average	$20,100–$69,200
Mortuary Assistant	1–2 years on-the-job training or 1-year HOE program	Above average	$12,200–$25,800

ADDITIONAL SOURCES OF INFORMATION

◆ American Board of Funeral Service Education
38 Florida Avenue
Portland, ME 04103
Internet address: *www.abfse.org*

◆ National Funeral Directors Association
13625 Bishop's Drive
Brookfield, WI 53005
Internet address: *www.nfda.org*

2:10 INFORMATION *Nursing Careers*

Those in the nursing careers provide care for patients as directed by physicians. Care focuses on the mental, emotional, and physical needs of the patient.

Hospitals are the major places of employment, but nursing workers are also employed in long-term care facilities, rehabilitation centers, physicians' offices, clinics, public health agencies, home health care agencies, health maintenance organizations (HMOs), schools, government agencies, and industry.

Levels include registered nurse, licensed practical/vocational nurse, and nurse assistant/technician (see table 2-12).

Registered nurses (RNs) (see figure 2-11), work under the direction of physicians and provide total care to patients. The RN observes patients; assesses patients' needs; reports to other health care personnel; administers prescribed medications and treatments; teaches health care; and supervises other nursing personnel. The type of facility determines specific job duties. Registered nurses with an advanced education can specialize. Examples include nurse practitioner (CRNP), nurse midwives (CNM), nurse educator, and nurse anesthetist. Nurse practitioners take health histories; perform basic

TABLE 2-12 Nursing Careers

OCCUPATION	EDUCATION REQUIRED	JOB OUTLOOK TO YEAR 2010	AVERAGE YEARLY EARNINGS
Registered Nurse (RN)	2–3-year diploma program in hospital school of nursing, or associate's degree or bachelor's degree; master's or doctor's for some administrative/educational positions; licensure in state of practice	Above average growth	$28,900–$69,200 / $60,300–$108,900 with advanced specialties
Licensed Practical/ Vocational Nurse (LPN/LVN)	1–2-year state-approved HOE practical/vocational nurse program; licensure in state of practice	Above average growth	$23,200–$43,100
Nurse Assistant / Geriatric Aide / Home Health Care Assistant / Certified Nurse Technician / Patient Care Technician (PCT)	HOE program; certification or registration required in all states for long-term care facilities—obtained by completing 75–120 hour state-approved program	Above average growth especially in geriatric or home care	$14,000–$27,200
Surgical Technician/ Technologist CST (certified)	1–2-year HOE program; certificate, diploma, or associate's degree; certification can be obtained from Liaison Council on Certification for Surgical Technologists	Above average growth	$22,800–$40,200

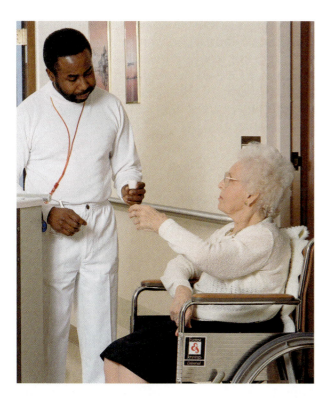

FIGURE 2-11 Registered nurses (RNs) administer prescribed medications to patients.

Nurse assistants (also called nurse aides, nurse technicians, **patient care technicians (PCTs)**, or orderlies) work under the supervision of RNs or LPNs/LVNs. They provide patient care such as baths, bedmaking, and feeding; assist in transfer and ambulation; and administer basic treatments. **Geriatric aides/assistants** acquire additional education to provide care for the elderly in work environments such as extended care facilities, nursing homes, retirement centers, adult day care agencies, and other similar agencies. **Home health care assistants** are trained to work in the patient's home and may perform additional duties such as meal preparation or cleaning.

OBRA Each nursing assistant working in a long-term care facility or home health care is now required under federal law to complete a mandatory, state-approved training program and pass a written and/or competency exam to obtain certification or registration. Health workers in these environments should check the requirements of their respective states.

Surgical technologists/technicians (STs), also called operating room technicians (see figure 2-12), working under the supervision of RNs

physical examinations; order laboratory tests and other procedures; refer patients to physicians; help establish treatment plans; treat common illnesses such as colds or sore throats; and teach and promote optimal health. Nurse midwives provide total care for normal pregnancies. The nurse midwife examines the pregnant woman at regular intervals; performs routine tests; teaches childbirth and childcare classes; monitors the infant and mother during childbirth; delivers the infant; and refers any problems to a physician. Nurse educators teach in HOE programs; schools of nursing; colleges and universities; wellness centers; and health care facilities. Nurse anesthetists administer anesthesia, monitor patients during surgery, and assist anesthesiologists (who are physicians).

Licensed practical/vocational nurses (LPNs/LVNs), working under the supervision of physicians or RNs, provide patient care requiring technical knowledge but not the level of education required of RNs. The type of care is determined by the work environment, which can include the home, hospital, long-term care facility, adult day-care center, physician's office, clinic, wellness center, and health maintenance organization. Care provided by LPN/LVNs is also determined by state laws regulating the extent of duties.

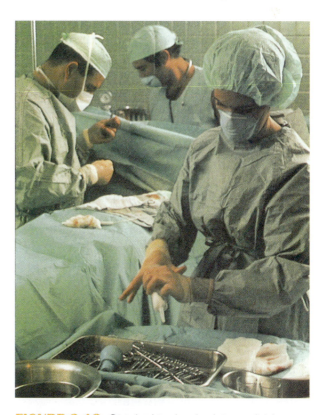

FIGURE 2-12 Surgical technologists assist by passing instruments and supplies to the surgeon. *(Photo courtesy of the U.S. Army)*

or physicians, prepare patients for surgery; set up instruments, equipment, and sterile supplies in the operating room; and assist during surgery by passing instruments and supplies to the surgeon. Although most surgical technologists/technicians work in hospital operating rooms, some are employed in outpatient surgical centers, emergency rooms, urgent care centers, physicians' offices, and other facilities.

◆ For information about specific tasks of a geriatric assistant/technician or nurse assistant/technician, ask your instructor for the Guideline for Clinical Rotations in the *Diversified Health Occupations Teacher's Resource Kit.* Additional career information is provided in the Career Highlight Section of Unit 20 in this textbook.

ADDITIONAL SOURCES OF INFORMATION

◆ American College of Nurse Practitioners
1111 19th Street NW, Suite 404
Washington, DC 20036
Internet address: *www.nurse.org/acnp/*

◆ American Health Care Association
1201 L Street NW
Washington, DC 20005
Internet address: *www.ahca.org*

◆ American Nurses' Association
600 Maryland Avenue SW
Washington, DC 20024
Internet address: *www.ana.org*

◆ Association of Surgical Technologists
7108-C S. Alton Way
Englewood, CO 80112
Internet address: *www.ast.org*

◆ National Association for Hospice and Homecare
228 Seventh Street SE
Washington, DC 20003
Internet address: *www.nahc.org*

◆ National Association for Practical Nurse Education and Service
1400 Spring Street, Suite 330
Silver Springs, MD 20910
Internet address: *www.napnes.org*

◆ National Federation of Licensed Practical Nurses
893 US Highway 70 West, Suite 202
Garner, NC 27529
Internet address: *www.nflpn.org*

◆ National League for Nursing
61 Broadway
New York, NY 10006
Internet address: *www.nln.org*

2:11 INFORMATION
Nutrition and Dietary Services

Health, nutrition, and physical fitness have become a way of life. Workers employed in the nutrition and dietary services recognize the importance of proper nutrition to good health. Using knowledge of nutrition, they promote wellness and optimum health by providing dietary guidelines used to treat various diseases, teaching proper nutrition, and preparing foods for health care facilities.

Places of employment include hospitals, long-term care facilities, child and adult daycare facilities, wellness centers, schools, home health care agencies, public health agencies, clinics, industry, and offices.

Levels include dietitian, dietetic technician, and dietetic assistant (see table 2-13).

Dietitians (RDs) or nutritionists (see figure 2-13) manage food service systems; assess patients'/residents' nutritional needs; plan menus; teach others proper nutrition and special diets; purchase food and equipment; enforce sanitary and safety rules; and supervise and/or train other personnel. Some dietitians specialize in the care of pediatric (child), renal (kidney), or diabetic patients; or in weight management.

Dietetic technicians (DTs), working under the supervision of dietitians, plan menus; order foods; standardize and test recipes; assist with food preparation; and provide basic dietary instruction.

Dietetic assistants, also called food service workers, work under the supervision of dietitians and assist with food preparation and service; help patients select menus; clean work areas; and assist other dietary workers.

TABLE 2-13 Nutrition and Dietary Services

OCCUPATION	EDUCATION REQUIRED	JOB OUTLOOK TO YEAR 2010	AVERAGE YEARLY EARNINGS
Dietitian, RD (registered)	Bachelor's degree; registration can be obtained from Commission on Dietetic Registration of the American Dietetic Association; licensure, certification, or registration required in many states	Average growth	$28,000–$59,600
Dietetic Technician, DTR (registered)	Associate's degree; licensure, certification, or registration required in some states; registration can be obtained from the Commission on Dietetic Registration	Above average growth	$20,200–$46,200
Dietetic Assistant	6–12 months on-the-job; 1 or more years HOE or food service vocational program	Average growth	$12,200–$21,000

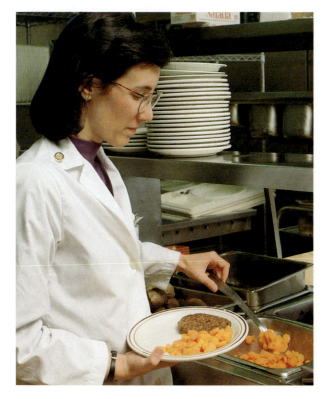

FIGURE 2-13 Dietitians manage food service systems, assess nutritional needs, and plan menus according to prescribed diets.

ADDITIONAL SOURCES OF INFORMATION

◆ American Dietetic Association
216 W. Jackson Boulevard
Chicago, IL 60606-6995
Internet address: *www.eatright.org*

◆ Dietary Managers Association
406 Surrey Woods Drive
St. Charles, IL 60174
Internet address: *www.dmaonline.org*

◆ Institute of Food Technologists
221 North LaSalle Street
Chicago, IL 60601-1291
Internet address: *www.ift.org*

◆ For information about specific tasks of a dietary assistant/food service worker, ask your instructor for the Guideline for Clinical Rotations in the *Diversified Health Occupations Teacher's Resource Kit.*

2:12 INFORMATION Therapeutic Services

Workers in the therapeutic services use a variety of treatments to help patients who are injured; physically or mentally disabled; or emotionally disturbed. All treatment is directed toward allowing patients to function at maximum capacity.

Places of employment include rehabilitation facilities, hospitals, clinics, mental health facilities, daycare facilities, long-term care facilities, home health care agencies, schools, and government agencies.

Most therapeutic occupations include levels of therapist, technician, and assistant/aide (see table 2-14).

Occupational therapists (OTs) (see figure 2-14) help people with physical, developmental, mental, or emotional disabilities to overcome,

TABLE 2-14 Therapeutic Services

OCCUPATION	EDUCATION REQUIRED	JOB OUTLOOK TO YEAR 2010	AVERAGE YEARLY EARNINGS
Occupational Therapist (OT) OTR (registered)	Bachelor's or master's degree and internship; licensure required in all states; certification can be obtained from American Occupational Therapy Association	Above average growth	$38,900–$87,500
Occupational Therapy Assistant COTA (certified)	1–2-year HOE certificate program or associate's degree and internship; licensure or certification required by most states; certification can be obtained from American Occupational Therapy Association	Above average growth	$20,800–$49,200
Pharmacist (PharmD)	5–6-year college program with Bachelor or Doctor of Pharmacy degree plus internship; licensure required in all states	Average growth	$48,300–$96,600
Pharmacy Technician	1 or more years on-the-job or 1–2-year HOE program or associate's degree; licensure required in a few states; certification can be obtained from the Pharmacy Technician Certification Board	Average growth	$14,200–$32,500
Physical Therapist (PT)	Bachelor's or master's degree; master's degree after 2002; licensure required in all states	Above average growth	$42,500–$89,600
Physical Therapist Assistant (PTA)	2-year HOE accredited program or associate's degree plus internship; licensure required in most states	Above average growth	$19,200–$44,800
Massage Therapist	3-month to 1-year accredited Massage Therapy Program; certification, registration, or licensure required in many states	Above average growth	$18,500–$44,600
Recreational Therapist (TR) **Certified Therapeutic Recreation Specialist (CTRS)**	Possibly associate's but usually bachelor's degree plus internship; licensure or certification required in a few states; certification can be obtained from National Council for Therapeutic Recreation Certification (NCTRC); registration can be obtained from Association for Rehabilitation Therapy	Average growth	$26,800–$52,500
Recreational Therapist Assistant (Activity Director)	1–2-year HOE certificate program or associate's degree; certification can be obtained from National Council for Therapeutic Recreation Certification	Average growth	$13,500–$32,800
Respiratory Therapist, RT RRT (registered)	Associate's or bachelor's degree; licensure required in most states; registration can be obtained from National Board for Respiratory Care	Above average growth	$29,900–$54,500
Respiratory Therapy Technician (RTT) CRTT (certified)	1–2-year HOE program or associate's degree; licensure or certification required in most states; certification can be obtained from National Board for Respiratory Care	Above average growth	$19,800–$34,500

(continued)

TABLE 2-14 Therapeutic Services *(Continued)*

OCCUPATION	EDUCATION REQUIRED	JOB OUTLOOK TO YEAR 2010	AVERAGE YEARLY EARNINGS
Speech–Language Therapist/Pathologist and/or Audiologist	Master's degree and 9 months postgraduate clinical experience; licensure required in most states; Certificate of Clinical Competence in Speech–Language Pathology (CCC–SLP) or Audiology (CCC–A) can be obtained from American Speech-Language-Hearing Association (ASHA)	Above average growth	$33,200–$80,500
Art, Music, Dance Therapist	Bachelor's or master's degree; certification for art therapist can be obtained from American Art Therapy Association; registration for music therapist can be obtained from National Association of Music Therapy and American Association for Music Therapy; registration for dance therapist can be obtained from American Dance Therapy Association	Average growth	$21,200–$56,800
Athletic Trainer ATC (certified)	Bachelor's or master's degree; licensure required in some states; certification can be obtained from National Athletic Trainers Association	Above average growth	$22,400–$58,600
Dialysis Technician	Varies with states; some states require RN or LPN license and state approved dialysis training; other states require 1–2-year HOE state approved dialysis program or associate's degree; certification can be obtained from National Association of Nephrology Technicians	Average growth	$14,200–$56,800
Perfusionist Extracorporeal Circulation Technologist (CCP)	Bachelor's degree and specialized extracorporeal circulation training and supervised clinical experience; licensure required in some states; certification can be obtained from American Board of Cardiovascular Perfusion	Above average growth	$36,200–$64,500

correct, or adjust to their particular problems. The occupational therapist uses various activities to assist the patient in learning skills or activities of daily living (ADL), adapting job skills, or preparing for return to work. Treatment is directed toward helping patients acquire independence, regain lost functions, adapt to disabilities, and lead productive and satisfying lives.

Occupational therapy assistants (OTAs), working under the guidance of occupational therapists, help patients carry out programs of prescribed treatment. They direct patients in arts and crafts projects, recreation, or social events; teach and help patients carry out rehabilitation activities and exercises; use games to develop balance and coordination; assist patients trying to master the activities of daily living; and inform therapists of patients' responses and progress.

Pharmacists (PharmDs) (see figure 2-15) dispense medications per written orders from physicians, dentists, and other health care professionals authorized to prescribe medications. They provide information on drugs and correct ways to use them; order and dispense other health care items such as surgical and sickroom supplies; recommend nonprescription items to customers/patients; ensure drug compatibility; maintain records on medications dispensed; and assess, plan, and monitor drug usage. Pharmacists can also either be entrepreneurs or work for one of the many drug manufacturers involved in researching, manufacturing, and selling drugs.

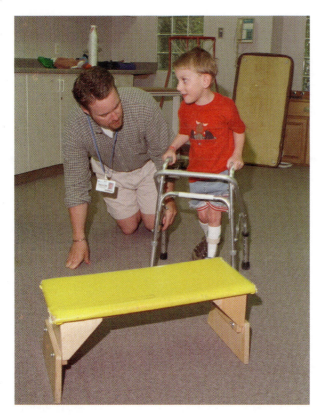

FIGURE 2-14 Occupational therapists (OTs) help patients with disabilities to overcome, correct, or adjust to the disabilities.

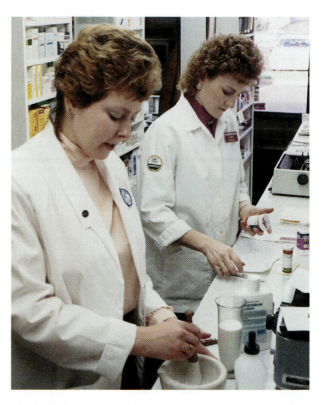

FIGURE 2-15 Pharmacists dispense medications and provide information on drugs. *(Courtesy of the Michigan Pharmacists Association and the Michigan Society of Pharmacy Technicians)*

Pharmacy technicians, working under the supervision of pharmacists, help prepare medications for dispensing to patients; label medications; perform inventories and order supplies; prepare intravenous solutions; help maintain records; and perform other duties as directed by pharmacists.

Physical therapists (PTs), see figure 2-16, provide treatment to improve mobility and prevent or limit permanent disability of patients with disabling joint, bone, muscle, and/or nerve injuries or diseases. Treatment may include exercise, massage, and/or applications of heat, cold, water, light, electricity, or ultrasound. Therapists assess the functional abilities of patients and use this information to plan treatment programs. They also promote health and prevent injuries by developing proper exercise programs and teaching patients correct use of muscles. Some physical therapists are entrepreneurs.

Physical therapist assistants (PTAs), working under the supervision of physical therapists, help carry out prescribed plans of treatment. They perform exercises and massages; administer applications of heat, cold, and/or water; assist patients to ambulate with canes, crutches, or braces; provide ultrasound or electrical stimulation treatments; inform therapists of patients' responses and progress; and perform other duties, as directed by therapists.

Massage therapists usually work under the supervision of physicians or physical therapists, and use many variations of massage, bodywork (manipulation or application of pressure to the muscular or skeletal structure of the body), and therapeutic touch to muscles to provide pain relief for chronic conditions (such as back pain) or inflammatory diseases; improve lymphatic circulation to decrease edema (swelling); and relieve stress and tension. Some massage therapists are entrepreneurs.

Recreational therapists (TRs), or *therapeutic recreation specialists,* use recreational and leisure activities as forms of treatment to minimize patients' symptoms and improve physical, emotional, and mental well-being. Activities might include organized athletic events; dances; arts and crafts; musical activities; drama; field trips to shopping centers or other places of interest; movies; or poetry or book readings. All activities are directed

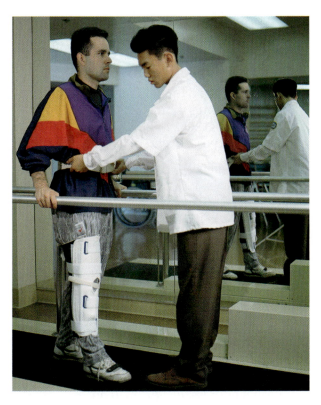

FIGURE 2-16 Physical therapists (PTs) provide treatment to improve mobility of patients with disabling injuries or diseases.

toward allowing the patient to gain independence, build self-confidence, and relieve anxiety. Some recreational therapists are entrepreneurs.

Recreational therapy assistants, also called *activity directors,* work under the supervision of recreational therapists or other health care professionals. They assist in carrying out the activities planned by therapists, and, at times, arrange activities or events. They note and inform therapists of patients' responses and progress.

Respiratory therapists (RTs), under physicians' orders, treat patients with heart and lung diseases by administering oxygen, gases, or medications; using exercise to improve breathing; monitoring ventilators; and performing diagnostic respiratory function tests (see figure 2-17). Some respiratory therapists are entrepreneurs.

Respiratory therapy technicians (RTTs) work under the supervision of respiratory therapists, and administer respiratory treatments; perform basic diagnostic tests; clean and maintain equipment; and note and inform therapists of patients' responses and progress.

Speech–language therapists, also called *speech pathologists,* identify, evaluate, and treat patients with speech and language disorders.

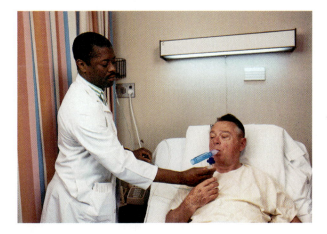

FIGURE 2-17 Respiratory therapists (RTs) provide treatments to patients with heart and lung diseases.

They help patients communicate as effectively as possible, and also teach patients to cope with the problems created by speech impairments.

Audiologists provide care to individuals who have hearing impairments. They test hearing, diagnose problems, and prescribe treatment, which may include hearing aids, auditory training, or instruction in speech or lip reading. They also test noise levels in workplaces and develop hearing protection programs.

Art, music, and **dance therapists** use the arts to help patients deal with social, physical, or emotional problems. Therapists usually work with individuals who are emotionally disturbed, mentally retarded, or physically disabled, but they may also work with adults and children who have no disabilities in an effort to promote physical and mental wellness.

Athletic trainers (ATs) prevent and treat athletic injuries and provide rehabilitative services to athletes. The athletic trainer frequently works with a physician who specializes in sports medicine. Athletic trainers teach proper nutrition; assess the physical condition of athletes; give advice regarding a physical conditioning program to increase strength and flexibility or correct weaknesses; put tape or padding on players to protect body parts; treat minor injuries; administer first aid for serious injuries; and help carry out any rehabilitation treatment prescribed by sports medicine physicians or other therapists.

Dialysis technicians operate the kidney hemodialysis machines used to treat patients with limited or no kidney function. Careful patient monitoring is critical during the dialysis process. The dialysis technician must also provide emotional support for the patient and teach proper nutrition (because many patients must follow restricted diets).

Perfusionists, also called *extracorporeal circulation technologists,* are members of open-heart surgical teams and operate the heart-lung machines used in coronary bypass surgery (surgery on the coronary arteries in the heart). This field is expanding to include new advances such as artificial hearts. Monitoring and operating these machines correctly is critical because the patient's life depends on the machines.

ADDITIONAL SOURCES OF INFORMATION

◆ American Alliance for Health, Physical Education, Recreation, and Dance
1900 Association Drive
Reston, VA 22091-1598
Internet address: *www.aahperd.org*

◆ American Art Therapy Association
1202 Allanson Road
Mundelheim, IL 60060
Internet address: *www.arttherapy.org*

◆ American Association for Respiratory Care
11030 Ables Lane
Dallas, TX 75229
Internet address: *www.aarc.org*

◆ American Association of Colleges of Pharmacy
1426 Prince Street
Alexandria, VA 22314
Internet address: *www.aacp.org*

◆ American Association of Pharmacy Technicians
P. O. Box 1447
Greensboro, NC 27402
Internet address:
www.pharmacytechnician.org

◆ American Dance Therapy Association
2000 Century Plaza
Columbia, MD 21044
Internet address: *www.adta.org*

◆ American Massage Therapy Association
820 Davis Street, Suite 100
Evanston, IL 60201-4444
Internet address: *www.amtamassage.org*

◆ American Pharmaceutical Association
2215 Constitution Avenue NW
Washington, DC 20037-2985
Internet address: *www.aphanet.org*

◆ American Physical Therapy Association
1111 N. Fairfax Street
Alexandria, VA 22314-1488
Internet address: *www.apta.org*

◆ American Occupational Therapy Association
4720 Montgomery Lane, P. O. Box 31220
Bethesda, MD 20824-1220
Internet address: *www.aota.org*

◆ American Society of Extracorporeal Technologists
503 Carlisle Drive
Herndon, VA 20170
Internet address: *www.amsect.org*

◆ American Speech–Language–Hearing Association
10801 Rockville Pike
Rockville, MD 20852
Internet address: *www.asha.org*

◆ American Therapeutic Recreation Association
1414 Prince Street, Suite 204
Alexandria, VA 22314
Internet address: *www.atra-tr.org*

◆ Associated Bodywork and Massage Professionals
1271 Sugarbush Drive
Evergreen, CO 80439-9766
Internet address: *www.abmp.com*

◆ Massage and Bodywork Resource Center
Internet address: *www.massageresource.com*

◆ National Association for Music Therapy
8455 Colesville Road
Silver Spring, MD 20910
Internet address: *www.namt.org*

◆ National Athletic Trainers Association
2952 Stemmons Freeway
Dallas, TX 75247
Internet address: *www.nata.org*

◆ National Therapeutic Recreation Society
22377 Belmont Ridge Road
Ashburn, VA 20148
Internet address: *www.nrpa.org*

◆ Pharmacy Technician Certification Board
2215 Constitution Avenue NW
Washington, DC 20037-2985
Internet address: *www.ptcb.org*

◆ For information about specific tasks of a pharmacy technician/assistant, physical therapy assistant/technician, or respiratory therapy assistant/technician, ask your instructor for the Guideline for Clinical Rotations in the

Diversified Health Occupations Teacher's Resource Kit. Additional career information for physical therapy is provided in the Career Highlight Section of Unit 21 in this textbook.

2:13 INFORMATION Veterinary Careers

Veterinary careers focus on providing care to all types of animals—from house pets to livestock to wildlife.

Places of employment include animal hospitals; veterinarian offices; laboratories; zoos; farms; animal shelters; aquariums; drug or animal food companies; and fish and wildlife services.

Levels of employment include veterinarian, animal health technician, and assistant (see table 2-15).

Veterinarians (DVMs or VMDs) work to prevent, diagnose, and treat diseases and injuries in animals. Specialties include surgery; small animal care; livestock; fish and wildlife; and research.

Veterinary technicians (VTs), also called *animal health technicians,* working under the supervision of veterinarians, assist with the handling and care of animals, collect specimens, assist with surgery, perform laboratory tests, take and develop X-rays, administer prescribed treatments, and maintain records.

Veterinary assistants, also called *animal caretakers,* feed, bathe, and groom animals;

exercise animals; prepare animals for treatment; assist with examinations; clean and sanitize cages, examination tables, and surgical areas; and maintain records.

ADDITIONAL SOURCES OF INFORMATION

◆ American Association for Laboratory Animal Science
9190 Crestwyn Hills Drive
Memphis, TN 38125
Internet address: *www.aalas.org*

◆ American Veterinary Medical Association
1931 N. Meacham Road, Suite 100
Schaumburg, IL 60173-4360
Internet address: *www.avma.org*

◆ Animal Caretakers Information
The Humane Society of the United States
2100 L Street NW
Washington, DC 20037
Internet address: *www.hsus.org*

◆ North America Veterinary Technician Association (NAVTA)
P. O. Box 224
Battle Ground, IN 47920
Internet address: *www.avma.org/navta*

◆ For information about specific tasks of a veterinary assistant, ask your instructor for the Guideline for Clinical Rotations in the *Diversified Health Occupations Teacher's Resource Kit.*

TABLE 2-15 Veterinary Careers

OCCUPATION	EDUCATION REQUIRED	JOB OUTLOOK TO YEAR 2010	AVERAGE YEARLY EARNINGS
Veterinarian (DVM or VMD)	3–4 years preveterinary college; 4 years veterinary college and Doctor of Veterinary Medicine degree; state licensure	Above average growth	$39,500–$92,800 or more
Veterinary (Animal Health) Technician VTR (registered)	Certificate, associate's, or bachelor's degree; registration, certification, or licensure required in most states	Above average growth	$17,400–$30,700
Veterinary Assistant (Animal Caretakers)	1–2 years on-the-job or 1–2-year HOE program	Above average growth	$13,200–$21,300

2:14 INFORMATION
Vision Services

Workers in the vision services provide care to prevent and treat vision disorders. Places of employment include offices, optical shops, department stores, hospitals, schools, health maintenance organizations (HMOs), government agencies, and clinics.

Levels include ophthalmologist; optometrist; ophthalmic technician and assistant; optician; and ophthalmic laboratory technician (see table 2-16). Many individuals in this field are entrepreneurs.

Ophthalmologists are medical doctors specializing in diseases and disorders of the eyes. They diagnose and treat disease; perform surgery; and correct vision problems or defects.

Optometrists (ODs), doctors of optometry, examine eyes for vision problems and defects; prescribe corrective lenses or eye exercises; and, in some states, use drugs for diagnosis and/or treatment. If eye disease is present or if eye surgery is needed, the optometrist refers the patient to an ophthalmologist.

Ophthalmic medical technologists (OMTs), working under the supervision of ophthalmologists, obtain patient histories, perform routine eye tests and measurements, fit patients for contacts, administer prescribed treatments, assist with eye surgery, perform advanced diagnostic tests such as ocular motility and biocular function tests, administer prescribed medications, and perform advanced microbiological procedures. In addition, they may perform any tasks that ophthalmic technicians or assistants perform.

Ophthalmic technicians (OTs) (see figure 2-18) work under the supervision of ophthalmologists and optometrists. Technicians prepare patients for examinations, obtain medical histories, take ocular measurements, administer basic

TABLE 2-16 Vision Services

OCCUPATION	EDUCATION REQUIRED	JOB OUTLOOK TO YEAR 2010	AVERAGE YEARLY EARNINGS
Ophthalmologist (MD)	Doctor's degree; 2–7 years postgraduate specialty training; state licensure; certification in ophthalmology	Average growth	$95,000–$218,000
Optometrist (OD)	3–4 years preoptometric college; 4 years at college of optometry; state licensure	Average growth	$48,500–$93,600
Ophthalmic Medical Technologist COMT (certified)	Associate's or bachelor's degree; certification can be obtained from the Joint Commission on Allied Health Personnel in Ophthalmology (JCAHPO)	Average growth	$23,000–$38,600
Ophthalmic Technician COT (certified)	Associate's degree; certification can be obtained from Joint Commission on Allied Health Personnel in Ophthalmology (JCAHPO)	Average growth	$20,100–$27,600
Ophthalmic Assistant COA (certified)	Some on-the-job training; 1 month to 1-year HOE program; certification can be obtained from the Joint Commission on Allied Health Personnel in Ophthalmology (JCAHPO)	Average growth	$13,200–$22,600
Optician	2–4 years on-the-job or 2–4-year apprenticeship or HOE program or associate's degree; licensure or certification required in some states; certification can be obtained from American Board of Opticianry and National Contact Lens Examiners	Average growth	$18,400–$42,500
Ophthalmic Laboratory Technician	2–3 years on-the-job or 1-year HOE certificate program	Below average growth	$14,400–$32,000

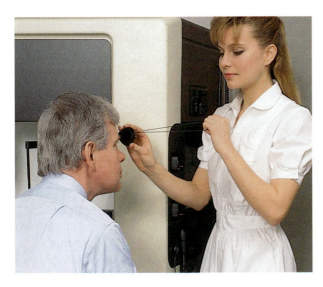

FIGURE 2-18 Ophthalmic technicians perform basic vision tests and teach eye exercises. *(Courtesy of the American Optometric Association, St. Louis, MO)*

vision tests, maintain ophthalmic and surgical instruments, adjust glasses, teach eye exercises, measure for contacts, instruct patients on the care and use of contacts, and perform receptionist duties.

Ophthalmic assistants (OAs) work under the supervision of ophthalmologists, optometrists, and/or ophthalmic technologists or technicians. Assistants prepare patients for examinations, measure visual acuity, perform receptionist duties, help patients with frame selections and fittings, order lenses, perform minor adjustments and repairs of glasses, and teach proper care and use of contact lenses.

Opticians make and fit the eyeglasses or lenses prescribed by ophthalmologists and optometrists. Some specialize in contact lenses.

Ophthalmic laboratory technicians cut, grind, finish, polish, and mount the lenses used in eyeglasses, contact lenses, and other optical instruments such as telescopes and binoculars.

ADDITIONAL SOURCES OF INFORMATION

◆ American Optometric Association
243 N. Lindbergh Boulevard
St. Louis, MO 63141
Internet address: *www.aoanet.org*

◆ Association of Schools and Colleges of Optometry
6110 Executive Boulevard, Suite 510
Rockville, MD 20852
Internet address: *www.opted.org*

◆ Commission on Opticianry Accreditation
10111 Martin Luther King Jr. Highway, Suite 100
Bowie, MD 20720
Internet address: *www.coaccreditation.com*

◆ Joint Commission on Allied Health Personnel in Ophthalmology
2025 Woodlane Drive
St. Paul, MN 55125-2995
Internet address: *www.jcahpo.org*

◆ National Federation of Opticianry Schools
9604 Escada Court
Chesterfield, VA 23832
Internet address: *ww.nfos.org*

◆ Opticians Association of America
7023 Little River Turnpike, Suite 207
Annandale, VA 22003
Internet address: *www.opticians.org*

STUDENT: *Go to the workbook and complete the assignment sheet for Unit 2, Careers in Health Care.*

UNIT 2 SUMMARY

Over 200 different careers in health care provide individuals with opportunities to find occupations they enjoy. Each health care career differs somewhat in the type of duties performed, the education required, the standards that must be met and maintained, and the salary earned.

This unit has described some of the major health care careers. For each career group, levels of workers, basic job duties, educational requirements, anticipated need for workers through the year 2010, and average yearly salaries were provided. Use this unit to evaluate the different health careers, and request additional information on specific careers from sources listed at the end of the respective career sections. In this way, you can research various occupational opportunities and determine which health care career is most appropriate for your interests and abilities.

INTERNET SEARCHES

Use the suggested search engines in Unit 11:4 of this textbook to search the Internet for additional information on the following topics:

1. *National Health Care Skill Standards (NHCSS).*

2. *Health care careers:* search for information on specific careers by entering the name of the career.

3. *Career organizations:* contact organizations at web addresses listed in each career cluster to determine the purpose of the organization, health careers it promotes, and advantages of membership.

4. *Accreditation Agencies:* Search the Commission on Accreditation of Allied Health Education Programs (CAAHEP) at *www.caahep.org* and the Accrediting Bureau of Health Education Schools (ABHES) at *www.abhes.org* to determine which health career programs are accredited by each agency. Research schools in your area that meet accreditation standards.

5. *Schools:* search for technical schools, colleges, and universities that offer educational programs for a specific career. Evaluate entrance requirements, financial aid, and programs of study.

REVIEW QUESTIONS

1. What is the difference between secondary and post-secondary health care education?

2. For each of the post-secondary degrees listed, state how many years of education are required to obtain the degree. For each degree, give three (3) examples of specific health care careers that require the degree for entry level workers.
   a. Associate's degree
   b. Bachelor's degree
   c. Master's degree
   d. Doctorate

3. Differentiate between certification, registration, and licensure.

4. What are CEUs? Why are they required in many health care careers?

5. Name at least four (4) specific careers within each cluster of the National Health Care Skill Standards.

6. What is an entrepreneur? Identify five (5) examples of health care careers that may be an entrepreneur.

7. Choose one health care career in which you have an interest. Use references or search the Internet to list ten (10) specific tasks performed by personnel in the career.

8. Choose one health care career in which you have an interest. Use references or search the Internet to identify three (3) different schools that offer accredited programs in the career.

UNIT 2

SUGGESTED REFERENCES

American Medical Association. *Handbook for Health Information Careers.* Clifton Park, NY: Delmar Learning, 1998.

American Medical Association. *Health Professions Education Directory.* Chicago, IL: American Medical Association, updated biannually.

Anderson, Shirley, and Jody Smith. *Delmar's Handbook for Health Information Careers.* Clifton Park, NY: Delmar Learning, 1998.

Baily, M. *Working: Career Success for the 21st Century.* 3rd ed. Cincinnati, OH: South-Western, 2003.

Burger, William, and Merill Youkeles. *The Helping Professions: A Career Sourcebook.* Pacific Grove, CA: Brooks/Cole, 2000.

Center for Nursing and Health Careers. *Health Careers.* Toledo, OH: Center for Nursing and Health Careers, 1994.

Colbert, Bruce. *Workplace Readiness for Health Occupations.* Clifton Park, NY: Delmar Learning, 2000.

Deem, Saitofi, and Joseph Deem. *Health Care Exploration.* Clifton Park, NY: Delmar Learning, 2000.

McCutcheon, Maureen. *Exploring Health Careers.* 2nd ed. Clifton Park, NY: Delmar Learning, 1999.

Mitchell, Joyce, and Lee Haroun. *Introduction to Health Care.* Clifton Park, NY: Delmar Learning, 2002.

National Health Council. *200 Ways to Put Your Talent to Work in the Health Field.* New York, NY: National Health Council, nd.

Thomson, Lois. *Clinical Rotations.* Clifton Park, NY: Delmar Learning, 1998.

U.S. Department of Labor. *Occupational Outlook Handbook.* Washington, D.C.: U.S. Government Printing Office, updated annually.

Williams, Stephen, and Paul Torrens. *Introduction to Health Services.* 6th ed. Clifton Park, NY: Delmar Learning, 2002.

Wischnitzer, Saul, and Edith Wischnitzer. *Health-Care Careers for the 21st Century.* Indianapolis, IN: Jist Works, Inc., 2000.

UNIT 3

Personal Qualities of a Health Care Worker

Unit Objectives

After completing this unit of study, you should be able to:

◆ Explain how diet, rest, exercise, good posture, and avoiding tobacco, alcohol, and drugs contribute to good health

◆ Demonstrate the standards of a professional appearance as they apply to uniforms, clothing, shoes, nails, hair, jewelry, and makeup

◆ Create a characteristic profile of a health care worker that includes at least eight personal/professional traits or attitudes

◆ Identify why teamwork is beneficial in health care

◆ Identify six basic characteristics of leaders

◆ Differentiate between democratic, laissez-faire, and autocratic leaders

◆ Differentiate between positive and negative stressors by identifying the emotional response to each type

◆ List six ways to eliminate or decrease stress

◆ Explain how time management, problem solving, and goal setting contribute to reducing stress

◆ Define, pronounce, and spell all the key terms

Observe Standard Precautions		Instructors Check—Call Instructor at This Point	
Safety—Proceed with Caution		 OBRA Requirement— Based on Federal Law	
Math Skill		Legal Responsibility	
Science Skill		Career Information	
Communications Skill		Technology	

KEY TERMS

acceptance of criticism	enthusiasm	responsibility
autocratic leader	goal	self-motivation
competence	honesty	stress
(kom'-peh-tense)	laissez-faire leader	tact
democratic leader	leader	team player
dependability	leadership	teamwork
discretion	patience	time management
empathy	personal hygiene	willingness to learn
(em'-path-ee")		

INTRODUCTION

Although health care workers are employed in many different career areas and in a variety of facilities, certain personal/professional characteristics, attitudes, and rules of appearance apply to all health care professionals. This unit discusses these basic requirements.

3:1 INFORMATION Personal Appearance

As a worker in any health career, it is important to present an appearance that inspires confidence and a positive self-image. Research has shown that within 20 seconds to 4 minutes people form an impression about another person based mainly on appearance. Although the rules of suitable appearance may vary, certain professional standards apply to most health careers and should be observed to create a positive impression.

GOOD HEALTH

Health care involves promoting health and preventing disease. Therefore, a health care worker should present a healthy appearance. Five main factors contribute to good health:

◆ *Diet*—Eating well-balanced meals and nutritious foods provides the body with the materials needed for optimum health. Foods from each of the five major food groups (milk; meat; vegetables; fruits; and bread, cereals, rice, and pasta) should be eaten daily. The Food Guide Pyramid, discussed in Unit 10:4, identifies the major food groups.

◆ *Rest*—Adequate rest and sleep help provide energy and the ability to deal with stress. The amount of sleep required varies from individual to individual.

◆ *Exercise*—Exercise maintains circulation and improves muscle tone. It also helps mental attitude and contributes to more restful sleep. Individuals should choose the form of exercise best suited to their own needs, but should exercise daily.

◆ *Good Posture*—Good posture helps prevent fatigue and puts less stress on muscles. Basic principles include standing straight with stomach muscles pulled in, shoulders relaxed, and weight balanced equally on each foot.

◆ *Avoid Use of Tobacco, Alcohol, and Drugs*—The use of tobacco, alcohol, and drugs can seriously affect good health. Tobacco affects the function of the heart, circulatory system, lungs, and digestive system. In addition, the odor of smoke is offensive to many individuals. For these reasons, most health care facilities are "smoke-free" environments. The use of alcohol and drugs impairs mental function, decreases ability to make decisions, and adversely affects many body systems. The use of alcohol or drugs can also result in job loss. Avoiding tobacco, alcohol, and drugs helps prevent damage to the body systems and contributes to good health.

PROFESSIONAL APPEARANCE

When you obtain a position in a health career, it is important to learn the rules or standards of dress and personal appearance that have been established by your place of employment. Abide by the rules, and make every effort to maintain a neat, clean, and professional appearance.

Uniform

Many health occupations require uniforms. A uniform should always be neat, well fitting, clean, and free from wrinkles (figure 3-1). Some agencies require a white uniform, but others allow pastel colors. In some facilities, the colors identify groups of workers. If white uniforms are required, white or neutral undergarments should be worn. A large variety of uniform styles is available. Extreme styles in any type of uniform should be avoided. It is important that the health care worker learn what type and color uniform is required or permitted and follow the standards established by the place of employment.

Clothing

If regular clothing is worn in place of a uniform, the clothing must be clean, neat, and in good repair (figure 3-2). The style should allow for freedom of body movement and should be appropriate for the job. For example, while clean, neat jeans might be appropriate at times for a recreational therapist, they are not proper attire for most other health professionals. Washable fabrics are usually best because frequent laundering is necessary.

Name Badge

Most health care facilities require personnel to wear name badges or photo identification tags at all times. The badge usually states the name, title, and department of the health care worker. In some health care settings, such as long-term care facilities, workers are required by law to wear identification badges.

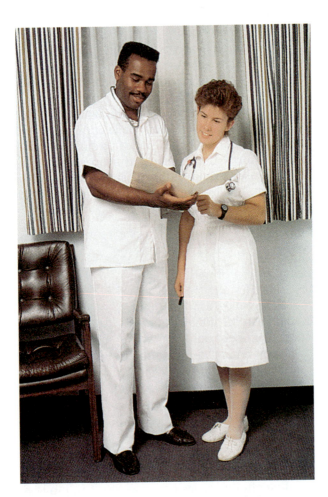

FIGURE 3-1 Uniform styles may vary, but a uniform should always be neat, well fitting, clean, and free from wrinkles.

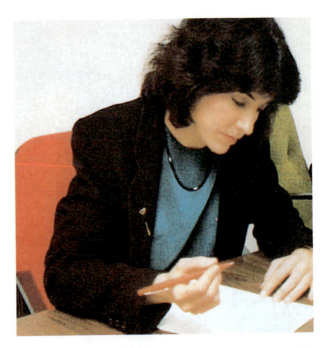

FIGURE 3-2 If regular clothing is worn in place of a uniform, the clothing should reflect a professional appearance.

Shoes

Although white shoes are frequently required, many occupations allow other types of shoes. Any shoes should fit well and provide good support to prevent fatigue. Low heels are usually best because they help prevent fatigue and accidents. Avoid wearing tennis shoes or sandals, unless they are standard dress for a particular occupation. Shoes should be cleaned daily. If shoelaces are part of the shoes, these must also be cleaned or replaced frequently. Women should wear white or beige stockings or pantyhose with dress uniforms; colored or patterned stockings should be avoided. White socks should be worn with white pants.

Personal Hygiene

Good **personal hygiene** is essential. Because health care workers typically work in close contact with others, body odor must be controlled. A daily bath or shower, use of deodorant or antiperspirant, good oral hygiene, and clean undergarments all help prevent body odor. Strong odors caused by tobacco, perfumes, scented hairsprays, and after-shave lotions can be offensive. In addition, certain scents can cause allergic reactions in some individuals. The use of these products should be avoided when working with patients and coworkers.

Nails

Nails should be kept short and clean. If fingernails are long and/or pointed, they can injure patients. They can also transmit germs, because dirt can collect under long nails. In addition, health care workers are now required to wear gloves for many procedures. Long nails can tear or puncture gloves. The use of colored nail polish is discouraged because the color can conceal any dirt that may collect under the nails. Further, because frequent handwashing causes polish to chip, germs can collect on the surfaces of nails. Finally, the flash of bright colors may bother a person who does not feel well. If nail polish is worn, it should be clear or colorless, and the nails must be kept scrupulously clean. Hand cream or lotion should be used to keep the hands from becoming chapped and dry from frequent handwashing.

Hair

Hair should be kept clean and neat. It should be styled attractively and be easy to care for. Fancy or extreme hairstyles and hair ornaments should be avoided. If the job requires close contact with patients, long hair must be pinned back and kept off the collar. This prevents the hair from touching the patient/resident, falling on a tray or on equipment, or blocking necessary vision during procedures.

Jewelry

Jewelry is usually not permitted with a uniform because it can cause injury to the patient and transmit germs or pathogens. Exceptions sometimes include a watch, wedding ring, and small, pierced earrings. Earrings with hoops or dangling earrings should be avoided. Body jewelry, such as nose, eyebrow, or tongue-piercing jewelry, detracts from a professional appearance and is prohibited in many health care facilities. When a uniform is not required, jewelry should still be limited. Excessive jewelry can interfere with patient care and detracts from the professional appearance of the health care worker.

Makeup

Excessive makeup should be avoided. The purpose of makeup is to create a natural appearance and add to the attractiveness of a person.

3:2	**INFORMATION** *Personal* **Characteristics**

Many personal/professional characteristics and attitudes are required in the health occupations. As a health care worker, you should make every effort to develop the following characteristics and attitudes and to incorporate them into your personality.

Empathy: Empathy means being able to identify with and understand another person's feelings, situation, and motives. As a health care worker, you may care for persons of all ages—from the newborn infant to the elderly individual. In order to be successful, you must be sincerely interested in working with people. You must care about others and be able to communicate and work with them. Understanding the needs of people and learning effective communication is one way to develop empathy. This topic is covered in greater detail in Unit 7 of this text.

Honesty: Truthfulness and integrity are important in any career field. Others must be able to trust you at all times. You must be willing to admit mistakes so they can be corrected.

Dependability: Employers and patients rely on you, so you must accept the responsibility required in your position. You must be prompt in reporting to work, and maintain a good attendance record (figure 3-3). You must perform assigned tasks on time and accurately.

Willingness to learn: You must be willing to learn and to adapt to changes. The field of health care changes because of research, new inventions, and technological advances. Change often requires learning new techniques or procedures. At times, additional education may be required to remain competent in a particular field. Be prepared for lifelong learning to maintain a competent level of knowledge and skills.

Patience: You must be tolerant and understanding. You must learn to control your temper and "count to ten" in difficult situations. Learning to deal with frustration and overcome obstacles is important.

Acceptance of criticism: Patients, employers, coworkers, and others may criticize you. Some criticism will be constructive and allow you to improve your work. Remember that everyone has some areas where performance can be improved. Instead of becoming resentful, you must be willing to accept criticism and learn from it.

Enthusiasm: You must enjoy your work and display a positive attitude. Enthusiasm is contagious; it helps you do your best and encourages others to do the same. If you do not like some aspects of your job, concentrating on the positive points can help diminish the importance of the negative points.

Self-motivation: Self-motivation, or self-initiative, is the ability to begin or to follow through with a task. You should be able to determine things that need to be done and do them without constant direction. You set goals for yourself and work to reach the goals.

Tact: Being tactful means having the ability to say or do the kindest or most fitting thing in a difficult situation. It requires constant practice. Tactfulness implies a consideration for the feelings of others. It is important to remember that all individuals have a right to their respective feelings, and that these feelings should not be judged as right or wrong.

Competence: Being competent means that you are qualified and capable of performing a task. You follow instructions, use approved procedures, and strive for accuracy in all you do. You know your limits and ask for help or guidance if you do not know how to perform a procedure.

Responsibility: Responsibility implies being willing to be held accountable for your actions. Others can rely on you and know that you will meet your obligations. Responsibility means that you do what you are supposed to do.

Discretion: You must always use good judgment in what you say and do. In any health care career, you will have access to confidential information. This information should not be told to anyone without proper authorization. A patient is entitled to confidential care; you must be discreet and ensure that the patient's rights are not violated.

Team player: In any health care field, you will become part of a team. It is essential that you become a team player and learn to work well with others. Each member of a health care team will have different responsibilities, but each member must do his or her part to provide the patient with quality care. By working together, a team can accomplish goals much faster than an individual.

Each of the preceding characteristics and attitudes must be practiced and learned. Some take more time to develop than do others. By being aware of these characteristics and striving constantly to improve, you will provide good patient/resident care and be a valuable asset to your employer and other members of the health care team.

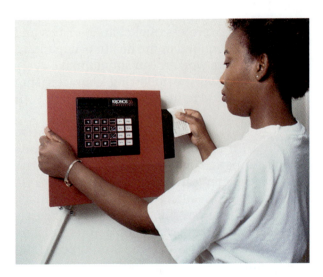

FIGURE 3-3 A health care worker must report to work on time and maintain a good attendance record.

3:3 INFORMATION
Teamwork

In almost any health care career, you will be a part of an interdisciplinary health care team. The team concept was created to provide quality holistic health care to every patient. **Teamwork** consists of many professionals, with different levels of education, ideas, backgrounds, and interests, working together for the benefit of the patient. For example, a surgical team might include the admitting clerk who collects admission information, an insurance representative who obtains approval for the surgery, nurses or patient care technicians who prepare the patient for surgery, one or more surgeons, an anesthesiologist, one or more operating room nurses, surgical technicians, housekeepers to clean and sanitize the area, sterile supply personnel to sterilize the instruments, and recovery room personnel. After the surgery is complete, a dietitian, social worker, physical therapist, occupational therapist, home health personnel, and other team members might be needed to assist the patient as he/she recuperates. Each team member has an important job to do. When the team members work well together, the patient receives quality care.

Teamwork improves communication and continuity of care. When a team is assigned to a particular patient, the patient knows his/her caregivers and support staff. All the team members can help to identify the needs of the patient, offer opinions on the best type of care, participate as decisions are made on options of care, and suggest additional professionals who might be able to assist with specific needs. This allows a patient to become more educated about health care options and to make informed decisions regarding treatment and care.

In order for a team to function properly, every person on the team must understand the role of each team member. This knowledge provides a picture of the patient's total care plan. It also helps clarify each person's responsibility and establishes the goals that the team wants to achieve. Most teams have frequent patient care conferences, and, in some instances, the patient is an active participant (see figure 3-4). Opinions are shared, options are discussed, decisions are made, and goals are established. During the conference, each team member must listen, be honest,

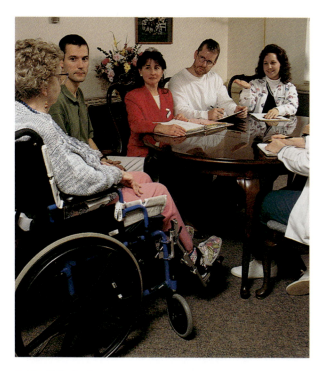

FIGURE 3-4 Most health care teams have frequent patient care conferences to establish team goals.

express his/her own opinion, and be willing to try different solutions.

A leader is an important part of any team. The leader is responsible for organizing and coordinating the team's activities, encouraging everyone to share ideas and give opinions, motivating all team members to work toward established goals, assisting with problems, monitoring the progress of the team, and providing reports and feedback to all team members on the effectiveness of the team. A good team leader will also allow others to assume the leadership role when circumstances indicate that another person can handle a particular situation more effectively. Leadership is discussed in more detail in Unit 3:4.

Good interpersonal relationships are also essential. Poor interpersonal relationships among team members can harm the quality of care and prevent the team from meeting its goals. In the same way, good interpersonal relationships can improve the quality of care. Members of a team will have different cultural and ethnic backgrounds, genders, ages, socioeconomic statuses, lifestyle preferences, beliefs, and levels of education. Each team member must understand that these differences affect the way a person thinks and acts. Each person must be sensitive to the hopes, feelings, and needs of other team members. The Golden Rule of "treat others as you would want to be treated" should be the main rule of teamwork. Some ways to develop good interpersonal relationships include:

◆ Maintain a positive attitude and learn to laugh at yourself

◆ Be friendly and cooperate with others

◆ Assist others when you see that they need help

◆ Listen carefully when another person is sharing ideas or beliefs

◆ Respect the opinions of others even though you may not agree with them

◆ Be open-minded and willing to compromise

◆ Avoid criticizing other team members

◆ Learn good communication skills so you can share ideas, concepts, and knowledge

◆ Support and encourage other team members

◆ Perform your duties to the best of your ability

Conflict among individuals with different personalities is a problem that can occur when a group of people is working as a team. When conflict occurs, it is essential for each person to deal with the conflict in a positive way. The people involved in the conflict should meet, talk with each other to identify the problem, listen to the other person's point of view, avoid accusations and hostility, try to determine a way to resolve the problem in a cooperative manner, and put the agreed-upon solution into action. If a situation occurs where two people do not feel comfortable talking privately with each other, a mediator may be able to assist with finding a solution to the problem. Some health care facilities have grievance committees to assist with conflicts that may occur. If a team is to meet its goals, conflict must be resolved.

Legal responsibilities are another important aspect of teamwork. Each member of a team must be aware of the legal limitations on duties that can be performed. All members must function within legal boundaries. No team member should ever attempt to solve a problem or perform a duty that is beyond the range of duties legally permitted.

Effective teams are the result of hard work, patience, commitment, and practice. When each individual participates fully in the team and makes every effort to contribute to the team, the team achieves success.

3:4 INFORMATION Professional Leadership

Leadership is an important concept in health occupations. **Leadership** is the skill or ability to encourage people to work together and do their best to achieve common goals. A **leader** is frequently defined as an individual who leads or guides others, or who is in charge or in command of others. A myth exists that leaders are born. In fact, leaders develop by their own efforts. Leaders combine visions of excellence with the ability to inspire others. They promote positive changes that benefit their professions and the people they serve. Anyone can learn to be a leader by making an effort to understand the principles of leadership. In a group, every member who makes a contribution to an idea can be considered a leader. The leadership in the group passes from person to person as each individual contributes to the achievement of the group's goals.

Many different characteristics are assigned to a leader. All the characteristics can be learned. In this way, leadership becomes a skill or function that can be learned, rather than an inherited set of characteristics.

Some common characteristics may include:

◆ Respects the rights, dignity, opinions, and abilities of others

◆ Understands the principles of democracy

◆ Works with a group and guides the group toward a goal

◆ Understands own strengths and weaknesses

◆ Displays self-confidence and willingness to take a stand

◆ Communicates effectively and verbalizes ideas clearly

◆ Shows self-initiative, a willingness to work, and completes tasks

◆ Shows optimism, is open-minded, and can compromise

◆ Praises others and gives credit to others

◆ Dedicated to meeting high standards

Leaders can often be classified into broad categories. Some of the categories include: religious, political, club or organizational, business, community, expertise in a particular area, and even informal or peer group. Leaders in these categories often develop based on their involvement with the particular category. An individual who joins a club or organization may become a leader when the group elects the individual to an office or position of leadership within the group.

Leaders are frequently classified as one of three types based on how they perform their leadership skills. The three main types are *democratic, laissez-faire,* and *autocratic.*

◆ **Democratic leader:** encourages the participation of all individuals in decisions that have to be made or problems that have to be solved. This leader listens to the opinions of others, and then bases decisions on what is best for the group as a whole. By guiding the individuals to a solution, the leader allows the group to take responsibility for the decision.

◆ **Laissez-faire leader:** more of an informal type of leader. This leader believes in noninterference in the affairs of others. A laissez-faire leader will strive for only minimal rules or regulations, and allow the individuals in a group to function in an independent manner with little or no direction. This leader almost has a "hands off" policy, and usually avoids making decisions until forced by circumstances to do so. The term laissez-faire comes from a French idiom meaning "to let alone" and can be translated to mean "allow to act," and therefore is an appropriate term to use for this type of leader.

◆ **Autocratic leader:** often called a "dictator." This individual maintains total rule, makes all of the decisions, and has difficulty delegating or sharing duties. This type of leader seldom asks for the opinions of others, emphasizes discipline, and expects others to follow directions at all times. Individuals usually follow this type of leader because of a fear of punishment or because of an extreme loyalty.

All types of leadership have advantages and disadvantages. In some rare situations, an autocratic leader may be beneficial. However, the democratic leader is the model frequently presented as most effective for group interactions. By allowing a group to share in deciding what, when, and how something is to be done, members of the group will usually do what has to be done because they want to do it. Respecting the rights and opinions of others becomes the most important guide for the leader.

3:5 INFORMATION Stress

Stress can be defined as the body's reaction to any stimulus that requires a person to adjust to a changing environment. Change always initiates stress. The stimuli to change, alter behavior, or adapt to a situation are called *stressors.* Stressors can be situations, events, or concepts. Stressors can also be external or internal forces. For example, a heart attack is an internal stressor and a new job is an external stressor. No matter what the cause, a stressor will cause the body to go into an alarm or warning mode. This mode is frequently called the "fight or flight" reaction because of the physical changes that occur in the body. When the warning is received from a stressor, the sympathetic nervous system prepares the body for action. Adrenaline, a hormone from the adrenal glands, is released into the bloodstream. It dilates blood vessels to the heart and brain to increase blood circulation to these areas. At the same time, it constricts blood vessels to the skin and other internal organs, resulting in cool skin, decreased movement in the digestive tract, and decreased production of urine. The pupils in the eyes dilate to improve vision. Saliva production decreases and the mouth becomes dry. The heart beats more rapidly, blood pressure rises, and the respiratory rate increases. These actions by the sympathetic nervous system help provide the body with a burst of energy and the stamina needed to respond to the stressor. After the individual responds to the stressor and adapts or changes as needed, the parasympathetic system slowly causes opposite reactions in the body. This results in fatigue or exhaustion while the body returns to normal and recuperates. If the body is subjected to continual stress with constant "up and down" nervous system reactions, the normal functions of the body will be disrupted. This can result in a serious illness or disease. Many diseases have stress-related origins. Examples include migraine headaches, anxiety reactions, depression, allergies, asthma, digestive disorders, hypertension (high blood pressure), insomnia (inability to sleep), and heart disease.

Everyone experiences a certain degree of stress on a daily basis. The amount of stress felt usually depends on the individual's reaction to and perception of the situation causing stress. For example, a blood test can be a routine event for some individuals, such as a diabetic who performs three or four blood tests on a daily basis. Another individual who is terrified of needles might feel extreme stress when a blood test is necessary. Many different things can cause stress. Examples include relationships with family, friends, and coworkers; job or school demands; foods such as caffeine, excessive sweets, and salt; illness; lifestyle; financial problems; family events such as birth, death, marriage, or divorce; overwork; boredom and negative feelings; time limitations (too much to do and not enough time to do it); and failure to achieve goals.

Not all stress is harmful. In fact, a small amount of stress is essential to an individual's well-being because it makes a person more alert and raises the energy level. The individual is able to make quick judgments and decisions, becomes more organized, and is motivated to accomplish tasks and achieve goals. The way in which an individual responds to stressors determines whether the situation is helpful or harmful. If stress causes positive feelings such as excitement, anticipation, self-confidence, and a sense of achievement, it is helpful. If stress causes negative feelings such as boredom, frustration, irritability, anger, depression, distrust of others, self-criticism, emotional and physical exhaustion, and emotional outbursts, it is harmful. Negative stress can also lead to substance abuse. An individual may smoke more, drink large amounts of alcohol, take drugs, or eat excessively to find comfort and escape from the negative feelings. Prolonged periods of harmful stress can lead to burnout or a mental breakdown. For this reason, an individual must become aware of the stressors in his/her life and learn methods to control them.

The first step in learning how to control stress is to identify stressors. Recognizing the symptoms of "fight or flight" can lead to an awareness of the factors that cause these symptoms. By keeping a list or diary of stressors, an individual can begin to evaluate ways to deal with the stressors and/or ways to eliminate them. When stressful events occur, note what the event was, why you feel stress, how much stress you experience, and how you deal with the stress. Do you tackle the cause of the stress or the symptom? This type of information allows you to understand the level of stress you are comfortable with, the type of stress that motivates you effectively, and the type of stress that is unpleasant. If

a chronic daily stressor is heavy traffic on the road to work, it may be time to evaluate the possibility of finding a new way to work, leaving earlier or later to avoid traffic, or finding a way to relax while stuck in traffic. Stressors are problems that must be solved or eliminated. One way to do this is to use the *problem-solving method*. It consists of the following steps:

- *Gather information or data:* assess the situation to obtain all facts and opinions
- *Identify the problem:* try to identify the real stressor and why it is causing a reaction
- *List possible solutions:* look at all ways to eliminate or adapt to the stressor; include both good and bad ideas; then, evaluate each of the ideas and try to determine how effective it will be
- *Make a plan:* after evaluating the solutions, choose one that you think will have the best outcome
- *Act on your solution:* use the solution to your problem to see if it has the expected outcome; does it allow you to eliminate or adapt to the stressor?
- *Evaluate the results:* determine if the action was effective; did it work or is another solution better?
- *Change the solution:* if necessary, use a different solution that might be more effective

Learning to manage a stress reaction is another important way of dealing with stressors. When you become aware that a stressor is causing a physical reaction in your body, use the following four-step plan to gain control:

- *Stop:* immediately stop what you are doing to break out of the stress response
- *Breathe:* take a slow deep breath to relieve the physical tension you are feeling
- *Reflect:* think about the problem at hand and the cause of the stress
- *Choose:* determine how you want to deal with the stress

The brief pause that the four-step method requires allows an individual to become more aware of the stressor, the physical reaction to the stressor, and the actual cause of the stress. This awareness can then be used to determine whether or not a problem exists. If a problem does exist, a solution to the problem must be found.

Many other stress reducing techniques can be used to manage stress. Some of the more common techniques include:

- *Live a healthy life:* eat balanced meals, get sufficient amounts of rest and sleep, and exercise on a regular basis
- *Take a break from stressors:* sit in a comfortable chair with your feet up
- *Relax:* take a warm bath
- *Escape:* listen to quiet soothing music
- *Relieve tension:* shut your eyes, take slow deep breaths, and concentrate on relaxing each muscle that is tense
- *Rely on others:* talk with a friend and reach out to your support system (see figure 3-5)
- *Meditate:* think about your values or beliefs in a higher power
- *Use imagery:* close your eyes and use all your senses to place yourself in a scene where you are at peace and relaxed
- *Enjoy yourself:* find an enjoyable leisure activity or hobby to provide "time outs"
- *Renew yourself:* learn new skills, take part in a professional organization, participate in community activities, and make every effort to continue growing as an individual
- *Think positively:* reflect on your accomplishments and be proud of yourself
- *Develop outside interests:* provide time for yourself; do not allow a job to dominate your life

- *Seek assistance or delegate tasks:* ask others for help or delegate some tasks to others; remember that no one can do everything all of the time
- *Avoid too many commitments:* learn to say "no"

It is important to remember that stress is a constant presence in every individual's life and cannot be avoided. However, by being aware of the causes of stress, by learning how to respond when a stress reaction occurs, by solving problems effectively to eliminate stress, and by practicing techniques to reduce the effect of stress, an individual can deal with the daily stressors in his/her life and even benefit from them. It is also important for every health care worker to remember that patients also experience stress, especially when they are dealing with an illness and/or disability. The same techniques can be used by the health care worker to help patients learn to deal with stress.

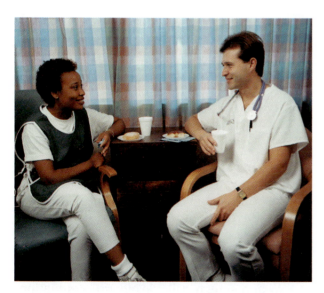

FIGURE 3-5 Relaxing and talking with a friend is one way to reduce stress.

3:6 INFORMATION Time Management

One way to help prevent stress is to use time management. **Time management** is a system of practical skills that allows an individual to use time in the most effective and productive way possible. Time management helps prevent or reduce stress by putting the individual in charge, keeping things in perspective when events are overwhelming, increasing productivity, using time more effectively, improving enjoyment of activities, and providing time for relaxing and enjoying life.

The first step of time management is to keep an activity record for a period of several days. This allows an individual to determine how he/she actually uses the time available. By noting activities as they are performed, listing the amount of time each activity takes, and noting how effective the activity was, an individual can see patterns emerging. Certain periods of the day will show higher energy levels and an improved quality of work. Other periods may indicate that accomplishments are limited because of fatigue. Wasted time will also become apparent. Time spent looking for objects, talking on the telephone, playing games on a computer, and doing things that are not worthwhile is time that can be put to more constructive use. After this information has been obtained, an individual can begin to organize time. Important projects can be scheduled during the periods of the day when energy levels are high. Rest or relaxation periods can be scheduled when energy levels are low.

Goal setting is another important factor of time management. A **goal** can be defined as a desired result or purpose toward which one is working. Goals can be compared to maps that help you find your direction and reach your destination. An old saying states "if you don't know where you are going, you will never get there." Goals allow you to know where you are going and provide direction to your life. Everyone should have both short- and long-term goals. Long-term goals are achievements that may take a period of years or even a lifetime to accomplish. Short-term goals usually take days, weeks, or months to accomplish. They are the smaller steps that are taken to reach the long-term goal. For example, a long-term goal might be to graduate from college with a health care degree. Short-term goals that have to be scheduled to reach this accomplishment might include researching and/or visiting various colleges, completing a college application form, obtaining financial aid, locating a place to live on or off campus, and starting your course of study. When you arrive at college, short-term goals for completing assignments in each course will have to be established. Short-term goals will change constantly as one set is completed and a new set is established. Completion of a goal, however, will lead to a sense of satisfaction and accomplishment and provide motivation to attempt other goals. To set goals effectively, certain points must be observed. These points include:

◆ *State goals in a positive manner:* use words such as "accomplish" rather than "avoid"

◆ *Define goals clearly and precisely:* if possible, set a time limit to accomplish the goal

◆ *Prioritize multiple goals:* determine which goals are the most important and complete them first

◆ *Write goals down:* this makes the goal seem real and attainable

◆ *Make sure each goal is at the right level:* goals should present a challenge, but not be too difficult or impossible to complete

After goals have been established, concentrate on ways to accomplish them. Review necessary skills, information that must be obtained, resources you can use, problems that may occur, and which goal should be completed first. Basically this is just organizing the steps that will lead to achieving the goal. After the goal has been achieved, enjoy your sense of accomplishment and satisfaction for a job well done. If you fail in obtaining the goal, evaluate the situation and determine why you failed. Was the goal unrealistic? Did you lack the skills or knowledge to obtain the goal? Is there another way to achieve the goal? Remember that failure can be a positive learning experience.

Time management is used to ensure success in meeting established goals. A daily planner and calendar are essential tools. These tools allow an individual to write everything down, organize all information, become aware of conflicts (two things to do at the same time), and provide an organized schedule to follow. An effective time management plan involves the following seven steps:

◆ *Analyze and prioritize:* review and list established goals; determine what tasks must be completed to achieve goals; list tasks in order, from the most important to the least important; decide if any tasks can be delegated to another person to complete and delegate whenever possible; eliminate unnecessary tasks

◆ *Identify habits and preferences:* know when you have the most energy to complete work and when it is best to schedule rest, exercise, or social activities

◆ *Schedule tasks:* use the daily planner and calendar to write down all events; be sure to include time for rest, exercise, meals, hobbies, and social activities; if a conflict arises with two things scheduled at the same time, prioritize and reschedule

◆ *Make a daily "to do" list:* list all tasks on a daily basis; as you complete each one, cross it off the list; enjoy the sense of satisfaction that occurs as you complete each job; if some things on the list are not completed at the end of the day, determine if they should be added to the next day's list or if they can be eliminated

◆ *Plan your work:* work at a comfortable pace; do one thing at a time whenever possible so you can complete it and cross it off the list; make sure you have everything you need to complete the task before you begin; ask for assistance when needed; work smarter, not harder

◆ *Avoid distractions:* make every effort to avoid interruptions; use a telephone answering system and screen calls; avoid procrastination; learn to say "no" when asked to interrupt your work for something that is not essential

◆ *Take credit for a job well done:* when a job is complete, recognize your achievement; cross the completed work off the list; if the task was a particularly hard one, reward yourself with a short break or other positive thing before going on to the next job on the list

These steps of time management provide for an organized and efficient use of time. However, even with careful planning, things do not always get done according to plan. Unexpected emergencies, a new assignment, a complication, and/or overscheduling are common events in the life of a health care worker. When a time management plan does not work, try to determine the reasons for failure. Reevaluate goals and revise the plan. Patience, practice, and an honest effort will eventually produce a plan that provides self-satisfaction for achieving goals, less stress, quality time for rest and relaxation, a sense of being in control, a healthier lifestyle, and increased productivity.

STUDENT: *Go to the workbook and complete the assignment sheet for Unit 3, Personal Qualities of a Health Care Worker.*

UNIT 3 SUMMARY

Certain personal characteristics, attitudes, and rules of appearance apply to health care workers in all health careers. Every health care worker must constantly strive to develop the necessary characteristics and to present a professional appearance.

A professional appearance helps inspire confidence and a positive self-image. Good health is an important part of appearance. By eating correctly, obtaining adequate rest, exercising daily, observing the rules of good posture, and avoiding the use of tobacco, alcohol, and drugs, a health care worker can strive to maintain good health. Wearing the appropriate uniform or appropriate clothing and shoes is essential to projecting the proper image. Proper hair and nail care, good personal hygiene, and limited makeup also help create a professional appearance.

Personal characteristics such as honesty, dependability, patience, enthusiasm, responsibility, discretion, and competence are essential. In addition, health care workers must be willing to learn and to accept criticism. These characteristics must be practiced and learned.

Teamwork is important in any health care career. Interdisciplinary health care teams provide quality holistic health care to every patient. Teamwork improves communication and continuity of care. A picture of the patient's total care plan is clear when the role of each team member is known. In order for a team to function effectively it needs a qualified leader, good interpersonal relationships, ways to avoid or deal with conflict, positive attitudes, and respect for legal responsibilities. Effective teams are the result of hard work, patience, commitment, and practice.

Leadership is a skill that can be learned by mastering the characteristics of a leader. A leader may or may not be a supervisor; any member of a group that contributes to the group's goals can be considered a leader. Of the three types of leaders, democratic, laissez-faire, and autocratic, the democratic leader is the most effective for group interaction.

Stress is a component in every individual's life. Stress can be good or bad, depending on the person's perception of and reaction to the stress. By being aware of the causes of stress, learning how to respond when a stress reaction occurs, solving problems to eliminate stress, and practicing techniques to reduce the effect of stress, an individual can deal with stress and even benefit from it.

Time management is a system of practical skills that allow an individual to use time in the most effective and productive way possible. It involves analyzing how one actually uses the time available, establishing short- and long-term goals, prioritizing tasks that must be accomplished, identifying habits and preferences, preparing written "to do" lists and crossing off work that has been completed, planning work carefully, avoiding distractions, and taking credit for a job well done. An effective time management plan will reduce stress, help an individual attain goals, increase self-confidence, lead to a healthier lifestyle, and provide quality time for rest and relaxation.

Health care workers must learn and follow the standards and requirements established by the health care facility in which they are employed.

INTERNET SEARCHES

Use the suggested search engine in Unit 11:4 of this textbook to search the Internet for additional information on the following topics:

1. *Uniform companies:* search "uniform suppliers" to locate companies that sell professional uniforms and compare styles, prices, and so forth.

2. *Professional characteristics:* choose a specific health care career and search for career descriptions; list the required personal qualities or characteristics necessary for the career you have chosen.

3. *Leadership:* search for information on types and characteristics of leaders; evaluate which types would be most effective in guiding a health care team.

4. *Stress:* search for information on stress and stress-reducing techniques.

5. *Time management:* search for information on time management.

REVIEW QUESTIONS

1. What five (5) main factors contribute to good health?

2. Identify eight (8) specific principles that must be followed for a professional appearance.

3. Create a personal description of yourself showing why you display at least six (6) of the personal characteristics desired in a health care worker.

4. A patient is admitted to a hospital to give birth to her baby. Identify at least ten (10) health care professionals who may be on the team that provide her care. Review the many careers in Unit 2 to prepare your list.

5. List six (6) characteristics of a leader.

6. Identify the three (3) types of leaders and describe their style of leadership.

7. Identify at least one major stress in your life. List the steps of the problem-solving method and then apply the stressor you have chosen to each of the steps. Identify at least three (3) courses of action that you can take.

8. List six (6) stress-reducing techniques that you find beneficial. State why they help you reduce stress.

9. Differentiate between short- and long-term goals. How are they related? How are they different?

10. What are the main goals of time management?

UNIT 3

SUGGESTED REFERENCES

Anspaugh, David, Michael Hamrick, and Frank Rosato. *Wellness-Concepts and Applications.* 4th ed. New York, NY: McGraw-Hill, 2001.

Boyle, Marie. *Personal Nutrition.* 4th ed. Clifton Park, NY: Delmar Learning, 2001.

Deem, Saitofi, and Joseph Deem. *Health Care Exploration.* Clifton Park, NY: Delmar Learning, 2000.

Kouzes, J. M., and B. Z. Posner. *The Leadership Challenge: How to Keep Getting Extraordinary Things Done in Organizations.* San Francisco, CA: Jossey-Bass Publishers, 1995.

Lindh, Wilburta, Marilyn Pooler, and Carol Tamparo. *Delmar's Comprehensive Medical Assisting.* 2nd ed. Clifton Park, NY: Delmar Learning, 2002.

Makely, Sherry. *Multiskilling: Team Building for The Health Care Provider.* Clifton Park, NY: Delmar Learning, 1999.

Maville, Janice. *Health Promotion in Nursing.* Clifton Park, NY: Delmar Learning, 2002.

McArdle, William, Frank Katch, and Victor Katch. *Exercise Physiology: Energy, Nutrition, and Human Performance.* 5th ed. Philadelphia, PA: Lippincott, Williams, & Wilkins, 2001.

McCutcheon, Maureen. *Exploring Health Careers.* 2nd ed. Clifton Park, NY: Delmar Learning, 1999.

Milliken, Mary Elizabeth. *Understanding Human Behavior.* 6th ed. Clifton Park, NY: Delmar Learning, 1998.

Mitchell, Joyce, and Lee Haroun. *Introduction to Health Care.* Clifton Park, NY: Delmar Learning, 2002.

O'Donnell, Michael. *Health Promotion in the Workplace.* 3rd ed. Clifton Park, NY: Delmar Learning, 2002.

Townsend, Carolynn E., and Ruth A. Roth. *Nutrition and Diet Therapy.* 7th ed. Clifton Park, NY: Delmar Learning, 2000.

Wallace, B., and J. Masters. *Personal Development for Life and Work.* 8th ed. Cincinnati, OH: South-Western, 2001.

White, Lois. *Foundations of Nursing: Caring for the Whole Person.* Clifton Park, NY: Delmar Learning, 2000.

Wray, J., L. Luft, and M. Highland. *Fundamentals of Human Relations: Applications for Life and Work.* Cincinnati, OH: South-Western, 1996.

UNIT 4

Legal and Ethical Responsibilities

Unit Objectives

After completing this unit of study, you should be able to:

◆ Provide one example of a situation that might result in legal action for each of the following: malpractice; negligence; assault and battery; invasion of privacy; false imprisonment; abuse; and defamation

◆ Describe how contract laws affect health care

◆ Define *privileged communications* and explain how they apply to health care

◆ State the legal regulations that apply to health care records

◆ List at least six basic rules of ethics for health care personnel

◆ List at least six rights of the patient who is receiving health care

◆ Justify at least eight professional standards by explaining how they help meet legal/ethical requirements

◆ Define, pronounce, and spell all the key terms

 Observe Standard Precautions

 Safety—Proceed with Caution

 Math Skill

 Science Skill

 Communications Skill

 Instructors Check—Call Instructor at This Point

 OBRA Requirement— Based on Federal Law

 Legal Responsibility

 Career Information

 Technology

KEY TERMS

abuse
advance directives
agent
assault and battery
civil law
confidentiality
 (con″-fih-den-chee″-ahl′-ih-tee)
contract
criminal law
defamation
 (deff″-ah-may′-shun)

Durable Power of Attorney (POA)
ethics
 (eth′-iks)
expressed contracts
false imprisonment
health care records
implied contracts
informed consent
invasion of privacy
legal
legal disability

libel
 (ly′-bull)
living wills
malpractice
negligence
 (neg′-lih-gents)
Patient Self-Determination Act
 (PSDA)
patients' rights
privileged communications
slander
torts

INTRODUCTION

In every aspect of life, there are certain laws and legal responsibilities formulated to protect you and society. An excellent example is the need to obey traffic laws when driving a motor vehicle. A worker in any health career also has certain responsibilities. Being aware of and following legal regulations is important for your own protection, the protection of your employer, and the safety and well-being of the patient.

4:1 INFORMATION Legal Responsibilities

Legal responsibilities are those that are authorized or based on law. This can include **civil law,** which focuses on legal relationships between people and the protection of a person's rights, and **criminal law,** which focuses on wrongs against a person, property, or society. Although health care is mainly affected by civil law, especially those aspects involving contracts and **torts** (wrongful acts that do not involve contracts), criminal laws can also apply. Examples of such criminal laws include practicing in a health profession without having the required license, misuse of narcotics, theft, and murder. In addition, *health care professionals/workers are also required to know and follow the state laws that regulate their respective licenses or registrations or set standards for their respective professions.*

TORTS

Failure to meet your legal responsibilities can result in legal action against you and your employer. A tort occurs when a person is harmed or injured because a health care provider does not meet the established or expected standards of care. Many different types of torts, or civil wrongs (as opposed to crimes), can lead to legal action. These offenses may be quite complex and may be open to different legal interpretations. Some of the more common torts include the following:

Malpractice: Malpractice can be interpreted as "bad practice" and is commonly called "professional negligence." It can be defined as the failure of a professional to use the degree of skill and learning commonly expected in that individual's profession, resulting in injury, loss, or damage to the person receiving care. Examples might include a physician not administering a tetanus injection when a patient has a puncture wound, or a nurse performing minor surgery without having any training.

Negligence: Negligence can be described as failure to give care that is normally expected of a person in a particular position, resulting in injury to another person. Examples include falls and injuries that occur when siderails are left down;

using or not reporting defective equipment; infections caused by the use of nonsterile instruments and/or supplies; and burns caused by improper heat or radiation treatments.

Assault and battery: Assault includes a threat or attempt to injure, and battery includes the unlawful touching of another person without consent. They are closely related and often used together. It is important to remember that patients must give consent for any care and that they have the right to refuse care. Some procedures or practices require written consent from the patient. Examples can include surgery, certain diagnostic tests, experimental procedures, treatment of minors (individuals below legal age, which varies from state to state), and even simple things such as siderail releases for a patient who wants siderails left down when other factors indicate siderails should be up to protect the patient. Verbal consent is permitted in other cases, but the law states that this must be "informed consent." **Informed consent** is permission granted voluntarily by a person who is of sound mind after the procedure and all risks involved have been explained in terms the person can understand. It is important to remember that a person has the right to withdraw consent at any time. Therefore, all procedures must be explained to the patient, and no procedure should be performed if the patient does not give consent. Examples of assault and battery include performing a procedure after a patient has refused to give permission and improper handling or rough treatment of a patient while providing care.

Invasion of privacy: Invasion of privacy includes unnecessarily exposing an individual or revealing personal information about an individual without that person's consent. Examples include improperly draping or covering a patient during a procedure so that other patients or personnel can see the patient exposed; sending information regarding a patient to an insurance company without the patient's written permission; or informing the news media of a patient's condition without the patient's permission.

False imprisonment: False imprisonment refers to restraining an individual or restricting an individual's freedom. Examples include keeping patients hospitalized against their will, or applying physical restraints without proper authorization or with no justification.

Abuse: Abuse includes any care that results in physical harm, pain, or mental anguish. Examples of the types of abuse include:

- Physical abuse: hitting, forcing people against their will, restraining movement, depriving people of food or water, and/or not providing physical care

- Verbal abuse: speaking harshly, swearing or shouting, using inappropriate words to describe a person's race or nationality, and/or writing threats or abusive statements

- Psychological abuse: threatening harm; denying rights; belittling, intimidating, or ridiculing the person; and/or threatening to reveal information about the person

- Sexual abuse: any unwanted sexual touching or act, using sexual gestures, and/or suggesting sexual behavior

Patients may experience abuse before entering a health care facility. Domestic abuse occurs when an intimate partner uses threatening, manipulative, aggressive, or violent behavior to maintain power and control over another person. If abuse is directed toward a child, it is child abuse. If it is directed toward an older person, it is elder abuse. Health care providers must be alert to the signs and symptoms that may indicate patients in their care are victims of abuse. These may include:

- unexplained bruises, fractures, burns, or injuries

- signs of neglect such as poor personal hygiene

- irrational fears or a change in personality

- aggressive or withdrawn behavior

- patient statements that indicate abuse or neglect

Many of the other torts can lead to charges of abuse, or a charge of abuse can occur alone. Laws in all states require that any form of abuse be reported to the proper authorities. Even though the signs and symptoms do not always mean a person is being abused, their presence indicates a need for further investigation. Health care workers are required to report any signs or symptoms of abuse to their immediate supervisor or to the individual in the health care facility responsible for reporting the suspicions to the proper authorities.

Defamation: Defamation occurs when false statements either cause a person to be ridiculed or damage the person's reputation. Incorrect information given out in error can result in defamation. If the information is spoken, it is

slander; if it is written, it is **libel.** Examples include reporting that a patient has an infectious disease to a government agency when lab results are inaccurate, or telling others that a person has a drug problem when another medical condition actually exists.

CONTRACTS

In addition to tort laws, contract laws also affect health care. A **contract** is an agreement between two or more parties. Most contracts have three parts:

◆ Offer: a competent individual enters into a relationship with a health care provider and offers to be a patient

◆ Acceptance: the health care provider gives an appointment or examines or treats the patient

◆ Consideration: the payment made by the patient for the services provided

Contracts in health care are implied or expressed. **Implied contracts** are those obligations that are understood without verbally expressed terms. For example, when a qualified health worker prepares a medication and a patient takes the medication, it is implied that the patient accepts this treatment. **Expressed contracts** are stated in distinct and clear language, either orally or in writing. An example is a surgery permit. Promises of care must be kept. Therefore, all risks associated with treatment must be explained completely to the patient (figure 4-1).

All parties entering into a contract must be free of **legal disability**. A person who has a legal disability does not have the legal capacity to form a contract. Examples of people with legal disabilities are minors (individuals under legal age), mentally incompetent persons, individuals under the influence of drugs that alter the mental state, and semiconscious or unconscious people. In such cases, parents, guardians, or others permitted by law must form the contract for the individual.

A contract requires that certain standards of care be provided by competent, qualified individuals. If the contract is not performed according to agreement, the contract is breached. Failure to provide care and/or giving improper care on the part of the health provider, or failure on the part of the patient to pay according to the

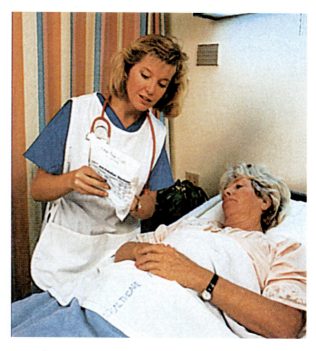

FIGURE 4-1 All risks of treatment must be explained to a patient before asking the patient for permission to administer treatment.

consideration, can be considered breach of contract and cause for legal action.

C In order to comply with legal mandates, a translator must be used when a contract is explained to a non-English-speaking individual. In addition, many states require the use of translator services for individuals who are deaf or hard of hearing. Most health care agencies have a list of translators that can be used in these situations. At times, an English-speaking relative or friend of the patient can also serve as a translator.

A final important consideration in contract law is the role of the **agent.** When a person works under the direction or control of another person, the employer is called the principal, and the person working under the employer is called the agent. The principal is responsible for the actions of the agent and can be required to pay or otherwise compensate people who have been injured by the agent. For example, if a dental assistant tells a patient "your dentures will look better than your real teeth," the dentist may have to compensate the patient financially should this statement prove false. Health care workers should therefore be aware of their role as agents of their employers and work to protect the interests of their employers.

PRIVILEGED COMMUNICATIONS

C **Privileged communications** are another important aspect of legal responsibility. Privileged communications comprise all information given to health care personnel by a patient; by law, this information must be kept confidential and shared only with other members of the patient's health care team. It cannot be told to anyone else without the written consent of the patient. The consent should state what information is to be released, to whom the information should be given, and any applicable time limits. Certain information is exempt by law and must be reported. Examples of exempt information are births and deaths; injuries caused by violence (such as assault and battery, abuse, stabbings) that may require police involvement; drug abuse; communicable diseases; and sexually transmitted diseases.

Health care records are also considered privileged communications. Such records contain information about the care provided to the patient. While such records belong to the health care provider (for example, the physician, dentist, hospital, long-term care facility), the patient has a right to obtain a copy of any information in the record. Health care records can be used as legal records in a court of law. Erasures are therefore not allowed on such records. Errors should be crossed out with a single line so material is still readable. Correct information should then be inserted, initialed, and dated. If necessary, an explanation for the correction should also be provided. Health care records must be properly maintained, kept confidential, and retained for the amount of time required by state law (figure 4-2). When records are destroyed after the legal time for retention, they should be burned or shredded to maintain confidentiality.

The growing use of computerized records has created a dilemma in maintaining confidentiality (figure 4-3). In a large health care facility such as a hospital, many different individuals may have access to a patient's records. For this reason, many health care providers are creating safeguards to maintain computer confidentiality. Some examples include limiting personnel who have access to such records; using codes to prevent access to certain information; requiring

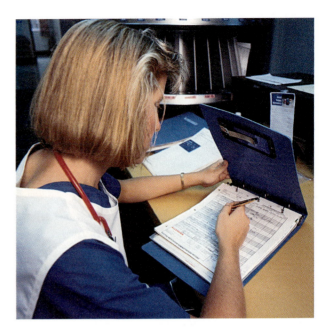

FIGURE 4-2 Confidentiality must be maintained with regard to health care records.

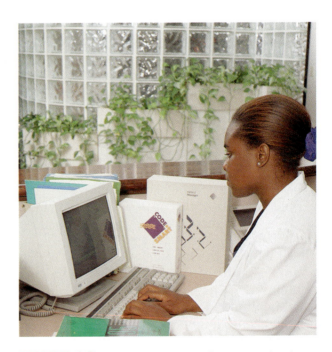

FIGURE 4-3 The growing use of computerized records has created the need for limiting access to computers in order to maintain confidentiality.

passwords in order to access specific information on records; and constantly monitoring and evaluating computer use.

Legal responsibilities are important aspects of health care. All states have rules and regulations governing health care. In addition, most health care agencies have specific rules, regulations, and standards that determine activities performed by individuals holding different positions of employment. Standards can vary from state to state, and even from agency to agency. It is important to remember that you are liable, or legally responsible, for your own actions regardless of what anyone tells you or what position you hold. Therefore, when you undertake a particular position of employment in a health agency, *it is your responsibility to learn exactly what you are legally permitted to do, and to familiarize yourself with your exact responsibilities.*

4:2 INFORMATION Ethics

Legal responsibilities are determined by law. **Ethics** are a set of principles relating to what is morally right or wrong. Ethics provide a standard of conduct or code of behavior. This allows a health care provider to analyze information and make decisions based on what people believe is right and good conduct. Modern health care advances, however, have created many ethical dilemmas for health care providers. Some of these dilemmas include:

- Is euthanasia (assisted death) justified in certain patients?

- Should a patient be told that a health care provider has AIDS?

- Should aborted fetuses be used for research?

- When should life support be discontinued?

- Do parents have a religious right to refuse a life-saving blood transfusion for their child?

- Can a health care facility refuse to provide expensive treatment such as a bone marrow transplant if a patient cannot pay for the treatment?

- Who decides whether a 75-year-old patient or a 56-year-old patient gets a single kidney available for transplant?

- Should people be allowed to sell organs for use in transplants?

- If a person can benefit from marijuana, should a physician be allowed to prescribe it as a treatment?

- Should animals be used in medical research even if it results in the death of the animal?

- Should genetic researchers be allowed to transplant specific genes to create the "perfect" human being?

- Should human beings be cloned?

- Should aborted embryos be used to obtain stem cells for research, especially since scientists may be able to use the stem cells to cure diseases such as diabetes, osteoporosis, and Parkinson's?

Although there are no easy answers to any of these questions, some guidelines are provided by an ethical code. Most of the national organizations affiliated with the different health care occupations have established ethical codes for personnel in their respective occupations. Although such codes differ slightly, most contain the same basic principles:

- Put the saving of life and the promotion of health above all else.

- Make every effort to keep the patient as comfortable as possible and to preserve life whenever possible.

- Respect the patient's choice to die peacefully and with dignity when all options have been discussed with the patient and family and/or predetermined by advance directives.

- Treat all patients equally, regardless of race, religion, social or economic status, sex, or nationality. Bias, prejudice, and discrimination have no place in health care.

- Provide care for *all* individuals to the best of your ability.

- Maintain a competent level of skill consistent with your particular occupation.

- Stay informed and up to date and pursue continuing education as necessary.

- **C** Maintain **confidentiality.** Confidentiality means that information about the patient must remain private and can be shared *only* with other members of the patient's health care team. A legal violation can occur if a patient suffers personal or financial damage when confidential information is shared with others, including family members. Information obtained from patients should not be repeated or used for personal gain. Gossiping about patients is ethically wrong.

- Refrain from immoral, unethical, and illegal practices. If you observe others taking part in illegal actions, report such actions to the proper authorities.

- ◆ Show loyalty to patients, coworkers, and employers. Avoid negative or derogatory statements and always express a positive attitude.

- ◆ Be sincere, honest, and caring. Treat others as you want to be treated. Show respect and concern for the feelings, dignity, and rights of others.

When you enter a health occupation, learn the code of ethics for that occupation. Make every effort to abide by the code so as to become a competent and ethical health care worker. In doing so, you will earn the respect and confidence of patients, coworkers, and employers.

4:3 INFORMATION Patients' Rights

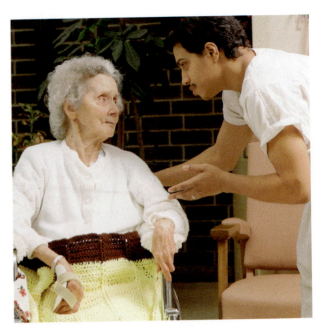

FIGURE 4-4 Patients have the right to refuse treatment.

OBRA Federal and state legislation requires health care agencies to have written policies concerning **patients' rights,** or the factors of care that patients can expect to receive. Agencies expect all personnel to respect and honor these rights.

The American Hospital Association has affirmed a "**Patient's Bill of Rights**" that is recognized and honored by many health care facilities. This bill of rights states, in part, that a patient has the right to:

1. considerate and respectful care;

2. obtain complete, current information concerning diagnosis, treatment, and prognosis (expected outcome);

3. receive information necessary to give informed consent prior to the start of any procedure or treatment;

4. have advance directives for health care and/or refuse treatment to the extent permitted under law (figure 4-4);

5. privacy concerning a medical care program;

6. confidential treatment of all communications and records;

7. reasonable response to a request for services;

8. obtain information regarding any relationship of the hospital to other health care and educational institutions;

9. be advised of and have the right to refuse to participate in any research project;

10. expect reasonable continuity of care;

11. review medical records and examine bills and receive an explanation of all care and charges;

12. be informed of any hospital rules, regulations, and/or policies and the resources available to resolve disputes or grievances.

OBRA Residents in long-term care facilities are guaranteed certain rights under the Omnibus Budget Reconciliation Act (OBRA) of 1987. Every long-term care facility must inform residents or their guardians of these rights and a copy must be posted in each facility. This is often called a "**Resident's Bill of Rights**" and states, in part, that a resident has a right to:

1. free choice regarding physician, treatment, care, and participation in research;

2. freedom from abuse and chemical or physical restraints;

3. privacy and confidentiality of personal and clinical records;

4. accommodation of needs and choice regarding activities, schedules, and health care;

5. voice grievances without fear of retaliation or discrimination;

6. organize and participate in family/resident groups and in social, religious, and community activities;

7. information on medical benefits, medical records, survey results, deficiencies of the facility, and advocacy groups including the ombudsman program (state representative who checks on resident care and violation of rights);

8. manage personal funds and use personal possessions;

9. unlimited access to immediate family or relatives and to share a room with his or her spouse, if both are residents (figure 4-5);

10. remain in the facility and not be transferred or discharged except for medical reasons; the welfare of the resident or others; failure to pay; or if the facility either cannot meet the resident's needs or ceases to operate.

All states have adopted these rights, and some have added additional rights. It is important to check state law and obtain a list of rights established in your state. Health care workers can face job loss, fines, and even imprisonment if they do not follow and grant established patients' or residents' rights. By observing these rights, the health care worker helps ensure the patient's safety, privacy, and well-being, and provides quality care at all times.

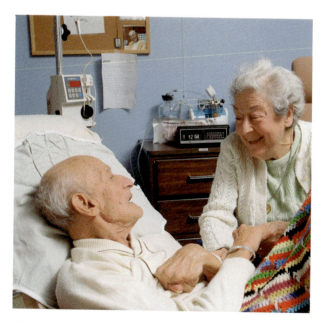

FIGURE 4-5 A married couple in a long-term care facility has the legal right to share a room if both members of the couple are residents in the facility.

4:4 INFORMATION Advance Directives for Health Care

Advance directives for health care, also known as legal directives, are legal documents that allow individuals to state what medical treatment they want or do not want in the event that they become incapacitated and are unable to express their wishes regarding medical care. Two main directives are a living will and a Durable Power of Attorney (POA) for Health Care.

Living wills (figure 4-6) are documents that allow individuals to state what measures should or should not be taken to prolong life when their conditions are terminal (death is expected). The document must be signed when the individual is competent and witnessed by two adults who cannot benefit from the death. Most states now have laws that allow the withholding of life-sustaining procedures and that honor living wills. A living will frequently results in a do not resuscitate (DNR) order for a terminally ill individual. The DNR order means that cardiopulmonary resuscitation is not performed when the patient stops breathing. The patient is allowed to die with peace and dignity. At times this is extremely difficult for health care workers to honor. It is important to remember that many individuals believe that the quality of life is important and a life on support systems has no meaning or purpose for them.

A **Durable Power of Attorney (POA)** for Health Care is a document that permits an individual (known as a principal) to appoint another person (known as an agent) to make any decisions regarding health care if the principal should become unable to make decisions (figure 4-7). This includes providing or withholding specific medical or surgical procedures; hiring or dismissing health care providers; spending or withholding funds for health care; and having access to medical records. Although they are most frequently given to spouses or adult children, POAs can be given to any qualified adult. To meet legal requirements, the POA must be signed by the principal, agent, and one or two adult witnesses.

A federal law, called the **Patient Self-Determination Act (PSDA)** of 1990, mandates

FLORIDA LIVING WILL

Declaration made this _____ day of _____, 19_____.

I, _____, willfully and voluntarily make known my desire that my dying not be artificially prolonged under the circumstances set forth below, and I do hereby declare:

If at any time I have a terminal condition and if my attending or treating physician and another consulting physician have determined that there is no medical probability of my recovery from such condition, I direct that life-prolonging procedures be withheld or withdrawn when the application of such procedures would serve only to prolong artificially the process of dying, and that I be permitted to die naturally with only the administration of medication or the performance of any medical procedure deemed necessary to provide me with comfort care or to alleviate pain.

It is my intention that this declaration be honored by my family and physician as the final expression of my legal right to refuse medical or surgical treatment and to accept the consequences for such refusal.

In the event that I have been determined to be unable to provide express and informed consent regarding the withholding, withdrawal, or continuation of life-prolonging procedures, I wish to designate, as my surrogate to carry out the provisions of this declaration:

Name: _____
Address: _____
_____ Zip Code: _____
Phone: _____

INSTRUCTIONS

PRINT THE DATE
PRINT YOUR NAME

PRINT THE NAME, HOME ADDRESS AND TELEPHONE NUMBER OF YOUR SURROGATE

© 1998
CHOICE IN DYING, INC.

FLORIDA LIVING WILL — PAGE 2 OF 2

I wish to designate the following person as my alternate surrogate, to carry out the provisions of this declaration should my surrogate be unwilling or unable to act on my behalf:

Name: _____
Address: _____
_____ Zip Code: _____
Phone: _____

Additional instructions (optional): _____

I understand the full import of this declaration, and I am emotionally and mentally competent to make this declaration.

Signed: _____

Witness 1:
  Signed: _____
  Address: _____
Witness 2:
  Signed: _____
  Address: _____

INSTRUCTIONS

PRINT NAME, HOME ADDRESS AND TELEPHONE NUMBER OF YOUR ALTERNATE SURROGATE

ADD PERSONAL INSTRUCTIONS (IF ANY)

SIGN THE DOCUMENT

WITNESSING PROCEDURE

TWO WITNESSES MUST SIGN AND PRINT THEIR ADDRESSES

© 1998
CHOICE IN DYING, INC.

Courtesy of **Choice In Dying, Inc.**
1035 30th Street, NW, Washington, DC 20007 800-989-9455   5/98

FIGURE 4-6 A living will is a legal document that allows an individual to state what measures should or should not be taken to prolong life. *(Reprinted by permission of Choice in Dying, Inc., 1035 30th Street, NW, Washington, DC 20007-3823, 1-800-989-WILL)*

FLORIDA DESIGNATION OF HEALTH CARE SURROGATE

Name: _____
  (Last)   *(First)*   *(Middle Initial)*

In the event that I have been determined to be incapacitated to provide informed consent for medical treatment and surgical and diagnostic procedures, I wish to designate as my surrogate for health care decisions:

Name: _____
Address: _____
_____ Zip Code: _____
Phone: _____

If my surrogate is unwilling or unable to perform his or her duties, I wish to designate as my alternate surrogate:

Name: _____
Address: _____
_____ Zip Code: _____
Phone: _____

I fully understand that this designation will permit my designee to make health care decisions and to provide, withhold, or withdraw consent on my behalf; to apply for public benefits to defray the cost of health care; and to authorize my admission to or transfer from a health care facility.

Additional instructions (optional):

INSTRUCTIONS

PRINT YOUR NAME

PRINT THE NAME, HOME ADDRESS AND TELEPHONE NUMBER OF YOUR SURROGATE

PRINT THE NAME, HOME ADDRESS AND TELEPHONE NUMBER OF YOUR ALTERNATE SURROGATE

ADD PERSONAL INSTRUCTIONS (IF ANY)

© 1998
CHOICE IN DYING, INC.

FLORIDA DESIGNATION OF HEALTH CARE SURROGATE — PAGE 2 OF 2

I further affirm that this designation is not being made as a condition of treatment or admission to a health care facility. I will notify and send a copy of this document to the following persons other than my surrogate, so they may know who my surrogate is:

Name: _____
Address: _____
Name: _____
Address: _____

Signed: _____
Date: _____

Witness 1:
  Signed: _____
  Address: _____
Witness 2:
  Signed: _____
  Address: _____

PRINT THE NAMES AND ADDRESSES OF THOSE WHO YOU WANT TO KEEP COPIES OF THIS DOCUMENT

SIGN AND DATE THE DOCUMENT

WITNESSING PROCEDURE

TWO WITNESSES MUST SIGN AND PRINT THEIR ADDRESSES

© 1998
CHOICE IN DYING, INC.

Courtesy of **Choice In Dying, Inc.**
1035 30th Street, NW Washington, DC 20007 800-989-9455   5/98

FIGURE 4-7 A durable power of attorney or designation of health care surrogate is a legal document that allows an individual to appoint another person to make health care decisions if the individual is unable to make his or her own decisions. *(Reprinted by permission of Choice in Dying, Inc., 1035 30th Street, NW, Washington, DC 20007-3823, 1-800-989-WILL)*

that all health care facilities receiving any type of federal aid comply with the following requirements:

◆ Inform every adult, both orally and in writing, of their right under state law to make decisions concerning medical care, including the right to refuse treatment and right-to-die options

◆ Provide information and assistance in preparing advance directives

◆ Document any advance directives on the patient's record

◆ Have written statements to implement the patient's rights in the decision-making process

◆ Affirm that there will be no discrimination or effect on care because of advance directives

◆ Educate the staff on the medical and legal issues of advance directives

The PSDA ensures that patients are informed of their rights and have the opportunity to determine the care they will receive.

All health care workers must be aware of and honor advance or legal directives. In addition, health care workers should give serious consideration to preparing their own advance directives.

4:5 INFORMATION Professional Standards

Legal responsibilities, ethics, patients' rights, and advance directives all help determine the type of care provided by health care workers. By following certain standards at all times, you can protect yourself, your employer, and the patient. Some of the basic standards are as follows:

1. **Perform only those procedures for which you have been trained and are legally permitted to do.** Never perform any procedure unless you are qualified. The necessary training may be obtained from an educational facility, from your employer, or in special classes provided by an agency. If you are asked to perform any procedure for which you are not qualified, it is your responsibility to state that you have not been trained and to refuse to do it until you receive the required instruction. If you are not legally permitted to either perform a procedure or to sign documents, it is your responsibility to refuse to do so because of legal limitations.

2. **Use approved, correct methods while performing any procedure.** Follow specific methods taught by qualified instructors in educational facilities or observe and learn procedures from your employer or authorized personnel. Most health care agencies have an approved procedure manual that explains the step-by-step methods for performing tasks. Use this manual or read the manufacturer's instructions on specific equipment or supplies.

3. **Obtain proper authorization before performing any procedure.** In some health careers, you will obtain authorization directly from the doctor, therapist, or individual in charge of a patient's care. In other careers, you will obtain authorization by checking written orders (figure 4-8). In careers where you have neither access to patients' records nor direct contact with the individuals in charge of care, an immediate supervisor will interpret orders and then direct you to perform procedures.

4. **Identify the patient and obtain the patient's consent before performing any procedure.** In some health care agencies, patients wear identification bands. If this is the case, check this name band (figure 4-9). In addition, state the patient's name clearly, repeating it if necessary.

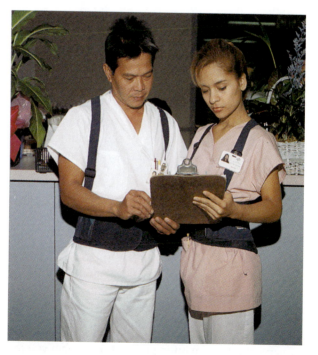

FIGURE 4-8 Obtain proper authorization before performing any procedure on a patient.

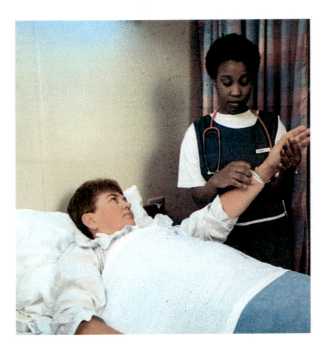

FIGURE 4-9 If a name band is present, use it to identify the patient.

For example, say "Miss Jones?" followed by "Miss Sandra Jones?" to be sure you have the correct patient. Always explain a procedure briefly or state what you are going to do, and obtain the patient's consent. It is best to avoid statements such as "May I take your blood pressure?" because the patient can say "No." By stating, "The doctor would like me to check your blood pressure," you are identifying the procedure and obtaining consent by the patient's acceptance and/or lack of objection. If a patient refuses to allow you to perform a procedure, check with your immediate supervisor. Some procedures require written consent from the patient. Follow the agency policy with regard to such procedures. Never sign your name as a witness to any written consent or document unless you are authorized to do so.

5. **Observe all safety precautions.** Handle equipment carefully. Be alert to all aspects of safety to protect the patient. Know and follow safety rules and regulations. Be alert to safety hazards in any area and make every effort to correct or eliminate such hazards as quickly as possible.

6. **Keep all information confidential.** This includes oral and written information. Ensure that you do not place patient records in any area where they can be seen by unauthorized individuals. Do not

reveal any information contained in the records without proper authorization and patient consent. If you are reporting specific information about a patient to your immediate supervisor, ensure that your conversation cannot be heard by others. Avoid discussing patients with others at home, in social situations, in public places, or anywhere outside the agency.

7. **Think before you speak and carefully consider everything you say.** Do not reveal information, such as a blood pressure reading, to the patient unless you are specifically instructed to do so.

8. **Treat all patients equally regardless of race; religion; social or economic status; sex; or nationality.** Provide care for *all* individuals to the best of your ability.

9. **Accept no tips or bribes for the care you provide.** You receive a salary for your services, and the care you provide should not be influenced by the amount of money a patient can afford to pay. A polite refusal such as "I'm sorry, I am not allowed to accept tips," is usually the best way to handle this situation.

10. **If any error occurs or you make a mistake, report it immediately to your supervisor.** Never try to hide or ignore an error. Make every effort to correct the situation as soon as possible, and take responsibility for your actions.

11. **Behave professionally in dress, language, manners, and actions.** Take pride in your occupation and in the work you do. Promote a positive attitude at all times.

Even when standards are followed, errors leading to legal action sometimes still occur. Liability insurance constitutes an additional form of protection in such cases. Many insurance companies offer policies at reasonable cost for health care workers and students. Some companies will even issue liability protection under a homeowner's policy or through a liability policy that protects the person against all liabilities, not just those related to occupation.

Again, remember that it is your responsibility to understand the legal and ethical implications of your particular health career. Never hesitate to ask specific questions or to request written policies from your employer. Contact your state board of health or state board of education to obtain information regarding regulations and guidelines for your occupation. By obtaining this information and by following the basic standards listed, you will protect yourself, your employer, and the patient to whom you provide health care.

STUDENT: *Go to the workbook and complete the assignment sheet for Unit 4, Legal and Ethical Responsibilities.*

UNIT 4 SUMMARY

All health care workers have legal and ethical responsibilities that exist to protect the health care worker and employer, and to provide for the safety and well-being of the patient.

Legal responsibilities in health care usually involve torts and contracts. Torts are wrongful acts that do not involve contracts. Examples of torts that can lead to legal action include malpractice; negligence; assault and battery; invasion of privacy; false imprisonment; abuse; and defamation. A contract is an agreement between two or more parties. Contracts create obligations that must be met by all involved individuals. If a contract is not performed according to agreement, the contract is breached, and legal action can occur.

Understanding privileged communications is another important aspect of legal responsibilities. A health care worker must be aware that all information given by a patient is confidential and should not be told to anyone other than members of the patient's health care team without the written consent of the patient. Health care records are also privileged communications and can be used as legal records in a court of law.

Ethical responsibilities are based not on law but, rather, on what is morally right or wrong. Most health care occupations each have an established code of ethics that provides a standard of conduct or code of behavior. Health care workers should make every effort to abide by the codes of ethics established for their given professions.

Health care workers must respect patients' rights. Health care agencies have written policies concerning the factors of care that patients can expect to receive. All personnel must respect and honor these rights.

Advance directives for health care are legal documents that allow individuals to state what medical treatment they want or do not want in the event that they become incapacitated. Two main examples are a living will and a Durable Power of Attorney for Health Care. As a result of a federal law called the Patient Self-Determination Act, any health care facility receiving federal funds must provide patients with information regarding and assistance in preparing advance or legal directives.

Professional standards of care help provide guidelines for meeting legal responsibilities, ethics, and patients' rights. Every health care worker should follow these standards at all times. In addition, all health care workers should know and follow the state laws that regulate their respective occupations.

INTERNET SEARCHES

Use the suggested search engines in Unit 11:4 of this textbook to search the Internet for additional information on the following topics:

1. *Torts:* search for additional information or actual legal cases involving malpractice, negligence, assault and battery, invasion of privacy, false imprisonment, and defamation.

2. *Abuse:* research domestic violence or abuse, child abuse, and elder abuse to determine how victims might react, signs and symptoms indicative of abuse, and information on how to help these victims.

3. *Contracts:* search for information on components of a contract and legal cases in health care caused by a breach of contract.

4. *Ethics:* use Internet addresses for professional organizations (see Unit 2) to find two or three different codes of ethics; compare and contrast the codes of ethics.

5. *Patient's rights:* search for complete copies of a patient's or resident's bill of rights; compare and contrast the different bills of rights (Hint: check American Hospital Association web site).

6. *Advance directives:* search for different examples of a living will and/or a durable power of attorney for health care; compare the different forms.

7. *Patient Self Determination Act of 1990:* locate a copy of this act or information on the purposes of this act (Hint: check federal legislation web sites).

8. *Insurance:* search for different types of liability insurance for health care providers; determine what different policies cover and their cost.

REVIEW QUESTIONS

1. Choose a specific health care profession (i.e., dental hygienist, physical therapist) and create a situation where this individual might be subject to legal action for each of the following torts: malpractice, negligence, assault, battery, invasion of privacy, false imprisonment, abuse, and defamation.

2. Differentiate between slander and libel.

3. What is the difference between an implied contract and an expressed contract?

4. You are employed as a geriatric assistant. A resident tells you that he is saving sleeping pills so he can commit suicide. He has terminal cancer and is in a great deal of pain. What should you do? Why?

5. Obtain at least two different codes of ethics for health professions by contacting professional organizations or searching the Internet. Compare the codes of ethics.

6. How does a living will differ from a Durable Power of Attorney for health care?

7. List five (5) different patient or resident rights.

8. Identify six (6) professional standards by explaining why they are important to meet legal responsibilities, ethics, and/or patient's rights.

UNIT 4
SUGGESTED REFERENCES

Brannigan, Michael. *Health Care Ethics in a Diverse Society.* New York, NY: McGraw-Hill, 2000.

Buckley, William, and Kathy Okrent. *Torts and Personal Injury Law.* Clifton Park, NY: Delmar Learning, 1997.

Burkhardt, Margaret, and Alvita Nathaniel. *Ethics and Issues in Contemporary Nursing.* 2nd ed. Clifton Park, NY: Delmar Learning, 2002.

Davidson, Judith Ann. *Legal and Ethical Considerations for Dental Hygienists and Assistants.* St. Louis, MO: Mosby, 1999.

Edge, Raymond, and John Grove. *Ethics of Health Care: A Guide for Clinical Practice.* 2nd ed. Clifton Park, NY: Delmar Learning, 1999.

Edge, Raymond, and John Kreiger. *Legal and Ethical Perspectives in Health Care: An Integrated Approach.* Clifton Park, NY: Delmar Learning, 1998.

Flight, Myrtle R. *Law, Liability and Ethics for Medical Office Personnel.* 3rd ed. Clifton Park, NY: Delmar Learning, 1998.

Hegner, Barbara, Esther Caldwell, and Joan Needham. *Nursing Assistant: A Nursing Process Approach.* 8th ed. Clifton Park, NY: Delmar Learning, 1999.

Hinderer, Drew, and Sara Hinderer. *A Multidisciplinary Approach to Health Care Ethics.* New York, NY: McGraw-Hill, 2000.

Keir, Lucille, Connie Krebs, and Barbara A. Wise. *Medical Assisting: Administrative and Clinical Competencies.* 5th ed. Clifton Park, NY: Delmar Learning, 2003.

Kenyon, Patricia. *What Would You Do? An Ethical Case Workbook for Human Services Professionals.* Pacific Grove, CA: Brooks/Cole, 1999.

Mappes, Thomas, and David DeGrazia. *Biomedical Ethics.* New York, NY: McGraw-Hill, 2000.

McWay, Dana. *Legal Aspects of Health Information Management.* Clifton Park, NY: Delmar Learning, 1997.

Quill, Timothy. *Death and Dignity.* New York, NY: W.W. Norton and Co., 1993.

Medical Terminology

Unit Objectives

After completing this unit of study, you should be able to:

◆ Identify basic medical abbreviations selected from a standard list
◆ Define prefixes, suffixes, and word roots selected from a list of words
◆ Spell and pronounce medical terms correctly
◆ Define, pronounce, and spell all the key terms

 Observe Standard Precautions

 Safety—Proceed with Caution

 Math Skill

 Science Skill

 Communications Skill

 Instructors Check—Call Instructor at This Point

 OBRA Requirement— Based on Federal Law

 Legal Responsibility

 Career Information

 Technology

KEY TERMS

abbreviations   suffix   word roots
prefix

5:1 INFORMATION Using Medical Abbreviations

As a health care worker, you will see many abbreviations. You will be expected to recognize the most common abbreviations. This section provides a basic list of these abbreviations.

Abbreviations are shortened forms of words, usually just letters. Common examples are AM, which means morning, and PM, which means afternoon or evening.

Abbreviations are used in many health fields. Sometimes they are used by themselves; other times, several abbreviations are combined to give orders or directions. Consider the following examples:

BR c̄ BRP, FFl qh, VS qid

NPO 8 PM, To Lab for CBC, BUN, and FBS

These examples are short forms for giving directions. The first example is interpreted as follows: bedrest with bathroom privileges, force fluids every hour, vital signs four times a day. The second example is interpreted as follows: nothing by mouth after eight o'clock in the evening, to the laboratory for a complete blood count, blood urea nitrogen, and fasting blood sugar. As these examples illustrate, it is much easier to write using abbreviations than it is to write the corresponding detailed messages.

A sample list of abbreviations and symbols follows. This list contains some of the most commonly used abbreviations. Different abbreviations may be used in different facilities and in different parts of the country. It is the responsibility of health care workers to learn the meanings of the abbreviations used in the agencies where they are employed.

NOTE: *There is a growing trend toward eliminating periods from most abbreviations. Although the following list does not show periods, you may work in* an agency that chooses to use them. When in doubt, follow the policy of your agency.

NOTE: Learn the abbreviations in the following way:

1. Use a set of index cards to make a set of flashcards of the abbreviations found on the abbreviation list. Print one abbreviation in big letters on each card. Put the abbreviation on the front of the card and the meaning on the back of the card.

2. Use the flashcards to study the abbreviations. A realistic goal is to learn all abbreviations for one letter per week. For example, learn all of the *A*s the first week, all of the *B*s the second week, all of the *C*s the third week, and so on until all are learned.

3. Prepare for weekly tests on the abbreviations. The tests will be cumulative. They will cover the letter of the week plus any letters learned in previous weeks.

A

@	at
ā	before
A&D	admission and discharge
A&P	anterior and posterior, anatomy and physiology
āā	of each
Ab	abortion
abd	abdomen, abdominal
ABG	arterial blood gas
ac	before meals
ACTH	adrenocorticotrophic hormone
AD	right ear
ADH	antidiuretic hormone
ad lib	as desired
ADL	activities of daily living
adm	admission
AHA	American Hospital Association

AIDS	acquired immune deficiency syndrome
am, AM	morning, before noon
AMA	American Medical Association, against medical advice
amal	amalgam
amb	ambulate, walk
amt	amount
ANA	American Nurses' Association
ANS	autonomic nervous system
ant	anterior
AP	apical pulse
approx	approximately
aq, aqua	aqueous (water base)
ARC	AIDS-related complex
ART	accredited records technician
AS	left ear
as tol	as tolerated
ASA	aspirin (acetylsalicylic acid)
ASAP	as soon as possible
ASCVD	arteriosclerotic cardiovascular disease
ASHD	arteriosclerotic heart disease
AU	both ears
av	average
AV	arteriovenous, atrioventricular
A&W	alive and well
Ax	axilla, axillary, armpit

B

Ba	barium
bacti	bacteriology
B&B	bowel and bladder training
BBB	bundle branch block
B&C	biopsy and conization
BE	barium enema
bid	twice a day
bil	bilateral
Bl	blood
Bl Wk	blood work
BM	bowel movement
BMR	basal metabolic rate
BP	blood pressure
BR	bed rest
BRP	bathroom privileges
BS	blood sugar
BSA	body surface area
BSC, bsc	bedside commode
BUN	blood urea nitrogen
Bx, bx	biopsy

C

°C	degrees Celsius (Centigrade)
c̄, w/	with
Ca	calcium
CA	cancer
cal	calorie
Cap	capsule
CAT	computerized axial tomography
Cath	catheter
CBC	complete blood count
CBET	certified biomedical equipment technician
CBR	complete bed rest
cc	cubic centimeter
CC	chief complaint
CCU	coronary care unit, critical care unit
CDA	certified dental assistant
CDC	Centers for Disease Control and Prevention
CEO	chief executive officer
CF	cystic fibrosis
CHD	coronary heart disease
CHF	congestive heart failure
CHO	carbohydrate
chol	cholesterol
CICU	cardiac intensive care unit
ck	check
Cl	chloride or chlorine
cl liq	clear liquids
cm	centimeter
CMA	certified medical assistant
CNP	certified nurse practitioner
CNS	central nervous system
co, c/o	complains of
CO	carbon monoxide, coronary occlusion
CO_2	carbon dioxide
Comp	complete, compound
cont	continued
COPD	chronic obstructive pulmonary disease
COTA	certified occupational therapy assistant
CP	cerebral palsy
CPK	creatine phosphokinase (cardiac enzyme)
CPR	cardiopulmonary resuscitation
CPT	current procedure terminology
CRTT	certified respiratory therapy technician

CS	central supply or service
C&S	culture and sensitivity
CSF	cerebral spinal fluid
CSR	central supply room
CST	certified surgical technologist
CT	computerized tomography
Cu	copper
CVA	cerebral vascular accident (stroke)
Cx	cervix, complication, complaint

D

d	day
D&C	dilatation and curettage
DA	dental assistant
DAT	diet as tolerated
DC	Doctor of Chiropractic
D/C, dc, disc	discontinue, discharge
DDS	Doctor of Dental Surgery
DEA	Drug Enforcement Agency
del	delivery
Dept	department
DH	dental hygienist
DHHS	Department of Health and Human Services
Diff	differential white blood cell count
dil	dilute, dissolve
DM	diabetes mellitus
DMD	Doctor of Dental Medicine
DMS	diagnostic medical sonography
DNA	deoxyribonucleic acid
DNR	do not resuscitate
DO	Doctor of Osteopathic Medicine
DOA	dead on arrival
DOB	date of birth
DOD	date of death
DON	director of nursing
DPM	Doctor of Podiatric Medicine
DPT	diphtheria, pertussis, tetanus
Dr	doctor
dr	dram, drainage
DRG	diagnostic related group
drg, drsg, dsg	dressing
D/S	dextrose in saline
DSD	dry sterile dressing
DTs	delirium tremors
DVM	Doctor of Veterinary Medicine
DW	distilled water
D/W	dextrose in water
Dx, dx	diagnosis

E

ea	each
EBL	estimated blood loss
ECG, EKG	electrocardiogram
ED	emergency department
EEG	electroencephalogram
EENT	ear, eye, nose, throat
elix	elixir
EMG	electromyogram
EMS	emergency medical services
EMT	emergency medical technician
ENT	ear, nose, throat
EPA	Environmental Protection Agency
ER	emergency room
ESR	erythrocyte sedimentation rate
et, etiol	etiology (cause of disease)
Ex, exam	examination
Exc	excision
Exp	exploratory
ext	extract, extraction, external

F

°F	degrees Fahrenheit
FBS	fasting blood sugar
FBW	fasting blood work
FC	Foley catheter
FDA	Food and Drug Administration
Fe	iron
FF, FFl	force fluids
FH, FHR	fetal heart rate
Fl, fl	fluid
Fr, Fx	fracture
FSH	follicle stimulating hormone
ft	foot
FUO	fever of unknown origin

G

GA	gastric analysis
gal	gallon
GB	gallbladder
Gc	gonococcus, gonorrhea
GH	growth hormone
GI	gastrointestinal
Gm, g	gram

gr	grain
gt, gtt, gtts	drop, drops
GTT	glucose tolerance test
GU	genitourinary
Gyn	gynecology

H

H	hydrogen
H_2O	water
H_2O_2	hydrogen peroxide
H, (h), hypo	hypodermic injection
HA	hearing aid, headache
HBP	high blood pressure
HBV	hepatitis B virus
HCG	human chorionic gonadotrophin hormone
HCl	hydrochloric acid
hct	hematocrit
HDL	high density lipoproteins (healthy type of cholesterol)
Hg	mercury
Hgb, Hb	hemoglobin
HHA	home health assistant/aide
HIV	human immunodeficiency virus (AIDS virus)
HMO	health maintenance organization
HOB	head of bed
HOH	hard of hearing
HOSA	Health Occupations Students of America
H&P	history and physical
Hr, hr, H, h	hour, hours
HS	hour of sleep (bedtime)
Ht	height
Hx, hx	history
hypo	hypodermic injection
Hyst	hysterectomy

I

I&D	incision and drainage
I&O	intake and output
ICCU	intensive coronary care unit
ICD	international classification of diseases
ICU	intensive care unit
ID	intradermal
IDDM	insulin-dependent diabetes mellitus

IH	infectious hepatitis
IM	intramuscular
imp	impression
in	inch
inf	infusion, inferior, infection
ing	inguinal
inj	injection
int	internal, interior
IPPB	intermittent positive pressure breathing
irr, irrig	irrigation
Isol, isol	isolation
IT	inhalation therapy
IUD	intrauterine device
IV	intravenous
IVP	intravenous pyelogram

J

jt	joint

K

K	potassium
KCl	potassium chloride
Kg, kg	kilogram
KUB	kidney, ureter, bladder X-ray

L

L	lumbar
L&D	labor and delivery
L&W	living and well
(L), lt, lft	left
L, l	liter (1,000 cc)
Lab	laboratory
Lap	laparotomy
lat	lateral
lb	pound
LCT	long-term care
LDH	lactose dehydrogenase (cardiac enzyme)
LDL	low density lipoprotein (unhealthy type of cholesterol)
lg	large
liq	liquid
LLQ	left lower quadrant
LMP	last menstrual period

LOC	laxative of choice, level of consciousness
LP	lumbar puncture
LPN	licensed practical nurse
LS	lumbar sacral
LUQ	left upper quadrant
LVN	licensed vocational nurse

M

m	minim
MA	medical assistant
Mat	maternity
mcg	microgram
MD	Medical Doctor, muscular dystrophy, myocardial disease
Med	medical, medicine
mEq	milliequivalent
mg	milligram
Mg	magnesium
MI	myocardial infarction (heart attack)
min	minute
mL, ml	milliliter
MLT	medical laboratory technician
mm	millimeter
MN	midnight
mod	moderate
MOM	milk of magnesia
MRI	magnetic resonance imaging
MS	multiple sclerosis, mitral stenosis, muscular–skeletal
MT	medical technologist

N

N	nitrogen
N/A	not applicable
Na	sodium
NA	nurse aide/assistant
NaCl	sodium chloride (salt)
NB	newborn
N/C	no complaints
neg	negative, none
Neur	neurology
NG, ng	nasogastric tube
NICU	neurological intensive care unit
NIDDM	non-insulin-dependent diabetes mellitus
NIH	National Institutes of Health

nil	none
no	number
NO	nursing office
noc, noct	at night, night
NP	nurse practitioner
NPN	nonprotein nitrogen
NPO	nothing by mouth
N/S, NS	normal saline
Nsy	nursery
N/V, N&V	nausea and vomiting
NVD	nausea, vomiting, diarrhea
NVS	neurological vital signs

O

O_2	oxygen
O&P	ova and parasites
Ob, Obs	obstetrics
OBRA	Omnibus Budget Reconciliation Act
od	overdose
OD	right eye, occular dextra, Doctor of Optometry
oint	ointment
OJ	orange juice
OOB	out of bed
OP	outpatient
OPD, OPC	outpatient department or clinic
opp	opposite
OR	operating room
Ord	orderly
Orth	orthopedics
os	mouth
OS	left eye, occular sinistra
OSHA	Occupational Safety and Health Administration
OT	occupational therapy/therapist
OTC	over the counter
OU	each eye
OV	office visit
oz	ounce

P

p̄	after
P	pulse, phosphorus
PA	physician's assistant
PAC	premature atrial contraction
PAP	Papanicolaou test (smear)

para	number of pregnancies
Path	pathology
Pb	lead
PBI	protein bound iodine
pc	after meals
PCA	patient controlled analgesia
PCC	poison control center
PCP	patient care plan
PCT	patient/personal care technician
PDR	*Physicians' Desk Reference*
PE	physical exam, pulmonary edema
Peds	pediatrics
per	by, through
PET	positron emission tomography
pH	measure of acidity/alkalinity
Pharm	pharmacy
PI	present illness
PID	pelvic inflammatory disease
PKU	phenylketonuria
PM, pm	after noon
PMC	postmortem (after death) care
PMS	premenstrual syndrome
PNS	peripheral nervous system
po	by mouth
PO	phone order
post	posterior, after
post-op	after an operation
PP	postpartum (after delivery)
PPE	personal protective equipment
PPO	preferred provider organization
pre-op	before an operation
prep	prepare
prn	whenever necessary, as needed
Psy	psychology, psychiatry
pt	patient, pint (500 mL or cc)
Pt	prothrombin time
PT	physical therapy/therapist
PTT	partial thromboplastin time
PVC	premature ventricular contraction
PVD	peripheral vascular disease
Px	prognosis, physical exam

Q

q, q̄	every
qd	every day

qh	every hour
q2h	every 2 hours
q3h	every 3 hours
q4h	every 4 hours
qhs	every night at bedtime
qid	four times a day
qns	quantity not sufficient
qod	every other day
qs	quantity sufficient
qt	quart

R

R	respiration, rectal
®, Rt	right
Ra	radium
RBC	red blood cell
RDA	recommended daily allowance
REM	rapid eye movement
RHD	rheumatic heart disease
RLQ	right lower quadrant
RN	registered nurse
RNA	ribonucleic acid
R/O	rule out
RO	reality orientation
ROM	range of motion
RR	recovery room
RRT	registered respiratory therapist, registered radiologic technologist
RT	respiratory therapy/therapist
RUQ	right upper quadrant
Rx	prescription, take, treatment

S

S	sacral
S&A	sugar and acetone
s̄, w/o	without
SA	sino atrial
sc, SC	subcutaneous
SGOT, SGPT	transaminase test
SICU	surgical intensive care unit
SIDS	sudden infant death syndrome
Sig	give the following directions
sm	small
SOB	short of breath
sol	solution
sos	if necessary
spec	specimen

SpGr, spgr	specific gravity
SPN	student practical nurse
spt	spirits, liquor
s̄s̄	one half
S/S, S&S	signs and symptoms
SSE	soap solution enema
staph	staphylococcus infection
stat	immediately, at once
STD	sexually transmitted disease
STH	somatotropic hormone
strep	streptococcus infection
supp	suppository
Surg	surgery, surgical
susp	suspension
Sx	symptom, sign
syp	syrup

T

T&A	tonsillectomy and adenoidectomy
T, Temp	temperature
tab	tablet
TB	tuberculosis
tbsp	tablespoon
TCDB	turn, cough, deep breathe
TH	thyroid hormone
TIA	transient ischemic attack
tid	three times a day
TLC	tender loving care
TO	telephone order
tol	tolerated
TPN	total parenteral nutrition
TPR	temperature, pulse, respiration
tr, tinct	tincture
TSH	thyroid stimulating hormone
tsp	teaspoon
TUR	transurethral resection
TWE	tap water enema
tx	traction, treatment, transplant

U

UA, U/A	urinalysis
ung	ointment
Ur, ur	urine
URI	upper respiratory infection

UTI	urinary tract infection
UV	ultraviolet

V

Vag	vaginal
VD	venereal disease
VDM	Veterinarian Degree of Medicine
VDRL	serology for syphilis, Venereal Disease Research Laboratory
VICA	Vocational Industrial Clubs of America
VO	verbal order
Vol	volume
VS	vital signs (TPR & BP)

W

WBC	white blood cell
WC	ward clerk/secretary
w/c	wheelchair
WHO	World Health Organization
WNL	within normal limits
W/P	whirlpool
wt	weight

X

x	times (2× means do 2 times)
x-match	cross match
XR	X-ray

Y

y/o	years old
YOB	year of birth
yr	year

Z

Zn	zinc

MISCELLANEOUS SYMBOLS

>	greater than
<	less than
↑	higher, elevate, or up
↓	lower or down
#	pound or number
ℨ	dram
℥	ounce
′	foot or minute
″	inch or second
°	degree
♀ or F	female
♂ or M	male
I or *i* or ī	one
II or *ii* or īī	two
V	five
X	ten
L	fifty
C	one hundred
D	five hundred
M	one thousand

STUDENT: *Go to the workbook and complete the assignment and evaluation sheets for 5:1, Using Medical Abbreviations.*

5:2 INFORMATION Interpreting Word Parts

Medical dictionaries have been written to include the many words used in health occupations. It would be impossible to memorize all such words. By breaking the words into parts, however, it is sometimes possible to figure out their meanings. This section provides basic information on doing just that.

A word is often a combination of different parts. The parts include prefixes, suffixes, and word roots (see figure 5-1).

A **prefix** can be defined as a syllable or word placed at the beginning of a word. A **suffix** can be defined as a syllable or word placed at the end of the word.

The meanings of prefixes and suffixes are set. For example, the suffix *itis* means "inflammation of." *Tonsillitis* means "an inflammation of the tonsils," and *appendicitis* means "an inflammation of the appendix." Note that the meaning of the suffix is usually placed first when the word is defined.

Word roots can be defined as main words or parts to which prefixes and suffixes can be added. In the example *appendicitis*, the word root is *appendix*. By adding the prefix *pseudo*, which means "false," and the suffix *itis*, which means "inflammation of," the word becomes *pseudoappendicitis*. This is interpreted as a "false inflammation of the appendix."

The prefix usually serves to further define the word root. The suffix usually describes what is happening to the word root.

When prefixes, suffixes, and/or word roots are joined together, vowels are frequently added. Common examples include a, e, i, ia, io, o, and u. These are listed in parentheses in the lists that follow. The vowels are not used if the word root or suffix begins with a vowel. For example, *encephal (o)* means brain. When it is combined with *itis* meaning inflammation of, the vowel is not used for *encephalitis*. When it is combined with *gram* meaning tracing or record, the vowel "o" is added for *encephalogram*. *Hepat (o)* means liver. When it is combined with *itis*, the vowel is not used for *hepatitis*. When it is combined with *megaly* meaning enlarged, the vowel "o" is added for *hepatomegaly*.

By learning basic prefixes, suffixes, and word roots, you will frequently be able to interpret the meaning of a word even when you have never before encountered the word. A list of common prefixes, suffixes, and word roots follows.

NOTE: Learn the prefixes, suffixes, and word roots in the following way:

1. Use a set of index cards to make flashcards of the word parts found on the prefix, suffix, and word root list. Place one prefix, suffix, or word root on each card. Put the word part on the front of the card and the meaning of the word part on the back of the card. Ensure that each is spelled correctly.

2. Use the flashcards to learn the meanings of the word parts. A realistic goal is to learn one letter per week. For example, learn all word parts starting with the letter *A* the first week, all of those starting with *B* the second week, all of those starting with *C* the third week, and so on until all are learned. Practice correct spelling of all of the word parts.

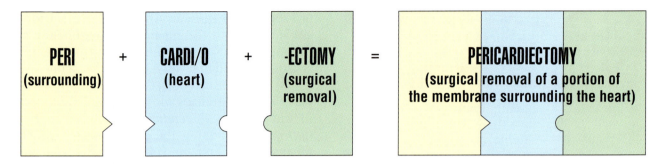

FIGURE 5-1 Prefixes, suffixes, and word roots can be used to interpret the meaning of a word.

3. Prepare for weekly tests on the word parts. The tests will be cumulative. They will cover the letter of the week plus any letters learned in previous weeks. Words will be presented that use the various word parts. In order to be considered correct, you must spell the words correctly.

A

a-, an-	without, lack of
ab-	from, away
-able	capable of
-ac, -ic	pertaining to
acr- (o)	extremities (arms and legs)
ad-	to, toward, near
aden- (o)	gland, glandular
adren- (o)	adrenal gland
aer- (o)	air
-al	like, similar, pertaining to
alba-	white
alges- (i, ia)	pain
-algia	pain
ambi-	both, both sides
an- (o, us)	anus (opening to rectum)
angi- (o)	vessel
ankyl-	crooked, looped, immovable, fixed
ante- (ro)	before, in front of, ahead of
anti-	against
append- (i, o)	appendix
arter- (io)	artery
arthr- (o)	joint
-ase	enzyme
-asis	condition of
-asthenia	weakness, lack of strength
ather- (o)	fatty, lipid
audi- (o)	sound, hearing
aur-	ear
auto-	self

B

bi- (s)	twice, double, both
bio-	life
-blast	germ/embryonic cell
blephar- (o)	eyelid
brachi-	arm
brachy-	short
brady-	slow
bronch- (i, o)	air tubes in lungs
bucc- (a)	cheek

C

calc- (u, ulus)	stone
carcin- (o)	cancer, malignancy
cardi- (a, o)	pertaining to heart
carp- (o)	wrist
-cele	swelling, tumor, cavity, hernia
cent- (i)	one hundred
-centesis	surgical puncture to remove fluid
cephal- (o)	head, pertaining to head
cerebro-	brain
cerv- (ic)	neck, neck of uterus
cheil- (o)	lip
chem- (o)	drug, chemical
chir- (o)	hand
chlor- (o)	green
chol- (e, o)	bile, gallbladder
chond- (i, r, ri)	cartilage
chrom- (o)	color
-cide	causing death
circum-	around, about
-cise	cut
-clysis	washing, irrigation
co- (n)	with, together
-coccus	round

-coele	chamber, enlarged space
col- (in, o)	colon, bowel, large intestine
colp- (i, o)	vagina
contra-	against, counter
cost- (a, i, o)	rib
crani- (o)	pertaining to the skull
-crine	secrete
cryo-	cold
crypt-	hidden
cut-	skin
cyan- (o)	blue
cyst- (i, o)	bladder, bag, sac
cyt- (e, o)	cell

D

dacry-	tear duct, tear
dactyl- (o)	finger, toe
dec- (a, i)	ten
demi-	half
dent- (i, o)	tooth
derm- (a, at, o)	pertaining to skin
-desis	surgical union or fixation
dextr- (i, o)	to the right
di- (plo)	double, twice
dia-	through, between, part
dis- (ti, to)	separation, away from
dors- (i, o)	to the back, back
duoden- (o)	duodenum
dyni- (a, c)	pain
dys-	difficult, painful, bad

E

e- (c)	without
-eal	pertaining to
ec- (ti, to)	outside, external
-ectasis	expansion, dilation, stretching
-ectomy	surgical removal of
electr- (o)	electrical
-emesis	vomit
-emia	blood
encephal- (o)	brain
endo-	within, innermost
enter- (i, o)	intestine
epi-	upon, over, upper
erythro-	red
-esis	condition of
-esthesia	sensation, perception, feel

eu-	well, easy, normal
ex- (o)	outside of, beyond

F

faci-	face
-fascia	fibrous band
-ferous	producing
fibr- (a, i, o)	fiber, connective tissue
fore-	in front of
-form	having the form of, shape
-fuge	driving away, expelling

G

galacto-	milk, galactose (milk sugar)
gast- (i, ro)	stomach
-genesis	development, production, creation
-genetic, -genic	origin, producing, causing
genito-	organs of reproduction
-genous	kind, type
geront- (o)	old age, elderly
gingiv-	gums, gingiva
gloss- (o)	tongue
gluc- (o)	sweetness, sugar, glucose
gly- (co)	sugar
-gram	tracing, picture, record
-graph	diagram, instrument for recording
gyn- (ec, o)	woman, female

H

hem- (a, ato, o)	blood
hemi-	half
hepat- (o)	liver
herni-	rupture
hetero-	other, unlike, different
hist- (o)	tissue
hom- (eo, o)	same, like
hydro-	water
hyper-	excessive, high, over, increased, more than normal
hypno-	sleep
hypo-	decreased, deficient, low, under, less than normal
hyster- (o)	uterus

I

-ia, -iasis	condition of, abnormal/pathological state
-ic, -ac	pertaining to
idio-	peculiar to an individual, self-originating
ile- (o, um)	ileum
infra-	beneath, below
inter-	between, among
intra-	within, into, inside
-ism	condition, theory, state of being
iso-	equal, alike, same
-itis	inflammation, inflammation of

K

kerat- (o)	cornea of eye
-kinesis, -kinetic	motion

L

labi- (a, o)	lip
lacrima-	tears
lact- (o)	milk
lapar- (o)	abdomen, abdominal wall
laryng- (o)	larynx (voicebox)
latero-	side
-lepsy	seizure, convulsion
leuco-, leuko-	white
lingu- (a, o)	tongue
lip- (o)	fat, lipids
lith- (o)	stone, calculus
-logy	study of, science of
lymph- (o)	lymph tissue
-lys (is, o)	destruction, dissolving of

M

macro-	large
mal-	bad, abnormal, disordered, poor
malac- (ia)	softening of a tissue
mamm- (o)	breast, mammary glands
-mania	insanity, mental disorder

mast- (o)	breast
med- (i)	middle, midline
-megaly, mega-	large, enlarged
melan- (o)	black
mening- (o)	membranes covering the brain and spinal cord
meno-	monthly, menstruation
mes- (o)	middle, midline
-meter	measuring instrument, measure
-metry	measurement
micro-	small
mono-	one, single
-mortem	death
muc- (o, us)	mucus, secretion of mucous membrane
multi-	many, much, a large amount
my- (o)	muscle
myc- (o)	fungus
myel- (o)	bone marrow, spinal cord
myring- (o)	eardrum, tympanic membrane

N

narc- (o)	sleep, numb, stupor
nas- (o)	nose
-natal	birth
necr- (o)	death
neo-	new
neph- (r, ro)	kidney
neur- (o)	nerve, nervous system
noct- (i)	night, at night
non-	no, none

O

ocul- (o)	eye
-ode, -oid	form, shape, like, resembling
odont- (o)	tooth
olig- (o)	few, less than normal, small
-ologist	person who does/studies
-ology	study of, science of
-oma	tumor, a swelling
onco-	mass, bulk, tumor
oophor- (o)	ovary, female egg cell
ophthalm- (o)	eye
-opia	vision
-opsy	to view
opt- (ic)	vision, eye

or- (o)	mouth
orch- (ido)	testicle, testes
-orrhea	flow, discharge
orth- (o)	normal, straight
ost- (e, eo)	bone
-oscopy	diagnostic examination
-osis	condition, state, process
ot- (o)	ear
-otic	pertaining to a condition
-otomy	cutting into
-ous	full of, containing, pertaining to, condition
ovi-, ovario-	egg, female sex gland, ovary

P

pan-	all, complete, entire
pancreat- (o)	pancreas
para-	near, beside, beyond, abnormal, lower half of the body
-paresis	paralysis
-partum	birth, labor
path- (ia, o, y)	disease, abnormal condition
ped- (ia)	child
-penia	lack of, abnormal reduction in number, deficiency
pent- (a)	five
-pepsia, -pepsis	digestion
per-	through, by, excessive
peri-	around
-pexy	fixation
phag- (o)	eat, ingest
-phage, -phagia	to eat, consuming, swallow
pharyng- (o)	pharynx, throat
-phas, -phasia	speech
-philia, -philic	affinity for, attracted to
phleb- (o)	vein
-phobia	fear
phon- (o)	sound, voice
-phylaxis	protection, prevention
-plasty	surgical correction or repair
-plegia	paralysis
pleuro-	side, rib
-pnea	breathing
pneum- (o, on)	lung, pertaining to the lungs, air
pod- (e, o)	foot
poly-	many, much
post-	after, behind
pre-	before, in front of
pro-	in front of, forward

proct- (o)	rectum, rectal, anus
psora-	itch
pseudo-	false
psych- (i, o)	pertaining to the mind
-ptosis	drooping down, sagging, downward displacement
pulmon- (o)	lung
py- (o)	pus
pyel- (o)	renal pelvis of kidney
pyr- (o)	heat, fever

Q

| quad- (ra, ri) | four |

R

radi- (o)	X-rays, radiation
re-	back, again
rect- (o)	rectum
ren- (o)	kidney
retro-	backward, in back, behind
rhin- (o)	nose, pertaining to the nose
-rraphy	suture of, sewing up of a gap or defect
-rrhagia	sudden or excessive flow
-rrhea	flow, discharge
-rrhexis	rupture of, bursting

S

salping- (i, o)	tube, fallopian tube
sanguin- (o)	blood
sarc- (o)	malignant (cancer) connective tissue
-sarcoma	tumor, cancer
scler- (o)	hardening
-sclerosis	dryness or hardness
-scope	examining instrument
-scopy	observation
-sect	cut
semi-	half, part
sep- (ti)	poison, rot, infection
sinistr- (o)	left
soma- (t)	body
son- (o)	sound
-spasm	involuntary contraction

sperm- (ato)	spermatozoa, male germ (sex) cell
splen- (o)	spleen
-stasis	stoppage, maintaining a constant level
steno-	contracted, narrow
stern- (o)	sternum, breast bone
stoma- (t)	mouth
-stomy	artificial opening
sub-	less, under, below
sup- (er, ra)	above, upon, over, higher in position
sym-, syn-	joined, fused, together

T

tach- (o, y)	rapid, fast
ten- (do, o)	tendon
tetra-	four
-therapy	treatment
therm- (o, y)	heat
thorac- (o)	thorax, chest
thromb- (o)	clot, thrombus
thym- (o)	thymus gland
thyr- (o)	thyroid gland
-tome	instrument that cuts
-tox (ic)	poison
trach- (e, i, o)	trachea, windpipe
trans-	across, over, beyond
tri-	three
trich- (o)	hair
-trips (y)	crushing by rubbing or grinding
-trophy	nutrition, growth, development
tympan- (o)	eardrum, tympanic membrane

U

ultra-	beyond, excess
uni-	one
ur- (o)	urine, urinary tract
ureter- (o)	ureter (tube from kidney to bladder)
urethr- (o)	urethra (tube from bladder to urinary meatus)
-uria	urine
uter- (o)	uterus, womb

V

vas- (o)	vessel, duct
ven- (a)	vein
ventro-	to the front, abdomen
vertebr- (o)	spine, vertebrae
vesic- (o)	urinary bladder
viscer- (o)	internal organs
vit- (a)	necessary for life

X

xanth- (o)	yellow
-xenia	strange, abnormal

Z

zoo-	animal
zymo-	enzymes

STUDENT: *Go to the workbook and complete the assignment and evaluation sheets for 5:2, Interpreting Word Parts.*

UNIT 5 SUMMARY

Medical abbreviations and terminology are used in all health care occupations and facilities. In order to communicate effectively, health care workers must be familiar with common abbreviations and terminology.

Medical abbreviations are shortened forms of words, usually just letters. Sometimes, they are used by themselves; other times, several abbreviations are combined to give orders or directions.

Medical terminology consists of the use of prefixes, suffixes, and word roots to create words. Entire dictionaries have been written to include the terminology used in health care. It would be impossible to memorize the meaning of every word. By learning common prefixes, suffixes, and word roots, however, a health care worker can break a word into parts and figure out the meaning of the word.

INTERNET SEARCHES

Use the suggested search engines in Unit 11:4 of this textbook to search the Internet for additional information on the following topics:

1. *Medical terminology resources:* search publishers such as Delmar Learning, Mosby, or McGraw-Hill, for medical terminology books, videos, and software. Evaluate different methods of learning medical terminology as presented in these resources.

2. *Diseases:* combine word parts to name diseases or conditions such as *cholecystitis.* Search for information on the diseases. Research the cause of the disease, signs and symptoms, and main forms of treatment.

3. *Cancer:* combine word parts to create words ending in "*oma.*" Then search for information on the different types of tumors. Research benign and malignant tumors and the signs and symptoms for each. (Hint: locate the web site for the American Cancer Society.)

REVIEW QUESTIONS

1. Determine the meaning of the abbreviations *bid, tid,* and *qid.* Find prefixes that define the first letters (b, t, and q) of the three abbreviations. Determining associations similar to these will make it easier to learn medical abbreviations.

2. List ten (10) abbreviations for diseases or disorders of the body.

3. List ten (10) abbreviations for diagnostic tests such as blood work or radiology (X-ray) studies.

4. Add the suffix "*oma*" to five different word roots for tissues or parts of the body. Check a medical dictionary to determine if the spelling is correct and to learn the full meaning of the word. One example is "*melanoma.*"

5. Choose five (5) word roots related to a part of the body. Add different prefixes and/or suffixes to the word root to create at least three different terms for each body part. For example: *cystitis, cystoscopy,* and *cystocoele.*

6. A patient is admitted to a hospital with a dx of pancreatitis, dysphagia, and gastralgia. Sx include NVD and a severe HA. The dr orders an abd MRI, CBC, NPO except for cl liq, VS q2h, and CBR. Interpret all the above medical abbreviations and terms to determine the patient's condition and plan of treatment.

UNIT 5

SUGGESTED REFERENCES

Collins, C. Edward, and Juanita Davies. *Modern Medical Language.* Clifton Park, NY: Delmar Learning, 1998.

Davies, Juanita. *Essentials of Medical Terminology.* 2nd ed. Clifton Park, NY: Delmar Learning, 2002.

Davies, Juanita. *Quick Reference for Medical Terminology.* Clifton Park, NY: Delmar Learning, 2002.

Delmar's Medical Terminology Flash! Computerized Flashcards. Clifton Park, NY: Delmar Learning, 2002.

Dennerll, Jean Tannis. *Medical Terminology Made Easy.* 2nd ed. Clifton Park, NY: Delmar Learning, 1998.

DeSousa, Luis. *Common Medical Abbreviations.* Clifton Park, NY: Delmar Learning, 1995.

Dofka, Charline. *Dental Terminology.* Clifton Park, NY: Delmar Learning, 2000.

Dorland's Illustrated Medical Dictionary. 29th ed. Philadelphia, PA: W. B. Saunders, 2000.

Ehrlich, Ann, and Carol L. Schroeder. *Medical Terminology for Health Professions.* 4th ed. Clifton Park, NY: Delmar Learning, 2001.

Jones, Betty Davis. *Delmar's Comprehensive Medical Terminology: A Competency Based Approach.* Clifton Park, NY: Delmar Learning, 1999.

Kelz, Rochelle. *Delmar's English–Spanish Pocket Dictionary for Health Professionals.* Clifton Park, NY: Delmar Learning, 1997.

Mosio, Marie. *Medical Terminology: A Student Centered Approach.* Clifton Park, NY: Delmar Learning, 2002.

Smith, Genevieve L., Phyllis E. Davis, and Jean Tannis Dennerll. *Medical Terminology: A Programmed Text.* 8th ed. Clifton Park, NY: Delmar Learning, 1999.

Sormunen, Carolee. *Terminology for Allied Health Professionals.* 4th ed. Clifton Park, NY: Delmar Learning, 1999.

Spilker, Bert. *Medical Dictionary in Six Languages.* Philadelphia, PA: Lippincott, Williams, & Wilkins, 1998.

Stedman's Medical Dictionary. 27th ed. Philadelphia, PA: Lippincott, Williams, & Wilkins, 2000.

UNIT 6

Anatomy and Physiology

Unit Objectives

After completing the 14 subunits in this unit of study, you should be able to:

◆ Apply the appropriate terminology to major organs and systems of the human body
◆ Identify the major functions of body systems
◆ Compare interrelationships of body systems
◆ Describe basic diseases affecting each of the body systems
◆ Define, pronounce, and spell all the key terms

NOTE: *This unit is meant to serve as a brief introduction to anatomy and physiology. For more detailed information, refer to the references listed at the end of the unit.*

 Observe Standard Precautions

 Safety—Proceed with Caution

 Math Skill

 Science Skill

 C Communications Skill

 Instructors Check—Call Instructor at This Point

 **OBRA** OBRA Requirement— Based on Federal Law

 Legal Responsibility

 Career Information

 Technology

6:1 Basic Structure of the Human Body

Objectives

After completing this section, you should be able to:

- Label a diagram of the main parts of a cell
- Describe the basic function of each part of a cell
- Compare the four main types of tissue by describing the basic function of each type
- Explain the relationship between cells, tissues, organs, and systems
- Define, pronounce, and spell all the key terms

KEY TERMS

anatomy

cell

cell membrane

centrosome
(sen'-troh-sohm)

chromatin
(crow'-ma-tin)

connective tissue

cytoplasm
(sy'-toe-plaz-um)

dehydration

edema
(eh-dee'-mah)

endoplasmic reticulum
(en'-doe-plaz-mik re-tik'-
you-lum)

epithelial tissue
(ep'-eh-thiel''-e-al tish'-u)

Golgi apparatus
(gawl'-jee ap-a-rat'-us)

lysosomes
(ly'-sah-soms)

meiosis
(my-o'-sis)

mitochondria
(my-toe-con'-dree-ah)

mitosis
(my-toe'-sis)

muscle tissue

nerve tissue

nucleolus
(new''-klee-oh'-lus)

nucleus

organ

organelles

pathophysiology

physiology
(fizz-ee-all'-oh-gee)

pinocytic vesicles

protoplasm
(pro'-toe-plaz-um)

system

tissue

RELATED HEALTH CAREERS

NOTE: A basic knowledge of human anatomy and physiology is essential for almost every health care provider. However, some health careers are related to specific body systems. As each body system is discussed, examples of related health careers are listed. The following health career categories require knowledge of the structure and function of the entire human body and will not be listed in specific body system units.

- Athletic Trainer
- Emergency Medical Careers
- Medical Laboratory Careers
- Medical Assistant
- Medical Illustrator
- Nursing Careers
- Pharmacy Careers
- Physician Assistant
- Physicians
- Surgical Technologist

6:1   INFORMATION

The human body is often described as an efficient, organized machine. When this machine does not function correctly, disease occurs. Before understanding the disease processes, however, the health worker must first understand the normal functioning of the body. A basic understanding of anatomy and physiology is therefore necessary. **Anatomy** is the study of the form and structure of an organism. **Physiology** is the study of the processes of living organisms, or why and how they work. **Pathophysiology** is the study of how disease occurs and the responses of living organisms to disease processes.

The basic substance of all life is **protoplasm**. This material makes up all living things. Although protoplasm is composed of ordinary elements such as carbon, oxygen, hydrogen, sulfur, nitrogen, and phosphorus, scientists are unable to combine such elements to create that characteristic called *life*.

CELLS

Protoplasm forms the basic unit of structure and function in all living things: the **cell**. Cells are microscopic structures that carry on all the functions of life. They take in food and oxygen; produce heat and energy; move and adapt to their environment; eliminate wastes; perform special functions; and reproduce to create new, identical cells. The human body contains trillions of cells. These cells vary in shape and size and perform many different functions.

Most cells have the following basic parts (see figure 6-1):

◆ **Cell membrane**—the outer protective covering of the cell. It is semipermeable, which means that it allows certain substances to enter and leave the cell while preventing the passage of other substances.

◆ **Cytoplasm**—a semi-fluid inside the cell. It contains water, proteins, lipids (fats), carbohydrates, minerals, and salts. It is the site for all chemical reactions that take place in the cell. **Organelles**, or cell structures that help a cell to function, are located in the cytoplasm. The main organelles are the nucleus, mitochondria, ribosomes, lysosomes, centrioles, Golgi apparatus, and endoplasmic reticulum.

◆ **Nucleus**—a mass in the cytoplasm. It is often called the "brain" of the cell because it controls many cell activities and is important in cell division.

◆ **Nucleolus**—located inside the nucleus, and important in cell reproduction. Ribosomes, made of ribonucleic acid (RNA) and protein, are manufactured in the nucleolus. The ribosomes move from the nucleus to the cytoplasm, where they aid in the synthesis (production) of protein. They can exist freely in the cytoplasm or be attached to the endoplasmic reticulum.

◆ **Chromatin**—located in the nucleus and made of deoxyribonucleic acid (DNA) and protein. During cell reproduction, the chromatin condenses to form rod-like structures called chromosomes. A human cell has 46 chromosomes or 23 pairs. The chromosomes contain about 100,000 genes, which carry inherited characteristics. Each gene has a specific and unique sequence of approximately 1,000 base pairs of DNA; the DNA sequence carries the genetic coding that allows for exact duplication of the cell. Since the DNA sequence on genes is unique for each individual, it is sometimes used as an identification tool similar to fingerprints, but much more exact.

◆ **Centrosome**—located in the cytoplasm and near the nucleus. It contains two centrioles. During mitosis, or cell division, the centrioles separate. Thin cytoplasmic spindle fibers form between the centrioles and attach to the chromosomes. This creates an even division of the chromosomes in the two new cells.

◆ **Mitochondria**—rod-shaped organelles located throughout the cytoplasm. These are often called the "furnaces" or "powerhouses" of the cell because they break down carbohydrates, proteins, and fats to produce adenosine triphosphate (ATP), the major energy source of the cell.

◆ **Golgi apparatus**—a stack of membrane layers located in the cytoplasm. This structure produces, stores, and packages secretions for discharge from the cell. Cells of the salivary, gastric, and pancreatic glands have large numbers of Golgi apparatus.

◆ **Endoplasmic reticulum**—a fine network of tubular structures located in the cytoplasm. This network allows for the transport

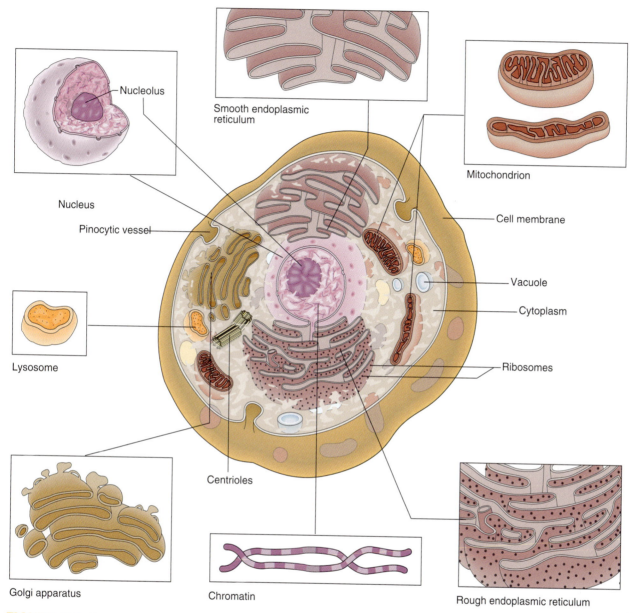

Nucleolus

Nucleus

Pinocytic vessel

Smooth endoplasmic reticulum

Mitochondrion

Cell membrane

Vacuole

Cytoplasm

Lysosome

Ribosomes

Golgi apparatus

Centrioles

Chromatin

Rough endoplasmic reticulum

FIGURE 6-1 Basic parts of a cell.

of materials into and out of the nucleus, and also aids in the synthesis and storage of proteins. Rough endoplasmic reticulum contains ribosomes, which are the sites for protein synthesis (production). Smooth endoplasmic reticulum does not contain ribosomes and is not present in all cells. It assists with cholesterol synthesis, fat metabolism, and detoxification of drugs.

◆ **Lysosomes**—oval or round bodies found throughout the cytoplasm. These structures contain digestive enzymes that digest and destroy old cells, bacteria, and foreign materials, an important function of the body's immune system.

◆ **Pinocytic vesicles**—pocketlike folds in the cell membrane. These folds allow large molecules such as proteins and fats to enter the cell. When such molecules are inside the cell, the folds close to form vacuoles or bubbles in the cytoplasm.

Cell Reproduction

Most cells reproduce by dividing into two identical cells. This process is called **mitosis**, a form of asexual reproduction (see figure 6-2). Skin cells, blood forming cells, and intestinal tract cells reproduce continuously. Muscle cells only reproduce every few years, but muscle tissue can be

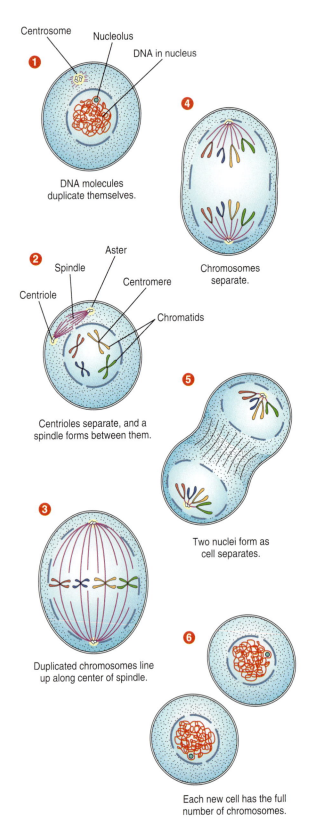

① Centrosome   Nucleolus   DNA in nucleus

DNA molecules
duplicate themselves.

② Aster   Spindle   Centriole   Centromere   Chromatids

Centrioles separate, and a
spindle forms between them.

③ Duplicated chromosomes line
up along center of spindle.

④ Chromosomes
separate.

⑤ Two nuclei form as
cell separates.

⑥ Each new cell has the full
number of chromosomes.

FIGURE 6-2 Mitosis is a form of asexual reproduction where a cell divides into two identical cells.

enlarged with exercise. Some specialized cells, such as nerve cells in the brain and spinal cord, do not reproduce after birth. If these cells are damaged or destroyed, others are not formed to replace them.

Prior to mitosis, the chromatin material in the nucleus condenses to form chromosomes, and an exact duplicate of each chromosome is made. Each chromosome then consists of two identical strands, called *chromatids,* joined together by a structure called a *centromere.* When mitosis begins, the two centrioles in the centrosome move to opposite ends of the cell. A spindle of threadlike fibers trails from the centrioles. The nuclear membrane disappears, and the pairs of duplicated chromosomes attach to the spindles at the center of the cell. The chromatids then split from their duplicated halves and move to opposite ends of the cell. Each end now has 46 chromosomes or 23 pairs. The cytoplasm divides, and a new cell membrane forms to create two new identical cells.

Sex cells (gametes) divide by a process known as **meiosis**. This process uses two separate cell divisions to produce four new cells. When female cells (ova) or male cells (spermatozoa or sperm) divide by meiosis, the number of chromosomes is reduced to 23, or one-half the number found in cells created by mitosis. When an ovum and sperm join to create a new life, the zygote, or new cell, has 46 chromosomes: 23 from the ovum and 23 from the sperm. Thus, the zygote has 46, or 23 pairs, of chromosomes, the normal number for all body cells except the sex cells.

Immediately after the ovum and sperm join to form a zygote, the zygote begins a period of rapid mitotic division. Within four to five days, the zygote is a hollow ball-like mass of cells called a *blastocyst.* Within this blastocyst are embryonic *stem cells.* These stem cells have the ability to transform themselves into any of the body's specialized cells and perform many different functions. A controversial area of research is now concentrated on these stem cells. Scientists are attempting to determine whether stem cells can be transplanted into the body and used to cure diseases such as diabetes mellitus, Parkinson's, heart disease, osteoporosis, and arthritis. The hope is that the stem cells can be programmed to produce new specialized cells that can replace a body's damaged cells and cure a disease. The controversy arises from the fact that a 4–5 day embryo, capable of creating a new life, is used to obtain the cells. Right-to-life advocates are strongly opposed to stem cell research if the cells are obtained from embryos. Stem cells also exist in adult tissues, such as bone marrow and the liver. Adult stem cells, however, do not have the ability to evolve into every kind of cell; these stem cells evolve into more cells of their own kind. This controversy will continue as scientists expand stem cell research.

TISSUE

Although most cells contain the same basic parts, cells vary greatly in shape, size, and special function. When cells of the same type join together for a common purpose, they form a **tissue**. Tissues are 60 percent to 99 percent water with various dissolved substances. This water is slightly salty in nature and is called *tissue fluid.* If there is an insufficient amount (not enough tissue fluid), a condition called **dehydration** occurs. When there is an excess amount (too much tissue fluid), a condition called **edema**, or swelling of the tissues, occurs.

There are four main groups of tissues: epithelial, connective, nerve, and muscle (see figure 6-3). **Epithelial tissue** covers the surface of the body and is the main tissue in the skin. It forms the lining of the intestinal, respiratory, circulatory, and urinary tracts, as well as that of other body cavities. Epithelial tissue also forms the body glands where it specializes to produce specific secretions for the body.

Connective tissue is the supporting fabric of organs and other body parts. There are two main classes of connective tissue: soft and hard. Soft connective tissue includes adipose, or fatty, tissue (which stores fat as a food reserve [or source of energy], insulates the body, and acts as padding) and fibrous connective tissue, such as ligaments and tendons (which help hold body structures together). Hard connective tissue includes cartilage and bone. Cartilage is a tough, elastic material that is found between the bones of the spine and at the end of long bones. It acts as a shock absorber and allows for flexibility. It is also found in the nose, ears, and larynx, or "voice box," to provide form or shaping. Bone is similar to cartilage but has calcium salts, nerves, and blood vessels; it is frequently called *osseous tissue.* Bone helps form the rigid structure of the human body. Blood and lymph are classified as liquid connective tissue or *vascular tissue.* Blood

Structure	Function
Nerve	Control and communicate
Epithelium	Secrete and protect
Muscle (cardiac)	Move and protect
Connective tissue	Support and connect

FIGURE 6-3 Four main groups of tissues and their functions.

carries nutrients and oxygen to the body cells and carries metabolic waste away from cells. Lymph transports tissue fluid, proteins, fats, and other materials from the tissues to the circulatory system.

Nerve tissue is made up of special cells called *neurons.* It controls and coordinates body activities by transmitting messages throughout the body. The nerves, brain, and spinal cord are composed of nerve tissue.

Muscle tissue produces power and movement by contraction of muscle fibers. There are three main types of muscle tissue: skeletal, cardiac, and visceral (smooth). Skeletal muscle attaches to the bones and provides for movement of the body. Cardiac muscle causes the heart to beat. Visceral muscle is present in the walls of the respiratory, digestive, urinary tract, and blood vessels.

ORGANS AND SYSTEMS

Two or more tissues joined together to perform a specific function are called an **organ**. Examples of organs include the heart, stomach, and lungs.

Organs and other body parts joined together to perform a particular function are called a **system**. The basic systems (discussed in more detail in succeeding sections) are the integumentary, skeletal, muscular, circulatory, lymphatic, nervous, respiratory, digestive, urinary (or excretory), endocrine, and reproductive. Their functions and main organs are shown in table 6-1.

In summary, cells combine to form tissues, tissues combine to form organs, and organs and

TABLE 6-1 Systems of the Body

SYSTEM	FUNCTIONS	MAJOR ORGANS/STRUCTURES
Integumentary	Protects body from injury, infection, and dehydration; helps regulate body temperature; eliminates some wastes; produces vitamin D	Skin, sweat and oil glands, nails, and hair
Skeletal	Creates framework of body, protects internal organs, produces blood cells, acts as levers for muscles	Bones and cartilage
Muscular	Produces movement, protects internal organs, produces body heat, maintains posture	Skeletal, smooth, and cardiac muscles
Nervous	Coordinates and controls body activities	Nerves, brain, spinal cord
Special Senses	Allow body to react to environment by providing sight, hearing, taste, smell, and balance	Eye, ear, tongue, nose, general sense receptors
Circulatory	Carries oxygen and nutrients to body cells; carries waste products away from cells; helps produce cells to fight infection	Heart, blood vessels, blood, spleen
Lymphatic	Carries some tissue fluid and wastes to blood, assists with fighting infection	Lymph nodes, lymph vessels, spleen, tonsils, and thymus gland
Respiratory	Breathes in oxygen and eliminates carbon dioxide	Nose, pharynx, larynx, trachea, bronchi, lungs
Digestive	Digests food physically and chemically, transports food, absorbs nutrients, eliminates wastes	Mouth, salivary glands, pharynx, esophagus, stomach, intestine, liver, gallbladder, pancreas
Urinary	Filters blood to maintain fluid and electrolyte balance in the body, produces & eliminates urine	Kidneys, ureters, urinary bladder, urethra
Endocrine	Produces and secretes hormones to regulate body processes	Pituitary, thyroid, parathyroid, adrenal, and thymus glands; pancreas, ovaries, testes
Reproductive	Provides for reproduction	Male: Testes, epididymis, vas deferens, ejaculatory duct, seminal vesicles, prostate gland, penis, urethra
		Female: Ovaries, fallopian tubes, uterus, vagina, breasts

other body parts combine to form systems. These systems working together help create the miracle called the human body (see figure 6-4).

STUDENT: *Go to the workbook and complete the assignment sheet for 6:1, Basic Structure of the Human Body.*

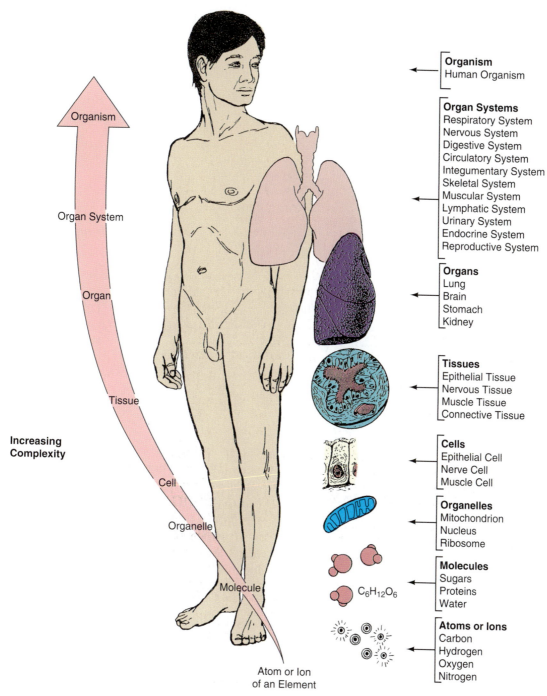

Organism
Human Organism

Organ Systems
Respiratory System
Nervous System
Digestive System
Circulatory System
Integumentary System
Skeletal System
Muscular System
Lymphatic System
Urinary System
Endocrine System
Reproductive System

Organs
Lung
Brain
Stomach
Kidney

Tissues
Epithelial Tissue
Nervous Tissue
Muscle Tissue
Connective Tissue

Cells
Epithelial Cell
Nerve Cell
Muscle Cell

Organelles
Mitochondrion
Nucleus
Ribosome

Molecules
Sugars
Proteins
Water

$C_6H_{12}O_6$

Atoms or Ions
Carbon
Hydrogen
Oxygen
Nitrogen

Organism

Organ System

Organ

Tissue

Increasing Complexity

Cell

Organelle

Molecule

Atom or Ion
of an Element

FIGURE 6-4 The levels of complexity in the human organism.

6:2 Body Planes, Directions, and Cavities

Objectives

After completing this section, you should be able to:

◆ Label the names of the planes and the directional terms related to these planes on a diagram of the three planes of the body

◆ Label a diagram of the main body cavities

◆ Identify the main organs located in each body cavity

◆ Locate the nine abdominal regions

◆ Define, pronounce, and spell all the key terms

KEY TERMS

abdominal cavity
abdominal regions
anterior
body cavities
body planes
buccal cavity
caudal
(kaw'-doll)
cranial
(kray'-nee-al)
cranial cavity
distal

dorsal
dorsal cavity
frontal (coronal) plane
inferior
lateral
(lat'-eh-ral)
medial
(me'-dee-al)
midsagittal (median) plane
(mid-saj'-ih-tahl)
nasal cavity
orbital cavity

pelvic cavity
posterior
proximal
(prox'-ih-mahl)
spinal cavity
superior
thoracic cavity
(tho-rass'-ik)
transverse plane
ventral
ventral cavity

6:2 INFORMATION

Because terms such as *south* and *east* would be difficult to apply to the human body, other directional terms have been developed. These terms are used to describe the relationship of one part of the body to another part.

BODY PLANES

Body planes are imaginary lines drawn through the body at various parts to separate the body into sections. Directional terms are created by these planes. The three main body planes are the transverse, midsagittal, and frontal (see figure 6-5).

The **transverse plane** is a horizontal plane that divides the body into a top half and a bottom half. Body parts above other parts are termed **superior**, and body parts below other parts are termed **inferior**. For instance, the knee is superior to the ankle, but inferior to the hip. Two other directional terms related to this plane include **cranial**, which means body parts located near the head, and **caudal**, which means body parts located near the sacral region of the spinal column (also known as the "tail").

The **midsagittal**, or **median, plane** divides the body into right and left sides. Body parts close to the midline, or plane, are called **medial**, and body parts away from the midline are called **lateral**.

The **frontal**, or **coronal, plane** divides the body into a front section and a back section. Body parts in front of the plane, or on the front of the body, are called **ventral**, or **anterior**. Body parts on the back of the body are called **dorsal**, or **posterior**.

Two other directional terms are **proximal** and **distal**. These are used to describe the location of

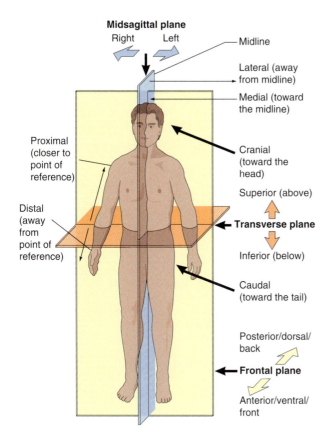

Midsagittal plane
Right   Left
— Midline

Lateral (away from midline)

Medial (toward the midline)

Cranial (toward the head)

Proximal (closer to point of reference)

Superior (above)

Distal (away from point of reference)

►Transverse plane

Inferior (below)

Caudal (toward the tail)

Posterior/dorsal/back

►Frontal plane

Anterior/ventral/front

FIGURE 6-5 Body planes and directional terms.

the extremities (arms and legs) in relation to the main trunk of the body, generally called the *point of reference*. Body parts close to the point of reference are called proximal, and body parts distant from the point of reference are called distal. For example, in describing the relationship of the wrist and elbow to the shoulder (or point of reference), the wrist is distal and the elbow is proximal to the shoulder.

BODY CAVITIES

Body cavities are spaces within the body that contain vital organs. There are two main body cavities; the dorsal, or posterior, cavity and the ventral, or anterior, cavity (see figure 6-6).

The **dorsal cavity** is one long, continuous cavity located on the back of the body. It is

divided into two sections: the **cranial cavity**, which contains the brain, and the **spinal cavity**, which contains the spinal cord.

The **ventral cavities** are larger than the dorsal cavities. The ventral cavity is separated into two distinct cavities by the dome-shaped muscle called the *diaphragm*, which is important for respiration (breathing). The **thoracic cavity** is located in the chest and contains the esophagus, trachea, bronchi, lungs, heart, and large blood vessels. The **abdominal cavity**, or abdomino-pelvic cavity, is divided into an upper part and a lower part. The upper abdominal cavity contains the stomach, small intestine, most of the large intestine, appendix, liver, gallbladder, pancreas, and spleen. The lower abdominal cavity, or **pelvic cavity**, contains the urinary bladder, the reproductive organs, and the last part of the large intestine.

Three small cavities are the **orbital cavity** (for the eyes), the **nasal cavity** (for the nose structures), and the **buccal cavity**, or mouth (for the teeth and tongue).

ABDOMINAL REGIONS

The abdominal cavity is so large that it is divided into regions or sections. One method of division is into quadrants, or four sections. As shown in figure 6-7, this results in a right upper quadrant (RUQ), left upper quadrant (LUQ), right lower quadrant (RLQ), and left lower quadrant (LLQ). Another method of division is into nine **abdominal regions** (see figure 6-8). The center regions are the epigastric (above the stomach), umbilical (near the umbilicus, or belly button), and hypogastric, or pelvic (below the stomach). On either side of the center the regions are the hypochondriac (below the ribs), lumbar (near the large bones of the spinal cord), and iliac, or inguinal (near the groin).

The terms relating to body planes, directions, and cavities are used frequently in the study of human anatomy.

STUDENT: *Go to the workbook and complete the assignment sheet for 6:2, Body Planes, Directions, and Cavities.*

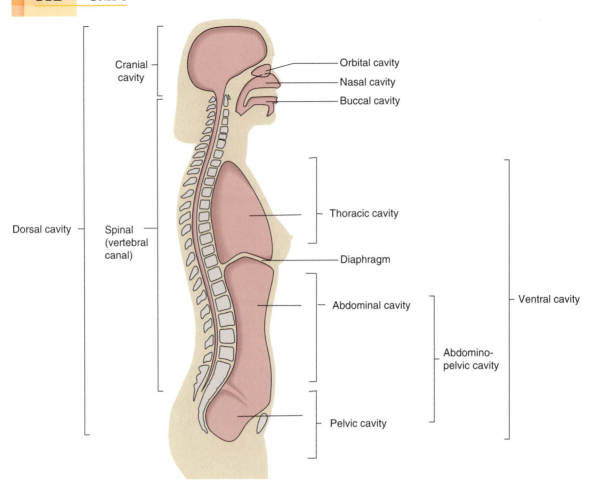

Cranial cavity

Orbital cavity

Nasal cavity

Buccal cavity

Thoracic cavity

Diaphragm

Dorsal cavity

Spinal (vertebral canal)

Abdominal cavity

Ventral cavity

Abdomino-pelvic cavity

Pelvic cavity

FIGURE 6-6 Body cavities.

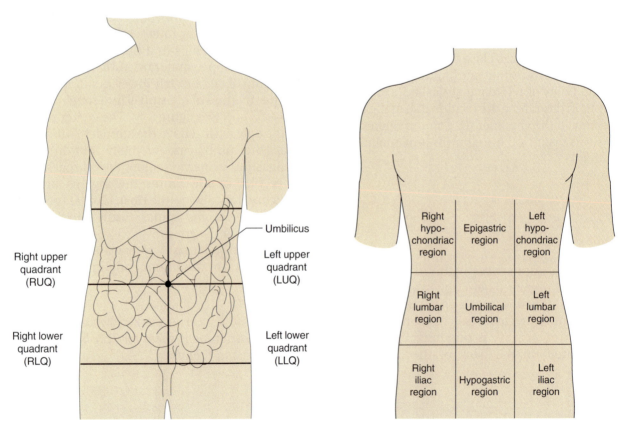

Umbilicus

Right upper quadrant (RUQ)

Left upper quadrant (LUQ)

Right lower quadrant (RLQ)

Left lower quadrant (LLQ)

Right hypo-chondriac region	Epigastric region	Left hypo-chondriac region
Right lumbar region	Umbilical region	Left lumbar region
Right iliac region	Hypogastric region	Left iliac region

FIGURE 6-7 Abdominal quadrants.

FIGURE 6-8 Nine abdominal regions.

6:3 Integumentary System

Objectives

After completing this section, you should be able to:

◆ Label a diagram of a cross section of the skin

◆ Differentiate between the two types of skin glands

◆ List six functions of the skin

◆ Provide the correct names for three abnormal colors of the skin and identify the cause of each abnormal color

◆ Describe at least four skin eruptions

◆ Describe at least four diseases of the integumentary system

◆ Define, pronounce, and spell all the key terms

KEY TERMS

albino

alopecia

constrict
(kun-strict′)

crusts

cyanosis
(sy″-eh-noh′-sis)

dermis

dilate
(die′-late)

epidermis
(eh-pih-der′-mis)

erythema
(err-ih-thee′-ma)

integumentary system
(in-teg-u-men′-tah-ree)

jaundice
(jawn′-diss)

macules
(mack′-youlz)

papules
(pap′-youlz)

pustules
(pus′-tyoulz)

sebaceous glands
(seh-bay′-shus)

subcutaneous fascia
(hypodermis)
(sub-q-tay′-nee-us fash′-ee-ah)

sudoriferous glands
(sue-de-rif′-eh-rus)

ulcer

vesicles
(ves′-i-kulz)

wheals

RELATED HEALTH CAREERS

◆ Allergist   ◆ Dermatologist   ◆ Plastic Surgeon

6:3 INFORMATION

The **integumentary system**, or skin, has been called both a membrane, because it covers the body, and an organ, because it contains several kinds of tissues. Most anatomy courses, however, refer to it as a system because it has organs and other parts that work together to perform a particular function.

Three main layers of tissue make up the skin (see figure 6-9):

◆ **Epidermis**—the outermost layer of skin. This layer is actually made of five smaller layers but

no blood vessels or nerve cells. Two main layers are the *stratum corneum*, the outermost layer, and the *stratum germinativum*, the innermost layer. The cells of the stratum corneum are constantly shed and replaced by new cells from the stratum germinativum.

◆ **Dermis**—also called *corium*, or "true skin." This layer has a framework of elastic connective tissue and contains blood vessels; lymph vessels; nerves; involuntary muscle; sweat and oil glands; and hair follicles. The top of the dermis is covered with papillae, which fit into ridges on the stratum germinativum of the epidermis. These ridges form lines, or striations, on the skin. Because the pattern of

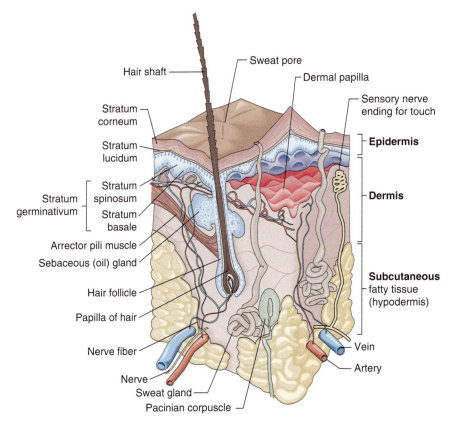

Hair shaft

Sweat pore

Dermal papilla

Sensory nerve ending for touch

Stratum corneum

Stratum lucidum

Stratum germinativum

Stratum spinosum

Stratum basale

Arrector pili muscle

Sebaceous (oil) gland

Hair follicle

Papilla of hair

Nerve fiber

Nerve

Sweat gland

Pacinian corpuscle

Epidermis

Dermis

Subcutaneous fatty tissue (hypodermis)

Vein

Artery

FIGURE 6-9 Cross-section of skin.

ridges is unique to each individual, fingerprints and footprints are often used as methods of identification.

◆ **Subcutaneous fascia** or **hypodermis**—the innermost layer. It is made of elastic and fibrous connective tissue and adipose (fatty) tissue, and connects the skin to underlying muscles.

The integumentary system has two main types of glands: sudoriferous and sebaceous. The **sudoriferous glands** (sweat glands) are coiled tubes that extend through the dermis and open on the surface of the skin at pores. The sweat, or perspiration, eliminated by these glands contains water, salts, and some body wastes. The **sebaceous glands** are oil glands that usually open onto hair follicles. They produce sebum, an oil that keeps the skin and hair from becoming dry and brittle. Because sebum is an antibacterial and antifungal secretion, it also helps prevent infections. When an oil gland becomes plugged, the accumulation of dirt and oil results in a blackhead or pimple.

Two other parts of the integumentary system are the hair and nails. Each hair consists of a root (which grows in a hollow tube, called a *follicle*) and a hair shaft. Hair helps protect the body and covers all body surfaces except for the palms of the hands

and the soles of the foot. Due to genetics, males (and some females) may experience **alopecia** or baldness, a permanent loss of hair on the scalp. Nails protect the fingers and toes from injury. They are made of dead, keratinized epidermal epithelial cells packed closely together to form a thick, dense surface. They are formed in the nail bed. If lost, nails will regrow if the nail bed is not damaged.

FUNCTIONS

The integumentary system performs the following important functions:

◆ *Protection*—It serves as a barrier to the sun's ultraviolet rays and the invasion of pathogens, or germs. It also holds moisture in and prevents deeper tissues from drying out.

◆ *Sensory perception*—The nerves in the skin help the body respond to pain, pressure, temperature (heat and cold), and touch sensations, figure 6-10.

◆ *Body temperature regulation*—The blood vessels in the skin help the body retain or lose heat. When the blood vessels **dilate** (get

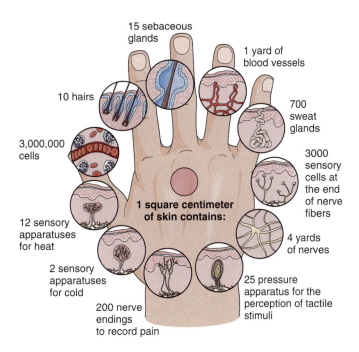

10 hairs

15 sebaceous glands

1 yard of blood vessels

700 sweat glands

3,000,000 cells

3000 sensory cells at the end of nerve fibers

1 square centimeter of skin contains:

12 sensory apparatuses for heat

4 yards of nerves

2 sensory apparatuses for cold

25 pressure apparatus for the perception of tactile stimuli

200 nerve endings to record pain

FIGURE 6-10 The nerves in the skin allow the body to respond to many different sensations.

larger), excess heat from the blood can escape through the skin. When the blood vessels **constrict** (get smaller), the heat is retained in the body. The sudoriferous glands also help cool the body through evaporation of perspiration.

◆ *Storage*—The skin has tissues for temporary storage of fat, glucose (sugar), water, vitamins, and salts. Adipose (fatty) tissue in the subcutaneous fascia is a source of energy.

◆ *Absorption*—Certain substances can be absorbed through the skin, such as motion sickness or heart disease medications and nicotine patches to help stop smoking. The medications are placed on sticky patches and applied to the skin. This is called a transdermal medication.

◆ *Excretion*—The skin helps the body eliminate salt, a minute amount of waste, and excess water and heat through perspiration.

◆ *Production*—The skin helps in the production of vitamin D by using ultraviolet rays from the sun to form an initial molecule of vitamin D that matures in the liver.

PIGMENTATION

Basic skin color is inherited and is determined by pigments in the epidermis of the skin. Melanin, a brownish-black pigment, can lead to a black, brown, or yellow skin tint, depending on racial origin. Melanin can also absorb ultraviolet light to tan the skin. Small concentrated areas of melanin pigment form freckles. Carotene, a yellowish-red pigment, also helps determine skin color. A person with an absence of color pigments is an **albino**. An albino's skin has a pinkish tint and the hair is pale yellow or white. The person's eyes also lack pigment and are red in color and very sensitive to light.

Abnormal colors of the skin can indicate disease. **Erythema** is a reddish color of the skin that can be caused by either burns or a congestion of blood in the vessels. **Jaundice**, a yellow discoloration of the skin, can indicate bile in the blood as a result of liver or gallbladder disease. Jaundice also occurs in conjunction with certain diseases that involve the destruction of red blood cells. **Cyanosis** is a bluish discoloration of the skin caused by insufficient oxygen. It can be associated with heart, lung, and circulatory diseases or disorders. Chronic poisoning may cause a gray or brown skin discoloration.

SKIN ERUPTIONS

Skin eruptions can also indicate disease. The most common eruptions include:

◆ **Macules**: (macular rash) flat spots on the skin, such as freckles.

◆ **Papules**: (papular rash) firm, raised areas such as pimples and the eruptions seen in some stages of chickenpox and syphilis.

◆ **Vesicles**: blisters, or fluid-filled sacs, such as those seen in chickenpox.

◆ **Pustules**: pus-filled sacs such as those seen in acne, or pimples.

◆ **Crusts**: areas of dried pus and blood, commonly called "scabs."

◆ **Wheals**: itchy, elevated areas with an irregular shape; hives and insect bites are examples.

◆ **Ulcer**: a deep loss of skin surface that may extend into the dermis; may cause periodic bleeding and the formation of scars.

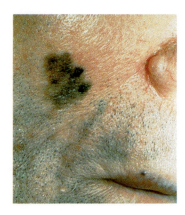

FIGURE 6-11 Melanoma is the most dangerous form of skin cancer. *(Courtesy of Robert A. Silverman, MD, Pediatric Dermatology, Georgetown University)*

DISEASES AND ABNORMAL CONDITIONS

Acne vulgaris is an inflammation of the sebaceous glands. Although the cause is unknown, acne usually occurs at adolescence. Hormonal changes and increased secretion of sebum are probably underlying causes. Symptoms include papules, pustules, and blackheads. These occur when the hair follicles become blocked with dirt, cosmetics, excess oil, and/or bacteria. Treatment methods include frequent, thorough skin washing; avoiding creams and heavy makeup; antibiotic or vitamin A ointments; oral antibiotics; and/or ultraviolet light treatments.

Athlete's foot is a contagious fungal infection that usually affects the feet. The skin itches, blisters, and cracks into open sores. Treatment involves applying an antifungal medication and keeping the area clean and dry.

Cancer of the skin occurs in different forms such as basal cell carcinoma, squamous cell carcinoma, and malignant melanoma, figure 6-11. Frequently, skin cancer develops from a mole or nevus that changes in color, shape, size, or texture. Bleeding or itching of a mole can also indicate cancer. Exposure to the sun, prolonged use of tanning beds, irritating chemicals, or radiation are the usual causes of skin cancer. Treatment involves surgical removal of the cancer and/or radiation.

Dermatitis, an inflammation of the skin, can be caused by any substance that irritates the skin. It is frequently an allergic reaction to detergents, cosmetics, pollen, or certain foods. One

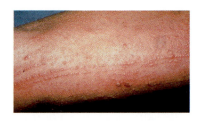

FIGURE 6-12 A contact dermatitis caused by contact with poison oak. *(Courtesy of the Centers for Disease Control and Prevention)*

example of contact dermatitis is the irritation caused by contact with poison ivy, poison sumac, or poison oak (see figure 6-12). Symptoms include dry skin, erythema, itching, edema, macular-papular rashes, and scaling. Treatment is directed at eliminating the cause, especially in the case of allergens. Anti-inflammatory ointments, antihistamines, and/or steroids are also used in treatment.

Eczema is a noncontagious, inflammatory skin disorder caused by an allergen or irritant. Diet, cosmetics, soaps, medications, and emotional stress can all cause eczema. Symptoms include dryness, erythema, edema, itching, vesicles, crusts, and scaling. Treatment involves removing the irritant and applying corticosteroids to reduce the inflammatory response.

Impetigo is a highly contagious skin infection usually caused by streptococci or staphylococci organisms. Symptoms include erythema, oozing vesicles, pustules, and the formation of a yellow crust. Lesions should be washed with soap and water and kept dry. Antibiotics, both topical and oral, are also used in treatment.

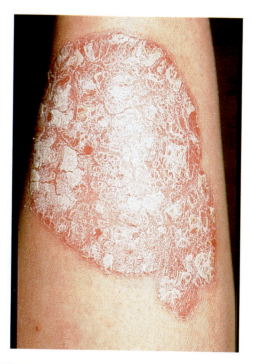

FIGURE 6-13 Psoriasis is characterized by white or silver scales. *(Courtesy of Robert A. Silverman, MD, Pediatric Dermatology, Georgetown University)*

Psoriasis is a chronic, noncontagious, inherited skin disease (see figure 6-13). Symptoms include thick, red areas covered with white or silver scales. Although there is no cure, treatment methods include coal/tar or cortisone ointments; ultraviolet light; and/or scale removal.

Ringworm is a highly contagious fungus infection of the skin or scalp. The characteristic symptom is the formation of a flat or raised circular area with a clear central area surrounded by an itchy, scaly, or crusty outer ring. Antifungal medications, both oral and topical, are used in treatment.

Verrucae, or warts, are caused by a viral infection of the skin. A rough, hard, elevated, rounded surface forms on the skin. Some warts disappear spontaneously, but others must be removed with electricity, liquid nitrogen, acid, chemicals, or laser.

STUDENT: *Go to the workbook and complete the assignment sheet for 6:3, Integumentary System.*

6:4 Skeletal System

Objectives

After completing this section, you should be able to:

◆ List five functions of bones

◆ Label the parts of a bone on a diagram of a long bone

◆ Name the two divisions of the skeletal system and the main groups of bones in each division

◆ Identify the main bones of the skeleton

◆ Compare the three classifications of joints by describing the type of motion allowed by each

◆ Give one example of each joint classification

◆ Describe at least four diseases of the skeletal system

◆ Define, pronounce, and spell all the key terms

KEY TERMS

appendicular skeleton
   (ap-pen-dick′-u-lar)
axial skeleton
carpals
clavicles
   (klav′-ih-kulz)
cranium
diaphysis
   (dy-af′-eh-sis)

endosteum
   (en-dos′-tee-um)
epiphysis
   (ih-pif′-eh-sis)
femur
   (fee′-mur)
fibula
   (fib′-you-la)
fontanels

foramina
   (for-ahm′-e-nah)
humerus
   (hue′-mer-us)
joints
ligaments
medullary canal
   (med′-hue-lair-ee)

(continued)

(Key Terms Continued)

metacarpals
(*met-ah-car'-pulz*)

metatarsals
(*met-ah-tar'-sulz*)

os coxae
(*ahs cock'-see*)

patella
(*pa-tell'-ah*)

periosteum
(*per-ee-os'-tee-um*)

phalanges
(*fa-lan'-jeez*)

radius

red marrow

ribs

scapula

sinuses
(*sigh'-nuss-ez*)

skeletal system

sternum

sutures

tarsals

tibia

ulna

vertebrae
(*vur'-teh-bray*)

yellow marrow

RELATED HEALTH CAREERS

- ◆ Athletic Trainer
- ◆ Chiropractor
- ◆ Orthopedist
- ◆ Osteopathic physician
- ◆ Physiatrist
- ◆ Physical Therapist
- ◆ Podiatrist
- ◆ Prosthetist
- ◆ Radiologic Technologist
- ◆ Sports Medicine

6:4 INFORMATION

The **skeletal system** is made of organs called *bones.* An adult human has 206 bones. These bones work as a system to perform the following functions:

- ◆ *Framework*—The bones form a framework to support the body's muscles, fat, and skin.

- ◆ *Protection*—Bones surround vital organs to protect them. Examples include the skull, which surrounds the brain, and the ribs, which protect the heart and lungs.

- ◆ *Levers*—Muscles attach to bones to help provide movement.

- ◆ *Production of blood cells*—Bones help produce red and white blood cells and platelets, a process called *hemopoiesis* or *hematopoiesis.*

- ◆ *Storage*—Bones store most of the calcium supply of the body.

Bones vary in shape and size depending on their locations within the body. Bones of the extremities (arms and legs) are called *long bones.* The basic parts of these bones are shown in figure 6-14. The long shaft is called the **diaphysis**, and the two extremities, or ends, are each called an **epiphysis**. The **medullary canal** is a cavity in the diaphysis. It is filled with **yellow marrow**, which is mainly fat cells. The **endosteum** is a membrane that lines the medullary canal and keeps the yellow marrow intact. It also produces some bone growth. **Red marrow** is found in certain bones such as the vertebrae, ribs, sternum, and cranium, and in the proximal ends of the humerus and femur. It produces red blood cells (erythrocytes), platelets (thrombocytes), and some white blood cells (leukocytes). Because bone marrow is important in the manufacture of blood cells and is involved with the body's immune response, the red marrow is used to diagnose blood diseases and is sometimes transplanted in people with defective immune systems. The outside of bone is covered with a tough membrane, called the **periosteum**, which contains blood vessels, lymph vessels, and *osteoblasts,* special cells that form new bone tissue. The periosteum is necessary for bone growth, repair, and nutrition. A thin layer of articular cartilage covers the epiphysis and acts as a shock absorber when two bones meet to form a joint.

The skeletal system is divided into two sections: the axial skeleton and the appendicular skeleton. The **axial skeleton** forms the main trunk of the body and is composed of the skull,

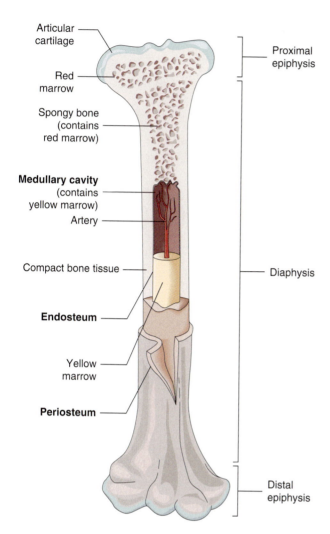

Articular cartilage

Red marrow

Spongy bone (contains red marrow)

Medullary cavity (contains yellow marrow)

Artery

Compact bone tissue

Endosteum

Yellow marrow

Periosteum

Proximal epiphysis

Diaphysis

Distal epiphysis

FIGURE 6-14 Anatomical parts of a long bone.

spinal column, ribs, and breastbone. The **appendicular skeleton** forms the extremities and is composed of the shoulder girdle, arm bones, pelvic girdle, and leg bones.

The skull is composed of the cranial and facial bones (see figure 6-15). The **cranium** is the spherical structure that surrounds and protects the brain. It is made of eight bones: one frontal, two parietal, two temporal, one occipital, one ethmoid, and one sphenoid. At birth, the cranium is not solid bone. Spaces called **fontanels**, or "soft spots," allow for the enlargement of the skull as brain growth occurs. The fontanels are made of membrane and cartilage and turn into solid bone by approximately 18 months of age. There are 14 facial bones: one mandible (lower jaw), two maxilla (upper jaw), two zygomatic (cheek), two lacrimal (inner aspect of eyes), five nasal, and two palatine (hard palate or roof of the mouth). **Sutures** are areas where the cranial bones have joined together. **Sinuses** are air spaces in the bones of the skull that act as resonating chambers for the voice. They are lined with mucous membranes. **Foramina** are openings in bones that allow nerves and blood vessels to enter or leave the bone.

The spinal column is made of 26 bones called **vertebrae** (see figure 6-16). These bones protect the spinal cord and provide support for the head and trunk. They include seven cervical (neck), twelve thoracic (chest), five lumbar

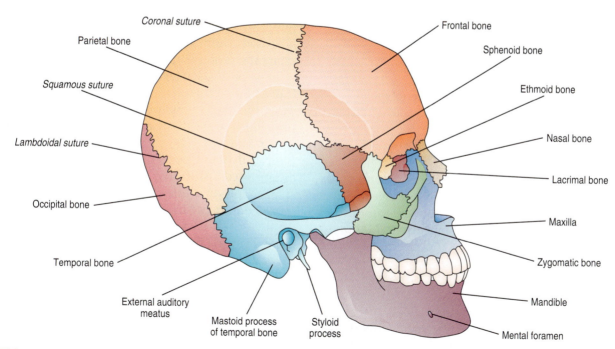

Coronal suture

Parietal bone

Squamous suture

Lambdoidal suture

Occipital bone

Temporal bone

External auditory meatus

Mastoid process of temporal bone

Styloid process

Frontal bone

Sphenoid bone

Ethmoid bone

Nasal bone

Lacrimal bone

Maxilla

Zygomatic bone

Mandible

Mental foramen

FIGURE 6-15 Bones of the skull.

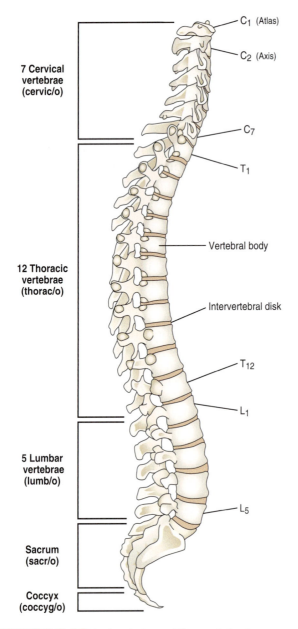

FIGURE 6-16 Lateral view of the vertebral, or spinal, column.

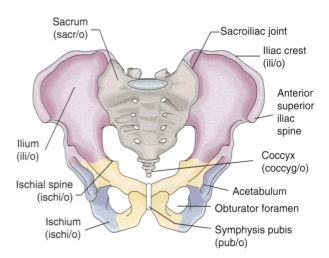

FIGURE 6-17 Anterior view of the pelvic girdle.

(waist), one sacrum (back of pelvic girdle), and one coccyx (tailbone). Pads of cartilage tissue, called *intervertebral disks,* separate the vertebrae. The disks act as shock absorbers and permit bending and twisting movements of the vertebral column.

There are 12 pairs of **ribs**, or costae. They attach to the thoracic vertebrae on the dorsal surface of the body. The first seven pairs are called *true ribs* because they attach directly to the sternum, or breastbone, on the front of the body. The next five pairs are called *false ribs.* The first three pairs of false ribs attach to the cartilage of the rib above. The last two pairs of false ribs are called *floating ribs* because they have no attachment on the front of the body.

The **sternum** or breastbone is the last bone of the axial skeleton. It consists of three parts: the manubrium (upper region), the gladiolus (body), and the xiphoid process (a small piece of cartilage at the bottom). The two collarbones, or clavicles, are attached to the manubrium by ligaments. The ribs are attached to the sternum with costal cartilages to form a "cage" that protects the heart and lungs.

The shoulder, or pectoral, girdle is made of two **clavicles** (collarbones) and two **scapulas** (shoulder bones). The scapulas provide for attachment of the upper arm bones.

Bones of each arm include one **humerus** (upper arm), one **radius** (lower arm on thumb side), one **ulna** (larger bone of lower arm with a projection called the *olecranon process* at its upper end, forming the elbow), eight **carpals** (wrist), five **metacarpals** (palm of the hand), and fourteen **phalanges** (fingers).

The pelvic girdle is made of two **os coxae** (coxal, or hip, bones), which join with the sacrum on the dorsal part of the body (see figure 6-17). On the ventral part of the body, the os coxae join together at a joint called the *symphysis pubis.* Each os coxae is made of three fused sections: the ilium, the ischium, and the pubis. The pelvic girdle contains two recessed areas, or sockets. These sockets, called *acetabula,* provide for the attachment of the leg bones. An opening between the ischium and pubis, called the *obturator foramen,*

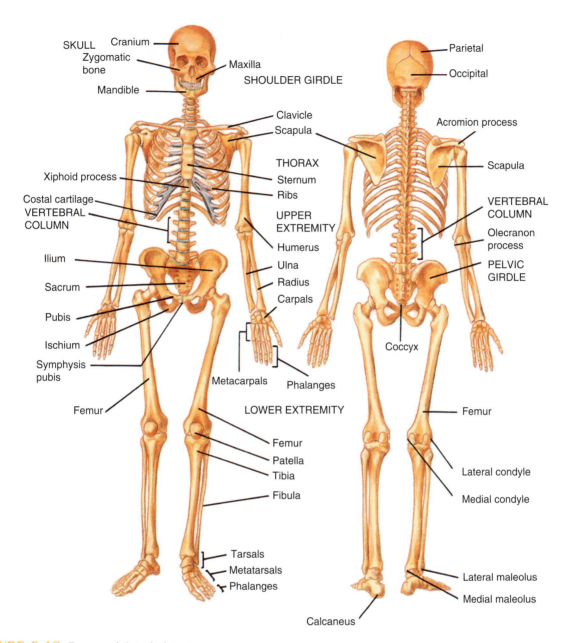

FIGURE 6-18 Bones of the skeleton.

allows for the passage of nerves and blood vessels to and from the legs.

Each leg consists of one **femur** (thigh); one **patella** (kneecap); one **tibia** and one **fibula** (lower leg); seven **tarsals** (ankle); five **metatarsals** (instep of foot); and fourteen **phalanges** (toes). The heel is formed by the large tarsal bone called the *calcaneous*. The bones of the skeleton are shown in figure 6-18.

Joints are areas where two or more bones join together. Connective tissue bands, called **ligaments**, help hold long bones to-

gether at joints. There are three main types of joints:

◆ *Diarthrosis:* freely movable; examples include the ball-and-socket joints of the shoulder and hip, or the hinge joints of the elbow and knee

◆ *Amphiarthrosis:* slightly movable; an example is the attachment of the ribs to the thoracic vertebrae

◆ *Synarthrosis:* immovable; an example is the cranium

DISEASES AND ABNORMAL CONDITIONS

Arthritis is actually a group of diseases involving inflammation of the joints. Two main types are osteoarthritis and rheumatoid arthritis. Osteoarthritis, the most common form, is a chronic disease that usually occurs as a result of aging. It frequently affects the hips and knees. Symptoms include joint pain, stiffness, aching, and limited range of motion. Although there is no cure, rest, applications of heat and cold, aspirin and anti-inflammatory medications, injection of steroids into the joints, and special exercises are used to relieve the symptoms. Rheumatoid arthritis is a chronic, inflammatory disease affecting the connective tissues and joints. It is three times more common in women than in men and onset often occurs between the ages of 35 and 45. Progressive attacks can cause scar tissue formation and atrophy of bone and muscle tissue, which result in permanent deformity and immobility. Early treatment is important to reduce pain and limit damage to joints. Rest, prescribed exercise, anti-inflammatory medications such as aspirin, and careful use of steroids are the main forms of treatment. Surgery, or arthroplasty, to replace damaged joints, such as those in the hips and knees, is sometimes performed when severe joint damage has occurred.

Bursitis is an inflammation of the bursae, small, fluid-filled sacs surrounding the joints. It frequently affects the shoulders, elbows, hips, or knees. Symptoms include severe pain, limited movement, and fluid accumulation in the joint. Treatment consists of administering pain medications; injecting steroids and anesthetics into the affected joint; rest; aspirating (withdrawing fluid with a needle) the joint; and physical therapy to preserve joint motion.

A *fracture* is a crack or break in a bone. Types of fractures, shown in figure 6-19, include:

- *Greenstick:* bone is bent and splits, causing a crack or incomplete break; common in children

- *Simple* or *closed:* complete break of the bone with no damage to the skin

- *Compound* or *open:* bone breaks and ruptures through the skin; creates an increased chance of infection

- *Impacted:* broken bone ends jam into each other

- *Comminuted:* bone fragments or splinters into more than two pieces

- *Spiral:* bone twists resulting in one or more breaks; common in skiing and skating accidents

- *Depressed:* a broken piece of skull bone moves inward; common with severe head injuries

- *Colles:* breaking and dislocation of the distal radius that causes a characteristic bulge at the wrist; caused by falling on an outstretched hand

Before a fracture can heal, the bone must be put back into its proper alignment. This process is called *reduction. Closed reduction* involves positioning the bone in correct alignment, usually with traction, and applying a cast or splint to maintain the position until the fracture heals. *Open reduction* involves surgical repair of the bone. In some cases, special pins, plates, or other devices are surgically implanted to maintain correct position of the bone.

A *dislocation* is when a bone is forcibly displaced from a joint. It frequently occurs in shoulders, fingers, knees, and hips. After the dislocation is reduced (the bone is replaced in the joint), the dislocation is immobilized with a splint, a cast, or traction.

A *sprain* is when a twisting action tears the ligaments at a joint. The wrists and ankles are common sites for sprains. Symptoms include pain, swelling, discoloration, and limited movement. Treatment methods include rest; elevation; immobilization with an elastic bandage or splint; and/or cold applications.

Osteomyelitis is a bone inflammation usually caused by a pathogenic organism. The infectious organisms cause the formation of an abscess within the bone and an accumulation of pus in the medullary canal. Symptoms include pain at the site, swelling, chills, and fever. Antibiotics are used to treat the infection.

Osteoporosis, or increased porosity or softening of the bones, is a metabolic disorder caused by a hormone deficiency (especially estrogen in females), prolonged lack of calcium in the diet, and a sedentary lifestyle. The loss of calcium and phosphate from the bones causes the bones to become porous, brittle, and prone to fracture. Bone density tests lead to early detection and preventative treatment for osteoporosis. Treatment methods include increased intake of calcium and vitamin D; medications to increase bone mass; exercise; and/or estrogen replacement.

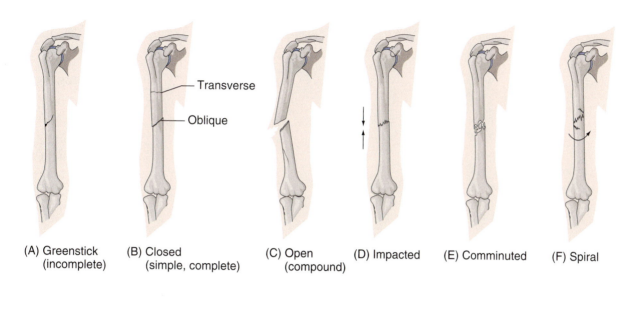

(A) Greenstick
(incomplete)

(B) Closed
(simple, complete)

(C) Open
(compound)

(D) Impacted

(E) Comminuted

(F) Spiral

Transverse

Oblique

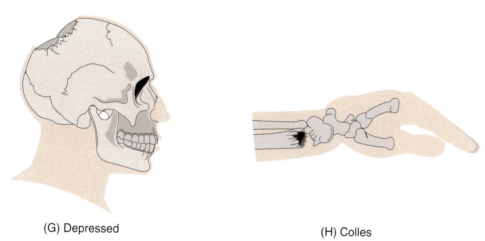

(G) Depressed

(H) Colles

FIGURE 6-19 Types of fractures.

A *ruptured disk,* also called a herniated or slipped disk, occurs when an intervertebral disk (pad of cartilage separating the vertebrae) ruptures or protrudes out of place and causes pressure on the spinal nerve. The most common site is at the lumbar–sacral area, but a ruptured disk can occur anywhere on the spinal column. Symptoms include severe pain, muscle spasm, impaired movement, and/or numbness. Pain, anti-inflammatory, and muscle relaxant medications may be used as initial forms of treatment. Other treatments include rest, traction, physical therapy, massage therapy, chiropractic treatment, and/or heat or cold applications. A laminectomy, surgical removal of the protruding disk, may be necessary in severe cases that do not respond to conservative treatment.

Abnormal curvatures of the spinal column include *kyphosis, scoliosis,* and *lordosis* (see figure 6-20). Kyphosis, or "hunchback," is a rounded bowing of the back at the thoracic area. Scoliosis is a side-to-side, or lateral, curvature of the spine. Lordosis, or "swayback," is an abnormal inward curvature of the lumbar region. Poor posture, congenital (at birth) defects, structural defects of the vertebrae, malnutrition, and degeneration of the vertebrae can all be causes of these defects. Therapeutic exercises, firm mattresses, and/or braces are the main forms of treatment. Severe deformities may require surgical repair.

STUDENT: *Go to the workbook and complete the assignment sheet for 6:4, Skeletal System.*

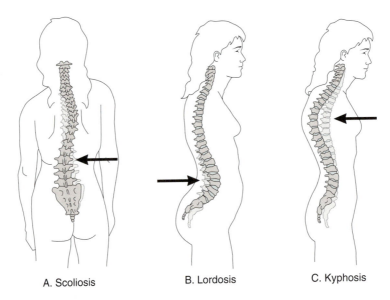

A. Scoliosis   B. Lordosis   C. Kyphosis

FIGURE 6-20 Abnormal curvatures of the spinal column.

6:5   Muscular System

Objectives

After completing this section, you should be able to:

◆ Compare the three main kinds of muscle by describing the action of each

◆ Differentiate between voluntary muscle and involuntary muscle

◆ List at least three functions of muscles

◆ Describe the two main ways muscles attach to bones

◆ Demonstrate the five major movements performed by muscles

◆ Describe at least three diseases of the muscular system

◆ Define, pronounce, and spell all the key terms

KEY TERMS

abduction
   (ab-duck'-shun)
adduction
   (ad-duck'-shun)
cardiac muscle
circumduction
contract
   (con-trackt')
contractibility
contracture
   (con-track'-shur)

elasticity
excitability
extensibility
extension
fascia
   (fash'-ee"-ah)
flexion
   (flek'-shun)
insertion
involuntary

muscle tone
muscular system
origin
rotation
skeletal muscle
tendons
visceral (smooth) muscle
voluntary

RELATED HEALTH CAREERS

- ◆ Athletic Trainer
- ◆ Chiropractor
- ◆ Doctor of Osteopathic Medicine
- ◆ Massage Therapist
- ◆ Myologist
- ◆ Orthopedist
- ◆ Physiatrist
- ◆ Physical Therapist
- ◆ Podiatrist
- ◆ Prosthetist
- ◆ Sports Medicine Physician

6:5 INFORMATION

Over 600 muscles make up the system known as the **muscular system**. Muscles are bundles of muscle fibers held together by connective tissue. All muscles have certain properties or characteristics:

- ◆ **excitability**: irritability, the ability to respond to a stimulus such as a nerve impulse
- ◆ **contractibility**: muscle fibers that are stimulated by nerves **contract**, or become short and thick, which causes movement
- ◆ **extensibility**: the ability to be stretched
- ◆ **elasticity**: allows the muscle to return to its original shape after it has contracted or stretched

There are three main kinds of muscle: cardiac, visceral, and skeletal (see figure 6-21). **Cardiac muscle** forms the walls of the heart and contracts to circulate blood. **Visceral**, or **smooth, muscle** is found in the internal organs of the body such as those of the digestive and respiratory systems, and the blood vessels and eyes. Visceral muscle contracts to cause movement in these organs. Cardiac muscle and visceral muscle are **involuntary**, meaning they function without conscious thought or control. **Skeletal muscle** is attached to bones and causes body movement. Skeletal muscle is **voluntary** because a person has control over its action. Because cardiac muscle and visceral muscle are discussed in sections on other systems, the following concentrates on skeletal muscle.

Skeletal muscles perform four important functions:

- ◆ attach to bones to provide voluntary movement
- ◆ produce heat and energy for the body
- ◆ help maintain posture
- ◆ protect internal organs

Skeletal muscles attach to bones in different ways. Some attach by **tendons**, strong, tough connective-tissue cords. An example is the gastrocnemius muscle on the calf of the leg, which attaches to the heelbone by the Achilles tendon. Other muscles attach by **fascia**, a tough, sheet-like membrane that covers and protects the tissue. Examples include the deep muscles of the trunk and back, which are surrounded by the lumbodorsal fascia. When a muscle attaches to a bone, the end that does not move is called the **origin**. The end that moves when the muscle contracts is called the **insertion**.

A variety of different actions or movements performed by muscles are shown in figure 6-22 and are described as follows:

- ◆ **Adduction**—moving a body part toward the midline
- ◆ **Abduction**—moving a body part away from the midline
- ◆ **Flexion**—decreasing the angle between two bones, or bending a body part
- ◆ **Extension**—increasing the angle between two bones, or straightening a body part
- ◆ **Rotation**—turning a body part around its own axis; for example, turning the head from side to side
- ◆ **Circumduction**—moving in a circle at a joint, or moving one end of a body part in a circle while the other end remains stationary, such as swinging arm in a circle

The major muscles of the body are shown in figure 6-23; the locations and actions of the major muscles are noted in table 6-2.

Muscles are partially contracted at all times, even when not in use. This state of partial contraction is called **muscle tone** and is sometimes described as a state of readiness to act. Loss of

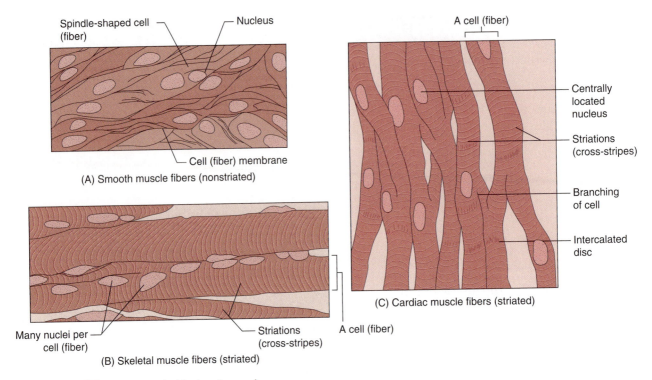

FIGURE 6-21   Three main kinds of muscle.

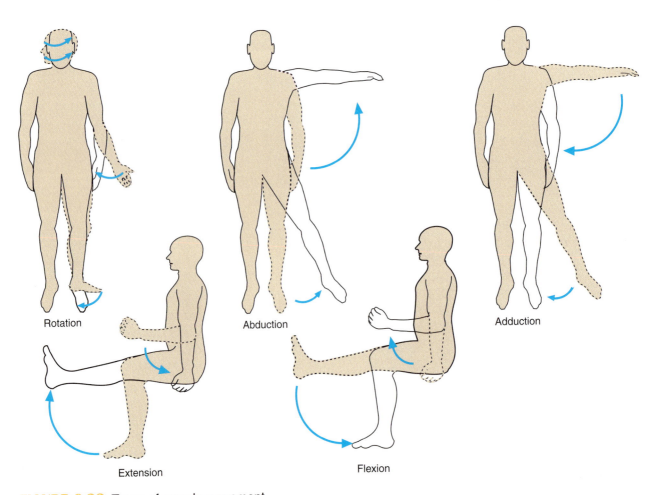

FIGURE 6-22   Types of muscle movement.

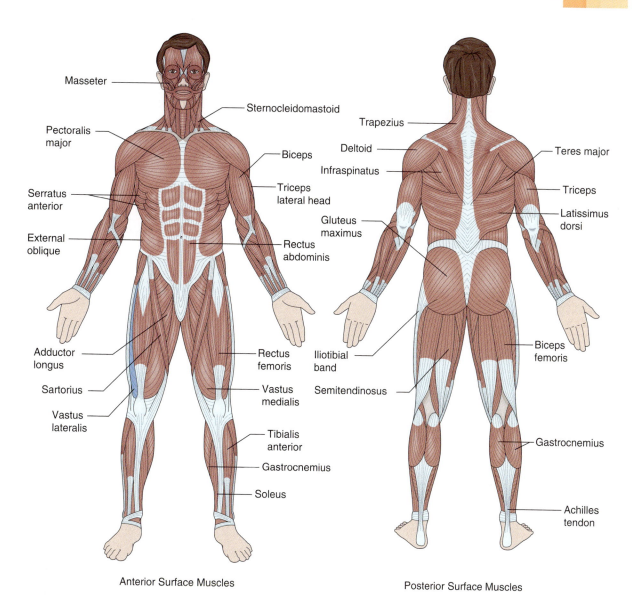

Anterior Surface Muscles   Posterior Surface Muscles

FIGURE 6-23 Major muscles of the body.

muscle tone can occur in severe illness such as paralysis. When muscles are not used for a long period of time, they can *atrophy* (shrink in size and lose strength). Lack of use can also result in a **contracture**, a severe tightening of a flexor muscle resulting in bending of a joint. Foot drop is a common contracture, but the fingers, wrists, knees, and other joints can also be affected.

DISEASES AND ABNORMAL CONDITIONS

Fibromyalgia is chronic, widespread pain in specific muscle sites. Other symptoms include muscle stiffness, numbness or tingling in the arms or legs, fatigue, sleep disturbances, headaches, and depression. The cause is unknown, but stress, weather, and poor physical fitness affect the condition. Treatment is directed toward pain relief and includes physical therapy, massage, exercise, stress reduction, and medication to relax muscles and relieve pain.

Muscular dystrophy is actually a group of inherited diseases that lead to chronic, progressive muscle atrophy. Muscular dystrophy usually appears in early childhood; most types result in total disability and early death. Although there is no cure, physical therapy is used to slow the progress of the disease.

Myasthenia gravis is a chronic condition where nerve impulses are not properly transmitted to the muscles. This leads to progressive muscular weakness and paralysis. If the condition affects the respiratory muscles, it can be fatal. While the cause is unknown, myasthenia gravis is thought to be an

TABLE 6-2 Locations and Functions of Major Muscles of the Body

MUSCLE	LOCATION	FUNCTION
Sternocleidomastoid	Side of neck	Turns and flexes head
Trapezius	Upper back and neck	Extends head, moves shoulder
Deltoid	Shoulder	Abducts arm, injection site
Biceps brachii	Upper arm	Flexes lower arm
Triceps brachii	Upper arm	Extends lower arm
Pectoralis major	Upper chest	Adducts and flexes upper arm
Intercostals	Between ribs	Moves ribs for breathing
Rectus abdominus	Ribs to pubis (pelvis)	Compresses abdomen
Latissimus dorsi	Spine around to chest	Extends and adducts upper arm
Gluteus maximus	Buttocks	Extends thigh, injection site
Sartorius	Front of thigh	Abducts thigh, flexes leg
Quadriceps femoris	Front of thigh	Extends leg
Tibialis anterior	Front of lower leg	Flexes and inverts foot
Gastrocnemius	Back of lower leg	Flexes sole of the foot

autoimmune disease, with antibodies attacking the body's own tissues. There is no cure, and treatment is supportive.

Muscle spasms, or cramps, are sudden, painful, involuntary muscle contractions. They usually occur in the legs or feet and may result from overexertion, low electrolyte levels, or poor circulation. Gentle pressure and stretching of the muscle are used to relieve the spasm.

A *strain* is an overstretching of or injury to a muscle and/or tendon. Frequent sites include the back, arms, and legs. Prolonged or sudden muscle exertion is usually the cause. Symptoms include myalgia (muscle pain), swelling, and limited movement. Treatment methods include rest; muscle relaxants or pain medications; elevating the extremity; and alternating hot and cold applications.

STUDENT: *Go to the workbook and complete the assignment sheet for 6:5, Muscular System.*

6:6 Nervous System

Objectives

After completing this section, you should be able to:

◆ Identify the four main parts of a neuron

◆ Name the two main divisions of the nervous system

◆ Describe the function of each of the five main parts of the brain

◆ Explain three functions of the spinal cord

◆ Name the three meninges

◆ Describe the circulation and function of cerebrospinal fluid

◆ Contrast the actions of the sympathetic and parasympathetic nervous systems

◆ Describe at least five diseases of the nervous system

◆ Define, pronounce, and spell all the key terms

KEY TERMS

autonomic nervous system

brain

central nervous system

cerebellum
(seh″-reh-bell′-um)

cerebrospinal fluid
(seh-ree″-broh-spy′-nal fluid)

cerebrum
(seh-ree′-brum)

diencephalon

hypothalamus

medulla oblongata
(meh-due′-la ob-lawn-got′-ah)

meninges (singular: meninx)
(meh-nin′-jeez)

midbrain

nerves

nervous system

neuron
(nur′-on)

parasympathetic
(par″-ah-sim″-pah-thet′-ik)

peripheral nervous system
(peh-rif′-eh-ral)

pons
(ponz)

spinal cord

sympathetic

thalamus

ventricles

RELATED HEALTH CAREERS

- Acupressurist
- Acupuncturist
- Anesthesiologist
- Chiropractor
- Diagnostic Imager
- Doctor of Osteopathic Medicine
- Electroencephalographic Technologist
- Electroneurodiagnostic Technologist
- Mental Health Technicians
- Neurologist
- Neurosurgeon
- Physical Therapist
- Polysomnographic Technologist
- Psychiatrist
- Psychologist

6:6 INFORMATION

The **nervous system** is a complex, highly organized system that coordinates all the activities of the body. This system enables the body to respond and adapt to changes that occur both inside and outside the body.

The basic structural unit of the nervous system is the **neuron**, or nerve cell (see figure 6-24). It consists of a cell body containing a nucleus; nerve fibers, called *dendrites* (which carry impulses toward the cell body); and a single nerve fiber, called an *axon* (which carries impulses away from the cell body). Many axons have a lipid (fat) covering called a *myelin sheath,* which increases the rate of impulse transmission and insulates and maintains the axon. The axon of one neuron lies close to the dendrites of many other neurons. The spaces between them are known as *synapses.* Impulses coming from one axon "jump" the synapse to get to the dendrite of another neuron, which will carry the impulse in the right direction. Special chemicals, called *neurotransmitters,* located at the end of each axon allow the nerve impulses to pass from one neuron to another. In this way, impulses can follow many different routes.

Nerves are a combination of many nerve fibers located outside the brain and spinal cord. *Afferent,* or sensory, nerves carry messages from all parts of the body to the brain and spinal cord. *Efferent,* or motor, nerves carry messages from the brain and spinal cord to the muscles and glands. *Associative,* or *internuncial,* nerves carry both sensory and motor messages.

There are two main divisions to the nervous system: the central nervous system and the peripheral nervous system. The **central nervous system** consists of the brain and spinal cord. The **peripheral nervous system** consists of the nerves. A separate division of the peripheral nervous system is the **autonomic nervous system**. This system controls involuntary body functions.

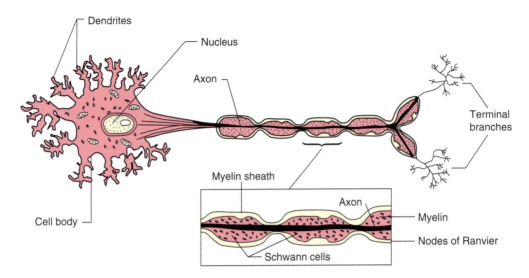

FIGURE 6-24 A neuron, the basic structural unit of the nervous system.

CENTRAL NERVOUS SYSTEM

The **brain** is a mass of nerve tissue well protected by membranes and the cranium, or skull (see figure 6-25). The main sections include:

◆ **Cerebrum**—the largest and highest section of the brain. The outer part is arranged in folds, called *convolutions,* and separated into lobes. The lobes include the frontal, parietal, temporal, and occipital, named from the skull bones that surround them, figure 6-26. The cerebrum is responsible for reasoning, thought, memory, speech, sensation, sight, smell, hearing, and voluntary body movement.

◆ **Cerebellum**—the section below the back of the cerebrum. It is responsible for muscle coordination; balance and posture; and muscle tone.

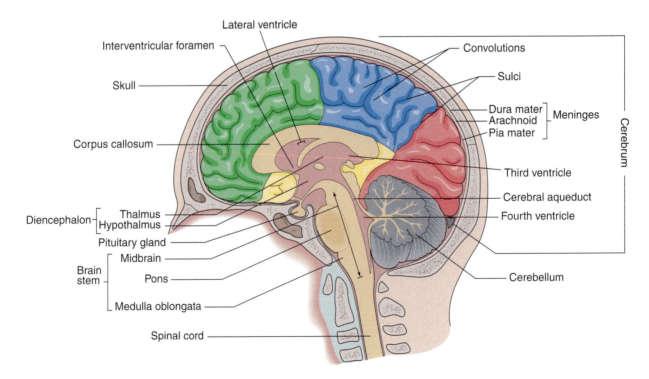

FIGURE 6-25 The brain and spinal cord.

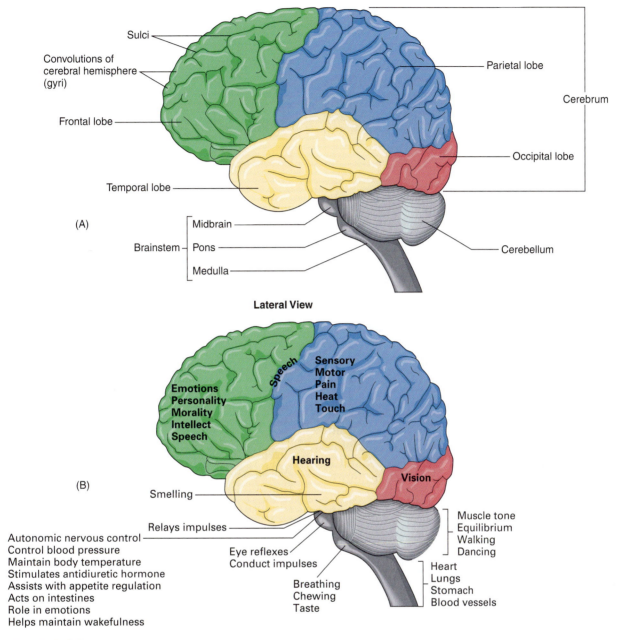

Sulci

Convolutions of
cerebral hemisphere
(gyri)

Frontal lobe

Temporal lobe

Parietal lobe

Cerebrum

Occipital lobe

(A)

Midbrain
Brainstem — Pons
Medulla

Cerebellum

Lateral View

Speech

Emotions
Personality
Morality
Intellect
Speech

Sensory
Motor
Pain
Heat
Touch

Hearing

Vision

(B)

Smelling

Relays impulses

Autonomic nervous control
Control blood pressure
Maintain body temperature
Stimulates antidiuretic hormone
Assists with appetite regulation
Acts on intestines
Role in emotions
Helps maintain wakefulness

Eye reflexes
Conduct impulses

Breathing
Chewing
Taste

Muscle tone
Equilibrium
Walking
Dancing

Heart
Lungs
Stomach
Blood vessels

FIGURE 6-26 Each lobe of the brain is responsible for different functions.

◆ **Diencephalon**—the section located between the cerebrum and midbrain. It contains two structures; the **thalamus** and **hypothalamus**. The thalamus acts as a relay center and directs sensory impulses to the cerebrum. The hypothalamus regulates and controls the autonomic nervous system, temperature, appetite, water balance, sleep, and blood vessel constriction and dilation. The hypothalamus is also involved in emotions such as anger, fear, pleasure, pain, and affection.

◆ **Midbrain**—the section located below the cerebrum at the top of the brain stem. It is responsi-

ble for conducting impulses between brain parts and for certain eye and auditory reflexes.

◆ **Pons**—the section located below the midbrain and in the brain stem. It is responsible for conducting messages to other parts of the brain; for certain reflex actions including chewing, tasting, and saliva production; and for assisting with respiration.

◆ **Medulla oblongata**—the lowest part of the brain stem. It connects with the spinal cord and is responsible for regulating heartbeat, respiration, swallowing, coughing, and blood pressure.

The **spinal cord** continues down from the medulla oblongata and ends at the first or second lumbar vertebrae (see figure 6-27). It is surrounded and protected by the vertebrae. The spinal cord is responsible for many reflex actions and for carrying sensory (afferent) messages up to the brain and motor (efferent) messages from the brain to the nerves that go to the muscles and glands.

The **meninges** are three membranes that cover and protect the brain and spinal cord. The *dura mater* is the thick, tough, outer layer. The middle layer is delicate and weblike and called the *arachnoid membrane*. The innermost layer, the *pia mater,* is closely attached to the brain and spinal cord and contains blood vessels that nourish the nerve tissue.

The brain has four **ventricles**, hollow spaces that connect with each other and with the space under the arachnoid membrane (the subarachnoid space). The ventricles are filled with a fluid called **cerebrospinal fluid**. This fluid circulates continually between the ventricles and through the subarachnoid space. It serves as a shock absorber to protect the brain and spinal cord. It also carries nutrients to some parts of the brain and spinal cord and helps remove metabolic products and wastes. The fluid is produced in the ventricles of the brain by the special structures called *choroid plexuses.* After circulating, it is absorbed into the blood vessels of the dura mater and returned to the bloodstream through special structures called *arachnoid villi.*

PERIPHERAL NERVOUS SYSTEM

The **peripheral nervous system** consists of the somatic and the autonomic nervous systems. The somatic nervous system consists of 12 pairs of cranial nerves and their branches, and 31 pairs of spinal nerves and their branches. Some of the cranial nerves are responsible for special senses such as sight, hearing, taste, and smell. Others receive general sensations such as touch, pressure, pain, and temperature and send out impulses for involuntary and voluntary muscle control. The spinal nerves carry messages to and from the spinal cord and are mixed nerves, both sensory (afferent) and motor (efferent). There are eight cervical, twelve thoracic, five lumbar, five sacral, and one pair of coccygeal spinal nerves. Each nerve goes directly to a particular part of the body or networks with other spinal nerves to form a plexus that supplies sensation to a larger segment of the body.

Autonomic Nervous System

The **autonomic nervous system** is an important part of the peripheral nervous system. It helps maintain a balance in the involuntary functions of the body and allows the body to react in times of emergency. There are two divisions to the autonomic nervous system: the **sympathetic** and **parasympathetic** nervous systems. These two systems usually work together to maintain a balanced state, or *homeostasis,* in the body and to control involuntary body functions at proper rates. In times of emergency, the sympathetic nervous system prepares the body to act by increasing heart rate, respiration, and blood pressure, and slowing activity in the digestive tract. This is known as the *fight or flight response.* After the emergency, the parasympathetic nervous system counteracts the actions of the sympathetic system by slowing heart rate, decreasing respiration, lowering blood pressure, and increasing activity in the digestive tract.

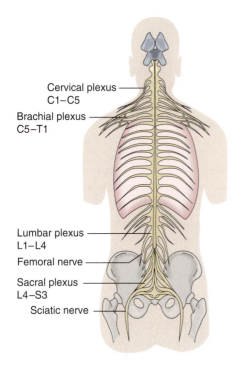

Cervical plexus
C1–C5

Brachial plexus
C5–T1

Lumbar plexus
L1–L4

Femoral nerve

Sacral plexus
L4–S3

Sciatic nerve

FIGURE 6-27 The spinal cord and nerves.

DISEASES AND ABNORMAL CONDITIONS

Cerebral palsy is a disturbance in voluntary muscle action and is caused by brain damage. Lack of oxygen to the brain, birth injuries, prenatal rubella (German measles), and infections can all cause cerebral palsy. Of the three forms—spastic, athetoid, and atactic—spastic is the most common. Symptoms include exaggerated reflexes, tense muscles, contracture development, seizures, speech impairment, spasms, tremors and, in some cases, mental retardation. Although there is no cure, physical, occupational, and speech therapy are important aspects of treatment. Muscle relaxants, anticonvulsive drugs, casts, braces, and/or orthopedic surgery (for severe contractures) are also used.

A *cerebrovascular accident (CVA),* also called a *stroke* or *apoplexy,* occurs when the blood flow to the brain is impaired, resulting in a lack of oxygen and a destruction of brain tissue. It can be caused by cerebral hemorrhage resulting from hypertension, an aneurysm, or a weak blood vessel; or by an occlusion, or blockage, caused by atherosclerosis or a thrombus (blood clot). Symptoms vary depending on the area and amount of brain tissue damaged. Some common symptoms of an acute CVA include loss of consciousness; weakness or paralysis on one side of the body (hemiplegia); dizziness; dysphagia (difficult swallowing); visual disturbances; mental confusion; aphasia (speech and language impairment); and incontinence. When a CVA occurs, immediate care during the first three hours can help prevent brain damage. Treatment with thrombolytic or "clot-busting" drugs such as TPA (tissue plasminogen activator) or angioplasty of the cerebral arteries can dissolve a blood clot and restore blood flow to the brain. Computerized tomography (CT) scans (noninvasive computerized X-rays that show cross-sectional views of body tissue) are used to determine the cause of the CVA. Clot-busting drugs cannot be used if the CVA is caused by a hemorrhage. Neuroprotective agents, or drugs that help prevent injury to neurons, are also used initially to prevent permanent brain damage. Additional treatment depends on symptoms and is directed toward helping the person recover from or adapt to the symptoms that are present. Physical, occupational, and speech therapy are the main forms of treatment.

Encephalitis is an inflammation of the brain and is caused by a virus, bacterium, or chemical agent. The virus is frequently contracted from a mosquito bite, because mosquitos can carry the encephalitis virus. Symptoms vary but may include fever; extreme weakness or lethargy; visual disturbances; headaches; vomiting; stiff neck and back; disorientation; seizures; and coma. Treatment methods are supportive and include antiviral drugs; maintenance of fluid and electrolyte balance; antiseizure medication; and monitoring of respiratory and kidney function.

Epilepsy, or seizure syndrome, is a brain disorder associated with abnormal electrical impulses in the neurons of the brain. Although causes can include brain injury, birth trauma, tumors, toxins such as lead or carbon monoxide, and infections, many cases of epilepsy are idiopathic (spontaneous, or primary). Absence, or petit mal, seizures are milder and characterized by a loss of consciousness lasting several seconds. They are common in children and frequently disappear by late adolescence. Generalized tonic-clonic, or grand mal, are the most severe seizures. They are characterized by a loss of consciousness lasting several minutes; convulsions accompanied by violent shaking and thrashing movements; hypersalivation causing foaming at the mouth; and loss of body functions. Anticonvulsant drugs are very effective in controlling epilepsy.

Hydrocephalus is an excessive accumulation of cerebrospinal fluid in the ventricles and, in some cases, the subarachnoid space of the brain. It is usually caused by a congenital (at birth) defect, infection, or tumor that obstructs the flow of cerebrospinal fluid out of the brain. Symptoms include an abnormally enlarged head, prominent forehead, bulging eyes, irritability, distended scalp veins, and, when pressure prevents proper development of the brain, retardation. The condition is treated by the surgical implantation of a shunt (tube) between the ventricles and the veins, heart, or abdominal peritoneal cavity to provide for drainage of the excess fluid.

Meningitis is an inflammation of the meninges of the brain and/or spinal cord and is caused by a bacterium, virus, fungus, or toxins such as lead and arsenic. Symptoms include high fever, headaches, back and neck pain and stiffness, nausea and vomiting, delirium, convulsions, and, if untreated, coma and death. Treatment methods include antibiotics, anticonvulsants, and/or medications for pain and cerebral edema.

Multiple sclerosis (MS) is a chronic, progressive, disabling condition resulting from a degeneration of the myelin sheath in the central nervous system. It usually occurs between the ages of 20 and 40, figure 6-28. The cause is unknown. The disease progresses at different rates and has periods of remission. Early symptoms include visual disturbances, weakness, fatigue, poor coordination, and tingling and numbness. As the disease progresses, tremors, muscle spasticity, paralysis, speech impairment, emotional swings, and incontinence occur. There is no cure. Treatment methods such as physical therapy, muscle relaxants, steroids, and psychological counseling are used to maintain functional ability as long as possible.

Neuralgia is nerve pain. It is caused by inflammation, pressure, toxins, and other disease. Treatment is directed toward eliminating the cause of the pain.

Paralysis usually results from a brain or spinal cord injury that destroys neurons and results in a loss of function and sensation below the level of injury. *Hemiplegia* is paralysis on one side of the body and is caused by a tumor, injury, or CVA. *Paraplegia* is paralysis in the lower extremities or lower part of the body and is caused by a spinal cord injury. *Quadriplegia* is paralysis of the arms, legs, and body below the spinal cord injury. There is currently no cure, although much research is being directed toward repairing spinal cord damage. Treatment methods are supportive and include physical and occupational therapy.

Parkinson's disease is a chronic, progressive condition involving degeneration of brain cells, usually in persons over 50 years of age. Symptoms include tremors; stiffness; muscular rigidity; a forward leaning position; a shuffling gait; difficulty in stopping while walking; loss of facial expression; drooling; mood swings and frequent depression; and behavioral changes. Although there is no cure, a drug called Levodopa is used to relieve the symptoms. In some cases, surgery can be performed to destroy selectively a small area of the brain and control involuntary movements. Physical therapy is also used to limit muscular rigidity.

Shingles, or herpes zoster, is an acute inflammation of nerve cells and is caused by the herpes virus, which also causes chicken pox. It characteristically occurs in the thoracic area on one side of the body and follows the path of the affected nerves (see figure 6-29). Fluid-filled vesicles appear on the skin, accompanied by severe pain, redness, itching, fever, and abnormal skin sensations. Treatment is directed toward relieving pain and itching until the inflammation subsides, usually in one to four weeks.

STUDENT: *Go to the workbook and complete the assignment sheet for 6:6, Nervous System.*

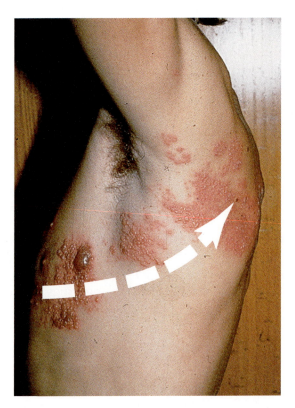

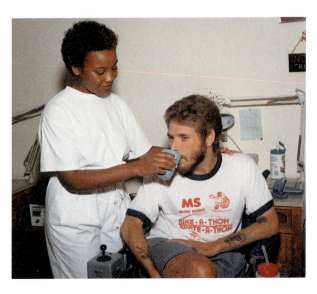

FIGURE 6-28 Multiple sclerosis usually occurs between the ages of 20 and 40.

FIGURE 6-29 The vesicles of shingles follow the path of the affected nerves.

6:7 Special Senses

Objectives

After completing this section, you should be able to:

- Identify five special senses
- Label the major parts on a diagram of the eye
- Trace the pathway of light rays as they pass through the eye
- Label the major parts on a diagram of the ear
- Trace the pathway of sound waves as they pass through the ear

- Explain how the ear helps maintain balance and equilibrium
- State the locations of the four main taste receptors
- List at least four general senses located throughout the body
- Describe at least six diseases of the eye and ear
- Define, pronounce, and spell all the key terms

KEY TERMS

aqueous humor
  (a´-kwee˝-us hue-more)
auditory canal
auricle
  (or´-eh-kul˝)
choroid coat
  (koh´-royd)
cochlea
  (co´-klee-ah)
conjunctiva
  (kon-junk˝-tye´-vah)
cornea

eustachian tube
  (you-stay´-she-en)
iris
lacrimal glands
  (lack´-rih˝-mal)
lens
organ of Corti
ossicles
  (os´-ick-uls)
pinna
  (pin´-nah)
pupil

refracts
retina
  (ret´-in-ah)
sclera
  (sklee´-rah)
semicircular canals
tympanic membrane
  (tim-pan´-ik)
vestibule
  (ves´-tih-bewl)
vitreous humor
  (vit´-ree-us hue´-more)

RELATED HEALTH CAREERS

- Allergist
- Audiologist
- Eye, Ear, Nose, and Throat Specialist
- Ophthalmic Assistant
- Ophthalmic Laboratory Technician

- Ophthalmic Medical Technologist
- Ophthalmic Technician
- Ophthalmologist
- Optician

- Optometrist
- Otolaryngologist
- Otologist

6:7 INFORMATION

Special senses allow the human body to react to the environment by providing for sight, hearing, taste, smell, and balance maintenance. These senses are possible because the body has structures that receive sensations, nerves that carry sensory messages to the brain, and a brain that interprets and responds to sensory messages.

THE EYE

The eye is the organ that controls the special sense of sight. It receives light rays and transmits impulses from the rays to the optic nerve, which carries the impulses to the brain, where they are interpreted as vision, or sight.

The eye (see figure 6-30A) is well protected. It is partially enclosed in a bony socket of the skull. Eyelids and eyelashes help keep out dirt and pathogens. **Lacrimal glands** in the eye produce tears, which constantly moisten and cleanse the eye. The tears flow across the eye and drain through the nasolacrimal duct into the nasal cavity. A mucous membrane, called the **conjunctiva**, lines the eyelids and covers the front of the eye to provide additional protection and lubrication.

There are three main layers to the eye (see figure 6-30B). The outermost layer is the tough connective tissue called the **sclera**. It is frequently referred to as the "white" of the eye. The sclera maintains the shape of the eye. Extrinsic muscles, responsible for moving the eye within the socket, are attached to the outside of the sclera. The **cornea** is a circular, transparent part of the front of the sclera. It allows light rays to enter the eye. The middle layer of the eye, the **choroid coat**, is interlaced with many blood vessels, which nourish the eyes. The innermost layer of the eye is the **retina**. It is made of many layers of nerve cells, which transmit the light impulses to the optic nerve. Two such special cells are *cones* and *rods*. Cones are sensitive to color and are used mainly for vision when it is light. Most of the cones are located in a depression located on the back surface of the retina and called the *fovea centralis;* this is the area of sharpest vision. Rods are used for vision when it is dark or dim.

The **iris** is the colored portion of the eye. It is located behind the cornea on the front of the choroid coat. The opening in the center of the iris is called the **pupil**. The iris contains two muscles, which control the size of the pupil and regulate the amount of light entering the eye.

Other special structures are also located in the eye. The **lens** is a circular structure located behind the pupil and suspended in position by ligaments.

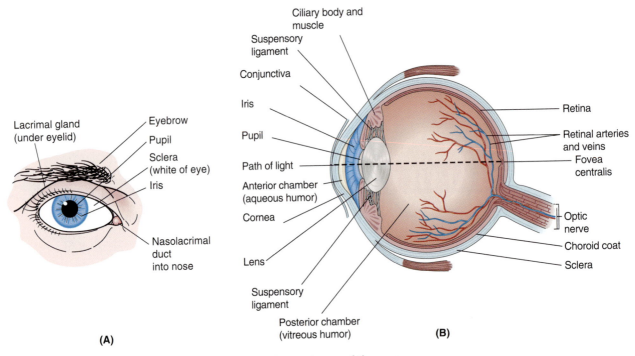

(A)   (B)

FIGURE 6-30 (A) External view of the eye; (B) structures of the eye.

It **refracts** (bends) light rays so the rays focus on the retina. The **aqueous humor** is a clear, watery fluid that fills the space between the cornea and iris. It helps maintain the forward curvature of the eyeball and refracts light rays. The **vitreous humor** is the jellylike substance that fills the area behind the lens. It helps maintain the shape of the eyeball and also refracts light rays. A series of muscles located in the eye provide for eye movement.

When light rays enter the eye, they pass through a series of parts that refract the rays so that the rays focus on the retina. These parts are the cornea, the aqueous humor, the pupil, the lens, and the vitreous humor. In the retina, the light rays (image) are picked up by the rods and cones, changed into nerve impulses, and transmitted by the optic nerve to the occipital lobe of the cerebrum, where sight is interpreted. If the rays are not refracted correctly by the various parts, vision can be distorted or blurred.

Diseases and Abnormal Conditions

Amblyopia, or lazy eye, commonly occurs in early childhood. It results in poor vision in one eye and is caused by the dominance of the other eye. Treatment methods include covering the good eye to stimulate development of the "lazy" eye, exercises to strengthen the weak eye, corrective lenses, and/or surgery. If the condition is not treated before eight to nine years of age, blindness of the affected eye may occur.

Astigmatism, figure 6-31, is an abnormal shape or curvature of the cornea that causes blurred vision. Corrective lenses (glasses or contact lenses) correct the condition.

A *cataract* occurs when the normally clear lens becomes cloudy, or opaque (see figure 6-32). This occurs gradually, usually as a result of aging, but may be the result of trauma. Symptoms include blurred vision, halos around lights, gradual vision loss, and, in later stages, a milky-white pupil. Sight is restored by the surgical removal of the lens. An implanted intraocular lens or prescription glasses or contact lenses correct the vision and compensate for the removed lens.

Conjunctivitis, or pink eye, is a contagious inflammation of the conjunctiva and is usually caused by a bacterium or virus. Symptoms include redness, swelling, pain, and, at times, pus formation in the eye. Antibiotics, frequently in the form of an eye ointment, are used to treat conjunctivitis.

Glaucoma is a condition of increased intraocular (within the eye) pressure caused by an excess amount of aqueous humor. It is common after age 40 and is a leading cause of blindness. A tonometer (instrument that measures intraocular pressure) is usually used during regular eye examinations to check for this condition. Symptoms include loss of peripheral (side) vision, halos around lights, limited night vision, and mild aching. Glaucoma is usually controlled with

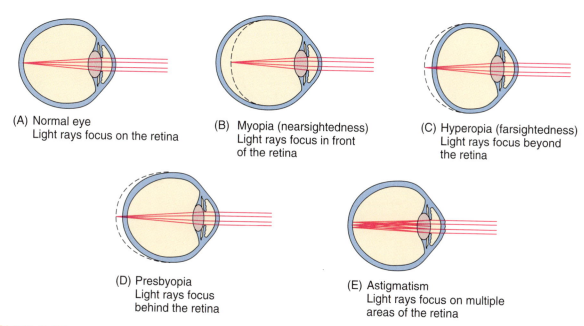

(A) Normal eye
Light rays focus on the retina

(B) Myopia (nearsightedness)
Light rays focus in front
of the retina

(C) Hyperopia (farsightedness)
Light rays focus beyond
the retina

(D) Presbyopia
Light rays focus
behind the retina

(E) Astigmatism
Light rays focus on multiple
areas of the retina

FIGURE 6-31 Improper refraction of light rays causes impaired vision.

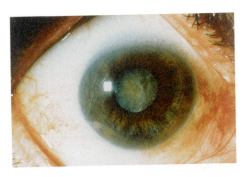

FIGURE 6-32 A cataract occurs when the lens of the eye becomes cloudy or opaque. (*Courtesy of National Eye Institute, NEH*)

medications that decrease the amount of fluid produced or improve the drainage. In severe cases, surgery is performed to create an opening for the flow of the aqueous humor.

Hyperopia is farsightedness. It occurs when the light rays are not refracted sharply enough, and the image focuses behind the retina, figure 6-31. Vision is corrected by the use of convex lenses.

Myopia is nearsightedness. It occurs when the light rays are refracted too sharply, and the image focuses in front of the retina. Vision is corrected by the use of concave lenses. A newer method of treatment is a surgical procedure called radial keratotomy (RK). Small incisions are made in the cornea to flatten it so it can refract light rays correctly. In some cases, a laser is used to flatten the cornea without cutting. RK can correct myopia and eliminate the need for corrective lenses.

Presbyopia is farsightedness caused by a loss of lens elasticity. It results from the normal aging process and is treated by the use of corrective lenses or "reading" glasses.

Strabismus is when the eyes do not move or focus together. The eyes may move inward (cross-eyed) or outward, or up or down. It is caused by muscle weakness in one or both eyes. Treatment methods include eye exercises, covering the good eye, corrective lenses, and/or surgery on the muscles that move the eye.

THE EAR

The ear is the organ that controls the special senses of hearing and balance. It transmits impulses from sound waves to the auditory nerve (vestibulocochlear), which carries the impulses to the brain for interpretation as hearing. The ear is divided into three main sections: the outer ear, the middle ear, and the inner ear (see figure 6-33).

The outer ear contains the visible part of the ear, called the **pinna**, or **auricle**. The pinna is elastic cartilage covered by skin. It leads to a canal, or tube, called the *external auditory meatus*, or **auditory canal**. Special glands in this canal produce *cerumen*, a wax that protects the ear. Sound waves

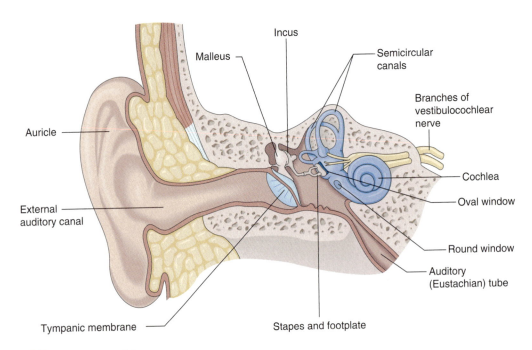

FIGURE 6-33 Structures of the ear.

travel through the auditory canal until they reach the eardrum, or **tympanic membrane**. The tympanic membrane separates the outer ear from the middle ear. It vibrates when sound waves hit it and transmits the sound waves to the middle ear.

The middle ear is a small space, or cavity, in the temporal bone. It contains three small bones **(ossicles)**: the malleus, the incus, and the stapes. The bones are connected and transmit sound waves from the tympanic membrane to the inner ear. The middle ear is connected to the pharynx, or throat, by a tube called the **eustachian tube**. This tube allows air to enter the middle ear and helps equalize air pressure on both sides of the tympanic membrane.

The inner ear is the most complex portion of the ear. It is separated from the middle ear by a membrane called the *oval window*. The first section is the **vestibule**, which acts as the entrance to the two other parts of the inner ear. The **cochlea**, shaped like a snail's shell, contains delicate, hair-like cells, which compose the **organ of Corti**, a receptor of sound waves. The organ of Corti transmits the impulses from sound waves to the auditory nerve. This nerve carries the impulses to the temporal lobe of the cerebrum, where they are interpreted as hearing. **Semicircular canals** are also located in the inner ear. These canals contain a liquid and delicate hair-like cells that bend when the liquid moves with head and body movements. Impulses sent from the semicircular canals to the cerebellum of the brain help to maintain our sense of balance and equilibrium.

Diseases and Abnormal Conditions

Hearing loss is classified as either conductive or sensory. Conductive hearing loss or deafness occurs when sound waves are not conducted to the inner ear. Possible causes include a wax (cerumen) plug, a foreign body obstruction, otosclerosis, an infection, or a ruptured tympanic membrane. Treatment is directed toward eliminating the cause. Surgery and the use of hearing aids are common forms of treatment. Sensory hearing loss or deafness occurs when there is damage to the inner ear or auditory nerve. This type of hearing loss usually cannot be corrected, but cochlear implants can improve severe hearing loss.

Meniere's disease results from a collection of fluid in the labyrinth of the inner ear and a degeneration of the hair cells in the cochlea and vestibule. Symptoms include severe vertigo (dizziness); tinnitus (ringing in the ears); nausea and vomiting; loss of balance; and a tendency to fall. Forms of treatment include drugs to reduce the fluid, draining the fluid, and antihistamines. In severe, chronic cases, surgery to destroy the cochlea may be performed; however, this causes permanent deafness.

Otitis externa is an inflammation of the external auditory canal. It is caused by a pathogenic organism such as a bacterium or virus. Swimmer's ear is one form. It is caused by swimming in contaminated water. Inserting bobby pins, fingernails, or cotton swabs into the ear can also cause this condition. Treatment methods include antibiotics; warm, moist compresses; and/or pain medications.

Otitis media is an inflammation or infection of the middle ear and is caused by a bacterium or virus. It frequently follows a sore throat because organisms from the throat can enter the middle ear through the eustachian tube. Infants and young children are very susceptible to otitis media because the eustachian tube is angled differently than in adults. Secretions from the nose and throat accumulate in the middle ear, resulting in an inflammatory response that causes the eustachian tube to swell shut. Symptoms include severe pain; fever; vertigo (dizziness); nausea and vomiting; and fluid buildup in the middle ear. Treatment usually consists of administering antibiotics and pain medications. At times, a *myringotomy* (incision of the tympanic membrane) is performed, and tubes are inserted to relieve pressure and allow fluid to drain.

Otosclerosis occurs when the stapes becomes immobile, causing conductive hearing loss. Symptoms include gradual hearing loss, tinnitus, and, at times, vertigo. Surgical removal of the stapes and insertion of an artificial stapes corrects the condition.

THE TONGUE AND SENSE OF TASTE

The tongue is a mass of muscle tissue with projections called papillae, figure 6-34. The papillae contain taste buds that are stimulated by the flavors of foods moistened by saliva. There are four

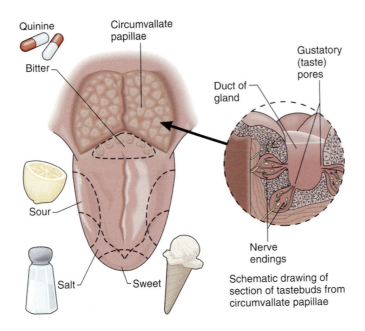

Quinine

Circumvallate papillae

Bitter

Gustatory (taste) pores

Duct of gland

Sour

Nerve endings

Salt

Sweet

Schematic drawing of section of tastebuds from circumvallate papillae

FIGURE 6-34 Locations of taste buds.

main tastes: sweet tastes and salty tastes at the tip of the tongue; sour tastes at the sides of the tongue; and bitter tastes at the back of the tongue. Taste is influenced by the sense of smell.

THE NOSE AND SENSE OF SMELL

The nose is the organ of smell, figure 6-35. The sense of smell is made possible by olfactory receptors, which are located in the upper part of the nasal cavity. Impulses from these receptors are carried to the brain by the olfactory nerve. The sense of smell is more sensitive than taste. The human nose can detect over 6,000 different smells. The sense of smell is closely related to the sense of taste. This is clearly illustrated by the fact that when you have a head cold and

your sense of smell is impaired, food does not taste as good.

THE SKIN AND GENERAL SENSES

General sense receptors for pressure, heat, cold, touch, and pain are located throughout the body in the skin and connective tissue. Each receptor perceives only one type of sense. For example, the skin contains special receptors for heat and different receptors for cold. Messages from these receptors allow the human body to respond to its environment and help it react to conditions that can cause injury.

STUDENT: *Go to the workbook and complete the assignment sheet for 6:7, Special Senses.*

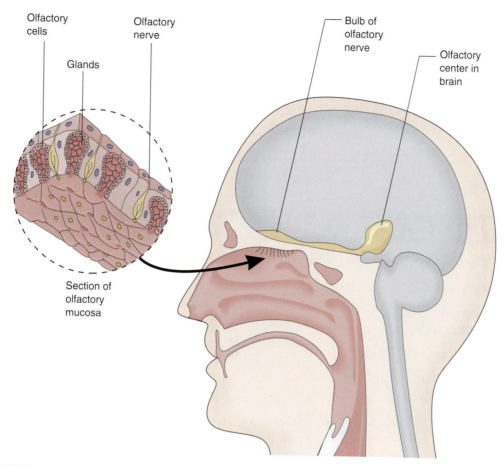

Olfactory cells

Olfactory nerve

Glands

Bulb of olfactory nerve

Olfactory center in brain

Section of olfactory mucosa

FIGURE 6-35 The sense of smell.

6:8 Circulatory System

Objectives

After completing this section, you should be able to:

◆ Label the layers, chambers, valves, and major blood vessels on a diagram of the heart

◆ Differentiate between systole and diastole by explaining what happens in the heart during each phase

◆ List the three major types of blood vessels and the action of each type

◆ Compare the three main types of blood cells by describing the function of each

◆ Describe at least five diseases of the circulatory system

◆ Define, pronounce, and spell all the key terms

KEY TERMS

aortic valve
   (ay-or′-tick)
arteries
blood
capillaries
   (cap′-ih-lair-eez)

circulatory system
diastole
   (dy-az′-tah-lee″)
endocardium
   (en-doe-car′-dee-um)

erythrocytes
   (eh-rith′-row-sitez)
hemoglobin
   (hee′-mow-glow″-bin)
left atrium
   (ay′-tree-um)

(continued)

(Key Terms Continued)
left ventricle
  (ven'tri"-kul)
leukocytes
  (lew'-coh-sitez")
mitral valve
  (my'-tral)

myocardium
pericardium
plasma
  (plaz'-ma)
pulmonary valve
right atrium
right ventricle

septum
systole
  (sis'-tah-lee")
thrombocytes
  (throm'-bow-sitez)
tricuspid valve
veins

RELATED HEALTH CAREERS

- Cardiac Surgeon
- Cardiologist
- Cardiovascular Technologist
- Echocardiographer
- Electrocardiographic Technician
- Hematologist
- Internist
- Medical Laboratory Technologist/ Technician
- Perfusionist
- Phlebotomist
- Radiology Technologist
- Thoracic Surgeon

6:8 INFORMATION

The **circulatory system**, also known as the cardiovascular system, is often referred to as the "transportation" system of the body. It consists of the heart, blood vessels, and blood. It transports oxygen and nutrients to the body cells, and carbon dioxide and metabolic materials away from the body cells.

THE HEART

The heart is a muscular, hollow organ often called the "pump" of the body (see figure 6-36). It is approximately the size of a closed fist and is located in the mediastinal cavity, between the lungs, behind the sternum, and above the diaphragm. Three layers of tissue form the heart. The **endocardium** is a smooth layer of cells that lines the inside of the heart and is continuous with the inside of blood vessels. It allows for the smooth flow of blood. The thickest layer is the **myocardium**, the muscular middle layer. The **pericardium** is a double-layered membrane, or

sac, that covers the outside of the heart. A lubricating fluid, pericardial fluid, fills the space between the two layers to prevent friction and damage to the membranes as the heart beats or contracts.

The **septum** is a muscular wall that separates the heart into a right side and a left side. It prevents blood from moving between the right and left sides of the heart. The upper part of the septum is called the *interatrial septum,* and the lower part is called the *interventricular septum.*

The heart is divided into four parts or chambers. The two upper chambers are called *atria,* and the two lower chambers are called *ventricles.* The **right atrium** receives blood as it returns from the body cells. The **right ventricle** receives blood from the right atrium and pumps the blood into the pulmonary artery, which carries the blood to the lungs for oxygen. The **left atrium** receives oxygenated blood from the lungs. The **left ventricle** receives blood from the left atrium and pumps the blood into the aorta for transport to the body cells.

One-way valves in the chambers of the heart keep the blood flowing in the right direction. The **tricuspid valve** is located between the right atrium and the right ventricle. It closes when the right ventricle contracts, allowing blood to flow to the lungs and preventing blood from flowing

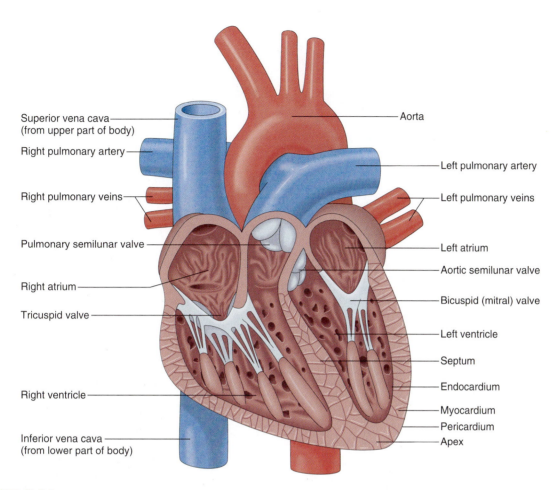

FIGURE 6-36 Basic structure of the heart.

back into the right atrium. The **pulmonary valve** is located between the right ventricle and the pulmonary artery, a blood vessel that carries blood to the lungs. It closes when the right ventricle has finished contracting, preventing blood from flowing back into the right ventricle. The **mitral valve** is located between the left atrium and left ventricle. It closes when the left ventricle is contracting, allowing blood to flow into the aorta (for transport to the body) and preventing blood from flowing back into the left atrium. The **aortic valve** is located between the left ventricle and the aorta, the largest artery in the body. It closes when the left ventricle is finished contracting, allowing blood to flow into the aorta and preventing blood from flowing back into the left ventricle.

Cardiac (Heartbeat) Cycle

Although they are separated by the septum, the right and left sides of the heart work together in a cyclic manner. The cycle consists of a brief period of rest, called **diastole**, followed by a period of ventricular contraction, called **systole** (see figure 6-37). At the start of the cycle, the atria contract and push blood into the ventricles. The atria then relax, and blood returning from the body enters the right atrium, while blood returning from the lungs enters the left atrium. As the atria are filling, systole begins, and the ventricles contract. The right ventricle pushes blood into the pulmonary artery, sending the blood to the lungs for oxygen. The left ventricle pushes blood into the aorta, sending the blood to all other parts of the body. The blood in the right side of the heart is low in oxygen and high in carbon dioxide. When this blood arrives in the lungs, the carbon dioxide is released into the lungs, and oxygen is taken into the blood. This oxygenated blood is then carried to the left side of the heart by the pulmonary veins. This blood in the left side of the heart, high in oxygen and low in carbon dioxide, is ready for transport to the body cells.

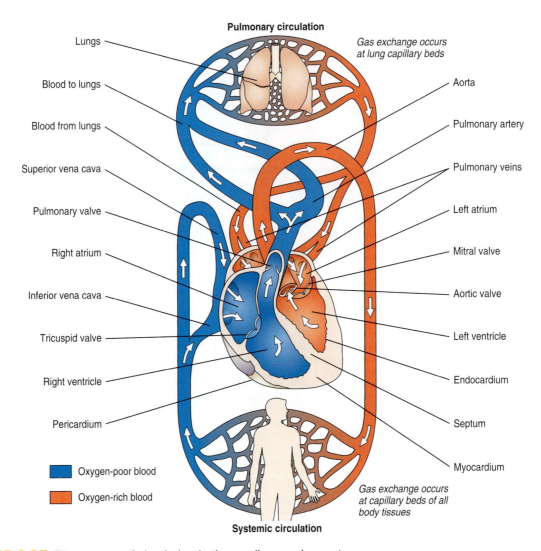

Pulmonary circulation

Gas exchange occurs at lung capillary beds

Lungs

Blood to lungs

Blood from lungs

Superior vena cava

Pulmonary valve

Right atrium

Inferior vena cava

Tricuspid valve

Right ventricle

Pericardium

Aorta

Pulmonary artery

Pulmonary veins

Left atrium

Mitral valve

Aortic valve

Left ventricle

Endocardium

Septum

Myocardium

■ Oxygen-poor blood

■ Oxygen-rich blood

Gas exchange occurs at capillary beds of all body tissues

Systemic circulation

FIGURE 6-37 The pattern of circulation in the cardiovascular system.

Conductive Pathway

Electrical impulses originating in the heart cause the cyclic contraction of the muscles (see figure 6-38). A group of nerve cells located in the right atrium and called the *sinoatrial (SA) node,* or the "pacemaker," sends out an electrical impulse, which spreads out over the muscles in the atria. The atrial muscles then contract and push blood into the ventricles. After the electrical impulse passes through the atria, it reaches the *atrioventricular (AV) node,* a group of nerve cells located between the atria and ventricles. The AV node sends the electrical impulse through the *bundle of His,* nerve fibers in the septum. The bundle of His divides into a *right bundle branch* and a *left bundle branch,* which carry the impulse down through the ventricles. The bundle branches further subdivide into the

Purkinje fibers, a network of nerve fibers throughout the ventricles. In this way, the electrical impulse reaches all the muscle tissue in the ventricles, and the ventricles contract. This electrical conduction pattern occurs approximately every 0.8 seconds. The movement of the electrical impulse can be recorded on an electrocardiogram (ECG) and used to detect abnormal activity or disease.

If something interferes with the normal electrical conduction pattern of the heart, arrhythmias occur. *Arrhythmias* are abnormal heart rhythms and can be mild to life-threatening. For example, an early contraction of the atria, or premature atrial contraction (PAC), can occur in anyone and usually goes unnoticed. Ventricle fibrillation, in which the ventricles contract at random without coordination, decreases or eliminates blood output and causes death if not

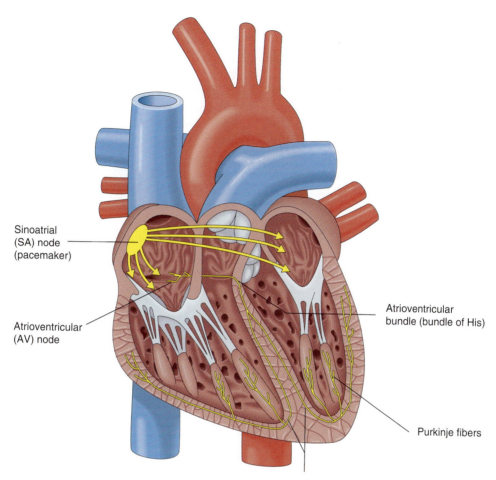

Sinoatrial (SA) node (pacemaker)

Atrioventricular (AV) node

Atrioventricular bundle (bundle of His)

Purkinje fibers

Left and right bundle branches

FIGURE 6-38 Electrical conduction pathways in the heart.

treated. Cardiac monitors and electrocardiograms are used to diagnose arrhythmias. Treatment depends on the type and severity of the arrhythmia. Life-threatening fibrillations are treated with a *defibrillator*, a device that shocks the heart with an electrical current to stop the uncoordinated contraction and allow the SA node to regain control.

At times it is necessary to use external or internal artificial pacemakers to regulate the heart's rhythm, figure 6-39. The *pacemaker* is a small battery-powered device with electrodes. The electrodes are threaded through a vein and positioned in the right atrium and in the apex of the right ventricle. The pacemaker monitors the heart's activity and delivers an electrical impulse through the electrodes to stimulate contraction. Fixed pacemakers deliver electrical impulses at a predetermined rate. Demand pacemakers, the most common type, deliver electrical impulses only when the heart's own conduction system is not responding correctly. Even though modern

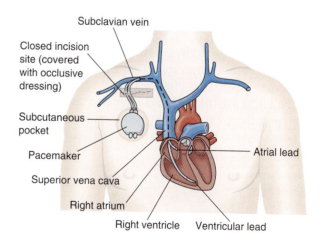

Subclavian vein

Closed incision site (covered with occlusive dressing)

Subcutaneous pocket

Pacemaker

Superior vena cava

Right atrium

Right ventricle

Atrial lead

Ventricular lead

FIGURE 6-39 Artificial pacemakers can help regulate the heart's rhythm.

pacemakers are protected from electromagnetic forces, such as microwave ovens, most manufacturers still recommend that people with pacemakers avoid close contact with digital cellular telephones.

BLOOD VESSELS

When the blood leaves the heart, it is carried throughout the body in blood vessels. The heart and blood vessels form a closed system for the flow of blood. There are three main types of blood vessels: arteries, capillaries, and veins.

Arteries (see figure 6-40) carry blood away from the heart. The aorta is the largest artery in the body; it receives the blood from the left ventricle of the heart. The aorta immediately begins branching into smaller arteries. The smallest branches of arteries are called *arterioles*. They join with capillaries. Arteries are more muscular and elastic than are the other blood vessels because they receive the blood as it is pumped from the heart.

Capillaries connect arterioles with *venules*, the smallest veins. Capillaries have thin walls containing only one layer of cells. These thin walls allow oxygen and nutrients to pass through to the cells and allow carbon dioxide and metabolic products from the cells to enter the capillaries.

Veins (see figure 6-41) are blood vessels that carry blood back to the heart. Venules, the smallest branches of veins, connect with the capillaries. The venules join together and, becoming larger, form veins. The veins continue to join together until they form the two largest veins: the superior vena cava and the inferior vena cava. The superior vena cava brings the blood from the upper part of the body, and the inferior vena cava brings the blood from the lower part of the body. Both vena cavae drain into the right atrium of the heart. Veins are thinner and have less muscle tissue than do arteries. Most veins contain valves, which keep the blood from flowing in a backward direction (see figure 6-42).

BLOOD COMPOSITION

The **blood** that flows through the circulatory system is often called a tissue because it contains many kinds of cells. There are approximately four to six quarts of blood in the average adult. This blood continuously circulates throughout the body. It transports oxygen from the lungs to the body cells; carbon dioxide from the body cells to the lungs; nutrients from the digestive tract to the body cells; metabolic and waste products from the body cells to the organs of excretion; heat produced by various body parts; and hormones produced by endocrine glands to the body organs.

Blood is made of the fluid called plasma and formed or solid elements called *blood cells* (see figure 6-43). **Plasma** is approximately 90 percent water, with many dissolved, or suspended, substances. Among these substances are blood proteins such as fibrinogen and prothrombin (both necessary for clotting); nutrients such as vitamins, carbohydrates, and proteins; mineral salts or electrolytes such as potassium, calcium, and sodium; gases such as carbon dioxide and oxygen; metabolic and waste products; hormones, and enzymes.

Blood Cells

There are three main kinds of blood cells: erythrocytes, leukocytes, and thrombocytes.

The **erythrocytes**, or red blood cells, are produced in the red bone marrow at a rate of approximately one million per minute. They live approximately 120 days before being broken down by the liver and spleen. There are 4.5 to 5.5 million erythrocytes per cubic millimeter (approximately one drop) of blood, or approximately 25 trillion in the body. The mature form circulating in the blood lacks a nucleus and is shaped like a disc with a thinner central area. The erythrocytes contain **hemoglobin**, a complex protein composed of the protein molecule called *globin* and the iron compound called *heme*. Hemoglobin carries both oxygen and carbon dioxide. When carrying oxygen, hemoglobin gives blood its characteristic red color. When blood contains a lot of oxygen, it is bright red; when blood contains less oxygen and more carbon dioxide, it is a much darker red with a bluish cast.

Leukocytes, or white blood cells, are not as numerous as are erythrocytes. They are formed in the bone marrow and lymph tissue and usually live about three to nine days. A normal count is 5,000 to 10,000 leukocytes per cubic millimeter of blood. Leukocytes can pass through capillary walls and enter body tissue. Their main function is to fight infection. Some do this by engulfing, ingesting, and destroying pathogens, or germs, by a process called *phagocytosis*. The five types of leukocytes and their functions include:

◆ *Neutrophils:* phagocytize bacteria by secreting an enzyme called lysozyme

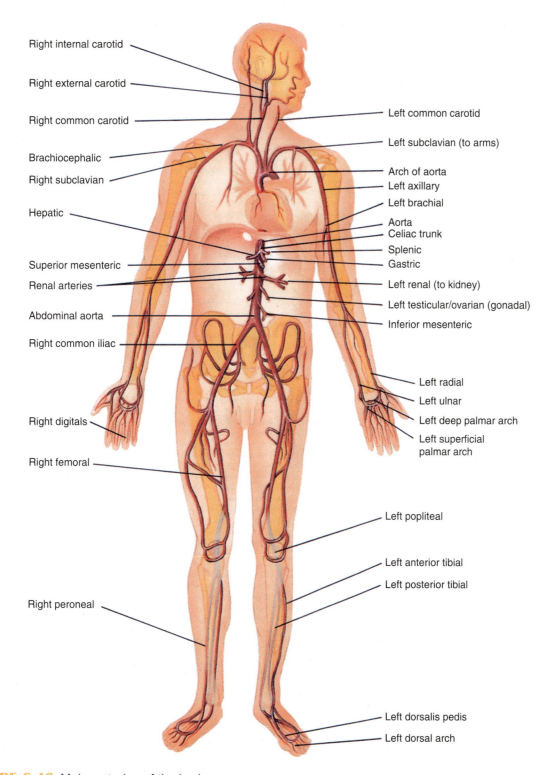

FIGURE 6-40 Major arteries of the body.

◆ *Eosinophils:* remove toxins and defend the body from allergic reactions by producing antihistamines

◆ *Basophils:* participate in the body's inflammatory response; produce histamine, a vasodilator, and heparin, an anticoagulant

◆ *Monocytes:* phagocytize bacteria and foreign materials

◆ *Lymphocytes:* provide immunity for the body by developing antibodies; protect against the formation of cancer cells

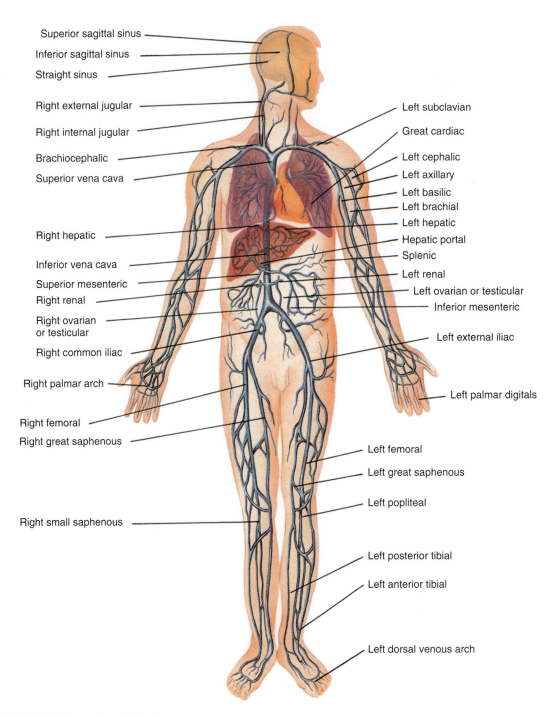

Superior sagittal sinus
Inferior sagittal sinus
Straight sinus
Right external jugular
Right internal jugular
Brachiocephalic
Superior vena cava
Right hepatic
Inferior vena cava
Superior mesenteric
Right renal
Right ovarian or testicular
Right common iliac
Right palmar arch
Right femoral
Right great saphenous
Right small saphenous

Left subclavian
Great cardiac
Left cephalic
Left axillary
Left basilic
Left brachial
Left hepatic
Hepatic portal
Splenic
Left renal
Left ovarian or testicular
Inferior mesenteric
Left external iliac
Left palmar digitals
Left femoral
Left great saphenous
Left popliteal
Left posterior tibial
Left anterior tibial
Left dorsal venous arch

FIGURE 6-41 Major veins of the body.

Thrombocytes, also called *platelets*, are usually described as fragments or pieces of cells because they lack nuclei and vary in shape and size. They are formed in the bone marrow and live for about five to nine days. A normal thrombocyte count is 250,000 to 400,000 per cubic millimeter of blood. Thrombocytes are important for the clotting process, which stops bleeding. When a blood vessel is cut, the thrombocytes collect at the site to form a sticky plug. They secrete a chemical, serotonin, which causes the blood vessel to spasm and narrow, decreasing the flow of blood. At the same time, the thrombocytes release an enzyme, thromboplastin, which acts with calcium and other substances in the plasma to form thrombin. Thrombin acts on the blood protein fibrinogen to form fibrin, a gel-like net of fine fibers that traps erythrocytes, platelets, and plasma to form a clot. This is a very effective method for controlling bleeding in smaller blood

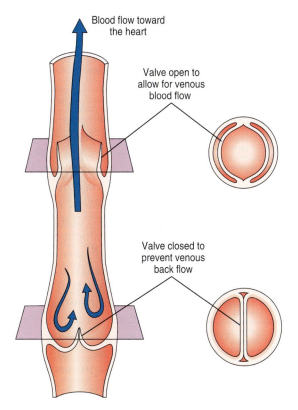

FIGURE 6-42 Most veins contain valves to prevent the backflow of blood.

vessels. If a large blood vessel is cut, the rapid flow of blood can interfere with the formation of fibrin. In these instances, a doctor may have to insert sutures (stitches) to close the opening and control the bleeding.

DISEASES AND ABNORMAL CONDITIONS

Anemia is an inadequate number of red blood cells, hemoglobin, or both. Symptoms include pallor (paleness), fatigue, dyspnea (difficult breathing), and rapid heart rate. Hemorrhage can cause rapid blood loss, and result in acute-blood-loss anemia. Blood transfusions are used to correct this form of anemia. *Iron deficiency anemia* results when there is an inadequate amount of iron to form hemoglobin in erythrocytes. Iron supplements and increased iron intake in the diet from green leafy vegetables and other foods can correct this condition. *Aplastic anemia* is a result of injury to or destruction of the bone marrow, leading to poor or no formation

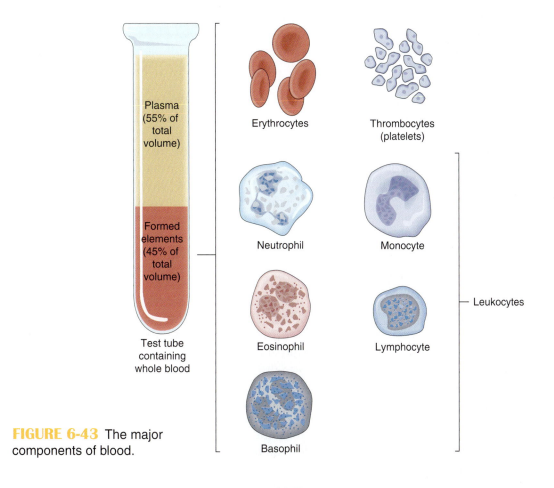

FIGURE 6-43 The major components of blood.

of red blood cells. Common causes include chemotherapy, radiation, toxic chemicals, and viruses. Treatment includes eliminating the cause, blood transfusions, and, in severe cases, a bone marrow transplant. Unless the damage can be reversed, it is frequently fatal. *Pernicious anemia* results in the formation of abnormally large and an inadequate number of erythrocytes. The cause is a lack of intrinsic factor (a substance normally present in the stomach), that results in inadequate absorption of vitamin B_{12}. Administering vitamin B_{12} injections can control and correct this condition. *Sickle cell anemia* is a chronic, inherited anemia. It results in the production of abnormal, crescent-shaped erythrocytes that carry less oxygen, break easily, and block blood vessels (see figure 6-44). Sickle cell anemia occurs almost exclusively among African Americans. Treatment methods include transfusions of packed cells and supportive therapy during crisis. Genetic counseling can lead to prevention of the disease if carriers make informed decisions not to have children.

An *aneurysm* is a ballooning out of, or saclike formation on, an artery wall. Disease, congenital defects, and injuries leading to weakened arterial wall structure can cause this defect. Although some aneurysms cause pain and pressure, others generate no symptoms. Common sites are the cerebral, aortal, and abdominal arteries. If an aneurysm ruptures, hemorrhage, which can cause death, occurs. Treatment usually involves surgically removing the damaged area of blood vessel and replacing it with a plastic graft or another blood vessel.

Arteriosclerosis is a hardening or thickening of the arterial walls, resulting in a loss of elasticity and contractility. It commonly occurs as a result of aging. Arteriosclerosis causes high blood pressure, or hypertension, and can lead to an aneurysm or cerebral hemorrhage.

Atherosclerosis occurs when fatty plaques (frequently cholesterol) are deposited on the walls of the arteries. This narrows the arterial opening, which reduces or eliminates blood flow. If plaques break loose, they can circulate through the bloodstream as *emboli*. A low-cholesterol diet, medications to lower cholesterol blood levels, and exercise are used to prevent atherosclerosis. Angioplasty, figure 6-45, may be used to remove or compress the deposits, or to insert a stent to allow blood flow. Bypass surgery is used when the arteries are completely blocked.

Congestive heart failure (CHF) is a condition that occurs when the heart muscles do not beat adequately to supply the blood needs of the body. It may involve either the right side or the left side of the heart. Symptoms include edema (swelling); dypsnea; pallor or cyanosis; distention of the neck veins; a weak, rapid pulse; and a cough accompanied by pink, frothy sputum. Cardiac drugs, diuretics (to remove retained body fluids), elastic support hose, oxygen therapy, bedrest, and/or a low-sodium diet are used as treatment methods.

An *embolus* is a foreign substance circulating in the bloodstream. It can be air, a blood clot, bacterial clumps, a fat globule, or other similar substances. When an embolus enters an artery or capillary too small for passage, blockage of the blood vessel occurs.

Hemophilia is an inherited disease that occurs almost exclusively in males but can be carried by females. Because of the lack of a plasma protein required for the clotting process, the blood is unable to clot. A minor cut can lead to prolonged bleeding, and a minor bump can cause internal bleeding. Treatment involves transfusing whole blood, or plasma, and administering the missing protein factor.

Hypertension is high blood pressure. A systolic pressure above 140 and a diastolic pressure above 90 millimeters of mercury is usually regarded as hypertension. Risk factors that increase the incidence of hypertension include family history, race (higher in African Americans), obesity, stress, smoking, aging (higher in postmenopausal women), and a diet high in saturated fat. Although there is no cure, hypertension can usually be controlled with antihypertensive drugs, diuretics (to remove retained body fluids), limited stress, avoidance of tobacco, and/or a low-sodium or low-fat diet. If hypertension is not treated, it can

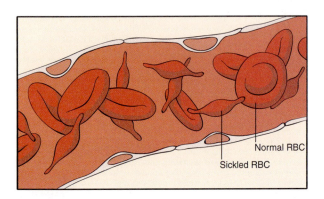

FIGURE 6-44 Sicke cell anemia is characterized by abnormal, crescent-shaped erythrocytes.

(A) Conventional balloon angioplasty

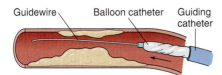

Guidewire   Balloon catheter   Guiding catheter

1. In conventional balloon angioplasty, a guiding catheter is positioned in the opening of the coronary artery. The physician then pushes a thin, flexible guidewire down the vessel and through the narrowing. The balloon catheter is then advanced over this guidewire.

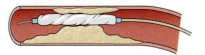

2. The balloon catheter is positioned next to the atherosclerotic plaque.

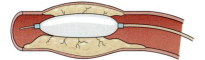

3. The balloon is inflated stretching and cracking the plaque.

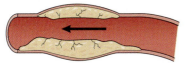

4. When the balloon is withdrawn, blood flow is re-established through the widened vessel.

(B) Coronary atherectomy

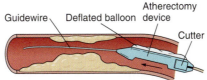

Guidewire   Deflated balloon   Atherectomy device   Cutter

1. In coronary atherectomy procedures, a special cutting device with a deflated balloon on one side and an opening on the other is pushed over a wire down the coronary artery.

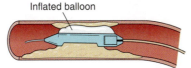

Inflated balloon

2. When the device is within a coronary artery narrowing, the balloon is inflated, so that part of the atherosclerotic plaque is "squeezed" into the opening of the device.

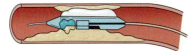

3. When the physician starts rotating the cutting blade, pieces of plaque are shaved off into the device.

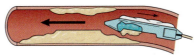

4. The catheter is withdrawn, leaving a larger opening for blood flow.

(C) Coronary stent

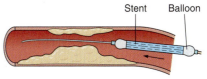

Stent   Balloon

1. To place a coronary stent within a vessel narrowing, physicians use a special catheter with a deflated balloon and the stent at the tip.

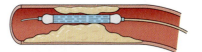

2. The catheter is positioned so that the stent is within the narrowed region of the coronary artery.

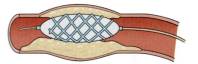

3. The balloon is then inflated, causing the stent to expand and stretch the coronary artery.

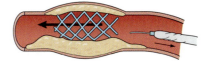

4. The balloon catheter is then withdrawn, leaving the stent behind to keep the vessel open.

FIGURE 6-45 Ways to open clogged arteries: (A) balloon angioplasty, (B) coronary atherectomy, (C) coronary stent.

cause permanent damage to the heart, blood vessels, and kidneys.

Leukemia is a malignant disease of the bone marrow or lymph tissue. It results in a high number of immature white blood cells. There are different types of leukemia, some acute and some chronic. Symptoms include fever, pallor, swelling of lymphoid tissues, fatigue, anemia, bleeding gums, excessive bruising, and joint pain. Treatment methods vary with the type of leukemia but can include chemotherapy, radiation, and/or bone marrow transplant.

A *myocardial infarction,* or heart attack, occurs when a blockage in the coronary arteries cuts off the supply of blood to the heart. The affected heart tissue dies and is known as an *infarct.* Death can occur immediately. Symptoms include severe crushing pain (angina pectoris) that radiates to the arm, neck, and jaw; pressure in the chest; perspiration and cold, clammy skin; dypsnea; and a change in blood pressure. If the heart stops, cardiopulmonary resuscitation should

be started immediately. Immediate treatment with a thrombolytic or "clot-busting" drug such as streptokinase or TPA, tissue plasminogen activator, may open the blood vessel and restore blood flow to the heart. However, the clot-busting drug must be used within the first several hours, and its use is prohibited if bleeding is present. Additional treatment methods include complete bed rest, pain medications, vasodilators, oxygen therapy, anticoagulants, and control of arrhythmias (abnormal heart rhythms). Long-term care includes control of blood pressure; a diet low in cholesterol and saturated fat; avoidance of tobacco and stress; regular exercise; and weight control.

Phlebitis is an inflammation of a vein, frequently in the leg. If a thrombus, or clot, forms, the condition is termed *thrombophlebitis.* Symptoms include pain, edema, redness, and discoloration at the site. Treatment methods include anticoagulants; pain medication; elevation of the affected area; antiembolism or support hose; and, if necessary, surgery to remove the clot.

Varicose veins are dilated, swollen veins that have lost elasticity and cause stasis, or decreased blood flow. They frequently occur in the legs and result from pregnancy, prolonged sitting or standing, and hereditary factors. Treatment methods include exercise; antiembolism or support hose; and avoidance of prolonged sitting or standing and tight-fitting or restrictive clothing. In severe cases, surgery can be performed to remove the vein.

STUDENT: *Go to the workbook and complete the assignment sheet for 6:8, Circulatory System.*

6:9 Lymphatic System

Objectives

After completing this section, you should be able to:

◆ Explain the function of lymphatic vessels

◆ List at least two functions of lymph nodes

◆ Identify the two lymphatic ducts and the areas of the body that each drains

◆ List at least three functions of the spleen

◆ Describe the function of the thymus

◆ Describe at least three diseases of the lymphatic system

◆ Define, pronounce, and spell all the key terms

KEY TERMS

cisterna chyli
 (sis-tern'-uh-kye'-lee)
lacteals
lymph
 (limf')
lymph nodes

lymphatic capillaries
 (lim-fat'-ik)
lymphatic system
lymphatic vessels
right lymphatic duct

spleen
thoracic duct
 (tho-rass'-ik)
thymus
tonsils

RELATED HEALTH CAREERS

◆ Immunologist   ◆ Internist

6:9 INFORMATION

The **lymphatic system** consists of lymph, lymph vessels, lymph nodes, and lymphatic tissue. This system works in conjunction with the circulatory system to remove wastes and excess fluids from the tissues (see figure 6-46).

Lymph is a thin, watery fluid composed of *intercellular,* or *interstitial,* fluid, which forms when plasma diffuses into tissue spaces. It is composed of water, digested nutrients, salts, hormones, oxygen, carbon dioxide, lymphocytes, and metabolic wastes such as urea. When this fluid enters the lymphatic system, it is known as lymph.

Lymphatic vessels are located throughout the body in almost all of the tissues that have blood vessels. Small, open-ended lymph vessels act like drainpipes and are called **lymphatic capillaries.** The lymphatic capillaries pick up lymph at tissues throughout the body. The capillaries then join together to form larger lymphatic vessels, which pass through the lymph nodes. Contractions of

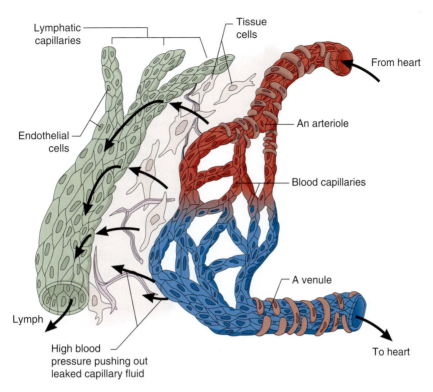

Lymphatic capillaries

Tissue cells

From heart

An arteriole

Endothelial cells

Blood capillaries

A venule

Lymph

To heart

High blood pressure pushing out leaked capillary fluid

FIGURE 6-46 The lymphatic system works with the circulatory system to remove metabolic waste and excess fluid from the tissues.

skeletal muscles against the lymph vessels cause the lymph to flow through the vessels. Lymphatic vessels also have valves that keep the lymph flowing in only one direction. In the area of the small intestine, specialized lymphatic capillaries, called **lacteals**, pick up digested fats or lipids. When lymph is mixed with the lipids it is called *chyle*. The lacteals transport the chyle to the bloodstream through the thoracic duct.

Lymph nodes, popularly called "glands," are located all over the body, usually in groups or clusters. They are small, round or oval masses ranging in size from that of a pinhead to that of an almond. Lymph vessels bring lymph to the nodes. The nodes filter the lymph and remove impurities such as carbon, cancer cells, pathogens (disease-producing organisms), and dead blood cells. In addition, the lymphatic tissue in the nodes produces lymphocytes (a type of leukocyte, or white blood cell) and antibodies (substances used to combat infection). The purified lymph, with lymphocytes and antibodies added, leaves the lymph node by a single lymphatic vessel.

As lymphatic vessels leave the lymph nodes, they continue to join together to form larger lymph vessels (see figure 6-47). Eventually, these vessels drain into one of two lymphatic ducts: the right lymphatic duct or the thoracic duct. The **right lymphatic duct** is the short tube that receives all

of the purified lymph from the right side of the head and neck, the right chest, and the right arm. It empties into the right subclavian vein, returning the purified lymph to the blood. The **thoracic duct**, a much larger tube, drains the lymph from the rest of the body. It empties into the left subclavian vein. At the start of the thoracic duct, an enlarged pouchlike structure called the **cisterna chyli** serves as a storage area for purified lymph before this lymph returns to the bloodstream. The cisterna chyli also receives chyle from the intestinal lacteals.

In addition to being found in the lymph nodes, lymphatic tissue is located throughout the body. The tonsils, spleen, and thymus are examples of lymphatic tissue.

The **tonsils** are masses of lymphatic tissue that filter interstitial fluid. There are three pairs of tonsils:

◆ *palatine tonsils:* located on each side of the soft palate

◆ *pharyngeal tonsils:* (also called adenoids) located in the nasopharynx (the upper part of the throat)

◆ *lingual tonsils:* located on the back of the tongue

The **spleen** is an organ located beneath the left side of the diaphragm and in back of the upper part of the stomach. It produces leukocytes

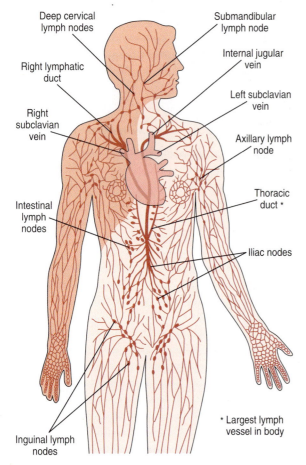

Deep cervical lymph nodes

Submandibular lymph node

Internal jugular vein

Right lymphatic duct

Left subclavian vein

Right subclavian vein

Axillary lymph node

Thoracic duct *

Intestinal lymph nodes

Iliac nodes

Inguinal lymph nodes

* Largest lymph vessel in body

FIGURE 6-47 Main components of the lymphatic system.

and antibodies; destroys old erythrocytes (red blood cells); stores erythrocytes to release into the bloodstream if excessive bleeding occurs; destroys thrombocytes (platelets); and filters metabolites and wastes from body tissues.

The **thymus** is a mass of lymph tissue located in the center of the upper chest. It atrophies (wastes away) after puberty and is replaced by fat and connective tissue. During early life, it produces antibodies and manufactures lymphocytes to fight infection. Its function is taken over by the lymph nodes.

DISEASES AND ABNORMAL CONDITIONS

Adenitis is an inflammation or infection of the lymph nodes. It occurs when large quantities of harmful substances, such as pathogens or cancer

cells, enter the lymph nodes and infect the tissue. Symptoms include fever and swollen, painful nodes. If the infection is not treated, an abscess may form in the node. Usually treatment methods are antibiotics and warm, moist compresses. If an abscess forms, it is sometimes necessary to incise and drain the node.

Hodgkin's disease is a chronic, malignant disease of the lymph nodes. It is the most common form of lymphoma (tumor of lymph tissue). Symptoms include painless swelling of the lymph nodes, fever, night sweats, weight loss, fatigue, and pruritus (itching). Chemotherapy and radiation are usually effective forms of treatment.

Lymphangitis is an inflammation of lymphatic vessels, usually resulting from an infection in an extremity. Symptoms include a characteristic red streak extending up an arm or leg from the source of infection; fever; chills; and tenderness or pain. Treatment methods include antibiotics, rest, elevation of the affected part, and/or warm, moist compresses.

Splenomegaly is an enlargement of the spleen. It can result from an abnormal accumulation of red blood cells; mononucleosis; and cirrhosis of the liver. The main symptoms are swelling and abdominal pain. An increased destruction of blood cells can lead to anemia (low red blood cell count), leukopenia (low white blood cell count), and thrombocytopenia (low thrombocyte count). If the spleen ruptures, intraperitoneal hemorrhage and shock can lead to death. In severe cases, where the underlying cause cannot be treated, a splenectomy (surgical removal of the spleen) is performed.

Tonsillitis is an inflammation or infection of the tonsils. It usually involves the pharyngeal (adenoid) and palatine tonsils. Symptoms include throat pain; dysphagia (difficulty swallowing); fever; white or yellow spots of exudate on the tonsils; and swollen lymph nodes near the mandible. Antibiotics, warm throat irrigations, rest, and analgesics for pain are the main forms of treatment. Chronic, frequent infections or hypertrophy (enlargement) that causes obstruction are indications for a tonsillectomy, or surgical removal of the tonsils.

STUDENT: *Go to the workbook and complete the assignment sheet for 6:9, Lymphatic System.*

6:10 Respiratory System

Objectives

After completing this section, you should be able to:

◆ Label a diagram of the respiratory system

◆ List five functions of the nasal cavity

◆ Identify the three sections of the pharynx

◆ Explain how the larynx helps create sound and speech

◆ Describe the function of the epiglottis

◆ Compare the processes of inspiration and expiration, including the muscle action that occurs during each process

◆ Differentiate between external and internal respiration

◆ Describe at least five diseases of the respiratory system

◆ Define, pronounce, and spell all the key terms

KEY TERMS

alveoli
  (ahl-vee′-oh″-lie)
bronchi
  (bron′-kie)
bronchioles
  (bron′-key″-ohlz)
cellular respiration
cilia
  (sil′-lee-ah)
epiglottis
  (ep-ih-glot′-tiss)

expiration
external respiration
inspiration
internal respiration
larynx
  (lar′-inks)
lungs
nasal cavities
nasal septum
nose

pharynx
  (far′-inks)
respiration
respiratory system
  (res′-peh-reh-tor′-ee)
sinuses
trachea
  (tray′-key″-ah)
ventilation

RELATED HEALTH CAREERS

◆ Internist

◆ Perfusionist

◆ Pulmonologist

◆ Respiratory Therapist

◆ Respiratory Therapy Technician

◆ Thoracic Surgeon

6:10 INFORMATION

The **respiratory system** consists of the lungs and air passages. This system is responsible for taking in oxygen, a gas needed by all body cells, and removing carbon dioxide, a gas that is a metabolic waste product produced by the cells. Because the body has only a four- to six-minute supply of oxygen, the respiratory system must work continuously to prevent death.

The parts of the respiratory system are the nose, pharynx, larynx, trachea, bronchi, alveoli, and lungs (see figure 6-48).

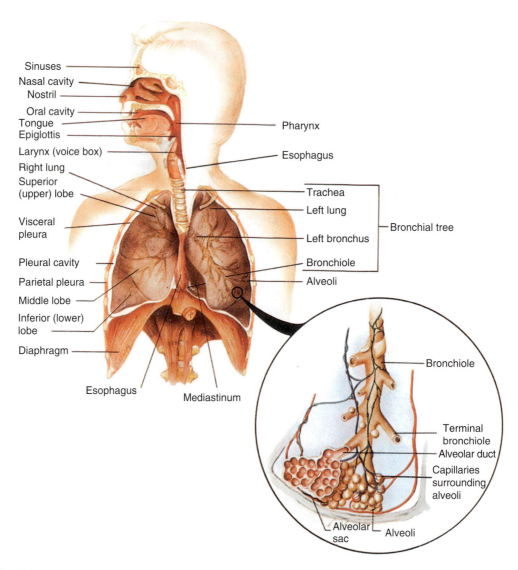

FIGURE 6-48 The respiratory system.

RESPIRATORY ORGANS AND STRUCTURES

The **nose** has two openings, called *nostrils* or *nares,* through which air enters. A wall of cartilage, called the **nasal septum**, divides the nose into two hollow spaces, called **nasal cavities**. The nasal cavities are lined with a mucous membrane and have a rich blood supply. As air enters the cavities, it is warmed, filtered, and moistened. Mucus, produced by the mucous membranes, moistens the air and helps trap pathogens and dirt. Tiny, hairlike structures, called **cilia**, help move the mucous layer that lines the airways pushing trapped particles toward the esophagus,

where they can be swallowed. The olfactory receptors for the sense of smell are also located in the nose. The nasolacrimal ducts drain tears from the eye into the nose to provide additional moisture for the air.

Sinuses are cavities in the skull that surround the nasal area. They are connected to the nasal cavity by short ducts. The sinuses are lined with a mucous membrane, which warms and moistens air. The sinuses also provide resonance for the voice.

The **pharynx**, or throat, lies directly behind the nasal cavities. As air leaves the nose, it enters the pharynx. The pharynx is divided into three sections. The *nasopharynx* is the upper portion, located behind the nasal cavities. The pharyngeal tonsils, or adenoids (lymphatic tissue), and the eustachian tube (tube to middle ear) openings are located in this section. The *oropharynx* is the middle section, located behind the oral cavity (mouth). This section receives both air from the nasopharynx and food and air from the mouth. The *laryngopharynx* is the bottom section of the pharynx. The esophagus, which carries food to the stomach, and the trachea, which carries air to and from the lungs, branch off the laryngopharynx.

The **larynx**, or voice box, lies between the pharynx and trachea. It has nine layers of cartilage. The largest, the thyroid cartilage, is commonly called the *Adam's apple.* The larynx contains two folds, called *vocal cords.* The opening between the vocal cords is called the *glottis.* As air leaves the lungs, the vocal cords vibrate and produce sound. The tongue and lips act on the sound to produce speech. The **epiglottis**, a special leaflike piece of cartilage, closes the opening into the larynx during swallowing. This prevents food and liquids from entering the respiratory tract.

The **trachea** (windpipe) is a tube extending from the larynx to the center of the chest. It carries air between the pharynx and the bronchi. A series of C-shaped cartilages (which are open on the dorsal, or back, surfaces) help keep the trachea open.

The trachea divides into two **bronchi** near the center of the chest, a right bronchus and a left bronchus. The right bronchus is shorter, wider, and extends more vertically than the left bronchus. Each bronchus enters a lung and carries air from the trachea to the lung. In the lungs, the bronchi continue to divide into smaller and smaller bronchi until, finally, they divide into the smallest branches, called **bronchioles**. The smallest bronchioles, called *terminal bronchioles,* end in air sacs, called *alveoli.*

The **alveoli** resemble a bunch of grapes. An adult lung contains approximately 500 million alveoli. They are made of one layer of squamous epithelial tissue and contain a rich network of blood capillaries. The capillaries allow oxygen and carbon dioxide to be exchanged between the blood and the lungs. The inner surfaces of the alveoli are covered with a lipid (fatty) substance, called surfactant, to help prevent them from collapsing.

The divisions of the bronchi and the alveoli are found in organs called **lungs**. The right lung has three sections or lobes: the superior, the middle, and the inferior. The left lung has only two lobes: the superior and the inferior. The left lung is smaller because the heart is located toward the left side of the chest. Each lung is enclosed in a membrane, or sac, called the *pleura.* The pleura consists of two layers: a visceral pleura attached to the surface of the lung, and a parietal pleura attached to the chest wall. A pleural space, located between the two layers, is filled with a thin layer of pleural fluid that lubricates the membranes and prevents friction as the lungs expand during breathing. Both of the lungs, along with the heart and major blood vessels, are located in the thoracic cavity.

PROCESS OF BREATHING

Ventilation is the process of breathing. It involves two phases: inspiration and expiration. **Inspiration** (inhalation) is the process of breathing in air. The diaphragm (dome-shaped muscle between the thoracic and abdominal cavities) and the intercostal muscles (between the ribs) contract and enlarge the thoracic cavity to create a vacuum. Air rushes in through the airways to the alveoli, where the exchange of gases takes place. This process is known as **respiration**. When the diaphragm and intercostal muscles relax, the process of **expiration** (exhalation) occurs. Air is forced out of the lungs and air passages. The process of respiration is controlled by the respiratory center in the medulla oblongata of the brain. An increased amount of carbon dioxide in the blood, or a decreased amount of oxygen as seen in certain diseases (asthma, congestive heart failure, or emphysema), causes the center to increase the rate of respiration. Although this process is usually involuntary, a person can control the rate of breathing by breathing faster or slower.

STAGES OF RESPIRATION

There are two main stages of respiration: external respiration and internal respiration (see figure 6-49). **External respiration** is the exchange of oxygen and carbon dioxide between the lungs and bloodstream. Oxygen, breathed in through the respiratory system, enters the alveoli. Since the oxygen concentration in the alveoli is higher than the oxygen concentration in the blood capillaries, oxygen leaves the alveoli and enters the capillaries and the bloodstream. Carbon dioxide,

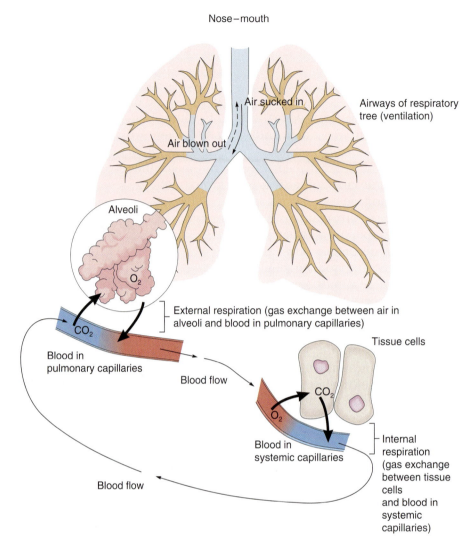

Nose–mouth

Air sucked in

Airways of respiratory tree (ventilation)

Air blown out

Alveoli

O_2

External respiration (gas exchange between air in alveoli and blood in pulmonary capillaries)

CO_2

Blood in pulmonary capillaries

Blood flow

Tissue cells

CO_2

O_2

Blood in systemic capillaries

Internal respiration (gas exchange between tissue cells and blood in systemic capillaries)

Blood flow

FIGURE 6-49 External and internal respiration.

a metabolic waste product, is carried in the bloodstream. Since the carbon dioxide concentration in the capillaries is higher than the carbon dioxide concentration in the alveoli, carbon dioxide leaves the capillaries and enters the alveoli, where it is expelled from the body during exhalation. **Internal respiration** is the exchange of carbon dioxide and oxygen between the tissue cells and the bloodstream. Oxygen is carried to the tissue cells by the blood. Since the oxygen concentration is higher in the blood than in the tissue cells, oxygen leaves the blood capillaries and enters the tissue cells. The cells then use the oxygen and nutrients to produce energy, water, and carbon dioxide. This process is called **cellular respiration**. Since the carbon dioxide concentration is higher in tissue cells than in the bloodstream, carbon dioxide leaves the cells and

enters the bloodstream to be transported back to the lungs, where external respiration takes place.

DISEASES AND ABNORMAL CONDITIONS

Asthma is a respiratory disorder usually caused by a sensitivity to an allergen such as dust, pollen, an animal, or a food. Stress, overexertion, and infection can also cause an asthma attack, during which bronchospasms narrow the openings of the bronchioles, mucus production increases, and edema develops in the mucosal lining. Symptoms of an asthma attack include dyspnea (difficult breathing), wheezing, coughing accompanied by expectoration of sputum, and tightness in the chest. Treatment methods include bronchodilators (to enlarge the bronchioles), anti-inflammatory medications, epinephrine, and oxygen therapy. Identification and elimination of or disensitization to allergens are important in preventing asthma attacks.

Bronchitis is an inflammation of the bronchi and bronchial tubes. *Acute bronchitis* is usually caused by infection and is characterized by a productive cough, dyspnea, chest pain, and fever. It is treated with antibiotics, expectorants (to remove excessive mucus), rest, and drinking large amounts of water. *Chronic bronchitis* results from frequent attacks of acute bronchitis and long-term exposure to pollutants or smoking. It is characterized by chronic inflammation, damaged cilia, and enlarged mucous glands. Symptoms include excessive mucus resulting in a productive cough, wheezing, dyspnea, chest pain, and prolonged air expiration. Although there is no cure, antibiotics, bronchodilators, and/or respiratory therapy are used in treatment.

Chronic obstructive pulmonary disease (COPD) is a term used to describe any chronic lung disease that results in obstruction of the airways. Disorders such as chronic asthma, chronic bronchitis, emphysema, and tuberculosis lead to COPD. Smoking is the primary cause, but allergies and chronic respiratory infections are also factors.

Emphysema is a noninfectious, chronic respiratory condition that occurs when the walls of the alveoli deteriorate and lose their elasticity, figure 6-50. Carbon dioxide remains trapped in the alveoli, and there is poor exchange of gases. The most common causes are heavy smoking and prolonged exposure to air pollutants. Symptoms include dyspnea, a feeling of suffocation, pain, barrel chest, chronic cough, cyanosis, rapid respirations accompanied by prolonged expirations, and eventual respiratory failure and death. Although there is no cure, treatment methods include bronchodilators, prompt treatment of respiratory infections, oxygen therapy, respiratory therapy, and avoidance of smoking.

Epistaxis, or a nosebleed, occurs when capillaries in the nose become congested and bleed. It can be caused by an injury or blow to the nose; hypertension; chronic infection; anticoagulant drugs; and blood diseases such as hemophilia and leukemia. Compressing the nostrils toward the septum; elevating the head and tilting it slightly forward; and applying cold compresses

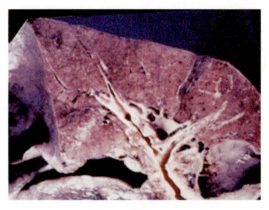

Normal lung

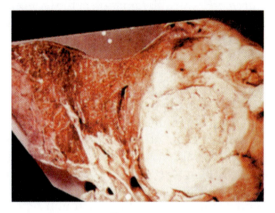

Cancer

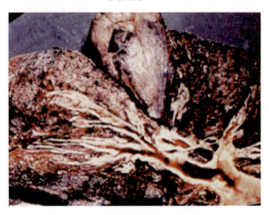

Emphysema

FIGURE 6-50 Two common lung diseases are emphysema and cancer. *(Courtesy of the American Cancer Society)*

will usually control epistaxis, although it is sometimes necessary to insert nasal packs or cauterize (burn and destroy) the bleeding vessels. Treatment of any underlying cause, such as hypertension, is important in preventing epistaxis.

Influenza, or flu, is a highly contagious, viral infection of the upper respiratory system. Onset is sudden, and symptoms include chills, fever, a cough, sore throat, runny nose, muscle pain, and fatigue. Treatment methods include bed rest, fluids, analgesics (for pain), and antipyretics (for fever). Antibiotics are not effective against the viruses causing influenza, but they are sometimes given to prevent secondary infections such as pneumonia. Immunization with a flu vaccine is recommended for the elderly, individuals with chronic diseases, pregnant women, and health care workers. Because many different viruses cause influenza, vaccines are developed each year to immunize against the most common viruses identified.

Laryngitis is an inflammation of the larynx and vocal cords. It frequently occurs in conjunction with other respiratory infections. Symptoms include hoarseness or loss of voice; sore throat; and dysphagia (difficult swallowing). Treatment methods include rest, limited voice use, fluids, and medication, if an infection is present.

Lung cancer is the leading cause of cancer death in both men and women (see figure 6-50). It is a preventable disease, because the main cause is exposure to carcinogens in tobacco, either through smoking or through exposure to "second-hand" smoke. Three common types of lung cancer include small cell, squamous cell, and adenocarcinoma. In the early stages, there are no symptoms. In later stages, symptoms include a chronic cough, hemoptysis (coughing up blood-tinged sputum), dyspnea, fatigue, weight loss, and chest pain. The prognosis (outcome) for lung cancer patients is poor since the disease is usually advanced before it is diagnosed. Treatment includes surgical removal of the cancerous sections of the lung, radiation, and/or chemotherapy.

Pleurisy is an inflammation of the pleura, or membranes, of the lungs. It usually occurs in conjunction with pneumonia or other lung infections. Symptoms include sharp, stabbing pain while breathing; crepitation (grating sounds in the lungs); dyspnea; and fever. Treatment methods include rest and medications to relieve pain and inflammation. If fluid collects in the pleural space, a thoracentesis (withdrawal of fluid through a needle) is performed to remove the fluid and prevent compression of the lungs.

Pneumonia is an inflammation or infection of the lungs characterized by exudate (a buildup of fluid) in the alveoli. It is usually caused by bacteria, viruses, or chemicals. Symptoms include chills, fever, chest pain, productive cough, dyspnea, and fatigue. Treatment methods include bed rest, fluids, antibiotics (if indicated), respiratory therapy, and/or pain medication.

Rhinitis is an inflammation of the nasal mucous membrane, resulting in a runny nose, soreness, and congestion. Common causes are infections and allergens. Treatment consists of administering fluids and medications to relieve congestion. Rhinitis is usually self limiting.

Sinusitis is an inflammation of the mucous membrane lining the sinuses. One or more sinuses may be affected. Sinusitis is usually caused by a bacterium or virus. Symptoms include headache or pressure; thick nasal discharge; congestion; and loss of voice resonance. Treatment methods include analgesics (for pain), antibiotics (if indicated), decongestants (medications to loosen secretions), and moist inhalations. Surgery is used in cases of chronic sinusitis to open the cavities and encourage drainage.

Tuberculosis (TB) is an infectious lung disease caused by the bacteria *Mycobacterium tuberculosis.* At times, white blood cells surround the invading TB organisms and wall them off creating nodules, called *tubercles,* in the lungs. The TB organisms remain dormant in the tubercles but can cause an active case of tuberculosis later, if body resistance is lowered. Symptoms of an active case of TB include fatigue, fever, night sweats, weight loss, hemoptysis (coughing up blood-tinged sputum), and chest pain. Treatment includes administering drugs for one or more years to destroy the bacteria. Good nutrition and rest are also important. In recent years, a new strain of the TB bacteria resistant to drug therapy has created concern that tuberculosis will become a widespread infectious disease.

An *upper respiratory infection (URI),* or common cold, is an inflammation of the mucous membrane lining the upper respiratory tract. Caused by viruses, URIs are highly contagious. Symptoms include fever, runny nose, watery eyes, congestion, sore throat, and hacking cough. There is no cure, and symptoms usually last approximately one week. Analgesics (for pain), antipyretics (for fever), rest, increased fluid intake, and antihistamines (to relieve congestion) are used to treat the symptoms.

STUDENT: *Go to the workbook and complete the assignment sheet for 6:10, Respiratory System.*

6:11 Digestive System

Objectives

After completing this section, you should be able to:

◆ Label the major organs on a diagram of the digestive system

◆ Identify at least three organs that are located in the mouth and aid in the initial breakdown of food

◆ Cite two functions of the salivary glands

◆ Describe how the gastric juices act on food in the stomach

◆ Explain how food is absorbed into the body by the villi in the small intestine

◆ List at least three functions of the large intestine

◆ List at least four functions of the liver

◆ Explain how the pancreas helps digest foods

◆ Describe at least five diseases of the digestive system

◆ Define, pronounce, and spell all the key terms

KEY TERMS

alimentary canal
  (ahl-ih-men'-tar"-ee)
anus
colon
  (coh'-lun)
digestive system
duodenum
  (dew-oh-deh'-num)
esophagus
  (ee"-sof-eh-gus)
gallbladder
hard palate
ileum
  (ill'-ee"-um)

jejunum
  (jeh-jew'-num)
large intestine
liver
mouth
pancreas
  (pan'-cree"-as)
peristalsis
  (pair"-ih-stall"-sis)
pharynx
  (far'-inks)

rectum
salivary glands
small intestine
soft palate
stomach
teeth
tongue
vermiform appendix
villi
  (vil'-lie)

RELATED HEALTH CAREERS

◆ Dental Assistant
◆ Dental Hygienist
◆ Dentist
◆ Dietetic Assistant
◆ Dietitian
◆ Enterostomal RN or Technician
◆ Gastroenterologist
◆ Hepatologist
◆ Internist
◆ Proctologist

6:11 INFORMATION

The **digestive system**, also known as the *gastrointestinal system,* is responsible for the physical and chemical breakdown of food so that it can be taken into the bloodstream and used by body cells and tissues. The system consists of the alimentary canal and accessory organs (see figure 6-51). The **alimentary canal** is a long, muscular tube that begins at the mouth and includes the mouth (oral cavity), pharynx, esophagus, stomach, small

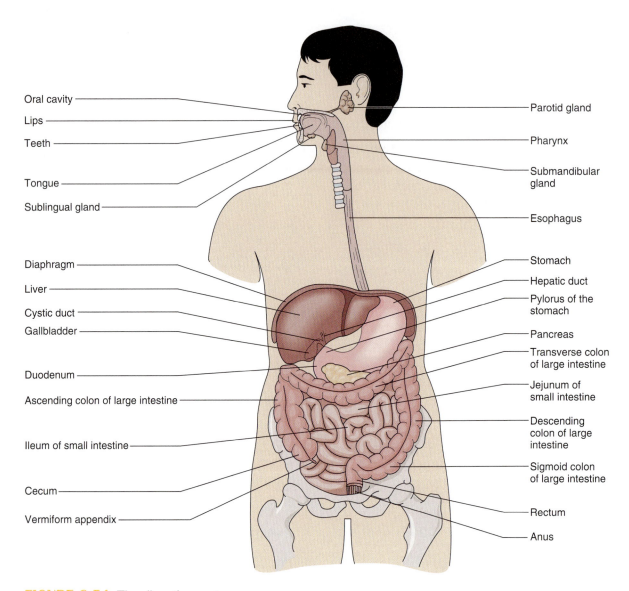

FIGURE 6-51 The digestive system.

intestine, large intestine, and anus. The accessory organs are the salivary glands, tongue, teeth, liver, gallbladder, and pancreas.

PARTS OF THE ALIMENTARY CANAL

The **mouth**, also called the buccal cavity, (see figure 6-52) receives food as it enters the body. While food is in the mouth, it is tasted, broken down physically by the teeth; lubricated and partially digested by saliva; and swallowed. The **teeth** are special structures in the mouth that physically break down food by chewing and grinding. This process is called *mastication.* The

tongue is a muscular organ that contains special receptors, called *taste buds.* The taste buds allow a person to taste sweet, salt, sour, and bitter sensations. The tongue also aids in chewing and swallowing food. The **hard palate** is the bony structure that forms the roof of the mouth and separates the mouth from the nasal cavities. Behind the hard palate is the **soft palate**, which separates the mouth from the nasopharynx. The *uvula,* a cone-shaped muscular structure, hangs from the middle of the soft palate. It prevents food from entering the nasopharynx during swallowing. Three pairs of **salivary glands**, the parotid, sublingual, and submandibular, produce a liquid called *saliva.* Saliva lubricates the mouth during speech and chewing and moistens food so that it can be swallowed easily. Saliva also contains the

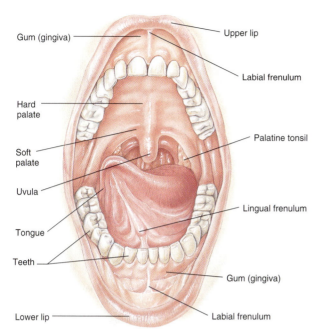

Gum (gingiva)

Upper lip

Labial frenulum

Hard palate

Soft palate

Palatine tonsil

Uvula

Tongue

Lingual frenulum

Teeth

Gum (gingiva)

Lower lip

Labial frenulum

FIGURE 6-52 Parts of the oral cavity, or mouth.

enzyme (substance that speeds up a chemical reaction) called *salivary amylase,* formerly known as *ptyalin.* Salivary amylase begins the chemical breakdown of carbohydrates, or starches, into sugars that can be taken into the body.

After the food is chewed and mixed with saliva, it is called a *bolus.* When the bolus is swallowed, it enters the **pharynx** (throat). The pharynx is a tube that carries both air and food. It carries the air to the trachea, or windpipe, and food to the esophagus. When a bolus is being swallowed, muscle action causes the epiglottis to close over the larynx preventing the bolus from entering the respiratory tract and causing it to enter the esophagus.

The **esophagus** is the muscular tube dorsal to (behind) the trachea. This tube receives the bolus from the pharynx and carries the bolus to the stomach. The esophagus, like the remaining part of the alimentary canal, relies on a rhythmic, wavelike, involuntary movement of its muscles, called **peristalsis**, to move the food in a forward direction.

The **stomach** is an enlarged part of the alimentary canal. It receives the food from the esophagus. The mucous membrane lining of the stomach contains folds, called *rugae.* These disappear as the stomach fills with food and expands. The cardiac sphincter, a circular muscle between the esophagus and stomach, closes after food enters the stomach and prevents food from going back up into the esophagus. The pyloric sphincter, a circular muscle between the stomach and small

intestine, keeps food in the stomach until the food is ready to enter the small intestine. Food usually remains in the stomach for approximately one to four hours. During this time, food is converted into a semifluid material, called *chyme,* by gastric juices produced by glands in the stomach. The gastric juices contain hydrochloric acid and enzymes. Hydrochloric acid kills bacteria, facilitates iron absorption, and activates the enzyme pepsin. The enzymes in gastric juices include lipase, which starts the chemical breakdown of fats, and pepsin, which starts protein digestion. In infants, the enzyme rennin is also secreted to aid in the digestion of milk. Rennin is not present in adults.

When the food, in the form of chyme, leaves the stomach, it enters the small intestine. The **small intestine** is a coiled section of the alimentary canal. It is approximately 20 feet in length and one inch in diameter, and is divided into three sections: the duodenum, the jejunum, and the ileum. The **duodenum** is the first nine to ten inches of the small intestine. Bile (from the gallbladder and liver) and pancreatic juice (from the pancreas) enter this section through ducts, or tubes. The **jejunum** is approximately eight feet in length and forms the middle section of the small intestine. The **ileum** is the final 12 feet of the small intestine, and it connects with the large intestine at the cecum. The circular muscle called the *ileocecal valve* separates the ileum and cecum and prevents food from returning to the ileum. While food is in the small intestine, the process of digestion is completed, and the products of digestion are absorbed into the bloodstream for use by the body cells. Intestinal juices, produced by the small intestine, contain the enzymes maltase, sucrase, and lactase, which break down sugars into simpler forms. The intestinal juices also contain enzymes known as *peptidases,* which complete the digestion of proteins, and steapsin, which aids in the digestion of fat. Bile, from the liver and gallbladder, emulsifies (physically breaks down) fats. Enzymes from the pancreatic juice complete the process of digestion. These enzymes include pancreatic amylase or amylopsin (which acts on sugars); trypsin and chymotrypsin (which act on proteins); and lipase or steapsin (which acts on fats). After food has been digested, it is absorbed into the bloodstream. The walls of the small intestine are lined with fingerlike projections called **villi** (see figure 6-53). The villi contain blood capillaries and lacteals. The blood capillaries absorb the digested nutrients and carry them to the liver, where they are either

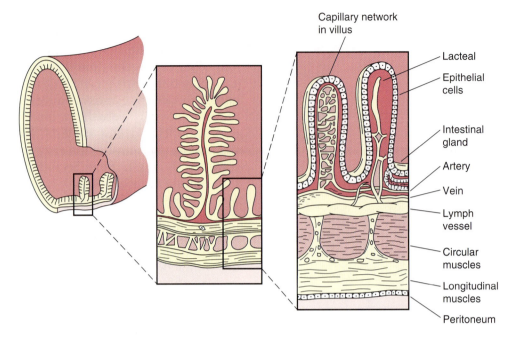

Capillary network in villus

Lacteal

Epithelial cells

Intestinal gland

Artery

Vein

Lymph vessel

Circular muscles

Longitudinal muscles

Peritoneum

FIGURE 6-53 Lymphatic and blood capillaries in the villi of the small intestine provide for the absorption of the products of digestion.

stored or released into general circulation for use by the body cells. The lacteals absorb most of the digested fats and carry them to the thoracic duct in the lymphatic system, which releases them into the circulatory system. When food has completed its passage through the small intestine, only wastes, indigestible materials, and excess water remain.

The **large intestine** is the final section of the alimentary canal. It is approximately five feet in length and two inches in diameter. Functions include absorption of water and any remaining nutrients; storage of indigestible materials before they are eliminated from the body; synthesis (formation) and absorption of some B-complex vitamins and vitamin K by bacteria present in the intestine; and transportation of waste products out of the alimentary canal. The large intestine is divided into a series of connected sections. The cecum is the first section and is connected to the ileum of the small intestine. It contains a small projection, called the **vermiform appendix**. The next section, the **colon**, has several divisions. The *ascending colon* continues up on the right side of the body from the cecum to the lower part of the liver. The *transverse colon* extends across the abdomen, below the liver and stomach and above the small intestine. The *descending colon* extends down the left side of the body. It connects with the *sigmoid colon,* an S-shaped section that joins with the rectum. The **rectum** is the final six to eight inches of the large intestine and is a storage area for indigestibles and wastes. It has a narrow canal, called the *anal canal,* which opens at a hole, called the **anus**. Fecal material, or stool, the final waste product of the digestive process, is expelled through this opening.

ACCESSORY ORGANS

The **liver** (see figure 6-54), is the largest gland in the body and is an accessory organ to the digestive system. It is located under the diaphragm and in the upper right quadrant of the abdomen. The liver secretes bile, which is used to emulsify fats in the digestive tract. Bile also makes fats water soluble, which is necessary for absorption. The liver stores sugar in the form of glycogen. The glycogen is converted to glucose and released into the bloodstream when additional blood sugar is needed. The liver also stores iron and certain vitamins. It produces heparin, which prevents clotting of the blood; blood proteins such as fibrinogen and prothrombin, which aid in clotting of the blood; and cholesterol. Finally, the liver detoxifies (renders less harmful) substances such as alcohol and pesticides, and destroys bacteria that have been taken into the blood from the intestine.

The **gallbladder** is a small, muscular sac located under the liver and attached to it by connective tissue. It stores and concentrates bile,

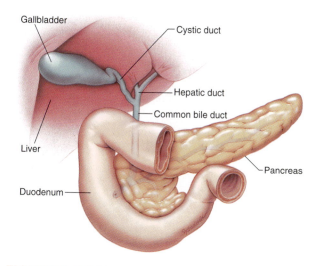

Gallbladder
Cystic duct
Hepatic duct
Common bile duct
Liver
Duodenum
Pancreas

FIGURE 6-54 The liver, gallbladder, and pancreas.

which it receives from the liver. When the bile is needed to emulsify fats in the digestive tract, the gallbladder contracts and pushes the bile through the common bile duct and into the duodenum.

The **pancreas** is a glandular organ located behind the stomach. It produces pancreatic juices, which contain enzymes to digest food. These juices enter the duodenum through the pancreatic duct. The enzymes in the juices include pancreatic amylase or amylopsin (to break down sugars); trypsin and chymotrypsin (to break down proteins); and lipase or steapsin (to act on fats). The pancreas also produces insulin, which is secreted into the bloodstream. Insulin regulates the metabolism, or burning, of carbohydrates to convert glucose (blood sugar) to energy.

DISEASES AND ABNORMAL CONDITIONS

Appendicitis is an acute inflammation of the appendix, usually resulting from an obstruction and infection. Symptoms include generalized abdominal pain that later localizes at the lower right quadrant; nausea and vomiting; mild fever; and elevated white blood cell count. If the appendix ruptures, the infectious material will spill into the peritoneal cavity and cause peritonitis, a serious condition. Appendicitis is treated by an appendectomy (surgical removal of the appendix).

Cholecystitis is an inflammation of the gallbladder. When gallstones form from crystallized cholesterol, bile salts, and bile pigments, the condition is known as *cholelithiasis.* Symptoms frequently occur after eating fatty foods and include indigestion; nausea and vomiting; and pain that starts under the rib cage and radiates to the right shoulder. If a gallstone blocks the bile ducts, the gallbladder can rupture and cause peritonitis. Treatment methods include low-fat diet, lithotripsy (shock waves that are used to shatter the gallstones), and/or a cholecystectomy (surgical removal of the gallbladder).

Cirrhosis is a chronic destruction of liver cells accompanied by the formation of fibrous connective and scar tissue. Causes include hepatitis, bile duct disease, chemical toxins, and malnutrition associated with alcoholism. Symptoms vary and become more severe as the disease progresses. Some common symptoms are liver enlargement; anemia; indigestion; nausea and vomiting, nosebleeds; jaundice (yellow discoloration); and ascites (an accumulation of fluid in the abdominal peritoneal cavity). When the liver fails, disorientation, hallucinations, hepatic coma, and death occur. Treatment is directed toward preventing further damage to the liver. Alcohol avoidance, proper nutrition, vitamin supplements, rest, infection prevention, and appropriate exercise are encouraged.

Constipation is when fecal material remains in the colon too long, causing excessive reabsorption of water. The feces or stool becomes hard, dry, and difficult to eliminate. Causes include poor bowel habits, chronic laxative use leading to a "lazy" bowel, a diet low in fiber, and certain digestive diseases. The condition is usually corrected by a high-fiber diet, adequate fluids, and exercise. Although laxatives are sometimes used to stimulate defecation, frequent laxative use may be habit forming and lead to chronic constipation.

Diarrhea is a condition characterized by frequent watery stools. Causes include infection, stress, diet, an irritated colon, and toxic substances. Diarrhea can be extremely dangerous in infants and small children because of the excessive fluid loss. Treatment is directed toward eliminating the cause, providing adequate fluid intake, and modifying the diet.

Diverticulitis is an inflammation of the diverticula, pouches (or sacs) that form in the intestine as the mucosal lining pushes through the surrounding muscle. When fecal material and bacteria become trapped in the diverticula, inflammation occurs. This can result in an abscess or rupture leading to peritonitis. Symptoms vary depending on the amount of inflammation but may include abdominal pain; irregular bowel movements; flatus (gas); constipation or diarrhea; abdominal distention (swelling); low-grade fever; nausea, and vomiting. Treatment methods include antibiotics, stool-softening medications, pain medications, and, in severe cases, surgery to remove the affected section of colon.

Gastroenteritis is an inflammation of the mucous membrane that lines the stomach and intestinal tract. Causes include food poisoning, infection, and toxins. Symptoms include abdominal cramping, nausea, vomiting, fever, and diarrhea. Usual treatment methods are rest and increased fluid intake. In severe cases, antibiotics, intravenous fluids, and medications to slow peristalsis may be used.

Hemorrhoids are painful, dilated or varicose veins of the rectum and/or anus. They may be caused by straining to defecate, constipation, pressure during pregnancy, insufficient fluid intake, laxative abuse, and prolonged sitting or standing. Symptoms include pain, itching, and bleeding. Treatment methods include a high-fiber diet; increased fluid intake; stool softeners; sitz baths or warm, moist compresses; and, in some cases, a hemorrhoidectomy (surgical removal of the hemorrhoids).

Hepatitis is a viral inflammation of the liver. Type A, HAV, or infectious hepatitis, is highly contagious and is transmitted in food or water contaminated by the feces of an infected person. A vaccine is available to prevent Hepatitis A. Type B, HBV, or serum hepatitis, is transmitted by blood and serum. It is more serious than type A and can lead to chronic hepatitis or to cirrhosis of the liver. A vaccine developed to prevent hepatitis B is recommended for all health care workers. Other strains of the hepatitis virus that have been identified include types C, D, and E. Symptoms include fever, anorexia (lack of appetite), nausea, vomiting, fatigue, dark-colored urine, clay-colored stool, enlarged liver, and jaundice. Treatment methods include rest and a diet high in protein and calories and low in fat. A liver transplant may be necessary if the liver is severely damaged.

A *hernia*, or rupture, occurs when an internal organ pushes through a weakened area or natural opening in a body wall. A hiatal hernia is when the stomach protrudes through the diaphragm and into the chest cavity through the opening for the esophagus, figure 6-55. Symptoms include heartburn, stomach distention, chest pain, and difficult swallowing. Treatment methods include

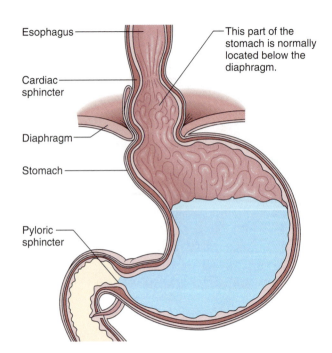

Esophagus

This part of the stomach is normally located below the diaphragm.

Cardiac sphincter

Diaphragm

Stomach

Pyloric sphincter

FIGURE 6-55 A hiatal hernia occurs when the stomach protrudes through the diaphragm.

a bland diet, small frequent meals, staying upright after eating, and surgical repair. An inguinal hernia is when a section of the small intestine protrudes through the inguinal rings of the lower abdominal wall. If the hernia cannot be reduced (pushed back in place), a herniorrhaphy (surgical repair) is performed.

Pancreatitis is an inflammation of the pancreas. The pancreatic enzymes begin to digest the pancreas itself, and the pancreas becomes necrotic, inflamed, and edematous. If the damage extends to blood vessels in the pancreas, hemorrhage and shock occur. Pancreatitis may be caused by excessive alcohol consumption or blockage of pancreatic ducts by gallstones. Many cases are *idiopathic,* or of unknown cause. Symptoms include severe abdominal pain that radiates to the back, nausea, vomiting, diaphoresis (excessive perspiration), and jaundice if swelling blocks the common bile duct. Treatment depends on the cause. A cholecystectomy, removal of the gall bladder, is performed if gallstones are the cause. Analgesics for pain and nutritional support are used if the cause of pancreatitis is alcoholism or idiopathic. This type of pancreatitis has a poor prognosis and often results in death.

Peritonitis, an inflammation of the abdominal peritoneal cavity, usually occurs when a rupture in the intestine allows the intestine contents to enter the peritoneal cavity. A ruptured appendix or gall-bladder can cause this condition. Symptoms include abdominal pain and distention; fever; nausea; and vomiting. Treatment methods include antibiotics and, if necessary, surgical repair of the damaged intestine.

An *ulcer* is an open sore on the lining of the digestive tract. Peptic ulcers include gastric (stomach) ulcers and duodenal ulcers. The major cause is a bacterium, *Helicobacter pylori (H. pylori)*, that burrows into the stomach membranes, allowing stomach acids and digestive juices to create an ulcer. Symptoms include burning pain, indigestion, hematemesis (bloody vomitus), and melena (dark, tarry stool). Usual treatment methods are antacids, a bland diet, decreased stress, and avoidance of irritants such as alcohol, fried foods, tobacco, and caffeine. If the *H. pylori* bacteria are present, treatment with antibiotics and a bismuth preparation, such as Pepto-Bismol, usually cures the condition. In severe cases, surgery is performed to remove the affected area.

Ulcerative colitis is a severe inflammation of the colon accompanied by the formation of ulcers and abscesses. It is thought to be caused by stress, food allergy, or an autoimmune reaction. The main symptom is diarrhea containing blood, pus, and mucus. Other symptoms include weight loss, weakness, abdominal pain, anemia, and anorexia. Periods of remission and exacerbation are common. Treatment is directed toward controlling inflammation, reducing stress with mild sedation, maintaining proper nutrition, and avoiding substances that aggravate the condition. In some cases, surgical removal of the affected colon and creation of a colostomy (an artificial opening in the colon that allows fecal material to be excreted through the abdominal wall) is necessary.

STUDENT: *Go to the workbook and complete the assignment sheet for 6:11, Digestive System.*

6:12 Urinary System

Objectives

After completing this section, you should be able to:

◆ Label a diagram of the urinary system

◆ Explain the action of the following parts of a nephron: glomerulus, Bowman's capsule, convoluted tubule, and collecting tubule

◆ State the functions of the ureter, bladder, and urethra

◆ Explain why the urethra is different in males and females

◆ Interpret at least five terms used to describe conditions affecting urination

◆ Describe at least three diseases of the urinary system

◆ Define, pronounce, and spell all the key terms

KEY TERMS

bladder
Bowman's capsule
cortex
  (core'-tex)
excretory system
  (ex'-kreh-tor"-ee)
glomerulus
  (glow"-mare'-you-luss)

hilum
kidneys
medulla
  (meh-due'-la)
nephrons
  (nef'-ronz)
renal pelvis

ureters
  (you'-reh"-turz)
urethra
  (you"-wreath'-rah)
urinary meatus
  (you'-rih-nah-ree" me-ate'-as)
urinary system
urine

6:12 INFORMATION

The **urinary system**, also known as the **excretory system**, is responsible for removing certain wastes and excess water from the body and for maintaining the body's acid-base balance. The parts of the urinary system are two kidneys, two ureters, one bladder, and one urethra (see figure 6-56).

The **kidneys** (see figure 6-57) are two bean-shaped organs located on either side of the vertebral column, behind the upper part of the abdominal cavity, and separated from this cavity by the peritoneum. The kidneys are protected by the ribs and a heavy cushion of fat. Connective tissue helps hold the kidneys in position. Each kidney is enclosed in a mass of fatty tissue, called an *adipose capsule,* and covered externally by a tough, fibrous tissue, called the *renal fascia,* or *fibrous capsule.*

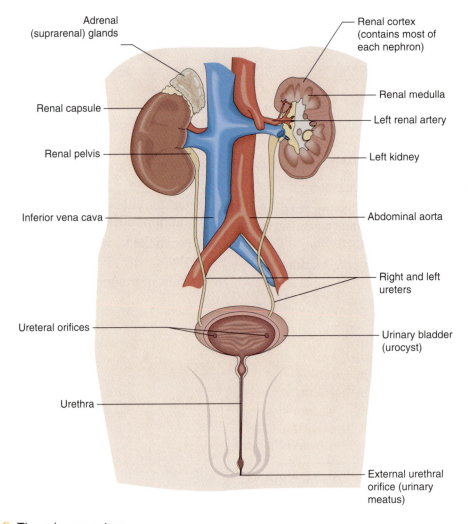

FIGURE 6-56 The urinary system.

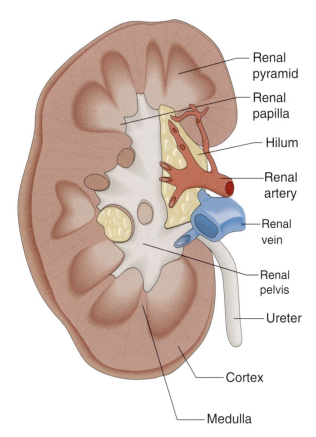

FIGURE 6-57 A cross-section of the kidney.

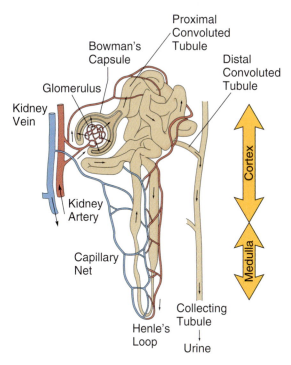

FIGURE 6-58 A nephron unit.

Each kidney is divided into two main sections: the cortex and the medulla. The **cortex** is the outer section of the kidney. It contains most of the nephrons, which aid in the production of urine. The **medulla** is the inner section of the kidney. It contains most of the collecting tubules, which carry the urine from the nephrons through the kidney. Each kidney has a **hilum**, a notched or indented area through which the ureter, nerves, blood vessels, and lymph vessels enter and leave the kidney.

Nephrons (figure 6-58) are microscopic filtering units located in the kidneys. There are more than one million nephrons per kidney. Each nephron consists of a glomerulus, a Bowman's capsule, a proximal convoluted tubule, a distal convoluted tubule, and a collecting duct (tubule). The renal artery carries blood to the kidney. Branches of the renal artery pass through the medulla to the cortex, where the blood enters the first part of the nephron, the **glomerulus** (a cluster of capillaries). As blood passes through the glomerulus, water, mineral salts, sugar, metabolic products, and other substances are filtered out of the blood. Red blood cells and proteins are

not filtered out. The filtered blood leaves the glomerulus and eventually makes its way to the renal vein, which carries it away from the kidney. The substances filtered out in the glomerulus enter the next section of the nephron, the **Bowman's capsule**. The Bowman's capsule is a C-shaped structure that surrounds the glomerulus and is the start of the convoluted tubule. It picks up the materials filtered from the blood in the glomerulus and passes them into the convoluted tubule. As these materials pass through the various sections of the tubule, substances needed by the body are reabsorbed and returned to the blood capillaries. By the time the filtered materials pass through the tubule, most of the water, sugar, vitamins, and mineral salts have been reabsorbed. Excess sugar and mineral salts; some water; and wastes (including urea, uric acid, and creatinine) remain in the tubule and become known as the concentrated liquid called *urine.* The urine then enters collecting ducts, or tubules, located in the medulla. These collecting ducts empty into the **renal pelvis** (renal basin), a funnel-shaped structure which is the first section of the ureter.

The **ureters** are two muscular tubes approximately 10 to 12 inches in length. One extends from the renal pelvis of each kidney to the bladder. Peristalsis (a rhythmic, wavelike motion of muscle) moves the urine through the ureter from the kidney to the bladder.

The **bladder** is a hollow, muscular sac that lies behind the symphysis pubis and at the midline of the pelvic cavity. It has a mucous membrane lining arranged in a series of folds, called *rugae*. The rugae disappear as the bladder expands to fill with urine. Three layers of visceral (smooth) muscle form the walls of the bladder, which receives the urine from the ureters and stores the urine until it is eliminated from the body. Although the urge to void (urinate, or micturate) occurs when the bladder contains approximately 250 cubic centimeters (1 cup) of urine, the bladder can hold much more. A circular sphincter muscle controls the opening to the bladder to prevent emptying. When the bladder is full, receptors in the bladder wall send out a reflex action, which opens the muscle. Infants cannot control this reflex action. As children age, however, they learn to control the reflex.

The **urethra** is the tube that carries the urine from the bladder to the outside. The external opening is called the **urinary meatus**. The urethra is different in females and males. In females, it is a tube approximately 3.75 cm (one and one-half inches) in length that opens in front of the vagina and carries only urine to the outside. In males, the urethra is approximately 20 cm (eight inches) in length and passes through the prostate gland and out through the penis. It carries both urine (from the urinary system) and semen (from the reproductive system), although not at the same time.

Urine is the liquid waste product produced by the urinary system. It is approximately 95 percent water. Waste products dissolved in this liquid are urea, uric acid, creatinine, mineral salts, and various pigments. Excess useful products, such as sugar, can also be found in the urine, but their presence usually indicates disease. Approximately 1,500 to 2,000 cubic centimeters (1½ to 2 quarts) of urine are produced daily from the approximately 150 quarts of liquid that is filtered through the kidneys.

Terms used to describe conditions affecting urination include:

◆ *polyuria:* excessive urination

◆ *oliguria:* below normal amounts of urination

◆ *anuria:* absence of urination

◆ *hematuria:* blood in the urine

◆ *pyuria:* pus in the urine

◆ *nocturia:* urination at night

◆ *dysuria:* painful urination

◆ *retention:* inability to empty the bladder

◆ *incontinence:* involuntary urination

DISEASES AND ABNORMAL CONDITIONS

Cystitis is an inflammation of the bladder, usually caused by pathogens entering the urinary meatus. It is more common in females because of the shortness of the urethra. Symptoms include frequent urination, dysuria, a burning sensation during urination, hematuria, bladder spasm, and fever. Treatment methods are antibiotics and increased fluid intake.

Glomerulonephritis, or nephritis, is an inflammation of the glomerulus of the kidney. *Acute glomerulonephritis* usually follows a streptococcal infection such as strep throat, scarlet fever, or rheumatic fever. Symptoms include chills, fever, fatigue, edema, oliguria, hematuria, and albuminuria (protein in the urine). Treatment methods include rest, restriction of salt, maintenance of fluid and electrolyte balance, antipyretics (for fever), and, at times, antibiotics. With treatment, kidney function is usually restored, and the prognosis is good. Repeated attacks can cause a chronic condition. *Chronic glomerulonephritis* is a progressive disease that causes scarring and sclerosing of the glomeruli. Early symptoms include hematuria, albuminuria, and hypertension. As the disease progresses and additional glomeruli are destroyed, edema, fatigue, anemia, hypertension, congestive heart failure, and, finally, renal failure and death occur. Treatment is directed at treating the symptoms, and treatment methods include a low-sodium diet, antihypertensive drugs, maintenance of fluids and electrolytes, and hemodialysis (removal of the waste products from the blood by a hemodialysis machine), figure 6-59. When both kidneys are severely damaged, a kidney transplant can be performed.

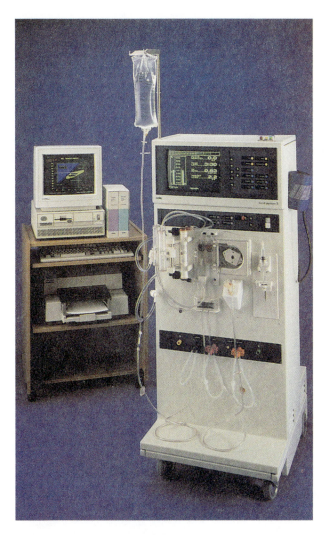

FIGURE 6-59 A hemodialysis machine helps remove waste products from the blood when the kidneys are not functioning correctly.

Pyelonephritis is an inflammation of the kidney tissue and renal pelvis (upper end of the ureter), usually caused by pyogenic (pus-forming) bacteria. Symptoms include chills, fever, back pain, dysuria, hematuria, and pyuria (pus in the urine). Treatment methods are antibiotics and increased fluid intake.

A *renal calculus,* or urinary calculus, is a kidney stone. A calculus is formed when salts in the urine precipitate (settle out of solution). Some small calculi may be eliminated in the urine, but larger stones often become lodged in the renal pelvis or ureter. Symptoms include sudden, intense pain (renal colic); hematuria; and, in some cases, urinary retention. Initial treatment consists of increasing fluids, providing pain medication, and straining all urine through gauze or filter paper to determine whether stones are being eliminated. Lithotripsy is a procedure where shock waves are used to crush the stones so that they can be eliminated through the urine. In some cases, surgery is required to remove the calculi.

Renal failure is when the kidneys stop functioning. *Acute renal failure (ARF)* can be caused by hemorrhage, shock, injury, poisoning, nephritis, or dehydration. Symptoms include oliguria or anuria, headache, an ammonia odor to the breath, edema, cardiac arrhythmia, and uremia. Prompt treatment involving dialysis, restricted fluid intake, and correction of the condition causing renal failure results in a good prognosis. *Chronic renal failure (CRF)* results from the progressive loss of kidney function. It can be caused by chronic glomerulonephritis, hypertension, toxins, and endocrine disease. Waste products accumulate in the blood and affect many body systems. Symptoms include nausea, vomiting, diarrhea, decreased mental ability, convulsions, muscle irritability, an ammonia odor to the breath, perspiration, and, in later stages, coma and death. Treatment methods are dialysis, diet modifications and restrictions, careful skin and mouth care, and control of fluid intake. A kidney transplant is the only cure.

Uremia is a toxic condition that occurs when the kidneys fail and urinary waste products are present in the bloodstream. It can result from any condition that affects the proper functioning of the kidneys, such as renal failure, chronic glomerulonephritis, and hypotension. Symptoms include headache, nausea, vomiting, an ammonia odor to the breath, oliguria or anuria, mental confusion, coma, and, eventually, death. Treatment consists of a restricted diet and dialysis until a kidney transplant can be performed.

Urethritis is an inflammation of the urethra, usually caused by bacteria (such as gonococcus), viruses, or chemicals (such as bubble bath solutions). Symptoms include frequent and painful urination, redness and itching at the urinary meatus, and a purulent (pus) discharge. Treatment methods include sitz baths or warm, moist compresses; antibiotics; and/or increased fluid intake.

STUDENT: *Go to the workbook and complete the assignment sheet for 6:12, Urinary System.*

6:13 Endocrine System

Objectives

After completing this section, you should be able to:

◆ Label a diagram of the main endocrine glands

◆ Describe how hormones influence various body functions

◆ Describe at least five diseases of the endocrine glands

◆ Define, pronounce, and spell all the key terms

KEY TERMS

adrenal glands
    (ah″-dree′-nal)
endocrine system
    (en′-doh″-krin)
hormones
ovaries

pancreas
    (pan-kree-as)
parathyroid glands
pineal body
    (pin′-knee″-ahl)
pituitary gland
    (pih″-too′-ih-tar-ee)

placenta
testes
    (tess′-tees)
thymus
thyroid gland

RELATED HEALTH CAREERS

◆ Endocrinologist

◆ Nuclear Medicine Technologist

6:13 INFORMATION

The **endocrine system** consists of a group of ductless (without tubes) glands that secrete substances directly into the bloodstream. These substances are called *hormones.* The endocrine system consists of the pituitary gland, thyroid gland, parathyroid gland, adrenal glands, pancreas, ovaries, testes, thymus, pineal body, and placenta (see figure 6-60).

Hormones, the substances produced and secreted by the endocrine glands, are frequently called "chemical messengers." They are transported throughout the body by the bloodstream and perform many functions, including stimulating exocrine glands (glands with ducts, or tubes) to produce secretions, stimulating other endocrine glands, regulating growth and development, regulating metabolism, maintaining fluid and chemical balance, and controlling various sex processes. Table 6-3 lists the main hormones produced by each endocrine gland and the actions they perform.

PITUITARY GLAND

The **pituitary gland** is often called the "master gland" of the body because it produces many hormones that affect other glands. It is located at the base of the brain in the sella turcica, a small, bony depression of the sphenoid bone. It is divided into two sections, or lobes: the anterior lobe and the posterior lobe. Each lobe secretes certain hormones, as shown in table 6-3.

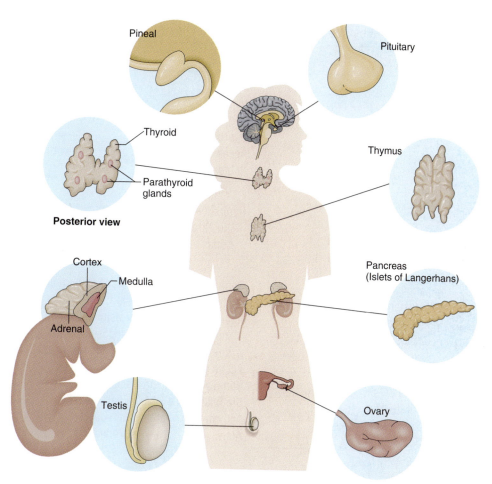

FIGURE 6-60 The endocrine system.

TABLE 6-3 Hormones Produced by the Endocrine Glands and Their Actions

GLAND	HORMONE	ACTION
Pituitary		
Anterior lobe	ACTH—adrenocorticotropic	Stimulates growth and secretion of the cortex of the adrenal gland
	TSH—thyrotropin	Stimulates growth and secretion of the thyroid gland
	GH—somatotropin	Growth hormone, stimulates normal body growth
	FSH—follicle stimulating	Stimulates growth and hormone production in the ovarian follicles of female, production of sperm in males
	LH—Luteinizing (female) *or*	Causes ovulation and secretion of progesterone in females
	ICSH—Interstitial cell-stimulating (male)	Stimulates testes to secrete testosterone
	LTH—Lactogenic or prolactin	Stimulates secretion of milk from mammary glands
	MSH—Melanocyte stimulating	Stimulates production and dispersion of melanin pigment in the skin
Posterior lobe	ADH—Vasopressin	Antidiuretic, promotes reabsorption of water in kidneys, constricts blood vessels
	Oxytocin (pitocin)	Cause contraction of uterus during childbirth, stimulates milk flow from the breasts

(continued)

TABLE 6-3 Hormones Produced by the Endocrine Glands and Their Actions *(Continued)*

GLAND	HORMONE	ACTION
Thyroid	Thyroxine and triiodothyronine	Increase metabolic rate, stimulate physical and mental growth, regulate metabolism of carbohydrates, fats, and proteins
	Thyrocalcitonin or calcitonin	Accelerates absorption of calcium by the bones and lowers blood calcium level
Parathyroid	Parathormone (PTH)	Regulates amount of calcium and phosphate in the blood, increases reabsorption of calcium and phosphates from bones
Adrenal Cortex	Mineralocorticoids Aldosterone	Regulate the reabsorption of sodium in the kidney and the elimination of potassium

	Glucocorticoids
	   Cortisol-hydrocortisone
	   Cortisone
		Aid in metabolism of proteins, fats, and carbohydrates; increase amount of glucose in blood; provide resistance to stress; and depress immune responses (anti-inflammatory)

	Gonadocorticoids
	   Estrogens
	   Androgens
		Act as sex hormones
		 Stimulate female sexual characteristics
		 Stimulate male sexual characteristics

Medulla	Epinephrine (adrenaline) Norepinephrine	Activates sympathetic nervous system, acts in stress Activates body in stress situations
Pancreas	Insulin	Used in metabolism of glucose (sugar) by promoting entry of glucose into cells
	Glucagon	Maintains blood level of glucose
Ovaries	Estrogen Progesterone	Promotes growth and development of sex organs in female Maintains lining of uterus
Testes	Testosterone	Stimulates growth and development of sex organs in the male
Thymus	Thymosin	Stimulates production of antibodies in early life
Pineal	Melatonin	May delay puberty by inhibiting gonadotropic (sex) hormones, may regulate sleep/wake cycles
	Adrenoglomerulotropin Serotonin	May stimulate adrenal cortex to secrete aldosterone May prevent vasoconstriction of blood vessels in the brain
Placenta	Estrogen	Stimulates growth of reproductive organs
	Chorionic gonadotropin	Causes corpus luteum of ovary to continue secretions
	Progesterone	Maintains lining of uterus to provide fetal nutrition

Diseases and Abnormal Conditions

Acromegaly results from an oversecretion of somatotropin (growth hormone) in an adult and is usually caused by a tumor of the pituitary. Bones of the hands, feet, and face enlarge and create a grotesque appearance. The skin and tongue thicken, and slurred speech develops. Surgical removal and/or radiation of the tumor is the usual treatment.

Giantism results from an oversecretion of somatotropin before puberty (see figure 6-61). It causes excessive growth of long bones, extreme tallness, decreased sexual development, and, at times, retarded mental development. If a tumor is involved, surgical removal or radiation is the treatment.

Diabetes insipidus is caused by decreased secretion of vasopressin, or antidiuretic hormone (ADH). A low level of ADH prevents water from being reabsorbed in the kidneys. Symptoms include polyuria (excessive urination), polydipsia (excessive thirst), dehydration, weakness, constipation, and dry skin. The condition is corrected by administering ADH.

Dwarfism results from an undersecretion of somatotropin and can be caused by a tumor, infection, genetic factors, or injury. It is characterized by small body size, short extremities, and lack of sexual development. Mental development is normal. If the condition is diagnosed early, it can be treated with injections of somatotropic

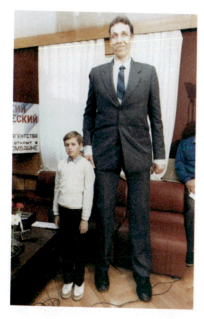

FIGURE 6-61 Giantism results when the pituitary gland secretes excessive amounts of somatotropin (growth hormone) before puberty.

hormone for five or more years until long bone growth is complete.

THYROID GLAND

The **thyroid gland** synthesizes hormones that regulate the body's metabolism and control the level of calcium in the blood. It is located in front of the upper part of the trachea (windpipe) in the neck. It has two lobes, one on either side of the larynx (voice box), connected by the isthmus, a small piece of tissue. In order to produce its hormones, the thyroid gland requires iodine, which is obtained from certain foods and iodized salt (see table 6-3).

Diseases and Abnormal Conditions

A *goiter* is an enlargement of the thyroid gland. Causes can include a hyperactive thyroid, an iodine deficiency, an oversecretion of thyroid stimulating hormone on the part of the pituitary gland, or a tumor. Symptoms include thyroid enlargement, dysphagia (difficult swallowing), a cough, and a choking sensation. Treatment is directed toward eliminating the cause. For example, iodine is given if a deficiency exists. Surgery may be performed to remove very large goiters.

Hyperthyroidism is an overactivity of the thyroid gland, which causes increased production of thyroid hormones and increased basal metabolic rate (BMR). Symptoms include extreme nervousness, tremors, irritability, rapid pulse, weight loss, goiter formation, and hypertension. Treatment consists of either radiation to destroy part of the thyroid or a thyroidectomy (surgical removal of the thyroid).

Graves' disease is a severe form of hyperthyroidism more common in women than men. Symptoms include a strained and tense facial expression, exophthalmia (protruding eyeballs), goiter, nervous irritability, emotional instability, tachycardia, a tremendous appetite accompanied by weight loss, and diarrhea. Treatment methods include medication to inhibit the synthesis of thyroxine, radioactive iodine to destroy thyroid tissue, and/or a thyroidectomy.

Hypothyroidism is an underactivity of the thyroid gland and a deficiency of thyroid hormones. Two main forms exist: *cretinism* and *myxedema*. Cretinism develops in infancy or early childhood and results in a lack of mental and physical growth, leading to mental retardation and an abnormal, dwarfed stature. If diagnosed early, oral thyroid hormone can be given to minimize mental and physical damage. Myxedema occurs in later childhood or adulthood. Symptoms include coarse, dry skin; slow mental function; fatigue; weakness; intolerance of cold; weight gain; edema; puffy eyes; and a slow pulse. Treatment consists of administering oral thyroid hormone to restore normal metabolism.

PARATHYROID GLANDS

The **parathyroid glands** are four small glands located behind and attached to the thyroid gland. Their hormone regulates the amount of calcium in the blood (see table 6-3). It stimulates bone cells to break down bone tissue and release calcium and phosphates into the blood, causes the kidneys to conserve and reabsorb calcium, and activates intestinal cells to absorb calcium from digested foods. Although most of the body's calcium is in the bones, the calcium circulating in the blood is very important for blood clotting, the tone of heart muscle, and muscle contraction. Because there is a constant exchange of calcium and phosphate between the bones and blood, the parathyroid hormone plays an important function in maintaining the proper level of circulating calcium.

Diseases and Abnormal Conditions

Hyperparathyroidism is an overactivity of the parathyroid gland, resulting in an overproduction of parathormone. This results in hypercalcemia (increased calcium in the blood), which leads to renal calculi (kidney stones) formation, lethargy, gastrointestinal disturbances, and calcium deposits on the walls of blood vessels and organs. Because the calcium is drawn from the bones, they become weak, deformed, and likely to fracture. This condition is often caused by an adenoma (glandular tumor), and removal of the tumor usually results in normal parathyroid function.

Hypoparathyroidism is an underactivity of the parathyroid gland, which causes a low level of calcium in the blood. Symptoms include tetany (a sustained muscular contraction), hyperirritability

of the nervous system, and convulsive twitching. Death can occur if the larynx and respiratory muscles are involved. The condition is easily treated with calcium, vitamin D (which increases the absorption of calcium from the digestive tract), and parathormone.

ADRENAL GLANDS

The **adrenal glands** are frequently called the "suprarenal" glands because one is located above each kidney. Each gland has two parts: the outer portion or cortex, and the inner portion, or medulla. The adrenal cortex secretes many steroid hormones, which are classified into three groups: mineralocorticoids, glucocorticoids, and gonadocorticoids. The groups and the main hormones in each group are listed in table 6-3. The adrenal medulla secretes two main hormones: epinephrine and norepinephrine. These hormones are sympathomimetic, meaning that they mimic the sympathetic nervous system and cause the fight or flight response.

Diseases and Abnormal Conditions

Addison's disease is caused by decreased secretion of aldosterone on the part of the adrenal cortex. This interferes with the reabsorption of sodium and water and causes an increased level of potassium in the blood. Symptoms include dehydration, hypotension (low blood pressure), mental lethargy, weight loss, muscle weakness, excessive pigmentation leading to a "bronzing" (yellow-brown color) of the skin, hypoglycemia (low blood sugar), and edema. Treatment methods include steroid hormones, controlled intake of sodium, and fluid regulation to combat dehydration.

Cushing's syndrome results from an oversecretion of glucocorticoids on the part of the adrenal cortex. It can be caused by either a tumor of the adrenal cortex or excess production of ACTH on the part of the pituitary gland. Symptoms include hyperglycemia (high blood sugar), hypertension, muscle weakness, poor wound healing, a tendency to bruise easily, a "moon" face, and obesity. If a tumor is causing the disease, treatment is removal of the tumor. If the glands are removed, hormonal therapy is required to replace the missing hormones.

PANCREAS

The **pancreas** is a fish-shaped organ located behind the stomach. It is both an exocrine gland and an endocrine gland. As an exocrine gland, it secretes pancreatic juices, which are carried to the small intestine by the pancreatic duct to aid in the digestion of food. Special B, or beta, cells located throughout the pancreas in patches of tissue called *islets of Langerhans* produce the hormone insulin, which is needed for the cells to absorb sugar from the blood. Alpha, or A, cells produce the hormone glucagon, which increases the glucose level in blood (see table 6-3).

Disease

Diabetes mellitus is a chronic disease caused by decreased secretion of insulin. The metabolism of carbohydrates, proteins, and fats is affected. There are two main types of diabetes mellitus named according to the age of onset and need for insulin. Insulin-dependent diabetes mellitus (IDDM), or Type 1, usually occurs early in life, is more severe, and requires insulin. Noninsulin-dependent diabetes mellitus (NIDDM), or Type 2, is the mature-onset form of diabetes mellitus. It frequently occurs in obese adults and is controlled with diet and/or oral hypoglycemic (lower-blood-sugar) medications. The main symptoms include hyperglycemia (high blood sugar), polyuria (excessive urination), polydipsia (thirst), polyphagia (hunger), glycosuria (sugar in the urine), weight loss, fatigue, slow healing of skin infections, and vision changes. If the condition is not treated, diabetic coma and death may occur. Treatment methods are a carefully regulated diet to control the blood sugar level, regulated exercise, and oral hypoglycemic drugs or insulin injections.

OTHER ENDOCRINE GLANDS

The **ovaries** are the gonads, or sex glands, of the female. They are located in the pelvic cavity, one on each side of the uterus. They secrete hormones that regulate menstruation and secondary sexual characteristics (see table 6-3).

The **testes** are the gonads of the male. They are located in the scrotal sac and are suspended outside the body. They produce hormones that regulate sexual characteristics of the male (see table 6-3).

The **thymus** is a mass of tissue located in the upper part of the chest and under the sternum. It contains lymphoid tissue. The thymus is active in early life, activating cells in the immune system, but atrophies (wastes away) during puberty, when it becomes a small mass of connective tissue and fat. It produces one hormone, thymosin (see table 6-3).

The **pineal body** is a small structure attached to the roof of the third ventricle in the brain. Knowledge regarding the physiology of this gland is limited. Three main hormones secreted by this gland are listed in table 6-3.

The **placenta** is a temporary endocrine gland produced during pregnancy. It acts as a link between the mother and infant, provides nutrition for the developing infant, and promotes lactation (the production of milk in the breasts). It is expelled after the birth of the child (when it is called *afterbirth*). Three hormones secreted by this gland are listed in table 6-3.

STUDENT: *Go to the workbook and complete the assignment sheet for 6:13, Endocrine System.*

6:14 Reproductive System

Objectives

After completing this section, you should be able to:

- Label a diagram of the male reproductive system
- Trace the pathway of sperm from where they are produced to where they are expelled from the body
- Identify at least three organs of the male reproductive system that secrete fluids added to semen

- Label a diagram of the female reproductive system
- Describe how an ovum is released from an ovary
- Explain the action of the endometrium
- Describe at least six diseases of the reproductive systems
- Define, pronounce, and spell all the key terms

KEY TERMS

Bartholin's glands
(Bar'-tha-lens)

breasts

Cowper's glands
(Cow'-purrs)

ejaculatory ducts
(ee-jack'-you-lah-tore''-ee)

endometrium
(en''-doe-me'-tree-um)

epididymis
(eh''-pih-did'-ih-muss)

fallopian tubes
(fah-low'-pea''-an)

fertilization
(fur''-til-ih-zay'-shun)

labia majora
(lay'-bee''-ah mah''-jore'-ah)

labia minora
(lay'-bee''-ah ma-nore'-ah)

ovaries

penis

perineum
(pear''-ih-knee'-um)

prostate gland

reproductive system

scrotum
(skrow'-tum)

seminal vesicles
(sem'-ih-null ves'-ik-ullz)

testes
(tes'-tees)

urethra

uterus

vagina
(vah-jie'-nah)

vas deferens
(vass deaf'-eh-rens)

vestibule

vulva
(vull'-vah)

RELATED HEALTH CAREERS

- Embryologist
- Genetic Counselor
- Gynecologist
- Midwife
- Obstetrician
- Ultrasound Technologist, (Sonographer)

6:14 INFORMATION

The function of the **reproductive system** is to produce new life. Although the anatomical parts differ in males and females, the reproductive systems of both have the same types of organs: gonads (sex glands); ducts (tubes) to carry the sex cells and secretions; and accessory organs.

MALE REPRODUCTIVE SYSTEM

The male reproductive system consists of the testes, epididymis, vas deferens, seminal vesicles, ejaculatory ducts, urethra, prostate gland, Cowper's glands, and penis (see figure 6-62).

The male gonads are the **testes**. The two testes are located in the **scrotum**, a sac suspended between the thighs. The testes produce the male sex cells called *sperm,* or *spermatozoa.* Because the scrotum is located outside the body, the temperature in the scrotum is lower than that inside the body. This lower temperature is essential for the production of sperm. The testes also produce male hormones. The main hormone is testosterone, which aids in the maturation of the sperm and also is responsible for the secondary male sex characteristics such as body hair, facial hair, large muscles, and a deep voice.

After the sperm develop in tubes in the testes, they enter the **epididymis**. The epididymis is a tightly coiled tube approximately 20 feet in length and located in the scrotum and above the testes. It stores the sperm while they mature and become motile (able to move by themselves). It also produces a fluid that becomes part of the semen (fluid released during ejaculation). The epididymis connects with the next tube, the vas deferens.

The **vas deferens**, also called the *ductus deferens,* receives the sperm and fluid from the epididymis. On each side, a vas deferens joins with

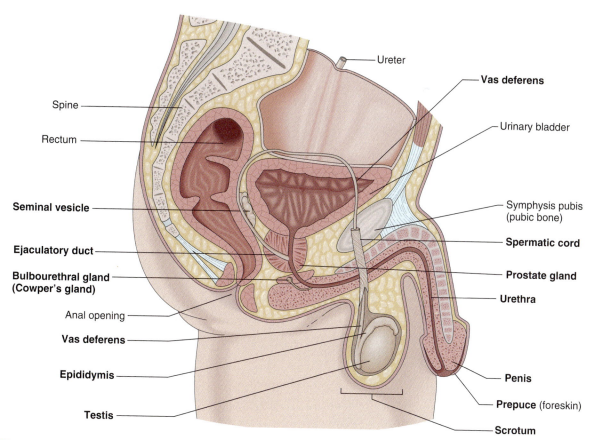

Spine

Rectum

Seminal vesicle

Ejaculatory duct

Bulbourethral gland (Cowper's gland)

Anal opening

Vas deferens

Epididymis

Testis

Ureter

Vas deferens

Urinary bladder

Symphysis pubis (pubic bone)

Spermatic cord

Prostate gland

Urethra

Penis

Prepuce (foreskin)

Scrotum

FIGURE 6-62 The male reproductive system.

the epididymis and extends up into the abdominal cavity, where it curves behind the urinary bladder and joins with a seminal vesicle. Each vas deferens acts as both a passageway and a temporary storage area for sperm. The vas deferens are also the tubes that are cut during a *vasectomy* (procedure to produce sterility in the male).

The **seminal vesicles** are two small pouch-like tubes located behind the bladder and near the junction of the vas deferens and the ejaculatory ducts. They contain a glandular lining. This lining produces a thick, yellow fluid that is rich in sugar and other substances and provides nourishment for the sperm. This fluid composes a large part of the semen.

The **ejaculatory ducts** are two short tubes formed by the union of the vas deferens and the seminal vesicles. They carry the sperm and fluids known collectively as *semen* through the prostate gland and into the urethra.

The **prostate gland** is a doughnut-shaped gland located below the urinary bladder and on either side of the urethra. It produces an alkaline secretion that both increases sperm motility and neutralizes the acidity in the vagina, providing a

more favorable environment for the sperm. The muscular tissue in the prostate contracts during ejaculation (expulsion of the semen from the body) to aid in the expulsion of the semen into the urethra. When the prostate contracts, it also closes off the urethra, preventing urine passage through the urethra.

Cowper's (or bulbourethral) **glands**, are two small glands located below the prostate and connected by small tubes to the urethra. They secrete mucus, which serves as a lubricant for intercourse, and an alkaline fluid, which decreases the acidity of the urine residue in the urethra, providing a more favorable environment for the sperm.

The **urethra** is the tube that extends from the urinary bladder, through the penis, and to the outside of the body. It carries urine, from the urinary bladder, and semen, from the reproductive tubes.

The **penis** is the external male reproductive organ and is located in front of the scrotum. At the distal end is an enlarged structure, called the *glans penis*. The glans penis is covered with a prepuce (foreskin), which is sometimes removed surgically in a procedure called a *circumcision*. The penis is made of spongy, erectile tissue. During sexual arousal, the spaces in this tissue fill with blood, causing the penis to become erect. The penis functions as the male organ of copulation, or intercourse; deposits the semen in the vagina; and provides for the elimination of urine from the bladder through the urethra.

Diseases and Abnormal Conditions

Epididymitis is an inflammation of the epididymis, usually caused by a pathogenic organism such as gonococcus, streptococcus, or staphylococcus. Symptoms include intense pain in the testes, swelling, and fever. Treatment methods include antibiotics, cold applications, scrotal support, and pain medication.

Orchitis is an inflammation of the testes, usually caused by mumps, pathogens, or injury. It can lead to atrophy of the testes and cause sterility. Symptoms include swelling of the scrotum, pain, and fever. Treatment methods include antibiotics (if indicated), antipyretics (for fever), scrotal support, and pain medication.

Prostatic hypertrophy, or hyperplasia, is an enlargement of the prostate gland. Common in men over age 50, prostatic hypertrophy can be a benign condition, caused by inflammation, a tumor, or a change in hormonal activity, or a malignant (cancerous) condition. A screening blood test, called a prostatic-specific antigen (PSA) test, can detect a substance released by cancer cells to aid in early diagnosis of prostatic cancer. Symptoms of prostatic hypertrophy include difficulty in starting to urinate, frequent urination, nocturia (voiding at night), dribbling, urinary infections, and, when the urethra is blocked, urinary retention. Initial treatment methods include fluid restriction, antibiotics (for infections), and prostatic massage. When hypertrophy causes urinary retention, a prostatectomy (surgical removal of all or part of the prostate) is necessary. A transurethral resection (TUR), removal of part of the prostate, is performed by inserting a scope into the urethra and resecting, or removing, the enlarged area. A prostatectomy can also be done by a perineal, or suprapubic (above the pubis bone), incision. If the condition is malignant, a prostatectomy, orchidectomy (removal of the testes), radiation, and estrogen therapy (to decrease the effects of testosterone) are the main treatments.

Testicular cancer, or cancer of the testes, occurs most frequently in men from age 20 to 35.

It is a highly malignant form of cancer and can metastasize, or spread, rapidly. Symptoms include a painless swelling of the testes, a heavy feeling, and an accumulation of fluid. Treatment includes an *orchiectomy*, or surgical removal of the testis, chemotherapy, and/or radiation. It has been recommended that men begin monthly testicular self-examinations at the age of 15. To perform the examination, the male should examine the testicles after a warm shower when scrotal skin is relaxed. Each testicle should be examined separately with both hands by placing the index and middle fingers under the testicle and the thumbs on top. The testicle should be rolled gently between the fingers to feel for lumps, nodules, or extreme tenderness. In addition, the male should examine the testes for any signs of swelling or changes in appearance. If any abnormalities are noted, the male should be examined by a physician as soon as possible.

FEMALE REPRODUCTIVE SYSTEM

The female reproductive system consists of the ovaries, fallopian tubes, uterus, vagina, Bartholin's glands, vulva, and breasts (see figure 6-63).

The **ovaries** are the female gonads (see figure 6-64). They are small, almond-shaped glands located in the pelvic cavity and attached to the uterus by ligaments. The ovaries contain thousands of small sacs called *follicles*. Each follicle contains an immature ovum, or female sex cell. When an ovum matures, the follicle enlarges and then ruptures to release the mature ovum. This process, called *ovulation*, usually occurs once every 28 days. The ovaries also produce hormones that aid in the development of the reproductive organs and produce secondary sexual characteristics.

The **fallopian tubes** are two tubes, each approximately five inches in length and attached to the upper part of the uterus. The lateral ends of these tubes are located above the ovaries but are not directly connected to the ovaries. These ends have fingerlike projections, called *fimbriae*. The fimbriae help move the ovum, which is released by the ovary, into the fallopian tube. Each fallopian tube serves as a passageway for the ovum as the ovum moves from the ovary to the uterus. The muscle layers of the tube move

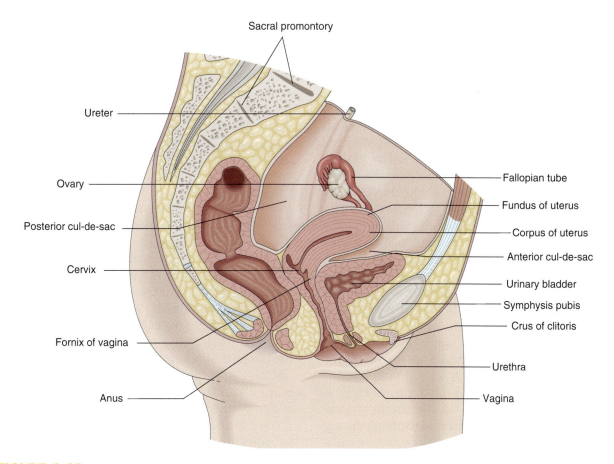

FIGURE 6-63 The female reproductive system.

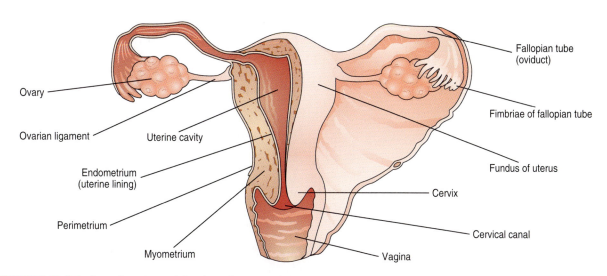

FIGURE 6-64 Anterior view of the female reproductive system.

the ovum by peristalsis. Cilia, hairlike structures on the lining of the tubes, also keep the ovum moving toward the uterus. **Fertilization**, the union of the ovum and a sperm to create a new life, usually takes place in the fallopian tubes.

The **uterus** is a hollow, muscular, pear-shaped organ located behind the urinary bladder and in front of the rectum. It is divided into three parts: the fundus (the top section, where the fallopian tubes attach); the body, or corpus (the middle section); and the cervix (the narrow, bottom section, which attaches to the vagina). The uterus is the organ of menstruation; allows for the development and growth of the fetus; and contracts to aid in expulsion of the fetus during birth. The uterus has three layers. The inner layer is called the **endometrium**. This layer of specialized epithelium provides for implantation of a fertilized ovum and aids in the development of the fetus. If fertilization does not occur, the endometrium deteriorates and causes the bleeding known as *menstruation*. The middle layer of the uterus, the *myometrium*, is a muscle layer. It allows for the expansion of the uterus during pregnancy and contracts to expel the fetus during birth. The outer layer, the *perimetrium*, is a serous membrane.

The **vagina** is a muscular tube that connects the cervix of the uterus to the outside of the body. It serves as a passageway for the menstrual flow; receives the sperm and semen from the male; is the female organ of copulation; and acts as the birth canal during delivery of the infant. The vagina is lined with a mucous membrane arranged in folds called rugae. The rugae allow the vagina to enlarge during childbirth and intercourse.

Bartholin's glands, also called *vestibular glands,* are two small glands located one on each side of the vaginal opening. They secrete mucus for lubrication during intercourse.

The **vulva** is the collective name for the structures that form the external female genital area (see figure 6-65). The mons veneris, or mons pubis, is the triangular pad of fat that is covered with hair and lies over the pubic area. The **labia majora** are the two large folds of fatty tissue that are covered with hair on their outer surfaces; they enclose and protect the vagina. The **labia minora** are the two smaller hairless folds of tissue that are located within the labia majora. The area of the vulva located inside the labia minora is called the **vestibule**. It contains the openings to the urethra and the vagina. An area of erectile

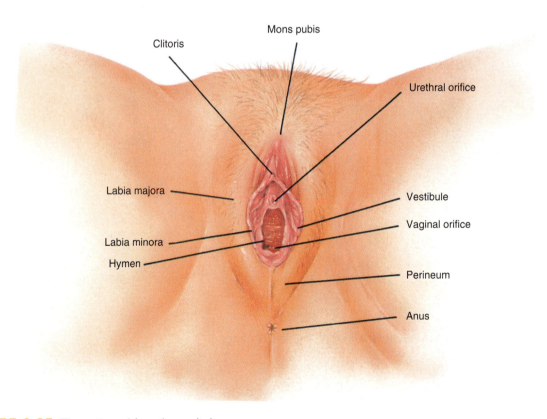

FIGURE 6-65 The external female genital area.

tissue, called the *clitoris,* is located at the junction of the labia minora. It produces sexual arousal when stimulated directly or indirectly during intercourse. The **perineum** is defined as the area between the vagina and anus in the female, although it can be used to describe the entire pelvic floor in both the male and female.

The **breasts**, or mammary glands, contain lobes separated into sections by connective and fatty tissue. Milk ducts located in the tissue exit on the surface at the nipples. The main function of the glands is to secrete milk (lactate) after childbirth.

Diseases and Abnormal Conditions

Breast tumors can be benign or malignant. Symptoms include a lump or mass in the breast tissue, a change in breast size or shape (flattening or bulging of tissue), and a discharge from the nipple. Breast self-examination (BSE) can often detect tumors early (see figure 6-66). The American Cancer Society recommends that an adult female should do a BSE every month at the end of menstruation, or on a scheduled day of the month after menopause. The breasts should be examined in front of a mirror to observe for changes in appearance, in a warm shower after soaping the breasts, and while lying flat in a supine position. A physician should be contacted immediately if any abnormalities are found. In addition, the American Cancer Society recommends that women between the ages of 35 to 40 years should have a baseline mammogram. Between ages 40 and 49, women should have a mammogram every one to two years, and after age 50, women should have a mammogram every year. Mammograms and ultrasonography can often detect tumors or masses up to two years before the tumor or mass could be felt. Treatment methods

HOW TO DO BSE

1. Lie down and put a pillow under your right shoulder. Place your right arm behind your head.
2. Use the finger pads of the three middle fingers on your left hand to feel for lumps or thickening. Your finger pads are the top third of each finger.

4. Move around the breast in a set way. You can choose either the circle (A), the up and down (B), or the wedge (C). Do it the same way every time. It will help you to make sure that you've gone over the entire breast area and to remember how your breast feels each month.

5. Now, examine your left breast using right hand finger pads.

   You might want to check your breasts while standing in front of a mirror right after you do your BSE each month. You might also want to do an extra BSE while you're in the shower. Your soapy hands will glide over the wet skin making it easy to check how your breasts feel.

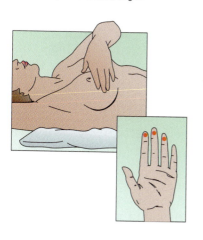

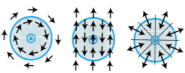

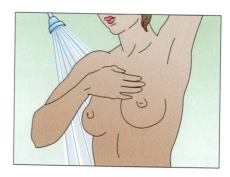

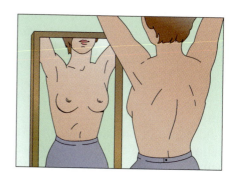

3. Press hard enough to know how your breast feels. If you are not sure how hard to press, ask your health care provider. Or try to copy the way your health care provider uses the finger pads during a breast exam. Learn what your breast feels like most of the time. A firm ridge in the lower curve of each breast is normal.

FIGURE 6-66 Breast self-examination (BSE) can often detect tumors early. *(Courtesy of the American Cancer Society)*

for breast tumors include a lumpectomy (removal of the tumor), a simple mastectomy (surgical removal of the breast), or a radical mastectomy (surgical removal of the tissue, underlying muscles, and axillary lymph nodes). If the tumor is malignant, chemotherapy and/or radiation are usually used in addition to surgery.

Cancer of the cervix and/or uterus is common in females. Cervical cancer can be detected early by a Pap smear. Symptoms of cervical cancer include abnormal vaginal discharge and bleeding. Symptoms of uterine cancer include an enlarged uterus, a watery discharge, and abnormal bleeding. Treatment methods include a hysterectomy (surgical removal of the uterus and cervix) or panhysterectomy (surgical removal of the uterus, ovaries, and fallopian tubes); chemotherapy; and/or radiation.

Endometriosis is the abnormal growth of endometrial tissue outside the uterus. The tissue can be transferred from the uterus by the fallopian tubes, blood, or lymph, or during surgery. It usually becomes embedded in a structure in the pelvic area, such as the ovaries or the peritoneal tissues, and constantly grows and sheds. Endometriosis can cause sterility if the fallopian tubes become blocked with scar tissue. Symptoms include pelvic pain, abnormal bleeding, and dysmenorrhea (painful menstruation). Treatment methods vary with the age of the patient and the degree of abnormal growth but can include hormonal therapy, pain medications, and/or surgical removal of affected organs.

Ovarian cancer is one of the most common causes of cancer deaths in women. It frequently occurs between ages 40 and 65. Initial symptoms are vague and include abdominal discomfort and mild gastrointestinal disturbances such as constipation and/or diarrhea. As the disease progresses, pain, abdominal distention, and urinary frequency occur. Treatment includes surgical removal of all of the reproductive organs and affected lymph nodes, chemotherapy, and radiation in some cases.

Pelvic inflammatory disease (PID) is an inflammation of the cervix, the endometrium of the uterus, fallopian tubes, and, at times, the ovaries. It is usually caused by pathogenic organisms such as bacteria, viruses, and fungi. Symptoms include pain in the lower abdomen, fever, and a purulent (pus) vaginal discharge. Treatment methods include antibiotics, increased fluid intake, rest, and/or pain medication.

Premenstrual syndrome (PMS) is actually a group of symptoms that appear three to fourteen days before menstruation. A large percentage of women experience some degree of PMS. The cause is unknown but may be related to a hormonal or biochemical imbalance; poor nutrition; or stress. Symptoms vary and may include nervousness, irritability, depression, headache, edema, backache, constipation, abdominal bloating, temporary weight gain, and breast tenderness and enlargement. Treatment is geared mainly toward relieving symptoms, and methods include diet modification, exercise, stress reduction, and/or medications to relieve the emotional symptoms.

SEXUALLY TRANSMITTED DISEASES

Sexually transmitted diseases (STDs), or venereal diseases, affect both males and females. The incidence of these diseases has increased greatly in recent years, especially among young people. If not treated, STDs can cause serious chronic conditions and, in some cases, sterility or death.

Acquired immune deficiency syndrome (AIDS) is caused by a virus called the *human immunodeficiency virus (HIV)*. This virus attacks the body's immune system, rendering the immune system unable to fight off certain infections and diseases, and, eventually, causing death. The virus is spread through sexual secretions or blood, and from an infected mother to her infant during pregnancy or childbirth.

The HIV virus does not live long outside the body and is not transmitted by casual, nonsexual contact. Individuals infected with HIV can remain free of any symptoms for years after infection. During this asymptomatic period, infected individuals can transmit the virus to any other individual with whom they exchange sexual secretions, blood, or blood products. After this initial asymptomatic period, many individuals develop HIV symptomatic infection, formerly called AIDS-related complex (ARC). Symptoms include a positive blood test for antibodies to the HIV virus, lack of infection resistance, appetite loss, weight loss, recurrent fever, night sweats, skin rashes, diarrhea, fatigue, and swollen lymph nodes. When the HIV virus causes a critical low level (below 200 cells per cubic millimeter of blood) of special leukocytes (white blood cells) called CD4 or T cells, and/or opportunistic diseases appear, AIDS is diagnosed. Three of the most common opportunistic diseases include the rare type of pneumonia called *Pneumocystis carinii*, a yeast infection called *Candidiasis,* and the slow-growing cancer called Kaposi's sarcoma (see figure 6-67).

At present, there is no cure for AIDS, although much research is being directed toward developing a vaccine to prevent and drugs to cure AIDS. One drug currently in use is Zidovudine (formerly AZT). Treatment with a combination of drugs, commonly called a "drug cocktail," is also used to slow the progression of the disease. These drugs, however, do not cure the disease. Although several other experimental drugs are currently being tested, many patients cannot tolerate the side effects and bone marrow toxicity of these drugs. Prevention is the best method in dealing with AIDS. Standard precautions should be followed while handling blood, body secretions, and sexual secretions. High-risk sexual activities, such as having multiple partners, should be avoided. A condom and an effective spermicide should be used to form a protective barrier during intercourse. The use of drugs and sharing of intravenous (IV) needles should be avoided. Females infected with HIV should avoid pregnancy. *Everyone* must concern themselves with eliminating the transmission of AIDS.

Chlamydia is one of the most frequently occurring STDs and is caused by several strains of the chlamydia organism, a specialized bacterium that lives as an intracellular parasite. Symptoms are similar to those of gonorrhea. Males experience burning when urinating and a mucoid discharge. Females are frequently asymptomatic, although some may have a vaginal discharge. The disease frequently causes pelvic inflammatory disease and sterility in females, if not treated. Chlamydia can be treated with tetracycline or erythromycin antibiotics.

Gonorrhea is caused by the gonococcus bacterium. Symptoms in males include a greenish-yellow discharge, burning when urinating, sore throat, and swollen glands. Females are frequently asymptomatic but may experience dysuria, pain in the lower abdomen, and vaginal discharge. An infected woman can transmit the gonococcus organism to her infant's eyes during childbirth, causing blindness. To prevent this, a drop of silver nitrate or antibiotic is routinely placed in the eyes of newborn babies. Gonorrhea is treated with large doses of penicillin or tetracycline antibiotics.

Herpes is a viral disease caused by the herpes simplex virus type II. Symptoms include a burning sensation, fluid-filled vesicles (blisterlike sores) that rupture and form painful ulcers, and painful urination. After the sores heal, the virus becomes dormant. Many people have repeated attacks, but the attacks are milder. There is no cure, and treatment is directed toward promoting healing and easing discomfort.

Pubic lice are parasites that are usually transmitted sexually, although they can be spread by contact with clothing, bed linen, or other items containing the lice. Symptoms include an intense itching and redness of the perineal area. Medications that kill the lice are used as treatment. To prevent a recurrence, it is essential to wash all clothing and bed linen to destroy any lice or nits (eggs).

Syphilis is caused by a spirochete bacterium. The symptoms occur in stages. During the primary stage, a painless chancre, or sore, appears, usually on the penis of the male and in the vulva or on the cervix of the female. This chancre heals within several weeks. During the second stage, which occurs if the chancre is not treated, the organism enters the bloodstream and causes a nonitching rash, a sore throat, a fever, and swollen glands. These symptoms also disappear within several weeks. The third stage occurs years later after the spirochete has damaged vital organs. Damage to the heart and blood vessels causes cardiovascular disease; damage to the spinal cord causes a characteristic gait and paralysis; and brain damage causes mental disorders, deafness, and blindness. At this stage, damage is irreversible, and death occurs. Early diagnosis and treatment with antibiotics can cure syphilis during the first two stages.

Trichomonas vaginalis is caused by a parasitic protozoan. The main symptom is a large amount of white or yellow, foul-smelling discharge. Males

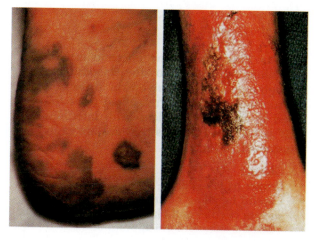

FIGURE 6-67 A common opportunistic disease that occurs in AIDS patients is Kaposi's sarcoma. *(Courtesy of the Centers for Disease Control and Prevention, Atlanta, GA)*

are frequently asymptomatic. The oral medication Flagyl is used to treat this disease; both sexual partners must be treated to prevent reinfection.

STUDENT: *Go to the workbook and complete the assignment sheet for 6:14, Reproductive System.*

UNIT 6 SUMMARY

A health care worker must understand normal functioning of the human body in order to understand disease processes. A study of anatomy, the form and structure of an organism, and physiology, the processes of living organisms, adds to this understanding.

The basic structural unit of the human body is the cell. Cells join together to form tissues. Tissues join together to form organs, which work together to form body systems.

Systems work together to provide for proper functioning of the human body. The integumentary system, or skin, provides a protective covering for the body. The skeletal and muscular systems provide structure and movement. The circulatory system transports oxygen and nutrients to all body cells, and carries carbon dioxide and metabolic materials away from the cells. The lymphatic system assists the circulatory system in removing wastes and excess fluid from the cells and tissues. The nervous system coordinates the many activities that occur in the body and allows the body to respond and adapt to changes. Special senses provided by organs such as the eyes and ears also allow the body to react to the environment. The respiratory system takes in oxygen for use by the body and eliminates carbon dioxide, a waste product produced by body cells. The digestive system is responsible for the physical and chemical breakdown of food so it can be used by body cells. The urinary system removes certain wastes and excess water from the body. The endocrine system, composed of a group of glands, controls many body functions. The reproductive system allows the human body to create new life.

All of the systems are interrelated, working as a unit to maintain a constant balance (homeostasis) within the human body. When disease occurs, this balance frequently is disturbed. Some of the major diseases and disorders of each system were also discussed in this unit.

INTERNET SEARCHES

Use the suggested search engines in Unit 11:4 of this textbook to search the Internet for additional information on the following topics:

1. *Anatomy and physiology:* search the name of a body system, organ, and/or tissue to obtain additional information on the structure and function of the system, organ, or tissue.

2. *Pathophysiology:* search the name of specific diseases discussed in each sub-unit to obtain additional information on occurrence, prognosis, signs and symptoms, and current methods of treatment.

3. *American Cancer Society:* search this information base to obtain information on cancer in various parts of the body, breast self-examination, testicular self-examination, and statistics on cancer.

4. *Tutorials:* search publishers, software providers, and bookstore sites to find a variety of materials that can be used to learn the anatomy and physiology of the human body.

REVIEW QUESTIONS

1. Differentiate between anatomy, physiology, and pathophysiology.

2. Name the four (4) main groups of tissues. By each tissue, list three (3) body systems that contain the tissue.

3. List at least ten (10) body systems and state the main function(s) of each system.

4. Identify the main bones or groups of bones in both the axial and the appendicular skeleton.

5. Describe the five (5) main actions or movements of muscles and provide a specific example for each type of movement.

6. Create a diagram showing the divisions of the nervous system and list the main parts in each division of the system.

7. List four (4) special senses and the organ that is required for each of the senses.

8. Trace a drop of blood as it enters the heart, goes through pulmonary circulation, returns to the heart, and goes to body cells. Name each chamber and valve in the heart, each blood vessel or type of vessel, and any organs blood passes through. Make sure all parts are in correct order.

9. Name all parts of the alimentary canal in correct order. Begin at the mouth and end at the anus.

10. Differentiate between endocrine and exocrine glands. Give five (5) examples of each type of gland and list the main function for each gland.

11. Evaluate three (3) sexually transmitted diseases (STDs) and describe how symptoms are the same or different in males versus females.

12. Body systems are interrelated and work together to perform specific functions. For example, the circulatory and respiratory systems perform a joint function of obtaining oxygen for the body and eliminating carbon dioxide. Describe five (5) other examples of interrelationships between body systems.

UNIT 6
SUGGESTED REFERENCES

Beebe, Richard, and Deborah Funk. *Functional Anatomy for Emergency Medical Services.* Clifton Park, NY: Delmar Learning, 2002

Beers, Mark, and Robert Berkow. *The Merck Manual of Diagnosis and Therapy.* 17th ed. Whitehouse Station, NJ: Merck and Company, 1999.

Borgstadt, Marcia. *Understanding and Caring for Human Diseases.* Clifton Park, NY: Delmar Learning, 1997.

Cohen, Barbara, and Dena Wood. *Memmler's Structure and Function of the Human Body.* 7th ed. Philadelphia, PA: Lippincott, Williams, & Wikins, 2000.

Colbert, Bruce, et al. *An Integrated Approach to Health Sciences: Anatomy and Physiology, Math, Physics, and Chemistry.* Clifton Park, NY: Delmar Learning, 1997.

Des Jardins, Terry. *Cardiopulmonary Anatomy and Physiology: Essentials for Respiratory Care.* 4th ed. Clifton Park, NY: Delmar Learning, 2002.

Gould, Barbara. *Pathophysiology for the Health Related Professions.* 2nd ed. Philadelphia, PA: W. B. Saunders, 2002.

Keir, Lucille, Connie Krebs, and Barbara A. Wise. *Medical Assisting: Administrative and Clinical Competencies.* 5th ed. Clifton Park, NY: Delmar Learning, 2003.

Mackie, Jennifer, and Joyce Greig. *Anatomy and Physiology Applied to Health Professions.* 7th ed. Philadelphia, PA: Harcourt Health Services, 2001.

McArdle, William, Frank Katch, and Victor Katch. *Exercise Physiology, Energy Nutrition, and Human Performance.* 5th ed. Philadelphia, PA: Lippincott, Williams, & Wilkins, 2001.

Myers, Jeffrey, Marianne Neighbors, and Ruth Tannehill-Jones. *Principles of Pathophysiology and Emergency Medical Care.* Clifton Park, NY: Delmar Learning, 2002.

Neighbors, Marianne, and Ruth Tannehill-Jones. *Human Diseases.* Clifton Park, NY: Delmar Learning, 2000.

Pucillo, John. *Delmar's Anatomy and Physiology Challenge CD-ROM.* Clifton Park, NY: Delmar Learning, 1998.

Rizzo, Donald. *Delmar's Fundamentals of Anatomy and Physiology.* Clifton Park, NY: Delmar Learning, 2001.

Scott, Ann, and Elizabeth Fong. *Body Structures and Functions.* 9th ed. Clifton Park, NY: Delmar Learning, 1998.

Scott, Ann Sensi, and Elizabeth Fong. *Functional Anatomy for EMS Providers.* Clifton Park, NY: Delmar Learning, 2002.

Short, Marjorie J. *Anatomy for Dental Assisting.* 3rd ed. Clifton Park, NY: Delmar Learning, 2002.

Thibodeau, Gary, and Kevin Patton. *Anatomy and Physiology.* 4th ed. St. Louis, MO: C. V. Mosby, 1999.

Thibodeau, Gary, and Kevin Patton. *Human Body in Health and Disease.* 3rd ed. St. Louis, MO: Mosby, 2001.

Thibodeau, Gary, and Kevin Patton. *Structure and Function of the Body.* 11th ed. St. Louis, MO: Mosby, 2000.

Woelfel, Julian, and Rickne Scheid. *Dental Anatomy.* Philadelphia, PA: Lippincott, Williams, & Wilkins, 2001.

UNIT 7

Human Growth and Development

Unit Objectives

After completing this unit of study, you should be able to:

- Identify at least two physical, mental, emotional, and social developments that occur during each of the seven main life stages
- Explain the causes and treatments for eating disorders and chemical abuse
- Identify methods used to prevent suicide and list common warning signs
- Recognize ways that life stages affect an individual's needs
- Describe the five stages of grieving that occur in the dying patient and the role of the health care worker during each stage
- List two purposes of hospice care and justify the "right to die"
- Create examples for each of Maslow's Hierarchy of Needs
- Name the two main methods people use to meet or satisfy needs
- Describe a situation that shows the use of each of the following defense mechanisms: rationalization, projection, displacement, compensation, daydreaming, repression, suppression, denial, and withdrawal
- Identify four factors that interfere with communication
- Explain the importance of listening, nonverbal behavior, reporting, and recording in the communication process
- Define, pronounce, and spell all the key terms

	Observe Standard Precautions		Instructors Check—Call Instructor at This Point
	Safety—Proceed with Caution	 OBRA	OBRA Requirement— Based on Federal Law
	Math Skill		Legal Responsibility
	Science Skill		Career Information
C	Communications Skill		Technology

KEY TERMS

acceptance
adolescence
affection
Alzheimer's disease
   (*Altz'-high-merz*)
anger
anorexia nervosa
   (*an-oh-rex'-see-ah ner-voh'-sah*)
arteriosclerosis
   (*ar-tear"-ee-oh-skleh-row'-sis*)
bargaining
bulimarexia
   (*byou-lee"-mah-rex'-ee-ah*)
bulimia
   (*byou-lee'-me-ah*)
chemical abuse
communication
compensation
   (*cahm"-pen-say'-shun*)
cultural diversity

daydreaming
defense mechanisms
denial
depression
displacement
early adulthood
early childhood
emotional
esteem
hospice
   (*hoss'-pis*)
infancy
late adulthood
late childhood
life stages
listening
mental
middle adulthood
motivated
needs
nonverbal

physical
physiological needs
   (*fizz"-ee-oh-lodg'-ih-kal*)
projection
puberty
   (*pew'-burr"-tee*)
rationalization
   (*rash"-en-nal-ih-zay'-shun*)
repression
right to die
safety
satisfaction
self-actualization
sexuality
social
suicide
suppression
tension
terminal illness
verbal
withdrawal

INTRODUCTION

Human growth and development is a process that begins at birth and does not end until death. During all stages of growth and development, individuals have needs that must be met. A health care worker must be aware of the various life stages and of individual needs in order to provide quality health care (see figure 7-1).

7:1 INFORMATION Life Stages

Even though individuals differ greatly, each person passes through certain stages of growth and development from birth to death. These stages are frequently called **life stages.** A common method of classifying life stages is as follows:

- ◆ **Infancy**—birth to 1 year
- ◆ **Early childhood**—1 to 6 years
- ◆ **Late childhood**—6 to 12 years
- ◆ **Adolescence**—12 to 20 years
- ◆ **Early adulthood**—20 to 40 years
- ◆ **Middle adulthood**—40 to 65 years
- ◆ **Late adulthood**—65 years and up

As individuals pass through these life stages, four main types of growth and development occur: physical, mental, emotional, and social. **Physical** refers to body growth and includes height and weight changes, muscle and nerve development, and changes in body organs. **Mental** refers to development of the mind and includes learning how to solve problems, make judgments, and deal with situations. **Emotional** refers to feelings and includes dealing with love, hate, joy, fear, excitement, and other similar feelings. **Social** refers to interactions and relationships with other people.

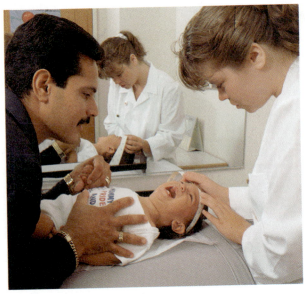
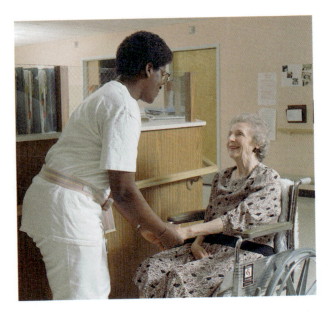

FIGURE 7-1 An understanding of life stages is important for the health care worker, who may provide care to individuals of all ages; from the very young (left) to the elderly (right).

Each stage of growth and development has its own characteristics and has specific developmental tasks that an individual must master. These tasks progress from the simple to the more complex. For example, an individual first learns to sit, then stand, then walk, and then, finally, run. Each stage establishes the foundation for the next stage. In this way, growth and development proceeds in an orderly pattern. It is important to remember, however, that the rate of progress varies among individuals. Some children master speech early, others master it later. Similarly, an individual may experience a sudden growth spurt and then maintain the same height for a period of time.

Erik Erikson, a psychoanalyst, has identified eight stages of psychosocial development. His eight stages of development, the basic conflict or need that must be resolved at each stage, and ways to resolve the conflict are shown in table 7-1. Erikson also believes that if an individual is not able to resolve a conflict at the appropriate stage, the individual will struggle with the same conflict later in life. For example, if a toddler is not allowed to learn by mastering basic tasks, the toddler may develop a sense of doubt in his or her abilities. This sense of doubt will interfere with later attempts at mastering independence.

Health care providers must understand that each life stage creates certain needs in individuals. Likewise, other factors can affect life stages and needs. An individual's sex, race, heredity (factors inherited from parents, such as hair color and body structure) culture, life experiences, and health status can influence needs. Injury or illness usually has a negative effect and can change needs or impair development.

INFANCY

Physical Development

The most dramatic and rapid changes in growth and development occur during the first year of life. A newborn baby usually weighs approximately 6 to 8 pounds (2.7 to 3.6 kg) and measures 18 to 22 inches (46 to 55 cm) (see figure 7-2). By the end of the first year of life, weight has usually tripled, to 21 to 24 pounds (9.5 to 11 kg), and height has increased to approximately 29 to 30 inches (74 to 76 cm).

Muscular system and nervous system developments are also dramatic. The muscular and nervous systems are very immature at birth. Certain reflex actions present at birth allow the infant to respond to the environment. These include the Moro, or startle, reflex to a loud noise or sudden movement; the rooting reflex, in which a slight touch on the cheek causes the mouth to open and the head to turn; the sucking reflex, caused by a slight touch on the lips; and the grasp reflex, in which infants can grasp an object placed in the hand. Muscle coordination develops in stages. At first, infants are able to lift the head slightly. By 2 months, they can usually roll from side to back.

TABLE 7-1 Erikson's Eight Stages of Psychosocial Development

STAGE OF DEVELOPMENT	BASIC CONFLICT	MAJOR LIFE EVENT	WAYS TO RESOLVE CONFLICT
Infancy Birth to 1 Year Oral–Sensory	Trust versus Mistrust	Feeding	Infant develops trust in self, others, and the environment when caregiver is responsive to basic needs and provides comfort; if needs not met, infant becomes uncooperative and aggressive, and shows a decreased interest in the environment
Toddler 1 to 3 Years Muscular–Anal	Autonomy versus Shame/Doubt	Toilet Training	Toddler learns control while mastering skills such as feeding, toileting, and dressing when caregivers provide reassurance but avoid overprotection; if needs not met, toddler feels ashamed and doubts own abilities, which leads to lack of self-confidence in later stages
Preschool 3 to 6 Years Locomotor	Initiative versus Guilt	Independence	Child begins to initiate activities in place of just imitating activities; uses imagination to play; learns what is allowed and what is not allowed to develop a conscience; caregivers must allow child to be responsible while providing reassurance; if needs not met, child feels guilty and thinks everything he or she does is wrong, which leads to a hesitancy to try new tasks in later stages
School-Age 6 to 12 Years Latency	Industry versus Inferiority	School	Child becomes productive by mastering learning and obtaining success; child learns to deal with academics, group activities, and friends when others show acceptance of actions and praise success; if needs not met, child develops a sense of inferiority and incompetence, which hinders future relationships and the ability to deal with life events
Adolescence 12 to 18 Years	Identity versus Role Confusion	Peer Relationships	Adolescent searches for self-identity by making choices about occupation, sexual orientation, lifestyle, and adult role; relies on peer group for support and reassurance to create a self-image separate from parents; if needs not met, adolescent experiences role confusion and loss of self-belief
Young Adulthood 19 to 40 Years	Intimacy versus Isolation	Love Relationships	Young adult learns to make a personal commitment to others and share life events with others; if self-identity is lacking, adult may fear relationships and isolate self from others
Middle Adulthood 40 to 65 Years	Generativity versus Stagnation	Parenting	Adult seeks satisfaction and obtains success in life by using career, family, and civic interests to provide for others and the next generation; if adult does not deal with life issues, feels lack of purpose to life and sense of failure
Older Adulthood 65 Years to Death	Ego Integrity versus Despair	Reflection on and Acceptance of Life	Adult reflects on life in a positive manner, feels fulfillment with his or her own life and accomplishments, deals with losses, and prepares for death; if not met, adult feels despair about life and fear of death

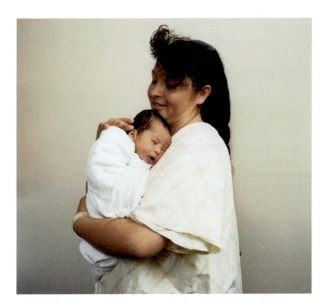

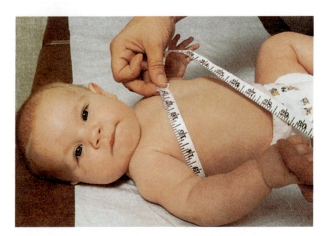

FIGURE 7-3 By 4 months of age, infants recognize their caregivers and stare intently at others.

FIGURE 7-2 A newborn baby usually weighs approximately 6 to 8 pounds and measures 18 to 22 inches in length.

By 4 to 5 months, they can turn the body completely around, accept objects handed to them, grasp stationary objects, and, with support, hold the head up while sitting. By 6 to 7 months, infants can sit unsupported for several minutes, grasp moving objects, and crawl on the stomach. By 12 months, infants frequently can walk without assistance, grasp objects with the thumb and fingers, and throw small objects.

Other physical developments are also dramatic. Most infants are born without teeth, but usually have 10 to 12 teeth by the end of the first year of life. At birth, vision is poor and may be limited to black and white, and eye movements are not coordinated. By 1 year of age, however, close vision is good, in color, and can readily focus on small objects. Sensory abilities such as those of smell, taste, sensitivity to hot and cold, and hearing, while good at birth, become more refined and exact.

Mental Development

Mental development is also rapid during the first year. Newborns respond to discomforts such as pain, cold, or hunger by crying. As their needs are met, they gradually become more aware of their surroundings and begin to recognize individuals associated with their care. As infants respond to stimuli in the environment, learning activities grow. At birth, they are unable to speak. By 6 months of age, however, infants understand some words and can make basic sounds; and by 12 months, infants understand many words and use many single words in their vocabularies.

Emotional Development

Emotional development is observed very early in life. Newborns show excitement. By 4 to 6 months of age, distress, delight, anger, disgust, and fear can often be seen. By 12 months of age, elation and affection for adults is evident. Events that occur in the first year of life when these emotions are first exhibited can have a strong influence on an individual's emotional behavior during adulthood.

Social Development

Social development progresses gradually from the self-centeredness concept of the newborn to the recognition of others in the environment. By 4 months of age, infants recognize their caregivers, smile readily, and stare intently at others (see figure 7-3). By 6 months of age, infants watch the activities of others, show signs of possessiveness, and may become shy or withdraw when in the presence of strangers. By 12 months of age, infants may still be shy with strangers, but they socialize freely with familiar people, and mimic and imitate gestures, facial expressions, and vocal sounds.

Infants are dependent on others for all needs. Food, cleanliness, and rest are essential for physical growth. Love and security are essential for emotional and social growth. Stimulation is essential for mental growth.

EARLY CHILDHOOD

Physical Development

During early childhood, from 1 to 6 years of age, physical growth is slower than during infancy. By age 6, the average weight is 45 pounds (20.4 kg), and the average height is 46 inches (116 cm). Skeletal and muscle development helps the child assume a more adult appearance. The legs and lower body tend to grow more rapidly than do the head, arms, and chest. Muscle coordination allows the child to run, climb, and move freely. As muscles of the fingers develop, the child learns to write, draw, and use a fork and knife. By age 2 or 3, most teeth have erupted, and the digestive system is mature enough to handle most adult foods. Between 2 and 4 years of age, most children learn bladder and bowel control.

Mental Development

Mental development advances rapidly during early childhood. Verbal growth progresses from the use of several words at age 1 to a vocabulary of 1,500 to 2,500 words at age 6. Two-year-olds have short attention spans but are interested in many different activities (see figure 7-4). They can remember details and begin to understand concepts. Four-year-olds ask frequent questions and usually recognize letters and some words. They begin to make decisions based on logic rather than on trial and error. By age 6, children are very verbal and want to learn how to read and write. Memory has developed to the point where the child can make decisions based on both past and present experiences.

Emotional Development

Emotional development also advances rapidly. At ages 1 to 2, children begin to develop self-awareness and to recognize the effect they have on other people and things. Limits are usually established for safety, leading the 1- or 2-year-old to either accept or defy such limits. Children feel impatience and frustration as they try to do things beyond their abilities. Anger, often in the form of "temper tantrums," occurs when they cannot perform as desired. Children at this age also like routine (see figure 7-5), and become stubborn, angry, or frustrated when changes occur. From ages 4 to 6, children begin to gain more control over their emotions. They understand the concept of right and wrong, and because they have achieved more independence, they are not frustrated as much by their lack of ability. By age 6, most children also show less anxiety when faced with new experiences, because they have learned they can deal with new situations.

Social Development

Social development expands from a self-centered 1-year-old to a very sociable 6-year-old. In the

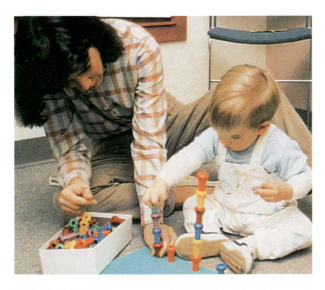

FIGURE 7-4 Two-year-olds are interested in many different activities, but they have short attention spans.

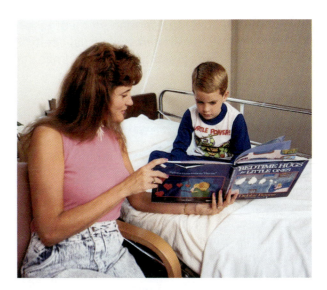

FIGURE 7-5 Two- to four-year-olds like routine, such as regular periods set aside for reading.

early years, children are usually strongly attached to their parents (or to the individuals who provide their care), and they fear any separation. They begin to enjoy the company of others, but are still very possessive. Playing alongside other children is more common than playing with other children. Gradually, children learn to put "self" aside and begin to take more of an interest in others. They learn to trust other people and make more of an effort to please others by becoming more agreeable and social. Friends of their own age are usually important to 6-year-olds.

The needs of early childhood still include food, rest, shelter, protection, love, and security. In addition, children need routine, order, and consistency in their daily lives. They must be taught to be responsible and must learn how to conform to rules. This can be accomplished by making reasonable demands based on the child's ability to comply.

LATE CHILDHOOD

Physical Development

This life stage, which covers ages 6 to 12, is also called *preadolescence*. Physical development is slow but steady. Weight gain averages 5 to 7 pounds (2.3 to 3.2 kg) per year, and height usually increases approximately 2 to 3 inches (5 to 7.5 cm) per year. Muscle coordination is well developed, and children can engage in physical activities that require complex motor-sensory coordination. During this age, most of the primary teeth are lost, and permanent teeth erupt. The eyes are well developed, and visual acuity is at its best. During ages 10 to 12, sexual maturation may begin in some children.

Mental Development

Mental development increases rapidly because much of the child's life centers around school. Speech skills develop more completely, and reading and writing skills are learned. Children learn to use information to solve problems and the memory becomes more complex. They begin to understand more abstract concepts such as loyalty, honesty, values, and morals. Children use more active thinking and become more adept at making judgments (see figure 7-6).

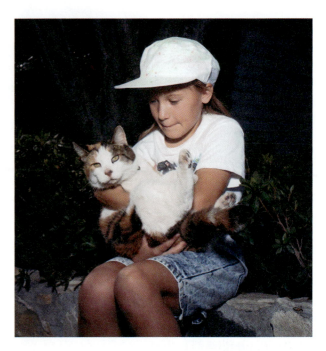

FIGURE 7-6 In late childhood (ages 6 to 12), children become more adept at making judgments.

Emotional Development

Emotional development continues to help the child achieve a greater independence and a more distinct personality. At age 6, children are often frightened and uncertain as they begin school. Reassuring parents and success in school help children gain self-confidence. Gradually, fears are replaced by the ability to cope. Emotions are slowly brought under control and dealt with in a more effective manner. By ages 10 to 12, sexual maturation and changes in body functions can lead to periods of depression followed by periods of joy. These emotional changes can cause children to be restless, anxious, and difficult to understand.

Social Development

Social changes are evident during these years. Seven-year-olds tend to like activities they can do by themselves and do not usually like group activities. However, they want the approval of others, especially their parents and friends. Children from ages 8 to 10 tend to be more group oriented, and they typically form groups with members of their own sex. They are more ready to accept the opinions of others and learn to conform to rules and standards of behavior followed by the group. Toward the end of this period, children tend to make friends more easily, and they begin to develop an increasing awareness of the opposite sex. As children spend more time with others their own age, their dependency on their parent(s) lessens, as does the time they spend with their parents.

Needs of children in this age group include the same basic needs of infancy and early childhood along with the need for reassurance, parental approval, and peer acceptance.

ADOLESCENCE

Physical Development

Adolescence, ages 12 to 20, is often a traumatic life stage. Physical changes occur most dramatically in the early period. A sudden "growth spurt" can cause rapid increases in weight and height. A weight gain of up to 25 pounds (11 kg) and a height increase of several inches can occur in a period of months. Muscle coordination does not advance as quickly. This can lead to awkwardness or clumsiness in motor coordination. This growth spurt usually occurs anywhere from ages 11 to 13 in girls and ages 13 to 15 in boys.

The most obvious physical changes in adolescents relate to the development of the sexual organs and the secondary sexual characteristics, frequently called **puberty.** Secretion of sex hormones leads to the onset of menstruation in girls and the production of sperm and semen in boys. Secondary sexual characteristics in females include growth of pubic hair, development of breasts and wider hips, and distribution of body fat leading to the female shape. The male develops a deeper voice; attains more muscle mass and broader shoulders; and grows pubic, facial, and body hair.

Mental Development

Since most of the foundations have already been established, mental development primarily involves an increase in knowledge and a sharpening of skills. Adolescents learn to make decisions and to accept responsibility for their actions. At times, this causes conflict because they are treated as both children and adults, or are told to "grow up" while being reminded that they are "still children."

Emotional Development

Emotional development is often stormy and in conflict. As adolescents try to establish their identities and independence, they are often uncertain and feel inadequate and insecure. They worry about their appearance, their abilities, and their relationships with others. They frequently respond more and more to peer group influences. At times, this leads to changes in attitude and behavior and conflict with values previously established. Toward the end of adolescence, self-identity has been established. At this point, teenagers feel more comfortable with who they are and turn attention toward what they may become. They gain more control of their feelings and become more mature emotionally.

Social Development

Social development usually involves spending less time with family and more time with peer groups. As adolescents attempt to develop self-identity and independence, they seek security in groups of people their own age who have similar problems and conflicts (see figure 7-7). If these peer relationships help develop self-confidence through the approval of others, adolescents become more secure and satisfied. Toward the end of this life stage, adolescents develop a more mature attitude and begin to develop patterns of behavior that they associate with adult behavior or status.

In addition to basic needs, adolescents need reassurance, support, and understanding. Many problems that develop during this life stage can

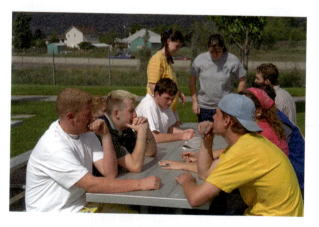

FIGURE 7-7 Adolescents use the peer group as a safety net as they try to establish their identities and independence.

be traced to the conflict and feelings of inadequacy and insecurity that adolescents experience. Examples include eating disorders, drug and alcohol abuse, and suicide. Even though these types of problems also occur in earlier and later life stages, they are frequently associated with adolescence.

Eating disorders often develop from an excessive concern with appearance. Two common eating disorders are anorexia nervosa and bulimia. **Anorexia nervosa,** commonly called *anorexia,* is a psychological disorder in which a person drastically reduces food intake or refuses to eat at all. This results in metabolic disturbances, excessive weight loss, weakness, and, if not treated, death. **Bulimia** is a psychological disorder in which a person alternately binges (eats excessively) and then fasts, or refuses to eat at all. When a person induces vomiting or uses laxatives to get rid of food that has been eaten, the condition is called **bulimarexia.** All three conditions are more common in females than males. Psychological or psychiatric help is usually needed to treat these conditions.

Chemical abuse is the use of substances such as alcohol or drugs and the development of a physical and/or mental dependence on these chemicals. Chemical abuse can occur in any life stage, but it frequently begins in adolescence. Reasons for using chemicals include anxiety or stress relief, peer pressure, escape from emotional or psychological problems, experimentation with feelings the chemicals produce, desire for "instant gratification," hereditary traits, and cultural influences. Chemical abuse can lead to physical and mental disorders and disease. Treatment is directed toward total rehabilitation that allows the chemical abuser to return to a productive and meaningful life.

Suicide, found in many life stages, is one of the leading causes of death in adolescents. Suicide is always a permanent solution to a temporary problem. Reasons for suicide include depression, grief over a loss or love affair, failure in school, inability to meet expectations, influence of suicidal friends, or lack of self-esteem. The risk of suicide increases with a family history of suicide, a major loss or disappointment, previous suicide attempts, and/or the recent suicide of friends, family, or role models (heroes or idols). The impulsive nature of adolescents also increases the possibility of suicide. Most individuals who are thinking of suicide give warning signs such as verbal statements like "I'd rather be dead" or "You'd be better off without me." Other warning signs include:

- sudden changes in appetite and sleep habits
- withdrawal, depression, and moodiness
- excessive fatigue or agitation
- neglect of personal hygiene
- alcohol or drug abuse
- losing interest in hobbies and other aspects of life
- injuring one's body
- giving away possessions
- saying goodbye to family and friends

These individuals are calling out for attention and help and usually respond to efforts of assistance. Their direct and indirect pleas should never be ignored. Support, understanding, and psychological or psychiatric counseling are used to prevent suicide.

EARLY ADULTHOOD

Physical Development

Early adulthood, ages 20 to 40, is frequently the most productive life stage. Physical development is basically complete, muscles are developed and strong, and motor coordination is at its peak. This is also the prime childbearing time and usually produces the healthiest babies (see figure 7-8). Both male and female sexual development is at its peak.

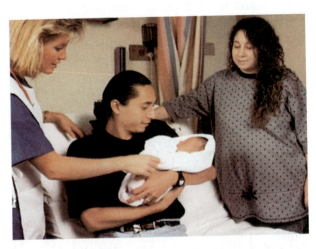

FIGURE 7-8 Early adulthood is the prime childbearing time and usually produces the healthiest babies.

Mental Development

Mental development usually continues throughout this stage. Many young adults pursue additional education to establish and progress in their chosen careers. Frequently, formal education continues for many years. The young adult often also deals with independence, makes career choices, establishes a lifestyle, selects a marital partner, starts a family, and establishes values, all of which involve making many decisions and forming many judgments.

Emotional Development

Emotional development usually involves preserving the stability established during previous stages. Young adults are subjected to many emotional stresses related to career, marriage, family, and other similar situations. If emotional structure is strong, most young adults can cope with these worries. They find satisfaction in their achievements, take responsibility for their actions, and learn to accept criticism and to profit from mistakes.

Social Development

Social development frequently involves moving away from the peer group, and young adults instead tend to associate with others who have similar ambitions and interests, regardless of age. The young adult often becomes involved with a mate and forms a family. Young adults do not necessarily accept traditional sex roles, and frequently adopt nontraditional roles. For example, males fill positions as nurses and secretaries, and females enter administrative or construction positions. Such choices have caused and will continue to cause changes in the traditional patterns of society.

MIDDLE ADULTHOOD

Physical Development

Middle adulthood, ages 40 to 65, is frequently called middle age. Physical changes begin to occur during these years. The hair tends to gray and thin, the skin begins to wrinkle, muscle tone tends to decrease, hearing loss starts, visual acuity declines, and weight gain occurs. Females experience *menopause,* or the end of menstruation, along with decreased hormone production that causes physical and emotional changes. Males also experience a slowing of hormone production. This can lead to physical and psychological changes, a period frequently referred to as the *male climacteric.* However, except in cases of injury, disease, or surgery, males never lose the ability to produce sperm or to reproduce.

Mental Development

Mental ability can continue to increase during middle age, a fact that has been proven by the many individuals in this life stage who seek formal education. Middle adulthood is a period when individuals have acquired an understanding of life and have learned to cope with many different stresses. This allows them to be more confident in decision making and excellent at analyzing situations.

Emotional Development

Emotionally, middle age can be a period of contentment and satisfaction, or it can be a time of crisis. The emotional foundation of previous life stages and the situations that occur during middle age determine emotional status during this period. Job stability, financial success, the end of child rearing, and good health from disease prevention can all contribute to emotional satisfaction (see figure 7-9). Stress, created by loss of job,

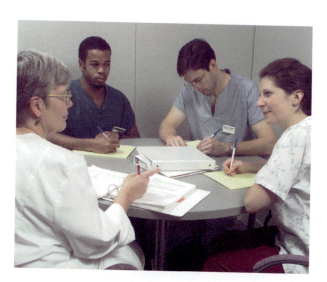

FIGURE 7-9 Job stability and enjoyment during middle adulthood contribute to emotional satisfaction.

fear of aging, loss of youth and vitality, illness, marital problems, or problems with children or aging parents, can contribute to emotional feelings of depression, insecurity, anxiety, and even anger. Therefore, emotional status varies in this age group and is largely determined by events that occur during this period.

Social Development

Social relationships also depend on many factors. Family relationships often see a decline as children begin lives of their own and parents die. Work relationships frequently replace family. Relationships between husband and wife can become stronger as they have more time together and opportunities to enjoy success. However, divorce rates are also high in this age group, as couples who have remained together "for the children's sake" now separate. Friendships are usually with people who have the same interests and lifestyles.

LATE ADULTHOOD

Physical Development

Late adulthood, age 65 and up, has many different terms associated with it. These include "elderly," "senior citizen," "golden ager," and "retired citizen." Much attention has been directed toward this life stage in recent years because people are living longer, and the number of people in this age group is increasing daily.

Physical development is on the decline. All body systems are usually affected. The skin becomes dry, wrinkled, and thinner. Brown or yellow spots (frequently called "age spots") appear. The hair becomes thin and frequently loses its luster or shine. Bones become more brittle and porous and are more likely to fracture or break. Cartilage between the vertebrae thins and can lead to a stooping posture. Muscles lose tone and strength, which can lead to fatigue and poor coordination. A decline in the function of the nervous system leads to hearing loss, decreased visual acuity, and decreased tolerance for temperatures that are too hot or too cold. Memory loss can occur, and reasoning ability can diminish. The heart is less efficient, and circulation decreases. The kidney and bladder are less efficient. Breathing capacity decreases and causes

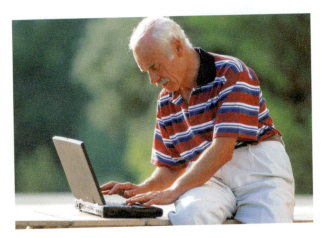

FIGURE 7-10 Elderly individuals who are willing to learn new things show fewer signs of decreased mental ability.

shortness of breath. However, it is important to note that these changes usually occur slowly over a long period of time. Many individuals, because of better health and living conditions, do not show physical changes of aging until their seventies and even eighties.

Mental Development

Mental abilities vary among individuals. Elderly people who remain mentally active and are willing to learn new things tend to show fewer signs of decreased mental ability (see figure 7-10). Although some 90-year-olds remain alert and well oriented, other elderly individuals show decreased mental capacities at much earlier ages. Short-term memory is usually first to decline. Many elderly individuals can clearly remember events that occurred 20 years ago, but do not remember yesterday's events. Diseases such as **Alzheimer's disease** can lead to irreversible loss of memory, deterioration of intellectual functions, speech and gait disturbances, and disorientation. **Arteriosclerosis,** a thickening and hardening of the walls of the arteries, can also decrease the blood supply to the brain and cause a decrease in mental abilities.

Emotional Development

Emotional stability also varies among individuals in this age group. Some elderly people cope well with the stresses presented by aging and remain happy and able to enjoy life. Others become lonely, frustrated, withdrawn, and depressed.

Emotional adjustment is necessary throughout this cycle. Retirement, death of a spouse and friends, physical disabilities, financial problems, loss of independence, and knowledge that life must end all can cause emotional distress. The adjustments that the individual makes during this life stage are similar to those made throughout life.

Social Development

Social adjustment also occurs during late adulthood. Retirement can lead to a loss of self-esteem, especially if work is strongly associated with self-identity: "I am a teacher," instead of "I am Sandra Jones." Less contact with co-workers and a more limited circle of friends usually occur. Many elderly individuals engage in other activities and continue to make new social contacts (see figure 7-11). Others limit their social relationships. Death of a spouse and friends, and moving to a new environment can also cause changes in social relationships. Development of new social contacts is important at this time. Senior centers, golden age groups, churches, and many other organizations help provide the elderly with the opportunity to find new social roles.

Needs of this life stage are the same as those of all other life stages. In addition to basic needs, the elderly need a sense of belonging, self-esteem, financial security, social acceptance, and love.

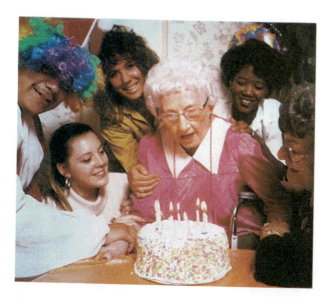

FIGURE 7-11 Social contacts and activities are important during late adulthood.

STUDENT: *Go to the workbook and complete the assignment sheet for 7:1, Life Stages.*

7:2 INFORMATION Death and Dying

Death is often referred to as "the final stage of growth." It is experienced by everyone and cannot be avoided. In our society, the young tend to ignore its existence. It is usually the elderly, having lost spouses and/or friends, who begin to think of their own deaths.

When a patient is told that he or she has a **terminal illness,** a disease that cannot be cured and will result in death, the patient may react in different ways. Some patients react with fear and anxiety. They fear pain, abandonment, and loneliness. They fear the unknown. They become anxious about their loved ones and about unfinished work or dreams. Anxiety diminishes in patients who feel they have had full lives and who have strong religious beliefs regarding life after death. Some patients view death as a final peace. They know it will bring an end to loneliness, pain, and suffering.

Dr. Elizabeth Kübler-Ross has done extensive research on the process of death and dying and is known as a leading expert on this topic. Because of her research, most medical personnel now feel patients should be told of their approaching deaths. However, patients should be left with "some hope" and the knowledge that they will "not be left alone." It is important that all staff members who provide care to the dying patient know both the extent of information given to the patient and how the patient reacted.

Dr. Kübler-Ross has identified five stages of grieving that dying patients and their families/friends may experience in preparation for death. The stages may not occur in order, and they may overlap or be repeated several times. Some patients may not progress through all of the stages before death occurs. Other patients may be in several stages at the same time. The stages are denial, anger, bargaining, depression, and acceptance.

Denial is the "No, not me!" stage, which usually occurs when a person is first told of a terminal illness. It occurs when the person cannot accept the reality of death or when the person feels loved ones cannot accept the truth. The person may make statements such as "The doctor does not know what he is talking about" or "The tests have to be wrong." Some patients seek second medical opinions or request additional tests. Others refuse to discuss their situations and avoid any references to their illnesses. It is important for patients to discuss these feelings. The health care worker should listen to a patient and try to provide support without confirming or denying. Statements such as "It must be hard for you" or "You feel additional tests will help?" will allow the patient to express feelings and move on to the next stage.

Anger occurs when the patient is no longer able to deny death. Statements such as "Why me?" or "It's your fault" are common. Patients may strike out at anyone who comes in contact with them and become very hostile and bitter. They may blame themselves, their loved ones, or health care personnel for their illnesses. It is important for the health care worker to understand that this anger is not a personal attack; the anger is caused by the situation the patient is experiencing. Providing understanding and support, listening, and making every attempt to respond to the patient's demands quickly and with kindness is essential during this stage. This stage continues until the anger is exhausted or the patient must attend to other concerns.

Bargaining occurs when patients accept death but want more time to live. Frequently, this is a period when patients turn to religion and spiritual beliefs. At this point, the will to live is strong, and patients fight hard to achieve goals set. They want to see their children graduate or get married; they want time to arrange care for their families; they want to hold new grandchildren; or other similar desires. Patients make promises to God to obtain more time. Health care workers must again be supportive and be good listeners. Whenever possible, they should help patients meet their goals.

Depression occurs when patients realize that death will come soon and they will no longer be with their families or be able to complete their goals. They may express these regrets, or they may withdraw and become quiet (see figure 7-12). They experience great sadness, and, at times, overwhelming despair. It is important for health care workers to let patients know that it is "OK" to be depressed. Providing quiet understanding, support, and/or a simple touch, and allowing patients to cry or express grief are important during this stage.

Acceptance is the final stage. Patients understand and accept the fact that they are going to

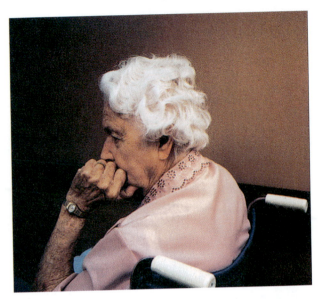

FIGURE 7-12 Depression can be a normal stage of grieving in a dying patient.

die. Patients may complete unfinished business and try to help those around them deal with the oncoming death. Gradually, patients separate themselves from the world and other people. At the end, they are at peace and can die with dignity. During this final stage, patients still need emotional support and the presence of others, even if it is just the touch of a hand (see figure 7-13).

Providing care to dying patients can be very difficult, but very rewarding. Providing supportive care when families and patients require it most can be one of the greatest satisfactions a health care worker can experience. In order to be able to provide this care, however, health care workers must first understand their own personal feelings about death and come to terms with these feelings. Feelings of fear, frustration, and uncertainty about death can cause workers to avoid dying patients or provide superficial, mechanical care. With experience, health care workers can find ways to deal with their feelings and learn to provide the supportive care needed by the dying.

Hospice care can play an important role in meeting the needs of the dying patient. Hospice care offers *palliative care,* or care that provides support and comfort. It can be offered in hospitals, medical centers, and special facilities, but most frequently it is offered in the patient's home. Hospice care is not limited to a specific time period in a patient's life. Usually it is not started until a physician declares that the patient has six months or less to live, but it can be started sooner. Most

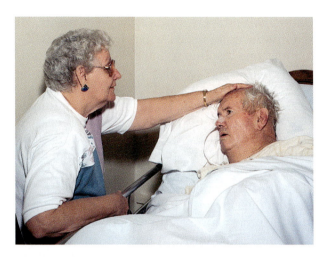

FIGURE 7-13 The support and presence of others is important to the dying person.

often patients and their families are reluctant to begin hospice care because they feel that this action recognizes the end of life. They seem to feel that if they do not use hospice care until later, death will not be as near as it actually is. The philosophy behind hospice care is to allow the patient to die with dignity and comfort. Using palliative measures of care and the philosophy of death with dignity provides patients and families with many comforts and provides an opportunity to find closure. Some of the comforts provided by hospice may include providing hospital equipment such as beds, wheelchairs, and bedside commodes; offering psychological, spiritual, social, and financial counseling; and providing free or less expensive pain medication. Pain is controlled so that the patient can remain active as long as possible. In medical facilities, personal care of the patient is provided by the staff; in the home situation, this care is provided by home health aides and other health care professionals. Specially trained volunteers are an important part of many hospice programs. They make regular visits to the patient and family, stay with the patient while the family leaves the home for brief periods of time, and help provide the support and understanding that the patient and family need. When the time for death arrives, the patient is allowed to die with dignity and in peace. After the death of the patient, hospice personnel often maintain contact with the family during the initial period of mourning.

The **right to die** is another issue that health care workers must understand. Because health care workers are ethically concerned with promoting life, allowing patients to die can cause conflict. However, a large number of surveys have shown that most people feel that an individual who has a terminal illness, with no hope of being cured, should be allowed to refuse measures that would prolong life. This is called the *right to die*. Most states have passed, or are now creating, laws that allow adults who have terminal illnesses to instruct their doctors, in writing, to withhold treatments that might prolong life. Most of the laws involve the use of advance directives, discussed in Unit 4:4. Under these laws, specific actions to end life cannot be taken. However, the use of respirators, pacemakers, and other medical devices can be withheld, and the person can be allowed to die with dignity.

Health care workers deal with death and with dying patients because death is a part of life. By understanding the process of death and by thinking about the needs of dying patients, the health care worker will be able to provide the special care needed by these individuals.

STUDENT: *Go to the workbook and complete the assignment sheet for 7:2, Death and Dying.*

7:3 INFORMATION
Human Needs

Needs are frequently defined as "a lack of something that is required or desired." From the moment of birth to the moment of death, every human being has needs. Needs motivate the individual to behave or act so that these needs will be met, if at all possible.

Certain needs have priority over other needs. For example, at times a need for food may take priority over a need for social approval, or the approval of others. If individuals have been without food for a period of time, they will direct most of their actions toward obtaining food. Even though they want social approval and the respect of others, they may steal for food, knowing that stealing may cause a loss of social approval or respect.

MASLOW'S HIERARCHY OF NEEDS

Abraham Maslow, a noted psychologist, developed a hierarchy of needs (see figure 7-14).

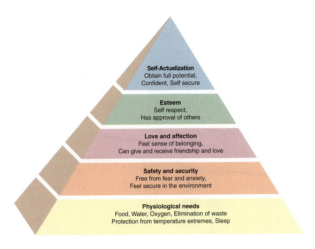

FIGURE 7-14 Maslow's Hierarchy of Needs: the lower needs should be met before the individual can try to meet higher needs.

According to Maslow, the lower needs should be met before an individual can strive to meet higher needs. Only when satisfaction has been obtained at one level is an individual motivated toward meeting needs at a higher level. The levels of needs include physiological needs, safety, affection, esteem, and self-actualization.

Physiological Needs

Physiological needs are often called "physical," "biological," or "basic" needs. These needs are required by every human being to sustain life. They include food, water, oxygen, elimination of waste materials, sleep, and protection from extreme temperatures. These needs must be met in order for life to continue. If any of these needs goes unmet, death will occur. Even among these needs, a priority exists. For example, because lack of oxygen will cause death in a matter of minutes, the need for oxygen has priority over the need for food. A patient with severe lung disease who is gasping for every breath will not be concerned with food intake. This individual's main concern will be to obtain enough oxygen to live through the next minute.

Other physiological needs include sensory and motor needs. If these needs are unmet, individuals may not die, but their body functions will be affected. Sensory needs include hearing, seeing, feeling, smelling, tasting, and mental stimulation. When these needs are met, they allow the individual to respond to the environment. If these needs are not met, the person may lose contact with the environment or with reality. An example is motor needs, which include the ability to move and respond to the individual's environment. If muscles are not stimulated, they will atrophy (waste away), and function will be lost.

Many of the physiological needs are automatically controlled by the body. The process of breathing is usually not part of the conscious thought process of the individual until something occurs to interfere with breathing. Another example is the functioning of the urinary bladder. The bladder fills automatically, and the individual only becomes aware of the bladder when it is full. If the individual does not respond and go to the restroom to empty the bladder, eventually control will be lost, and the bladder will empty itself.

Health care workers must be aware of how an illness interferes with meeting physiological needs. A patient scheduled for surgery or laboratory tests may not be allowed to eat or drink prior to the procedure. Anxiety about an illness may interfere with a patient's sleep or elimination patterns. Medications may affect a patient's appetite. Elderly individuals are even more likely to have difficulty meeting physiological needs. A loss of vision or hearing due to aging may make it difficult for an elderly person to communicate with others. A decreased sense of smell and taste can affect appetite. Deterioration of muscles and joints can lead to poor coordination and difficulty in walking. Any of these factors can cause a change in a person's behavior. If health care workers are aware that physiological needs are not being met, they can provide understanding and support to the patient and make every effort to help the patient satisfy the needs.

Safety

Safety becomes important when physiological needs have been met. Safety needs include the need to be free from anxiety and fear and the need to feel secure in the environment. The need for order and routine is another example of an individual's effort to remain safe and secure. Individuals often prefer the familiar over the unknown. New environments, a change in routine, marital problems, job loss, injury, disease, and other similar events can threaten an individual's safety.

Illness is a major threat to an individual's security and well being. Health care workers are familiar with laboratory tests, surgeries, medications, and therapeutic treatments. Patients are usually frightened when they are exposed to them and their sense of security is threatened. If health care workers explain the reason for the tests or treatments and the expected outcomes to the patient, this can frequently alleviate the patient's anxieties. Patients admitted to a health care facility or long-term care facility must adapt to a strange and new environment. They frequently experience anxiety or depression. Patients may also experience depression over the loss of health or loss of a body function. Health care workers must be aware of the threats to safety and security that patients are experiencing, and make every effort to explain procedures, provide support and understanding, and help patients adapt to the situation.

Love and Affection

The need for love and **affection,** a warm and tender feeling for another person, occupies the third level of Maslow's Hierarchy of Needs. When an individual feels safe and secure, and after all physiological needs have been met, the individual next strives for social acceptance, friendship, and to be loved. The need to belong, to relate to others, and to win approval of others motivates an individual's actions at this point. The individual may now attend a social function that was avoided when safety was more of a priority. Individuals who feel safe and secure are more willing to accept and adapt to change and more willing to face unknown situations. The need for love and affection is satisfied when friends are made, social contacts are established, acceptance by others is received, and the individual is able to both give and receive affection and love (see figure 7-15).

Maslow states that sexuality is both a part of the need for love and affection as well as a physiological need. **Sexuality** in this context is defined by people's feelings concerning their masculine/feminine natures, their abilities to give and receive love and affection, and, finally, their roles in reproduction of the species. It is important to note that in all three of these areas, sexuality involves a person's feelings and attitudes, not just the person's sexual relationships.

It is equally important to note that a person's sexuality extends throughout the life cycle. At conception, a person's sexual organs are determined. Following birth, a person is given a name, at least generally associated with the person's sex.

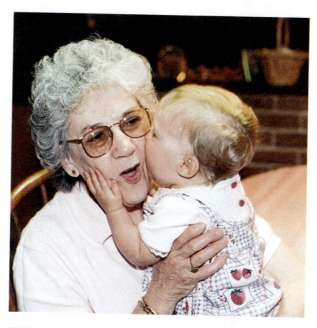

FIGURE 7-15 Individuals of all ages need love and affection. *(Courtesy of Sandy Clark)*

Studies have shown that children receive treatment according to gender from early childhood and frequently are rewarded for behavior that is deemed "gender appropriate." With the onset of puberty, adolescents become more aware of their emerging sexuality and of the standards that society places on them. During both childhood and adolescence, much of what is learned about sexuality comes from observing adult role models. As the adolescent grows into young adulthood, society encourages a reexamination of sexuality and the role it plays in helping to fulfill the need for love and affection. In adulthood, sexuality develops new meanings according to the roles that the adult takes on. Sexuality needs do not cease in late adulthood. Long-term care facilities are recognizing this fact by allowing married couples to each share a room, instead of separating people according to sex. Even after the death of a spouse, an individual may develop new relationships. Determining what role sexuality will play in a person's life is a dynamic process that allows people to meet their need for love and affection throughout their life.

Sexuality, in addition to being related to the satisfaction of needs, is also directly related to an individual's moral values. Issues such as the appropriateness of sex before marriage, the use of birth control, how to deal with pregnancy, and how to deal with sexually transmitted diseases all require individuals to evaluate their moral beliefs.

These beliefs then serve as guidelines to help people reach decisions on their behaviors.

Some individuals use sexual relationships as substitutes for love and affection. Individuals who seek to meet their needs only in this fashion cannot successfully complete Maslow's third level.

Esteem

Maslow's fourth level includes the need for **esteem.** Esteem includes feeling important and worthwhile. When others show respect, approval, and appreciation, an individual begins to feel esteem and gains self-respect. The self-concept, or beliefs, values, and feelings people have about themselves, becomes positive. Individuals will engage in activities that bring achievement, success, and recognition in an effort to maintain their need for esteem. Failure in an activity can cause a loss of confidence and lack of esteem. When esteem needs are met, individuals gain confidence in themselves and begin to direct their actions toward becoming what they want to be.

Illness can have a major effect on esteem. When self-reliant individuals, competent at making decisions, find themselves in a health care facility dependent on others for basic care such as bathing, eating, and elimination, they can experience a severe loss of esteem. They may also worry about a lack of income, possible job loss, the well being of their family, and/or the possibility of permanent disability or death. Patients may become angry and frustrated or quiet and withdrawn. Health care workers must recognize this loss of esteem and make every attempt to listen to the patient, encourage as much independence as possible, provide supportive care, and allow the person to express anger or fear.

Self-Actualization

Self-actualization, frequently called *self-realization,* is the final need in Maslow's hierarchy. All other needs must be met, at least in part, before self-actualization can occur. Self-actualization means that people have obtained their full potentials, or that they are what they want to be. People at this level are confident and willing to express their beliefs and stick to them. They feel so strongly about themselves that they are willing to reach out to others to provide assistance and support.

MEETING NEEDS

When needs are felt, individuals are **motivated** (stimulated) to act. If the action is successful and the need is met, **satisfaction,** or a feeling of pleasure or fulfillment, occurs. If the need is not met, **tension,** or frustration, an uncomfortable inner sensation or feeling, occurs. Several needs can be felt at the same time, so individuals must decide which needs are stronger. For example, if individuals need both food and sleep, they must decide which need is most important, because an individual cannot eat and sleep at the same time.

Individuals feel needs at different levels of intensity. The more intense a need, the greater the desire to meet or reduce the need. Also, when an individual first experiences a need, the individual may deal with it by trying different actions in a trial-and-error manner, a type of behavior frequently seen in very young children. As they grow older, children learn more effective means of meeting the need, and are able to satisfy the need easily.

METHODS OF SATISFYING HUMAN NEEDS

Needs can be satisfied by direct or indirect methods. Direct methods work at meeting the need and obtaining satisfaction. Indirect methods work at reducing the need or relieving the tension and frustration created by the unmet need.

Direct Methods

Direct methods include:

- hard work
- realistic goals
- situation evaluation
- cooperation with others

All these methods are directed toward meeting the need. Students who constantly fail tests but who want to pass a course have a need for success. They can work harder by listening more in class, asking questions on points they do not understand, and studying longer for the tests. They can set realistic goals that will allow them to find success. By working on one aspect of the course at a time, by concentrating on new material for the next test, by planning to study a little each night rather than studying only the night before a test, and by working on other things that will enable them to pass, they can establish goals they can achieve. They can evaluate the situation to determine why they are failing and to try to find other ways to pass the course. They may determine that they are always tired in class and that by getting more sleep, they will be able to learn the material. They can cooperate with others. By asking the teacher to provide extra assistance, by having parents or friends question them on the material, by asking a counselor to help them learn better study habits, or by having a tutor provide extra help, they may learn the material, pass the tests, and achieve satisfaction by meeting their need.

Indirect Methods

Indirect methods of dealing with needs usually reduce the need and help relieve the tension created by the unmet need. The need is still present, but its intensity decreases. **Defense mechanisms,** unconscious acts that help a person deal with an unpleasant situation or socially unacceptable behavior, are the main indirect methods used. Everyone uses defense mechanisms to some degree. Defense mechanisms provide methods for maintaining self-esteem and relieving discomfort. Some use of defense mechanisms is helpful because it allows individuals to cope with certain situations. However, defense mechanisms can be unhealthy if they are used all the time and individuals substitute them for more effective ways of dealing with situations. Being aware of the use of defense mechanisms and the reason for using them is a healthy use. This allows the individual to relieve tension while modifying habits, learning to accept reality, and striving to find more efficient ways to meet needs.

Examples of defense mechanisms include:

◆ **Rationalization**—This involves using a reasonable excuse or acceptable explanation for behavior in order to avoid the real reason or true motivation. For example, a patient who fears having laboratory tests performed may tell the health worker, "I can't take time off from my job," rather than admit fear.

◆ **Projection**—This involves placing the blame for one's own actions or inadequacies on someone else or on circumstances rather than accepting responsibility for the actions. Examples include, "The teacher failed me because she doesn't like me," rather than, "I failed because I didn't do the work"; and, "I'm late because the alarm clock didn't go off," rather than, "I forgot to set the alarm clock, and I overslept." When people use projection to blame others, they avoid having to admit that they have made mistakes.

◆ **Displacement**—This involves transferring feelings about one person to someone else. Displacement usually occurs because individuals cannot direct the feelings toward the person who is responsible. Many people fear directing hostile or negative feelings toward their bosses or supervisors because they fear job loss. They then direct this anger toward coworkers and/or family members. The classic example is the man who is mad at his boss. When the man gets home, he yells at his wife or children. In such a case, a constructive talk with the boss may solve the problem. If not, or if this is not possible, physical activity can help work off hostile or negative feelings.

◆ **Compensation**—This involves the substitution of one goal for another goal in order to achieve success. If a substitute goal meets needs, this can be a healthy defense mechanism. For example, Joan wanted to be a doctor, but she did not have enough money for a medical education. So she changed her educational plans and became a physician's assistant. Compensation was an efficient defense mechanism because she enjoyed her work and found satisfaction.

◆ **Daydreaming**—This is a dreamlike thought process that occurs when a person is awake. Daydreaming provides a means of escape when a person is not satisfied with reality. If it allows a person to establish goals for the future and leads to a course of action to accomplish those goals, it is a good defense mechanism. If daydreaming is a substitute for reality, and the dreams become more satisfying than actual life experiences, it can contribute to a poor adjustment to life. For example, if a person dreams about becoming a dental hygienist and takes courses and works toward this goal, daydreaming is effective. If the person dreams about the goal but is satisfied by the thoughts and takes no action, the person will not achieve the goal and is simply escaping from reality.

◆ **Repression**—This involves the transfer of unacceptable or painful ideas, feelings, and thoughts into the unconscious mind. An individual is not aware that this is occurring. When feelings or emotions become too painful or frightening for the mind to deal with, repression allows the individual to continue functioning and to "forget" the fear or feeling. Repressed feelings do not vanish, however. They can resurface in dreams or affect behavior. For example, a person is terrified of heights but does not know why. It is possible that a frightening experience regarding heights happened in early childhood and that the experience was repressed.

◆ **Suppression**—This is similar to repression, but the individual is aware of the unacceptable feelings or thoughts and refuses to deal with them. The individual may substitute work, a hobby, or a project to avoid the situation. For example, a woman ignores a lump in her breast and refuses to go to a doctor. She avoids thinking about the lump by working overtime and joining a health club to exercise during her spare time. This type of behavior creates excessive stress and eventually the individual will be forced to deal with the situation.

◆ **Denial**—This involves disbelief of an event or idea that is too frightening or shocking for a person to cope with. Often, an individual is not aware that denial is occurring. Denial frequently occurs when a terminal illness is diagnosed. The individual will say that the doctor is wrong and seek another opinion. When the individual is ready to deal with the event or idea, denial becomes acceptance.

◆ **Withdrawal**—There are two main ways withdrawal can occur: individuals can either cease to communicate or remove themselves physically from a situation (see figure 7-16). Withdrawal is sometimes a satisfactory means of avoiding conflict or an unhappy situation. For example, if you are forced to work with an individual you dislike and who is constantly criticizing your work, you can withdraw by avoiding any and all communication with this individual, quitting your job, or asking for a transfer to another area. At times, interpersonal conflict cannot be avoided, however. In these cases, an open and honest communication with the

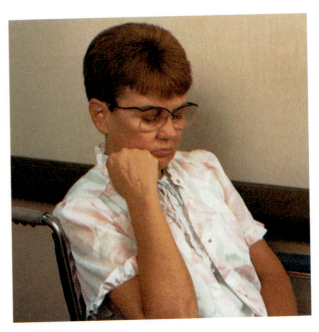

FIGURE 7-16 Refusing to communicate is a sign of withdrawal.

individual may lead to improved understanding in the relationship.

It is important for health care workers to be aware of both their own and patients' needs. By recognizing needs and understanding the actions individuals take to meet needs, more efficient and higher quality care can be provided. Health care workers will be better able to understand their own behavior and the behavior of others.

STUDENT: *Go to the workbook and complete the assignment sheet for 7:3, Human Needs.*

7:4 INFORMATION Effective Communications

C   Communicating effectively with others is an important part of any health career. The health care worker must be able to relate to patients and their families, to coworkers, and to other professionals. An understanding of communication skills will assist the health care worker who is trying to relate effectively.

Communication is the exchange of information, thoughts, ideas, and feelings. It can occur through **verbal** means (spoken words), written communications, and **nonverbal** behavior such as facial expressions, body language, and touch.

COMMUNICATION PROCESS

The communication process involves three essential elements:

◆ *sender:* an individual who creates a message to convey information or an idea to another person

◆ *message:* information, ideas, or thoughts

◆ *receiver:* an individual who receives the message from the sender

Without a sender, message, and receiver, communication cannot occur.

Feedback is a method that can be used to determine if communication was successful. This occurs when the receiver responds to the message. It allows the original sender to evaluate how the message was interpreted and to make any necessary adjustments or clarification. Feedback can be verbal or nonverbal.

Even though the communication process seems simple, many factors can interfere with the completion of the process. Important elements of effective communication include:

◆ *The message must be clear:* The message must be in terms that both the sender and receiver understand. Health care workers learn and use terminology that is frequently not understood by those people who are not in health care. Even though these terms are familiar to the health care worker, they must be modified, defined, or substituted with other words when messages are conveyed to people not in health care. For example, if a health care worker needs a urine specimen, some patients can be told to urinate in a container. Others, such as very small children or individuals with limited education, may have to be told to "pee" or "do number one." Even a term such as *apical pulse* is not understood by many individuals. Instead of telling a patient, "I am going to take your apical pulse," say, "I am going to listen to your heart." It requires experience and constant practice to learn to create a message that can be clearly understood.

◆ *The sender must deliver the message in a clear and concise manner:* Correct pronunciation and the use of good grammar are essential. The use of slang words or words with double meanings should be avoided. Meaningless phrases or terms such as "you know," "all that stuff," "um," and "OK," distract from the message and also must be avoided. In verbal communications, the tone and pitch of voice is important. A moderate level, neither too soft nor too loud, and good inflection, to avoid monotone, are essential. Think of the many different ways the sentence "I really like this job" can be said and the different meanings that can be interpreted depending on the tone and pitch of the voice. The proper rate, or speed, of delivering a message is also important. If a message is delivered too quickly, the receiver may not have enough time to hear all parts of the message. In written communications, the message should be spelled correctly, contain correct grammar and punctuation, and be concise but thorough.

◆ *The receiver must be able to hear and receive the message:* Patients who are heavily medicated or are weak may nod their heads as if messages are heard, when, in reality, the patients are not receiving the information. They may hear it, but it is not being interpreted and understood because of their physical states. Patients with hearing or visual impairments or patients with limited English-speaking abilities are other examples of individuals who may not be able to easily receive messages (see figure 7-17). Repeating the message, changing the form of the message, and getting others to interpret or clarify the message are some ways to help the receiver receive and respond to the message.

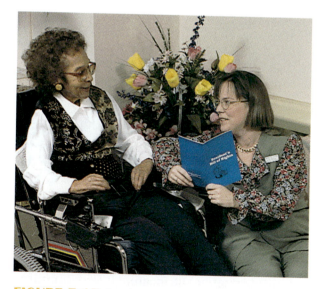

FIGURE 7-17 In communicating with a person who has a hearing impairment, face the individual and speak slowly and distinctly.

◆ *The receiver must be able to understand the message:* Using unfamiliar terminology can cause a breakdown in communication. Many people do not want to admit that they do not understand terms because they think others will think they are dumb. The health care worker should ask questions or repeat information in different terms if it appears that the patient does not understand the information. The receiver's attitude and prejudices can also interfere with understanding. If a patient feels that health care workers do not know what they are talking about, the patient will not accept the information presented. Receivers must have some confidence and belief in the sender before they will accept and understand a message. It is important that health care workers are willing to say, "I don't know, but I will try to find out that information for you" when they are asked a question about which they do not have correct knowledge. It is also important for health care workers to be aware of their own prejudices and attitudes when they are receiving messages from patients. If health care workers feel that certain patients are lazy, ignorant, or uncooperative, they will not respond correctly to messages sent by these patients. Health care workers must be aware of these feelings and work to overcome them so they can accept patients as they are.

◆ *Interruptions or distractions must be avoided:* Interruptions or distractions can interfere with any communication. Trying to talk with others while answering the phone or writing a message can decrease the effectiveness of spoken and/or written communication. Loud noises, or distractions in the form of bright light or uncomfortable temperature can interrupt communication. When two people are talking outside in freezing temperatures, for example, the conversation will be limited because of the discomfort from the cold. A small child jumping around or climbing up and down off a mother's lap will distract the mother as she is getting instructions from a health care worker. A loud television or radio interferes with verbal messages, because receivers may pay more attention to the radio or television than to the person speaking to them. It is important to eliminate or at least limit distractions if meaningful communication is to take place.

LISTENING

Listening is another essential part of effective communication. Listening means paying attention to and making an effort to hear what the other person is saying. Good listening skills require constant practice. Techniques that can be used to learn good listening skills include:

◆ Show interest and concern for what the speaker is saying.

◆ Be alert and maintain eye contact with the speaker.

◆ Avoid interrupting the speaker.

◆ Pay attention to what the speaker is saying.

◆ Avoid thinking about how you are going to respond.

◆ Try to eliminate your own prejudices and see the other person's point of view.

◆ Eliminate distractions by moving to a quiet area for the conversation.

◆ Watch the speaker closely to observe actions that may contradict what the person is saying.

◆ Reflect statements back to the speaker to let the speaker know that statements are being heard.

◆ Ask for clarification if you do not understand part of a message.

◆ Keep your temper under control and maintain a positive attitude.

Good listening skills will allow you to receive the entire message a person is trying to convey to you. For example, if a patient says, "I'm not worried about this surgery," but is very restless and seems nervous, the patient's body movements may indicate fear that is being denied by words. The health care worker could reflect the patient's statement by saying, "You're not at all worried about this surgery?" The patient may respond by saying, "Well, not really. It's just that I worry about my family if something should happen to me." Good listening allowed the patient to express fears and opened the way to more effective communication. In this same case, the entire pattern of communication could have been blocked if the health care worker had instead responded, "That's good."

NONVERBAL COMMUNICATION

Nonverbal communication involves the use of facial expressions, body language, gestures, eye contact, and touch to convey messages or ideas (see figure 7-18). If a person is smiling and sitting in a very relaxed position while saying, "I am very angry about this entire situation," two different messages are being conveyed. A smile, a frown, a wink, a shrug of the shoulders, a bored expression, a tapping of fingers or feet, and other similar body gestures or actions all convey messages to the receiver. It is important for health care workers to be aware of both their own and patients' nonverbal behaviors because these are an important part of any communication process. A touch of the hand, a pat on the back, a firm handshake, and a hug can convey more interest and caring than words could ever do. When verbal and nonverbal messages agree, the receiver is more likely to understand the message being sent.

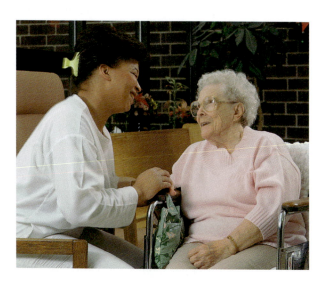

FIGURE 7-18 What aspects of listening and nonverbal behavior can you see in this picture?

BARRIERS TO COMMUNICATION

A communication barrier is something that gets in the way of clear communication. Three common

barriers are physical disabilities, psychological attitudes and prejudice, and cultural diversity.

Physical disabilities may include:

◆ Deafness or hearing loss: People who are deaf or hearing impaired have difficulty receiving messages. To improve communication, it is essential to use body language such as gestures and signs, speak clearly in short sentences, face the individual to improve the potential for lip reading, write messages if necessary, and make sure that any hearing aids have good batteries and are inserted correctly (see figure 7-19).

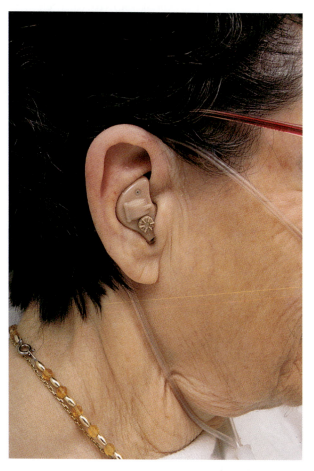

FIGURE 7-19 In order to be effective, hearing aids must be inserted correctly and have good batteries.

◆ Blindness or impaired vision: People who are blind or visually impaired may be able to hear what is being said, but they will not see body language, gestures, or facial expressions. To improve communication, use a soft tone of voice, describe events that are occurring, announce your presence as you enter a room, explain sounds or noises, and use touch when appropriate.

- ◆ Aphasia or speech impairments: Individuals with aphasia or speech impairments can have difficulty with not only the spoken word but also written communications. They may know what they want to say but have difficulty remembering the correct words, may not be able to pronounce certain words, or may have slurred and distorted speech. Patience is essential while working with these individuals. Allow them to try to speak, encourage them to take their time, ask questions that require only short responses, speak slowly and clearly, repeat messages to be sure they are correct, encourage them to use gestures or point to objects, provide writing materials if they can write messages, or use pictures with key messages to communicate (see figure 7-20).

Psychological barriers to communication are often caused by prejudice, attitudes, and personality. Examples include closed-mindedness, judging,

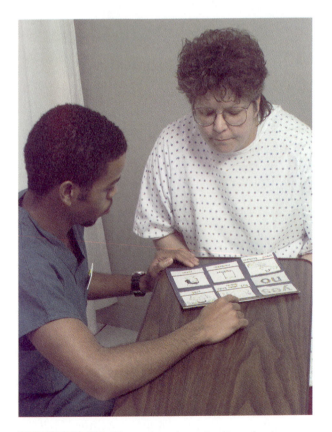

FIGURE 7-20 Picture cards make it easier to communicate with a patient who has aphasia or a speech impairment.

preaching, moralizing, lecturing, over-reacting, arguing, advising, and prejudging. Our judgments of others are too often based on appearance, lifestyle, and social or economic status. Stereotypes such as "dumb blonde," "lazy bum," or "fat slob" cause us to make snap judgments about an individual and affect the communication process. Health care workers must learn to put prejudice aside and show respect to all individuals. A homeless person deserves the same quality of health care as the president of the United States. It is important to respect each person as an individual and to remember that each person has the right to good care and considerate treatment. At times, this can be extremely difficult, and patience and practice are essential. When individuals have negative attitudes or constantly complain or criticize your work, it can be difficult to show them respect. The health care worker must learn to see beyond the surface attitude to the human being underneath. Frequently, fear is the cause of anger or a negative attitude. Allow patients to express their fears or anger, encourage them to talk about their feelings, avoid arguing, remain calm, talk in a soft and non-threatening tone of voice, and provide quality care. If other health care workers seem to be able to communicate more effectively with patients, watch these workers to learn how they handle difficult or angry patients. This is often the most effective means of learning good communication skills.

Cultural diversity, discussed in detail in Unit 8, is another possible communication barrier. Culture consists of the values, beliefs, attitudes, and customs shared by a group of people and passed from one generation to the next. It is often defined as a set of rules, because culture allows an individual to interpret the environment and actions of others and behave appropriately. The main barriers created by cultural diversity include:

- ◆ *Beliefs and practices regarding health and illness:* Individuals from different cultures may have their own beliefs about the cause of an illness and the type of treatment required. It is important to remember that they have the right to determine their treatment plans and even to refuse traditional treatments. At times, these individuals may accept traditional health care but add their own cultural remedies to the treatment plan.

- ◆ *Language differences:* Language differences can create major barriers. In the United States,

English is a primary language used in health care. If a person has difficulty communicating in English, and a health care worker is not fluent in another language, a barrier exists. When providing care to people who have limited English-speaking abilities, speak slowly, use simple words, use gestures or pictures to clarify the meaning of words, use nonverbal communication in the form of a smile or gentle touch, and avoid the tendency to speak louder because this does not improve comprehension. Whenever possible, try to find an interpreter who speaks the language of the patient. Frequently, another health care worker, a consultant, or a family member may be able to assist in the communication process.

◆ *Eye contact:* In some cultures, direct eye-to-eye contact while communicating is not acceptable. These cultures believe that looking down shows proper respect for another individual. A health care worker who feels that eye contact is important must learn to accept and respect this cultural difference and a person's inability to engage in eye contact while communicating.

◆ *Ways of dealing with terminal illness and/or severe disability:* In the United States, a traditional health care belief is that the patient should be told the truth about his or her diagnosis and informed about the expected outcome. Some cultural groups believe that a person should not be told of a fatal diagnosis or be burdened with making decisions about treatment. In these cultures, the family, the mother or father, or another designated individual is expected to make decisions about care, treatment, and information given to the patient. In such instances, it is important for health care workers to recognize and respect this and to involve these individuals in the patient's care. At times, it may be necessary for a patient to use legal means, such as power of attorney for health care, in order to designate responsibility for his or her care to another person.

◆ *Touch:* In some cultures, it is inappropriate to touch someone on the head. Other cultures have clearly defined areas of the body that can be touched or that should be avoided. Even a simple handshake can be regarded as showing lack of respect. In some cultures, only family members provide personal care. For this reason, health care workers should always get permission from the patient before providing care and should avoid any use of touch that seems to be inappropriate for the individual.

Respect for and acceptance of cultural diversity is essential for any health care worker. When beliefs, ideas, concepts, and ways of life are different, communication barriers can result. By making every attempt to learn about cultural differences and by showing respect for an individual's right to cultural beliefs, a health care worker can provide quality health care.

RECORDING AND REPORTING

In health care, an important part of effective communication is reporting or recording all observations while providing care. In order to do this, it is important to not only listen to what the patient is saying, but to make observations about the patient. All senses are used to make observations:

◆ *Sense of sight:* notes the color of skin, swelling or edema, the presence of a rash or sore, the color of urine or stool, the amount of food eaten, and other similar factors

◆ *Sense of smell:* alerts a health care worker to body odor or unusual odors of breath, wounds, urine, or stool

◆ *Sense of touch:* used to feel the pulse, dryness or temperature of the skin, perspiration, and swelling

◆ *Sense of hearing:* used while listening to respirations, abnormal body sounds, coughs, and speech

By using all senses, the health care worker can learn a great deal about a patient's condition and be able to report observations objectively.

Observations should be reported promptly and accurately to an immediate supervisor. There are two types of observations:

◆ *Subjective observations:* these cannot be seen or felt, and are commonly called symptoms. They are usually statements or complaints made by the patient. They should be reported in the exact words the patient used.

◆ *Objective observations:* these can be seen or measured, and are commonly called signs. A bruise, cut, rash, or swelling can be seen. Blood pressure and temperature are measurable.

For example, the health care worker should not state, "I think Mr. B. has a fever." The report should state, "Mr. B. is complaining of feeling hot. His skin is red and flushed, and his temperature is 102°."

In some health care facilities, observations are recorded on a patient's health care record. Effective communication requires these written observations to be accurate, concise, and complete (see figure 7-21). The writing should be neat and legible, and spelling and grammar should be correct. Only objective observations should be noted. Subjective observations that the health care worker feels or thinks should be avoided. If a patient's statement is recorded, the statement should be written in the patient's own words and enclosed in quotation marks. All information should be signed with the name and title of the person recording the information. Errors should be crossed out neatly with a straight line, have

"error" recorded by them, and show the initials of the person making the error. In this way, recorded communication will be effective communication.

Good communication skills allow health care workers to develop good interpersonal relationships. Patients feel accepted, they feel that others have an interest and concern in them, they feel free to express their ideas and fears, they develop confidence in the health care workers, and they feel they are receiving quality health care. In addition, the health care worker will relate more effectively with coworkers and other individuals.

STUDENT: *Go to the workbook and complete the assignment sheet for 7:4, Effective Communications.*

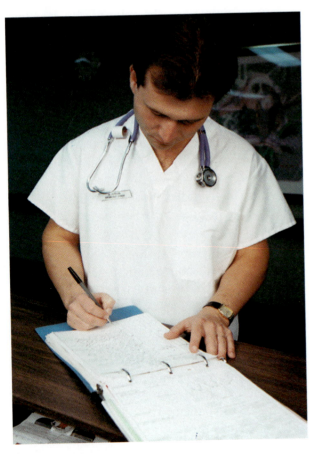

FIGURE 7-21 Information recorded on health care records must be accurate, concise, and complete.

UNIT 7 SUMMARY

Human growth and development is a process that begins at birth and does not end until death. Each individual passes through certain stages of growth and development, frequently called life stages. Each stage has its own characteristics and has specific developmental tasks that an individual must master. Each stage also establishes the foundation for the next stage.

Death is often called "the final stage of growth." Dr. Elizabeth Kübler-Ross has identified five stages that dying patients and their families may experience prior to death. These stages are denial, anger, bargaining, depression, and acceptance. The health care worker must be aware of these stages in order to provide supportive care to the dying patient. In addition, the health care worker must understand the concepts represented by hospice care and the right to die.

Each life stage creates needs that must be met by the individual. Abraham Maslow, a noted psychologist, developed a hierarchy of needs that is frequently used to classify and define the needs experienced by human beings. The needs are classified into five levels, and according to Maslow, the lower needs must be met before an individual can strive to meet the higher needs. The needs, beginning at the lowest level and progressing to the highest, are physiological, or physical, needs; safety and security; love and affection; esteem; and self-actualization.

Needs are met or satisfied by direct and indirect methods. Direct methods meet and eliminate a need. Indirect methods, usually the use of defense mechanisms, reduce the need and help relieve the tension created by the unmet need.

Effective communication is an important aspect of helping individuals through stages of growth and development and in meeting needs. A health care worker must have an understanding of the communication process, factors that interfere with communication, the importance of listening, and verbal and nonverbal communication. Another important aspect of communication is the proper reporting or recording of all observations noted while providing care.

Communication barriers such as physical disabilities, psychological attitudes, and cultural diversity can interfere with the communication process. Special consideration must be given to these barriers to improve communication. Some cultural groups have beliefs and practices that may relate to health and illness. Because individuals will respond to health care according to their cultural beliefs, a health care worker must be aware of and show respect for different cultural values in order to provide optimal patient care.

Mastering these concepts will allow health care workers to develop good interpersonal relationships and provide more effective health care.

INTERNET SEARCHES

Use the suggested search engines in Unit 11:4 of this textbook to search the Internet for additional information on the following topics:

1. *Erikson's stages of psychosocial development:* search for more details and examples of the stages of development.

2. *Stages of human growth and development:* search words such as infancy, childhood, adolescence, puberty, and adulthood to obtain information on each stage.

3. *Eating disorders:* search for statistics, signs and symptoms, and treatment of anorexia nervosa, bulimia, and bulimarexia.

4. *Chemical or drug abuse:* search for statistics, signs/symptoms, and treatment of chemical and drug abuse (*Hint:* use words such as alcoholism and cocaine).

5. *Suicide:* search for statistics, signs/symptoms, and ways to prevent suicide.

6. *Death and dying:* search for information on Dr. Kübler-Ross, hospice care, palliative treatment, advance directives, and the right to die.

7. *Maslow's hierarchy of needs:* search for additional information on each of the five levels of needs.

8. *Defense mechanisms:* search for specific information on rationalization, projection, displacement, compensation, daydreaming, repression, suppression, denial, and withdrawal.

9. *Communication:* search for information on listening skills, nonverbal communication, and the communication process.

REVIEW QUESTIONS

1. List the seven (7) life stages and at least two (2) physical, mental, emotional, and social developments that occur in each stage.

2. Create an example for what a patient and/or family member might say or do during each of the five (5) stages of death and dying.

3. Explain what is meant by the "right to die." Do you believe in this right? Why or why not?

4. Identify each level of Maslow's hierarchy of needs and give examples of specific needs at each level.

5. Create a specific example for each of the following defense mechanisms: rationalization, projection, displacement, compensation, daydreaming, repression, suppression, denial, and withdrawal.

6. Why is it important to observe both verbal and nonverbal communication?

7. List five (5) factors that can interfere with the communication process. Give two (2) specific examples for each factor.

8. Differentiate between objective and subjective observations. Provide two (2) examples for each type of observation.

UNIT 7

SUGGESTED REFERENCES

Agency for Instructional Technology. *Communication 2000: Classroom to Career.* Cincinnati, OH: South-Western, 1998.

Allen, K. Eileen, and Lynn Marotz. *Developmental Profiles: Pre-Birth to Eight.* 3rd ed. Clifton Park, NY: Delmar Learning, 1999.

Browning, Doreen, and Lorriane Villemaire. *Writing Skills for Health Care Professionals.* Clifton Park, NY: Delmar Learning, 2001.

Johns, Merida. *Information Management for Health Professions.* 2nd ed. Clifton Park, NY: Delmar Learning, 2002.

Kelz, Rochelle. *Delmar's English–Spanish Pocket Dictionary for Health Professions.* Clifton Park, NY: Delmar Learning, 1997.

Kübler-Ross, Elizabeth. *Death: The Final Stage of Growth.* Englewood Cliffs, NJ: Prentice-Hall, 1975.

Kübler-Ross, Elizabeth. *On Death and Dying.* New York, NY: Macmillan, 1977.

Kübler-Ross, Elizabeth. *Questions and Answers to Death and Dying.* New York, NY: Macmillan, 1974.

Marotz, Lynn, Marie Cross, and Jeanettia Rush. *Health, Safety, and Nutrition for the Young Child.* Clifton Park, NY: Delmar Learning, 1997.

McWay, Dana. *Legal Aspects of Health Information Management.* 2nd ed. Clifton Park, NY: Delmar Learning, 2003.

Means, Tom. *Communication for the Workplace.* Cincinnati, OH: South-Western, 2001.

Milliken, Mary Elizabeth. *Understanding Human Behavior.* 6th ed. Clifton Park, NY: Delmar Learning, 1998.

Olson, Melodie. *Healing the Dying.* 2nd ed. Clifton Park, NY: Delmar Learning, 2002.

Papalia, Diane, Harvey Sterns, and Ruth Feldman. *Adult Development and Aging.* 2nd ed. New York, NY: McGraw-Hill, 2001.

Potts, Nicki, and Barbara Mandleco. *Pediatric Nursing: Caring for Children and Their Families.* Clifton Park, NY: Delmar Learning, 2002.

Quill, Timothy. *Death and Dignity.* New York, NY: W.W. Norton and Co., 1993.

Roach, Sally, and Beatriz Nieto. *Healing and the Grief Process.* Clifton Park, NY: Delmar Learning, 1997.

Rybash, John. *Adult Development and Aging.* 3rd ed. Dubuque, IA: Wm. C. Brown Publishers, 1996.

Spiegel, David. *Living Beyond Limits.* New York, NY: Random House, 1993.

Tamparo, Carol, and Wilburta Lindh. *Therapeutic Communications for Health Professionals.* 2nd ed. Clifton Park, NY: Delmar Learning, 2000.

Villemarie, Doreen, and Lorraine Villemarie. *Grammar and Writing Skills for the Health Professional.* Clifton Park, NY: Delmar Learning, 2001.

Watson, Linda, Michael Watson, and LaVisa Wilson. *Infants and Toddlers.* 3rd ed. Clifton Park, NY: Delmar Learning, 1998.

Waughfield, Claire. *Mental Health Concepts.* Clifton Park, NY: Delmar Learning, 2001.

Wray, J., L. Luft, and M. Highland. *Fundamentals of Human Relations: Applications for Life and Work.* Cincinnati, OH: South-Western, 1996.

Cultural Diversity

Unit Objectives

After completing this unit of study, you should be able to:

- List the four basic characteristics of culture
- Differentiate between culture, ethnicity, and race
- Identify some of the major ethnic groups in the United States
- Provide an example of acculturation in the United States
- Create an example of how a bias, prejudice, or stereotype can cause a barrier to effective relationships with others
- Describe at least five ways to avoid bias, prejudice, and stereotyping
- Differentiate between a nuclear family and an extended family
- Identify ways in which language, personal space, touching, eye contact, and gestures are affected by cultural diversity
- Compare and contrast the diverse health beliefs of different ethnic/cultural groups
- List five ways health care providers can show respect for an individual's religious beliefs
- Identify methods that can be used to show respect for cultural diversity
- Define, pronounce, and spell all the key terms

 Observe Standard Precautions

 Safety—Proceed with Caution

 Math Skill

 Science Skill

 C Communications Skill

 Instructors Check—Call Instructor at This Point

 **OBRA** OBRA Requirement— Based on Federal Law

 Legal Responsibility

 Career Information

 Technology

215

KEY TERMS

acculturation
agnostic
atheist
bias
cultural assimilation
cultural diversity
culture
ethnicity

ethnocentric
extended family
holistic care
matriarchal
    (may′-tree-ar″-kel)
nuclear family
patriarchal
    (pay′-tree-ar″-kel)

personal space
prejudice
race
religion
sensitivity
spirituality
stereotyping

8:1 INFORMATION Culture, Ethnicity, and Race

Health care providers must work with and provide care to many different people. At the same time, they must respect the individuality of each person. Therefore, every health care provider must be aware of the factors that cause each individual to be unique. Uniqueness is influenced by many things including physical characteristics (gender, body size, and hair, nail, and skin color), family life, socioeconomic status, religious beliefs, geographical location, education, occupation, and life experiences. A major influence on any individual's uniqueness is the person's cultural/ethnic heritage.

Culture is defined as the values, beliefs, attitudes, languages, symbols, rituals, behaviors, and customs unique to a particular group of people and passed from one generation to the next. It is often defined as a set of rules, because culture provides an individual with a blueprint or general design for living. Family relations, child rearing, education, occupational choice, social interactions, spirituality, religious beliefs, food preferences, health beliefs, and health care are all influenced by culture. Culture is not uniform among all members within a cultural group, but it does provide a foundation for behavior. Even though differences exist between cultural groups and in individuals within a cultural group, all cultures have four basic characteristics:

◆ *Culture is learned:* Culture does not just happen. It is taught to others. For example, children learn patterns of behavior by imitating adults and developing attitudes accepted by others.

◆ *Culture is shared:* Common practices and beliefs are shared with others in a cultural group.

◆ *Culture is social in nature:* Individuals in the cultural group understand appropriate behavior based on traditions that have been passed from generation to generation.

◆ *Culture is dynamic and constantly changing:* New ideas may generate different standards for behavior. This allows a cultural group to meet the needs of the group by adapting to environmental changes.

Ethnicity is a classification of people based on national origin and/or culture. Members of an ethnic group may share a common heritage, geographic location, social customs, language, and beliefs. Even though every individual in an ethnic group may not practice all of the beliefs of the group, the individual is still influenced by other members of the group. There are many different ethnic groups in the United States (see figure 8-1). Some of the common ethnic groups and their countries of origin include:

◆ African American: Central and South African countries, Dominican Republic, Haiti, and Jamaica

◆ Asian American: Cambodia, China, India, Indonesia and Pacific Island countries, Japan, Korea, Laos, Philippines, Samoa, and Vietnam

◆ European American: England, France, Germany, Ireland, Italy, Poland, Russia, Scandinavia, and Scotland

◆ Hispanic American: Cuba, Mexico, Puerto Rico, Spain, and Spanish-speaking countries in Central and South America

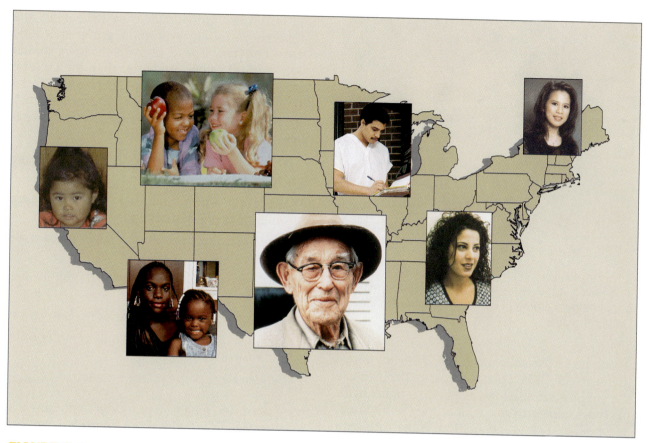

FIGURE 8-1 The many faces of the United States.

◆ Middle Eastern/Arabic Americans: Egypt, Iran, Jordan, Kuwait, Lebanon, Palestine, Saudi Arabia, Yemen, and other North African and Middle Eastern countries

◆ Native American: Over 500 tribes of American Indians and Eskimos

It is important to recognize that within each of the ethnic groups, there are numerous subgroups, each with its own lifestyle and beliefs. For example, the European American group includes Italians and Germans, two groups with different languages and lifestyles.

Race is a classification of people based on physical or biological characteristics such as the color of skin, hair, and eyes; facial features; blood type; and bone structure. Race is frequently used to label a group of people and explain patterns of behavior. In reality, race cuts across multiple ethnic/cultural groups, and it is the values, beliefs, and behaviors learned from the ethnic/cultural group that generally account for the behaviors attributed to race. For example, blacks from Africa and blacks from the Caribbean both share many of the same physical characteristics, but they have different cultural beliefs and values. In addition, there are different races present in

most ethnic groups. For example, there are white and black Hispanics, white Africans and Caribbeans, and white and black Asians.

Culture, ethnicity, and race do influence an individual's behavior, self-perception, judgment of others, and interpersonal relationships. These differences based on cultural, ethnic, and racial factors are called **cultural diversity.** It is important to remember that differences exist within ethnic/cultural groups and in individuals within a group. In previous times, the United States has often been called a "melting pot" to represent the absorption of many cultures into the dominant culture through a process called **cultural assimilation.** Cultural assimilation requires that the newly arrived cultural group alter unique beliefs and behaviors and adopt the ways of the dominant culture. In reality, the United States is striving to be more like a "salad bowl" where cultural differences are appreciated and respected. The simultaneous existence of various ethnic/cultural groups gives rise to a "multicultural" society that must recognize and respect many different beliefs. **Acculturation,** or the process of learning the beliefs and behaviors of a dominant culture and assuming some of the characteristics, does occur. However, acculturation occurs slowly over

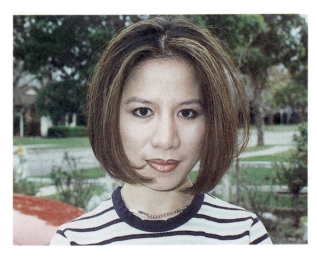

FIGURE 8-2 Second- or third-generation individuals in the same ethnic/cultural group will adopt many patterns of behavior dominant in the United States.

a long period, usually many years. Recent immigrants to the United States are more likely to use the language and follow the patterns of behavior of the country from which they emigrated. Second- and third-generation Americans are more likely to use English as their main language and follow the patterns of behavior prevalent in the United States (see figure 8-2).

Because they provide care to culturally diverse patients in a variety of settings, health care providers must be aware of these factors and remember that no individual is one hundred percent anything! Every individual has and will continue to create new and changing blends of values and beliefs. **Sensitivity,** the ability to recognize and appreciate the personal characteristics of others, is essential in health care. For example, in some cultures such as Native Americans or Asians, calling an adult by a first name is not acceptable except for close friends or relatives. Sensitive health care workers will address patients by their last names unless they are asked to use a patient's first name.

8:2 INFORMATION Bias, Prejudice, and Stereotyping

Bias, prejudice, and stereotyping can interfere with acceptance of cultural diversity. A **bias** is a preference that inhibits impartial judgment.

For example, individuals who believe in the supremacy of their own ethnic group are called **ethnocentric.** These individuals believe that their cultural values are better than the cultural values of others, and may antagonize and alienate people from other cultures. Individuals may also be biased with regard to other factors. Examples of common biases include:

◆ *Age:* Young people are physically and mentally superior to older people.

◆ *Education:* College-educated individuals are superior to uneducated individuals.

◆ *Economic:* Rich people are superior to poor people.

◆ *Physical size:* Obese and short people are inferior.

◆ *Occupation:* Nurses are inferior to doctors.

◆ *Sexual preference:* Homosexuals are inferior to heterosexuals.

◆ *Gender:* Women are inferior to men.

Prejudice means to pre-judge. A prejudice is a strong feeling or belief about a person or subject that is formed without reviewing facts or information. Prejudiced individuals regard their ideas or behavior as right and other ideas or behavior as wrong. They are frequently afraid of things that are different. Prejudice causes fear and distrust and interferes with interpersonal relationships. Every individual is prejudiced to some degree. We all want to feel that our beliefs are correct. In health care, however, it is important to be aware of our prejudices and to make every effort to obtain as much information about a situation as possible. This allows us to learn about other individuals, understand their beliefs, and communicate successfully.

Stereotyping occurs when an assumption is made that everyone in a particular group is the same. A stereotype ignores individual characteristics and "labels" an individual. A classic example is, "All blondes are dumb." This stereotype has been perpetuated by "blonde jokes" detrimental to individuals who have light colored hair. Similar stereotypes exist with regard to race, gender, body size (thin, obese, short, or tall), occupation, and ethnic/cultural group. It is essential to remember that everyone is a unique individual. Each person will have different life experiences and exposure to other cultures and ideas. This allows a person to develop a unique personality and lifestyle.

Bias, prejudice, and stereotyping are barriers to effective relationships with others. Health care providers must be alert to these barriers and make every effort to avoid them. Some ways to avoid bias, prejudice, and stereotyping include:

◆ Know and be consciously aware of your own personal and professional values and beliefs.

◆ Obtain as much information as possible about different ethnic/cultural groups.

◆ Be sensitive to behaviors and practices different from your own.

◆ Remember that you are not being pressured to adopt other beliefs, but that you must respect them.

◆ Develop friendships with a wide variety of people from different ethnic/cultural groups.

◆ Ask questions and encourage questions from others to share ideas and beliefs.

◆ Evaluate all information before you form an opinion.

◆ Be open to differences.

◆ Avoid jokes that may offend.

◆ Remember that mistakes happen. Apologize if you hurt another person, and forgive if another person hurts you.

8:3 INFORMATION Understanding Cultural Diversity

The cultural and ethnic beliefs of an individual will affect the behavior of the individual. Health care providers must be aware of these beliefs in order to provide **holistic care,** care that provides for the well-being of the whole person and meets not only physical needs, but also social, emotional, and mental needs. Some areas of cultural diversity include family organization, language, personal space, touching, eye contact, gestures, health care beliefs, spirituality, and religion.

FAMILY ORGANIZATION

Family organization refers to the structure of a family and the dominant or decision-making person in a family. Families vary in their composition and in the roles assumed by family

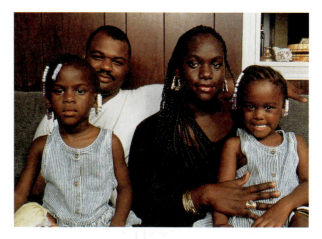

FIGURE 8-3 A nuclear family usually consists of a mother, father, and children.

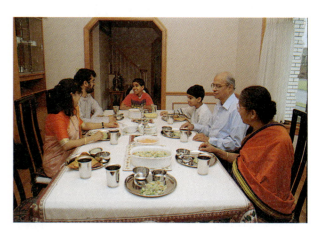

FIGURE 8-4 An extended family includes grandparents, aunts, uncles, and cousins in addition to the nuclear family.

members. A **nuclear family** usually consists of a mother, father, and children (see figure 8-3). It may also consist of a single parent and child(ren). An **extended family** includes the nuclear family plus grandparents, aunts, uncles, and cousins (see figure 8-4). The nuclear family is usually the basic unit in European American families, but the extended family is important. The basic unit for Asian, Hispanic, and Native Americans is generally the extended family, and frequently, several different generations live in the same household. This affects care of children, the sick, and the elderly. In extended family cultures, families tend to take care of their children and sick or elderly relatives in their home. For example, most Asian families have great respect for their elders and consider it a privilege to care for them. In some nuclear family cultures, people outside the family frequently care for children and sick or elderly relatives. Never assume anything about a family's organization. It is important to ask questions and observe the family.

Some families are **patriarchal** and the father or oldest male is the authority figure. In a **matriarchal** family, the mother or oldest female is the authority figure. This also affects health care. In a patriarchal family, the dominant male will make most health care decisions for all family members. For example, in some Asian and Middle Eastern families, men have the power and authority, and women are expected to be obedient. Husbands frequently accompany their wives to medical appointments and expect to make all the medical care decisions. In a matriarchal family, the dominant female may assume this responsibility. For example, if the mother or other female is the dominant figure in a family, she will make all the health decisions for all members of the family. In many families, both the mother and father share the decisions. Regardless of who the decision maker is, respect for the individual and the family must be the primary concern for the health care worker. Health care providers must respect patients who state, "I have to check with my husband (wife) before I decide if I should have the surgery."

Recognition and acceptance of family organization is essential for health care providers. Patients who have extended families as basic units may have many visitors in a hospital or long-term care center. Everyone will be concerned with the care provided, and all family members may help make decisions regarding care. At times, family members may even insist on providing basic personal care to the patient, such as bathing or hair care. Health care providers must adapt to these situations and allow the family to assist as much as possible.

C To determine a patient's family structure and learn about a patient's preferences, the health care provider should talk with the patient or ask questions. Examples of questions that can be asked include:

◆ Who are the members of your family?

◆ Do you have any children? Who will care for them while you are sick?

◆ Do you have extended family? For example, aunts, uncles, cousins, nephews, nieces?

◆ Who will be caring for you while you are sick?

◆ Who is the head of the household?

◆ Where do you and your family live?

◆ Was your entire family born in the United States?

◆ What do you and your family do together for recreation?

◆ Do you have family members who will be visiting you? (If patient is admitted to a health care facility)

LANGUAGE

C In the United States, the dominant language is English, but many other languages are also spoken. Statistics from the U. S. Census Bureau, based on Census 2000, verified that almost 20 percent of the population under age 65 speaks a language other than English at home. There are even variations within a language caused by different dialects. For example, the German taught in school may differ from the language spoken by Germans from different areas of Germany. Health care providers frequently encounter patients who do not use English as a dominant language. The health care provider must determine the patient's ability to communicate by talking with the patient or a relative and asking questions such as:

◆ Do you speak English as your primary language?

◆ What language is spoken at home?

◆ Do you read English? Do you read another language?

◆ Do you have a family member or friend who can interpret information for you?

Whenever possible, try to find a translator who speaks the language of the patient (see figure 8-5). Frequently another health care worker, a consultant, or a family member may be able to assist in the communication process. Most health care facilities have a roster of employees who speak other languages.

C When providing care to people who have limited English-speaking abilities, speak slowly, use simple words, use gestures or pictures to clarify the meaning of words, and use nonverbal communication in the form of a smile or

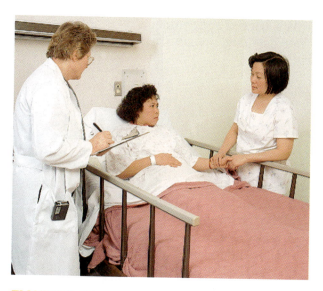

FIGURE 8-5 Whenever possible, try to find a translator to assist in communicating with a non-English-speaking patient.

gentle touch if it is culturally appropriate. Avoid the tendency to speak louder because this does not improve comprehension. Try to learn some words or phrases in the patient's language. Even a few words allow you to show the patient that you are trying to communicate. If you work with many patients who speak a common language, such as Spanish, try to master the basics of that language by taking an introductory course or by using an audiotape.

Other resources are also available to help a health care provider meet the needs of a non-English-speaking patient. Many health care facilities have health care information or questions printed in several languages. Cards can be purchased that explain basic health care procedures or treatments in many other languages.

Most states require that any medical permit requiring a written signature be printed in the patient's language to ensure that the patient understands what he or she is signing. Health care providers must be aware of legal requirements for non-English-speaking patients and make sure that these requirements are met.

PERSONAL SPACE AND TOUCH

Personal space, often called territorial space, describes the distance people require to feel comfortable while interacting with others. This varies greatly among different ethnic/cultural groups. Some cultures are called "close contact" and others are called "distant contact." Individuals from close-contact cultures are comfortable standing very close to and even touching the person with whom they are interacting. For example, Arabs are a very close contact group; they touch, feel, and smell people with whom they interact. French and Latin Americans tend to stand very close together while talking. Hispanic Americans are also comfortable with close contact and use hugs and handshakes to greet others. Even within a cultural group, there are variations. For example, women tend to stand closer together than men do and children stand closer together than adults do. European and African Americans prefer some space (approximately 2 to 6 feet) during interactions, but do not hesitate to shake hands as a greeting. Asian Americans will stand closer, but usually do not touch during a conversation. Kissing or hugging is reserved for intimate relationships and never done in public view. In Cambodia, members of the opposite sex may never touch each other in public, not even brothers and sisters. In addition, only a parent can touch the head of a child. The Vietnamese allow only the elderly to touch the head of a child because the head is considered sacred. In some Middle Eastern countries, men may not touch females who are not immediate family members, and only men may shake hands with other men. This may cause a female from one of these countries to refuse personal health care provided by a male health care provider. For Native Americans, personal space is important, but they will lightly touch another person's hand during greetings. It is important to understand that these situations are examples. You must never assume anything about an individual's personal space and touch preferences. You need to question the individual. Sample questions can be found at the end of this section.

Health care providers have to use touch and invade personal space to give many types of care. For example, taking blood pressure involves palpation of arteries, wrapping a cuff around a person's arm, and placing a stethoscope on the skin. If a health care provider uses a slow, relaxed approach, explains the procedure, and encourages the patient to relax, this may help alleviate fear and eliminate the discomfort and panic that can occur when personal space is invaded.

Always be alert to the patient's verbal and non-verbal communication as well as inconsistencies between them. For example, a patient may give verbal permission for a procedure, but may seem anxious when personal space is invaded and demonstrate nonverbal behavior such as tensing muscles, turning or pulling away, or shaking when touched. An alert health care provider can try to move away from the patient periodically to give the patient "breathing room" and encourage the patient to relax.

C When personal care must be provided to a patient, the health care provider should determine the patient's preferences by talking with the patient or asking questions. Examples of questions may include:

◆ Do you prefer to do as much of your own personal care as possible or would you like assistance?

◆ Would you like a family member to assist with your personal care?

◆ Are there any special routines you would like followed while receiving personal care?

◆ Do you prefer to bathe in the morning or evening?

◆ Is there anything I can do to make you more comfortable?

EYE CONTACT

Eye contact is also affected by different cultural beliefs. Most European Americans regard eye contact during a conversation as indicative of interest and trustworthiness. They feel that individuals who look away are either not trustworthy or not paying attention. Some Asian Americans consider direct eye contact to be rude. Native Americans may use peripheral (side) vision and avoid direct eye contact. They may regard direct stares as hostile and threatening. Hispanic and African Americans may use brief eye contact, but then look away to indicate respect and attentiveness. Muslim women may avoid eye contact as a sign of modesty. In India, people of different socioeconomic classes may avoid eye contact with each other. The many different beliefs regarding eye contact can lead to misunderstandings when people of different cultures interact.

Health care providers must be alert to the comfort levels of patients while using direct eye contact and recognize the cultural diversity that exists. Lack of eye contact is often interpreted as "not listening," when in reality it can indicate respect.

GESTURES

Gestures are used to communicate many things. A common gesture in the United States is nodding the head up and down for "yes," and side to side for "no." In India, the head motions for "yes" and "no" are the exact opposite. Pointing at someone is also a common gesture in the United States and is frequently used to stress a specific idea. To Asian and Native Americans, this can represent a strong threat. Even the hand gesture for "OK" can be found insulting to some Asians.

Again, health care providers must be aware of how patients respond to hand gestures. If a patient seems uncomfortable with hand gestures, they should be avoided.

HEALTH CARE BELIEFS

The most common health care system in the United States is the biomedical health care system or the "Western" system. This system of health care bases the cause of disease on such things as microorganisms, diseased cells, and the process of aging. When the cause of disease is determined, heath care is directed toward eliminating the microorganisms, conquering the disease process, and/or preventing the effects of aging. Health care providers in the United States receive biomedical training and are licensed to practice as professionals. Some beliefs of this system of care include encouraging patients to learn as much as possible about their illnesses, informing patients about terminal diseases, teaching self-care, using medications and technology to cure or decrease the effects of a disease or illness, and teaching preventive care.

Health care beliefs vary greatly. These beliefs can affect an individual's response to health care. Most cultures have common conceptions regarding the cause of illness, ways to maintain health, appropriate response to pain, and effective methods of treatment. Some of the common beliefs are shown in table 8-1. It is important to remember that not all individuals in a specific ethnic/cultural group will believe and follow all of the customs. The customs, however, might still

TABLE 8-1 Health Care Beliefs

CULTURE	HEALTH CONCEPTS	CAUSE OF ILLNESS	TRADITIONAL HEALERS	METHODS OF TREATMENT	RESPONSE TO PAIN
South African	Maintain harmony of body, mind, and spirit Harmony with nature Illness can be prevented by diet, rest, and cleanliness	Supernatural cause Spirits and demons Punishment from God Conflict or disharmony in life	Root doctor Folk practitioners (community "mother" healer, spiritualist)	Restore harmony Prayer or meditation Herbs, roots, poultices, and oils Religious rituals Charms, talismans, and amulets	Tolerating pain is a sign of strength; some may express pain
Asian	Health is a state of physical and spiritual harmony with nature Balance of two energy forces: yin (cold) and yang (hot)	Imbalance between yin and yang Supernatural forces such as God, evil spirits, or ancestral spirits Unhealthy environment	Herbalist Physician Shaman healer (physician–priest)	Cold remedies if yang is over-powering and hot remedies if yin is overpowering Herbal remedies Acupuncture and acupressure Energy to restore balance between yin and yang	Pain must be accepted and endured silently; displaying pain in public brings disgrace; may refuse pain medication
European	Health can be maintained by diet, rest, and exercise Immunizations and preventive practices help maintain health Good health is a personal responsibility	Outside sources such as germs, pollutants, or contaminants Punishment for sins Lack of cleanliness	Physician Nurse	Medications and surgery Diet and exercise Home remedies and self-care for minor illnesses Prayer and religious rituals	Some express pain loudly and emotionally; others value self-control in response to pain; pain can be helped by medications
Hispanic	Health is a reward from God Health is good luck Balance between "hot" and "cold" forces	Punishment from God for sins Susto (fright), mal ojo (evil eye), or envidia (envy) Imbalance between hot and cold	Native healers (Curandero, Espiritualista, Yerbero or herbalist, Brujo)	Hot and cold remedies to restore balance Prayers, medals, candles, and religious rituals Herbal remedies, especially teas Massage Anointing with oil Wearing an Azabache (black stone) to ward off the evil eye	Many will express pain verbally and accept treatment; others feel pain is a part of life and must be endured

(continued)

TABLE 8-1 Health Care Beliefs *(Continued)*

CULTURE	HEALTH CONCEPTS	CAUSE OF ILLNESS	TRADITIONAL HEALERS	METHODS OF TREATMENT	RESPONSE TO PAIN
Middle Eastern	Health is caused by spiritual causes Cleanliness essential for health Males dominate and make decisions on health care	Spiritual causes Punishment for sins Evil spirits or evil "eye"	Traditional healers Physician	Meditation Charms and amulets Medications and surgery	Tolerating pain is a sign of strength; self-inflicted pain is used as a sign of grief
Native American	Health is harmony between man and nature Balance between body, mind, and spirit Spiritual powers control body's harmony	Supernatural forces and evil spirits Violation of a taboo Imbalance between man and nature	Shaman Medicine Man	Rituals, charms, and masks Prayer and meditation to restore harmony with nature Plants and herbs Medicine bag or bundle filled with herbs and blessed by medicine man	Pain is a normal part of life and tolerance of pain signifies strength and power

influence an individual's response to a different type of care.

Health care providers must understand that every culture has a system for health care based on values and beliefs that have existed for generations. Individuals may use herbal remedies, religious rites, and other forms of ethnic/cultural health care even while receiving biomedical health care. A major change in the practice of health care in the United States is the increase in the use of alternative health care methods. Many individuals are using alternative health care in addition to, or as a replacement for, biomedical care. Alternative health care providers include chiropractors, homeopaths, naturopaths, and hypnotists. Some types of treatments, discussed in more detail in table 1-2 of Unit 1:7, include:

◆ *Nutritional methods:* organic foods, herbs, vitamins, and antioxidants

◆ *Mind and body control methods:* relaxation, meditation, biofeedback, hypnotherapy, and imagery

◆ *Energetic touch therapy:* massage, acupuncture, acupressure, and therapeutic touch

◆ *Body-movement methods:* chiropractic, yoga, and tai chi

◆ *Spiritual methods:* faith healing, prayer, and spiritual counseling

C Every individual has the right to choose the type health care system and method of treatment he or she feels is best. Health care providers must respect this right. To determine a patient's health care preferences, the health care provider should talk with the patient and ask questions. Examples of questions may include:

◆ What do you do to stay healthy?

◆ Except for this current illness, do you feel that you are reasonably healthy?

◆ What do you feel is a healthy diet? Do you try to follow this diet?

◆ What do you do for exercise?

◆ Is there anything else that you do to stay healthy?

◆ Why do you think people become ill?

◆ What health care treatment method do you use when you are ill?

◆ Why do you think you have become ill?

◆ Were you born in the United States? Were your parents born in the United States?

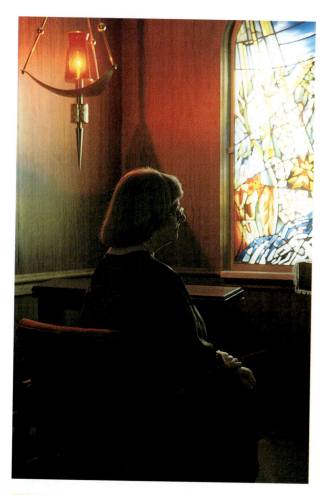

FIGURE 8-6 Spirituality is an individual's need to find meaning and purpose in life.

◆ Do you or your parents still follow the traditions of your native land (or culture)? (If a patient and/or parents were not born in the United States)

SPIRITUALITY AND RELIGION

Spirituality and religion are an inherent part of every ethnic or cultural group. **Spirituality** is defined as the beliefs individuals have about themselves, their connections with others, and their relationship with a higher power. It is also described as an individual's need to find meaning and purpose in life (see figure 8-6). When a person's spiritual beliefs are firmly established, the individual has a basis for understanding life,

finding sources of support when they are needed, and drawing on inner and/or external resources and strength to deal with situations that arise. Spirituality is often expressed through religious practices, but spirituality and religion are *not* the same. Spirituality is an individualized and personal set of beliefs and practices that evolves and changes throughout an individual's life. **Religion** is an organized system of belief in a superhuman power or higher power. Religious beliefs and practices are associated with a particular form or place of worship. Beliefs about birth, life, illness, and death usually have a religious origin. Some of the more common religious beliefs are shown in table 8-2. Religious beliefs that affect dietary practices are discussed in Unit 10 in table 10-6.

Even though a religion may establish certain beliefs and rituals, it is important to remember that not everyone follows all of the beliefs or rituals of their own religion. In addition, some individuals are non-believers. For example, an **atheist** is a person who does not believe in any deity. An **agnostic** is an individual who believes that the existence of God cannot be proved or disproved. Health care providers must determine what an individual personally believes to be important and respect that individual's beliefs.

C To determine an individual's spiritual and religious needs, the health care provider should talk with the patient and ask questions. Examples of questions that may be asked include:

◆ Do you have a religious affiliation?

◆ Are there any spiritual practices that help you feel better (prayer, meditation, reading scriptures)?

◆ Do you normally pray at certain times of the day?

◆ Would you like a visit from a representative of your religion?

◆ Do you consult a religious healer?

◆ Do you observe any special religious days?

◆ Do you wear clothing or jewelry with a religious significance?

◆ Do you have any religious objects that require special care?

◆ Do your beliefs restrict any specific food or drink?

◆ Do you fast or abstain from eating certain foods?

TABLE 8-2 Major Religious Beliefs

RELIGION	BELIEFS ABOUT BIRTH	BELIEFS ABOUT DEATH	HEALTH CARE BELIEFS	SPECIAL SYMBOLS, BOOKS, RELIGIOUS PRACTICES
Baptist (Christian)*	No infant baptism Baptism after person reaches age of under-standing	Clergy provides prayer and counseling to patient and family Autopsy, organ donation, and cremation are an individual's choice No last rites	Oppose abortion Some believe in the healing power of "laying on of hands" May respond passively to medical treatment if believe that illness is "God's will" Physician is instrument for God's intervention	Bible is holy book Rite of Communion important Baptism by full immersion in water after a person reaches an age of understanding and accepts Jesus Christ Some use cross as symbol
Buddhism	No infant baptism but have infant presentation	Believe in reincarnation Buddhist priest must be present at death Last rites chanted at bedside immediately after death Autopsy, cremation, and organ donation are an individual's choice	Suffering is an inevitable part of life Illness is the result of negative Karma (a person's acts and their ethical consequences) Cleanliness is very important to maintain health	Belief in Buddha, the "enlightened one" Tipitaka, three collections of writings, are Buddhist canon Nirvana, the state of greater inner freedom, is the goal of existence Emphasize practice and personal enlightenment rather than doctrine or study of scripture
Christian Scientist (Christian)*	No infant baptism	No last rites Autopsy only when required by law Organ donation discouraged but can be an individual's decision	Illness can be eliminated through prayer and spiritual understanding May not use medicine or surgical procedures May refuse blood transfusions Will accept legally mandated immunizations	Bible is holy book Rite of Communion important *Science and Health* by Mary Baker Eddy is basic textbook of Christian Science Prayer and faith will maintain health and prevent disease
Episcopal (Christian)*	Infant baptism (may be performed by anyone in an emergency)	Some observe last rites by priest Autopsy and organ donation encouraged Cremation is an individual's choice	May use Holy Unction or anointing of the sick with oil as a healing sacrament	Bible is holy book Rite of Communion important Book of Common Prayer Use cross as symbol

(continued)

TABLE 8-2 Major Religious Beliefs *(Continued)*

RELIGION	BELIEFS ABOUT BIRTH	BELIEFS ABOUT DEATH	HEALTH CARE BELIEFS	SPECIAL SYMBOLS, BOOKS, RELIGIOUS PRACTICES
Hinduism	No ritual at birth	Believe in reincarnation as humans, animals, or even plants Ultimate goal is freedom from the cycle of rebirth and death Priest ties thread around the neck or wrist of the deceased and may pour water in the mouth Only family and friends may touch and wash the body Autopsy and organ donation regarded as individual's decision Cremation preferred	Some believe illness is punishment for sins Some believe in faith healing Will accept most medical interventions	Vedas, four books, are the sacred scripture Brahma is principal source of universe and center of all things All forms of nature and life are sacred Person's karma is determined by accumulated merits and demerits that result from all the actions the soul has committed in its past life or lives
Islam (Muslim)	No ritual at birth Circumcision performed when 7 days old	Family must be with dying person Dying person must confess sins and ask forgiveness Only family touches or washes body after death Body is turned toward Mecca after death Autopsy only when required by law Organ donation is permitted if donor consents in writing Cremation not permitted	Illness is an atonement for sins May face city of Mecca (southeast direction if in United States) 5 times a day to pray to Allah Ritual washing before and after prayer Must take medications with right hand since left hand considered dirty	Allah is supreme deity Mohammed, founder of Islam, is chief prophet Holy Day of Worship is sunset Thursday to sunset Friday Koran is holy book of Islam (do not touch or place anything on top) Prayer rug is sacred Fast during daylight hours in month of Ramadan and during other religious holidays May wear item with words from Koran on arm, neck, or waist; do not remove or allow item to get wet

(continued)

TABLE 8-2 Major Religious Beliefs *(Continued)*

RELIGION	BELIEFS ABOUT BIRTH	BELIEFS ABOUT DEATH	HEALTH CARE BELIEFS	SPECIAL SYMBOLS, BOOKS, RELIGIOUS PRACTICES
Jehovah's Witness (Christian)*	No infant baptism	No last rites Autopsy only when required by law and body parts may not be removed Organ donation discouraged but decision is an individual's choice All organs and tissues must be drained of blood before transplantation Cremation permitted	Prohibited from receiving blood or blood products Elders of church will pray and read scriptures to promote healing Medications accepted if not derived from blood products	Bible is holy book: New World Bible Rite of Communion important Church elders provide guidance Each witness is a minister who must spread the group's teachings Acknowledge allegiance only to kingdom of Jesus Christ and refuse allegiance to any government
Judaism (**Orthodox**)	No infant baptism Male circumcision performed on 8th day after birth by Mohel (circumcisor), child's father, or Jewish physician	Person should never die alone Body is ritually cleaned after death May bury dead before sundown on day of death and usually within 24 hours Autopsy only when required by law Organ donation only after consultation with rabbi Cremation forbidden	May refuse surgical procedure or diagnostic tests on Sabbath or holy days Family may want surgically removed body parts for burial Ritual handwashing upon awakening and prior to eating	Lord God Jehovah is one Sabbath is sunset Friday to sunset Saturday Sabbath is devoted to prayer, study, and rest Torah is basis of religion (5 books of Moses) Rabbi is spiritual leader Star of David is symbol of Judaism Fast (no food or drink) during some holy days
Lutheran (Christian)*	Infant baptism by sprinkling (may be performed by any baptized Christian in an emergency)	No last rites Autopsy and organ donation allowed Cremation permitted	Communion often administered by clergy to sick or prior to surgery	Bible is holy book Rite of Communion important Use cross as symbol
Methodist (**United**) (Christian)*	Infant baptism	No last rites Organ donations encouraged Cremation permitted	May request communion before surgery or while ill	Bible is holy book Rite of Communion important Religion is a matter of personal belief and provides a guide for living Use cross as symbol

(continued)

TABLE 8-2 Major Religious Beliefs *(Continued)*

RELIGION	BELIEFS ABOUT BIRTH	BELIEFS ABOUT DEATH	HEALTH CARE BELIEFS	SPECIAL SYMBOLS, BOOKS, RELIGIOUS PRACTICES
Mormon (Latter Day Saints)	Infant blessed by clergy in church as soon as possible after birth Baptism at 8 years of age	May want church elders present at death No last rites Autopsy and organ donation is individual's decision Cremation discouraged	May believe in divine healing with "laying on of hands" by church elders Anointing with oil can promote healing	Special undergarment may be worn to symbolize dedication to God and should not be removed unless absolutely necessary Fast on first Sunday of each month Avoid medications containing alcohol or caffeine
Presbyterian (Christian)*	Infant baptism	No last rites Autopsy and organ donation permitted Cremation permitted	Prayer and counseling an important part of healing May request communion while ill or before surgery	Bible is holy book Rite of Communion important Salvation is a gift from God Use cross as symbol
Roman Catholic (Christian)*	Infant baptism mandatory Baptism necessary for salvation (any baptized Christian may perform an emergency baptism)	Sacrament of the Sick (last rites) performed by priest Autopsy and organ donation permitted Cremation permitted	Sacrament of the Sick and anointing with oil Life is sacred: abortion and contraceptive use prohibited	Bible is holy book Rite of Communion important May use prayer books, crucifix, rosary beads, religious medals, pictures and statues of saints Confession used as a rite for forgiveness of sins Use cross as symbol
Russian Orthodox (Christian)*	Infant baptism by priest	Last rites by ordained priest mandatory Arms of deceased are crossed Autopsy only if required by law Organ donations not encouraged Cremation prohibited	Holy Unction and anointing body with oil used for healing Will accept most medical treatments but believe in divine healing	Bible is holy book Rite of Communion important May wear a cross necklace which should not be removed unless absolutely necessary Use cross as symbol
Seventh Day Adventist (Christian)*	No infant baptism (baptize individuals when they reach the age of accountability)	No last rites Autopsy only when required by law Organ donation is an individual's decision	May avoid over-the-counter medications and caffeine May anoint body with oil Use prayer for healing Some believe only in divine healing Will accept required immunizations	Literal acceptance of Holy Bible Rite of Communion important Sabbath worship is sunset on Friday to sunset on Saturday

*Any religion that is designated as "Christian" has the following beliefs:
God is one in three parts: Father, Son, and Holy Spirit
Jesus Christ is the Son of God
By accepting Jesus Christ, a person may be saved and inherit eternal life

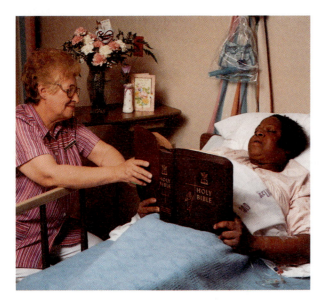

FIGURE 8-7 Always respect the patient's religious symbols and books.

◆ Should food be prepared in a certain way?

◆ Do you prefer certain types of foods (vegetarian diet, diet free from pork)?

As long as it will not cause harm, every effort must be made to allow an individual to express his or her beliefs, practice any rituals, and/or follow a special diet. To show respect for an individual's beliefs and practices, the health care worker should:

◆ Be a willing listener.

◆ Provide support for spiritual and religious practices.

◆ Respect religious symbols and books (see figure 8-7).

◆ Allow privacy for the patient during clergy visits or while the patient is observing religious customs such as communion, prayer, and meditation.

◆ Refrain from imposing your own beliefs on the patient.

8:4 INFORMATION Respecting Cultural Diversity

The key to respecting cultural diversity is to regard each person as a unique individual. Every individual adopts beliefs and forms a pattern of behavior based on culture, ethnicity, race, life experiences, spirituality, and religion. Even though this pattern of behavior and beliefs may change based on new exposures and experiences, they are still an inherent part of the individual.

Health care workers must be aware of the needs of each individual in order to provide total care. They must learn to appreciate and respect the personal characteristics of others. Some ways to achieve this goal include:

◆ Listen to patients as they express their beliefs.

◆ Appreciate differences in people.

◆ Learn more about the cultural and ethnic groups that you see frequently.

◆ Recognize and avoid bias, prejudice, and stereotyping.

◆ Ask questions to determine a person's beliefs.

◆ Evaluate all information before forming an opinion.

◆ Allow patients to practice and express their beliefs as much as possible.

◆ Remember that you are not expected to adopt another's beliefs, just accept and respect them.

◆ Recognize and promote the patient's interactions with family.

◆ Be sensitive to how patients respond to eye contact, touch, and invasion of personal space.

◆ Respect spirituality, religious beliefs, symbols, and rituals.

STUDENT: *Go to the workbook and complete the assignment sheet for Unit 8, Cultural Diversity.*

UNIT 8 SUMMARY

Because health care providers work with and care for many different people, they must be aware of the factors that cause each individual to be unique. These factors include culture, ethnicity, and race. Culture is defined as the values, beliefs, attitudes, languages, symbols, rituals, behaviors, and customs unique to a group of people and passed from one generation to the next.

Ethnicity is a classification of people based on national origin and/or culture. Race is a classification of people based on physical or biological characteristics. The differences among people resulting from cultural, ethnic, and racial factors are called cultural diversity. Health care providers must show sensitivity, or recognize and appreciate the personal characteristics of others, because America is a multicultural society.

Bias, prejudice, and stereotyping can interfere with acceptance of cultural diversity. A bias is a preference that inhibits impartial judgment. A prejudice is a strong feeling or belief about a person or subject that is formed without reviewing facts or information. Stereotyping occurs when an assumption is made that everyone in a particular group is the same. Bias, prejudice, and stereotyping are barriers to effective relationships with others. Health care providers must be alert to these barriers and make every effort to avoid them.

An understanding of cultural diversity allows health care providers to give holistic care, care that provides for the well-being of the whole person and meets not only physical, but also social, emotional, and mental needs. Some areas of cultural diversity include family organization, language, personal space, touching, eye contact, gestures, health care beliefs, spirituality, and religion.

The key to respecting cultural diversity is to regard each person as a unique individual. Health care providers must learn to appreciate and respect the personal characteristics of others.

INTERNET SEARCHES

Use the suggested search engines in Unit 11:4 of this textbook to search the Internet for additional information on the following topics:

1. *Cultural diversity:* search words such as culture, ethnicity, and race to obtain additional information on characteristics and examples for each.

2. *Ethnic groups:* search countries of origin for information on different ethic groups or on your own ethnic group; for example, if you are German–Irish, search for information on both Germany and Ireland.

3. *Cultural assimilation and acculturation:* search for additional information on these two topics.

4. *Bias, prejudice, and stereotyping:* use these key words to search for more detailed information.

5. *Family structure:* search words such as extended or nuclear family, patriarchal, and/or matriarchal.

6. *Health care beliefs:* search by country of origin for health care beliefs, or search words such as yin and yang or shaman.

7. *Alternative health care:* search for additional information on chiropractor, homeopath, naturopath, hypnotist, hypnotherapy, meditation, biofeedback, acupuncture, acupressure, therapeutic touch, yoga, tai chi, and/or faith healing.

8. *Spirituality and religion:* search for additional information on spirituality; use the name of a religion to obtain more information about the beliefs and practices of the religion.

REVIEW QUESTIONS

1. Differentiate between culture, ethnicity, and race.

2. Name five (5) common ethnic groups and at least two (2) countries of origin for each group.

3. Create examples of how a bias, prejudice, and stereotype may interfere with providing quality health care.

4. Describe your family structure. Is it a nuclear or extended family? Is it patriarchal or matriarchal or neither? Why?

5. Do you feel acculturation occurs in the United States? Why or why not?

6. Describe at least three (3) different health care practices that you have seen or heard about. Do you feel they are beneficial or harmful? Why?

7. Differentiate between spirituality and religion.

8. List six (6) specific ways to respect cultural diversity.

UNIT 8

SUGGESTED REFERENCES

Alternative Link Systems, Inc. *The State Legal Guide to Complementary and Alternative Medicine and Nursing.* Clifton Park, NY: Delmar Learning, 2001.

American Medical Association. *Alternative Health Methods.* Chicago, IL: American Medical Association, 1995.

Andrews, Margaret, and Joyceen Boyle. *Transcultural Concepts in Nursing Care.* 3rd ed. Philadelphia, PA: Lippincott, Williams, & Wilkins, 1999.

Brannigan, Michael. *Health Care Ethics in a Diverse Society.* New York, NY: McGraw–Hill, 2000.

Burkhardt, Margaret, and Mary Nagai-Jacobson. *Spirituality: Living Our Connectedness.* Clifton Park, NY: Delmar Learning, 2002.

DeLaune, Sue C., and Patricia K. Ladner. *Fundamentals of Nursing: Standards and Practices.* 2nd ed. Clifton Park, NY: Delmar Learning, 2002.

Diller, Jerry. *Cultural Diversity: A Primer for the Human Services.* Pacific Grove, CA: Brooks/Cole, 1999.

Fugh-Berman, Adriane. *Alternative Medicine— What Works.* Philadelphia, PA: Lippincott, Williams, & Wilkins, 1998.

Geissler, Elaine. *Pocket Guide to Cultural Assessment.* 2nd ed. St. Louis, MO: Mosby, 1998.

Giger, Joyce Newman, and Ruth Elaine Davidhizar. *Transcultural Nursing: Assessment and Intervention.* 3rd ed. St. Louis, MO: Mosby, 1999.

Hegner, Barbara, Esther Caldwell, and Joan Needham. *Nursing Assistant: A Nursing Process Approach.* 8th ed. Clifton Park, NY: Delmar Learning, 1999.

Hogan-Garcia, Mikel. *Four Skills of Cultural Diversity Competency: A Process for Understanding and Practice.* Pacific Grove, CA: Brooks/Cole, 1999.

Hoover-Kramer, Dorothea. *Healing Touch: A Resource for Health Professions.* Clifton Park, NY: Delmar Learning, 2002.

Jonas, Wayne, and Jeffrey Levin. *Essentials of Complementary and Alternative Medicine.* Philadelphia, PA: Lippincott, Williams, & Wilkins, 1999.

Keegan, Lynn. *Healing and Complementary and Alternative Therapies.* Clifton Park, NY: Delmar Learning, 1999.

Kelz, Rochelle. *Conversational Spanish for Health Professions.* 3rd ed. Clifton Park, NY: Delmar Learning, 1999.

Libster, Martha. *Delmar's Integrative Herb Guide for Nurses.* Clifton Park, NY: Delmar Learning, 2002.

Luckmann, Joan. *Transcultural Communication in Health Care.* Clifton Park, NY: Delmar Learning, 2000.

Milliken, Mary Elizabeth. *Understanding Human Behavior.* 6th ed. Clifton Park, NY: Delmar Learning, 1998.

Rios, JoAnna, and Jose Fernandez. *ProSpanish Healthcare: Spanish for Medical Service Providers.* New York, NY: McGraw–Hill, 2001.

Segen, Joseph. *Dictionary of Alternative Medicine.* Norwalk, CT: Appleton–Lange, 1998.

Spiker, Bert. *Medical Dictionary in Six Languages.* Philadelphia, PA: Lippincott, Williams, & Wilkins, 1998.

White, Lois, and Gena Duncan. *Medical–Surgical Nursing: An Integrated Approach.* Clifton Park, NY: Delmar Learning, 1998.

NOTE: The cultural assessment questions presented in this unit were adapted from Joan Luckmann's *Transcultural Communication in Health Care,* which adapted them from Fong's CONFHER model and Rosenbaum.

UNIT 9

Geriatric Care

Unit Objectives

After completing this unit of study, you should be able to:

◆ Differentiate between the myths and facts of six aspects of aging
◆ Identify at least two physical changes of aging in each body system
◆ Demonstrate at least ten methods of providing care to the elderly person who is experiencing physical changes of aging
◆ List five factors that cause psychosocial changes of aging
◆ Describe at least six methods to assist an elderly individual in adjusting to psychosocial changes
◆ Recognize the causes and effects of confusion and disorientation in the elderly
◆ Create a reality orientation program
◆ Justify the importance of respecting cultural and religious differences
◆ Explain the role of an ombudsman
◆ Define, pronounce, and spell all the key terms

 Observe Standard Precautions

 Safety—Proceed with Caution

 Math Skill

 Science Skill

C Communications Skill

 Instructors Check—Call Instructor at This Point

 OBRA Requirement— Based on Federal Law

 Legal Responsibility

 Career Information

 Technology

233

KEY TERMS

Alzheimer's disease
  (Altz'-high-merz")
arteriosclerosis
  (r-tear-ee-o-skleh-row'-sis)
arthritis
atherosclerosis
  (ath-eh-row"-skleh-row'-sis)
cataracts
cerebrovascular accident
culture
dementia
  (d-men'-she-a)
disability

disease
dysphagia
  (dis-fay'-gee-ah)
geriatric care
gerontology
  (jer-un-tahl'-oh-gee)
glaucoma
  (glaw-ko'-mah)
incontinence
myths
nocturia
  (nok-tur'-ee-ah)

ombudsman
osteoporosis
  (os-tee'-oh-pour-oh'-sis)
reality orientation (RO)
religion
senile lentigines
  (seen'-ile len-ti'-jeans)
thrombus
transient ischemic attacks
  (TIAs)
  (tran'-z-ent is-ke'mik)

INTRODUCTION

Just as they experienced the "baby boom," the United States and most other countries are now experiencing an "aging boom." In the 1900s, most individuals died before age 60. Today, most individuals can expect to live into their 70s, and many individuals enjoy healthy and happy lives as 80- and 90-year-olds. This age group uses health care services frequently, so it is essential for a health care worker to understand the special needs of the elderly population.

9:1 INFORMATION Myths on Aging

Aging is a process that begins at birth and ends at death. It is a normal process and leads to normal changes in body structure and function. Even though few people want to grow old, it is a natural event in everyone's life. **Gerontology** is the scientific study of aging and the problems of the old. **Geriatric care** is care provided to elderly individuals. Through the study of the aging process and the elderly, many facts on aging have been established. However, many **myths**, or false beliefs, still exist regarding aging and elderly individuals. It is essential for the health care worker to

be able to distinguish fact from myth when providing geriatric care.

◆ *Myth:* Most elderly individuals are cared for in institutions or long-term care facilities.

◆ *Fact:* Only approximately 5 percent of the elderly population lives in long-term care facilities. Most elderly individuals live in their own homes or apartments or with other family members (see figure 9-1). Others may choose to live in retirement communities or in independent-living or assisted-living facilities. These facilities provide assistance with meals, transportation, housekeeping, social activities, and medical care. By purchasing or renting a home or apartment in one of these

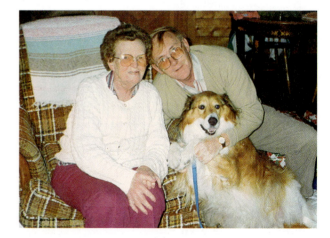

FIGURE 9-1 Most elderly individuals live in their own homes or apartments.

facilities, the individual can obtain the degree of assistance needed while still living independently.

- *Myth:* Anyone over a certain set age, such as 65, is "old."

- *Fact:* Old is determined less by the number of years lived and more by how an individual thinks, feels, and behaves. For example, to a 10-year-old, a 35-year-old is old. It is important to remember that many individuals are active, productive, and self-sufficient into their 80s and even 90s. Too often the term *old* becomes synonymous with *worthless* or *worn-out*. A better term would be *experienced* or *mature*.

- *Myth:* Elderly people are incompetent and incapable of making decisions or handling their own affairs.

- *Fact:* Even though some experience confusion and disorientation, the majority of elderly individuals remain mentally competent until they die. In fact, older individuals may make better decisions and judgments because they frequently base their decisions on many years of experience and knowledge. In addition, studies have proven that older people are able to concentrate, learn new skills, and evaluate new information. Colleges and adult education programs recognize this fact and often provide tuition-free access that allows elderly individuals to participate in a wide variety of educational programs.

- *Myth:* All elderly people live in poverty.

- *Fact:* Even though many older individuals have limited incomes, most also have comparatively low expenses. Many own their own homes, and their children are raised and out on their own. With social security, savings, retirement pensions, and other sources of income, some elderly individuals are financially secure and enjoy comfortable lifestyles. Although it is true that some elderly individuals live in poverty, this is true of some individuals in all age groups. The financial status of the elderly varies just as the financial status of young or middle-aged people varies.

- *Myth:* Older people are unhappy and lonely.

- *Fact:* Studies have shown that most elderly individuals live with someone and/or associate frequently with friends or family members. Many elderly individuals are active in civic

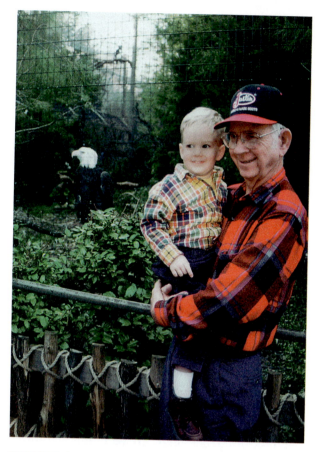

FIGURE 9-2 Caring for grandchildren is a very satisfying social relationship for many elderly individuals.

groups, charities, social activities, and volunteer programs. Others provide care for grandchildren and remain active as heads of extended families (see figure 9-2). Although it is true that some elderly individuals are lonely and unhappy, the percentage is small, and many social agencies exist to assist these individuals.

- *Myth:* Elderly individuals do not want to work—that the goal of the elderly is to retire and, prior to retirement, they lose interest in work.

- *Fact:* Many individuals remain employed and productive into their 70s and even 80s (see figure 9-3). Studies have shown that the older worker has good attendance, performs efficiently, readily learns new skills, and shows job satisfaction. Employers, desiring good work ethics and experience, frequently recruit and hire older workers. Many retired individuals return to part-time positions or serve as consultants or volunteer workers.

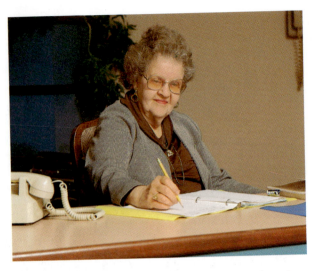

FIGURE 9-3 Many individuals remain employed and productive into their 70s and even 80s.

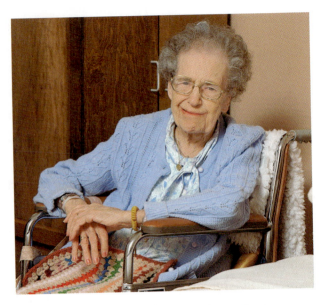

FIGURE 9-4 Note the physical signs of aging.

♦ *Myth:* Retired people are bored and have nothing to do with their lives.

♦ *Fact:* Many retired people enjoy full and active lives. They engage in travel, hobbies, sports, social activities, family events, and church or community activities. In fact, many retired individuals say, "I don't know how I found time to work."

Many other myths also exist. It is important for the health care worker both to recognize problems that do exist for the elderly and to understand that the needs of the elderly vary according to many circumstances. Even the fact that only 5 percent of the elderly are in long-term care facilities means that over 2 million people will be in these facilities by the year 2008. Many health care workers at all levels will provide needed services for these individuals. Geriatric care is and will continue to be a major aspect of health care.

STUDENT: *Go to the workbook and complete the assignment sheet for 9:1, Myths on Aging.*

9:2 INFORMATION Physical Changes of Aging

As aging occurs, certain physical changes also occur in all individuals (see figure-9-4). These changes are a normal part of the aging process. It is important to note that most of the changes are gradual and take place over a long period of time. In addition, the rate and degree of change varies among individuals. Factors such as disease can increase the speed and degree of the changes. Lifestyle, nutrition, economic status, social environment, and limited access to medical care can also have effects.

Most physical changes of aging involve a decrease in the function of body systems. Body processes slow down. There is a corresponding decrease in energy level. If an individual can recognize these changes as a normal part of aging, the individual can usually learn to adapt to and cope with the changes.

INTEGUMENTARY SYSTEM

Some of the most obvious effects of aging are seen in the integumentary system (see figure 9-5). Production of new skin cells decreases with age. The sebaceous (oil) and sudoriferous (sweat) glands become less active. Circulation to the skin decreases and causes coldness, dryness, and poor healing of injured tissue. The hair loses color, and hair loss occurs.

The decreases in body function lead to the physical changes. The skin becomes less elastic and dry. Itching is common. Dark yellow- or brown-colored spots, called **senile lentigines,** appear. Although these are frequently called "liver spots," they are not related to the liver. When the fatty tissue layer of the skin diminishes,

Proper diet, exercise, good hygiene, decreased sun exposure, and careful skin care can help slow and even decrease the normal physical changes in the integumentary system.

MUSCULOSKELETAL SYSTEM

As aging occurs, muscles lose tone, volume, and strength. **Osteoporosis,** a condition in which calcium and other minerals are lost from the bones, causes the bones to become brittle and more likely to fracture or break. **Arthritis,** an inflammation of the joints, causes the joints to become stiff, less flexible, and painful. The rib cage becomes more rigid, and the bones in the vertebral column press closer together (compress).

These changes cause the elderly individual to experience a gradual loss in height, decreased mobility, and weakness. Movement is slower, and the sense of balance is less sure. Falls occur easily and often result in fractures of the hips, arms, and/or legs. Fine finger movements, such as those required when buttoning clothes or tying shoes, are often difficult for the elderly individual.

Elderly individuals should be encouraged to exercise as much as their physical conditions permit (see figure 9-6). This helps keep muscles active and joints as flexible as possible. Even slow, daily walks help maintain muscle tone. Range-of-motion exercises can also maintain muscle strength. A diet rich in protein, calcium, and vitamins can slow the loss of minerals from the bones and maintain muscle structure. Extra attention must be paid to the environment so it is safer for the elderly person. Grab bars in the bathroom, hand rails in halls and on stairs, and other similar devices aid in ambulation. When the sense of balance is poor, an elderly person may need assistance and support during ambulation. The use of walkers and quad canes is frequently recommended. In addition, well-fitting shoes with non-slip soles and flat heels can help prevent falls. Self-stick strips and bands can replace buttons and shoestrings to make dressing easier. A consultation with a physician, physical therapist, and/or occupational therapist can provide an elderly individual with information on the latest and most effective adaptive devices to maintain independence.

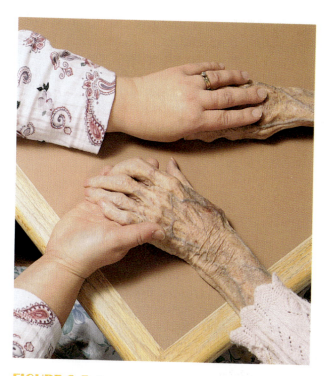

FIGURE 9-5 Some of the most obvious effects of aging are seen on the skin.

lines and wrinkles develop. The nails become thick, tough, and brittle. An increased sensitivity to temperature develops, and the elderly individual frequently feels cold. Hypothermia, a below normal body temperature, can be a serious problem for the elderly.

Good skin, nail, and hair care are essential. Mild soaps should be used because many soaps cause dryness. Frequently, bath oils or lanolin lotions are recommended to combat dryness and itching. Daily baths can also contribute to dry, itchy skin; baths or showers two or three times a week with partial baths on other days are recommended. Brushing of the hair helps stimulate circulation and production of oil. Shampooing is usually done less frequently, but should be done as often as needed for cleanliness and comfort. Any sores or injuries to the skin should be cared for immediately. It is important to keep injured areas clean and free from infection. When elderly people notice sores or injuries that do not heal, they should get medical help. Frequently, the elderly person requires a room temperature that is higher than normal and free from drafts. Socks, sweaters, lap blankets, and layers of clothing can all help alleviate the feeling of coldness. The use of hot water bottles or heating pads is not recommended because the decreased sensitivity to temperature can result in burns.

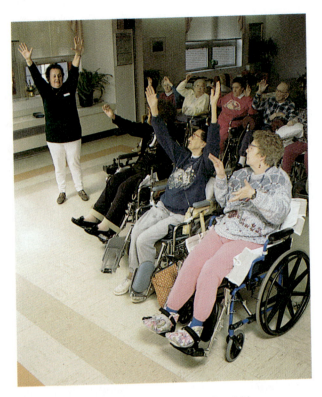

FIGURE 9-6 Elderly individuals should be encouraged to exercise as much as their physical condition permits.

CIRCULATORY SYSTEM

In the circulatory system, the heart muscle becomes less efficient at pushing blood into the arteries, and cardiac output decreases with aging. The blood vessels narrow and become less elastic. Blood flow to the brain and other vital organs may decrease. Blood pressure may increase or decrease.

Many elderly individuals do not notice any changes while at rest. They are more aware of changes when exercise, stress, excitement, illness, and other similar events call for increases in the body's need for oxygen and nutrients. During these periods, they experience weakness, dizziness, numbness in the hands and/or feet, and a rapid heart rate.

Elderly individuals who experience circulatory changes should avoid strenuous exercise or overexertion. They need periods of rest during the day. Moderate exercise, according to the individual's ability to tolerate it, does stimulate circulation and help prevent the formation of a **thrombus,** or blood clot. Support stockings, anti-embolism hose, and not using garters or tight bands around the legs also help prevent blood clots. If an individual is confined to bed, range-of-motion exercises help circulation. If high blood pressure is present, a diet low in salt or sodium and, in some cases, fat may be recommended. Individuals with circulatory system disease should follow the diet and exercise plans recommended by their doctors.

RESPIRATORY SYSTEM

Respiratory muscles become weaker with age. The rib cage becomes more rigid. The alveoli, or air sacs in the lungs, become thinner and less elastic, which decreases the exchange of gases between the lungs and bloodstream. The bronchioles, or air tubes in the lungs, also lose elasticity. Changes in the larynx lead to a higher-pitched and weaker voice. Chronic conditions such as *emphysema*, in which the alveoli lose their elasticity, or *bronchitis*, in which the bronchioles become inflamed, decrease the efficiency of the respiratory system even more severely.

These changes frequently cause the elderly individual to experience *dyspnea*, or difficult breathing. Breathing becomes more rapid, and they have difficulty coughing up secretions from the lungs. This makes them more susceptible to respiratory infections such as colds and pneumonia.

Learning to alternate activity with periods of rest is important to avoid dyspnea. Proper body alignment and positioning can also ease breathing difficulties. The elderly individual with respiratory problems frequently sleeps in a semi-Fowler's position with two or three pillows elevating the upper body to make breathing easier. Avoiding polluted air, such as that in smoke-filled rooms, is essential. Breathing deeply and coughing at frequent intervals helps clear the lung passages and increase lung capacity. Elderly individuals with chronic respiratory problems often use oxygen on a continuous basis. Portable oxygen units allow many individuals to continue to lead active lives.

NERVOUS SYSTEM

Physical changes in the nervous system affect many body functions. Blood flow to the brain decreases, and there is a progressive loss of brain cells. This interferes with thinking, reacting,

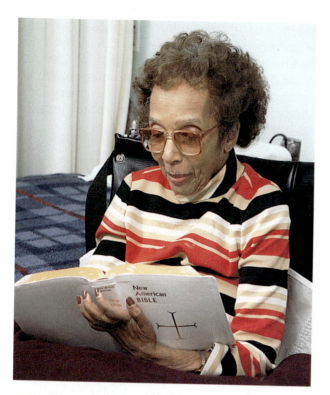

FIGURE 9-7 Individuals who remain mentally active usually show fewer mental changes.

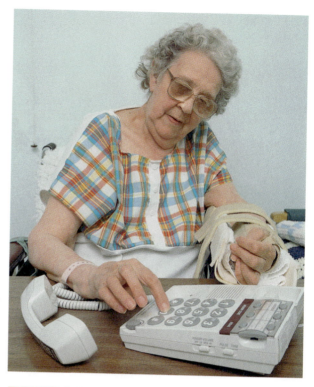

FIGURE 9-8 Good lighting and large numbers on a telephone can help improve vision.

interpreting, and remembering. The senses of taste, smell, vision, and hearing diminish. Nerve endings are less sensitive, and there is a decreased ability to respond to pain and other stimuli.

As these physical changes occur, the elderly individual may experience memory loss. Short-term memory is usually affected. For example, an individual may not remember what he or she ate for breakfast, but does remember the entire menu from his or her retirement party. Long-term memory and intelligence do not always decrease. It may take elderly individuals longer to react, but given enough time, they can think and react appropriately. Individuals who remain mentally active and involved in current events usually show fewer mental changes (see figure 9-7).

Changes in vision cause problems in reading small print or seeing objects at a distance. There is a decrease in peripheral (side) vision and night vision. The eyes take longer to adjust from light to dark, and there is an increased sensitivity to glare. Elderly individuals are also more prone to the development of **cataracts,** where the normally transparent lens of the eye becomes cloudy or opaque. **Glaucoma,** a condition in which the intraocular pressure of the eye increases and interferes with vision, is also more common in

the elderly. Proper eye care, prescription glasses/lenses, medical treatment of cataract or glaucoma, and proper lighting can all improve vision (see figure 9-8).

Hearing loss usually occurs gradually in the elderly. The individual may speak more loudly than usual, ask for words to be repeated, and not hear high-frequency sounds such as the ringing of a telephone. Problems may be more apparent when there is a lot of background noise. For example, an elderly person may not hear well in a crowded restaurant where music is playing and many other people are talking. A hearing aid can help resolve some hearing problems. However, in cases of severe nerve damage, a hearing aid will not eliminate the problem. In addition, many individuals resist using hearing aids. If a person wears a hearing aid, it is important to keep the aid in good working condition by changing batteries, keeping the aid clean, and checking to make sure the individual is wearing it correctly. When a person has a hearing impairment, it is important to talk slowly and clearly. Avoid yelling or speaking excessively loudly. Facing individuals while talking to them also helps in many situations. Eliminating background noise, such as that produced by a radio or television, also increases the ability to hear.

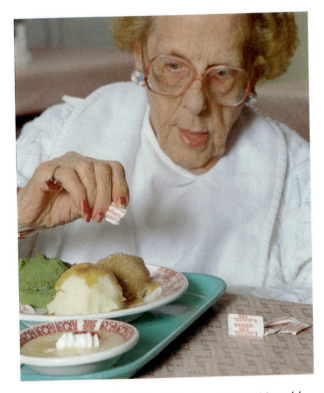

FIGURE 9-9 Elderly individuals may want to add salt to food because of their decreased sense of taste.

The decrease in the sense of taste and smell frequently affects the appetite. Elderly individuals often complain that food is tasteless and add sugar, salt, or pepper (see figure 9-9). Attractive foods with a variety of textures and tastes may help stimulate the appetite. The decrease in the sense of smell may also make the elderly individual less sensitive to the smell of gas, chemicals, smoke, and other dangerous odors. A smoke detector, chemical detectors, and careful monitoring of the environment can help eliminate this danger.

Decreased sensation of pain and other stimuli can lead to injuries. The elderly are more susceptible to burns, frostbite, cuts, fractures, muscle strain, and many other injuries. At times, elderly people are not even aware of injury or disease because they do not sense pain. It is important for elderly individuals to handle hot or cold items with extreme care, and to be aware of dangers in the environment.

Changes in the nervous system usually occur gradually over a long period of time. This allows an individual time to adapt to the changes and learn to accommodate them. However, it is sometimes necessary for someone else to assist when the changes become severe. For example, many elderly individuals continue to drive cars. Because of slower reaction times, however, these individuals may be more prone to having automobile accidents. When an elderly person shows impaired driving ability, it often becomes necessary for a family member or the law to prevent the individual from driving.

DIGESTIVE SYSTEM

Physical changes in the digestive system occur when fewer digestive juices and enzymes are produced, muscle action becomes slower and peristalsis decreases, teeth are lost, and liver function decreases.

Dysphagia, or difficult swallowing, is a frequent complaint of the elderly. Less saliva and a slower gag reflex contribute to this problem. In addition, the loss of teeth or use of poor-fitting dentures makes it more difficult to chew food properly. Another common complaint is indigestion, which results from slower digestion of foods caused by decreased digestive juices. Flatulence (gas) and constipation are common because of decreased peristalsis and poor diet. The decreased sensation of taste also contributes to a poor appetite and diet.

Good oral hygiene, repair or replacement of damaged teeth, and a relaxed eating atmosphere can contribute to better chewing and digestion of food. Most elderly people find it is best to avoid dry, fried, and/or fatty foods because such foods are difficult to chew and digest. High-fiber and high-protein foods with different tastes and textures are recommended. Careful use of seasonings to improve taste also increases appetite. It is important to avoid excessive seasonings because they can cause indigestion. Increasing fluid intake makes swallowing easier, helps prevent constipation, and aids kidney function.

URINARY SYSTEM

With aging, the kidneys decrease in size and become less efficient at producing urine. Poor circulation to the kidneys and a decrease in the number of nephrons result in a loss of ability to concentrate the urine, which causes a loss of electrolytes and fluids. The ability of the bladder to hold urine decreases. Sometimes the bladder does not empty completely and urine is retained in the bladder, a major cause of bladder infections.

The elderly person may find it necessary to urinate more frequently. **Nocturia,** or urination at night, is common and disrupts the sleep pattern. Retention of urine in the bladder causes bladder infections. Males frequently experience enlargement of the prostate gland, which makes urination difficult and causes urinary retention. Loss of muscle tone results in **incontinence,** or the inability to control urination. Incontinence may also result from treatment for prostatic hypertrophy (enlargement) or cancer.

Many elderly individuals decrease fluid intake to cut down on the frequent need to urinate. This can cause dehydration, kidney disease, and infection. Elderly individuals should be encouraged to increase fluid intake to improve kidney function. To decrease incidents of nocturia, most fluids should be taken before evening. Regular trips to the bathroom, wearing easy-to-remove clothing, and using absorbent pads as needed can help the individual who has mild incontinence. Bladder training programs can also help increase bladder capacity and lead to more control over urination in incontinent persons. An indwelling catheter may be needed if all urinary control is lost.

When changes in the urinary system cause poor functioning of the kidneys, waste substances can build up in the bloodstream and cause serious illness. Therefore, it is important to keep the kidneys functioning as efficiently as possible.

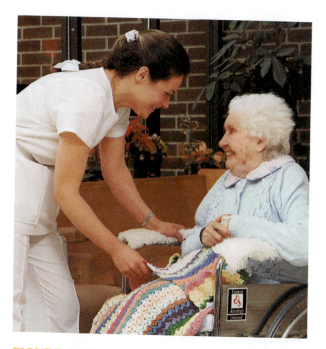

FIGURE 9-10 A lap blanket can help when an elderly person complains of feeling cold.

As with the other body systems, changes in the endocrine system occur slowly over a long period of time. Many elderly individuals are not as aware of changes in this system. Proper exercise, adequate rest, medical care for illness, a balanced diet, and a healthy lifestyle all help decrease the effects caused by changes in hormone activity.

ENDOCRINE SYSTEM

Changes in the endocrine system result in increased production of some hormones, such as parathormone and thyroid stimulating hormone, and decreased production of other hormones, such as thyroxin, estrogen, progesterone, and insulin. The actions of these hormones are listed in Unit 6:13 of this text.

Because hormones affect many body functions, several physical changes may occur. The immune system of the body is less effective, and elderly individuals are more prone to disease. The basal metabolic rate decreases, resulting in complaints of feeling cold, tired, and less alert (see figure 9-10). Intolerance to glucose can develop, resulting in increased blood glucose levels.

REPRODUCTIVE SYSTEM

In the reproductive system, the decrease of estrogen and progesterone in the female causes a thinning of the vaginal walls and a decrease in vaginal secretions. Vaginal infections or inflammations become more common. In some cases, a weakness in its supporting tissues causes the uterus to sag downward, a condition known as *prolapsed uterus.* The breasts sag when fat is redistributed.

Slowly decreasing levels of testosterone in the male slow the production of sperm. Response to sexual stimulation of the penis is slower, and ejaculation may take longer. The testes become smaller and less firm. The seminal fluid becomes thinner, and smaller amounts are produced.

Sexual desire and need do not necessarily diminish with age (see figure 9-11). Many elderly individuals are sexually active. Studies have

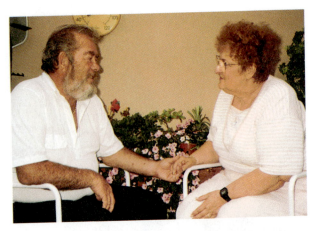

FIGURE 9-11 Elderly individuals still experience a need for companionship and sexuality.

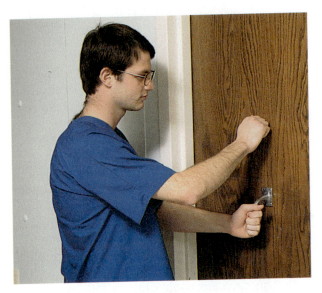

FIGURE 9-12 To respect the right to privacy, always knock before entering a resident's room.

shown that sex improves muscle tone and circulation. Even pain from arthritis seems to decrease after sexual activity, probably because of increased hormone levels. When elderly individuals are in long-term care facilities, it is important for the health care worker to understand both the physical and psychological sexual needs of the resident. Long-term care facilities now allow married couples to live together in the same room. The health care worker must respect the privacy of these residents and allow them to meet their sexual needs (see figure 9-12).

Aging causes many physical changes in all body systems. The rate and degree of the changes vary in different individuals, but all elderly individuals experience some degree of change. Providing means of adapting to and coping with changes allows elderly people to enjoy life even with physical limitations. It is important for all health care workers to learn to recognize changes and provide methods for dealing with them. Tolerance, patience, and empathy are essential.

STUDENT: *Go to the workbook and complete the assignment sheet for 9:2, Physical Changes of Aging.*

9:3 INFORMATION Psychosocial Changes of Aging

In addition to physical changes, elderly individuals also experience psychological and social changes. Some individuals cope with these changes effectively, but others experience extreme frustration and mental distress. It is important for the health care worker to be aware of the psychosocial changes and stresses experienced by the elderly.

WORK AND RETIREMENT

Most adults spend a large portion of their days working. Many associate their feelings of self-worth with the jobs they perform. They are proud to state that they are nurses, electricians, teachers, lawyers, or secretaries. In addition, social contact while working is a major form of interaction with others.

Retirement is often viewed as an end to the working years. Many individuals are able to enjoy retirement and find other activities to replace job roles. Some individuals find part-time or consultant-type jobs after retirement from their primary jobs. Other individuals become active in volunteer work or take part in community or club activities. These individuals find satisfactory replacements for the feelings of self-worth once provided by their jobs.

However, some elderly individuals feel a major sense of loss upon retirement. They lose social contacts, develop feelings of uselessness, and, in some cases, experience financial difficulties. This causes them to experience stress, and they frequently become depressed. Until other sources of restoring the individual's sense of self-worth are found, these elderly individuals can have difficulty coping with life.

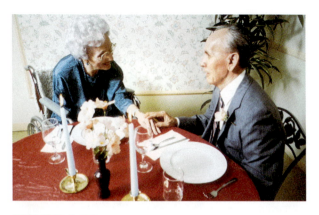

FIGURE 9-13 After the death of a spouse, the elderly individual sometimes can adjust by making new social contacts.

SOCIAL RELATIONSHIPS

Social relationships change throughout life. Among the elderly, these changes may occur more frequently. Often, children marry and move away. This brings about a loss of contact with the family. If a spouse dies, the "couple" image is replaced by one of "widow" or "widower." As a person ages, more friends and relatives die, and social contacts decrease.

Some elderly individuals are able to adjust to these changes by making new friends and establishing new social contacts (see figure 9-13). Church and community groups provide many social activities for the elderly. By taking part in these activities, individuals who made friends readily throughout their lives can continue to do so as they grow older.

Some elderly individuals cannot cope with the continuous loss of friends and relatives. They become withdrawn and depressed. They avoid social events and isolate themselves from others. The death of a spouse is frequently devastating to an elderly individual, especially when a couple has had a close relationship for many years. A surviving spouse may even attempt suicide. Psychological help is essential in these cases.

LIVING ENVIRONMENTS

Changes in living environments create psychosocial changes. Most elderly individuals prefer to remain in their own homes. They feel secure surrounded by familiar environments. Many elderly individuals express fear at the thought of losing their homes.

Some elderly people leave their homes by personal choice. They find the burden of maintaining their homes too great, and move to apartments or retirement communities. The elderly individual may even move to another state with a better climate. These individuals often cope well with the change in living environment and feel the change is beneficial.

Financial problems or physical disabilities may force some people to move from their homes, sometimes to retirement communities or apartments. If they can maintain their independence, coping is usually good. In other cases, an elderly individual may be forced to move in with a son or daughter. This move creates a change in roles, where the child becomes the caretaker of the parent. If the elderly person feels secure in this situation, coping occurs. However, if the elderly person feels unwanted or useless, conflicts and tension may develop.

Moving to a long-term care facility often creates stress in elderly individuals. They feel a loss of independence and become frightened by their lack of control over environment. Many elderly individuals view long-term care facilities as "places to die," even when they may only require the use of the facility for a short period of time. For this reason, it is important to allow individuals to create their own "home" environments in the facility (see figure 9-14). Most long-term care facilities refer to the individuals as "residents." They allow the residents to bring favorite pieces

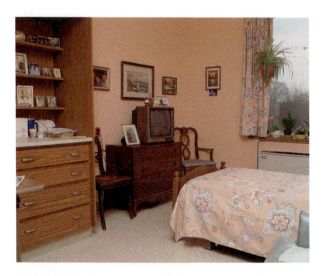

FIGURE 9-14 It is important to allow residents to create their own "home" environments in the long-term care facility.

of furniture, pictures, televisions, radios, and personal items. By being allowed choices in the arrangement of their items, residents are able to create comfortable, homelike environments. Factors such as these allow the elderly individual to adjust to the new environment and to cope with the changes it brings.

INDEPENDENCE

Most individuals want to be independent and self-sufficient. Even 2-year-olds begin to assert their right to choose and strive to be independent. Just as children learn that there are limits to independence, the elderly learn that independence can be threatened with age. Physical disability, illness, decreased mental ability, and other factors can all lead to a loss of independence in the elderly.

Individuals who once took care of themselves find it necessary to ask others for assistance. After driving for a lifetime, elderly individuals might find that they can no longer drive safely. They have to depend on others to take them where they need to go. Physical limitations prevent them from mowing lawns, cooking meals, washing, cleaning, and, in some cases, even taking care of themselves. Frustration, anger, and depression can develop.

Any care provided to elderly individuals should allow as much independence as possible. Assistance should be provided as needed for the individual's safety, but the individual should be allowed to do as much as possible. For example, a health care worker should encourage elderly persons to choose their clothing and dress themselves, even if this takes longer (see figure 9-15). Self-stick strips can replace buttons to make the task of dressing easier and to provide more independence. This helps the elderly individual adapt to the situation and maintain a sense of self-worth. At all times, elderly individuals should be allowed as much choice as possible to help them maintain individuality.

DISEASE AND DISABILITY

Elderly people are more prone to disease and disability. **Disease** is usually defined as "any condition that interferes with the normal function of the body." Common examples in the elderly

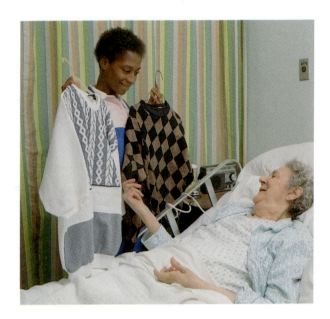

FIGURE 9-15 To encourage independence, encourage elderly individuals to make as many decisions as possible.

include diabetes, heart disease, emphysema, arthritis, and osteoporosis. A **disability** is defined as "a physical or mental defect or handicap that interferes with normal functions." Hearing impairments, visual defects, or the inability to walk caused by a fractured hip are examples. Diseases sometimes cause permanent disabilities. For example, a cerebrovascular accident, or stroke, can result in permanent paralysis of one side of the body, or *hemiplegia*.

When disease or disability affects the functioning of the body, an individual may experience psychological problems. When this occurs in an elderly individual already stressed by other changes or circumstances, it can be traumatic. A fractured hip can cause an elderly individual who had been living independently in his or her own home to be admitted to a long-term care facility. Disease or disability frequently occurs suddenly and does not allow for gradual adjustment to and coping with change.

Sick people often have fears of death, chronic illness, loss of function, and pain. These are normal fears, and these individuals need time to adjust to their situations. Listen to them as they express these fears and be patient and understanding. If they cannot discuss their feelings, accept this and provide supportive care (see figure 9-16).

Psychosocial changes can be major sources of stress in the elderly. As changes occur, the individual must learn to accommodate the changes

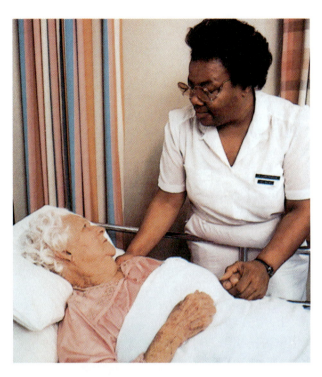

FIGURE 9-16 Provide supportive care and listen to sick individuals as they express their fears.

and function in new situations. With support, understanding, and patience, the health care worker can assist elderly individuals as they learn to adapt.

STUDENT: *Go to the workbook and complete the assignment sheet for 9:3, Psychosocial Changes of Aging.*

9:4 INFORMATION
Confusion and Disorientation in the Elderly

Although most elderly individuals remain mentally alert until death, some experience periods of confusion and disorientation. Signs of confusion or disorientation include talking incoherently, not knowing their own names, not recognizing others, wandering aimlessly, lacking awareness of time or place, displaying hostile and combative behavior (see figure 9-17), hallucinating, regressing in behavior, paying less attention to personal hygiene, and being unable to respond to simple commands or follow instructions.

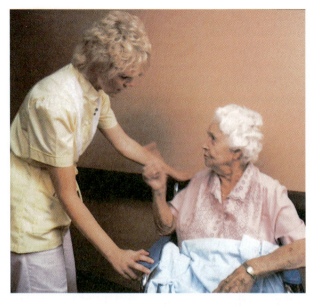

FIGURE 9-17 Hostile or combative behavior often signals feelings of frustration or confusion.

Confusion or disorientation is sometimes a temporary condition. Stress and/or depression caused by physical or psychosocial changes is one possible cause. Use of alcohol or chemicals is another. Kidney disease, which interferes with electrolyte balance; respiratory disease, which decreases oxygen; or liver disease, which interferes with metabolism, are other causes. Elderly individuals are also more sensitive to medications, and drugs can sometimes accumulate in the body and cause confusion and disorientation. Even poor nutrition or lack of fluid intake can interfere with mental ability. Frequently, identification and treatment of any of these conditions decreases and even eliminates the confusion and disorientation. For example, changing a medication or giving it in smaller doses may restore normal function.

Disease and/or damage to the brain can sometimes result in chronic confusion or disorientation. A **cerebrovascular accident,** or stroke, which damages brain cells, is one possible cause. A blood clot can obstruct blood flow to the brain, or a vessel can rupture and cause hemorrhaging in the brain. **Arteriosclerosis,** a condition in which the walls of blood vessels become thick and lose their elasticity, is common in elderly individuals. If the vessels become narrow because of deposits of fat and minerals, such as calcium, the condition is called **atherosclerosis.** These conditions can cause **transient ischemic attacks (TIAs),** or ministrokes, which result in temporary periods of diminished blood flow to the brain. Each time an attack occurs, more damage to brain cells results.

Dementia, also called *brain syndrome,* is a loss of mental ability characterized by a decrease in intellectual ability, loss of memory, impaired judgment, personality change, and disorientation. When the symptoms are caused by high fever, kidney infection, dehydration, hypoxia (lack of oxygen), drug toxicity, or other treatable conditions, the condition is called *acute.* When the symptoms are caused by permanent, irreversible damage to brain cells, the condition is called *chronic.* Cerebral vascular accidents, arteriosclerosis, and TIAs can be contributing causes to chronic dementia. One modern theory suggests that chronic dementia is caused by either a complete lack or an inadequate amount of an enzyme. Whatever the cause, chronic dementia is usually regarded as a progressive, irreversible disease.

Alzheimer's disease is a form of dementia that causes progressive changes in brain cells. Individuals with Alzheimer's lack a neurotransmitter, or chemical, that allows messages to pass between nerve cells in the brain. This results in the death of neurons and the development of neuritic plaques (deposits of protein) and neurofibrillary tangles. Alzheimer's disease can occur in individuals as young as 40 years of age, but frequently occurs in those in their 60s. The cause is unknown, but there are many theories currently being researched. A genetic defect, a missing enzyme, toxic effects of aluminum, a virus, and the faulty metabolism of glucose have all been implicated as possible causes. Whatever the cause, Alzheimer's disease is viewed as a terminal, incurable brain disease usually lasting from 3 to 10 years. In the early stages, the individual exhibits self-centeredness, a decreased interest in social activities, memory loss, mood and personality changes, depression, poor judgment, confusion regarding time and place, and an inability to plan and follow through with many activities of daily living (see figure 9-18). As the disease progresses, nighttime restlessness and wandering occur, mood swings become frequent, personal hygiene is ignored, confusion and forgetfulness become severe, perseveration or repetitious behavior occurs, the ability to understand others and/or speak coherently decreases, weight fluctuates, paranoia and hallucinations increase, and full-time supervision becomes necessary. In the terminal stages, the individual experiences total disorientation regarding person, time, and place;

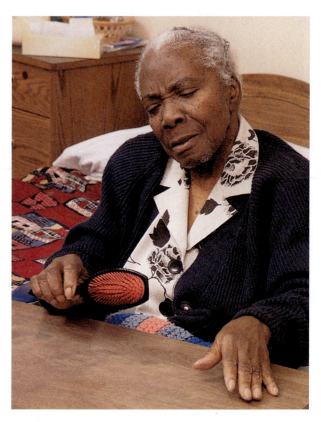

FIGURE 9-18 A patient with Alzheimer's disease may forget how common objects are used and have problems with normal activities of daily living.

becomes incoherent and is unable to communicate with words; loses control of bladder and bowel functions; develops seizures; loses weight despite eating a balanced diet; becomes totally dependent; and, finally, lapses into a coma and dies. Death is frequently caused by pneumonia, infections, and kidney failure. Progress through the various stages of this disease varies among individuals.

Whatever the cause of confusion or disorientation, certain courses of care should be followed. A primary concern is to provide a safe and secure environment. Dangerous objects such as drugs, poisons, scissors, knives, razors, guns, power tools, cleaning solutions, and matches and lighters should be kept out of reach and in a locked area. If the individual tends to wander, doors and windows should be secure. In severe cases, special sensors may be attached to the leg or wrist of the disoriented individual (see figure 9-19). The sensors alert others if the individual starts to leave a specific area.

Following the same routine is also important. Meals, baths, dressing, walks, and bedtime should each occur at approximately the same time each

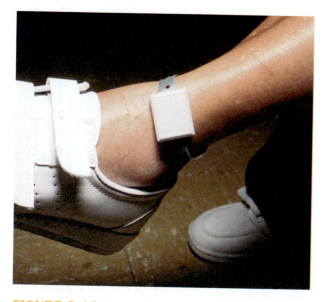

FIGURE 9-19 Special sensors may be attached to the leg or wrist of a wandering or disoriented individual.

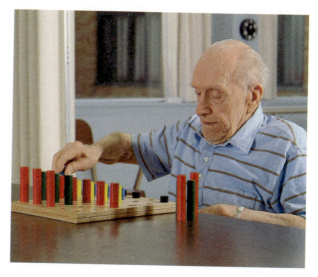

FIGURE 9-20 Activities for an individual who is confused or disoriented should be kept simple and last for short periods of time.

day. Any change in routine can cause stress and confusion. Even though the individual should be encouraged to be as active as possible, activities should be kept simple and last for short periods of time (see figure 9-20). A calm, quiet environment is also important. Loud noises, crowded rooms, and excessive commotion can cause the individual to become agitated and even more disoriented.

Reality orientation (RO) consists of activities that help promote awareness of person, time, and place. The activities can be followed by anyone caring for the confused individual, whether the care is in the home or in a long-term care facility. Some aspects of reality orientation are the following:

1. Be calm and gentle when approaching the individual.

2. Address the person by the name they prefer, for example, "Mr. Smith" or "Mike."

3. Avoid terms such as "sweetie," "baby," and "honey."

4. State your name and correct the person if he or she calls you a wrong name. For example, if a patient thinks you are his or her daughter, say, "I am not your daughter Lisa. I am Mrs. Simmers, your nurse for today."

5. Make constant references to day, time, and place. "It is 8:00 Tuesday morning and time for breakfast."

6. Use clocks, calendars, and information boards to point out time, day, and activities (see figure 9-21).

7. Maintain a constant, limited routine.

8. Keep the individual oriented to day-night cycles. During the day, encourage the person to wear regular clothes. Also, open the curtains and point out the sunshine. At night, close the curtains, use night lights if necessary, and promote quiet and rest.

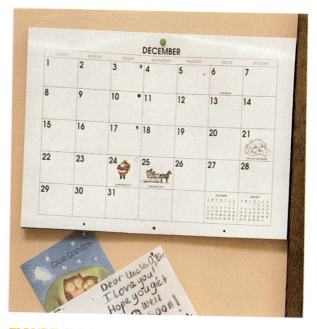

FIGURE 9-21 A large calendar may help orient a person to days and special events.

9. Speak slowly and clearly and ask clear and simple questions.

10. Never rush or hurry the individual.

11. Repeat instructions patiently. Allow time for the individual to respond.

12. Encourage conversations about familiar things or current events.

13. Encourage the use of a television or radio, but avoid overstimulating the individual.

14. Make sure the individual uses sensory aids such as glasses and hearing aids (if needed), and that the devices are in good working order.

15. Keep familiar objects and pictures within view. Avoid moving the person's furniture or belongings.

16. Do not argue with incorrect statements. Gently provide correct information if the person is able to accept the information without agitation. For example, when a person states it is time to dress for work, say, "You don't have to go to work today. You retired 7 years ago."

17. Do not hesitate to use touch, if culturally appropriate, to communicate with the person, unless this causes agitation (see figure 9-22).

18. Avoid arguments or recriminations. When you find an elderly resident in the wrong area, do not say, "You know you are not supposed to be here." Instead, say, "Let me show you how to get to your room."

19. Encourage independence and self-help whenever possible.

20. Always treat the person with respect and dignity.

Reality orientation is usually effective during the early stages of confusion or disorientation. In later stages, when the individual is not able to respond, it can cause increased anxiety and agitation. When patient assessment shows that this is occurring, avoid confronting the patient with reality. For example, do not tell a patient, who wants to see her husband, that her husband died 10 years ago. Instead, ask her to tell you about her husband and allow her to reminisce. Provide supportive care to allow the patient to maintain dignity and express feelings.

Caring for a confused or disoriented individual can be frustrating and even frightening at times. Continual assessment of the individual's abilities and problems is needed to design a health care program that will allow the individual to function within the level of his or her ability. Patience, consistency, and sincere caring are essential on the part of the health care provider.

STUDENT: *Go to the workbook and complete the assignment sheet for 9:4, Confusion and Disorientation in the Elderly.*

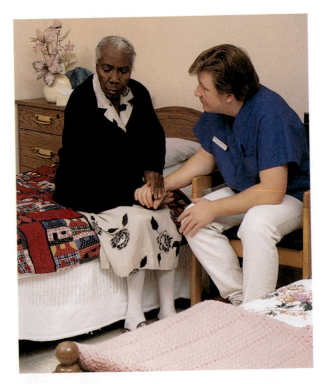

FIGURE 9-22 Do not hesitate to use touch, if culturally appropriate, to communicate with an individual who is disoriented.

9:5 INFORMATION Meeting the Needs of the Elderly

Providing care to the elderly can be a challenging but rewarding experience. It is important to remember that the needs of the elderly do not differ greatly from the needs of any other individual. They have the same physical and psychological needs as any person at any age. However, these needs are sometimes intensified by physical or psychosocial changes that disrupt the normal life pattern. When this occurs, the elderly individual needs understanding, acceptance, and the knowledge that someone cares.

A few other factors must be considered when caring for elderly individuals. One is the importance of meeting cultural needs. **Culture** can be defined as "the values, beliefs, ideas, customs, and characteristics that are passed from one generation to the next." An individual's culture can affect language, food habits, dress, work, leisure activities, and health care. Culture creates differences in individuals. For example, a person may speak a different language or have specific likes or dislikes about food or dress. It is important for the health care worker to learn about a person's culture, and about the person's likes, dislikes, and beliefs. This allows the health care worker to provide care that shows a respect and acceptance of the cultural differences. (Cultural diversity is also discussed in Unit 8 of this text.)

Religious needs are another important aspect of care. **Religion** can be defined as "the spiritual beliefs and practices of an individual." Like culture, religious or spiritual beliefs can affect the lifestyle of an individual. Diet, days of worship, practices relating to birth and death, and even acceptance of medical care can be affected. The beliefs of specific religions are discussed in table 8-2 in Unit 8:3 of this text. It is important to accept an individual's beliefs without bias. It is equally important that health care workers do not force their own religious beliefs on the individuals for whom they provide care. For example, if a patient asks, "Do you believe in life after death?" a health care worker may respond by saying, "How do you feel?" or "You have been thinking about the meaning of life." This allows patients to express their own feelings and thoughts. Other ways the health care worker can show respect and consideration for a person's religious beliefs include proper treatment of religious articles, such as a Bible or Koran; allowing a person to practice religion with prayer, observance of religious holidays, or participation in religious services; honoring a patient's requests for special foods; and providing privacy during clergy visits (see figure 9-23).

Freedom from abuse is another important aspect of care. Abuse of the elderly can be physical, verbal, psychological, or sexual. Handling the individual roughly; denying food, water, or medication; yelling or screaming at the person; or causing fear are all forms of abuse. Abuse is sometimes difficult to prove. Frequently, the abuser is a family member or caretaker. Elderly individuals may want to protect the abuser or may even feel that they deserve the abuse. All states have laws requiring the reporting of any

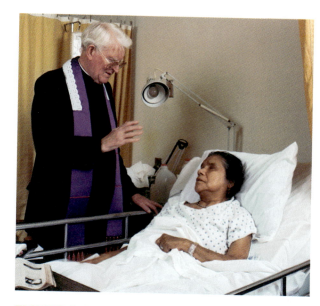

FIGURE 9-23 Respect religious needs and provide privacy while a resident is visiting with a member of the clergy.

suspected abuse. It is important for any health care worker who sees or suspects abuse of the elderly to report it to the proper agency.

A final aspect of meeting the needs of the elderly is to respect and follow the patient's rights. Patients' rights are discussed in Unit 4:3 of this textbook. These rights assure the elderly individual of "kind and considerate care" and provide for meeting individual needs. One program that exists to ensure the rights of the elderly is the Ombudsman Program. It was developed by the federal government in its Older American Act. Each state has its own program designed to meet federal standards. Basically, an **ombudsman** is a specially trained individual who works with the elderly and their families, health care providers, and other concerned individuals to improve quality of care and quality of life. The ombudsman may investigate and try to resolve complaints, suggest improvements for health care, monitor and enforce state and/or federal regulations, report problems to the correct agency, and provide education for individuals involved in the care of the elderly. Although the role of the ombudsman may vary from state to state, it is important for the health care worker to cooperate and work effectively with the ombudsman in order to ensure that the needs of the elderly are met.

STUDENT: *Go to the workbook and complete the assignment sheet for 9:5, Meeting the Needs of the Elderly.*

UNIT 9 SUMMARY

Geriatric care is care provided to elderly individuals. Because this age group uses health care services frequently, and many individuals are now living longer, it is important for the health care worker to understand the special needs of the elderly population.

Many myths, or false beliefs, exist regarding elderly individuals. Examples include the belief that most elderly individuals are cared for in long-term care facilities, are incompetent and incapable of making decisions, live in poverty, do not want to work, and are unhappy and lonely. Although these beliefs may be true for some elderly individuals, they are not true for the majority.

Physical changes occur in all individuals as a normal part of the aging process. It is important to remember that most of the changes are gradual and occur over a long period of time. The physical changes may impose some limitations on the activities of the individual. If the health care worker is aware of these changes and is able to provide individuals with ways to adapt to and cope with the changes, many elderly individuals can enjoy life even with physical limitations.

Psychosocial changes also create special needs in the elderly. Retirement, death of a spouse and of friends, changes in social relationships, new living environments, loss of independence, and disease and disability can all cause stress and crisis for an individual. With support, understanding, and patience, health care workers can assist elderly individuals as they learn to accommodate the changes and to function in new situations.

Although most elderly individuals remain mentally alert until death, some have periods of confusion and disorientation. This is sometimes a temporary condition that can be corrected. Other times, disease and/or damage to the brain results in chronic confusion or disorientation. Special techniques should be used in dealing with these individuals. Providing a safe and secure environment, following a set routine, promoting reality orientation, and giving supportive care can allow individuals to function to the best of their abilities.

Meeting the cultural and religious needs of the elderly is also essential. In addition, it is important for health care workers to respect and follow the "rights" of elderly individuals and to protect the elderly from abuse.

INTERNET SEARCHES

Use the suggested search engines in Unit 11:4 of this textbook to search the Internet for additional information on the following topics:

1. *Gerontology:* search words such as gerontology, geriatrics, and geriatric assistant for additional information on aging.

2. *Long-term care facilities:* search for information on assisted-living, independent living, extended-care, and adult day-care facilities, meals on wheels, and other resources for the elderly.

3. *Diseases:* search for additional information on senile lentigines, osteoporosis, arthritis, emphysema, bronchitis, cerebrovascular accident, arteriosclerosis, atherosclerosis, transient ischemic attack, dementia, and Alzheimer's disease.

4. *Disabilities:* search for information on different types of assistive devices for individuals with disabilities.

5. *Federal government programs:* search for information on the Older American Act, Omnibus Budget Reconciliation Act of 1987, and an ombudsman.

REVIEW QUESTIONS

1. Define *gerontology.*

2. Why is it important for a health care worker to differentiate between myths and facts of aging?

3. Identify factors that can decrease the speed and degree of physical changes of aging. Identify factors that can cause an increase.

4. What measures can be taken to help an individual adapt or cope with the following physical changes of aging?
a. dry, itching skin
b. increased sensitivity to cold
c. hearing loss and the inability to hear high frequency sounds
d. difficulty in chewing and a decreased sense of taste
e. indigestion, flatulence, and constipation
f. weakness, dizziness, and dyspnea while exercising

5. Differentiate between disease and disability.

6. List four (4) factors that cause psychosocial changes in aging. For each factor, provide at least two (2) examples of ways an individual can be helped to adapt or cope with the change.

7. Differentiate between acute and chronic dementia. Identify four (4) causes for each type of dementia.

8. Why is it important to respect an individual's cultural and religious beliefs?

UNIT 9

SUGGESTED REFERENCES

Acello, Barbara. *Nursing Assisting: Essentials of Long-Term Care.* Clifton Park, NY: Delmar Learning, 1999.

Acello, Barbara. *Patient Care: Basic Skills for the Health Care Provider.* Clifton Park, NY: Delmar Learning, 1998.

Acello, Barbara. *The OBRA Guidelines for Quality Improvement.* 2nd ed. Clifton Park, NY: Delmar Learning, 2002.

Beers, Mark, and Robert Berkow. *The Merck Manual of Geriatrics.* 3rd ed. Whitehouse Station, NJ: McGraw-Hill, 2000.

Evashwick, Connie. *The Continuum of Long-Term Care.* 2nd ed. Clifton Park, NY: Delmar Learning, 2001.

Hegner, Barbara R., and Joan Needham. *Assisting in Long-Term Care.* 4th ed. Clifton Park, NY: Delmar Learning, 2002.

Hegner, Barbara, and Joan Needham. *Long-Term Care Survival Handbook.* Clifton Park, NY: Delmar Learning, 2002.

Hogstel, Mildred. *Nursing Care of the Older Adult.* Clifton Park, NY: Delmar Learning, 2001.

Huber, Helen, and Audree Spatz. *Homemaker–Home Health Aide.* 5th ed. Clifton Park, NY: Delmar Learning, 1998.

Jaffe, Marie. *Geriatric Nutrition and Diet.* Clifton Park, NY: Delmar Learning, 1998.

Milliken, Mary Elizabeth. *Understanding Human Behavior.* 6th ed. Clifton Park, NY: Delmar Learning, 1998.

Papalia, Diane, Harvey Sterns, and Ruth Feldman. *Adult Development and Aging.* 2nd ed. New York, NY: McGraw-Hill, 2001.

Rybash, John. *Adult Development and Aging.* 3rd ed. Dubuque, IA: Wm. C. Brown Publishers, 1996.

UNIT 10

Nutrition and Diets

Unit Objectives

After completing this unit of study, you should be able to:

◆ Define the term *nutrition* and list the effects of good and bad nutrition
◆ Name the six groups of essential nutrients and their functions and sources
◆ Create a sample daily menu using the five major food groups
◆ Differentiate between the processes of digestion, absorption, and metabolism
◆ Name, describe, and explain the purposes of at least eight therapeutic diets
◆ Define, pronounce, and spell all the key terms

 Observe Standard Precautions

 Safety—Proceed with Caution

 Math Skill

 Science Skill

 C Communications Skill

 Instructors Check—Call Instructor at This Point

 OBRA OBRA Requirement— Based on Federal Law

 Legal Responsibility

 Career Information

 Technology

252

KEY TERMS

absorption

anorexia
  (an-oh-rex'-ee"-ah)

antioxidants

atherosclerosis
  (ath-eh-row"-skleh-row'-sis)

basal metabolic rate (BMR)
  (base'-al met"-ah-ball'-ik)

bland diet

calorie

calorie-controlled diets

carbohydrates

cellulose

cholesterol
  (co"-less'-ter-all)

diabetic diet

digestion

essential nutrients

fat-restricted diets

fats

hypertension
  (high"-purr-ten'-shun)

kilocalorie (kcal)
  (kill'-oh-kall"-oh-ree)

lipids

liquid diets

low-cholesterol diet

low-residue diet

malnutrition

metabolism
  (meh-tab'-oh-liz"-em)

minerals

nutrition

nutritional status

osteoporosis
  (os-tee"-oh-pour-oh'-sis)

peristalsis
  (per-eh-stall"-sis)

protein diets

proteins

regular diet

sodium-restricted diets

soft diet

therapeutic diets
  (ther"-ah-pew'-tick)

vitamins

wellness

10:1 INFORMATION Fundamentals of Nutrition

People enjoy food and like to discuss it. Most people know that there is an important relationship between food and good health. However, many people do not know which nutrients are needed or why they are necessary. They are not able to select proper foods in their daily diets in order to promote optimum health. Therefore, it is important for every health care worker to have a solid understanding of basic nutrition. With this understanding, the health care worker can both practice and promote good nutrition.

Nutrition includes all body processes relating to food. These include digestion, absorption, metabolism, circulation, and elimination. These processes allow the body to use food for energy, maintenance of health, and growth. **Nutritional status** refers to the state or condition of one's nutrition. The goal is, of course, to be in a state of good nutrition and to maintain **wellness,** a state of good health with optimal body function. To do this, one must choose foods that are needed by the body, and not just foods that taste good.

Nutrition plays a large role in determining height, weight, strength, skeletal and muscular development, physical agility, resistance to disease, appetite, posture, complexion, mental ability, and emotional and psychological health. The immediate effects of good nutrition include a healthy appearance, a good attitude, proper sleep and bowel habits, a high energy level, enthusiasm, and freedom from anxiety. In addition, the effects of good nutrition accumulate throughout life and may prevent or delay diseases or conditions such as the following:

◆ **Hypertension**—high blood pressure; may be caused by an excess amount of fat or salt in the diet; can lead to diseases of the heart, blood vessels, and kidneys.

◆ **Atherosclerosis**—condition in which arteries are narrowed by the accumulation of fatty substances on their inner surfaces; thought to be caused by a diet high in saturated fats and cholesterol; can lead to heart attack or stroke.

◆ **Osteoporosis**—condition in which bones become porous (full of tiny openings) and break easily; one cause is long-term deficiencies of calcium, magnesium, and vitamin D.

◆ **Malnutrition**—the state of poor nutrition; may be caused by poor diet or illness. Symptoms include fatigue, depression, poor posture, being overweight or underweight, poor complexion, lifeless hair, and irritability. It can cause deficiency diseases, poor muscular and skeletal development, reduced mental abilities, and even death. Malnutrition is most likely to affect individuals living in extreme poverty, patients undergoing drug therapy such as treatment for cancer, infants, young children, adolescents, and the elderly. Obesity is also a form of malnutrition, caused by excess food consumption.

10:2 INFORMATION *Essential Nutrients*

Essential nutrients are composed of chemical elements found in food. They are used by the body to perform many different body functions. As the body uses the elements, they are replaced by elements in the food one eats. The essential nutrients are divided into six groups. The six groups and the specific functions of each group are shown in table 10-1.

TABLE 10-1 The Six Essential Nutrient Groups

NUTRIENT GROUPS	FUNCTIONS
Carbohydrates	Provide heat and energy; supply fiber for good digestion and elimination
Lipids (Fats)	Provide fatty acids needed for growth and development; provide heat and energy; carry fat-soluble vitamins (A, D, E, and K) to body cells
Proteins	Build and repair body tissue; provide heat and energy; help produce antibodies
Vitamins	Regulate body functions; build and repair body tissue
Minerals	Regulate body functions; build and repair body tissue
Water	Carries nutrients and wastes to and from body cells; regulates body functions

CARBOHYDRATES

Carbohydrates are the major source of readily usable human energy. They are commonly called "starches" or "sugars." Carbohydrates are a cheaper source of energy than are proteins and fats, because they are mainly produced by plants. They are easily digested, grow well in most climates, and keep well without refrigeration. They are made of carbon, hydrogen, and oxygen.

The main sources of carbohydrates are breads, cereals, noodles or pastas, crackers, potatoes, corn, peas, beans, grains, fruits, sugar, and syrups.

Cellulose is the fibrous, indigestible form of plant carbohydrate. It is important because it provides bulk in the digestive tract and causes regular bowel movements. The best sources of cellulose are bran, whole-grain cereals, and fibrous fruits and vegetables.

LIPIDS (FATS)

Lipids, commonly called **fats** and oils, are organic compounds. Three of the most common lipids found in both food and the human body are *triglycerides* (fats and fatty acids), *phospholipids* (lecithin), and *sterols* (cholesterol). Lipids are also made of carbon, hydrogen, and oxygen, but they contain more oxygen than carbohydrates. Fats provide the most concentrated form of energy but are a more expensive source of energy than carbohydrates. Fats also maintain body temperature by providing insulation, cushion organs and bones, aid in the absorption of fat-soluble vitamins, and provide flavor to meals. The main sources of fats include butter, margarine, oils, cream, fatty meats, cheeses, and egg yolk.

Fats are also classified as saturated or polyunsaturated. *Saturated fats* are usually solid at room temperature. Examples include the fats in meats, eggs, whole milk, cream, butter, and cheeses. *Polyunsaturated fats* are usually soft or oily at room temperature. Examples include vegetable oils, margarines and other products made from vegetable oils, fish, and peanuts.

Cholesterol is a sterol lipid found in body cells and animal products. It is used in the production of steroid hormones, vitamin D, and bile acids. Cholesterol is also a component of cell membranes. Common sources are egg yolk, fatty meats, shellfish, butter, cream, cheeses, whole milk, and organ meats (liver, kidney, and brains). In addition, cholesterol is synthesized (manufactured) by the liver. Cholesterol is transported in the bloodstream mainly by two carrier molecules called lipoproteins. They are known as HDL and LDL, or high-density and low-density lipoprotein. HDL, commonly called "good" cholesterol, tends to transport cholesterol back to the liver and prevents plaque from accumulating on the walls of arteries. LDL, commonly called "bad" cholesterol, tends to contribute to plaque buildup and an excess amount leads to atherosclerosis. Consequently, it is advisable to limit the intake of foods containing fats from animal sources.

PROTEINS

Proteins are the basic components of all body cells. They are essential for building and repairing tissue, regulating body functions, and providing energy and heat. They are made of carbon, hydrogen, oxygen, and nitrogen, and some also contain sulfur, phosphorus, iron, and iodine.

Proteins are made up of 22 "building blocks" called *amino acids*. Nine of these amino acids are essential to life. The proteins that contain these nine are called *complete proteins*. The best sources of complete proteins are animal foods such as meats, fish, milk, cheeses, and eggs. Proteins that contain any of the remaining 13 amino acids and some of the nine essential amino acids are called *incomplete proteins*. Sources of incomplete proteins are usually vegetable foods such as cereals, soybeans, dry beans, peas, corn, and nuts. Choosing plant foods carefully can provide a mixture of amino acids from incomplete proteins that contain all the essential amino acids. It is very important for a vegetarian to select foods that meet these dietary needs.

VITAMINS

Vitamins are organic compounds that are essential to life. They are important for metabolism, tissue building, and regulation of body processes. They allow the body to use the energy provided by carbohydrates, fats, and proteins. Only small amounts of vitamins are required, and a well-balanced diet usually provides the required vitamins. An excess amount of vitamins or a deficiency of vitamins can cause poor health.

Some vitamins are **antioxidants,** organic molecules that help protect the body from harmful chemicals called free radicals. In the body, oxygen used during metabolism causes free radicals to form. Free radicals can damage tissues, cells, and even genes in the same way that oxygen causes metals to rust or apples to become brown. Research is indicating that free radicals can lead to the development of chronic diseases such as cancer, heart disease, and arthritis. Antioxidants, found mainly in fruits and vegetables, deactivate the free radicals and prevent them from damaging body cells. The main antioxidant vitamins are vitamins A, C, and E.

Vitamins are usually classified as water soluble or fat soluble. *Water-soluble* vitamins dissolve in water, are not normally stored in the body, and are easily destroyed by cooking, air, and light. *Fat-soluble* vitamins dissolve in fat, can be stored in the body, and are not easily destroyed by cooking, air, and light. Some of the vitamins along with their sources and functions are listed in table 10-2.

MINERALS

Minerals are inorganic (nonliving) elements found in all body tissues. They regulate body fluids, assist in various body functions, contribute to growth, and aid in building tissues. Some minerals, such as selenium, zinc, copper, and manganese, are antioxidants. Table 10-3 lists some of the minerals essential to life, their sources, and their main functions.

WATER

Water is found in all body tissues. It is essential for the digestion (breakdown) of food, makes up most of the blood plasma and cytoplasm of cells, helps body tissues absorb nutrients, and helps move waste material through the body. Although water is found in almost all foods, the average person should still drink six to eight glasses of water each day to provide the body with the water it needs.

TABLE 10-2 Vitamins

VITAMINS	BEST SOURCES	FUNCTIONS
Fat-Soluble Vitamins		
Vitamin A (Retinol)	Liver Butter, margarine Whole milk, cream, cheese Egg yolk Leafy green and yellow vegetables	Growth and development Health of eyes Structure and functioning of the cells of the skin and mucous membranes Antioxidant to protect cells from free radicals
Vitamin D (Calciferol)	Sunshine (stimulates production in skin) Fatty fish, liver Egg yolk Butter, cream, fortified milk	Growth Regulates calcium and phosphorous absorption and metabolism Builds and maintains bones and teeth
Vitamin E (Tocopherol)	Vegetable oils, butter, margarine Peanuts Egg yolk Dark-green leafy vegetables Soybeans and wheat germ	Necessary for protection of cell structure, especially red blood cells and epithelial cells Antioxidant to inhibit breakdown of vitamin A and some unsaturated fatty acids
Vitamin K	Spinach, kale, cabbage, broccoli Liver Soybean oil Cereals	Normal clotting of blood Formation of prothrombin
Water-Soluble Vitamins		
Thiamine (B_1)	Enriched bread and cereals Liver, heart, kidney, lean pork Potatoes, legumes	Carbohydrate metabolism Promotes normal appetite and digestion Normal function of nervous system
Riboflavin (B_2)	Milk, cheese, yogurt, eggs Enriched breads and cereals Green leafy vegetables Liver, kidney, heart	Carbohydrate, fat, and protein metabolism Health of mouth tissue Healthy eyes
Niacin (Nicotinic Acid)	Meats (especially organ meats) Poultry and fish Enriched breads and cereals Peanuts and legumes	Carbohydrate, fat, and protein metabolism Healthy skin, nerves, and digestive tract
Pyridoxine (B_6)	Liver, kidney, pork Poultry and fish Enriched breads and cereals	Protein synthesis and metabolism Production of antibodies
Vitamin B_{12} (Cobalamin)	Liver, kidney, muscle meats Milk, cheese Eggs	Metabolism of proteins Production of healthy red blood cells Maintains nerve tissue
Vitamin C (Ascorbic Acid)	Citrus fruits, pineapple Melons, berries, tomatoes Cabbage, broccoli, green peppers	Healthy gums Aids in wound healing Aids in absorption of iron Formation of collagen
Folic Acid (Folacin)	Green leafy vegetables Citrus fruits Organ meats, liver Whole-grain cereals, yeast	Protein metabolism Maturation of red blood cells Formation of hemoglobin Synthesis of DNA Reduces risk of neural tube defect (spina bifida) in fetus—important for pregnant women to consume recommended daily amount

TABLE 10-3 Minerals

MINERALS	BEST SOURCES	FUNCTIONS
Calcium (Ca)	Milk and milk products Cheese Some dark-green leafy vegetables	Develops/maintains bones and teeth Clotting of the blood Normal heart and muscle action Nerve function
Phosphorus (P)	Milk and cheese Meat, poultry, fish Nuts, legumes Whole-grain cereals	Develops/maintains bones and teeth Maintains blood acid-base balance Metabolism of carbohydrates, fats, and proteins Constituent of body cells
Magnesium (Mg)	Meat, seafood Nuts and legumes Milk and milk products Cereal grains Fresh green vegetables	Constituent of bones, muscles, and red blood cells Healthy muscles and nerves Metabolism
Sodium (Na)	Salt Meat and fish Poultry and eggs Milk, cheese	Fluid balance, acid-base balance Regulates muscles and nerves Glucose (sugar) absorption
Potassium (K)	Meat Milk and milk products Vegetables Oranges, bananas, prunes, raisins Cereals	Fluid balance Regular heart rhythm Cell metabolism Proper nerve function
Chlorine (Cl) (Chloride)	Salt Meat, fish, poultry Milk, eggs	Fluid balance Acid–base balance Formation of hydrochloric acid
Sulfur (S)	Meat, poultry, fish Eggs	Healthy skin, hair, and nails Activates energy-producing enzymes
Iron (Fe)	Liver, muscle meats Dried fruits Egg yolk Enriched breads and cereals Dark-green leafy vegetables	Formation of hemoglobin in red blood cells Part of cell enzymes Aids in production of energy
Iodine (I)	Saltwater fish Iodized salt	Formation of hormones in thyroid gland
Copper (Cu)	Liver, organ meats Nuts, legumes Whole-grain cereals	Utilization of iron Component of enzymes
Fluorine (Fl) (Fluoride)	Fluoridated water Fish, meat, seafood	Healthy teeth and bones
Zinc (Zn)	Seafood, especially oysters Eggs Milk and milk products	Component of enzymes and insulin Essential for growth and wound healing

10:3 INFORMATION Utilization of Nutrients

Before the body is able to use nutrients, it must break down the foods that are eaten to obtain the nutrients and then absorb them into the circulatory system. These processes are called *digestion* and *absorption* (see figure 10-1). The actual use of the nutrients by the body is called *metabolism*.

DIGESTION

Digestion is the process by which the body breaks down food into smaller parts, changes the food chemically, and moves the food through the digestive system. There are two types of digestive action: mechanical and chemical. During mechanical digestion, food is broken down by the teeth and moved through the digestive tract by a process called **peristalsis,** a rhythmic, wavelike motion of the muscles. During chemical digestion, food is mixed with digestive juices secreted by the mouth, stomach, small intestine, and pancreas.

The digestive juices contain enzymes, which break down the food chemically so the nutrients can be absorbed into the blood.

ABSORPTION

After the food is digested, absorption occurs. **Absorption** is the process in which blood or lymph capillaries pick up the digested nutrients. The nutrients are then carried by the circulatory system to every cell in the body. Most absorption occurs in the small intestine, but water, salts, and some vitamins are absorbed in the large intestine.

METABOLISM

After nutrients have been absorbed and carried to the body cells, **metabolism** occurs. This is the process in which nutrients are used by the cells for building tissue, providing energy, and regulating various body functions. During this process, nutrients are combined with oxygen, and energy and heat are released. Energy is required for voluntary work, such as swimming or housecleaning, and for involuntary work, such as breathing and digestion.

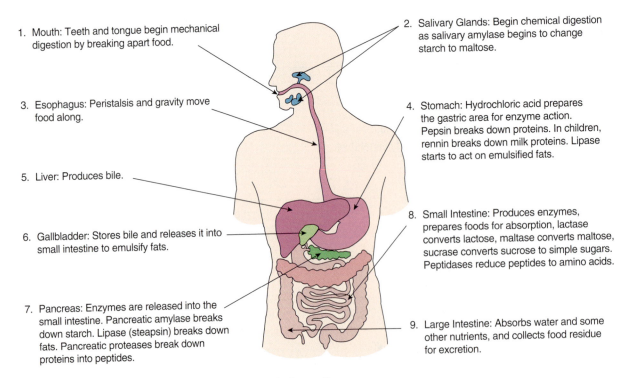

1. Mouth: Teeth and tongue begin mechanical digestion by breaking apart food.

2. Salivary Glands: Begin chemical digestion as salivary amylase begins to change starch to maltose.

3. Esophagus: Peristalsis and gravity move food along.

4. Stomach: Hydrochloric acid prepares the gastric area for enzyme action. Pepsin breaks down proteins. In children, rennin breaks down milk proteins. Lipase starts to act on emulsified fats.

5. Liver: Produces bile.

6. Gallbladder: Stores bile and releases it into small intestine to emulsify fats.

7. Pancreas: Enzymes are released into the small intestine. Pancreatic amylase breaks down starch. Lipase (steapsin) breaks down fats. Pancreatic proteases break down proteins into peptides.

8. Small Intestine: Produces enzymes, prepares foods for absorption, lactase converts lactose, maltase converts maltose, sucrase converts sucrose to simple sugars. Peptidases reduce peptides to amino acids.

9. Large Intestine: Absorbs water and some other nutrients, and collects food residue for excretion.

FIGURE 10-1 The processes of digestion and absorption.

The rate at which the body uses energy just for maintaining its own tissue, without doing any voluntary work, is called the **basal metabolic rate,** or **BMR.** The body needs energy continuously, so it stores some nutrients for future use. These stored nutrients are used to provide energy when food intake is not adequate for energy needs.

MEASURING FOOD ENERGY

Foods vary in the amount of energy they contain. For example, a candy bar provides more energy than does an apple. When the body metabolizes nutrients to produce energy, heat is also released. The amount of heat produced during metabolism is the way the energy content of food is measured. This heat is measured by a unit called a **kilocalorie (kcal),** or just **calorie.** The number of kilocalories, or calories, in a certain food is known as that food's *caloric value.* Carbohydrates and proteins provide four calories per gram. Fat provides nine calories per gram. Vitamins, minerals, and water do not provide any calories.

An individual's caloric requirement is the number of kilocalories, or calories, needed by the body during a 24-hour period. Caloric requirements vary from person to person, depending on activity, age, size, sex, physical condition, and climate. The amount of physical activity or exercise is usually the main factor determining caloric requirement, because energy used must be replaced. An individual who wants to gain weight can decrease activity and increase caloric intake. An individual who wants to lose weight can increase activity and decrease caloric intake. A general guideline for weight loss or gain is that 1 pound of body fat equals approximately 3,500 calories. To lose 1 pound, a decrease of 3,500 calories is required, either by consuming 3,500 fewer calories or by using 3,500 calories through increased exercise. To gain 1 pound, an increase of 3,500 calories is required. A general guideline to maintain weight is that a person consume 15 calories per pound per day. For example, if a person weighs 120 pounds, maintaining this weight would require a daily intake of 15×120, or 1,800, calories daily. By decreasing caloric intake by 500 calories per day, a person would lose 1 pound per week (500 calories per day times 7 days equals 3,500 calories, or 1 pound of fat). By increasing caloric intake by 500 calories per day, a person would gain 1 pound per week. It is important to note that increasing or decreasing exercise along with controlling calorie intake is essential. Also, a slow, steady gain or loss of 1 to 2 pounds per week is an efficient and safe form of weight control.

10:4 INFORMATION Maintenance of Good Nutrition

Good health is everyone's goal, and good nutrition is the best way of achieving and maintaining it. Normally, this is accomplished by eating a balanced diet in which all of the required nutrients are included in correct amounts. The simplest guide for planning healthy meals is the *U.S. Department of Agriculture (USDA) Food Guide,* which classifies foods into five major food groups. Foods are arranged in groups containing similar nutrients. This is known as the Food Guide Pyramid (see figure 10-2). Portion sizes are small, and the number of servings will vary according to the caloric requirements of individuals.

The five major food groups, number of daily recommended servings, average serving size, and nutrient contents of the foods are shown in table 10-4. A sample menu using the five major food groups is shown in table 10-5.

Although the major food groups are a key to healthy meal plans, variety, taste, color, aroma, texture, and general food likes and dislikes must also be considered. If food is not appealing, people will usually not eat it even though it is healthy.

Sound and sensible nutritional principles can be found in the booklet published by the USDA and entitled *Nutrition and Your Health: Dietary Guidelines for Americans.* This booklet lists the following seven guidelines to help establish good eating habits based on moderation and variety:

1. Eat a variety of foods. Choose different foods from each of the five major food groups each day. Adjust the number and size of portions based on body weight and nutritional needs. This helps provide the wide variety of nutrients required for good health.

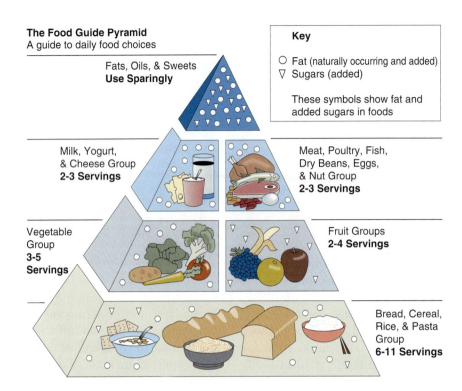

The Food Guide Pyramid
A guide to daily food choices

Fats, Oils, & Sweets
Use Sparingly

Key

○ Fat (naturally occurring and added)
▽ Sugars (added)

These symbols show fat and
added sugars in foods

Milk, Yogurt,
& Cheese Group
2-3 Servings

Meat, Poultry, Fish,
Dry Beans, Eggs,
& Nut Group
2-3 Servings

Vegetable
Group
**3-5
Servings**

Fruit Groups
2-4 Servings

Bread, Cereal,
Rice, & Pasta
Group
6-11 Servings

FIGURE 10-2 The Food Guide Pyramid shows the five major food groups and recommended daily servings. *(Courtesy of the U.S. Department of Agriculture).*

TABLE 10-4 The Five Major Food Groups

FOOD GROUP	NUMBER OF SERVINGS	AVERAGE RECOMMENDED PORTION SIZE	NUTRIENT CONTENT
Breads, Cereals, Rice, & Pasta	6–11	1 slice bread 1/2 bagel or English muffin 1/2 cup cooked cereal or rice 2–3 ounces pasta (cooked) 1 ounce dry cereal	Carbohydrates; phosphorus; magnesium; potassium; iron; vitamins B, K, and folic acid
Vegetables	3–5	1 cup salad greens 1/2 cup cooked vegetables 3/4 cup vegetable juice	Carbohydrates; iron; calcium; potassium; magnesium; vitamins A, B, C, E, K, and folic acid
Fruits	2–4	1 medium size fruit 1/2 cup canned/cooked fruit 1/4 cup dried fruit 3/4 cup fruit juice	Carbohydrates; potassium; vitamin C and folic acid
Milk, Milk Products, Yogurt, & Cheese	2–3	1 cup milk, yogurt, pudding 1–2 ounces cheese 8 ounces cottage cheese 1 1/2 cups ice cream	Protein; carbohydrate; fat; calcium; potassium; sodium; magnesium; phosphorus; vitamins A, B_{12}, D, and riboflavin
Meats, Fish, Poultry, Dry Beans, Eggs, & Nuts	2–3	2–3 ounces meat, fish, or poultry 1 cup cooked beans 2 eggs 4 tablespoons peanut butter 1 ounce nuts	Proteins; fats; iron; sulfur; copper; iodine; sodium; magnesium; zinc; potassium; phosphorus; chlorine; fluorine; vitamins A, B, and D

TABLE 10-5 Sample Menu Using the Five Major Food Groups

BREAKFAST	LUNCH	DINNER
Orange juice	Tuna sandwich	Roast chicken
Cereal	with	Rice
Toast	Lettuce and tomato	Broccoli
Margarine	Carrot and celery sticks	Green salad
Milk	Cookies	Oil dressing
	Milk	Rolls and margarine
	Fresh fruit	Milk
		Fruit sherbet

Suggested snacks: fresh fruit, pizza, milkshake

2. Maintain healthy weight. Determine your proper body weight and try to maintain this weight by proper eating habits and exercise.

3. Choose a diet low in fat, saturated fat, and cholesterol. Eat lean meat, poultry without skin, fish, and low-fat dairy products. Use fats and oils sparingly and limit fried foods.

4. Choose a diet with plenty of vegetables, fruits, and grain products.

5. Use sugars only in moderation. Limit cookies, candy, cakes, and soft drinks. Brush and floss your teeth after eating sweet foods.

6. Use salt and sodium only in moderation. Flavor foods with herbs and spices. Reduce the amount of salty foods.

7. If alcohol is consumed, it should be in moderation. Alcohol should be avoided by pregnant women, individuals using medications, children and adolescents, and individuals who are driving or engaging in an activity that requires attention or skill.

Following the preceding guidelines will result in a diet that will maintain and may even improve health.

Food habits also affect nutrition. At times, habits are based on cultural or religious beliefs. Different cultures and races have certain food preferences. Some religions require certain dietary restrictions that must be observed (see table 10-6). Unusual habits are not necessarily bad. They should be evaluated using the five major food groups as a guide. When habits do require changing in order to improve nutrition, the person making suggestions must use tact, patience, and imagination. Many food habits are formed during youth, and changing them is a difficult and slow process.

10:5 INFORMATION
Therapeutic Diets

Therapeutic diets are modifications of the normal diet and are used to improve specific health conditions. They are normally prescribed by a doctor and planned by a dietitian. These diets may change the nutrients, caloric content, and/or texture of the normal diet. They may seem strange and even unpleasant to patients. In addition, a patient's appetite may be affected by **anorexia** (loss of appetite), weakness, illness, loneliness, self-pity, and other factors. Therefore, it is essential that the health care worker use patience and tact to convince the patient to eat the foods on the diet. An understanding of the purposes of the various diets will also help the health care worker provide simple explanations to patients.

REGULAR DIET

A **regular diet** is a balanced diet usually used for the ambulatory patient. At times, it has a slightly reduced calorie content. Foods such as rich desserts, cream sauces, salad dressings, and fried foods may be decreased or omitted.

LIQUID DIETS

Liquid diets include both clear liquids and full liquids. Both are nutritionally inadequate and should be used only for short periods of time. All foods served must be liquid at body temperature. Foods included on the clear-liquid diet are

TABLE 10-6 Religious Dietary Restrictions

RELIGION	COFFEE & TEA	ALCOHOL	DAIRY PRODUCTS	PORK & PORK PRODUCTS	MEAT	SPECIAL RESTRICTIONS
Baptist (Strict)	*	*				Some groups drink coffee and tea Many are ovolactovegetarians (use eggs and milk, but no meat)
Buddhist	Some sects	Some sects		*	*	Many sects are vegetarians; some sects eat beef and pork
Roman Catholic					Ash Wednesday and Fridays during Lent	Many avoid food and beverages 1 hour prior to communion
Christian Scientist	*	*				
Greek Orthodox (Eastern Orthodox)			Wednesdays and Fridays during Lent and other Holy Days		Wednesdays and Fridays during Lent and other Holy Days	Avoid food and beverages before communion
Hindu	*			*	*	Most are vegetarians; many do not use eggs as they represent life; never eat beef since cows considered sacred
Islamic, Muslim	*			*		Do not eat or drink during daylight hours in month of Ramadan; shellfish forbidden; meat must be slaughtered according to specific rules
Jewish (Orthodox)				*		Forbids serving of milk with meat; forbids cooking on Sabbath; shellfish forbidden; food must be prepared according to Kosher rules; may fast on certain holy days
Mormon (Latter Day Saints)	*	*				Cola and other caffeine drinks prohibited Some fast on the first Sunday of each month
Seventh Day Adventist	*	*		*		Vegetarian diet is encouraged; avoid shellfish; prohibit foods containing caffeine

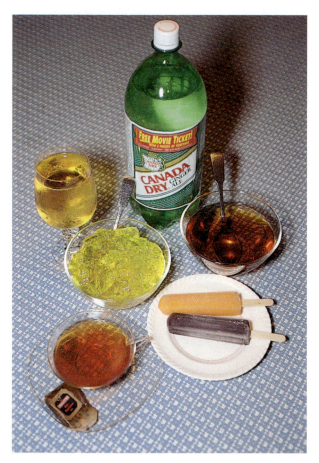

FIGURE 10-3 Foods included on the clear-liquid diet are mainly carbohydrates and water.

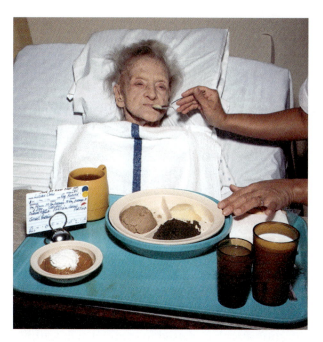

FIGURE 10-4 Soft diets include foods that require little chewing and are easy to digest.

may be used following surgery, or for patients with infections, digestive disorders, or chewing problems.

DIABETIC DIET

A **diabetic diet** is used for patients with diabetes mellitus. In this condition, the body does not produce enough of the hormone insulin to metabolize carbohydrates. Patients frequently take insulin by injection. The diet contains exchange lists that group foods according to type, nutrients, and caloric content. Patients are allowed a certain number of items from each exchange list according to their individual needs. Sugar-heavy foods such as candy, soft drinks, desserts, cookies, syrup, honey, condensed milk, chewing gum, and jams and jellies are usually avoided.

CALORIE-CONTROLLED DIETS

Calorie-controlled diets include both low-calorie and high-calorie diets. Low-calorie diets are frequently used for patients who are overweight. High-calorie foods are either avoided or very

mainly carbohydrates and water, including apple or grape juice, fat-free broths, plain gelatin, fruit ice, ginger ale, and tea or black coffee with sugar (see figure 10-3). The full-liquid diet includes the liquids allowed on the clear-liquid diet plus strained soups and cereals, fruit and vegetable juices, yogurt, hot cocoa, custard, ice cream, pudding, sherbet, and eggnog. These diets may be used after surgery, for patients with acute infections or digestive problems, to replace fluids lost by vomiting or diarrhea, and before some X-rays of the digestive tract.

SOFT DIET

A **soft diet** is similar to the regular diet, but foods must require little chewing and be easy to digest (see figure 10-4). Foods to avoid include meat and shellfish with tough connective tissue, coarse cereals, spicy foods, rich desserts, fried foods, raw fruits and vegetables, nuts, and coconut. This diet

limited. Examples of such foods include butter, cream, whole milk, cream soups or gravies, sweet soft drinks, alcoholic beverages, salad dressings, fatty meats, candy, and rich desserts. High-calorie diets are used for patients who are underweight or have anorexia nervosa, hyperthyroidism (overactivity of thyroid gland), or cancer. Extra proteins and carbohydrates are included. High-bulk foods such as green salads, watermelon, and fibrous fruits are avoided because they fill up the patient too soon. High-fat foods such as fried foods, rich pastries, and cheese cake are avoided because they digest slowly and spoil the appetite.

LOW-CHOLESTEROL DIET

A **low-cholesterol diet** restricts foods containing cholesterol. It is used for patients with atherosclerosis and heart disease. Foods high in saturated fat, such as beef, liver, pork, lamb, egg yolk, cream cheese, natural cheeses, shellfish (crab, shrimp, lobster), and whole milk, are limited, as are coconut and palm oil products.

FAT-RESTRICTED DIETS

Fat-restricted diets are also called *low-fat diets*. Examples of foods to avoid include cream, whole milk, cheeses, fats, fatty meats, rich desserts, chocolate, nuts, coconut, fried foods, and salad dressings. Fat-restricted diets may be used for obese patients or patients with gallbladder and liver disease or atherosclerosis.

SODIUM-RESTRICTED DIETS

Sodium-restricted diets are also called *low-sodium* or *low-salt diets*. Frequently, patients use low-sodium-diet lists similar to the carbohydrate-exchange lists used by diabetic patients. Patients should avoid or limit adding salt to food, smoked meats or fish, processed foods, pickles, olives, sauerkraut, and some processed cheeses. This diet reduces salt intake for patients with cardiovascular diseases (such as hypertension or congestive heart failure), kidney disease, and edema (retention of fluids).

PROTEIN DIETS

Protein diets include both low-protein and high-protein diets. Protein-rich foods include meats, fish, milk, cheeses, and eggs. These foods would be limited or decreased in low-protein diets and increased in high-protein diets. Low-protein diets are ordered for patients with certain kidney or renal diseases and certain allergic conditions. High-protein diets may be ordered for children and adolescents, if growth is delayed; for pregnant or lactating (milk-producing) women; before and/or after surgery; and for patients suffering from burns, fevers, or infections.

BLAND DIET

A **bland diet** consists of easily digested foods that do not irritate the digestive tract. Foods to be avoided include coarse foods, fried foods, highly seasoned foods, pastries, candies, raw fruits and vegetables, alcoholic and carbonated beverages, smoked and salted meats or fish, nuts, olives, avocados, coconut, whole-grain breads and cereals, and, usually, coffee and tea. It is used for patients with ulcers, colitis, and other diseases of the digestive system.

LOW-RESIDUE DIET

A **low-residue diet** eliminates or limits foods that are high in bulk and fiber. Examples of such foods include raw fruits and vegetables, whole-grain breads and cereals, nuts, seeds, beans, peas, coconut, and fried foods. It is used for patients with digestive and rectal diseases, such as colitis or diarrhea.

OTHER DIETS

Other therapeutic diets that restrict or increase certain nutrients may also be ordered. The health care worker should always check the prescribed diet and ask questions if foods seem incorrect. Every effort should be made to include foods the patient likes if they are allowed on a particular diet. If a patient will not eat the foods on a prescribed therapeutic diet, the diet will not contribute to good nutrition.

STUDENT: *Go to the workbook and complete the assignment sheet for Unit 10, Nutrition and Diets.*

UNIT 10 SUMMARY

An understanding of basic nutrition is essential for health care workers. Good nutrition helps maintain wellness, a state of good health with optimal body function.

Essential nutrients are used by the body to perform many different functions. There are six groups of essential nutrients: carbohydrates, fats, proteins, vitamins, minerals, and water. Daily food intake should provide an individual with proper amounts of the essential nutrients.

Before the body can obtain the essential nutrients from food, the body must digest the food. After digestion, the nutrients are absorbed and carried by the circulatory system to every cell in the body. Metabolism then occurs, and the nutrients are used by cells for body functions.

The simplest guide for planning healthy meals that provide the required essential nutrients is to eat a variety of foods from the five major food groups. Portion sizes should vary according to the individual's caloric requirements. Maintaining healthy weight, choosing foods low in fat, using sugar and salt in moderation, and limiting alcoholic beverages are also important aspects of proper nutrition.

Therapeutic diets are modifications of the normal diet. They are used to improve specific health conditions. Examples of therapeutic diets include liquid, diabetic, calorie-controlled, low-cholesterol, fat- or sodium- restricted, high- or low-protein, and bland diets. An understanding of these diets will allow the health care worker to encourage patients to follow prescribed diets.

INTERNET SEARCHES

Use the suggested search engines in Unit 11:4 of this textbook to search the Internet for additional information on the following topics:

1. *Nutritional status:* search words such as nutrition, diet, and nutritional status.

2. *Diseases:* search for more detailed information on nutritional diseases such as hypertension, atherosclerosis, osteoporosis, and malnutrition.

3. *Essential nutrients:* search for information on daily nutritional requirements for nutrients such as carbohydrates, proteins, lipids or fats, vitamins, and minerals.

4. *Utilization of nutrients:* search for information on the processes of digestion, absorption, and metabolism.

5. *Food energy:* use words such as weight loss, weight gain, and diet to learn more about weight control by proper nutrition.

6. *Organizations:* obtain additional information on nutrition from organizations such as the U. S. Department of Agriculture and the American Dietetic Association.

7. *Therapeutic diets:* determine foods allowed or foods that must be avoided in diabetic, calorie-controlled, low-cholesterol, fat-restricted, sodium-restricted, low-residue, bland, and high- or low-protein diets.

REVIEW QUESTIONS

1. List the six (6) essential nutrients and the main function of each nutrient.

2. Differentiate between digestion, absorption, and metabolism.

3. What is BMR?

4. List all of the foods you have eaten today. Be sure to include all snacks. Compare your list with the recommended daily intake of various foods on the food pyramid. Is your diet adequate or deficient? Explain why.

5. Calculate the number of calories you require per day to maintain your present weight. How many calories should you ingest per day to gain one pound per week? How many calories

should you ingest per day to lose one pound per week?

6. Identify the type of therapeutic diet that may be ordered for patients with the following conditions:
   a. gallbladder or liver disease
   b. diabetes mellitus
   c. hypertension or heart disease
   d. ulcers, colitis, or diseases of the digestive tract
   e. pregnant or lactating women
   f. severe nausea, vomiting, and/or diarrhea

UNIT 10

SUGGESTED REFERENCES

Airaghi, Jo-Ann, and Rebecca S. Galvin. *Multiskilling: Dietary Assisting for the Health Care Provider.* Clifton Park, NY: Delmar Learning, 1999.

Boyle, Marie. *Personal Nutrition.* Clifton Park, NY: Delmar Learning, 2001.

Cataldo, Corrine Balog, Linda Kelly DeBruyne, and Eleanor Ross Whitney. *Nutrition and Diet Therapy: Principles and Practices.* 5th ed. Clifton Park, NY: Delmar Learning, 2000.

Jaffe, Marie. *Geriatric Nutrition and Diet.* 3rd ed. Clifton Park, NY: Delmar Learning, 1998.

Keegan, Lynn. *Healing Nutrition.* 2nd ed. Clifton Park, NY: Delmar Learning, 2000.

Libster, Martha. *Delmar's Integrative Herb Guide for Nurses.* Clifton Park, NY: Delmar Learning, 2002.

Marotz, Lynn, Marie Cross, and Jeanettia Rush. *Health, Safety, and Nutrition for the Young Child.* Clifton Park, NY: Delmar Learning, 1997.

McArdle, William, Frank Katch, and Victor Katch. *Exercise and Physiology: Energy, Nutrition, and Human Performance.* 5th ed. Philadelphia, PA: Lippincott, Williams, & Wilkins, 2001.

Mitchell, Mary Kay. *Nutrition Across the Life Span.* 2nd ed. Philadelphia, PA: W.B. Saunders, 2002.

Townsend, Carolynn E., and Ruth A. Roth. *Nutrition and Diet Therapy.* 7th ed. Clifton Park, NY: Delmar Learning, 2000.

U.S. Department of Agriculture. *Nutrition and Your Health: Dietary Guidelines for Americans.* Washington, D.C.: U. S. Government Printing Office, n.d.

Whitney, Eleanor Ross, Corrine Balog Cataldo, Linda Kelly DeBruyne, and Sharon Rady Rolfes. *Nutrition for Health and Health Care.* Clifton Park, NY: Delmar Learning, 2001.

Williams, Sue. *Basic Nutrition and Diet Therapy.* 11th ed. St. Louis, MO: Mosby, 2000.

Computers in Health Care

After completing this unit of study, you should be able to:

♦ Identify the three major components of a computer system
♦ Compare computer capabilities and limitations
♦ Describe computer applications currently being used in today's health care computer systems
♦ Search the Internet for information on a specific topic
♦ Define, pronounce, and spell all the key terms

 Observe Standard Precautions

 Safety—Proceed with Caution

 Math Skill

 Science Skill

 C Communications Skill

 Instructors Check—Call Instructor at This Point

 OBRA OBRA Requirement— Based on Federal Law

 Legal Responsibility

 Career Information

 Technology

KEY TERMS

central processing unit (CPU)
computer literacy
    (come-pew'-tur lit'-er-ass-see)
computer-assisted
    instruction (CAI)
computerized tomography (CT)
    (com-pew'-tur-eyesd toe-mawg'-rah-fee)
database
echocardiograph
hardware

input
interactive video (computer-assisted video)
magnetic resonance
    imaging (MRI)
    (mag-net'-ik rez'-oh-nance im'-adj-ing)
mainframe computer
microcomputer
output
personal computer

positron emission
    tomography (PET)
    (pahs'-ih'-tron ee-miss'-shun toe-mawg'-rah-fee)
random access memory (RAM)
read only memory (ROM)
software
spreadsheet
stress test
ultrasonography
    (ul-trah-sawn-ahg'-rah-fee)

11:1 INFORMATION
Introduction

Computer technology has been called the greatest advance in information processing since Gutenberg invented the printing press. The rapid advances in health care and the explosion of information needed for health care workers to provide quality patient care have made the use of the computer a necessity. Today, it is as common to see a computer terminal in the admissions office of your local hospital or clinic as it is to see a bar code reader being used to add up a grocery bill in your neighborhood supermarket. In fact, many hospitals use this same bar coding method to control inventories and patient costs for hospital supplies.

The computer has become essential in almost every aspect of health care. Computers are used in four general areas:

◆ *hospital information systems (HIS) or medical information systems (MIS):* managing budgets, equipment inventories, patient information, laboratory reports, operating room and personnel scheduling, and general records

◆ *diagnostic testing:* analyzing blood and scanning or viewing body parts by computerized tomography (CT scan), magnetic resonance imaging (MRI), positron emission tomography (PET), and ultrasonography

◆ *educational tools:* computer-assisted instruction (CAI) and computer-assisted video

instruction (interactive video) for professional nurses, physicians, and other allied health personnel

◆ *basic and applied research:* statistical analysis of data

It is estimated that the health care industry will spend approximately one billion dollars on computer technology within the next few years. Whether you want to be a physician, registered nurse, lab technician, nurse's aide, radiology technician, dietitian, pharmacist, occupational therapist, physical therapist, or any other type of allied health professional, a working knowledge of the computer is essential. This working knowledge is sometimes called *computer literacy.* **Computer literacy** means a basic understanding of how the computer works and a basic understanding of the applications used in your field or profession. Computer literacy also means feeling comfortable using a computer for your job needs. Practice and experience in using a computer are essential in order to develop computer literacy.

HISTORY OF THE COMPUTER

The first computers were installed in hospitals in the late 1950s and early 1960s. Some of these hospitals had some form of assistance from the International Business Machines (IBM) Corporation.

Today's computers have come a long way from the Electronic Numerical Integrator and Computer (ENIAC) built in 1946 by J. P. Eckert and J. W. Mauchly at the University of Pennsylvania. This huge computer had to be housed in a room that measured 20 by 40 feet. The ENIAC contained approximately 18,000 vacuum tubes. With the invention of the silicon chip in the 1970s, hundreds of thousands of electronic components were able to fit on a single chip smaller in size than a fingernail. These microchips paved the way for the introduction of the microcomputer.

Computer chips are found in many commonly used items such as watches, cameras, telephones, thermometers, blood pressure gauges, cars, satellite navigation equipment, stoves, burglar alarm systems, and personal desktop computers.

Computers vary in size. Computer size can range anywhere from a **microcomputer** such as a hand-held calculator or personal digital assistant (PDA), which can be held in one hand, to a laptop in a compact case (see figure 11-1), to a **personal computer,** which can sit on a desktop, to a very large **mainframe computer,** which can control the launching of a rocket to outer space.

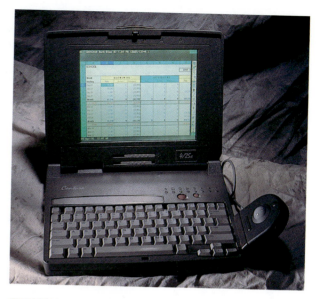

FIGURE 11-1 Today's microcomputers fit easily on a lap or desktop.

screen. The **software** consists of the programs, or instructions, that run the hardware and allow the computer to perform specific tasks.

There are three major components to a computer system (see figure 11-2):

◆ **Input:** information that is entered into the computer by means of an input device.

◆ **Central processing unit (CPU):** processes the input and performs the operations of the computer by following the instructions in the software.

◆ **Output:** the processed information, or final product. It can be displayed on a screen, printed as hard copy, stored on magnetic tape or disks, or transmitted to another user or users.

INFORMATION

11:2 What is a Computer System?

A computer system is an electronic device that can be thought of as a complete information-processing center. It can calculate, store, sort, update, manipulate, sequence, organize, and process data. It also controls logic operations and can rapidly communicate in graphics, numbers, words, and sound.

COMPONENTS OF A COMPUTER SYSTEM

All computer systems contain essentially the same parts, the hardware and the software. The **hardware** consists of the machine components, including the keyboard, central processing unit (CPU), disk drive, and monitor with display

Input Devices

In order for the computer to work, instructions and data, or input, must be entered into it using some form of input device. One of the most popular input devices is the computer keyboard. This device is similar to the familiar typewriter keyboard. Other input devices include:

◆ *Magnetic tape*—usually used to enter data on large, mainframe computers.

◆ *Touch screen monitor*—a monitor with touch-sensitive areas built into the screen. Examples are the touch screens found in many fast food outlets and on many microwave ovens.

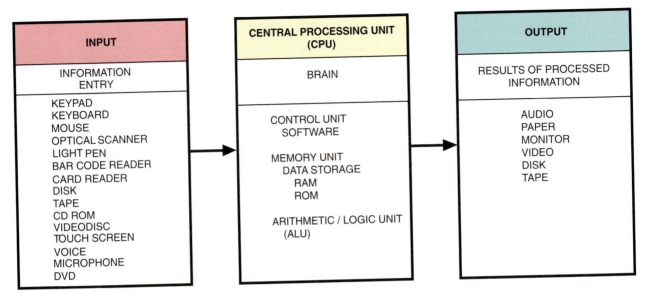

INPUT	CENTRAL PROCESSING UNIT (CPU)	OUTPUT
INFORMATION ENTRY	BRAIN	RESULTS OF PROCESSED INFORMATION
KEYPAD KEYBOARD MOUSE OPTICAL SCANNER LIGHT PEN BAR CODE READER CARD READER DISK TAPE CD ROM VIDEODISC TOUCH SCREEN VOICE MICROPHONE DVD	CONTROL UNIT SOFTWARE MEMORY UNIT DATA STORAGE RAM ROM ARITHMETIC / LOGIC UNIT (ALU)	AUDIO PAPER MONITOR VIDEO DISK TAPE

FIGURE 11-2 Components of a computer system.

◆ *Optical scanner*—a machine that can scan a document and read the printed text. An example is the bar code readers found in many supermarkets and used to record and total grocery items.

◆ *Mouse*—a small device that sits on a desktop or is built into the keyboard of a laptop computer; it controls the cursor, and performs other functions such as creating graphics.

◆ *Light pen*—a device that looks like a pen and is used to perform functions such as selecting menus and drawing graphics on a cathode ray tube, or CRT, which is similar to a television screen (see figure 11-3).

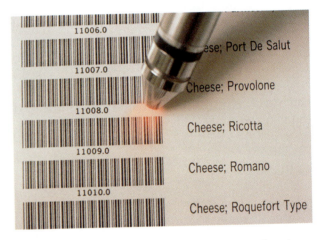

FIGURE 11-3 The light pen is a common input device. *(Courtesy of USDA/ARS #K-2656-2)*

Central Processing Unit

The central processing unit, or CPU, processes all information or data entering the computer. It acts as the "brain" of the computer. The CPU is divided into three main units: the internal memory unit, the arithmetic and logic unit, and the control unit (see figure 11-4).

◆ *Internal Memory Unit:* This unit is controlled by two types of memory. A permanent program already built and stored in the computer system by the manufacturer of the computer is called **read only memory (ROM).** A program that is *NOT* permanent because data can be stored, changed, and/or retrieved is called **random access memory (RAM),** or read/write memory.

◆ *Arithmetic and Logic Unit (ALU):* This performs all of the calculations, such as addition, subtraction, multiplication, and division. It also provides for a logical, step-by-step handling of data or information as the data or information enters or leaves the computer.

◆ *Control Unit:* This unit communicates with the input and output units of the computer system. It initiates, interprets, directs, and controls the processing of information.

Output Devices

Output is the finished work of the computer. Output occurs after the data has been processed by the CPU. The most common output devices are

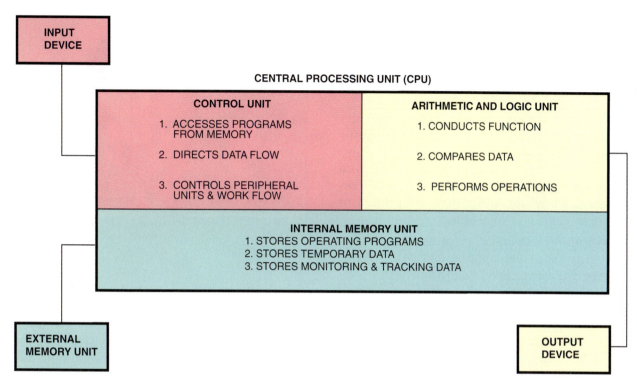

FIGURE 11-4 The central processing unit (CPU) is the "brain" of the computer.

the printer (see figure 11-5), which is similar to a typewriter, and the video display monitor, such as the *cathode-ray tube* (CRT) or flat-screen monitor.

Output can take the form of a hard copy (paper printout) from a printer or plotter. Output can also appear on a computer monitor display screen. Data can be stored or transferred to magnetic tapes, to disks, or to CD–ROM. Data can also be displayed on a video monitor or heard as music or sound through an audio speaker.

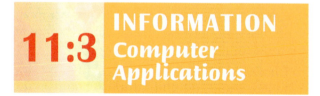

11:3 INFORMATION
Computer Applications

INFORMATION SYSTEMS

Computers were first introduced into hospitals to simplify accounting procedures such as payrolls and inventories. The introduction of computers saved both money and time. The Medical Information System (MIS)—or Hospital Information System (HIS), as it is sometimes called when used in a hospital environment—used expensive, large, mainframe computers. The software, or computer programs needed to run the hardware, was also very expensive to produce and took time to develop. Because of the expense, other departments in the hospital—such as the pharmacy (medications), hematology (blood and blood-forming tissues), clinical chemistry (chemical

FIGURE 11-5 The printer is a common output device that produces a paper printout called *hard copy. (Courtesy of Photodisc)*

laboratory methods to aid in the diagnosis and treatment of disease), microbiology, dietary, and nursing—were slowly added to the system.

Today's health care providers use computers in every health care facility. Computers are used for:

◆ *Word processing:* writing letters, memos, reports, policies, and procedures; creating patient care plans; and documenting care on a patient's record. Documents created by word processing software can be edited and corrected, stored for future use, and printed or sent by electronic mail or fax.

◆ *Compiling databases:* creating information records for patients and employees. A **database** is an organized collection of information. Information is entered into areas called *fields.* For example, the database may contain information such as name, address, telephone, insurance information, social security number, place of employment, and medical history. Each type of information is a *field.* Within the database, each collection of related information is called a *record.* For example, when all of the fields for a particular patient are combined, the information on the patient is the record. All records can be edited and corrected, stored for future use, and printed or sent by electronic mail or fax. Most databases that contain patient records are access limited or password protected to maintain patient confidentiality.

◆ *Scheduling:* recording appointments for patients and creating work schedules for employees

◆ *Maintaining financial records:* processing charges, billing patients, recording payments, completing insurance forms, maintaining accounts, and calculating payrolls for employees

◆ *Monitoring patients:* recording heart rhythms, pulse, blood pressure, blood oxygen levels, and fetal movements (see figure 11-6)

◆ *Performing diagnostic tests:* performing radiological imaging (CT, PET, MRI), blood tests, urine tests, and cardiac and respiratory functions

◆ *Maintaining inventories:* ordering and tracking supplies and equipment; coding supplies with bar codes for billing purposes

◆ *Developing spreadsheets:* A **spreadsheet** uses special software to access a computer's ability

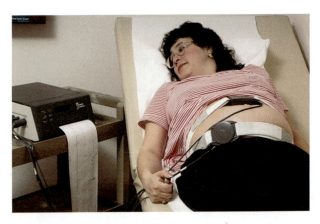

FIGURE 11-6 Computers are used to monitor fetal movements.

to perform high-speed math calculations. The user enters formulas to tell the computer to perform specific math functions (addition, subtraction, multiplication, division, percentage) with numerical data. This allows the user to process bills, maintain accounts, create budgets, develop statistical reports, analyze finances, tabulate nutritional value of foods, evaluate treatments, and project future needs.

◆ *Communicating:* using modems or high-speed data transmission networks to communicate with other departments or different facilities, send or receive information by electronic mail (e-mail), order supplies or equipment, and operate security systems

A typical example of how computers are used in hospitals might be as follows. When a patient enters the hospital, the admission is recorded by an admissions clerk. The patient's name, age, and all other vital information are entered, processed, and stored in the computer's memory. An electronic database is established so that the information about the patient can be retrieved whenever it is needed. For example, while sitting at a computer terminal with a typewriterlike keyboard, the physician can use word processing to enter all the findings of the initial admitting physical examination; order all of the patient's medications from the pharmacy; order laboratory tests, including blood and urine studies; and/or order an electrocardiogram, X-rays, dietary restrictions, and specific nursing care. A pharmacist in the pharmacy department both checks the computer regularly for new orders and supplies the nursing departments with ordered medications. The pharmacist also uses the computer to warn physicians of drug interactions and to monitor pharmacy inventory

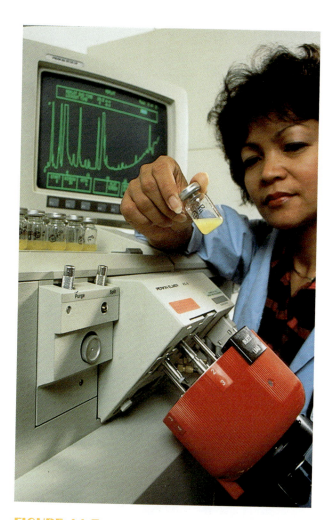

FIGURE 11-7 Pharmacists can use the computer to monitor medications and maintain inventories. *(Courtesy of USDA/ARS #K-3512-3)*

(see figure 11-7). A dietitian may check the dietary restrictions and create a spreadsheet to show a nutritional analysis of the prescribed diet. Laboratory technicians check the computers for their new or revised orders. When any test or procedure is completed, the laboratory technician records the results in the patient's computerized record. Environmental service workers, such as central supply/central processing workers, use the computer to maintain an inventory of all supplies in the facility, order required supplies, and provide information for billing supplies. Many facilities use bar codes on each supply item. When the item is used for a particular patient, the bar code is scanned into the patient's record for automatic billing to the patient. All current information is then immediately accessible to the medical, nursing, and allied health teams. These teams no longer have to wait for the results of tests to be typed on a typewriter and hand delivered to the

patient care area. Nurses no longer have to manually transcribe physicians' orders or nurses' notes. Because patient care plans are computerized, they can be easily updated. This use of the computer decreases the time nurses spend on paperwork and away from patient care.

Hand-held portable computers are used in many hospitals. The terminal device contains a miniature keyboard and is linked remotely to the nurse's station. With this small terminal, the health care worker is able to record data at a patient's bedside. Patient information, such as temperature, heart rate, and respirations, is recorded and immediately available to other health care providers. Updated data is also received from other parts of the hospital. Other health care workers can then retrieve this information from the computer.

Confidentiality of patient information must be strictly enforced. This is usually done by means of access codes or special passwords. Computer users must enter the special access code or password to enter or retrieve information. Only authorized workers are given access to the system. Health care workers must keep their code or password confidential to protect themselves and the patient.

A contingency backup plan is always essential when computers are used. At times, a computer must be shut down for reprogramming or adding additional or new software. At other times, power or computer failure will shut down the computer system. When the computer is not functioning, manual recording of all information is required and an alternative plan must be used to avoid losing essential information. Most facilities make frequent backup tapes or disks to prevent a loss of information when computer failure occurs.

DIAGNOSTICS

The major goal of health care and medicine is determining exactly what is wrong with the patient. The first step in the process is taking a medical history and doing a physical examination. Based on these findings, several tests may be ordered to diagnose or rule out disease.

Several computer-related diagnostic tests have had a real impact on patient care. These diagnostic aids or specialized technological tools are quite varied. They may be invasive, such as a

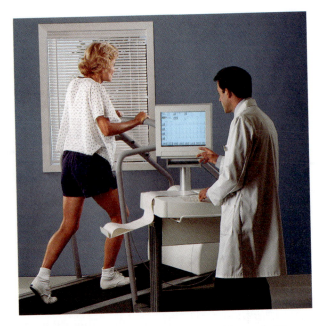

FIGURE 11-8 Computers are used to perform stress tests to evaluate the function of a patient's heart during exercise. *(Courtesy of Spacelabs Medical Inc.)*

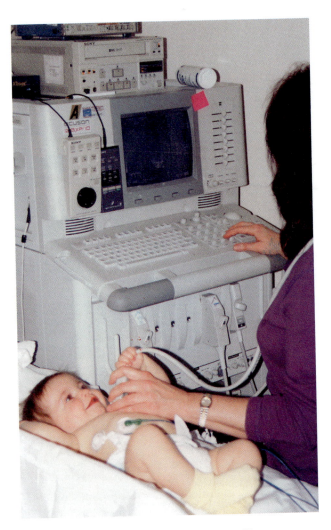

FIGURE 11-9 An echocardiograph utilizes a computer to evaluate cardiac function, reveal heart valve irregularity, and show defects or diseases of the heart.

blood test where a syringe is inserted into a vein and blood is removed, or noninvasive, such as an X-ray procedure where no opening into the body is required.

Some computerized instruments automate the step-by-step manual procedure of analyzing blood, urine, serum, and other body-fluid samples. Most laboratories rely heavily on computers for both blood and urine analysis. Smaller units are now used in many medical offices and other health care facilities. The computerized instruments can analyze a drop of serum, blood, urine, or body fluid placed on a slide at rates of over 500 specimens an hour. Such systems have proven to be reliable for clinical chemistry evaluations.

An electrocardiogram (ECG) computerized interpretation system produces visual pictures on a computer monitor and a printout of the electrical activity of a patient's heart. The ECG gives important information concerning the spread of electrical impulses to the heart chambers. It is very important in diagnosing heart disease. An ECG run while the patient is exercising is known as a **stress test** (see figure 11-8). This allows the physician to evaluate the function of the patient's heart during activity. An **echocardiograph** utilizes a computer to direct ultrahigh-frequency sound waves through the chest wall and into the heart (see figure 11-9). The computer then converts the reflection of the waves into an image of

the heart. This test can be used to evaluate cardiac function, reveal valve irregularities, show defects in the heart walls, and visualize the presence of fluid between the layers of the pericardium (membrane that surrounds the outside of the heart). Computers are also used to monitor a patient's pulse and to determine the oxygen level in the blood (see figure 11-10).

One advance in medical imaging is the **computerized tomography (CT)** scanner, introduced in 1972. The CT scanner was the first computer-based body and brain scanner. This noninvasive, computerized X-ray permits physicians to see clear, cross-sectional views of both bone and body tissues and to find abnormalities such as tumors (see figure 11-11). The CT scanner shoots a pencil-thin beam of X-rays through any part of the body and from many different

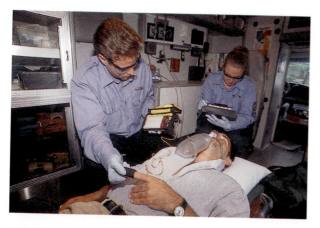

FIGURE 11-10 Pulse oximeters use computer technology to monitor a patient's pulse and determine the oxygen level in the blood.

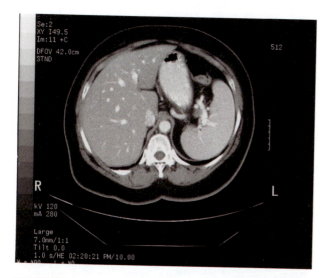

FIGURE 11-11 This CT scan highlights the blood vessels of the liver, heart, and spleen.

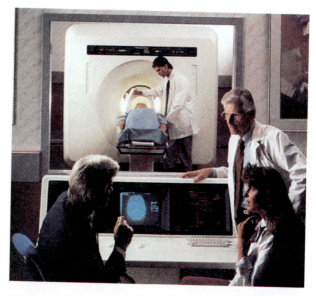

FIGURE 11-12 For magnetic resonance imaging (MRI), the patient is placed in the center of a large magnet that measures the activity of hydrogen ions inside the body and creates an image of the body. (*Courtesy of GE Medical Systems*)

angles. The device's computer then creates a cross-sectional image of the body part on a screen. A CT scan provides a clear image of the soft tissues inside the body and exposes the patient to less radiation than a conventional X-ray. In addition, a regular X-ray shows little depth, and the soft tissue does not appear clearly.

Another powerful advance in medical imaging is **magnetic resonance imaging (MRI).** This computerized, body-scanning method uses nuclear magnetic resonance instead of X-ray radiation. Magnetic resonance imaging is the alteration of the magnetic position of hydrogen atoms to produce an image. The patient is placed in a large circular magnet, which uses the magnetic field to measure activity of hydrogen atoms within the body (see figure 11-12). A computer

translates that activity into cross-sectional images of the body (see figure 11-13). For example, a lung tumor can be more easily detected by scanning with MRI than by scanning with X-rays or CT. Magnetic resonance imaging allows physicians to see blood moving through veins and arteries, to see a swollen joint shrink in response to medication, and to see the reaction of cancerous tumors to treatment.

Positron emission tomography (PET) is another scanning procedure. A slightly radioactive substance is injected into the patient and detected by the PET scanner. The device's computer then composes a three-dimensional image from the radiation detected. The image allows the doctor to see an organ or bone from all sides. In this way, a PET image is similar to a model that can be picked up and examined.

Ultrasonography, figure 11-14, is another noninvasive scanning method. It uses high-frequency sound waves that bounce back as an echo when they hit different tissues and organs inside the body. A computer then uses the sound wave signals to create a picture of the body part, which can be viewed on a computer screen or processed on a photographic film that resembles an X-ray. Ultrasonography can be used to detect tumors, locate aneurysms and blood vessel abnormalities, and examine the shape and size of internal organs. During pregnancy, when radiation

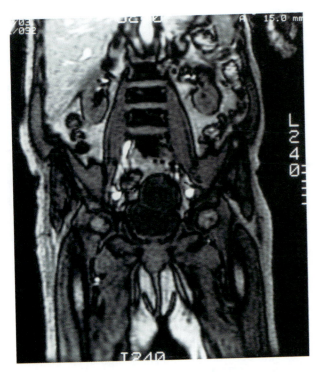

FIGURE 11-13 This MRI scan shows a coronal image of the abdomen.

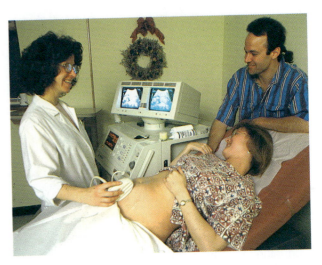

FIGURE 11-14 Ultrasonography is used during pregnancy to determine the size, position, sex, and even abnormalities of the fetus.

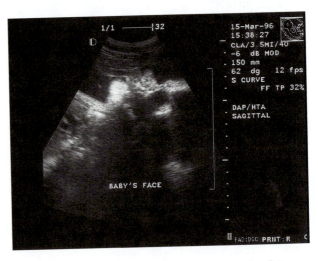

FIGURE 11-15 This ultrasound shows the fetus inside the uterus. *(Courtesy of Sandy Clark)*

can harm the fetus, ultrasonography is used to detect multiple pregnancies, and to determine the size, position, sex, and even abnormalities of the fetus (see figure 11-15). A more recent development in sonography is the 3-D sonogram. This type of ultrasound uses a specialized machine that allows technicians to store five seconds worth of images in a computer. The technician can then create a 3-D colored picture similar to a portrait of the infant in the uterus. Physicians use the 3-D ultrasound to detect birth defects that are not always visible on a standard sonogram, and to determine the severity of a birth defect.

Computers play a major role in oncology (malignancy or cancer) radiology departments. Computers are used to convert information from various scanners to exact data on the location of a tumor. The computer then directs the power of therapeutic radiation precisely to the tumor being irradiated.

EDUCATION

Computers have become commonplace as educational tools. They can be found in elementary, middle, junior high, and high schools, in addition to post-secondary education institutions, such as colleges and universities. Research has shown that computer-based learning decreases time on the task and increases achievement and retention of knowledge. Therefore, it comes as no surprise to find computer-based learning in most schools of medicine, nursing, and allied health.

Computer-assisted instruction (CAI) is educational computer programming designed for individualized use. It is user paced, user friendly, and proceeds in an orderly, organized fashion from topic to topic. It may use animated graphics, color, and sound. It may be a drill-and-practice program for learning to calculate medication doses, or may take the form of a tutorial for learning concepts about the heart. In addition, it can be a simulation that allows the learner to do a clinical procedure, such as taking a patient's blood pressure or drawing blood from a vein (venipuncture), while sitting in front of the computer. Computer programs have even been developed to allow a user to perform a simulated operation on a patient.

Patient-education software is available for the patient with osteoarthritis (inflammation of the joints), obesity (overweight), and many other diseases. Software is even available to teach people how to manage stress.

Another advance in computer learning technology is **interactive video,** or **computer-assisted video.** Interactive video is the integration of computer and video technology. It combines the advantages of video (color, sound, and motion) with the advantages of computer-assisted instruction to provide a dynamic new learning medium. Research has shown that this technology greatly enhances learning and retention. Programs available include those that teach medical terminology to health care workers, clinical skills to nurses, physical examination techniques to physicians, and anatomy and physiology to students. Programs are stored on compact disks or CD–ROM that are inserted into a videodisc player.

RESEARCH

Today, health care research without the use of computers is almost nonexistent. A major source used to help health care professionals analyze statistics and obtain information is the National Library of Medicine database, which is the largest research library in the scientific community. It serves as a national resource for all United States health science libraries. It is located at the National Institutes of Health in Bethesda, Maryland, where it occupies two buildings, one of which is ten stories high.

The library's computer-based MEDical Literature Analysis and Retrieval System (MEDLARS) is a bibliographic biomedical information database. It can be easily accessed by computer through the Regional Medical Library Network. The MEDLARS includes twenty other databases, including Index Medicus, a monthly subject/author guide to over 3,000 journal articles, and Medline, which currently contains over 5 million references as well as information about audiovisual materials.

Statistical Package for the Social Sciences (SPSS) is a program used in many universities to prepare and analyze research data. Other programs score and analyze student test scores. Some programs can draw graphs and charts, and others help the user learn how to use the program in a step-by-step fashion.

Research using computer technology is being conducted in the areas of diabetes, arthritis, patient management systems, and speech recognition patterns. Interactive videodiscs are used to teach anatomy to medical students, and to teach health care personnel and patients about AIDS.

In addition, clinical researchers are now using microcomputers in several areas. For example, in people who have had severe spinal cord injuries, microcomputers are used to initiate the electrical impulses that stimulate skeletal muscles. This exciting application of computing was used to develop a computer-controlled walking system. This system enables paraplegics and quadriplegics to stand, sit, and walk. Electrodes are applied above the hamstring, quadriceps, and gluteus maximus muscles. These electrodes allow control of flexion and extension of the knees and hips. Sensors applied to the knee provide information to coordinate movement of the knee when the patient is standing or walking. Electrical impulses (controlled by the microcomputer) are delivered through these electrodes to stimulate the muscles through a preprogrammed exercise workout. The computer is programmed to automatically stop the exercise program when the sensors detect that the muscles have become fatigued.

SUMMARY

Today, computers are used as cost-effective and efficient tools to enhance quality patient care. They are used to analyze blood; regulate electrical impulses to muscles; take pictures of the body; collect patient data; analyze electrocardiograms; schedule hospital personnel; keep hospital and clinic records, inventories, and budgets; and provide information on wellness to the general public. Computer technology has truly invaded the health care field.

11:4 INFORMATION Using the Internet

A network of computer users can be found on the Internet. By using a modem attached to a computer, telephone or cable lines, and specialized software, one computer operator can readily contact other operators. Many types of services and sources of information are offered on the Internet. Through the Internet, health care professionals can readily contact others for medical updates, information on new procedures, aid in making diagnoses, and many other kinds of information.

One major use of the Internet in health care relates to organ transplants. When an individual needs a transplant, vital information regarding the individual is recorded on the transplant network. The computer monitors all organs as they become available, and can immediately notify the on-line facility when an organ is suitable for a particular patient. This allows the most expedient use of donor organs and ensures that organs are given to the most compatible recipient. It is another example of modern technology providing a service that saves lives.

Since the Internet contains a wealth of information, every health care provider should be familiar with how to use the Internet as a research tool. In order to do this, the health care provider must first become familiar with search engines. A search engine, or search service, can be defined as a database of Internet files. It usually consists of three parts:

◆ *Search program:* commonly called a spider, wanderer, crawler, robot, or worm, the search program explores different sites and identifies and reads pages

◆ *Index:* the search program creates a main database that contains copies of all the information obtained

◆ *Retrieval program:* a program that searches the database for specific information, lists all sources of the information, and, in most cases, ranks the sources with the most relevant first

There are three main types of search engines:

◆ *Crawler-based:* creates an index by exploring different sites on the web and indexing the sites

◆ *Human-powered:* creates an index when a description of the information and key words are entered into the index by an individual

◆ *Mixed:* combines results of both crawler-based and human-powered indexes

There are many different search engines available to an Internet user. Many of them use a variety of indexes or directories to provide sources of information. In addition, different search engines partner together to share index listings. Some of the more popular search engines that provide dependable results, are constantly upgraded with new information, and are available to all Internet users include:

◆ *All the Web (FAST search): www.alltheweb.com,* one of the largest indexes of the web

◆ *Alta Vista: www.altavista.com;* one of the oldest and largest crawler-based directories; also offers news search, shopping search, multimedia search, and human-powered directory results from other search engines

◆ *America On Line (AOL): http://search.aol.com,* provides web search services to AOL subscribers by using both crawler-based and human-powered directories of other search engines

◆ *Ask Jeeves: www.askjeeves.com,* human-powered search that attempts to provide an exact page of information in response to a question

◆ *Google: www.google.com,* has the largest collection of web pages for a crawler-based search engine, provides links to other sites, provides web page search results to other search engines

◆ *Look Smart: www.looksmart.com,* human-powered directory of web sites, provides search results to many other search engines

◆ *Lycos: www.lycos.com,* began as crawler-based but switched to human-powered directory, obtains search results from other search engines

◆ *MSN: http://search.msn.com,* Microsoft's search service that uses results from many other search engines

◆ *Yahoo: www.yahoo.com*, most popular search service, largest human-powered directory on the web with over 1 million sites listed, also uses results from other search engines

In order to find relevant material on the Internet, it is important to develop a strategy to locate information on a specific topic in an efficient and effective way. Searching for information on a topic such as "Does smoking or drinking alcohol during pregnancy increase the chance of a premature birth?" can result in hundreds or even thousands of listings. Some of the listings may be relevant; others will not be. Various techniques can be used to limit the search and produce only information that is specific to the topic. Basic steps that should be followed include:

◆ *Identify key words:* Always try to determine the main words that pertain to the information you desire. In the example above, the key words are *smoking, alcohol, pregnancy,* and *premature birth.* Other words that are alternative ways of expressing the key words might include *cigarettes, premature infants,* and *alcoholism.*

◆ *Combine key words:* If any of the above key words are entered as separate searches, a large amount of information generated would not be pertinent. More specific information can be obtained by telling the search engine to limit the search. This can be accomplished in several ways. One of the easiest methods, recognized by most major search engines, is to use math symbols:

a. *Plus (+) symbol:* tells an engine that you want all words entered; for example: *+ pregnancy +alcohol +premature birth* will produce only listings that contain all three words

b. *Minus (−) symbol:* tells the search engine that you want to find information with one word but not another word; for example: *search +engines −car −automobile* will eliminate information on car or automobile engines

c. *Quotation marks ("):* placed around a phrase or group of words tell a search engine to locate pages that contain the exact same phrase in the order specified; for example: *"hearing aids"* will only provide information on hearing aids, not the disease AIDS.

Boolean operators/connectors are also used to tell a search engine how to limit a search.

Common connectors include *AND* (used like the plus sign), *NOT* used like the minus sign, *OR* used to present an alternative word such as *cigarettes OR smoking,* and *NEAR* to indicate words that should be used close to one another. Most search engines that recognize Boolean operators require that the word be keyed in capital letters.

◆ *Vary your search:* To obtain as much information as possible on a specific topic, it is wise to use a variety of key word combinations. For example, to obtain information on the relationship of smoking and alcohol during pregnancy on premature births, one search could be: *+smoking OR cigarettes +alcohol OR alcoholism +pregnancy +premature births.* This search would bring up all information that contains all the terms. A second search such as *+alcohol OR alcoholism +pregnancy + premature births* or even *+alcohol OR alcoholism + pregnancy* would provide additional information on just the effects of alcohol. Many articles might discuss the effects of alcohol on pregnancy and not discuss smoking. Similarly, other articles might discuss the effects of smoking, but not alcohol. By changing key words, additional pertinent information can be located.

◆ *Use different search engines:* If one search engine does not locate pertinent information, try different search engines. No search engine has access to all the information on the Internet.

◆ *Evaluate the source of all information:* The Internet can provide a wealth of information to health care providers, but individuals using it must also evaluate the information. Not all data is accurate or current. It is important to check the source of any information (universities, government agencies, and national organizations are usually reliable sources), the author (the person should have the proper education and credentials), the date of publication if provided (information should be recent and up-to-date), and references if they are listed. For example, a search for *diabetes mellitus* will provide many journal articles, newsletters, organizational reports, and similar data. If material is published by an organization such as The American Diabetic Association, the information should be accurate. If material is published by an individual who states he has diabetes but can eat any and all sweets, it would be wise to discount this information.

Health care providers can research many topics on the Internet. They can obtain current health care information; learn about new diagnostic tests; research diseases, medications, therapies, and other health concerns; and communicate with other health care providers. The Internet is an excellent learning tool and another example of how technology has enhanced health care.

STUDENT: *Go to the workbook and complete the assignment sheet for Unit 11, Computers in Health Care.*

UNIT 11 SUMMARY

The use of computers in health care has almost become a necessity. All health care workers should have basic computer literacy, meaning an understanding of how the computer works and an understanding of the applications used in their particular health careers.

A computer system is a complete information-processing center. All computer systems contain essentially the same parts: hardware and software. The hardware consists of the machine components. The software consists of the programs, or instructions, that run the hardware and allow the computer to perform specific tasks. Each computer system also requires input, or the information entered into the computer, and a central processing unit (CPU), which performs the operations of the computer by following the directions in the software. This results in output (the processed information, or final product), which can be displayed on a screen, printed, stored, or transmitted to another user.

Computers are used in many aspects of health care. They serve as information centers to provide patient information, schedule personnel, and maintain records and inventory. Computers are also used as diagnostic tools by performing blood tests or viewing

body parts. They are major educational tools, and many computer-assisted instructional programs exist to teach both health care workers and patients. Another major use is in research. The use of computers in health care has proven they are efficient tools that enhance the quality of patient care.

INTERNET SEARCHES

Use the suggested search engines in Unit 11:4 of this textbook to search the Internet for additional information on the following topics:

1. *Computer hardware:* obtain information about different computer systems and compare and contrast the systems by searching the sites of computer manufacturers such as Gateway, Dell, Compaq, and IBM.

2. *Computer software:* search for different types of software for health care providers.

3. *Diagnostic devices:* search for additional information on blood analyzers, echocardiographs, computerized tomography, magnetic resonance imaging, positron emission tomography, and ultrasonography.

4. *Organizations:* search for additional information and Internet links to the National Library of Medicine, National Institutes of Health, Medical Literature Analysis and Retrieval System (MEDLARS), and the Statistical Package for Social Sciences (SPSS).

5. *Search engines:* search for information on the main search engines, advantages and disadvantages of the engines, and ways to use the engines most effectively.

REVIEW QUESTIONS

1. Define *computer literacy.*

2. Differentiate between hardware and software.

3. List five (5) examples of input devices and two (2) examples of output devices.

4. Identify ways confidentiality of patient information can be maintained while using computers.

5. Why is a contingency backup plan essential when computers are used to record information?

6. Briefly describe the main uses of the following imaging techniques:
   a. computerized tomography (CT)
   b. magnetic resonance imaging (MRI)
   c. positron emission tomography (PET)
   d. ultrasonography

7. You are conducting an Internet search for information on the research question "Does hypertension affect some cultures and/or races more readily than others?"
   a. Identify the key words in the question.
   b. List at least three (3) possible search phrases using math symbols and/or Boolean connectors.
   c. Which search engine will you use? Why?

UNIT 11

SUGGESTED REFERENCES

Burke, L., and Weill, B. *Information Technology for the Health Professions.* Upper Saddle River, NJ: Brady/Prentice Hall Health, 2000.

Carlton, Richard R., and Arlene McKenna-Adler. *Principles of Radiographic Imaging.* 3rd ed. Clifton Park, NY: Delmar Learning, 2001.

Davis, T. *Computerizing Health Care Information.* New York, NY: McGraw-Hill Book Company, 1998.

Griffin, Attrices. *Delmar's Dictionary of Internet Sources for Health Professionals.* Clifton Park, NY: Delmar Learning, 1999.

Hall, A., and D. Allen. *Internet Guide for Business Communications.* Cincinnati, OH: South-Western Publishers, 1997.

Kramer, Candice. *Success in On-Line Learning.* Clifton Park, NY: Delmar Learning, 2002.

Mitchell, Joyce, and Lee Haroun. *Introduction to Health Care.* Clifton Park, NY: Delmar Learning, 2002.

Nicoll, Leslie. *Computers in Nursing: Nurse's Guide to the Internet.* Philadelphia, PA: Lippincott, Williams, & Wilkins, 2000.

Saba, Virginia, and Kathleen McCormick. *Essentials of Computers for Nurses: Informatics for the New Millennium.* New York, NY: McGraw-Hill, 2001.

Shelly, Gary B., Thomas Cashman, and Gloria Waggoner. *Using Computers: A Gateway to Information.* Clifton Park, NY: Delmar Learning, 1995.

UNIT 12 Promotion of Safety

Unit Objectives

After completing this unit of study, you should be able to:

- Define the term *body mechanics* as it is used
- Use correct body mechanics while performing procedures in the laboratory or clinical area
- Observe all safety standards established by the Occupational Safety and Health Administration (OSHA), especially the Occupational Exposure to Hazardous Chemicals Standard and the Bloodborne Pathogen Standard
- Follow safety regulations stated in the information sections while performing in the laboratory area
- Observe all regulations for patient safety while performing procedures on a student partner in the laboratory or clinical area or on a patient in any area
- List the four main classes of fire extinguishers
- Relate each class of fire extinguisher to the specific fire(s) for which it is used
- Simulate the operation of a fire extinguisher by following the directions on the extinguisher and specific measures for observing fire safety
- Locate and describe the operation of the nearest fire alarm
- Describe in detail the evacuation plan for the laboratory area according to established school policy
- Define, pronounce, and spell all the key terms

Observe Standard Precautions		Instructors Check—Call Instructor at This Point
Safety—Proceed with Caution		 OBRA Requirement— Based on Federal Law
Math Skill		Legal Responsibility
Science Skill		Career Information
Communications Skill		Technology

282

KEY TERMS

base of support
Bloodborne Pathogen Standard
body mechanics
ergonomics
fire extinguishers

Material Safety Data Sheet
  (MSDS)
Occupational Exposure to
  Hazardous Chemicals
  Standard

Occupational Safety and
  Health Administration
  (OSHA)
safety standards

12:1 INFORMATION Using Body Mechanics

In order to prevent injury to yourself and others while working in the health field, it is important that you observe good body mechanics. **Body mechanics** refers to the way in which the body moves and maintains balance while making the most efficient use of all its parts. Basic rules for body mechanics are provided as guidelines to prevent strain and help maintain muscle strength.

There are four main reasons for using good body mechanics:

◆ Muscles work best when used correctly.

◆ Correct use of muscles makes lifting, pulling, and pushing easier.

◆ Correct application of body mechanics prevents unnecessary fatigue and strain, and saves energy.

◆ Correct application of body mechanics prevents injury to self and others.

Eight basic rules of good body mechanics include:

◆ Maintain a broad **base of support** by keeping the feet 8 to 10 inches apart, placing one foot slightly forward, balancing weight on both feet, and pointing the toes in the direction of movement (see figure 12-1).

◆ Bend from the hips and knees to get close to an object, and keep your back straight (see figure 12-2). Do not bend at the waist.

◆ Use the strongest muscles to do the job. The larger and stronger muscles are located in the

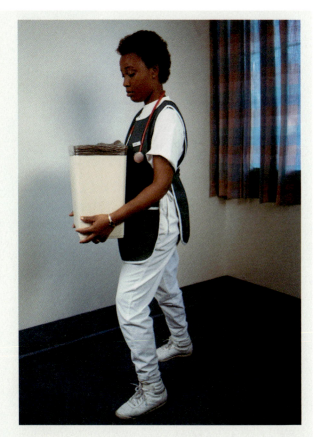

FIGURE 12-1 Maintain a broad base of support by keeping the feet 8 to 10 inches apart.

shoulders, upper arms, hips, and thighs. Back muscles are weak.

◆ Use the weight of your body to help push or pull an object. Whenever possible, push, slide, or pull rather than lift.

◆ Carry heavy objects close to the body. Also, stand close to the object or person being moved.

◆ Avoid twisting your body as you work. Turn with your feet and entire body when you change direction of movement.

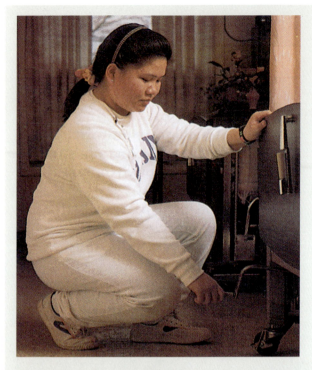

FIGURE 12-2 Bend from the hips and knees to get close to an object.

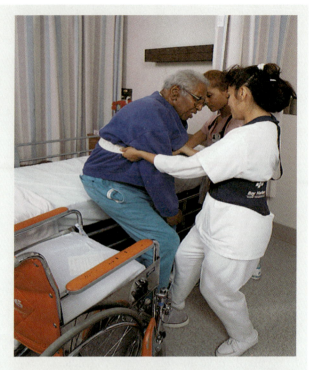

FIGURE 12-3 Many health care facilities now require workers to wear back supports while lifting or moving patients.

◆ Avoid bending for long periods of time.

◆ If a patient or object is too heavy for you to lift alone, always get help. Mechanical lifts, transfer (gait) belts, wheelchairs, and other similar types of equipment are also available to help lift and move patients.

Many health care facilities now require health care workers to wear back supports while lifting or moving patients (see figure 12-3). The supports are supposed to help prevent back injuries, but their use is controversial. They do remind the wearer to use good body mechanics.

If a back support is used, it should be the correct size to provide the maximum benefit. When the worker is performing strenuous tasks, the support should fit snugly. At other times, it can be loosened; but it should be worn at all times, so it is in place when needed.

STUDENT: *Go to the workbook and complete the assignment sheet for 12:1, Using Body Mechanics. Then return and continue with the procedure.*

PROCEDURE 12:1

Using Body Mechanics

Equipment and Supplies

Heavy book, bedside stand, bed with wheel locks

Procedure

1. Assemble equipment.

2. Compare using a narrow base of support to using a broad base of support. Stand on your toes, with your feet close together. Next, stand on your toes with your feet further apart. Then, stand with your feet flat on the floor but close together. Finally, stand with your feet flat on the floor but approximately

8 to 10 inches apart and with one foot slightly forward. Balance your weight on both feet. You should feel the best support in the final position because the broad base supports your body weight.

3. Place the book on the floor. Bend from the hips and knees (not the waist) and keep your back straight to pick up the book. Return to the standing position.

4. Place the book between your thumb and fingers, but not touching the palm of your hand, and hold your hand straight out in front of your body. Slowly move your hand toward your body, stopping several times to feel the weight of the book in different positions. Finally, hold the book with your entire hand and bring your hand close to your body. The final position should be the most comfortable.

   NOTE: This illustrates the need to carry heavy objects close to your body and to use the strongest muscles to do the job.

5. Stand at either end of the bed. Release the wheel locks on the bed. Position your feet to provide a broad base of support. Get close to the bed. Use the weight of your body to push the bed forward.

6. Place the book on the bed. Pick up the book and place it on the bedside stand. Avoid twisting your body. Turn with your feet to place the book on the stand.

   NOTE: Remember that holding the book close to your body allows you to use the strongest muscles.

7. Practice the rules of body mechanics by setting up situations similar to those listed in the previous steps. Continue until the movements feel natural to you.

8. Replace all equipment used.

Practice *Use the evaluation sheet for 12:1, Using Body Mechanics to practice this procedure. When you feel you have mastered this skill, sign the sheet and give it to your instructor for further action.*

Final Checkpoint Using the criteria listed on the evaluation sheet, your instructor will grade your performance.

INFORMATION
12:2 Preventing Accidents and Injuries

The **Occupational Safety and Health Administration (OSHA),** a division of the Department of Labor, establishes and enforces **safety standards** for the workplace. Two main standards affect health care workers:

◆ The Occupational Exposure to Hazardous Chemicals Standard

◆ The Bloodborne Pathogen Standard

The **Occupational Exposure to Hazardous Chemicals Standard** requires that employers inform employees of all chemicals and hazards in the workplace. In addition, all manufacturers must provide **Material Safety Data Sheets (MSDSs)** with any hazardous products they sell (see figure 12-4). The MSDSs must provide the following information:

◆ Product identification information about the chemical

◆ Protection or precautions that should be used while handling the chemical (for example, wearing protective equipment or using only in a well-ventilated area)

◆ Instructions for the safe use of the chemical

◆ Procedures for handling spills, clean-up, and disposal of the product

◆ Emergency first aid procedures to use if injury occurs

The Occupational Exposure to Hazardous Chemicals Standard also mandates that all

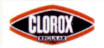

The Clorox Company
1221 Broadway
Oakland, CA 94612
Tel. (510) 271-7000

Material Safety Data Sheet

I Product:	ULTRA CLOROX REGULAR BLEACH
Description:	CLEAR, LIGHT YELLOW LIQUID WITH A CHLORINE ODOR

Other Designations	**Distributor**	**Emergency Telephone Nos.**
Laundry Bleach US EPA Registration # 5813-50	Clorox Sales Company 1221 Broadway Oakland, CA 94612	For Medical Emergencies call: (800) 446-1014 For Transportation Emergencies Chemtrec (800) 424-9300

II Health Hazard Data

CORROSIVE to the eyes. May cause severe irritation or damage to eyes and skin. Harmful if swallowed; nausea, vomiting, and burning sensation of the mouth and throat may occur. The following medical conditions may be aggravated by exposure to high concentrations of vapor or mist: heart conditions, or chronic respiratory problems such as asthma, chronic bronchitis or obstructive lung disease. Some clinical reports suggest a low potential for skin sensitization upon exaggerated exposure to sodium hypochlorite, particularly on damaged or irritated skin. Routine clinical tests conducted on intact skin with Clorox Liquid Bleach found no sensitization in the test subjects. No adverse health effects are expected with recommended use.

FIRST AID: <u>EYE CONTACT:</u> Immediately flush eyes with water for 15 minutes. Contact a physician.
<u>INGESTION:</u> Drink a glassful of water. <u>DO NOT</u> induce vomiting. Immediately contact a physician or Poison Control Center.
<u>SKIN CONTACT:</u> Remove contaminated clothing. Flush skin with water. Contact a physician if irritation or discomfort persists.
<u>INHALATION:</u> Remove from exposure to fresh air.

III Hazardous Ingredients

Ingredient Exposure Limit	Concentration	Worker
Sodium hydroxide CAS #1310-73-2	<0.2%	2 mg/m^3 TLV-C
Sodium hypochlorite CAS #7681-52-9	6-7.35%	not established

None of the ingredients in this product [are on] the IARC, [O]SHA or NTP carcinogen lists.
TLV-C=Threshold Limit Value-Ceiling. Th[e] [exposure] exposure limit should not be exceeded at any ti[me.] Source: ACGIH.

IV Special Protection and Precautions

The following recommendations are given f[or production facil]ity and other conditions and situations where the[re is increa]sed potential for accidental, large-scale, or prolonged expo[sure.]

<u>Hygienic Practices:</u> W[ear g]lasses an[d nit]rile [or] [or] butyl rubber gloves. Th[e availa]bility of an eye wa[sh and sh]ower [is] recommended in a [m]anufacturing environme[nt.]
<u>Engineering Contro[ls:]</u> [Use ventil]ation [to mi]nimize exposure to vapors.
<u>Work Practices:</u> Avoid eye and skin [cont]act and inhalation of vapor or mist.

KEEP OUT OF REACH OF C[HILDREN.]

V Transportation and Regulatory Data

<u>U.S. [DO]T Hazard Class:</u> Not restricted per 49 CFR 172.101(c)(12)(iv).
<u>U.S. Proper Shipping Name:</u> None
<u>IMDG:</u> Not restricted per IMDG Code Page 40 Paragraph 2.3.1.3.
<u>IATA:</u> Not restricted per IATA DGR special provision A3 and ICAO special provision 223.

<u>EPA - SARA TITLE III/CERCLA:</u> Bottled product is not reportable under Sections 311/312 and contains no chemicals reportable under Section 313. This product does contain chemicals (sodium hydroxide <0.2% and sodium hypochlorite <7.35%) that are regulated under Section 304/CERCLA.

<u>TSCA/DSL STATUS:</u> All components of this product are on the U.S. TSCA Inventory and Canadian DSL.

VI Spill Procedures/Waste Disposal

<u>Spill Procedures:</u> Control spill. Containerize liquid and use absorbents on residual liquid; dispose appropriately. Wash area and let dry. For spills of multiple products, responders should evaluate the MSDS's of the products for incompatibility with sodium hypochlorite. Breathing protection should be worn in enclosed, and/or poorly ventilated areas until hazard assessment is complete.
<u>Waste Disposal:</u> Dispose of in accordance with all applicable federal, state, and local regulations.

VII Reactivity Data

Stable under normal use and storage conditions. Strong oxidizing agent. Reacts with other household chemicals such as toilet bowl cleaners, rust removers, vinegar, acids or ammonia containing products to produce hazardous gases, such as chlorine and other chlorinated species. Prolonged contact with metal may cause pitting or discoloration.

VIII Fire and Explosion Data

<u>Flash Point:</u> None
<u>Special Firefighting Procedures:</u> None
<u>Unusual Fire/Explosion Hazards:</u> None. Not flammable or explosive. Product does not ignite when exposed to open flame.

IX Physical Data

Boiling point...approx. 212°F/100°C
Specific Gravity (H$_2$0=1)...............................~ 1.1 at 70°F
Solubility in Water ....complete
pH ....~11.4

© 1963, 1991 THE CLOROX COMPANY

DATA SUPPLIED IS FOR USE ONLY IN CONNECTION WITH OCCUPATIONAL SAFETY AND HEALTH DATE PREPARED <u>10/19/01</u>

FIGURE 12-4 Read the Material Safety Data Sheet (MSDS) before using any chemical product. *(Courtesy of the Clorox Company, Oakland, CA)*

employers train employees on the proper procedures or policies to follow with regard to:

◆ Identifying the types and locations of all chemicals or hazards

◆ Locating and using the MSDS manual containing all of the safety data sheets

◆ Reading and interpreting chemical labels and hazard signs

◆ Using personal protective equipment (PPE) such as masks, gowns, gloves, and goggles

◆ Locating cleaning equipment and following correct methods for managing spills and/or disposal of the chemicals

◆ Reporting accidents or exposures and documenting any incidents that occur

The **Bloodborne Pathogen Standard** has mandates to protect health care providers from diseases caused by exposure to body fluids. Examples of body fluids include blood and blood components, urine, stool, semen, vaginal secretions, cerebrospinal fluid, saliva, mucus, and other similar fluids. Three diseases that can be contracted by exposure to body fluids include hepatitis B, caused by the HBV, or hepatitis B virus, hepatitis C, caused by the HCV, or hepatitis C virus, and acquired immune deficiency syndrome (AIDS), caused by the HIV, or human immunodeficiency virus. The mandates of this standard are discussed in detail in Unit 13:3.

Ergonomics is an applied science used to promote the safety and well-being of a person by adapting the environment and using techniques to prevent injuries. Ergonomics includes the correct placement of furniture and equipment, training in required muscle movements, efforts to avoid repetitive motions, and an awareness of the environment to prevent injuries. The prevention of accidents and injury centers around people and the immediate environment. The health worker must be conscious of personal and patient/resident safety and must exercise care in handling equipment and solutions that may be used.

In addition, every health care worker must accept the responsibility for using good judgment in all situations, asking questions when in doubt, and following approved policies and procedures to create a safe environment. Always remember that a health care worker has a legal responsibility to protect the patient from harm and injury.

Equipment and Solutions

◆ Do *not* operate or use any equipment until you have been instructed on how to use it.

◆ Read and follow the operating instructions for all major pieces of equipment. If you do not understand the instructions, ask for assistance.

◆ Do *not* operate any equipment if your instructor/immediate supervisor is not in the room.

◆ Report any damaged or malfunctioning equipment immediately. Make no attempt to use it. Some facilities use a lockout tag system for damaged electrical or mechanical equipment. A locking device is placed on the equipment to prevent the equipment from being used (see figure 12-5).

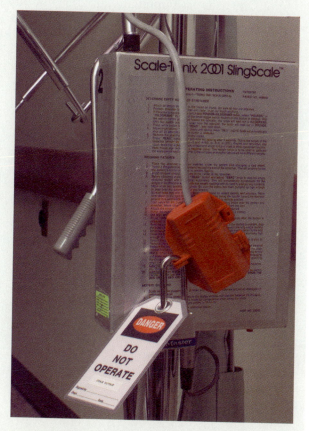

FIGURE 12-5 Some facilities use a lockout tag system for damaged equipment to prevent anyone from using the equipment.

◆ Do not use frayed or damaged electrical cords. Do not use a plug if the third prong for grounding has been broken off.

◆ When handling any equipment, observe all safety precautions that have been taught.

◆ Read Material Safety Data Sheets (MSDSs) before using any hazardous chemical solutions.

◆ Never use solutions from bottles that are not labeled.

◆ Read the labels of solution bottles at least three times during use to be sure you have the correct solution (see figure 12-6).

◆ Do *not* mix any solutions together unless instructed to do so by your instructor/immediate supervisor.

◆ Some solutions can be injurious or poisonous. Avoid contact with your eyes and skin. Use only as directed.

◆ If you break any equipment or spill any solutions, immediately report the incident to your instructor/immediate supervisor. You will be told how to dispose of the equipment or how to remove the spilled solution (see figure 12-7).

Patient/Resident Safety

◆ Do *not* perform any procedure on patients unless you have been instructed to do so. Make sure you have the proper authorization. Follow instructions carefully. Ask questions if you do not understand. Use correct or approved methods while performing any procedure. Avoid shortcuts or incorrect techniques.

◆ Provide privacy for all patients. Knock on the door before entering any room (see figure 12-8A). Speak to the patient and identify yourself. Ask for permission to enter before going behind closed privacy curtains. Close the door and/or draw curtains for privacy before beginning a procedure on the patient (see figure 12-8B).

◆ Always identify your patient. Be absolutely positive that you have the correct patient. Check the identification wristband, if present. Repeat the patient's name at least twice. Check the name on the patient's bed and on the patient's record.

◆ Always explain the procedure so the patient knows what you are going to do (see figure

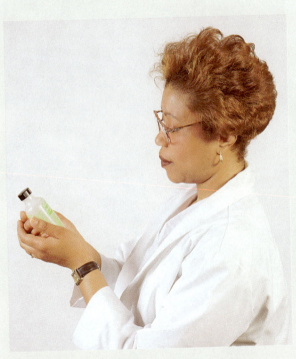

FIGURE 12-6 Read the label on a solution bottle at least three times to be sure you have the correct solution.

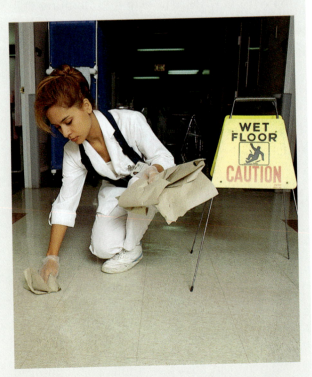

FIGURE 12-7 Follow proper procedure to clean up spilled solutions.

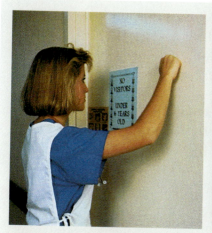

FIGURE 12-8A Always knock on the door or speak before entering a patient's room.

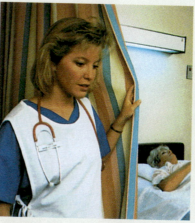

FIGURE 12-8B Close the door and draw curtains for privacy before beginning a procedure.

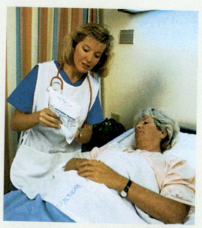

FIGURE 12-8C Explain the procedure and answer any questions to make sure you have the patient's consent.

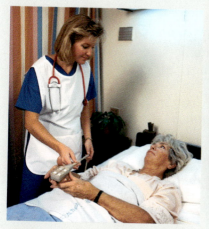

FIGURE 12-9A Lower the bed and place the call signal within easy reach of the patient before leaving a patient.

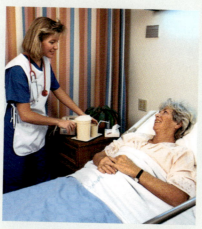

FIGURE 12-9B Make sure other supplies and equipment are conveniently placed within the patient's reach.

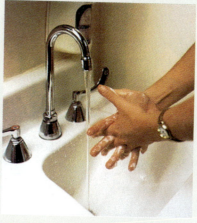

FIGURE 12-10 Wash your hands before and after any procedure, and any time they become contaminated during a procedure.

12-8C). Answer any questions and make sure you have the patient's consent before performing any procedure. Never perform a procedure if a patient refuses to allow you to do so.

◆ Observe the patient closely during any procedure. If you notice any change, immediately report this. Be alert to the patient's condition at all times.

◆ Frequently check the patient area, waiting room, office rooms, bed areas, or home environment for safety hazards. Report all unsafe situations immediately to the proper person or correct the safety hazard.

◆ Before leaving a patient/resident in a bed, observe all safety checkpoints. Make sure the patient is positioned in a comfortable position. Check the bed to be sure that the side rails are elevated, if indicated; the bed is at the lowest level to the floor; and the wheels on the bed are locked to prevent movement of the bed. Place the call signal (a bell can be used in a home situation) (see figure 12-9A), and other supplies within easy reach of the patient/resident (see figure 12-9B). Open the privacy curtains if they were closed. Leave the area neat and clean and make sure no safety hazards are present.

Personal Safety

- Remember, it is your responsibility to protect yourself and others from injury.

- Use correct body mechanics while performing any procedure.

- Wear the required uniform.

- Walk—do *not* run—in the laboratory area or clinical area, in hallways, and especially on stairs. Keep to the right and watch carefully at intersections to avoid collisions. Use handrails on stairways.

- Report any personal injury or accident, no matter how minor, to your instructor/immediate supervisor promptly.

- If you see an unsafe situation or a violation of a safety practice, report it to your instructor/immediate supervisor promptly.

- Keep all areas clean and neat with all equipment and supplies in their proper locations at all times.

- Wash your hands frequently. Hands should always be washed before and after any procedure, and any time they become contaminated during a procedure (see figure 12-10).

Keep your hands away from your face, eyes, mouth, and hair.

- Dry your hands thoroughly before handling any electrical equipment.

- Wear safety glasses when instructed to do so and in situations that might result in possible eye injury.

- While working with your partner in patient simulations, observe all safety precautions taught in caring for a patient. Review the role each of you will have before you begin practicing a procedure so each person knows his or her responsibilities. Avoid horseplay and practical jokes; they cause accidents.

- If any solutions come in contact with your skin or eyes, immediately flush the area with water. Inform your instructor/immediate supervisor.

- If a particle gets in your eye, inform your instructor/immediate supervisor. Do *not* try to remove the particle or rub your eye.

STUDENT: *Go to the workbook and complete the assignment sheet for 12:2, Preventing Accidents and Injuries. Then return and continue with the procedure.*

PROCEDURE 12:2

Preventing Accidents and Injuries

Equipment and Supplies

Information section on Preventing Accidents and Injuries, several bottles of solutions, laboratory area with equipment

Procedure

1. Assemble equipment.

2. Review the safety standards in the information section for Preventing Accidents and Injuries. Note standards that are not clear and ask your instructor for an explanation.

3. Examine several bottles of solutions. Read the labels carefully. Read the safety or danger warnings on the bottles. Read Material Safety Data Sheets provided with hazardous chemicals.

4. Practice reading the label three times to be sure you have the correct solution. Read the label before taking the bottle off the shelf, before pouring from the bottle, and after you have poured from the bottle.

5. Look at major pieces of equipment in the laboratory. Read the operating instructions for the equipment. Do *not* operate the

equipment until you are taught how to do it correctly.

6. Role play the following situations by using another student as a patient.

   ◆ Show ways to provide privacy for the patient.

   ◆ Identify the patient.

   ◆ Explain a procedure to the patient.

   ◆ Check various patient areas in the laboratory. Note any safety hazards that may be present. Discuss how you can correct the problems. Report your findings to your instructor.

   ◆ Observe the patient during a procedure. List points you should observe to note a change in the patient's condition.

7. Discuss the following situations with another student and decide how you would handle them:

   ◆ You see an unsafe situation or a violation of a safety practice.

   ◆ You see a wet area on the laboratory counter.

   ◆ You get a small cut on your hand while using a glass slide.

   ◆ A solution splashes on your arm.

   ◆ A particle gets in your eye.

   ◆ A piece of equipment is not working correctly.

   ◆ A bottle of solution does not have a label.

   ◆ You break a glass thermometer.

8. Observe and practice all of the safety regulations as you work in the laboratory.

9. Study the regulations in preparation for the safety examination. You must pass the safety examination.

10. Replace all equipment used.

Practice *Use the evaluation sheet for 12:2, Preventing Accidents and Injuries, to practice this procedure. When you feel you have mastered this skill, sign the sheet and give it to your instructor for further action.*

Final Checkpoint Using the criteria listed on the evaluation sheet, your instructor will grade your performance.

12:3 INFORMATION
Observing Fire Safety

This information section provides you with basic facts about fires, how they start, and how to prevent them. This information is important for fire safety in the laboratory and work environment.

Fires need three things in order to start: oxygen or air, fuel (any material that will burn), and heat (sparks, matches, flames) (see figure 12-11).

The major cause of fires is carelessness with smoking and with matches. Other causes include

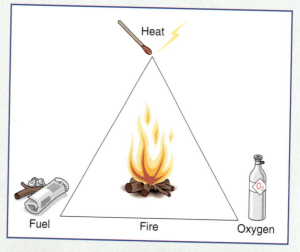

FIGURE 12-11 The fire triangle shows the three things needed to start a fire.

misuse of electricity (overloaded circuits, frayed electrical wires, and/or improperly grounded plugs), defects in heating systems, spontaneous ignition, improper rubbish disposal, and arson.

Fire extinguishers are classified according to the kind of fire they extinguish. There are many different fire extinguishers. The main ones are:

◆ *Class A:* This extinguisher contains pressurized water. It is used on fires involving combustibles such as paper, cloth, and wood.

◆ *Class B:* This extinguisher contains carbon dioxide (CO_2). It is used on gasoline, oil, paint, liquid, and cooking fat fires. These types of fire spread if water is used to put them out. Carbon dioxide provides a smothering action. A Class B extinguisher does leave a powdery, snowlike residue that irritates the skin and eyes. The residue is also dangerous if inhaled.

◆ *Class C:* This extinguisher is a dry-chemical type. It contains potassium bicarbonate or potassium chloride. The chemical is a nonconducting agent, so it is used on electrical fires. It can also be used on burning liquids for a smothering action.

◆ *Class ABC,* or *Combination:* This extinguisher contains a graphite-type chemical. It is a multipurpose extinguisher and can be used on all fires. This type also leaves a residue irritating to skin and eyes.

In case of fire, the main rule is to remain calm. If your personal safety is endangered, evacuate the area according to the stated method and sound the alarm. If the fire is small, confined to one area, and your safety is not endangered, determine what type of fire it is and use the proper extinguisher.

While working in a health care facility, know and follow the fire emergency plan established by the facility (see figure 12-12). The plan usually states that all patients and personnel in immediate danger should be moved from the area. The alarm should be activated as quickly as possible. All doors and windows should be closed, if possible, to prevent drafts, which cause fire to spread more rapidly. Electrical equipment and oxygen should be shut off. Elevators should never be used during a fire. The acronym *RACE* is frequently used to remember the important steps. RACE stands for:

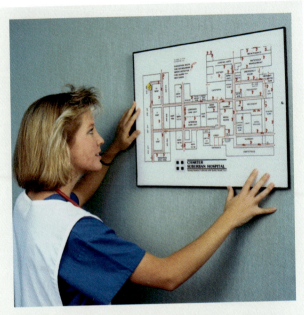

FIGURE 12-12 All personnel must be familiar with the fire emergency plan established by the facility in which they work.

◆ *R* = Rescue anyone in immediate danger. Move patients to a safe area. If the patient can walk, escort him or her to a safe area. At times it may be necessary to move a patient in a bed or use the bed sheets as lift sheets to carry a patient to a safe area.

◆ *A* = Activate the alarm. Sound the alarm and give the location and type of fire.

◆ *C* = Confine the fire. Close windows and doors to prevent drafts. Shut off electrical equipment and oxygen if your safety is not endangered.

◆ *E* = Extinguish the fire. If the fire is small and contained, and you are not in danger, locate the correct fire extinguisher to extinguish the fire.

By following the fire emergency plan, knowing the location of fire extinguishers and exit doors, and remaining calm, the health care worker can help prevent loss of life or serious injury during a fire.

Preventing fires is everyone's job. Constantly be alert to causes of fires, and correct all situations that can lead to fires. Some rules for preventing fires are:

◆ Obey all "No Smoking" signs. Many health care facilities are now "smoke-free" environments and do not permit smoking anywhere on the premises.

◆ Extinguish matches, cigarettes, and any other flammable items completely. Do not empty ashtrays into trash cans or plastic bags that can burn. Always empty ashtrays into separate metal cans or containers partially filled with sand or water.

◆ Dispose of all waste materials in proper containers.

◆ Before using electrical equipment, check for damaged cords or improper grounding. Avoid overloading electrical outlets.

◆ Store flammable materials such as kerosene or gasoline in proper containers and in a safe area. If you spill a flammable liquid, wipe it up immediately.

◆ Do not allow clutter to accumulate in rooms, closets, doorways, or traffic areas. Make sure no equipment or supplies block any fire exits.

◆ When oxygen is in use, observe special precautions. Post a "No Smoking—Oxygen in Use" sign. Remove all smoking materials, candles, lighters, and matches from the room. Avoid the use of electrically operated equipment whenever possible. Do not use flammable liquids such as alcohol, nail polish, and oils. Avoid static electricity by using cotton blankets, sheets, and gowns.

In addition to fires, other types of disasters may occur. Examples include tornadoes, hurricanes, earthquakes, floods, and bomb threats. In any type of disaster, stay calm, follow the policy of the health care facility, and provide for the safety of yourself and the patient. It is important to note that health care workers are legally responsible for familiarizing themselves with disaster policies so appropriate action can be taken when a disaster strikes.

STUDENT: *Go to the workbook and complete the assignment sheet for 12:3, Observing Fire Safety. Then return and continue with the procedure.*

PROCEDURE 12:3
Observing Fire Safety

Equipment and Supplies
Fire alarm box, fire extinguishers

Procedure

1. Read the information section on Observing Fire Safety.

2. Learn the four classes of fire extinguishers and know what kind of fire each type is used for.

3. Locate the nearest fire alarm box. Read the instructions on how to operate the alarm. Be sure you could set off the alarm in case of a fire.

4. Locate any fire extinguishers in the laboratory area. Look for extinguishers in both the room and surrounding building. Identify each extinguisher and the kind of fire for which it is meant to be used.

5. Learn how to operate a fire extinguisher. Read the manufacturer's operating instructions carefully. Work with a practice extinguisher or do a mock demonstration.

CAUTION: Do *not* discharge a real extinguisher in the laboratory.

a. Check the extinguisher type to be sure it is the proper one to use for the mock fire (see figure 12-13A).

b. Locate the lock or pin at the top handle. Release the lock following the manufacturer's instructions, then grasp the handle (see figure 12-13B).

NOTE: During a mock demonstration, only pretend to release the lock.

c. Hold the extinguisher firmly in an upright position.

d. Stand approximately 6 to 10 feet from the near edge of the fire.

e. Aim the nozzle at the fire.

f. Discharge the extinguisher. Use a side-to-side motion. Spray toward the near edge of the fire at the bottom of the fire.

> ⚠ **CAUTION:** Do not spray into the center or top of the fire, because this will cause the fire to spread in an outward direction.

g. Continue with the same motion until the fire is extinguished.

> **NOTE:** The word *PASS* can help you remember the correct steps:
>
> *P* = Pull the pin.
>
> *A* = Aim the extinguisher at the near edge and bottom of the fire.
>
> *S* = Squeeze the handle to discharge the extinguisher.
>
> *S* = Sweep the extinguisher from side to side.

h. At all times, stay a safe distance from the fire to avoid personal injury.

> ⚠ **CAUTION:** Avoid contact with residues from chemical extinguishers.

i. After an extinguisher has been used, it must be recharged or replaced. Another usable extinguisher must be put in position when the extinguisher is removed.

6. Check the policy in your area for evacuating the laboratory area during a fire. Practice the method and know the locations of all exits.

> **NOTE:** Remember to remain calm and avoid panic.

7. Replace all equipment used.

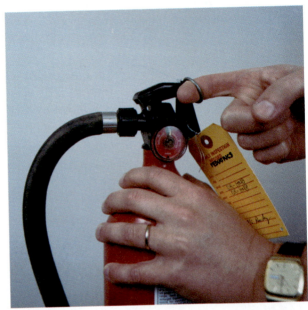

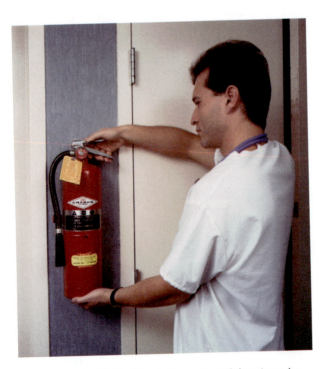

FIGURE 12-13A Check the extinguisher type to make sure it is the correct one to use.

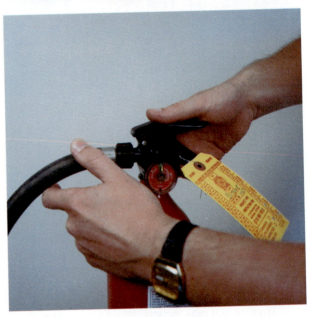

FIGURE 12-13B Release the pin, aim the nozzle at the near edge of the fire, and push the handle to discharge the extinguisher.

Practice *Use the evaluation sheet for 12:3, Observing Fire Safety, to practice this procedure. When you feel you have mastered this skill, sign the sheet and give it to your instructor for further action.*

 Final Checkpoint Using the criteria listed on the evaluation sheet, your instructor will grade your performance.

Practice *Study the safety regulations throughout Unit 12 in preparation for the safety examination.*

 Final Checkpoint Take the safety examination and obtain a passing grade to demonstrate your knowledge of safety.

UNIT 12 SUMMARY

Safety is the responsibility of every health care worker. It is essential that established safety standards be observed by everyone. This protects the worker, the employer, and the patient.

One important aspect of safety is the correct use of body mechanics. Body mechanics refer to the way the body moves and maintains balance while making the most efficient use of all its parts. Practicing basic principles of good body mechanics prevents strain and maintains muscle strength. In addition, correct body mechanics make lifting, pulling, and pushing easier.

Knowing and following basic safety standards is also important. In this unit, basic standards are listed in regard to the use of equipment and solutions, patient safety, and personal safety. It is important for everyone to learn and follow the established standards at all times.

An awareness of the causes and prevention of fires is essential. Every health care worker should be familiar with the types and use of fire extinguishers. In addition, every facility has a fire emergency plan. By following the fire emergency plan, knowing the location of fire extinguishers and exit doors, and remaining calm, the health care worker can help prevent loss of life or serious injury during a fire.

INTERNET SEARCHES

Use the suggested search engines in Unit 11:4 of this textbook to search the Internet for additional information on the following topics:

1. *Federal regulations:* obtain more information on federal safety regulations by searching sites of the Occupational Safety and Health Administration (OSHA), Occupational Exposure to Hazardous Chemicals Standard, Bloodborne Pathogen Standard, and Material Safety Data Sheets (MSDSs).

2. *Ergonomics:* search for additional information on ergonomics and environmental safety.

3. *Diseases:* obtain information on the causative agents and methods of transmission for hepatitis B and C and acquired immune deficiency syndrome (AIDS).

4. *Fire safety:* search for information on fire prevention and fire safety.

5. *Fire extinguishers:* search for various manufacturers of fire extinguishers and obtain information on the types of extinguishers, their main uses, precautions for handling, and safety rules that must be observed while using extinguishers.

6. *Disasters:* obtain information on safety procedures that must be followed for tornadoes, floods, hurricanes, and earthquakes.

REVIEW QUESTIONS

1. Define *body mechanics* and list four (4) reasons why it is important to use good body mechanics.

2. You are using an electrical microhematocrit centrifuge to spin blood. You see smoke coming from the back of the machine. What should you do?

3. List four (4) safety precautions that must be followed while using solutions.

4. Identify three (3) things that must be done before performing any procedure on a patient.

5. State five (5) checkpoints that must be observed before leaving a patient/resident in bed.

6. List five (5) rules that must be followed while oxygen is in use.

7. What does the acronym *RACE* stand for?

8. Create a chart showing the four (4) main types of fire extinguishers, what each extinguisher contains, and the type of fire for which it is effective.

UNIT 12
SUGGESTED REFERENCES

Acello, Barbara. *Patient Care: Basic Skills for the Health Care Provider.* Clifton Park, NY: Delmar Learning, 1998.

Acello, Barbara. *The OSHA Handbook: Guidelines to Compliance in Health Care Facilities.* 3rd ed. Clifton Park, NY: Delmar Learning, 2002.

Hegner, Barbara, Esther Caldwell, and Joan Needham. *Nursing Assistant: A Nursing Process Approach.* 8th ed. Clifton Park, NY: Delmar Learning, 1999.

Klinoff, Robert. *Introduction to Fire Protection.* Clifton Park, NY: Delmar Learning, 1997.

Marotz, Lynn, Marie Cross, and Jeanettia Rush. *Health, Safety, and Nutrition for the Young Child.* Clifton Park, NY: Delmar Learning, 1997.

Nielson, Ronald. *OSHA Regulations and Guidelines: A Guide for Health Care Providers.* Clifton Park, NY: Delmar Learning, 2000.

Infection Control

Introduction

After completing this unit of study, you should be able to:

◆ Identify five classes of microorganisms by describing the characteristics of each class
◆ List the six components of the chain of infection
◆ Differentiate between antisepsis, disinfection, and sterilization
◆ Wash hands according to recommended aseptic technique
◆ Observe standard precautions while working in the laboratory or clinical area
◆ Wash, wrap, and autoclave instruments, linen, and equipment
◆ Operate an autoclave with accuracy and safety
◆ Follow basic principles on using chemicals for disinfection
◆ Clean instruments with an ultrasonic unit
◆ Open sterile packages without contaminating the contents
◆ Don sterile gloves without contaminating the gloves
◆ Prepare a sterile dressing tray without contaminating the supplies
◆ Change a sterile dressing without contaminating the materials
◆ Don and remove a transmission-based isolation mask, gloves, and gown
◆ Relate specific basic tasks to the care of a patient in a transmission-based isolation unit
◆ Define, pronounce, and spell all the key terms

 Observe Standard Precautions

 Safety—Proceed with Caution

 Math Skill

 Science Skill

 C Communications Skill

 Instructors Check—Call Instructor at This Point

 **OBRA** OBRA Requirement— Based on Federal Law

 Legal Responsibility

 Career Information

 Technology

KEY TERMS

acquired immune deficiency
  syndrome (AIDS)
aerobic
airborne precautions
anaerobic
antisepsis
  (ant"-ih-sep'-sis)
asepsis
  (a-sep'-sis)
autoclave
bacteria
causative agent
cavitation
  (kav"-ih-tay'-shun)
chain of infection
chemical disinfection
clean
communicable disease
contact precautions

contaminated
disinfection
droplet precautions
endogenous
exogenous
fomites
fungi
  (fun'-guy)
hepatitis B
hepatitis C
microorganism
  (my-crow-or'-gan-izm)
mode of transmission
nonpathogens
nosocomial
opportunistic
pathogens
  (path'-oh-jenz")

personal protective equipment
  (PPE)
portal of entry
portal of exit
protective (reverse) isolation
protozoa
  (pro-toe-zo'-ah)
reservoir
rickettsiae
  (rik-et'-z-ah)
standard precautions
sterile
sterile field
sterilization
susceptible host
transmission-based isolation
  precautions
ultrasonic
viruses

13:1 INFORMATION
Understanding the Principles of Infection Control

OBRA Understanding the basic principles of infection control is essential for any health care worker in any field of health care. The principles described in this unit provide a basic knowledge of how disease is transmitted and the main ways to prevent disease transmission.

A **microorganism,** or microbe, is a small, living organism that is not visible to the naked eye. It must be viewed under a microscope. Microorganisms are found everywhere in the environment, including on and in the human body. Many microorganisms are part of the normal flora (plant life adapted for living in a specific environment) of the body and are beneficial in

maintaining certain body processes. These are called **nonpathogens.** Other microorganisms cause infection and disease and are called **pathogens,** or germs. At times, a microorganism that is beneficial in one body system can become pathogenic when it is present in another body system. For example, a bacterium called *Escherichia coli* (*E. coli*) is part of the natural flora of the large intestine. If *E. coli* enters the urinary system, however, it causes an infection.

There are many different classes of microorganisms. In each class, some of the microorganisms are pathogenic to humans. The main classes include:

◆ **Bacteria**—These are simple, one-celled organisms that multiply rapidly. They are classified by shape and arrangement. *Cocci* are round or spherical in shape (see figure 13-1). If cocci occur in pairs, they are diplococci. Diplococci bacteria cause diseases such as gonorrhea, meningitis, and pneumonia. If cocci occur in chains, they are streptococci. A common streptococcus causes a severe sore throat (strep throat) and rheumatic fever. If

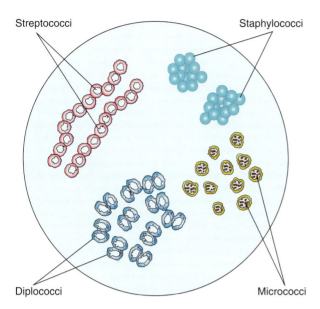

FIGURE 13-1 Kinds of cocci bacteria.

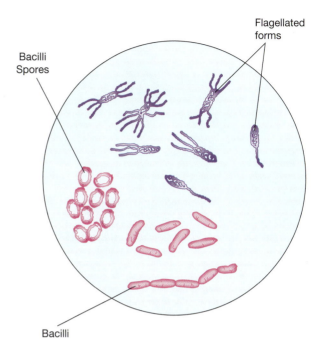

FIGURE 13-2 Bacilli bacteria.

cocci occur in clusters or groups, they are staphylococci. These are the most common pyogenic (pus-producing) microorganisms. Staphylococci cause infections such as boils, wound infections, and toxic shock. Rod-shaped bacteria are called *bacilli* (see figure 13-2). They can occur singly, in pairs, or in chains. Many bacilli contain flagella, which are threadlike projections that are similar to tails and allow the organisms to move. Bacilli also have the ability to form spores, or thick-walled capsules, when conditions for growth are poor. In the spore form, bacilli are extremely difficult to kill. Diseases caused by different types of bacilli include tuberculosis; tetanus; pertussis, or whooping cough; botulism; diphtheria; and typhoid. Bacteria that are spiral or corkscrew in shape are called *spirilla* (see figure 13-3). These include the comma-shaped vibrio and the corkscrew-shaped spirochete. Diseases caused by spirilla include syphilis and cholera. Antibiotics are used to kill bacteria. However, some strains of bacteria have become antibiotic-resistant, which means that the antibiotic is no longer effective against the bacteria.

◆ **Protozoa**—These are one-celled animal-like organisms often found in decayed materials and contaminated water (see figure 13-4). Many contain flagella which allow them to move freely. Some protozoa are pathogenic and cause diseases such as malaria, amebic

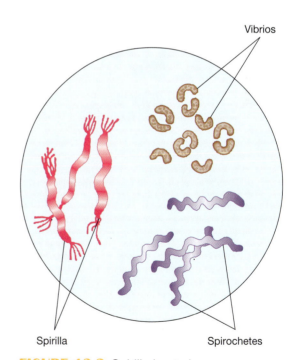

FIGURE 13-3 Spirilla bacteria.

dysentery, trichomonas, and African sleeping sickness.

◆ **Fungi**—These are simple, plant-like organisms that live on dead organic matter. Yeasts and molds are two common forms that can be

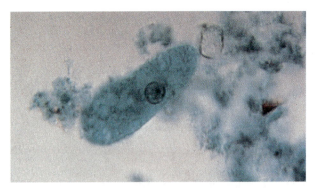

FIGURE 13-4 An intestinal protozoan, *Entamoeba coli. (Courtesy of the Centers for Disease Control and Prevention, Atlanta, GA)*

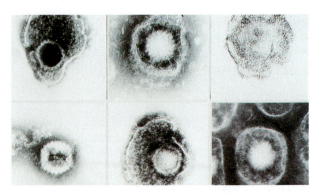

FIGURE 13-6A Electron micrographs of the various types of herpes simplex virus. *(Courtesy of the Centers for Disease Control and Prevention, Atlanta, GA)*

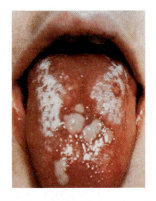

FIGURE 13-5 The yeast (fungus) called thrush causes these characteristic white patches on the tongue.

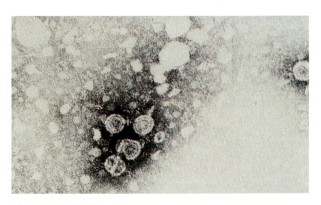

FIGURE 13-6B Electron micrograph of the hepatitis B virus. *(Courtesy of the Centers for Disease Control and Prevention, Atlanta, GA)*

pathogenic. They cause diseases such as ringworm, athlete's foot, histoplasmosis, yeast vaginitis, and thrush (see figure 13-5). Antibiotics do not kill fungi. Antifungal medications are available for many of the pathogenic fungi, but they are expensive, must be taken internally for a long period of time, and may cause liver damage.

◆ **Rickettsiae**—These are parasitic microorganisms, which means they cannot live outside the cells of another living organism. They are commonly found in fleas, lice, ticks, and mites and are transmitted to humans by the bites of these insects. Rickettsiae cause diseases such as typhus fever and Rocky Mountain spotted fever. Antibiotics are effective against many different rickettsiae.

◆ **OBRA** **Viruses**—These are the smallest microorganisms, visible only using an electron microscope (see figure 13-6A and B). They cannot reproduce unless they are inside another living cell. They are spread from human to human by blood and other body secretions. It is important to note that viruses are more difficult to kill because they are resistant to many disinfectants and are not affected by antibiotics. Viruses cause many diseases including the common cold, measles, mumps, chicken pox, herpes, warts, influenza, and polio. Three diseases of major concern to the health care worker are hepatitis B, hepatitis C, and acquired immune deficiency syndrome (AIDS). **Hepatitis B,** or serum hepatitis, is caused by the HBV virus and is transmitted by blood, serum, and other body secretions. It affects the liver and can lead to the destruction and scarring of liver cells. A vaccine has been developed to protect individuals from this disease. The vaccine is expensive and involves a series of three injections. Under federal law, employers must provide the vaccination at no cost to any health care worker with occupational exposure to blood or other body secretions that may carry the HBV virus. An individual does have the right to refuse the vaccination, but a written record must be kept proving that the vaccine was offered. **Hepatitis C** is caused by the hepatitis C virus, or HCV, and is transmitted by blood and blood-containing body fluids. Many individuals who contact the disease are asymptomatic (display no symptoms); others have mild symptoms that are often diagnosed as influenza or flu. In either case, HCV can cause serious liver damage. At present there is no preventive immunization, but a vaccine is being developed. Both HBV and HCV are extremely difficult to destroy. These viruses can even remain active for several days in dried blood. Health care workers must take every precaution to protect themselves from hepatitis viruses. **Acquired immune deficiency syndrome** is caused by the human immunodeficiency virus (HIV) and suppresses the immune system. An individual with AIDS cannot fight off many cancers and infections that would not affect a healthy person. Presently there is no cure and no vaccine available, so it is important for the health care worker to take precautions to prevent the spread of this disease.

In order to grow and reproduce, microorganisms need certain things. Most microorganisms prefer a warm environment, and body temperature is ideal. Darkness is also preferred by most microorganisms, and many are killed quickly by sunlight. In addition, a source of food and moisture is needed. Some microorganisms, called **aerobic** organisms, require oxygen to live. Others, called **anaerobic** organisms, live and reproduce in the absence of oxygen. The human body is the ideal supplier of all the requirements of microorganisms.

Pathogenic microorganisms cause infection and disease in different ways. Some pathogens produce poisons, called *toxins,* which harm the body. An example is the bacillus that causes tetanus, which produces toxins that damage the central nervous system. Some pathogens cause an allergic reaction in the body, resulting in a runny nose, watery eyes, and sneezing. Other pathogens attack and destroy the living cells they

invade. An example is the protozoan that causes malaria. It invades red blood cells and causes them to rupture.

Infections and diseases are also classified as endogenous, exogenous, nosocomial, or opportunistic. **Endogenous** means the infection or disease originates within the body. These include metabolic disorders, congenital abnormalities, tumors, and infections caused by microorganisms within the body. **Exogenous** means the infection or disease originates outside the body. Examples include pathogenic organisms that invade the body, radiation, chemical agents, trauma, electric shock, and temperature extremes. A **nosocomial** infection is one acquired by an individual in a health care facility such as a hospital or long-term care facility. Nosocomial infections are usually present in the facility and transmitted by health care workers to the patient. Many of the pathogens transmitted in this manner are antibiotic-resistant and can cause serious and even life-threatening infections in patients. Common examples are staphylococcus, pseudomonas, and enterococci. Infection-control programs are used in health care facilities to prevent and deal with nosocomial infections. **Opportunistic** infections are those that occur when the body's defenses are weak. These diseases do not usually occur in individuals with intact immune systems. Examples include the development of Kaposi's sarcoma (a rare type of cancer) or *Pneumocystis carinii* pneumonia in individuals with AIDS.

In order for disease to occur and spread from one individual to another, certain conditions must be met. First, there must be a **causative agent,** or pathogen, such as a bacterium or virus. Second, the causative agent must find a **reservoir** where it can live. Some common reservoirs include the human body, animals, the environment, and **fomites,** or objects contaminated with infectious material that contains the pathogens. Common fomites include doorknobs, bedpans, urinals, linens, instruments, and specimen containers. The pathogen must then have a **portal of exit,** or a way to escape from the reservoir in which it has been growing. In the human body, pathogens can leave the body through urine, feces, saliva, blood, tears, mucous discharge, sexual secretions, and draining wounds. When the pathogen leaves the reservoir, it must have a **mode of transmission,** or way in which it can be transmitted to another reservoir or host where it can live. The pathogen can be transmitted in different ways. One way is by direct person-to-person contact (physical or sexual contact), or direct contact with a body secretion containing the pathogen. Contaminated hands are one of the most common sources of direct transmission. Another way is by indirect contact, when the pathogen is transmitted from contaminated substances such as food, air, soil, insects, feces, clothing, instruments, and equipment. Examples include touching contaminated equipment and spreading the pathogen on the hands, breathing in droplets carrying airborne infections, and being bitten by an insect carrying a pathogen. A **portal of entry,** or a way to enter a new reservoir or host, is also essential. Some ways pathogens can enter the body are through breaks in the skin, breaks in the mucous membrane, the respiratory tract, the digestive tract, the genitourinary tract, and the circulatory system. If the defense mechanisms of the body are intact and the immune system is functioning, a human can frequently fight off the causative agent and not contract the disease. Body defenses include:

◆ *mucous membrane:* lines the respiratory, digestive, and reproductive tracts and traps pathogens;

◆ *cilia:* tiny, hairlike structures that line the respiratory tract and propel pathogens out of the body;

◆ *coughing and sneezing;*

◆ *hydrochloric acid:* destroys pathogens in the stomach;

◆ *tears in the eye:* contain bacteriocidal (killing bacteria) chemicals;

◆ *fever;*

◆ *inflammation:* leukocytes, or white blood cells, destroy pathogens;

◆ *immune response:* body produces antibodies, protective proteins that combat pathogens, and protective chemicals secreted by cells, such as interferon and complement.

However, if large numbers of a pathogen invade the body, or if the body defenses are weak, the individual can contract the infection or disease. This individual is called a **susceptible host,** or a person likely to get an infection or disease. These factors—a causative agent, a reservoir, a portal of exit, a mode of transmission, a portal of entry, and a susceptible host—form what is commonly called the **chain of infection** (see figure 13-7). If any part of the chain is eliminated, the spread of disease or infection will be stopped. A health care worker who is aware of this can follow practices to interrupt or break this chain and prevent the transmission of disease. It is important to remember that pathogens are everywhere and that preventing their transmission is a continuous process.

A major way to break the chain of infection is to use aseptic techniques while providing health care. **Asepsis** is defined as the absence of disease-producing microorganisms, or pathogens. Any object or area that may contain pathogens is considered to be contaminated. Aseptic techniques are directed toward maintaining cleanliness and eliminating or preventing contamination. Common aseptic techniques include handwashing, good personal hygiene, use of disposable gloves when contacting body secretions or contaminated objects, proper cleaning of instruments and equipment, and thorough cleaning of the environment.

Various levels of aseptic control are possible. These include:

◆ **Antisepsis**—Antiseptics prevent or inhibit growth of pathogenic organisms but are not effective against spores and viruses. They can usually be used on the skin. Common examples include alcohol and betadine.

◆ **Disinfection**—This is a process that destroys or kills pathogenic organisms. It is not always effective against spores and viruses. Chemical disinfectants are used in this process. Disinfectants can irritate or damage the skin and are used mainly on objects, not people. Some common disinfectants are bleach solutions and zephirin.

◆ **Sterilization**—This is a process that destroys all microorganisms, both pathogenic and non-pathogenic, including spores and viruses. Steam under pressure, gas, radiation, and chemicals can be used to sterilize objects. An autoclave is the most common piece of equipment used for sterilization.

In the sections that follow, correct methods of aseptic techniques are described. It is important for the health care worker to know and use these methods in every aspect of providing health care in order to prevent the spread and transmission of disease.

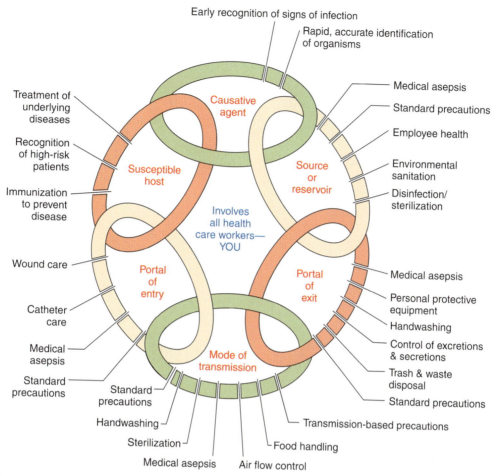

Early recognition of signs of infection

Rapid, accurate identification of organisms

Treatment of underlying diseases

Recognition of high-risk patients

Immunization to prevent disease

Medical asepsis

Standard precautions

Employee health

Environmental sanitation

Disinfection/ sterilization

Causative agent

Susceptible host

Source or reservoir

Involves all health care workers— YOU

Portal of entry

Portal of exit

Wound care

Catheter care

Medical asepsis

Standard precautions

Mode of transmission

Standard precautions

Handwashing

Sterilization

Medical asepsis

Air flow control

Food handling

Transmission-based precautions

Standard precautions

Trash & waste disposal

Control of excretions & secretions

Handwashing

Personal protective equipment

Medical asepsis

FIGURE 13-7 Note the components in the chain of infection and the ways in which the chain can be broken.

STUDENT: *Go to the workbook and complete the assignment sheet for 13:1, Understanding the Principles of Infection Control.*

13:2 INFORMATION *Washing Hands*

OBRA Handwashing is a basic task required in any health occupation. The method described in this unit has been developed to ensure that a thorough cleansing occurs. An aseptic technique is a method followed to prevent the spread of germs or pathogens. *Handwashing is the most important method used to practice aseptic technique.* Handwashing is also the most effective way to prevent the spread of infection.

The hands are a perfect medium for the spread of pathogens. Thoroughly washing the hands helps prevent and control the spread of pathogens from one person to another. It also helps protect the health worker from disease and illness.

Handwashing should be performed frequently. It should be done:

◆ When you arrive at the facility and immediately before leaving the facility

◆ Before and after every patient contact

◆ Any time the hands become contaminated during a procedure

◆ Before applying and immediately after removing gloves

◆ Before and after handling any specimen

◆ After contact with any soiled or contaminated item

◆ After picking up any item off the floor

◆ After personal use of the bathroom

◆ After you cough, sneeze, or use a tissue

◆ Before and after any contact with your mouth or mucous membrane, such as eating, drinking, smoking, applying lip balm, or inserting or removing contact lenses

The recommended method for handwashing is based on the following principles; they should be observed whenever hands are washed:

◆ Soap is used as a cleansing agent because it aids in the removal of germs through its sudsy action and alkali content. Pathogens are trapped in the soapsuds and rinsed away. Use liquid soap from a dispenser whenever possible because bar soap can contain microorganisms.

◆ Warm water should be used. This is less damaging to the skin than hot water. It also creates a better lather with soap than does cold water.

◆ Friction must be used in addition to soap and water. This action helps rub off pathogens from the surface of the skin.

◆ All surfaces on the hands must be cleaned. This includes the palms, the backs/tops of the hands, and the areas between the fingers.

◆ Fingertips must be pointed downward. The downward direction prevents water from getting on the forearms and then running down to contaminate the clean hands.

◆ Dry paper towels must be used to turn the faucet on and off. This action prevents contamination of the hands from pathogens on the faucet. A dry towel must be used because pathogens can travel more readily through a wet towel.

Nails also harbor dirt and must be cleaned during the handwashing process. An orange/cuticle stick can be used. Care must be taken to use the blunt end of the stick because the pointed end can injure the nailbeds. A brush can also be used to clean the nails. If a brush or orange stick is not available, the nails can be rubbed against the palm of the opposite hand. Keep the nails short to prevent scratching the skin.

STUDENT: *Go to the workbook and complete the assignment sheet for 13:2, Washing Hands. Then return and continue with the procedure.*

PROCEDURE 13:2

Washing Hands

Equipment and Supplies

Paper towels, running water, waste container, hand brush or orange/cuticle stick, soap

Procedure

1. Assemble all equipment. Stand back slightly from the sink so you do not contaminate

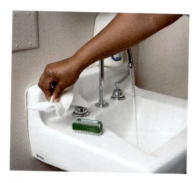

FIGURE 13-8A Use a dry towel to turn the faucet on.

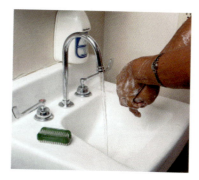

FIGURE 13-8B Point the fingertips downward and use the palm of one hand to clean the back of the other hand.

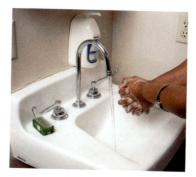

FIGURE 13-8C Interlace the fingers to clean between the fingers.

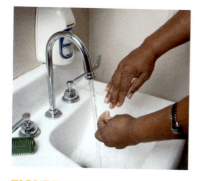

FIGURE 13-8D The blunt end of an orange stick can be used to clean the nails.

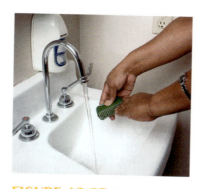

FIGURE 13-8E A hand brush can also be used to clean the nails.

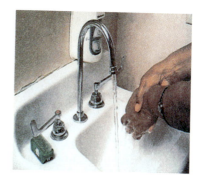

FIGURE 13-8F With the fingertips pointing downward, rinse the hands thoroughly.

your uniform or clothing. Avoid touching the inside of the sink with your hands since it is considered contaminated.

2. Turn the faucet on by holding a paper towel between your hand and the faucet (see figure 13-8A). Regulate the temperature of the water and let water flow over your hands. Discard the towel in the waste container.
   NOTE: Water should be warm.
   ⬡! **CAUTION:** Hot water will burn your hands.

3. With your fingertips pointing downward, wet your hands.
   NOTE: Washing in a downward direction prevents water from getting on the forearms and then running back down to contaminate hands.

4. Use soap to get a lather on your hands.

5. Put the palms of your hands together and rub them using friction and a circular motion for approximately 10 to 15 seconds.

6. Put the palm of one hand on the back of the other hand. Rub together several times.

Repeat this after reversing position of hands (see figure 13-8B).

7. Interlace the fingers on both hands and rub them back and forth (see figure 13-8C).

8. Clean the nails with an orange/cuticle stick and/or hand brush (see figures 13-8D and E).
   ⬡! **CAUTION:** Use the blunt end of orange/cuticle stick to avoid injury.
   NOTE: Steps 3 through 8 ensure that all parts of both hands are clean.

9. Rinse your hands, keeping fingertips pointed downward (see figure 13-8F).

10. Use a clean paper towel to dry hands thoroughly, from tips of fingers to wrist. Discard the towel in the waste container.

11. Use another dry paper towel to turn off the faucet.
    ⬡! **CAUTION:** Wet towels allow passage of pathogens.

12. Discard all used towels in the waste container. Leave the area neat and clean.

Practice *Go to the workbook and use the evaluation sheet for 13:2, Washing Hands, to practice this procedure. When you feel you have mastered this skill, sign the sheet and give it to your instructor for further action.*

 Final Checkpoint Using the criteria listed on the evaluation sheet, your instructor will grade your performance.

13:3 INFORMATION Observing Standard Precautions

OBRA In order to prevent the spread of pathogens and disease, the chain of infection must be broken. The standard precautions discussed in this unit are an important way health care workers can break this chain.

One of the main ways that pathogens are spread is by blood and body fluids. Three pathogens of major concern are the hepatitis B virus (HBV), the hepatitis C virus (HCV), and the human immunodeficiency virus (HIV), which causes AIDS. Consequently, extreme care must be taken at all times when an area, object, or person is contaminated with blood or body fluids. In 1991, the Occupational Safety and Health Administration (OSHA) established *Bloodborne Pathogen Standards* that must be followed by all health care facilities. The employer faces civil penalties if the regulations are not implemented by the employer and followed by the employees. These regulations require all health care facility employers to:

- Develop a written exposure control plan, and update it annually, to minimize or eliminate employee exposure to bloodborne pathogens.
- Identify all employees who have occupational exposure to blood or potentially infectious materials such as semen, vaginal secretions, and other body fluids.
- Provide hepatitis B vaccine free of charge to all employees who have occupational exposure, and obtain a written release form signed by any employee who does not want the vaccine.

- Provide **personal protective equipment (PPE)** such as gloves, gowns, lab coats, masks, and face shields in appropriate sizes and in accessible locations.
- Provide adequate handwashing facilities and supplies.
- Ensure that the worksite is maintained in a clean and sanitary condition, follow measures for immediate decontamination of any surface that comes in contact with blood or infectious materials, and dispose of infectious waste correctly.
- Enforce rules of no eating, drinking, smoking, applying cosmetics or lip balm, handling contact lenses, and mouth pipetting or suctioning in any area that can be potentially contaminated by blood or other body fluids.
- Provide appropriate containers that are color coded (fluorescent orange or orange-red) and labeled for contaminated sharps (needles, scalpels) and other infectious or biohazard wastes.
- Post signs at the entrance to work areas where there is occupational exposure to biohazardous materials.
- Provide a confidential medical evaluation and follow-up for any employee who has an exposure incident. Examples might include an accidental needle stick or the splashing of blood or body fluids on the skin, eyes, or mucous membranes.
- Provide training about the regulations and all potential biohazards to all employees at no cost during working hours, and provide additional education as needed when procedures or working conditions are changed or modified.

In 2001, OSHA revised its Bloodborne Pathogen Standards in response to Congress passing the *Needlestick Safety and Prevention*

Act in November, 2000. This act was passed after the Centers for Disease Control and Prevention (CDC) estimated that 600,000 to 800,000 needle sticks occur each year, exposing health care workers to bloodborne pathogens. Employers are required to:

♦ *Identify and use effective and safer medical devices:* OSHA defines safer devices as sharps with engineered injury protections and includes, but is not limited to, devices such as syringes with a sliding sheath that shields the needle after use, needles that retract into a syringe after use, shielded or retracting catheters that can be used to administer intravenous medications or fluids, and intravenous systems that administer medication or fluids through a catheter port or connector site using a needle housed in a protective covering (see figure 13-9). OSHA also encourages the use of needleless systems which include, but are not limited to, intravenous medication delivery systems that administer medication or fluids through a catheter port or connector site using a blunt cannula or other non-needle connection, and jet injection systems that deliver subcutaneous or intramuscular injections through the skin without using a needle.

♦ *Incorporate changes in annual update of Exposure Control Plan:* Employers must include changes in technology that eliminate or reduce exposure to bloodborne pathogens in the annual update and document the implementation of any safer medical devices.

♦ *Solicit input from nonmanagerial employees who are responsible for direct patient care:* Employees who provide patient care, and are exposed to injuries from contaminated sharps, must be included in a multidisciplinary team that identifies, evaluates, and selects safer medical devices, and determines safer work practice controls.

♦ *Maintain a sharps injury log:* Employers with more than 11 employees must maintain a sharps injury log to help identify high risk areas and evaluate ways of decreasing injuries. Each injury recorded must protect the confidentiality of the injured employee, but must state the type and brand of device involved in the incident, the work area or department where the exposure injury

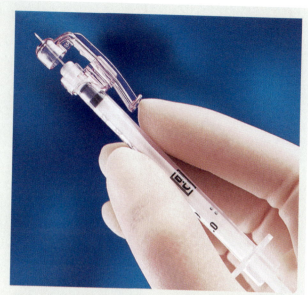

FIGURE 13-9 The Safety-Glide syringe is one example of a safer device to prevent needlesticks. *(Photo reprinted courtesy of BD [Becton Dickinson and Company])*

occurred, and a description of how the incident occurred.

Employers are also required to make sure that every employee uses standard precautions at all times to prevent contact with blood or other potentially infectious materials. **Standard precautions** (see figure 13-10) are rules developed by the Centers for Disease Control and Prevention (CDC). According to standard precautions, every body fluid must be considered a potentially infectious material, and all patients must be considered potential sources of infection, regardless of their disease or diagnosis. Standard precautions must be used in any situation where health care providers may contact:

♦ Blood or any fluid that may contain blood

♦ Body fluids, secretions, and excretions, such as mucus, sputum, saliva, cerebrospinal fluid, urine, feces, vomitus, amniotic fluid (surrounding a fetus), synovial (joint) fluid, pleural (lung) fluid, pericardial (heart) fluid, peritoneal (abdominal cavity) fluid, semen, and vaginal secretions

♦ Mucous membranes

♦ Nonintact skin

♦ Tissue or cell specimens

STANDARD PRECAUTIONS

FOR INFECTION CONTROL

Wash Hands (Plain soap)
Wash after touching **blood**, **body fluids**, **secretions**, **excretions**, and **contaminated items**.
Wash immediately **after gloves are removed** and **between patient contacts**.
Avoid transfer of microorganisms to other patients or environments.

Wear Gloves
Wear when touching **blood**, **body fluids**, **secretions**, **excretions**, and **contaminated items**.
Put on **clean** gloves just **before touching mucous membranes** and **nonintact skin**.
Change gloves between tasks and procedures on the same patient after contact with material that may contain high concentrations of microorganisms. Remove gloves promptly after use, before touching noncontaminated items and environmental surfaces, and before going to another patient, and wash hands immediately to avoid transfer of microorganisms to other patients or environments.

Wear Mask and Eye Protection or Face Shield
Protect mucous membranes of the eyes, nose and mouth during procedures and patient–care activities that are likely to generate **splashes** or **sprays** of **blood**, **body fluids**, **secretions**, or **excretions**.

Wear Gown
Protect skin and prevent soiling of clothing during procedures that are likely to generate **splashes** or **sprays** of **blood**, **body fluids**, **secretions**, or **excretions**. Remove a soiled gown as promptly as possible and wash hands to avoid transfer of microorganisms to other patients or environments.

Patient-Care Equipment
Handle used patient–care equipment soiled with **blood**, **body fluids**, **secretions**, or **excretions** in a manner that prevents skin and mucous membrane exposures, contamination of clothing, and transfer of microorganisms to other patients and environments. Ensure that reusable equipment is not used for the care of another patient until it has been appropriately cleaned and reprocessed and single use items are properly discarded.

Environmental Control
Follow hospital procedures for routine care, cleaning, and disinfection of environmental surfaces, beds, bedrails, bedside equipment and other frequently touched surfaces.

Linen
Handle, transport, and process used linen soiled with **blood**, **body fluids**, **secretions**, or **excretions** in a manner that prevents exposures and contamination of clothing, and avoids transfer of microorganisms to other patients and environments.

Occupational Health and Bloodborne Pathogens
Prevent injuries when using needles, scalpels, and other sharp instruments or devices; when handling sharp instruments after procedures; when cleaning used instruments; and when disposing of used needles.

Never recap used needles using both hands or any other technique that involves directing the point of a needle toward any part of the body; rather, use either a one-handed "scoop" technique or a mechanical device designed for holding the needle sheath.

Do not remove used needles from disposable syringes by hand, and do not bend, break, or otherwise manipulate used needles by hand. Place used disposable syringes and needles, scalpel blades, and other sharp items in puncture–resistant sharps containers located as close as practical to the area in which the items were used, and place reusable syringes and needles in a puncture–resistant container for transport to the reprocessing area.

Use **resuscitation devices** as an alternative to mouth–to–mouth resuscitation.

Patient Placement
Use a **private room** for a patient who contaminates the environment or who does not (or cannot be expected to) assist in maintaining appropriate hygiene or environmental control. Consult Infection Control if a private room is not available.

The information on this sign is abbreviated from the HICPAC Recommendations for Isolation Precautions in Hospitals.

Form No. **SPR**   BREVIS CORP., 3310 S 2700 E, SLC, UT 84109   © 1996 Brevis Corp.

FIGURE 13-10 Standard precautions must be observed while working with all patients. *(Courtesy of Brevis Corporation)*

A major precaution is to wash your hands before and after contact with any patient. If your hands or other skin surfaces are contaminated with blood, body fluids, secretions, or excretions, they must be washed immediately and thoroughly with soap and water. Hands must always be washed immediately after removal of gloves.

Gloves (see figure 13-11) must be worn whenever contact with blood, body fluids, secretions, excretions, mucous membranes, tissue specimens, or nonintact skin is possible; when handling or cleaning any contaminated items or surfaces; when performing any invasive (entering the body) procedure; and when performing venipuncture or blood tests. Rings must be removed before putting on gloves to avoid puncturing the gloves. Gloves must be changed after contact with each patient, and hands must be washed immediately after removal of gloves. Care must be taken while removing gloves to avoid contamination of the skin. Gloves must *not* be washed or disinfected for reuse because washing may allow penetration of liquids through undetected holes, and disinfecting agents may cause deterioration of gloves.

Gowns must be worn during any procedure that is likely to cause splashing or spraying of blood, body fluids, secretions, or excretions. This helps prevent contamination of clothing or uniforms. Contaminated gowns must be handled according to agency policy and local and state laws. Wash hands immediately after removing a gown.

Masks and protective eyewear or face shields (see figure 13-12) must be worn during procedures that may produce splashes or sprays of blood, body fluids, secretions, or excretions. Examples include irrigation of wounds, suctioning, dental procedures, delivery of a baby, and surgical procedures. This prevents exposure of the mucous membranes of the mouth, nose,

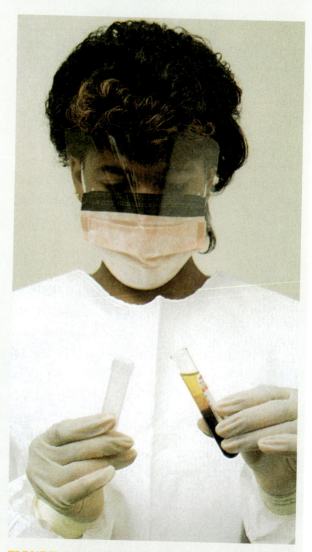

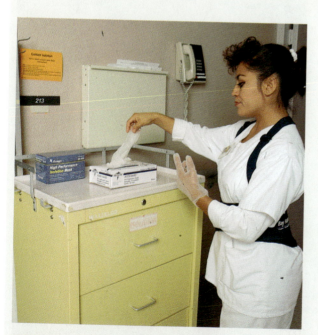

FIGURE 13-11 Gloves must be worn whenever contact with blood, body fluids, secretions, excretions, mucous membranes, or nonintact skin is possible.

FIGURE 13-12 Gloves, a gown, a mask, and protective eyewear must be worn during any procedure that may produce droplets or cause splashing of blood, body fluids, secretions, or excretions.

and eyes to any pathogens. Masks must be used once and then discarded. In addition, masks should be changed every 30 minutes or anytime they become moist or wet. They should be removed by grasping the ties or elastic strap. Hands must be washed immediately after the mask is removed. Protective eyewear or face shields should provide protection for the front, top, bottom, and sides of the eyes. If eyewear is not disposable, it must be cleaned and disinfected before it is reused.

To avoid accidental cuts or punctures, extreme care must be taken while handling sharp objects. Whenever possible, safe needles or needleless devices must be used. Disposable needles must never be bent or broken after use. They must be left uncapped and attached to the syringe and placed in a leakproof puncture-resistant sharps container (see figure 13-13). The sharps container must be labeled with a red biohazard symbol (see figure 13-14). Surgical blades, razors, and other sharp objects must also be discarded in the sharps container. The containers must *not* be emptied or reused. Federal, state, and local laws establish regulations for the disposal of sharps containers. In some areas, the filled container is placed in a special oven and melted. The material remaining is packaged as biohazard or infectious waste

and disposed of according to legal requirements for infectious waste.

Spills or splashes of blood, body fluids, secretions, or excretions must be wiped up immediately (see figure 13-15). Gloves must be worn while wiping up the area with disposable cleaning cloths. The area must then be cleaned with a disinfectant solution such as a 10-percent bleach solution. Furniture or equipment contaminated by the spill or splash must be cleaned and disinfected immediately. For large spills, an

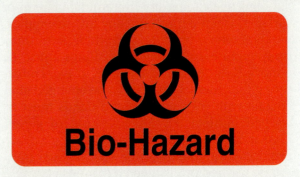

FIGURE 13-14 The universal biohazard symbol indicates a potential source of infection.

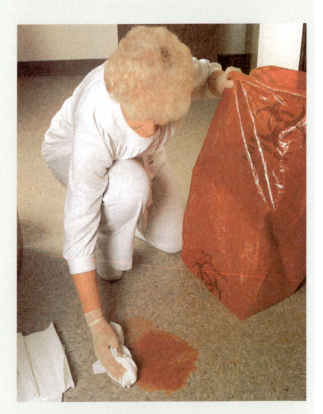

FIGURE 13-15 Gloves must be worn while wiping up any spills of blood, body fluids, secretions, or excretions.

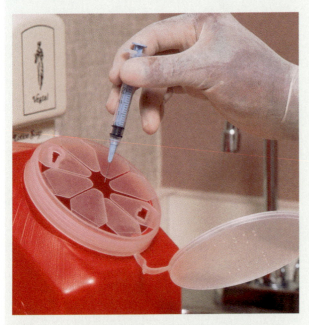

FIGURE 13-13 All needles and sharp objects must be discarded immediately in a leakproof puncture-resistant sharps container.

absorbent powder may be used to soak up the fluid. After the fluid is absorbed, it is swept up and placed in an infectious waste container.

Whenever possible, mouthpieces or resuscitation devices should be used to avoid the need for mouth-to-mouth resuscitation. These devices should be placed in convenient locations and be readily accessible for use.

To dispose of waste and soiled linen, wear gloves and follow the agency policy developed according to law. Infectious wastes such as contaminated dressings; gloves; urinary drainage bags; incontinent pads; vaginal pads; disposable emesis basins, bedpans, and/or urinals; and body tissues must be placed in special infectious waste or biohazardous material bags (see figure 13-16) according to law. Other trash is frequently placed in plastic bags and incinerated. The health care worker must dispose of waste in the proper container (see figure 13-17) and know the requirements for disposal. Soiled linen should be placed in laundry bags to prevent any contamination. Linen soiled with blood, body fluids, or excretions is placed in a special bag for contaminated linen and is usually soaked in a disinfectant prior to being laundered. Gloves must be worn while handling any contaminated linen, and any bag containing contaminated linen must be clearly labeled and color coded.

Any cut, injury, needle stick, or splashing of blood or body fluids must be reported immediately. Agency policy must be followed to deal with the injury or contamination. Every health care facility must have a policy for documenting any exposure incident, recording the care given, noting follow-up to the exposure incident, and identifying ways to prevent a similar incident.

Standard precautions must be followed at all times by all health care workers. By observing these precautions, health care workers can help break the chain of infection and protect themselves, their patients, and all other individuals.

STUDENT: *Go to the workbook and complete the assignment sheet for 13:3, Observing Standard Precautions. Then return and continue with the procedure.*

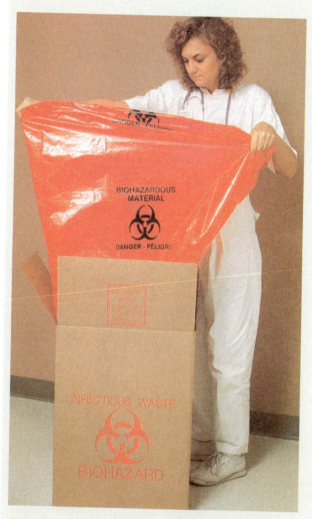

FIGURE 13-16 All infectious wastes must be placed in special infectious waste or biohazardous material bags.

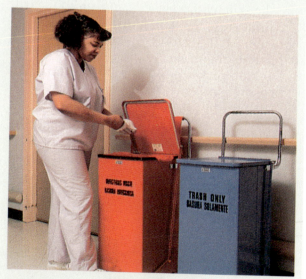

FIGURE 13-17 The health care worker must know the requirements for disposal of waste materials and dispose of wastes in the proper containers.

PROCEDURE 13:3
Observing Standard Precautions

Equipment and Supplies

Disposable gloves, infectious waste bags, needle and syringe, sharps container, gown, masks, protective eyewear, resuscitation devices

NOTE: This procedure will help you learn standard precautions. It is important for you to observe these precautions at all times while working in the laboratory or clinical area.

Procedure

1. Assemble equipment.
2. Review the precautions in the information section for Observing Standard Precautions. Note points that are not clear, and ask your instructor for an explanation.
3. Practice handwashing according to Procedure 13:2. Identify at least six times that hands must be washed according to standard precautions.
4. Name four instances when gloves must be worn to observe standard precautions. Put on a pair of disposable gloves. Practice removing the gloves without contaminating the skin. With a gloved hand, grasp the cuff of the glove on the opposite hand, handling only the outside of the glove (see figure 13-18A). Pull the glove down and turn it inside out while removing it. Take care not to touch the skin with the gloved hand. Using the ungloved hand, slip the fingers under the cuff of the glove on the opposite hand (see figure 13-18B). Touching only the inside of the glove and taking care not to touch the skin, pull the glove down and turn it inside out while removing it. Place the gloves in an infectious waste container. Wash your hands immediately.
5. Practice putting on a gown. State when a gown is to be worn. To remove the gown, touch only the inside. Fold the contaminated gown so the outside is folded inward. Roll it into a bundle and place it in an infectious waste container if it is disposable, or in a bag for contaminated linen if it is not disposable.

   CAUTION: If a gown is contaminated, gloves should be worn while removing the gown.

   NOTE: Folding the gown and rolling it prevents transmission of pathogens.
6. Practice putting on a mask and protective eyewear. To remove the mask, handle it by

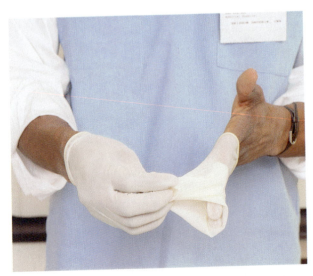

FIGURE 13-18A To remove the first glove, use a gloved hand to grasp the outside of the glove on the opposite hand. Pull the glove down and turn it inside out while removing it.

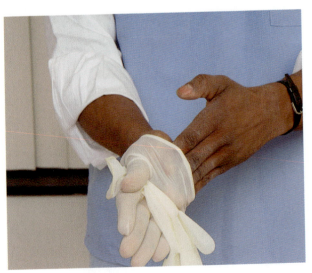

FIGURE 13-18B To remove the second glove, slip the fingers of the ungloved hand inside the cuff of the glove. Touch only the inside of the glove while pulling it down and turning it inside out.

the ties only. Clean and disinfect protective eyewear after use.

7. Practice proper disposal of sharps. Uncap a needle attached to a syringe, taking care not to stick yourself with the needle. Place the entire needle and syringe in a sharps container. State the rules regarding disposal of the sharps container.

8. Spill a small amount of water on a counter. Pretend that it is blood. Put on gloves and use disposable cloths or gauze to wipe up the spill. Put the contaminated cloths or gauze in an infectious waste bag. Use clean disposable cloths or gauze to wipe the area thoroughly with a disinfectant agent. Put the cloths or gauze in the infectious waste bag, remove your gloves, and wash your hands.

9. Practice handling an infectious waste bag. Fold down the top edge of the bag to form a cuff at the top of the bag. Wear gloves to close the bag after contaminated wastes have been placed in it. Put your hands under the folded cuff (see figure 13-19A) and gently expel excess air from the bag. Twist the top of the bag shut and fold down the top edges to seal the bag. Secure the fold with tape or a tie according to agency policy (see figure 13-19B).

10. Examine mouthpieces and resuscitation devices that can be used in place of mouth-to-mouth resuscitation. You will be taught to use these devices when you learn cardiopulmonary resuscitation (CPR).

11. Discuss the following situations with another student and determine which standard precautions should be observed:

    ◆ A patient has an open sore on the skin and pus is seeping from the area. You are going to bathe the patient.

    ◆ You are cleaning a tray of instruments that contains a disposable surgical blade and needle with syringe.

    ◆ A tube of blood drops to the floor and breaks, spilling the blood on the floor.

    ◆ Drainage from dressings on an infected wound has soiled the linen on the bed you are changing.

    ◆ You work in a dental office and are assisting a dentist while a tooth is being extracted (removed).

12. Replace all equipment used.

Practice *Go to the workbook and use the evaluation sheet for 13:3, Observing Standard Precautions. When you feel you have mastered this skill, sign the sheet and give it to your instructor for further action.*

 Final Checkpoint Using the criteria listed on the evaluation sheet, your instructor will grade your performance.

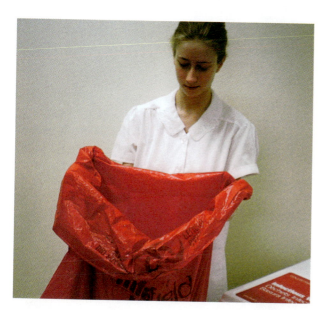

FIGURE 13-19A To close an infectious waste bag, wear gloves and place your hands under the cuff to gently expel excess air.

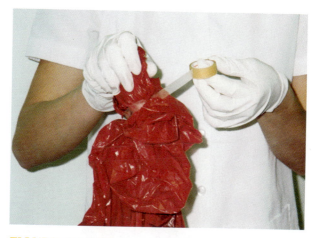

FIGURE 13-19B After folding down the top edge of the infectious waste bag, tie or tape it securely.

13:4 INFORMATION
Sterilizing with an Autoclave

Sterilization of instruments and equipment is essential in preventing the spread of infection. In any of the health fields, you may be responsible for proper sterilization. The following basic principles relate to sterilization methods. The autoclave is the safest, most efficient sterilization method.

An **autoclave** is a piece of equipment that uses steam under pressure or gas to sterilize equipment and supplies (see figure 13-20). It is the most efficient method of sterilizing most articles, and it will destroy all microorganisms, both pathogenic and nonpathogenic, including spores and viruses.

Autoclaves are available in various sizes and types. Offices and health clinics usually have smaller units, and hospitals or surgical areas have large floor model units. A pressure cooker can be used in home situations.

Before any equipment or supplies are sterilized in an autoclave, they must be prepared properly. All items must be washed thoroughly and then rinsed. Oily substances can often be removed with alcohol or ether. Any residue left on articles will tend to bake and stick to the article during the autoclaving process.

Items that are to remain sterile must be wrapped before they are autoclaved. A wide variety of wraps are available. The wrap must be a material that will allow for the penetration of steam during the autoclaving process. Samples of wraps include muslin, autoclave paper, special plastic or paper bags, and autoclave containers (see figure 13-21).

Autoclave indicators are used to ensure that articles have been sterilized (see figure 13-22). Examples of indicators include autoclave tape, sensitivity marks on bags or wraps, and indicator capsules. The indicator is usually placed on or near the article when the article is put into the autoclave. Indicators can also be placed in the center of a package, such as a tray of instruments, to show that sterilization of the entire package has occurred. The indicator will change appearance during the autoclaving process because of time and temperature, which leads to sterilization. Learn how to recognize that an article is sterile by reading the directions provided with indicators.

The autoclave must be loaded correctly in order for all parts of an article to be sterilized. Steam builds at the top of the chamber and moves downward. As it moves down, it pushes cool, dry air out of the bottom of the chamber. Therefore, materials must be placed so the

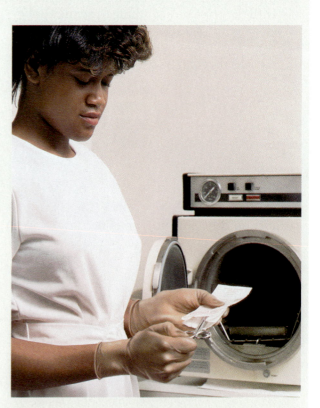

FIGURE 13-21 Special plastic or paper autoclave bags can be used to sterilize instruments.

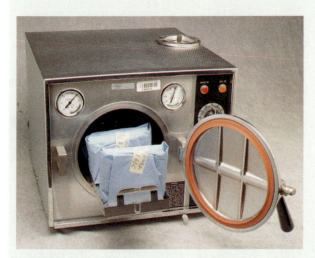

FIGURE 13-20 An autoclave uses steam under pressure to sterilize items.

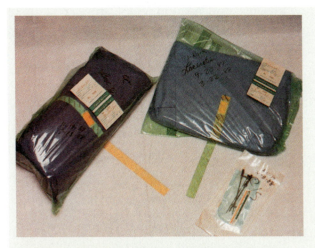

FIGURE 13-22 Autoclave indicators change color to show that sterilization has occurred. The strips below each package show how the indicators looked before sterilization.

steam can penetrate along the natural planes between the packages of articles in the autoclave. Place the articles in such a way that there is space between all pieces. Packages should be placed on the sides, not flat. Jars, basins, and cans should be placed on their sides, not flat, so that steam can enter and air can flow out. No articles should come in contact with the sides, top, or door of the autoclave.

The length of time and amount of pressure required to sterilize different items varies (see figure 13-23). *It is important to check the directions that come with the autoclave.* Because different types of articles require different times and pressures, it is important to separate loads so that all articles sterilized at one time require the same time and pressure. For example, rubber tubings usually require a relatively short period of time and can be damaged by long exposure. Certain instruments and needles require a longer period of time to ensure sterilization; so, items of this type should not be sterilized in the same load as are rubber tubings.

Wet surfaces permit rapid infiltration of organisms, so it is important that all items are thoroughly dry before being removed from the autoclave. The length of time for drying varies. Follow the manufacturer's instructions.

Sterilized items must be stored in clean, dustproof areas. Items usually remain sterile for 30 days after autoclaving. However, if the wraps loosen or tear, if they become wet, or if any chance of contamination occurs, the items should be rewrapped and autoclaved again.

ARTICLES	TIME AT 250° TO 254°F (121° TO 123°C)
Glassware: empty, inverted	15 minutes
Instruments: metal in covered or open, padded or unpadded tray	
Needles, unwrapped	
Syringes: unassembled, unwrapped	
Instruments, metal combined with other materials in covered and/or padded tray	
Instruments wrapped in double-thickness muslin	20 minutes
Flasked solutions, 75–250 mL	
Needles, individually packaged in glass tubes or paper	
Syringes: unassembled, individually packed in muslin or paper	30 minutes
Dressings wrapped in paper or muslin (small packs only)	
Flasked solutions, 500–1,000 mL	
Sutures: silk, cotton, or nylon; wrapped in paper or muslin	
Treatment trays wrapped in muslin or paper	

FIGURE 13-23 The length of time required to sterilize different items varies.

NOTE: At the end of the 30-day sterile period—providing that the wrap has not loosened, been torn, or gotten wet—remove the old autoclave tape from the package, replace with a new, dated tape, and resterilize according to correct procedure.

Some autoclaves are equipped with a special door that allows the autoclave to be used as a dry-heat sterilizer. Dry heat involves the use of a high temperature for a long period of time. The temperature is usually a minimum of 320°F to 350°F (160°C to 177°C). The minimum time is usually 60 minutes. Dry-heat sterilization is a good method for sterilizing instruments that may corrode, such as knife blades, or items that would be destroyed by the moisture in steam sterilization, such as powders. Dry heat should never be used on soft rubber goods because the heat will destroy the rubber. Some types of plastic will also melt in dry heat. An oven can be used for dry-heat sterilization in home situations.

Procedures 13:4A and 13:4B, following, describe wrapping articles for autoclaving and autoclaving techniques. These procedures vary in different agencies and areas, but the same principles apply. In some facilities, many supplies are purchased as sterile, disposable items; needles and syringes are purchased in sterilized wraps, used once, and then destroyed. In other facilities, however, special treatment trays are sterilized and used more than one time.

It is important that you follow the directions specific to the autoclave with which you are working, and the agency policy for sterile supplies. Careless autoclaving permits the transmission of disease-producing organisms. Infection control is everyone's responsibility.

STUDENT: *Go to the workbook and complete the assignment sheet for 13:4, Sterilizing with an Autoclave. Then return and continue with the procedures.*

PROCEDURE 13:4A
Wrapping Items for Autoclaving

Equipment and Supplies

Items to wrap: instrument, towel, bowl; autoclave wrap: paper, muslin, plastic or paper bag; autoclave tape or indicator; disposable or utility gloves; pen or autoclave marker; masking tape (if autoclave tape is not used)

Procedure

1. Assemble equipment.
2. Wash hands. Put on gloves.

   ⚠️ ❗ **CAUTION:** If the items to be autoclaved are contaminated with blood, body fluids, or tissues, gloves must be worn while cleaning the items.

3. Sanitize the items to be sterilized. Instruments, bowls, and similar items should be cleaned thoroughly in soapy water (see figure 13-24). Rinse the items well in cool water to remove any soapy residue. Then rinse well with hot water. Dry the items with a towel. After the items are sanitized and dry, remove the gloves and wash hands.

   NOTE: If stubborn stains are present, it may be necessary to soak the items.

   NOTE: Check the teeth on serrated (notched like a saw) instruments. Scrub with a brush as necessary.

4. To prepare linen for wrapping, check first to make sure it is clean and dry. Fold the linen in half lengthwise. If it is very wide, fold lengthwise again. Fanfold or accordion pleat the linen from end to end until a compact package is formed (see figure 13-25A). All folds should be the same size. Fold back

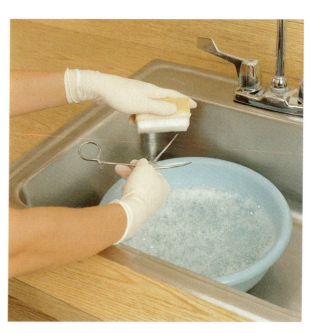

FIGURE 13-24 Wear gloves to scrub instruments thoroughly with soapy water.

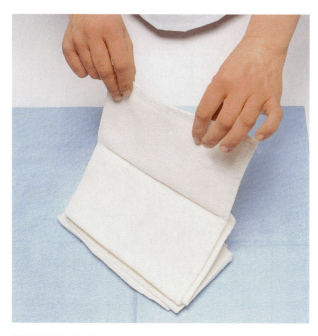

FIGURE 13-25A Fanfold clean, dry linen so all the folds are the same size.

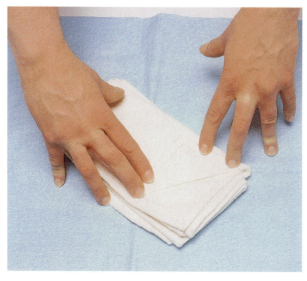

FIGURE 13-25B Fold back one corner on the top fold of the linen.

one corner on the top fold (see figure 13-25B). This provides a piece to grab when opening the linen.

NOTE: Fanfolding linens allows for easy handling after sterilization.

5. Select the correct wrap for the item. Make sure the wrap is large enough to enclose the item to be wrapped.

NOTE: Double-thickness muslin, disposable paper wraps, and plastic or paper bags are the most common wraps.

6. With the wrap positioned at a diagonal angle and one corner pointing toward you, place the item to be sterilized in the center of the wrap.

NOTE: Make sure that hinged instruments are open so the steam can sterilize all edges.

7. Fold up the bottom corner to the center (see figure 13-26A). Double back a small corner (see figure 13-26B).

8. Fold a side corner over to the center. Make sure the edges are sealed and that there are no air pockets. Bring back a small corner (see figure 13-26C).

⚠ **CAUTION:** Any open areas at corners will allow pathogens to enter.

9. Fold in the other side corner. Again, watch for and avoid open edges. Bring back a small corner (see figure 13-26D).

10. Bring the final corner up and over the top of the package. Check the two edges to be sure they are sealed and tight. Tuck this under the pocket created by the previous folds. Leave a small corner exposed so it can be used when unwrapping the package (see figure 13-26E).

NOTE: This is frequently called an "envelope" wrap, because the final corner is tucked into the wrap similar to the way the flap is tucked into an envelope.

11. Secure with autoclave or pressure-sensitive indicator tape.

NOTE: If regular masking tape is used, attach an autoclave indicator to reflect when contents are sterilized.

12. Label the package by marking the tape with the date and contents (see figure 13-26F). Some health care agencies may require you to initial the label.

NOTE: For certain items, the type or size of item should be noted, for example, curved hemostat or mosquito hemostat, hand towel or bath towel, small bowl or large bowl.

NOTE: Contents will not be sterile after 30 days, so the date of sterilization must be noted on the package.

13. Check the package. It should be firm enough for handling but loose enough for proper circulation of steam.

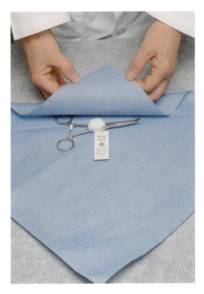

FIGURE 13-26A Place the instrument in the center of the wrap. Fold the bottom corner in to the center.

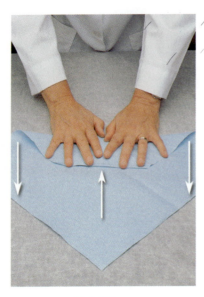

FIGURE 13-26B Turn a small corner back to form a tab.

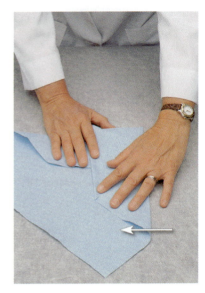

FIGURE 13-26C Fold in one side and fold back a tab.

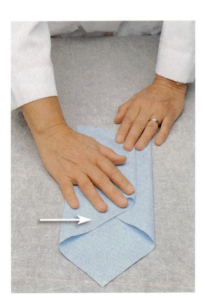

FIGURE 13-26D Fold in the opposite side and fold back a tab.

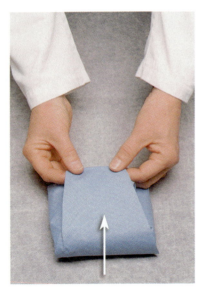

FIGURE 13-26E Bring the final corner up and over the top of the pack and tuck it in, leaving a small corner exposed.

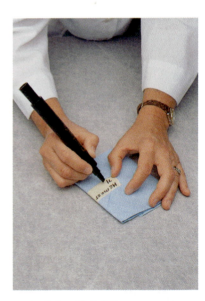

FIGURE 13-26F Secure the package with autoclave tape. Label it with the date, contents, and your initials.

14. To use a plastic or paper autoclave bag (refer to figure 13-21), select or cut the correct size for the item to be sterilized. Place the clean item inside the bag. Double fold the open end(s) and tape or secure with autoclave tape. Check the package to make sure it is secure.

NOTE: In some agencies, the ends are sealed with heat prior to autoclaving.

NOTE: If the bag has an autoclave indicator, regular masking tape can be used to seal the ends.

15. Replace all equipment used.
16. Wash hands.

PROCEDURE 13:4B

Loading and Operating an Autoclave

NOTE: Follow the operating instructions for your autoclave. The basic principles of loading apply to all autoclaves. Basic controls for one autoclave are shown in figure 13-27.

Equipment and Supplies

Autoclave, distilled water, small pitcher or measuring cup, items wrapped or prepared for autoclaving, time chart for autoclave, 13:4 Information section

Procedure

Review the Information section for 13:4, Sterilizing with an Autoclave. Then proceed with the following activities. You should read through the

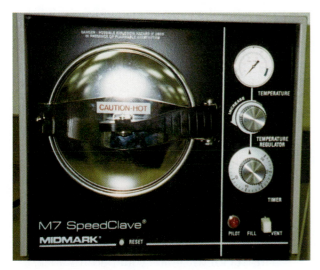

FIGURE 13-27 Autoclave control valves vary, but most contain the same basic controls.

procedure first, checking against the diagram. Then practice with an autoclave.

1. Assemble equipment.
2. Wash and dry hands thoroughly.
3. Check the three-prong plug and the electrical cord. If either is damaged or prongs are missing, do not use the autoclave. If no problems are present, plug the cord into a wall outlet.
4. Use distilled water to fill the reservoir to within 2 1/2 inches below the opening or to the level indicated on the autoclave.
   NOTE: Distilled water prevents the collection of mineral deposits and prolongs the life and effectiveness of the autoclave.
5. Check the pressure gauge to make sure it is at zero.
   CAUTION: Never open the door unless the pressure is zero.
6. Open the safety door by following the manufacturer's instructions. Some door handles require an upward and inward pressure; others require a side-pressure technique.
7. Load the autoclave. Make sure all articles have been prepared correctly. Check for autoclave indicators, secure wraps, and correct labels. Separate loads so all items require the same time, temperature, and pressure. Place packages on their sides. Place bowls or basins on their sides so air and steam can flow in and out of the container (see figure 13-28). Make sure there is space between the packages so the steam can circulate.
   NOTE: Check to make sure no large packages block the steam flow to smaller packages. Place large packages on the bottom.

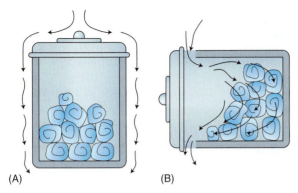

(A)   (B)

FIGURE 13-28 Bowls or basins should be placed on their sides in the autoclave so air and steam can flow in and out of the container: **(A)** shows incorrect placement, while **(B)** shows correct placement.

> ⚠ **CAUTION:** Make sure no item comes in contact with the sides, top, or door of the autoclave chamber.

8. Follow the instructions for filling the chamber with the correct amount of water. Most autoclaves have a "Fill" setting on the control. Allow water to enter the chamber until the water covers the fill plate inside the chamber.

9. When the correct amount of water is in the chamber, follow the instructions for stopping the flow of water. In many autoclaves, turning the control valve to "Sterilize" stops the flow of water from the reservoir.

10. Check the load in the chamber to be sure it is properly spaced. The chamber can also be loaded at this point, if this has not been done previously.

11. Close and lock the door.

> ⚠ **CAUTION:** Be sure the door is securely locked; check by pulling slightly.

12. Read the time chart for the specific time and temperature required for sterilization of items that were placed in the autoclave.

13. After referring to the chart provided with the autoclave or reviewing figure 13-23, set the control valves to allow the temperature and pressure to increase in the autoclave.

14. When the desired temperature (usually 250° to 255°F or 121° to 123°C) and pressure (usually 15 pounds) have been reached, set the controls to maintain the desired temperature during the sterilization process. Follow the manufacturer's instructions.

15. Based on the information in the time chart, set the timer to the correct time.

NOTE: Many autoclaves require you to rotate the timer past 10 (minutes) before setting the time.

16. Check the pressure and temperature gauges at intervals to make sure they remain as originally set.

NOTE: Most autoclaves automatically shut off when pressure reaches 35 pounds.

17. When the required time has passed, set the controls so the autoclave will vent the steam from the chamber.

18. Put on safety glasses.

> ⚠ **CAUTION:** *Never* open the door without glasses. The escaping steam can burn the eyes.

19. Check the pressure and temperature gauges. When the pressure gauge is at zero, and the temperature gauge is at or below 212°F, open the door about 1/2 to 1 inch to permit thorough drying of contents.

> ⚠ **CAUTION:** Do not open the door until pressure is zero.

20. After the autoclaved items are dry, remove and store them in a dry, dust-free area.

> ⚠ **CAUTION:** Handle supplies and equipment carefully. They may be hot.

21. If there are additional loads to run, leave the main valve in the vent position. This will keep the autoclave ready for immediate use.

22. If this is the final load, turn the autoclave off. Unplug the cord from the wall outlet; do not pull on the cord.

NOTE: The autoclave must be cleaned on a regular basis. Follow manufacturer's instructions.

23. Replace all equipment used.

24. Wash hands.

Practice *Go to the workbook and use the evaluation sheet for 13:4B, Loading and Operating an Autoclave, to practice this procedure. When you feel you have mastered this skill, sign the sheet and give it to your instructor for further action.*

 Final Checkpoint Using the criteria listed on the evaluation sheet, your instructor will grade your performance.

13:5 INFORMATION Using Chemicals for Disinfection

Many health fields require the use of chemicals for aseptic control. Certain points that must be observed while using the chemicals are discussed in the following information.

Chemicals are frequently used for aseptic control. Many chemicals do not kill spores and viruses; therefore, chemicals are not a method of sterilization. Because sterilization does not occur, **chemical disinfection** is the appropriate term (rather than cold sterilization, a term sometimes used). A few chemicals will kill spores and viruses, but these chemicals frequently require that instruments be submerged in the chemical for ten or more hours. It is essential to read an entire label to determine the effectiveness of the product before using any chemical.

Chemicals are used to disinfect instruments that do not penetrate body tissue. Many dental instruments, percussion hammers, scissors, and similar items are examples. In addition, chemicals are used to disinfect thermometers and other items that would be destroyed by the high heat used in the autoclave.

Proper cleaning of all instruments or articles is essential. Particles or debris on items may contaminate the chemicals and reduce their effectiveness. In addition, all items must be rinsed thoroughly because the presence of soap can also reduce the effectiveness of chemicals. The articles must be dry before being placed in the disinfectant in order to keep the chemical at its most effective strength.

Some chemical solutions used as disinfectants are 90-percent isopropyl alcohol, formaldehyde–alcohol, 2-percent phenolic germicide, 10-percent bleach (sodium hypochlorite) solution, glutaraldehyde, iodophor, Lysol, Cidex, and benzalkonium (zephiran). The manufacturer's directions should be read completely before using any solution. Some solutions must be diluted or mixed before use. The directions will also specify the recommended time for the most thorough disinfection.

Chemical solutions can cause rust to form on certain instruments, so antirust tablets or solutions are frequently added to the chemicals. Again, it is important to read the directions provided with the tablets or solution. If improperly used, antirust substances may cause a chemical reaction with a solution and reduce the effectiveness of the chemical disinfectant.

The container used for chemical disinfection must be large enough to accommodate the items. In addition, the items should be separate so each one will come in contact with the chemical. A tight-fitting lid must be placed on the container while the articles are in the solution.

The chemical disinfectant must completely cover the article. This is the only way to be sure that all parts of the article will be disinfected.

Before removing items from solutions, health workers must wash their hands. Sterile pick-ups or transfer forceps may be used to remove the instruments from the solution. The instruments are placed on a sterile or clean towel to dry, and then stored in a drawer or dust-free closet.

Solutions must be changed frequently. Some solutions can be used over a period of time, but others must be discarded after one use. Follow the manufacturer's instructions. However, any time contamination occurs or dirt is present in the solution, discard it. A fresh solution must be used.

STUDENT: *Go to the Workbook and complete the assignment sheet for 13:5, Using Chemicals for disinfection. Then return and continue with the procedure.*

PROCEDURE 13:5

Using Chemicals for Disinfection

Equipment and Supplies

Chemicals, container with tight-fitting lid, basin, soap, water, instruments, brush, sterile pick-ups or transfer forceps, sterile towel, disposable gloves

Procedure

1. Assemble equipment.
2. Wash hands. Put on gloves.
   NOTE: Wear gloves if any of the instruments or equipment are contaminated with blood or body fluids.
3. Wash all instruments or equipment thoroughly. Use warm soapy water. Use the brush on serrated edges of instruments.
4. Rinse in cool water to remove soapy residue. Then rinse well with hot water. Dry all instruments or equipment thoroughly.
   NOTE: Water on the instruments or equipment will dilute the chemical disinfectant.
5. Check container. Make sure lid fits securely.
   NOTE: A loose cover will permit entrance of pathogens.
6. Place instruments in the container. Make sure there is a space between instruments. Leave hinged edges open so the solution can flow between the surfaces.
7. Carefully read label instructions about the chemical solution. Some solutions must be diluted. Check the manufacturer's recommended soaking time.
   CAUTION: Reread instructions to be sure solution is safe to use on instruments.
   NOTE: An antirust substance must be added to some solutions.
8. Pour solution into the container slowly to avoid splashing. Make sure that all instruments are covered (see figure 13-29). Close the lid of the container.
   NOTE: Read label three times: before pouring, while pouring, and after pouring.
   CAUTION: Avoid splashing the chemical on your skin. Improper handling of chemicals may cause burns and/or injuries.

9. Remove gloves. Wash hands.
10. Leave the instruments in the solution for the length of time recommended by the manufacturer.
    NOTE: Twenty to thirty minutes is the usual soaking time.
11. When instruments have soaked the correct amount of time, use sterile pick-ups or transfer forceps to remove the instruments from the solution. Place them on a sterile towel to dry. A second sterile towel is sometimes used to cover the instruments while they are drying. Store the instruments in special drawers, containers, or dust-free closets.
    NOTE: Some contamination occurs when instruments are exposed to the air. In some cases, such as with external instruments, this minimal contamination will not affect usage.
12. Replace all equipment used.
    CAUTION: If the disinfectant solution can be used again, label the container with the name of the disinfectant, date, and number of days it can be used according to manufacturer's instructions. When solutions cannot be reused, dispose of the solution according to manufacturer's instructions.
13. Wash hands.

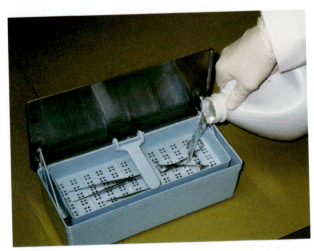

FIGURE 13-29 Pour the chemical disinfectant into the container until all instruments are covered with solution.

Practice *Go to the workbook and use the evaluation sheet for 13:5, Using Chemicals for Disinfection, to practice this procedure. When you feel you have mastered this skill, sign the sheet and give it to your instructor for further action.*

 Final Checkpoint Using the criteria listed on the evaluation sheet, your instructor will grade your performance.

13:6 INFORMATION
Cleaning with an Ultrasonic Unit

Ultrasonic units are used in many dental and medical offices and other health agencies to clean a large variety of instruments prior to sterilizing them. The following information explains operation of the unit.

Ultrasonic cleaning is used on a large variety of instruments and items in health care agencies. An ultrasonic unit uses sound waves to clean. When the unit is turned on, the sound waves produce millions of microscopic bubbles in a cleaning solution. When the bubbles strike the items being cleaned, they explode, a process known as **cavitation,** and drive the cleaning solution onto the article. Accumulated dirt and residue are easily and gently removed from the article.

Ultrasonic cleaning is not sterilization because spores and viruses remain on the articles. If sterilization is desired, other methods must be used after the ultrasonic cleaning.

Only ultrasonic solutions should be used in the unit. Different solutions are available for different materials. A general, all-purpose cleaning solution is usually used in the permanent tank and to clean many items. There are other specific solutions for alginate, plaster and stone removal, and tartar removal. The solution chart provided with the ultrasonic unit will state which solution should be used. It is important to read labels carefully before using any solutions. Some solutions must be diluted before use. Some can be used only on specific materials. All solutions are toxic. They can also cause skin irritation, so contact with the skin and eyes should be avoided. Solutions should be discarded when they become cloudy or contaminated, or if cleaning results are poor.

The permanent tank of the ultrasonic unit (figure 13-30) must contain a solution at all times. A general, all-purpose cleaning solution is used most of the time. Glass beakers or auxiliary pans or baskets can then be placed in the permanent tank. The items to be cleaned and the proper

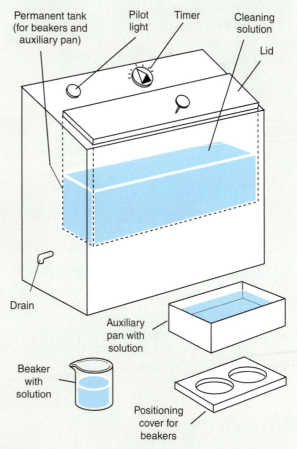

FIGURE 13-30 Parts of an ultrasonic cleaning unit.

cleaning solution are then put in the beakers or pans. The bottoms of the beakers or pans must always be positioned below the level of the solution present in the permanent tank. In this way, cavitation can be transmitted from the main tank and through the solution to the items being cleaned in the beakers or pans. Never run the ultrasonic unit unless solutions are in both containers. In addition, the items being cleaned must be submerged in the cleaning solution.

Many different items can be cleaned in an ultrasonic unit. Examples include instruments, impression trays, glass products, and most jewelry. Do not use the ultrasonic unit on jewelry with pearls or pasted stones. The sound waves can destroy the pearls or the paste holding the stones. Prior to cleaning, most of the dirt or particles should be brushed off the items being cleaned. It is better to clean a few articles at a time and avoid overloading the unit. If items are close together, the process of cavitation is poor because the bubbles cannot strike all parts of the items being cleaned.

The glass beakers used in the ultrasonic unit are made of a type of glass that allows the passage of sound waves. After continual use, the sound waves etch the bottom of the beakers. A white, opaque coating forms. The beakers must be discarded and replaced when this occurs.

After each use, the beakers should be washed with soap and water and rinsed thoroughly to remove any soapy residue. They must be dry before being filled with solution because water in the beaker can dilute the solution.

The permanent tank of the unit must be drained and cleaned at intervals based on tank use or appearance of the solution in the tank. A drain valve on the side of the tank is opened to allow the solution to drain. The tank is then wiped with a damp cloth or disinfectant. Another damp cloth or disinfectant is used to wipe off the outside of the unit. Never submerge the unit in water to clean it. After cleaning, a fresh solution should be placed in the permanent tank.

Read the manufacturer's instructions carefully before using any ultrasonic unit. Most manufacturers provide cleaning charts that state the type of solution and time required for a variety of cleaning problems. Each time an item is cleaned in an ultrasonic unit, the chart should be used to determine the correct cleaning solution and time required.

STUDENT: *Go to the workbook and complete the assignment sheet for 13:6, Cleaning with an Ultrasonic Unit. Then return and continue with the procedure.*

PROCEDURE 13:6

Cleaning with an Ultrasonic Unit

Equipment and Supplies

Ultrasonic unit, permanent tank with solution, beakers, auxiliary pan or basket with covers, beaker bands, cleaning solutions, transfer forceps or pick-ups, paper towels, brush, soap, water for rinsing, articles for cleaning, solution chart

Procedure

1. Assemble all equipment.
2. Wash hands. Put on gloves if any items are contaminated with blood, body fluids, secretions, or excretions.
3. Use a brush and soap and water to remove any large particles of dirt from articles to be cleaned. Rinse articles thoroughly. Dry items.

   NOTE: Rinsing is important because soap may interact with the cleaning solution.
4. Check the permanent tank to be sure it has enough cleaning solution. An all-purpose cleaning solution is usually used in this tank.

   CAUTION: Never run the unit without solution in the permanent tank.

   NOTE: Many solutions must be diluted before use; if new solution is needed, read the instructions on the bottle.

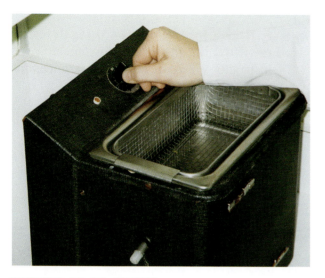

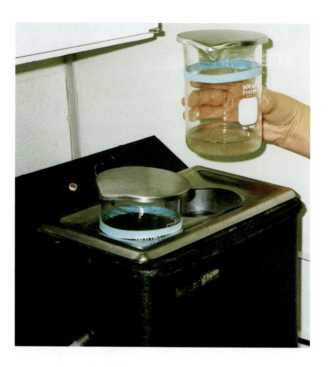

FIGURE 13-31 ABOVE The auxiliary basket can be used to clean larger items in an ultrasonic unit.
FIGURE 13-31 RIGHT Glass beakers can be used to clean smaller items in an ultrasonic unit.

5. Pour the proper cleaning solution into the auxiliary pan or beakers.
   NOTE: Use the cleaning chart to determine which solution to use.
   ⚠ **CAUTION:** Read label before using.

   ⚠ **CAUTION:** Handle solutions carefully. Avoid contact with skin and eyes.

6. Place the beakers, basket, or auxiliary pan into the permanent tank (see figure 13-31). Use beaker positioning covers and beaker bands. Beaker bands are large bands that circle the beakers to hold them in position and keep them from hitting the bottom of the permanent tank.

7. Check to be sure that the bottoms of the beakers, basket, or pan are below the level of solution in the permanent tank.
   NOTE: In order for sonic waves to flow through solutions in beakers, basket, or pan, the two solution levels must overlap.

8. Place articles to be cleaned in the beakers, basket, or pan. Be sure the solution completely covers the articles. Do not get solution on your hands.
   NOTE: Remember that pearls or pasted stones cannot be cleaned in an ultrasonic unit.

9. Turn the timer past 5 (minutes) and then set the proper cleaning time. Use the cleaning chart to determine the correct amount of time required for the items. Most articles are cleaned in 2 to 5 minutes.

10. Check that the unit is working. You should see a series of bubbles in both solutions. This is called cavitation.
    ⚠ **CAUTION:** Do not get too close. Solution can spray into your face and eyes. Use beaker lids to prevent spray.

11. When the timer stops, cleaning is complete. Use transfer forceps or pick-ups to lift articles from the basket, pan, or beakers. Place the articles on paper towels. Then rinse articles thoroughly under running water.
    ⚠ **CAUTION:** Avoid contact with skin. Solutions are toxic.

12. Allow articles to air dry or dry them with paper towels. Inspect the articles for cleanliness. If they are not clean, repeat the process.

13. Periodically change solutions in the permanent tank and auxiliary containers. Do this when solutions become cloudy or cleaning has not been effective. To clean the permanent tank, place a container under the side drain to collect the solution. Then open the valve and drain solution from the tank. Wash the inside with a damp cloth or disinfectant. To clean the auxiliary pans or beakers, discard the solution. (It can be poured down the sink, but allow water to run for a time after disposing of the solution.) Then wash the containers and rinse thoroughly.
    NOTE: If the bottoms of beakers are etched and white, the beakers must be discarded and replaced.

14. Clean and replace all equipment used. Make sure all beakers are covered with lids.
15. Wash hands.

Practice *Go to the workbook and use the evaluation sheet for 13:6, Cleaning with an Ultrasonic Unit, to practice this procedure. When you feel you have mastered this skill, sign the sheet and give it to your instructor for further action.*

 Final Checkpoint Using the criteria listed on the evaluation sheet, your instructor will grade your performance.

13:7 INFORMATION Using Sterile Techniques

Many procedures require the use of sterile techniques to protect the patient from further infection. *Surgical asepsis* refers to procedures that keep an object or area free from living organisms. The main facts are presented here.

Sterile means "free from all organisms," including spores and viruses. **Contaminated** means that organisms and pathogens are present. While working with sterile supplies, it is important that correct techniques be followed to maintain sterility and avoid contamination. It is also important that you are able to recognize sterile surfaces and contaminated surfaces.

A clean, uncluttered working area is required when working with sterile supplies. If other objects are in the way, it is easy to contaminate sterile articles. If sterile articles touch the skin or any part of your clothing, they are no longer sterile. Because any area below the waist is considered contaminated, sterile articles must be held away from and in front of the body and above the waist.

Once a **sterile field** has been set up (for example, a sterile towel has been placed on a tray), never reach across the top of the field. Microorganisms can drop from your arm or clothing and contaminate the field. Always reach in from either side to place additional articles on the field. Never turn your back to a sterile field.

The 2-inch border around the sterile field (towel-covered tray) is considered contaminated. Therefore, 2 inches around the outside of the field must not be used when sterile articles are placed on the sterile field.

Various techniques can be used to remove articles from sterile wraps, depending on the article being unwrapped. Some common techniques are the drop, mitten, and transfer-forceps techniques:

◆ *Drop technique:* for gauze pads, dressings, small items. The wrapper is partially opened and then held upside down over the sterile field. The item drops out of the wrapper and onto the sterile field (see figure 13-32A). It is important to keep fingers back so the article does not touch the skin as it falls out of the wrapper. It is also important to avoid touching the inside of the wrapper.

◆ *Mitten technique:* for bowls, drapes, linen, and other similar items. The wrapper is opened and its loose ends are grasped around the wrist with the opposite hand (see figure 13-32B). In this way, a mitten is formed around the hand that is still holding the item (for example, a bowl). With the mitten hand, the item can be placed on the sterile tray.

◆ *Transfer forceps:* for cotton balls, small items, or articles that cannot be removed by the drop or mitten techniques. Either sterile gloves or sterile transfer forceps (pick-ups) are used. Sterile transfer forceps or pick-ups are removed from their container of disinfectant solution and used to grasp the article from the opened package. Remove the item from the

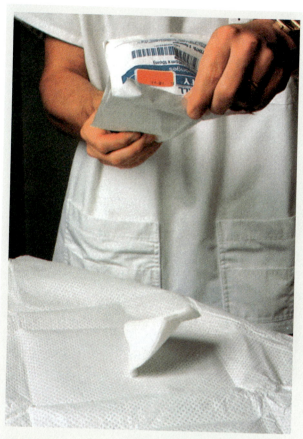

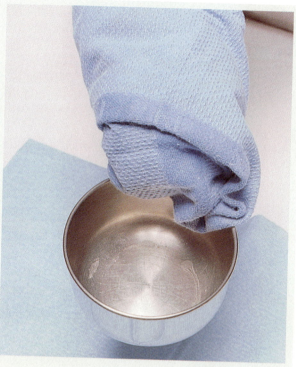

FIGURE 13-32B By using the wrap as a mitten, sterile supplies can be placed on a sterile field.

FIGURE 13-32A Sterile items can be dropped from the wrapper onto the sterile field.

opened, sterile wrap and place it on the sterile field (see figure 13-32C). It is important to keep the transfer forceps pointed in a downward direction. If they are pointed upward, the solution will flow back to the handle, become contaminated, and return to contaminate the sterile tips when they are being used to pick up items. In addition, care must be taken not to touch the sides or rim of the forceps container while removing or inserting the transfer forceps. Also, before using the transfer forceps, carefully shake them to get rid of excess disinfectant solution.

Organisms and pathogens travel quickly through a wet surface, so the sterile field must be kept dry. If a sterile towel or article gets wet, contamination has occurred. It is very important to use care when pouring solutions into sterile bowls or using solutions around a sterile field.

Make sure your sterile tray is open and you are ready to do the sterile procedure *before* putting the sterile gloves on your hands. Sterile

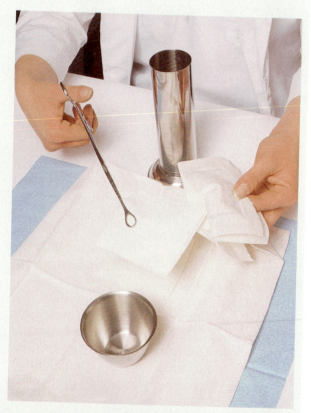

FIGURE 13-32C Sterile transfer forceps or pickups can be used to grasp sterile items and place them on a sterile field.

gloves are considered sterile on the outside and contaminated on the inside (side against the skin). Once they have been placed on the hands, it is important to hold the hands away from the body and above the waist to avoid contamination. You must handle only sterile objects while wearing sterile gloves.

If at any time during a procedure there is any suspicion that you have contaminated any article, start over. Never take a chance on using contaminated equipment or supplies.

A wide variety of commercially prepared sterile supplies is available. Packaged units are often set up for special procedures, such as changing dressings. Many agencies use these units instead of setting up special trays. Observe all sterile principles while using these units and read any directions provided with the units.

STUDENT: *Go to the workbook and complete the assignment sheet for 13:7, Using Sterile Techniques. Then return and continue with the procedures.*

PROCEDURE 13:7A

Opening Sterile Packages

Equipment and Supplies

Sterile package of equipment or supplies, a table or other flat surface, sterile field (tray with sterile towel)

Procedures

1. Assemble equipment.
2. Wash hands.
3. Take equipment to the area where it will be used. Check the autoclave indicator and date on the package.
   NOTE: Contents are not considered sterile if 30 days have elapsed since autoclaving.
4. Pick up the package with the tab or sealed edge pointing toward you. If the item is small, it can be held in the hand while being unwrapped. If it is large, place it on a table or other flat surface.
5. Loosen the wrapper fastener (usually tape).
6. Check to be sure the package is away from your body. If it is on a table, make sure it is not close to other objects.
   NOTE: Avoid possible contamination by keeping sterile supplies away from other objects.
7. Open the distal (furthest) flap of the wrapper by grasping the outside of the wrapper and pulling it away from you (see figure 13-33A).

   ⊘ **CAUTION:** Do not reach across the top of the package. Reach around the package to open it.

8. With one hand, raise a side flap and pull laterally (sideways) away from the package (see figure 13-33B).

   ⊘ **CAUTION:** Do *not* touch the inside of the wrapper at any time.

9. With the opposite hand, open the other side flap by pulling the tab to the side (see figure 13-33C).
   NOTE: Always reach in from the side. Never reach across the top of the sterile field or across any opened edges.

10. Open the proximal (closest) flap by lifting the flap up and toward you. Then drop it over the front of your hand (or the table) (see figure 13-33D).

    ⊘ **CAUTION:** Be careful not to touch the inside of the package or the contents of the package.

11. Transfer the contents of the sterile package using one of the following techniques:
    a. Drop: Separate the ends of the wrap and pull apart gently (see figure 13-34). Avoid touching the inside of the wrap. Secure the loose ends of the wrap and hold the package upside down over the sterile field. Allow the contents to drop onto the sterile tray.

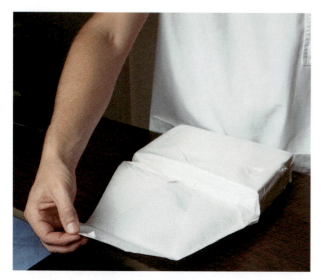

FIGURE 13-33A To open a sterile package, open the top flap away from you, handling only the outside of the wrap.

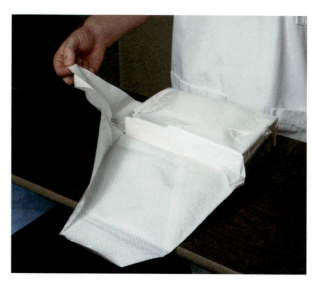

FIGURE 13-33B Open one side by pulling the wrap out to the side.

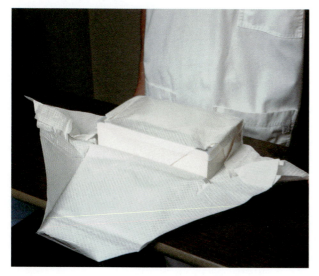

FIGURE 13-33C Open the opposite side by pulling the wrap out to the opposite side.

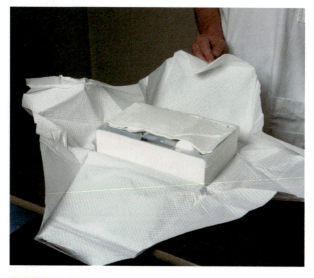

FIGURE 13-33D Open the side nearest to you by pulling back on the wrap.

b. Mitten: Grasp the contents securely by holding on to the outside of the wrapper as you unwrap it. With your free hand, gather the loose edges of the wrapper together and hold them securely around your wrist. This can be compared to making a mitten of the wrapper (with the sterile equipment on the outside of the mitten). Place the item on the sterile tray or hand it to someone who is wearing sterile gloves (refer to figure 13-32B).

c. Transfer forceps: Remove forceps from their sterile container, taking care not to touch the side or rim of the container with the forceps (see figure 13-35). Hold the forceps pointed downward. Shake them to remove excess disinfectant solution. Take care not to touch anything with the forceps. Use the forceps to grasp the item in the package and then place the item on the sterile tray.

NOTE: The method of transfer depends on the sterile item being transferred.

NOTE: If at any time during the procedure there is any suspicion that you have contaminated any article, start over. Never take a chance on using equipment for a sterile

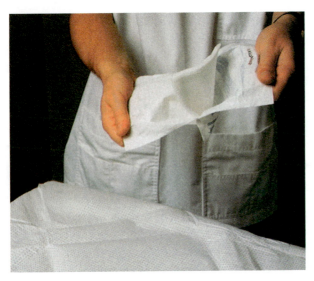

FIGURE 13-34 Separate the ends of the wrap and pull the edges apart gently without touching the contents.

procedure if there is any possibility that the equipment is contaminated.

12. Replace all equipment used.
13. Wash hands.

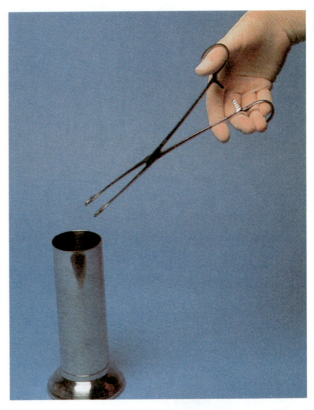

FIGURE 13-35 Remove the transfer or pick-up forceps without touching the sides or rim of the container and point them in a downward direction.

> *Practice* *Go to the workbook and use the evaluation sheet for 13:7A, Opening Sterile Packages, to practice this procedure. When you feel you have mastered this skill, sign the sheet and give it to your instructor for further action.*

 Final Checkpoint Using the criteria listed on the evaluation sheet, your instructor will grade your performance.

PROCEDURE 13:7B

Preparing a Sterile Dressing Tray

Equipment and Supplies

Tray, sterile towels, sterile basin, sterile cotton balls or gauze sponges, sterile dressings (different sizes), antiseptic solution, forceps in disinfectant solution

Procedure

1. Assemble all equipment.
2. Wash hands.

3. Check the date and autoclave indicator for sterility. If more than 30 days have elapsed, use another package with a more recent date. Put the unsterile package aside for resterilization.

4. Place the tray on a flat surface or a Mayo stand.

   NOTE: Make sure the work area is clean and dry and there is sufficient room to work.

5. Open the package that contains the sterile towel. Be sure it is held away from your

body. Place the wrapper on a surface away from the tray or work area. Touch only the outside of the towel. Pick up the towel at its outer edge. Allow it to open by releasing the fanfolds. Place the towel with the outer side (side you have touched) on the tray. The untouched, or sterile, side will be facing up. Holding onto the outside edges of the towel, fanfold the back of the towel so the towel can be used later to cover the supplies.

⚠ **CAUTION:** Do not reach across the top of the towel. Reach in from either side.

NOTE: If you are setting up a relatively large work area, one towel may not be large enough when fanfolded to cover the supplies. In such a case, you will need a second sterile towel (later) to cover your sterile field.

⚠ **CAUTION:** At all times, make sure that you do *not* touch the sterile side of the towel. Avoid letting the towel come in contact with your uniform, other objects, or contaminated areas.

6. Correctly unwrap the package containing the sterile basin. Place the basin on the tray. Do not place it close to the edge of the towel.

NOTE: A 2-inch border around the outside edges of the towel is considered to be contaminated. No equipment should come in contact with this border.

⚠ **CAUTION:** Make sure that the wrapper does *not* touch the towel while placing the basin in position.

7. Unwrap the package containing the sterile cotton balls or gauze sponges. Use a dropping motion to place them in the basin. Do not touch the basin with the wrapper.

8. Unwrap the package containing the larger dressing. Use the sterile forceps to remove the dressing from the package and place it on the tray. Make sure the dressing is not too close to the edge of the towel.

NOTE: The larger, outside dressing is placed on the tray first (before other dressings). In this way, the supplies will be in the order of use. For example, gauze dressings placed directly on the skin will be on top of the pile, and a thick abdominal pad used on top of the gauze pads will be on the bottom of the pile.

NOTE: The forceps must be lifted straight up out of the container and must *not* touch the side or rim of the container. Keep the tips pointed down and above the waist at all times. Shake off excess disinfectant solution.

9. Unwrap the inner dressings correctly. Use the sterile forceps to place them on top of the other dressings on the sterile towel, or use a drop technique.

NOTE: Dressings are now in a pile; the dressing that will be used first is on the top of the pile.

NOTE: The number and type of dressings needed is determined by checking the patient being treated.

10. Open the bottle containing the correct antiseptic solution. Place the cap on the table, with the inside of the cap facing up. Pour a small amount of the solution into the sink to clean the lip of the bottle. Then hold the bottle over the basin and pour a sufficient amount of solution into the basin (see figure 13-36).

⚠ **CAUTION:** Make sure that no part of the bottle touches the basin or the sterile tray. Pour carefully to avoid splashing. If the tray gets wet, the entire tray will be contaminated, and you must begin again.

11. Check the tray to make sure all needed equipment is on it.

12. Pick up the fanfolded edge of the towel by placing one hand on each side edge of the towel on the underside, or contaminated side. Do not touch the sterile side. Keep your hands and arms to the side of the tray, and bring the towel forward to cover the supplies.

NOTE: A second sterile towel may be used to cover the supplies if the table or sterile field

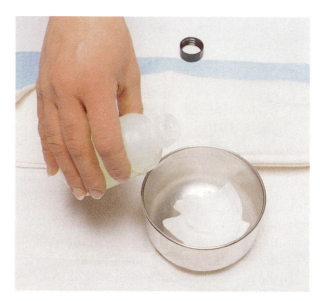

FIGURE 13-36 Avoid splashing the solution onto the sterile field while pouring it into the basin.

area is too large to be covered by the one fanfolded towel.

> ⚠ **CAUTION:** Never reach across the top of the sterile tray.

13. Once the sterile tray is ready, never allow it out of your sight. Take it to the patient area and use it immediately. If you need more equipment, you must take the tray with you. This is the only way to be completely positive that the tray does not become contaminated.

14. Replace equipment.

15. Wash hands.

 Final Checkpoint Using the criteria listed on the evaluation sheet, your instructor will grade your performance.

PROCEDURE 13:7C
Donning and Removing Sterile Gloves

Equipment and Supplies

Sterile gloves

Procedure

1. Assemble equipment and take it to the area where it is to be used. Check the date and/or autoclave indicator on the package to be sure gloves are still sterile. If they are not, put the package aside for re-sterilization and select a package with a current sterilization date.

2. Remove rings. Wash hands. Dry hands thoroughly.

3. Open the package of gloves, taking care not to touch the inside of the inner wrapper. The inner wrapper contains the gloves. Gently open it. The folded cuffs will be nearest you.

    > ⚠ **CAUTION:** If you touch the *inside* of the package (where the gloves are), get a new package and start again.

4. The glove for the right hand will be on the right side and the glove for the left hand will be on the left side of the package. With the thumb and forefinger of the nondominant hand pick up the top edge of the folded-down cuff (inside of glove) of the glove for the dominant hand. Remove the glove carefully (see figure 13-37A).

    > ⚠ **CAUTION:** Do *not* touch the outside of the glove. This is sterile. Only the part

that will be next to the skin can be touched. Remember, unsterile touches unsterile and sterile touches sterile.

5. Hold the glove by the inside cuff and slip the fingers and thumb of your other hand into the glove. Pull it on carefully (see figure 13-37B).

    NOTE: Hold the glove away from the body. Pull gently to avoid tearing the glove.

6. Insert your gloved hand under the cuff (outside) of the other glove and lift the glove from the package (see figure 13-37C). Do not touch any other area with your gloved hand while removing the glove from the package.

    > ⚠ **CAUTION:** If contamination occurs, discard the gloves and start again.

7. Holding your gloved hand under the cuff of the glove, insert your other hand into the glove (see figure 13-37D). Keep the thumb of your gloved hand tucked in to avoid possible contamination.

8. Turn the cuffs up by manipulating only the sterile surface of the gloves (sterile touches sterile). Go up under the folded cuffs, pull out slightly, and turn cuffs over and up (see figure 13-37E.) Do not touch the inside of the gloves or the skin with your gloved hand.

9. Interlace the fingers to position the gloves correctly, taking care not to touch the skin with the gloved hands (see figure 13-37F).

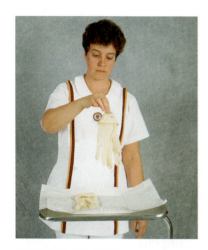

FIGURE 13-37A Pick up the first glove by grasping the glove on the top edge of the folded-down cuff.

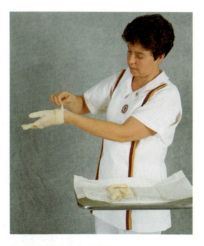

FIGURE 13-37B Hold the glove securely by the cuff and slip the opposite hand into the glove.

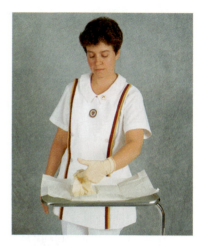

FIGURE 13-37C Slip the gloved fingers under the cuff of the second glove to lift it from the package.

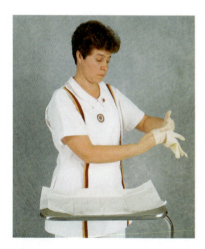

FIGURE 13-37D Hold the gloved hand under the cuff while inserting the other hand into the glove.

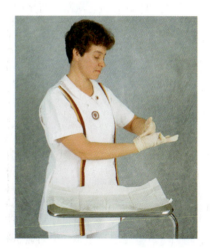

FIGURE 13-37E Insert the gloved fingers under the cuff, pull out slightly, and turn the cuffs over and up without touching the inside of the gloves or the skin.

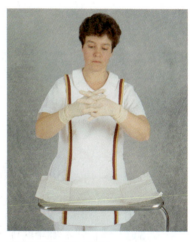

FIGURE 13-37F Interlace the fingers to position the gloves correctly, taking care not to touch the skin with the gloved hands.

⚠ **CAUTION:** If contamination occurs, start again with a new pair of gloves.

10. Do not touch anything that is not sterile once the gloves are in place. Gloves are applied for the purpose of performing procedures requiring sterile technique. During any procedure they become contaminated with organisms related to the patient's condition, for example, wound drainage, blood, or other body discharges. Even a clean, dry wound may contaminate gloves.

NOTE: Gloved hands should remain in position above the waist. Do *not* allow them to fall below waist.

11. After the procedure requiring sterile gloves is completed, dispose of all contaminated supplies before removing gloves.
NOTE: This reduces the danger of cross-infection caused by handling contaminated supplies without glove protection.

12. To remove the gloves, use one gloved hand to grasp the other glove by the outside of the

cuff. Taking care not to touch the skin, remove the glove by pulling it down over the hand. It will be wrong side out when removed.

NOTE: This prevents contamination of your hands by organisms picked up during performance of the procedure. Now you must consider the outside of the gloves contaminated, and the area inside, next to your skin, clean.

13. Insert your bare fingers on the inside of the second glove. Remove the glove by pulling it down gently, taking care not to touch the outside of the glove with your bare fingers. It will be wrong side out when removed.

    ! CAUTION: Avoid touching your uniform or any other object with the contaminated gloves.

14. Put the contaminated gloves in an infectious waste container immediately after removal.

15. Wash your hands immediately and thoroughly after removing gloves.

16. Once the gloves have been removed, do not handle any contaminated equipment or supplies such as soiled dressings or drainage basins. Protect yourself.

17. Replace equipment if necessary.

18. Wash hands thoroughly.

Practice *Go to the workbook and use the evaluation sheet for 13:7C, Donning and Removing Sterile Gloves, to practice this procedure. When you feel you have mastered this skill, sign the sheet and give it to your instructor for further action.*

 Final Checkpoint Using the criteria listed on the evaluation sheet, your instructor will grade your performance.

PROCEDURE 13:7D

Changing a Sterile Dressing

Equipment and Supplies

Sterile tray with basin, solution, gauze sponges and pads (or a prepared sterile dressing package); sterile gloves; adhesive or nonallergic tape; disposable gloves; infectious waste bag

Procedure

1. Check doctor's written orders or obtain orders from immediate supervisor.

   NOTE: Dressings should *not* be changed without orders.

   NOTE: The policy of your agency will determine how you obtain orders for procedures.

2. Assemble equipment. Check autoclave indicator and date on all equipment. If more than 30 days have elapsed, use another package with a more recent date. Put the unsterile package aside for resterilization.

3. Wash hands thoroughly.

4. Prepare a sterile tray as previously taught (in Procedure 13:7B) or obtain a commercially prepared sterile dressing package.

   NOTE: Prepared packages are used in some agencies.

   ! CAUTION: Never let the tray out of your sight once it has been prepared.

5. Take all necessary equipment to the patient area. Place it where it will be convenient for use yet free from possible contamination by other equipment, for example, an uncluttered bedside tray or stand.

6. Introduce yourself. Identify the patient. Explain the procedure. Close the door and/or windows to avoid drafts and flow of organisms into the room.

7. Screen the unit or draw curtains to provide privacy for the patient. If the patient is in a bed, elevate the bed to a comfortable working height and lower the siderail. Expose the body area needing the dressing change. Use

sheets or drapes as necessary to prevent unnecessary exposure of the patient.

8. Fold down a 2- to 3-inch cuff on the top of the infectious waste bag. Position it in a convenient location. Tear off the tape you will need later to secure the clean dressing. Place it in an area where it will be available for easy access.

9. Put on disposable, nonsterile gloves. Gently but firmly remove the tape from the soiled dressing. Discard it in the infectious waste bag. Hold the skin taut and then lift the dressing carefully, taking care not to pull on any surgical drains. Note the type, color, and amount of drainage on the dressing. Discard dressing in the infectious waste bag.

    NOTE: Surgical drains are placed in some surgical incisions to aid the removal of secretions. Care must be taken to avoid moving the drains when the dressing is removed.

10. Check the incision site. Observe the type and amount of remaining drainage, color of drainage, and degree of healing.

    CAUTION: Report any unusual observations immediately to your supervisor. Examples are bright-red blood, pus, swelling, or abnormal discharges at the wound site or patient complaints of pain or dizziness.

11. Remove disposable gloves and place in infectious waste bag. Immediately wash your hands.

    CAUTION: Nonsterile disposable gloves should be worn while removing dressings to avoid contamination of the hands or skin by blood or body discharge.

12. Fanfold the towel back to uncover the sterile tray.

    CAUTION: Handle only the contaminated (outside) side of the towel. The side in contact with the tray's contents is the sterile side.

    NOTE: If a prepared package is used, open it at this time.

13. Don sterile gloves as previously taught in Procedure 13:7C.

14. Using thumb and forefinger, pick up a gauze sponge from the basin. Squeeze it slightly to remove any excess solution. Warn the patient that the solution may be cool.

15. Cleanse the wound. Use a circular motion (see figure 13-38).

NOTE: Begin near the center of the wound and move outward or away from the wound. Make an ever-widening circle. Discard the wet gauze sponge after use. Never go back over the same area with the same gauze sponge. Repeat this procedure until the area is clean, using a new gauze sponge each time.

16. Do not cleanse directly over the wound unless there is a great deal of drainage or it is specifically ordered by the physician. If this is to be done, use sterile gauze and wipe with a single stroke from the top to the bottom. Discard the soiled gauze. Repeat as necessary, using a new sterile gauze sponge each time.

17. The wound is now ready for clean dressings. Lift the sterile dressings from the tray and place them lightly on the wound. Make sure they are centered over the wound.

    NOTE: The inner dressing is usually made up of 4- by 4-inch gauze sponges.

18. Apply outer dressings until the wound is sufficiently protected.

    NOTE: Heavier dressings such as abdominal pads are usually used.

    NOTE: The number and size of dressings needed to dress the wound will depend on the amount of drainage and the size of the wound.

19. Remove the sterile gloves as previously taught. Discard them in the infectious waste bag. Immediately wash your hands.

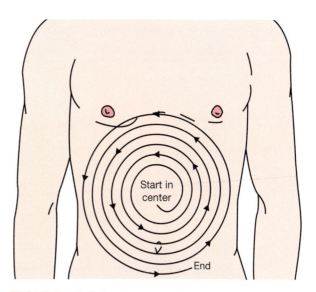

FIGURE 13-38 Use a circular motion to clean the wound, starting at the center of the wound and moving in an outward direction.

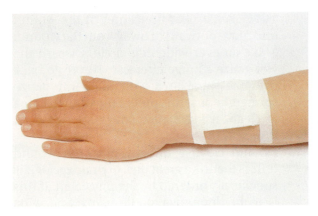

FIGURE 13-39 Tape should be applied so that it runs opposite to body action or movement.

20. Place the precut tape over the dressing at the proper angle. Check to make sure that the dressing is secure and the ends are closed.

    NOTE: Tape should be applied so it runs opposite from body action or movement (see figure 13-39). It should be the correct width for the dressing. It should be long enough to support the dressing, but it should not be too long because it will irritate the patient's skin.

21. Check to be sure the patient is comfortable and that safety precautions have been observed before leaving the area.

22. Put on disposable, nonsterile gloves. Clean and replace all equipment used. Tie or tape the infectious waste bag securely. Dispose of it according to agency policy.

     CAUTION: Disposable, nonsterile gloves should be worn to provide a protective barrier while cleaning equipment or supplies that may be contaminated by blood or body fluids.

23. Remove disposable gloves. Wash hands thoroughly. Protect yourself from possible contamination.

24. **C** Record the following information on the patient's chart or agency form: date, time, dressing change, amount and type of drainage, and any other pertinent information, or tell this information to your immediate supervisor.

    Example: 1/8/—, 9:00 A.M. Dressing changed on right abdominal area. Small amount of thick, light-yellow discharge noted on dressings. No swelling or inflammation apparent at incision site. Sterile dressing applied. Your signature and title.

    NOTE: Report any unusual observations immediately.

Practice *Go to the workbook and use the evaluation sheet for 13:7D, Changing a Sterile Dressing, to practice this procedure. When you feel you have mastered this skill, sign the sheet and give it to your instructor for further action.*

✔ **Final Checkpoint** Using the criteria listed on the evaluation sheet, your instructor will grade your performance.

13:8 INFORMATION
Maintaining Transmission-Based Isolation Precautions

OBRA In health occupations, you will deal with many different diseases/disorders. Some diseases are communicable and require isolation. A **communicable disease** is caused by a pathogenic organism that can be easily transmitted to others.

Transmission-based isolation precautions are a method or technique of caring for patients who have communicable diseases. Examples of communicable diseases are tuberculosis, wound infections, and pertussis (whooping cough). Standard precautions, discussed in Information Section 13:3, do not eliminate the need for specific transmission-based isolation precautions. Standard precautions are used on all patients. Transmission-based isolation techniques are used to provide extra protection against specific diseases or pathogens to prevent their spread.

Communicable diseases are spread in many ways. Some examples include direct contact with the patient; contact with dirty linen, equipment, and/or supplies; and contact with blood, body fluids, secretions, and excretions such as urine, feces, droplets (from sneezing, coughing, or spitting), and discharges from wounds. Transmission-based isolation precautions are used to limit contact with pathogenic organisms. These techniques help prevent the spread of the disease to other people and protect patients, their families, and health care providers.

The type of transmission-based isolation used depends on the causative organism of the disease, the way the organism is transmitted, and whether or not the pathogen is antibiotic-resistant (not affected by antibiotics). Personal protective equipment (PPE) is used to provide protection from the pathogen. Some transmission-based isolation precautions require the use of gowns, gloves, face shields, and masks (see figure 13-40), while others only require the use of a mask.

Two terms are extensively used in transmission-based isolation: *contaminated* and *clean*. These words refer to the presence of organisms on objects.

◆ **Contaminated,** or dirty, means that objects contain disease-producing organisms. These objects must not be touched, unless the health worker is protected by gloves, gown, and other required items.
NOTE: The outside and waist ties of the gown, protective gloves, and mask are considered contaminated.

◆ **Clean** means that objects or parts of objects do *not* contain disease-producing organisms and therefore have minimal chance of spreading the disease. Every effort must be made to prevent contamination of these objects or parts of objects.
NOTE: The insides of the gloves and gown are clean, as are the neckband, its ties, and the mask ties.

The Centers for Disease Control and Prevention (CDC) in conjunction with the National Center for Infectious Diseases (NCID) and the Hospital Infection Control Practices Advisory Committee (HICPAC) has recommended four

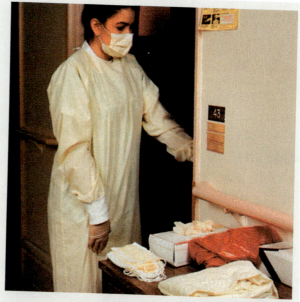

FIGURE 13-40 Some transmission-based isolation precautions require the use of gowns, gloves, and a mask, while others only require the use of a mask.

main classifications of precautions that must be followed: standard, airborne, droplet, and contact. Health care facilities are provided with a list of infections/conditions that shows the type and duration of precautions needed for each specific disease. In this way, facilities can follow the guidelines to determine the type of transmission-based isolation that should be used along with the specific precautions that must be followed.

Standard precautions (discussed in Information Section 13:3), are used on all patients. In addition, a patient must be placed in a private room if the patient contaminates the environment or does not (or cannot be expected to) assist in maintaining appropriate hygiene. Every health care worker must be well informed about standard precautions and follow the recommendations for the use of gloves, gowns, and face masks when conditions indicate their use.

Airborne precautions (see figure 13-41), are used for patients known or suspected to be infected with pathogens transmitted by airborne droplet nuclei, small particles of evaporated droplets that contain microorganisms and remain suspended in the air or on dust particles. Examples of diseases requiring these isolation precautions are rubella (measles), varicella (chicken pox), tuberculosis, and shingles or herpes zoster (varicella-zoster). In addition to using standard precautions, several other precautions are required. The patient must be placed in a private room, and the door should be kept closed. Air in the room must be discharged to outdoor air or filtered before being circulated to other areas. Each person who enters the room must wear respiratory protection in the form of a N95, P100 or more powerful filtering mask such as a high-efficiency particulate air (HEPA) mask (see figure 13-42A, B). These masks contain special filters to prevent the entrance of the small airborne pathogens. The masks must be fit tested to make sure they create a tight seal each time they are worn by a health care provider. Men with facial hair cannot wear a standard filtering mask because a beard prevents an airtight

AIRBORNE PRECAUTIONS
In Addition to Standard Precautions

Visitors - Report to Nurses' Station Before Entering Room

BEFORE CARE	DURING CARE	AFTER CARE

BEFORE CARE

1. Private room and closed door with monitored negative air pressure, frequent air exchanges, and high-efficiency filtration.

2. Wash hands.

3. Wear respiratory protection appropriate for disease.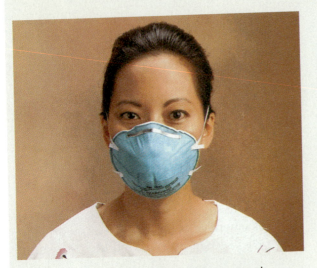

DURING CARE

1. Limit transport of patient/resident to essential purposes only. Patient resident must wear mask appropriate for disease.

2. Limit use of noncritical care equipment to a single patient/resident.

AFTER CARE

1. Bag linen to prevent contamination of self, environment, or outside of bag.

2. Discard infectious trash to prevent contamination of self, environment, or outside of bag.

3. Wash hands.

FIGURE 13-41 Airborne precautions. *(Courtesy of Brevis Corporation)*

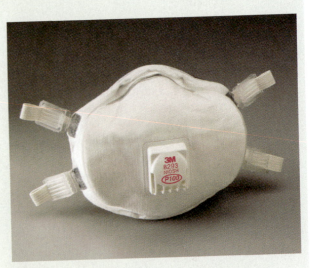

FIGURE 13-42A The N95 respirator mask. *(Courtesy of 3M Company, St. Paul, MN)*

FIGURE 13-42B The P100 respirator mask. *(Courtesy of 3M Company, St. Paul, MN)*

seal. Men with facial hair can use a special HEPA-filtered hood. People susceptible to measles or chicken pox should not enter the room. If at all possible, the patient should not be moved from the room. If transport is essential, however, the patient must wear a surgical mask during transport to minimize the release of droplets into the air.

Droplet precautions (see figure 13-43), must be followed for a patient known or suspected to be infected with pathogens transmitted by large-particle droplets expelled during coughing, sneezing, talking, or laughing. Examples of diseases requiring these isolation precautions include *Haemophilus influenzae* meningitis and pneumonia; *Neisseria* meningitis and pneumonia; multidrug-resistant *Streptococcus* meningitis, pneumonia, sinusitis, and otitis media; diphtheria; *Mycoplasma* pneumonia; pertussis; adenovirus; mumps; and severe viral influenza. In addition to using standard precautions, the patient should be placed in a private room. If a private room is not available and the patient cannot be placed in a room with a patient who has the same infection, a distance of at least 3 feet should separate the infected patient and other patients or visitors. Masks must be worn when working within three feet of the patient, and the use of masks anywhere in the room is strongly recommended. If transport or movement of the patient is essential, the patient must wear a surgical mask.

Contact precautions (see figure 13-44), must be followed for any patients known or suspected to be infected with *epidemiologically* (capable of spreading rapidly from person to person, an epidemic) important microorganisms that can be transmitted by either direct or indirect contact. Examples of diseases requiring these precautions include any gastrointestinal, respiratory, skin, or wound infections caused by multidrug-resistant organisms; diapered or incontinent patients with enterohemorrhagic *E. coli*, *Shigella*, hepatitis A, or rotavirus; viral or hemorrhagic conjunctivitis or fevers; and any skin infections that are highly contagious or that may occur on dry skin, such as diphtheria, herpes simplex virus, impetigo, pediculosis (head or body lice), scabies, and staphylococcal infections. In addition to using standard precautions, the patient should be placed in a private room or, if a private room is not available, in a room with a patient who has an active infection caused by the same organism. Gloves must be

DROPLET PRECAUTIONS
In Addition to Standard Precautions

Visitors - Report to Nurses' Station Before Entering Room

BEFORE CARE

1. Private room. Maintain 3 feet of spacing between patient/resident and visitors.

2. Mask/face shield for staff and visitors within 3 feet of patient/resident.

DURING CARE

1. Limit transport of patient/resident to essential purposes only. Patient/resident must wear mask appropriate for disease.

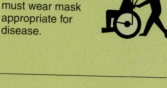

2. Limit use of noncritical care equipment to a single patient/resident.

AFTER CARE

1. Bag linen to prevent contamination of self, environment, or outside of bag.

2. Discard infectious trash to prevent contamination of self, environment, or outside of bag.

3. Wash hands.

FIGURE 13-43 Droplet precautions. *(Courtesy of Brevis Corporation)*

worn when entering the room. Gloves must be changed after having contact with any material that may contain high concentrations of the microorganism, such as wound drainage or fecal material. Gloves must be removed before leaving the room, and the hands must be washed with an antimicrobial agent. A gown must be worn in the room if there is any chance of contact with the patient, environmental surfaces, or items in the room. The gown must be removed before leaving the room and care must be taken to ensure that clothing is not contaminated after gown removal. Movement and transport of the patient from the room should be for essential purposes only. The room and items in it must receive daily cleaning and disinfection as needed. If possible, patient-care equipment (bedside commode, stethoscope, sphygmomanometer, thermometer) should be left in the room and used only for this patient. If this is not possible, all equipment must be cleaned and disinfected before being used on another patient.

Protective or **reverse isolation** refers to methods used to protect certain patients from organisms present in the environment. Protective isolation is used mainly for *immunocom-promised* patients, or those whose body defenses are not capable of protecting them from infections and disease. Examples of patients requiring this protection are patients whose immune systems have been depressed prior to receiving transplants (such as bone marrow transplants), severely burned patients, patients receiving chemotherapy or radiation treatments, or patients whose immune systems have failed. Precautions vary depending on the patient's condition. The patient is usually placed in a room that has been cleaned and disinfected. Frequent disinfection occurs while the patient occupies the room. Many facilities require anyone entering the room to wear clean or sterile gowns, gloves, and masks. All equipment or supplies brought into the room are clean, disinfected, and/or sterile. Special filters may be used to purify air that enters the room. Every effort is made to protect the patient from microorganisms that cause infection or disease.

Exact procedures for maintaining transmission-based isolation precautions vary from one facility to another. The procedures used depend on the type of units provided for isolation patients, and on the kind of supplies or special isolation equipment available. Most facilities

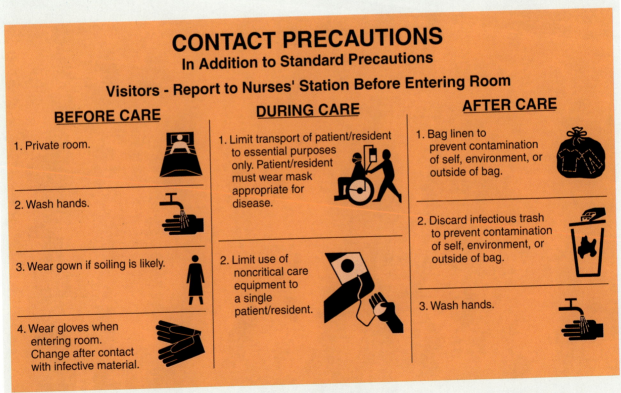

CONTACT PRECAUTIONS
In Addition to Standard Precautions

Visitors - Report to Nurses' Station Before Entering Room

BEFORE CARE

1. Private room.

2. Wash hands.

3. Wear gown if soiling is likely.

4. Wear gloves when entering room. Change after contact with infective material.

DURING CARE

1. Limit transport of patient/resident to essential purposes only. Patient/resident must wear mask appropriate for disease.

2. Limit use of noncritical care equipment to a single patient/resident.

AFTER CARE

1. Bag linen to prevent contamination of self, environment, or outside of bag.

2. Discard infectious trash to prevent contamination of self, environment, or outside of bag.

3. Wash hands.

FIGURE 13-44 Contact precautions. *(Courtesy of Brevis Corporation)*

convert a regular patient room into an isolation room, but some facilities use special, two-room isolation units. Some facilities use disposable supplies such as gloves, gowns, and treatment packages. Therefore, it is essential that you learn the isolation procedure followed by your agency. However, the basic principles for maintaining transmission-based isolation are the same regardless of the facility. Therefore, if you know these basic principles, you will be able to adjust to any setting.

STUDENT: *Go to the workbook and complete the assignment sheet for 13:8, Maintaining Transmission-Based Isolation Precautions. Then return and continue with the procedures.*

PROCEDURE 13:8A

Donning and Removing Transmission-Based Isolation Garments

OBRA **NOTE:** The following procedure deals with contact transmission-based isolation precautions. For other types of transmission-based isolation, follow only the steps that apply.

Equipment and Supplies

Isolation gown, surgical mask, gloves, small plastic bag, linen cart or container, infectious waste container, paper towels, sink with running water

Procedure

1. Assemble equipment.
   NOTE: In many agencies, clean isolation garments and supplies are kept available on a cart outside the isolation unit, or in the outer room of a two-room unit. A waste container should be positioned just inside the door.
2. Wash hands.
3. Remove rings and place them in your pocket or pin them to your uniform.
4. Remove your watch and place it in a small plastic bag or centered on a clean paper towel. If placed on a towel, handle only the bottom part of the towel; do not touch the top.
   NOTE: The watch will be taken into the room and placed on the bedside stand for taking vital signs. Because it cannot be sterilized, it must be kept clean.
   NOTE: In some agencies, a plastic-covered watch is left in the isolation room.

5. Put on the mask. Secure it under your chin. Make sure to cover your mouth and nose. Handle the mask as little as possible. Tie the mask securely behind your head and neck. Tie the top ties first and the bottom ties second.
   NOTE: The tie bands on the mask are considered clean. The mask is considered contaminated.
   NOTE: The mask is considered to be contaminated after 30 minutes in isolation or anytime it gets wet. If you remain in isolation longer than 30 minutes, or if the mask gets wet, you must wash your hands, and remove and discard the old mask. Then wash your hands again, and put on a clean mask.
6. If uniform sleeves are long, roll them up above the elbows before putting on the gown.
7. Lift the gown by placing your hands inside the shoulders (see figure 13-45A).
   NOTE: The inside of the gown and the ties at the neck are considered clean.
   NOTE: Most agencies use disposable gowns that are discarded after use.
8. Work your arms into the sleeves of the gown by gentle twisting. Take care not to touch your face with the sleeves of the gown.
9. Place your hands *inside* the neckband, adjust until it is in position, and then tie the bands at the back of your neck (see figure 13-45B).
10. Reach behind and fold the edges of the gown over so that the uniform is completely

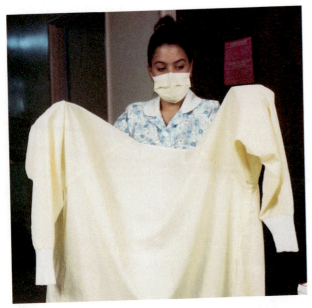

FIGURE 13-45A After tying the mask in place, put on the gown by placing your hands inside the shoulders.

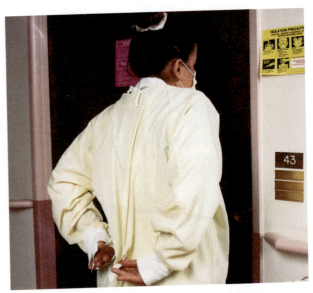

FIGURE 13-45C Overlap the back edges of the gown so your uniform is completely covered before tying the waist ties.

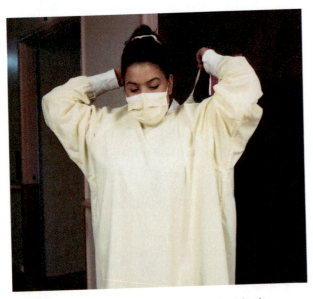

FIGURE 13-45B Slip your fingers inside the neckband to tie the gown at the neck.

covered. Tie the waistbands (see figure 13-45C). Some waistbands are long enough to wrap around your body before tying.

11. If gloves are to be worn, put them on. Make sure that the cuff of the glove comes over the top of the cuff of the gown. In this way, there are no open areas for entrance of organisms.

12. You are now ready to enter the isolation room. Double check to be sure you have all

equipment and supplies that you will need for patient care before you enter the room.

13. When patient care is complete, you will be ready to remove isolation garments. In a two-room isolation unit, go to the outer room. In a one-room unit, remove garments while you are standing close to the inside of the door. Take care to avoid touching the room's contaminated articles.

14. Untie the waist ties. Loosen the gown at the waist.
NOTE: The waist ties are considered contaminated.

15. If gloves are worn, remove the first glove by grasping the outside of the cuff with the opposite gloved hand. Pull the glove over the hand so that the glove is inside out. Remove the second glove by placing the bare hand inside the cuff. Pull the glove off so it is inside out. Place the disposable gloves in the infectious waste container.

16. To avoid unnecessary transmission of organisms, use paper towels to turn on the water faucet. Wash and dry your hands thoroughly. When they are dry, use a clean, dry paper towel to turn off the faucet.
⚠ CAUTION: Organisms travel rapidly through wet towels.

17. Untie the mask. Holding the mask by the ties only, drop it into the infectious waste container.

NOTE: The ties of the mask are considered clean. Do not touch any other part of the mask because it is considered contaminated.

18. Untie the neck ties. Loosen the gown at the shoulders, handling only the inside of the gown.

    NOTE: The neck ties are considered clean.

19. Slip the fingers of one hand inside the opposite cuff. Do *not* touch the outside. Pull the sleeve down over the hand (see figure 13-46A).

    ⚠ **CAUTION:** The outside of the gown is considered contaminated and should not be touched.

20. Using the gown-covered hand, pull the sleeve down over the opposite hand (see figure 13-46B).

21. Ease your arms and hands out of the gown. Keep the gown in front of your body and keep your hands away from the outside of the gown. Use as gentle a motion as possible.

    NOTE: Excessive flapping of the gown will spread organisms.

22. With your hands inside the gown at the shoulders, bring the shoulders together and turn the gown so that it is inside out (see figure 13-46C). In this manner, the outside of the contaminated gown is on the inside. Fold the gown in half and then roll it together. Place it in the infectious waste container.

    NOTE: Avoid excess motion during this procedure because motion causes the spread of organisms.

23. Wash hands thoroughly. Use dry, clean paper towels to operate the faucets.

24. Touch only the inside of the plastic bag to remove your watch. Discard the bag in the waste container. If the watch is on a paper towel, handle only the "clean," top portion (if necessary). Discard the towel in the infectious waste container.

25. Use a clean paper towel to open the door. Discard the towel in the waste container before leaving the room.

    ⚠ **CAUTION:** The inside of the door is considered contaminated.

    NOTE: The waste container should be positioned just inside the door of the room.

26. After leaving the isolation room, wash hands thoroughly. This will help prevent spread of the disease. It also protects you from the illness.

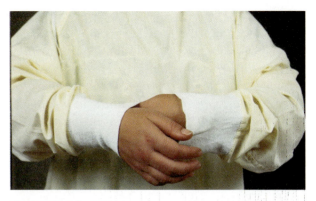

FIGURE 13-46A To remove the gown, slip the fingers of one hand under the cuff of the opposite arm to pull the gown down over the opposite hand.

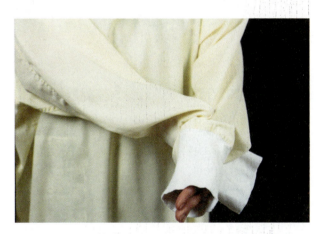

FIGURE 13-46B Using the gown-covered hand, grasp the outside of the gown on the opposite arm and pull the gown down over the hand.

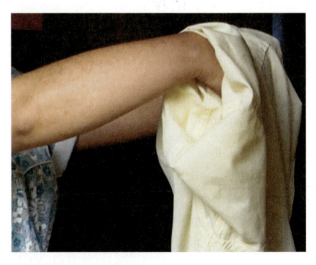

FIGURE 13-46C With your hands inside the gown at the shoulders, bring the shoulders together and turn the gown so that it is inside out, with the contaminated side on the inside.

Practice *Go to the workbook and use the evaluation sheet for 13:8A, Donning and Removing Transmission-Based Isolation Garments, to practice this procedure. When you feel you have mastered this skill, sign the sheet and give it to your instructor for further action.*

 Final Checkpoint Using the criteria listed on the evaluation sheet, your instructor will grade your performance.

PROCEDURE 13:8B

Working in a Hospital Transmission-Based Isolation Unit

Equipment and Supplies

Clothes hamper, two laundry bags, two trays, dishes, cups, bowls, waste container lined with a plastic bag, infectious waste bags, bags, tape, pencil, pen, paper

Procedure

1. Assemble all equipment.
   NOTE: Any equipment or supplies to be used in the isolation room must be assembled prior to entering the room.
2. Wash hands.
3. Put on appropriate isolation garments as previously instructed.
4. Tape paper to the outside of the isolation door. This will be used to record vital signs.
5. Enter the isolation room. Take all needed equipment into the room.
6. Introduce yourself. Greet and identify patient. Provide patient care as needed.
   NOTE: All care is provided in a routine manner. However, transmission-based isolation garments must be worn as ordered.
7. To record vital signs:
   a. Take vital signs using the watch in the plastic bag. (If the watch is not in a plastic bag, hold it with the bottom part of a paper towel.) Use other equipment in the room as needed.
   b. Open the door touching only the inside, or contaminated side.

   c. Using a pencil, record the vital signs on the paper taped to the door. Do *not* touch the outside of the door at any time.
   NOTE: The pencil remains in the room because it is contaminated.
8. To transfer food into the isolation unit:
   a. Transfer of food requires two people; one person must stay outside the unit and one inside.
   b. The person inside the isolation unit picks up the empty tray in the room and opens door, touching only the inside of the door.
   c. The person outside hands in the cups, bowls, and plates of food.
   d. When transferring food, the two people should handle the opposite sides of the dishes. In this manner, one person will not touch the other person.
   e. Glasses should be held near the top by the transfer person on the outside. The transfer person on the inside should receive the glasses by holding them on the bottom.
9. To dispose of leftover food or waste:
   a. Liquids can be poured down the sink or flushed down the toilet.
   b. Soft foods such as mashed potatoes or cooked vegetables can be flushed down the toilet.
   c. Hard particles of food, such as bone, should be placed in the plastic-lined trash container.
   d. Disposable utensils or dishes should be placed in the plastic-lined trash container.

e. Metal utensils should be washed and kept in the isolation room to be used as needed for other meals. These utensils, however, are contaminated. When they are removed from the isolation room, they must be disinfected or double bagged and labeled before being sent for decontamination and reprocessing.

10. To transfer soiled linen from the unit, two people are required:
   a. All dirty linen should be folded and rolled.
   b. Place linen in the linen hamper.
   c. Person outside the unit should cuff the top of a clean infectious waste laundry bag and hold it. Hands should be kept on the inside of the bag's cuff to avoid contamination.
   d. Person in isolation should seal the isolation bag. The bag is then placed inside the outer bag, which is being held by the person outside.
   e. Outer bag should be folded over at the top and taped by the person outside. The bag should be labeled as "BIOHAZARDOUS LINEN."
   f. At all times, no direct contact should occur between the two people transferring linen.
   NOTE: Many agencies use special isolation linen bags. Hot water dissolves the bags during the washing process. Therefore, no other personnel handle the contaminated linen after it leaves the isolation unit.

11. To transfer trash from the isolation unit, two people are required:
   a. Any trash in the isolation room should be in plastic bags. Any trash or disposable items contaminated with blood, body fluids, secretions, or excretions should be placed in infectious waste bags.
   b. When the bag is full, expel excess air by pushing gently on the bag.
   c. Tie a knot at the top of the bag to seal it or fold the top edge twice and tape it securely.
   d. Place this bag inside a cuffed biohazardous waste bag held by a "clean" person outside the unit.
   e. The outside person then ties the outer bag securely or tapes the outer bag shut.
   f. The double-bagged trash should then be burned. Double-bagged infectious waste is autoclaved prior to incineration or disposal as infectious waste according to legal requirements.

   g. At all times, direct contact between the two people transferring trash must be avoided.
12. To transfer equipment from the isolation unit two people are required:
   a. Thoroughly clean and disinfect all equipment in the unit.
   b. After cleaning, place equipment in a plastic bag or special isolation bag. Label the bag with the contents and the word "ISOLATION."
   c. After folding the bag down twice at the top, tape the bag shut.
   d. A second person outside the isolation room should hold a second, cuffed infectious waste bag.
   e. The person in isolation places the sealed, contaminated bag inside the bag being held outside the unit. The person in isolation should have no direct contact with the clean bag.
   f. The person outside the unit turns down the top of the infectious waste bag twice and securely tapes the bag. The outside person then labels the bag with the contents, for example, "ISOLATION DISHES."
   g. The double-bagged material is then sent to Central Supply or another designated area for sterilization and/or decontamination.
13. The transmission-based isolation unit must be kept clean and neat at all times. Equipment no longer needed should be transferred out of the unit using the appropriate isolation technique.
14. Before leaving an isolation room, ask the patient whether a urinal or bedpan is needed. This will save time and energy by reducing the need to return to provide additional patient care shortly after leaving. Also, prior to leaving, check all safety and comfort points to make sure patient care is complete.
15. Remove isolation garments as previously instructed (in Procedure 13:8A).
16. Wash hands thoroughly.

Practice *Go to the workbook and use the evaluation sheet for 13:8B, Working in a Hospital Transmission-Based Isolation Unit, to practice this procedure. When you feel you have mastered this skill, sign the sheet and give it to your instructor for further action.*

Final Checkpoint Using the criteria listed on the evaluation sheet, your instructor will grade your performance.

UNIT 13 SUMMARY

Understanding the basic principles of infection control is essential for any health care worker in any health care field. Disease is caused by a wide variety of pathogens, or germs. An understanding of the types of pathogens, methods of transmission, and the chain of infection allows health care workers to take precautions to prevent the spread of disease.

Asepsis is defined as "the absence of disease-producing microorganisms, or pathogens." Various levels of aseptic control are possible. Antisepsis refers to methods that prevent or inhibit the growth of pathogenic organisms. Proper handwashing and using an ultrasonic unit to clean instruments and supplies are examples. Disinfection is a process that destroys or kills pathogenic organisms, but is not always effective against spores and viruses. Chemical disinfectants are used for this purpose. Sterilization is a process that destroys all microorganisms, including spores and viruses. The use of an autoclave is an example. Instruments and equipment are properly prepared, and then processed in the autoclave to achieve sterilization.

Following the standard precautions established by the Centers for Disease Control and Prevention helps prevent the spread of pathogens by way of blood, body fluids, secretions, and excretions. The standard precautions provide guidelines for handwashing; wearing gloves; using gowns, masks, and protective eyewear, when splashing is likely; proper handling and disposal of contaminated sharp objects; proper disposal of contaminated waste; and proper methods to wipe up spills of blood, body fluids, secretions, and excretions. Every health care worker must be familiar with and follow the recommended standard precautions while working with all patients.

Sterile techniques are used in specific procedures, such as changing dressings. Health care workers must learn and follow sterile techniques when they are required to perform these procedures.

Transmission-based isolation precautions are used for patients who have communicable diseases, or diseases that are easily transmitted from one person to another. An awareness of the major types of transmission-based isolation presented in this unit will help the health care worker prevent the transmission of communicable diseases.

Infection control must be followed when performing any and every health care procedure. By learning and following the principles discussed in this unit, health care workers will protect themselves, patients, and others from disease.

INTERNET SEARCHES

Use the suggested search engines in Unit 11:4 of this textbook to search the Internet for additional information on the following topics:

1. *Organizations regulating infection control:* find the organization sites for the Occupational Safety and Health Administration (OSHA), Centers for Disease Control and Prevention (CDC), National Center for Infectious Diseases (NCID), and the Hospital Infection Control Practices Advisory Committee (HICPAC) to obtain information on regulations governing infection control.

2. *Microbiology:* search for specific information on bacteria (can also search for specific types

such as *Escherichia coli*), protozoa, fungi, rickettsiae, and viruses.

3. *Diseases:* obtain information on the method of transmission, signs and symptoms, treatment, and complications for diseases such as hepatitis B, hepatitis C, acquired immune deficiency syndrome, and specific diseases listed by the discussion on microorganisms in this unit.

4. *Infections:* research endogenous infections, exogenous infections, nosocomial infections, and opportunistic infections.

5. *Infection control:* locate and read the Bloodborne Pathogen Standards, Needlestick Safety and Prevention Act, Standard Precautions, and Transmission-Based Isolation Precautions (airborne precautions, droplet precautions, and contact precautions).

6. *Medical supply companies:* search for names of specific medical supply companies to research products available such as autoclaves, chemical disinfectants, and spill clean-up kits.

REVIEW QUESTIONS

1. List the classifications of bacteria by shape and give two (2) examples of diseases caused by each class.

2. Draw the chain of infection and identify three (3) ways to break each section of the chain.

3. Differentiate between antisepsis, disinfection, and sterilization.

4. List eight (8) times the hands must be washed.

5. Name the different types of personal protective equipment (PPE) and state when each type must be worn to meet the requirements of standard precautions.

6. What level of infection control is achieved by an ultrasonic cleaner? chemicals? an autoclave?

7. Name three (3) methods that can be used to place sterile items on a sterile field. Identify the types of items that can be transferred by each method.

8. List the three (3) types of transmission-based isolation precautions and the basic principles that must be followed for each type.

UNIT 13
SUGGESTED REFERENCES

Acello, Barbara. *Patient Care: Basic Skills for the Health Care Provider.* Clifton Park, NY: Delmar Learning, 1998.

Acello, Barbara. *The OSHA Handbook: The Guidelines for Compliance in Health Care Facilities.* 3rd ed. Clifton Park, NY: Delmar Learning, 2002.

Burhoe, Steven. *Bloodborne Pathogens: An Overview of OSHA's Standards.* Columbia, MO: Instructional Materials Laboratory, 1992.

Dietz, Ellen. *Safety Standards and Infection Control for Dental Assistants.* Clifton Park, NY: Delmar Learning, 2002.

Grover-Lakomia, Lynne, and Elizabeth Fong. *Microbiology for Health Careers.* 6th ed. Clifton Park, NY: Delmar Learning, 1999.

Hegner, Barbara, Esther Caldwell, and Joan Needham. *Nursing Assistant: A Nursing Process Approach.* 8th ed. Clifton Park, NY: Delmar Learning, 1999.

Keir, Lucille, Connie Krebs, and Barbara A. Wise. *Medical Assisting: Administrative and Clinical Competencies.* 5th ed. Clifton Park, NY: Delmar Learning, 2003.

Kennamer, Michael. *Basic Infection Control for the Health Care Profession.* Clifton Park, NY: Delmar Learning, 2002.

Nielson, Ronal. *OSHA Regulations and Guidelines: A Guide for Health Care Providers.* Clifton Park, NY: Delmar Learning, 2000.

Palmer, Darwin, Sue Palmer, and Jean Giddens. *Infection Control.* Clifton Park, NY: Delmar Learning, 1996.

Schaffer, Susan, Laurel Garzon, and Denise Korniewicz. *Pocket Guide to Infection Control.* St. Louis, MO: Mosby, 1995.

Shimeld, Lisa. *Essentials of Diagnostic Microbiology.* Clifton Park, NY: Delmar Learning, 1999.

U.S. Department of Health and Human Services. "Guidelines for Isolation Precautions in Hospitals." *Federal Register.* Vol. 59, No. 214, November 7, 1994.

For information on federal recommendations, contact the Centers for Disease Control and Prevention, Atlanta, Georgia 30333 or use the Internet Address: *www.cdc.gov*

Descriptive literature supplied with equipment such as autoclave or ultrasonic cleaners.

UNIT 14

Vital Signs

Introduction

After completing this unit of study, you should be able to:

◆ List the four main vital signs
◆ Convert Fahrenheit temperatures to Celsius, or Celsius to Fahrenheit
◆ Read a clinical thermometer to the nearest two-tenths of a degree
◆ Measure and record oral temperature accurately
◆ Measure and record rectal temperature accurately
◆ Measure and record axillary temperature accurately
◆ Measure and record tympanic (aural) temperature accurately
◆ Measure and record radial pulse to an accuracy within ± 2 beats per minute
◆ Count and record respirations to an accuracy within ± 1 respiration per minute
◆ Measure and record apical pulse to an accuracy within ± 2 beats per minute
◆ Measure and record blood pressure to an accuracy within ± 2 mm of actual mercury reading
◆ State the normal range for oral temperature, axillary temperature, rectal temperature, pulse, respirations, systolic pressure, and diastolic pressure
◆ Define, pronounce, and spell all the key terms

 Observe Standard Precautions

 Safety—Proceed with Caution

 Math Skill

 Science Skill

 Communications Skill

 Instructors Check—Call Instructor at This Point

 OBRA Requirement— Based on Federal Law

 Legal Responsibility

 Career Information

 Technology

KEY TERMS

apical pulse
  (ape'-ih-kal)

apnea
  (ap'-nee"-ah)

arrhythmia
  (ah-rith'-me-ah)

aural

axillary

blood pressure

bradycardia
  (bray"-dee-car'-dee-ah)

bradypnea
  (brad"-ip-nee'-ah)

character

Cheyne–Stokes
  (chain' stokes")

clinical thermometers

cyanosis

diastolic
  (die"-ah-stall'-ik)

dyspnea
  (dis(p)'-nee"-ah)

electronic thermometers

fever

homeostasis
  (home"-ee-oh-stay'-sis)

hypertension

hyperthermia
  (high-pur-therm'-ee-ah)

hypotension

hypothermia
  (high-po-therm'-ee-ah)

oral

orthopnea
  (or"-thop-nee'-ah)

pulse

pulse deficit

pulse pressure

pyrexia

rale *(rawl)*

rate

rectal

respirations

rhythm

sphygmomanometer
  (sfig"-moh-ma-nam'-eh-ter)

stethoscope
  (steth'-uh-scope)

systolic
  (sis"-tall'-ik)

tachycardia
  (tack"-eh-car'-dee-ah)

tachypnea
  (tack"-ip-nee'-ah)

temperature

tympanic thermometers

vital signs

volume

wheezing

INFORMATION

14:1 Measuring and Recording Vital Signs

Vital signs are important indicators of health states of the body. This unit discusses all of the vital signs in detail. The basic information that follows serves as an introduction for this topic.

Vital signs are defined as various determinations that provide information about the basic body conditions of the patient. The four main vital signs are temperature, pulse, respirations, and blood pressure. Many health care professionals are now regarding the degree of pain as the fifth vital sign. Patients are asked to rate their level of pain on a scale of 1 to 10, with 1 being minimal pain and 10 being severe pain. Other important vital signs that provide information about the patient's condition include the color of the skin, the size of the pupils in the eyes and their reaction to light, the level of consciousness, and the patient's response to stimuli. As a health care worker, it will be your responsibility to measure and record the vital signs of patients. However, it is not in your realm of duties to reveal this information to the patient. The physician will decide if the patient should be given this information. It is essential that vital signs be accurate. They are often the first indication of a disease or abnormality in the patient.

Temperature is a measurement of the balance between heat lost and heat produced by the body. Temperature can be

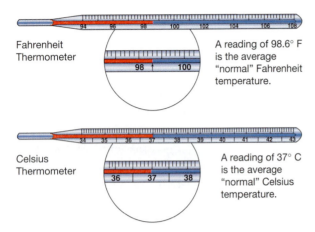

FIGURE 14-1 Normal oral body temperature on Fahrenheit and Celsius thermometers.

measured in the mouth (oral), rectum (rectal), armpit (axillary), or ear (aural). A low or high reading can indicate disease. Most temperatures are measured in degrees on a thermometer that has a Fahrenheit scale. However, some health care facilities are now measuring temperature in degrees on a Celsius (centigrade) scale. A comparison of the two scales is shown in figure 14-1 and in Appendix B. At times, it may be necessary to convert Fahrenheit temperatures to Celsius, or Celsius to Fahrenheit. The formulas for the conversion are as follows:

◆ To convert Fahrenheit (F) temperatures to Celsius (C) temperatures, subtract 32 from the Fahrenheit temperature and then multiply the result by 5/9, or 0.5556. For example, to convert a Fahrenheit temperature of 212 to Celsius, subtract 32 from 212 to get 180. Then multiply 180 by 5/9, or 0.5556, to get the Celsius temperature of 100.0.

◆ To convert Celsius (C) temperatures to Fahrenheit (F) temperatures, multiply the Celsius temperature by 9/5, or 1.8, and then add 32 to the total. For example, to convert a Celsius temperature of 37 to Fahrenheit, multiply 37 by 9/5, or 1.8, to get 66.6. Then add 32 to 66.6 to get the Fahrenheit temperature of 98.6.

Pulse is the pressure of the blood felt against the wall of an artery as the heart contracts and relaxes, or beats. The rate, rhythm, and volume are recorded. **Rate** refers to the number of beats per minute, **rhythm** refers to regularity, and **volume** refers to strength. The pulse is usually taken over the radial artery, although it may be felt over any superficial artery that has a bone behind it. Any abnormality can indicate disease.

Respirations reflect the breathing rate of the patient. In addition to the respiration count, the rhythm (regularity) and character (type) of respirations are noted. Abnormal respirations usually indicate that a health problem or disease is present.

Blood pressure is the force exerted by the blood against the arterial walls when the heart contracts or relaxes. Two readings (systolic and diastolic) are noted to show the greatest pressure and the least pressure. Both are very important. Abnormal blood pressure is often the first indication of disease.

Another vital sign is the **apical pulse.** This pulse is taken with a stethoscope at the apex of the heart. The actual heartbeat is heard and counted. At times, because of illness, hardening of the arteries, a weak or very rapid radial pulse, or doctor's orders, you will be required to take an apical pulse. Also, because infants and small children have a very rapid radial pulse that is difficult to count, apical pulses are usually taken.

C If you note any abnormality or change in any vital sign, it is your responsibility to report this immediately to your supervisor. If you have difficulty obtaining a correct reading, ask another individual to check the patient. Never guess, or report an inaccurate reading.

STUDENT: *Go to the workbook and complete the assignment sheet for 14:1, Measuring and Recording Vital Signs.*

14:2 INFORMATION Measuring and Recording Temperature

OBRA Body temperature is one of the main vital signs. This section provides the basic guidelines for taking and recording temperature.

Temperature is defined as "the balance between heat lost and heat produced by the body." Heat is lost through perspiration, respiration, and excretion (urine and feces). Heat is produced by the metabolism of food, and by muscle and gland activity. A constant state of fluid balance, known as **homeostasis,** is the ideal health state in the human body. The rates of chemical reactions in the body are regulated by body temperature. Therefore, if body temperature is too high or too low, the body's fluid balance is affected.

The normal range for body temperature is 97° to 100° Fahrenheit, or 36.1° to 37.8° Celsius (sometimes called centigrade). However, variations in body temperature can occur, as noted in the following information:

◆ Individuals have different body temperatures. Some people have accelerated body processes and, thus, usually have higher temperatures. Others have slower body processes and, thus, lower temperatures.

◆ Time of day also affects body temperature. Body temperature is usually lower in the morning, after the body has rested. It is higher in the evening, after muscular activity and daily food intake have taken place.

◆ Parts of the body where temperatures are taken lead to variations. Temperature variations by body site are shown in table 14-1.

(1) **Oral** temperatures are taken in the mouth. The clinical thermometer is left in place for 3 to 5 minutes. This is usually the most common, convenient, and comfortable method of obtaining a temperature.

(2) **Rectal** temperatures are taken in the rectum. The clinical thermometer is left in place for 3 to 5 minutes. This is an internal measurement and is the most accurate of all methods.

(3) An **axillary** temperature is taken in the armpit, under the upper arm. The arm is held close to the body, and the thermometer is inserted between the two folds of skin. A *groin* temperature is taken between the two folds of skin formed by the inner part of the thigh and the lower abdomen. Both axillary and groin are external temperatures and, thus, less accurate. The clinical thermometer is held in place for 10 minutes.

(4) An **aural** temperature is taken with a special thermometer that is placed in the ear or auditory canal. The thermometer detects and measures the thermal, infrared energy radiating from blood vessels in the tympanic membrane, or eardrum. Because this provides a measurement of body core temperature, there is no normal range. Instead, the temperature is calculated by the thermometer into an equivalent of one of four usual settings: equal mode, oral equivalent, rectal equivalent, or core equivalent. The equal mode provides no offset (adjustment) and is recommended for newborns, for whom axillary temperature is often taken. The oral equivalent is calculated with an offset; this mode is used for adults and children over 3 years of age, for whom oral readings are commonly used. The rectal mode is calculated with an offset and is used mainly for infants up to 3 years of age, for whom rectal temperatures are commonly taken. When the rectal mode is used on adults, the temperature

TABLE 14-1 Temperature Variations by Body Site

	ORAL	RECTAL	AXILLARY OR GROIN
Average Temperature	98.6°F (37°C)	99.6°F (37.6°C)	97.6°F (36.4°C)
Normal Range of Temperature	97.6–99.6°F (36.5–37.5°C)	98.6–100.6°F (37–38.1°C)	96.6–98.6°F (36–37°C)

may read higher than average. The core equivalent is calculated with an offset and measures core body temperatures such as those found in the bladder or pulmonary artery. The core equivalent mode should only be used where adult "core" temperatures are commonly used and should not be used for routine vital sign measurements. Most aural thermometers record temperature in less than 2 seconds; so this is a fast and convenient method for obtaining temperature.

◆ Factors that lead to increased body temperature include illness, infection, exercise, excitement, and high temperatures in the environment.

◆ Factors that lead to decreased body temperature include starvation or fasting, sleep, decreased muscle activity, mouth breathing, exposure to cold temperatures in the environment, and certain diseases.

Very low or very high body temperatures are indicative of abnormal conditions. **Hypothermia** is a low body temperature, below 95°F (35°C) measured rectally. It can be caused by prolonged exposure to cold. Death usually occurs if body temperature drops below 93°F (33.9°C) for a period of time. A **fever** is an elevated body temperature, usually above 101°F (38.3°C) measured rectally. **Pyrexia** is another term for fever. The term *febrile* means a fever is present; *afebrile* means no fever is present or the temperature is within the normal range. Fevers are usually caused by infection or injury. **Hyperthermia** occurs when the body temperature exceeds 104°F (40°C) measured rectally. It can be caused by prolonged exposure to hot temperatures, brain damage, and serious infections. Immediate actions must be taken to lower body temperature, because temperatures above 106°F (41.1°C) can quickly lead to convulsions, brain damage, and death.

Clinical thermometers may be used to record temperatures. A clinical thermometer consists of a slender glass tube containing mercury or alcohol with red dye, which expands when exposed to heat. There are different types of clinical thermometers (see figure 14-2). The glass oral thermometer has a long, slender bulb or a blue tip. A security oral thermometer has a shorter, rounder bulb and is usually marked with a blue tip. A rectal thermometer has a short,

stubby, rounded bulb and may be marked with a red tip. In addition, some clinical thermometers have the word "oral" or "rectal" written on their stems. Disposable plastic sheaths may be used to cover the thermometer when it is used on a patient.

If a clinical thermometer containing mercury breaks, the mercury can evaporate and create a toxic vapor that can harm both humans and the environment. Mercury poisoning attacks the central nervous system in humans. Children, especially those under the age of six, are very susceptible. Mercury can contaminate water supplies and build up in the tissues of fish and animals. Therefore, proper cleanup of a broken clinical thermometer is essential. *Never* use a vacuum cleaner or broom to clean up mercury because this will break up the beads of mercury and allow them to vaporize more quickly. *Never* pour mercury down a drain or discard it in a toilet because this causes contamination of the water supply. If a clinical thermometer breaks, close doors to other indoor areas and open the windows in the room with the mercury spill to vent any vapors outside. Put on gloves and use two cards or stiff paper to push the droplets of mercury and broken glass into a plastic container with a tight-fitting lid. If necessary, use an eyedropper to pick up the balls of mercury. Shine a flashlight in the area of the spill because the light will reflect off the shiny mercury beads and make them easier to see. Wipe the entire area with a damp sponge. Then place all cleanup material, including the paper, eyedropper, gloves, and sponge, in the plastic container and label it "Mercury for Recycling." Seal the lid tightly and take the container to a mercury recycling center. Most waste disposal companies will accept mercury for recycling. To discard unbroken mercury thermometers, place the intact thermometer in a

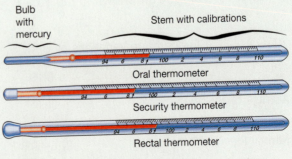

FIGURE 14-2 Types of clinical thermometers.

plastic container with a tight-fitting lid, label it, and take it to a mercury recycling center. To avoid the chance of mercury contamination, the Occupational Health and Safety Administration (OSHA), the Environment Protection Agency (EPA), and the American Medical Association (AMA) recommend the use of alcohol-filled thermometers or digital thermometers.

Electronic thermometers are also used in many facilities. This type of thermometer registers the temperature on a viewer in a few seconds (see figure 14-3). Electronic thermometers can be used to take oral, rectal, axillary, and/or groin temperatures. Most facilities have electronic thermometers with blue probes for oral use and red probes for axillary or rectal use. To prevent cross-contamination, a disposable cover is placed over the thermometer probe

before the temperature is taken. By changing the disposable cover after each use, one unit can be used on many patients. Electronic digital thermometers are excellent for home use because they eliminate the hazard of a mercury spill that occurs when a clinical thermometer is broken (see figure 14-4). The small battery-operated unit usually will register the temperature in about 60 seconds on a digital display screen. Disposable probe covers prevent contamination of the probe. **Tympanic thermometers** are specialized electronic thermometers that record the aural temperature in the ear (see figure 14-5). A disposable plastic cover is placed on the ear probe. By inserting the probe into the auditory canal and pushing a scan button, the temperature is recorded on the screen within 1 to 2 seconds. It is important to read and follow instructions while using this thermometer to obtain an accurate reading.

Plastic or paper thermometers are used in some health care facilities (see figure 14-6). These thermometers contain special chemical dots or strips that change color when exposed to specific temperatures. Some types are placed on the forehead and skin temperature is recorded. Other types are used orally. Both types are used once and discarded.

Electronic and tympanic thermometers are easy to read because they have digital displays. Reading a glass clinical thermometer is a procedure that must be practiced. Hold it at eye level and rotate it slowly to find the solid column of mercury or alcohol (see figure 14-7). Read the thermometer at the point where the mercury or alcohol line ends. Each long line on a

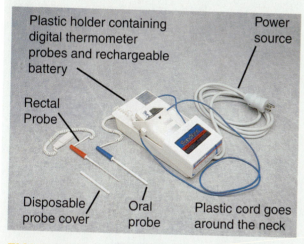

Plastic holder containing digital thermometer probes and rechargeable battery

Power source

Rectal Probe

Disposable probe cover

Oral probe

Plastic cord goes around the neck

FIGURE 14-3 An electronic thermometer registers the temperature in easy-to-read numbers on a viewer.

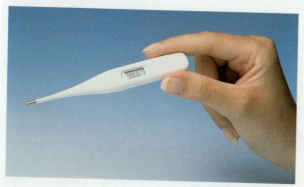

FIGURE 14-4 Electronic digital thermometers are excellent for home use. *(Courtesy of Omron Healthcare Inc., Vernon Hills, IL)*

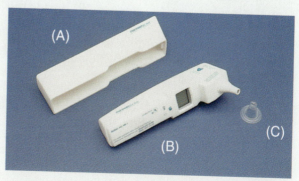

(A)

(B)

(C)

FIGURE 14-5 Tympanic thermometers record the aural temperature in the ear. *Parts include: (A) holder, (B) thermometer, and (C) disposable cover.*

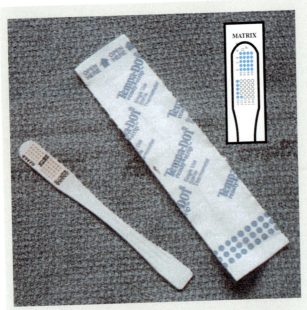

FIGURE 14-6 Plastic disposable thermometers have chemical dots that change color to register body temperature. The matrix shown reads 101°F.

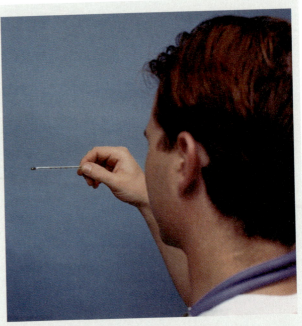

FIGURE 14-7 Hold a clinical thermometer at eye level to find the solid column of mercury or alcohol.

thermometer is read as one degree. An exception to this is the long line for 98.6°F (37°C), which is the normal oral body temperature. Each short line represents 0.2 (two-tenths) of a degree. Temperature is always recorded to the next nearest two-tenths of a degree. In figure 14-8, the line ends at 98.6°F. Top figures explain the markings for each line.

C To record the temperature, write 98^6 instead of 98.6. This reduces the possibility of making an error in reading. For example, a temperature of 100.2 could easily be read as 102. By writing 100^2, the chance of error decreases. If a temperature is taken orally, it is not necessary to indicate that it is an oral reading. If it is taken rectally, place an (R) beside the recording. If it is taken in the axillary area, place an (Ax) beside the recording. If it is taken tympanically (aurally), place a (T) beside the recording. For example:

- 98^6 is an oral reading
- 99^6 (R) is a rectal reading
- 97^6 (Ax) is an axillary reading
- 98^6 (T) is an aural reading

Eating, drinking hot or cold liquids, and/or smoking can alter the temperature in the mouth. It is important to make sure the patient has *not* had anything to eat or drink, or has *not*

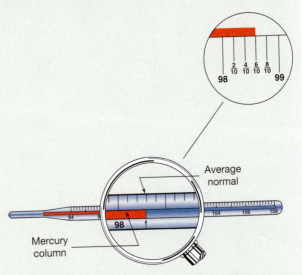

FIGURE 14-8 Each line on a thermometer equals two-tenths of a degree, so the thermometer shown reads 98.6°F.

smoked for at least 15 minutes prior to taking the patient's oral temperature. If the patient has done any of these things, explain why you cannot take the temperature and that you will return to do so.

Thermometers must be cleaned thoroughly after use. The procedure used varies with different agencies. In some agencies, the glass thermometer is washed and rinsed. Cool water is used to prevent breakage and to avoid destroying the column of mercury. The thermometer is then soaked in a disinfectant solution (frequently 70-percent alcohol) for a minimum of 30 minutes before it is used again. Other agencies cover the glass thermometer with a plastic sheath that is discarded after use (see figure 14-9). The probe on electronic thermometers is covered with a plastic sheath that is discarded after each use. These covers prevent the thermometers from coming into contact with each patient's mouth or skin and prevent transmission of germs. Follow your agency's policy for cleaning and care of thermometers.

STUDENT: *Go to the workbook and complete the assignment sheet for 14:2, Measuring and Recording Temperature. Then return and continue with the procedures.*

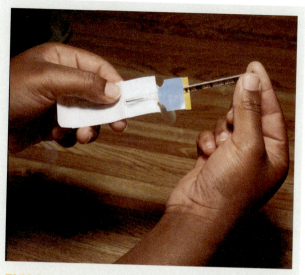

FIGURE 14-9 A clinical thermometer can be covered with a plastic sheath that is discarded after each use.

PROCEDURE 14:2A

OBRA

Cleaning a Clinical Thermometer

Equipment and Supplies

Thermometers, soapy cotton balls, small trash bag or waste can, running water, soaking basin with 70-percent alcohol, alcohol sponges or cotton balls, dry cotton balls or gauze pads, thermometer holder, disposable gloves

Procedure

1. Assemble equipment.
2. Wash hands. Put on gloves if needed.
   CAUTION: Follow standard precautions. Wear gloves if the thermometer was used for an oral or rectal temperature and was not covered with a plastic sheath.
3. After using the thermometer, use a soapy cotton ball or gauze pad to wipe the thermometer once from the top toward the tip or bulb (see figure 14-10A). Discard the soiled cotton ball in trash bag or waste can.
   NOTE: Rotate the thermometer while wiping it to clean all sides and parts.

4. With the bulb pointed downward, hold the thermometer by the stem and rinse the thermometer in cool water.
   CAUTION: Hot water will break the thermometer or destroy the mercury column.
5. Shake the thermometer down to 96°F (35.6°C) or lower.
   CAUTION: Hold the thermometer securely between your thumb and index finger. Use a snapping motion of the wrist. Avoid countertops, tables, and other surfaces.
6. Place the thermometer in a small basin or container filled with disinfectant solution (usually 70-percent alcohol). Make sure the thermometer is completely covered by the solution (see figure 14-10B).
   NOTE: Thirty minutes is usually the minimum time recommended for soaking.
7. Remove gloves and wash hands.
8. After 30 minutes, remove the thermometer from the soaking solution and use an alcohol

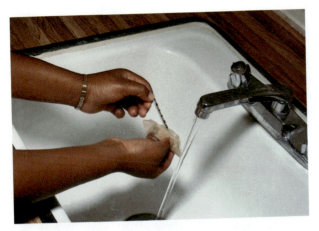

FIGURE 14-10A After each use, use a soapy cotton ball or gauze to wipe the thermometer in a circular motion from the stem to the bulb.

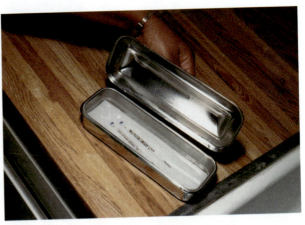

FIGURE 14-10B Soak the thermometer in a disinfectant solution for a minimum of 30 minutes.

cotton ball or alcohol sponge to wipe it from the stem toward the bulb. This removes any sediment from the thermometer.

9. Rinse the thermometer in cool water. Examine it carefully for any signs of breakage. Discard any broken thermometers according to the agency policy for disposal of mercury or mercury-containing items.

10. Read the thermometer to be sure it reads 96°F (35.6°C) or lower. Place it in a clean gauze-lined container. It is now ready for use.

    NOTE: Many health care agencies fill the container or thermometer holder with a disinfectant, usually 70-percent alcohol.

11. Replace all equipment used.

12. Remove gloves and discard in infectious container. Wash hands.

    NOTE: This procedure may vary according to agency policy.

Practice *Go to the workbook and use the evaluation sheet for 14:2A, Cleaning a Clinical Thermometer, to practice this procedure. When you feel you have mastered this skill, sign the sheet and give it to your instructor for further action.*

 Final Checkpoint   Using the criteria listed on the evaluation sheet, your instructor will grade your performance.

PROCEDURE 14:2B   OBRA

Measuring and Recording Oral Temperature

Equipment and Supplies

Oral thermometer, plastic sheath (if used), holder with disinfectant solution, tissues or dry cotton balls, container for used tissues, watch with second hand, soapy cotton balls, disposable gloves, notepaper, pencil/pen

Procedure

1. Assemble equipment.
2. Wash hands and put on gloves.

   CAUTION: Follow standard precautions for contact with saliva or the mucous membrane of the mouth.

3. Introduce yourself. Identify the patient. Explain the procedure.

4. Position the patient comfortably. Ask the patient if he/she has eaten, has had hot or cold fluids, or has smoked in the past 15 minutes.
   NOTE: Eating, drinking liquids, or smoking can affect the temperature in the mouth. Wait at least 15 minutes if the patient says "yes" to your question.

5. Remove the clean thermometer by the upper end. Use a clean tissue or dry cotton ball to wipe the thermometer from stem to bulb.
   NOTE: If the thermometer was soaking in a disinfectant, rinse first in cool water.
   (!) CAUTION: Hold the thermometer securely to avoid breaking.

6. Read the thermometer to be sure it reads 96°F (35.6°C) or lower. Check carefully for chips or breaks.
   (!) CAUTION: Never use a cracked thermometer because it may injure the patient.
   NOTE: If a plastic sheath is used, place it on the thermometer after checking for damage.

7. Insert the bulb under the patient's tongue, toward the side of the mouth (see figure 14-11). Ask the patient to hold it in place with the lips, and caution against biting it.
   NOTE: Check to be sure patient's mouth is closed.

8. Leave the thermometer in place for 3 to 5 minutes.
   NOTE: Some agencies require that the thermometer be left in place for 5 to 8 minutes. Follow your agency's policy.

9. Remove the thermometer. Hold it by the stem and use a tissue or cotton ball to wipe toward the bulb.
   NOTE: If a plastic sheath was used to cover the thermometer, there is no need to wipe the thermometer. Simply remove the sheath, taking care not to touch the part that was in the patient's mouth.
   (!) CAUTION: Do *not* hold the bulb end. This could alter the reading because of the warmth of your hand.

10. Read the thermometer. Record the reading on notepaper.
    NOTE: Recheck the reading and your notation for accuracy.
    NOTE: If the reading is less than 97°F, reinsert the thermometer in the patient's mouth for 1 to 2 minutes.

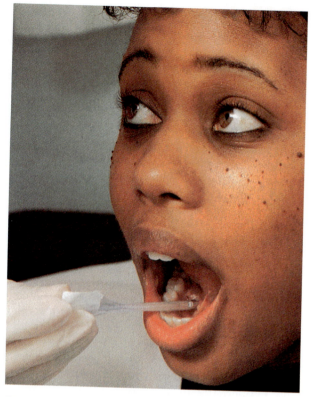

FIGURE 14-11 Insert the bulb of the thermometer under the patient's tongue (sublingually).

11. Clean the thermometer as instructed. Shake down to 96°F (35.6°C) or lower for next use.

12. Check the patient for comfort and safety before leaving.

13. Replace all equipment.

14. Remove gloves and discard in infectious waste container. Wash hands.

15. **C** Record required information on the patient's chart or agency form, for example, date and time, T 98^6, your signature and title. Report any abnormal reading to your supervisor immediately.

Practice *Go to the workbook and use the evaluation sheet for 14:2B, Measuring and Recording Oral Temperature, to practice this procedure. When you feel you have mastered this skill, sign the sheet and give it to your instructor for further action.*

 Final Checkpoint Using the criteria listed on the evaluation sheet, your instructor will grade your performance.

PROCEDURE 14:2C

OBRA

Measuring and Recording Rectal Temperature

Equipment and Supplies

Rectal thermometer, plastic sheath (if used), lubricant, tissues/cotton balls, waste bag or container, watch with second hand, paper, pencil/pen, soapy cotton ball, disposable gloves
NOTE: A manikin is frequently used to practice this procedure.

Procedure

1. Assemble equipment.
2. Wash hands and put on gloves.

   CAUTION: Follow standard precautions if contact with rectal discharge is possible.
3. Introduce yourself. Identify the patient. Explain the procedure. Screen unit, draw curtains, and/or close door to provide privacy for the patient.
4. Remove rectal thermometer from its container. If the thermometer was soaking in a disinfectant, hold it by the stem end and rinse in cool water. Use a dry tissue/cotton ball to wipe from stem to bulb. Check that the thermometer reads 96°F (35.6°C) or lower. Check condition of thermometer. If a plastic sheath is used, position it on the thermometer.

   CAUTION: Breaks in a thermometer can injure the patient. Never use a cracked thermometer.
5. Place a small amount of lubricant on the tissue. Roll the bulb end of the thermometer in the lubricant to coat it. Leave the lubricated thermometer on the tissue until the patient is properly positioned.
6. Turn the patient on his or her side. If possible, use Sims' position (lying on left side with right leg bent up near the abdomen). Infants are usually placed on their backs, with legs raised and held securely, or on their abdomens (see figure 14-12).
7. Fold back covers just enough to expose the anal area.

   NOTE: Avoid exposing the patient unnecessarily.

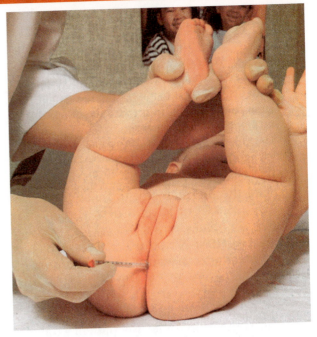

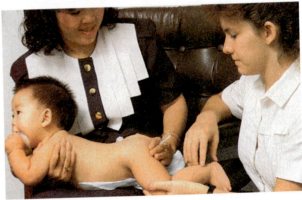

FIGURE 4-12 The infant can be positioned on the back or abdomen for a rectal temperature.

8. With one hand, raise the upper buttock gently. With the other hand, insert the lubricated thermometer approximately 1 to 1½ inches (½ to 1 inch for an infant) into the rectum. Tell the patient what you are doing.

   NOTE: At times, rotating the thermometer slightly will make it easier to insert.

   CAUTION: Never force the thermometer. It can break. If you are unable to insert it, obtain assistance.

9. Replace the covers. Keep your hand on the thermometer the entire time it is in place.

   ⚠ CAUTION: *Never* let go of the thermometer. It could slide further into the rectum or break.

10. Hold the thermometer in place for 3 to 5 minutes.

11. Remove the thermometer gently. Tell the patient what you are doing.

12. Remove plastic sheath, if used, and discard it or use a tissue to remove excess lubricant from the thermometer. Wipe from stem to bulb. Hold by the stem area only. Discard the tissue into a waste container.

13. Read and record. Recheck your reading for accuracy. Remember to place an (R) next to the recording to indicate a rectal temperature was taken.

14. Reposition the patient. Observe all safety checkpoints before leaving the patient.

15. Clean the thermometer as instructed in Procedure 14:2A, Cleaning a Clinical Thermometer.

16. Replace all equipment.

17. Remove gloves and discard in infectious waste container. Wash hands.

18. **C** Record required information on the patient's chart or agency form, for example, date and time, T 99^6 (R), your signature and title. Report any abnormal reading immediately to your supervisor.

Practice *Go to the workbook and use the evaluation sheet for 14:2C, Measuring and Recording Rectal Temperature, to practice this procedure. When you feel you have mastered this skill, sign the sheet and give it to your instructor for further action.*

 Final Checkpoint Using the criteria listed on the evaluation sheet, your instructor will grade your performance.

PROCEDURE 14:2D
OBRA

Measuring and Recording Axillary Temperature

Equipment and Supplies

Oral thermometer, plastic sheath (if used), disposable gloves (if needed), tissues/cotton balls, towel, waste container, watch with second hand, paper, pencil/pen, soapy cotton ball

Procedure

1. Assemble equipment.

2. Wash hands. Put on gloves if necessary.

   ⚠ CAUTION: Follow standard precautions if contact with open sores or body fluids is possible.

3. Introduce yourself. Identify the patient. Explain the procedure.

4. Remove oral thermometer from its container. Use a tissue to wipe from stem to bulb. Check thermometer for damaged areas. Read the thermometer to be sure it reads below 96°F (36.5°C). Place a plastic sheath on the thermometer, if used.

5. Expose the axilla and use a towel to pat the armpit dry.

   NOTE: Moisture can alter a temperature reading. Do not rub area hard because this too can alter the reading.

6. Raise the patient's arm and place the bulb end of the thermometer in the hollow of the axilla (see figure 14-13). Bring the arm over the chest and rest the hand on the opposite shoulder.

   NOTE: This position holds the thermometer in place.

7. Leave the thermometer in place for 10 minutes.

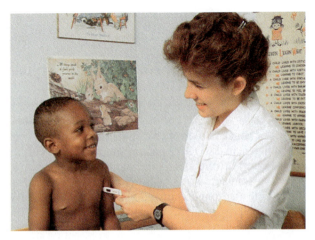

FIGURE 14-13 To take an axillary temperature, insert the bulb end of the thermometer in the hollow of the axilla or armpit.

8. Remove the thermometer. Remove sheath, if used, and discard. Wipe from stem to bulb to remove moisture. Hold by the stem end only.
   ⚠ **CAUTION:** Holding the bulb end will change the reading.

9. Read and record. Check your reading for accuracy. Remember to mark (Ax) by the recording to indicate axillary temperature.

10. Reposition the patient. Be sure to check for safety and comfort before leaving.

11. Clean the thermometer as instructed.

12. Replace all equipment used.

13. Remove gloves and discard in an infectious waste container. Wash hands.

14. Ⓒ Record required information on the patient's chart or agency form, for example, date and time, T 97^6 (Ax), your signature and title. Report any abnormal reading immediately to your supervisor.

Practice *Go to the workbook and use the evaluation sheet for 14:2D, Measuring and Recording Axillary Temperature, to practice this procedure. When you feel you have mastered this skill, sign the sheet and give it to your instructor for further action.*

✔ **Final Checkpoint** Using the criteria listed on the evaluation sheet, your instructor will grade your performance.

PROCEDURE 14:2E   OBRA

Measuring and Recording Tympanic (Aural) Temperature

Equipment and Supplies

Tympanic thermometer, probe cover, paper, pencil/pen, container for soiled probe cover

Procedure

1. Assemble equipment.
   NOTE: Read the operating instructions so you understand exactly how the thermometer must be used.

2. Wash hands. Put on gloves if needed.
   ☣ **CAUTION:** Follow standard precautions if contact with open sores or body fluids is possible.

3. Introduce yourself. Identify the patient. Explain the procedure.

4. Remove the thermometer from its base. Set the thermometer on the proper mode according to operating instructions. The equal mode is usually used for newborn infants, the rectal mode for children under

3 years of age, and the oral mode for children over 3 years of age and all adults. In areas where core body temperatures are recorded, such as critical care units, the core mode may be used.

5. Install a probe cover according to instructions. This will usually activate the thermometer, showing the mode selected and the word *ready,* indicating the thermometer is ready for use.

   ! **CAUTION:** Do not use the thermometer until *ready* is displayed because inaccurate readings will result.

6. Position the patient. Infants under 1 year of age should be positioned lying flat with the head turned for easy access to the ear. Small children can be held on the parent's lap, with the head held against the parent's chest for support. Adults who can cooperate and hold the head steady can either sit or lie flat. Patients in bed should have the head turned to the side, and stabilized against the pillow.

7. Hold the thermometer in your right hand to take a temperature in the right ear, and in your left hand to take a temperature in the left ear. With your other hand, pull the ear pinna (external lobe) up and back on any child over 1 year of age and on adults. Pull the ear pinna straight back for infants under 1 year of age.

   NOTE: Pulling the pinna correctly straightens the auditory canal so the probe tip will point directly at the tympanic membrane.

8. Insert the covered probe into the ear canal as far as possible to seal the canal (see figure 14-14).

9. Hold the thermometer steady and press the scan or activation button. Hold it for the required amount of time, usually 1 to 2 seconds, until the reading is displayed on the screen.

10. Remove the thermometer from the patient's ear. Read and record the temperature. Place a (T) by the recording to indicate tympanic temperature.

    NOTE: The temperature will remain on the screen until the probe cover is removed.

    ! **CAUTION:** If the temperature reading is low or does not appear to be accurate,

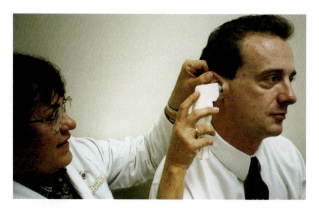

FIGURE 14-14 Insert the covered probe of the tympanic thermometer into the ear canal as far as possible to seal the canal.

change the probe cover and repeat the procedure. The opposite ear can be used for comparison.

11. Press the eject button on the thermometer to discard the probe cover into a waste container.

12. Return the thermometer to its base.

13. Reposition the patient. Observe all safety checkpoints before leaving the patient.

14. Remove gloves and discard in an infectious waste container. Wash hands.

15. **C** Record required information on the patient's chart or agency form, for example, date and time, T 98⁰ (T), your signature and title. Report any abnormal reading immediately to your supervisor.

Practice *Go to the workbook and use the evaluation sheet for 14:2E, Measuring and Recording Tympanic (Aural) Temperature, to practice this procedure. When you feel you have mastered this skill, sign the sheet and give it to your instructor for further action.*

 Final Checkpoint Using the criteria listed on the evaluation sheet, your instructor will grade your performance.

PROCEDURE 14:2F

OBRA

Measuring Temperature with an Electronic Thermometer

Equipment and Supplies

Electronic thermometer with probe, sheath (probe cover), paper, pen/pencil, container for soiled sheath

Procedure

1. Assemble equipment.
   NOTE: Read the operating instructions for the electronic thermometer so you understand how the particular model operates.
2. Wash hands. Put on gloves.
   CAUTION: Follow standard precautions and wear gloves if you are taking a rectal or oral temperature.
3. Introduce yourself. Identify the patient. Explain the procedure.
4. Position the patient comfortably and correctly.
   NOTE: For an oral temperature, ask the patient if he/she has eaten, has had hot or cold fluids, or has smoked in the past 15 minutes. Wait at least 15 minutes if the patient answers "yes."
   NOTE: For a rectal temperature, position the patient in Sims' position if possible.
5. If the probe has to be connected to the thermometer unit, insert the probe into the correct receptacle. If the thermometer has an "on" or "activate" button, push the button to turn on the thermometer.
6. Cover the probe with the sheath or probe cover.
   NOTE: For a rectal temperature, the sheath must be lubricated.
7. Insert the covered probe into the desired location. Most probes are heavy, so it is usually necessary to hold the probe in position (see figure 14-15A).
   CAUTION: Hold on to the probe at all times for a rectal temperature.
8. When the unit signals that the temperature has been recorded, remove the probe.
   NOTE: Many electronic thermometers have an audible "beep." Others indicate that tem-perature has been recorded when the numbers stop flashing and become stationary.
9. Read and record the temperature. Recheck your reading for accuracy.
   NOTE: Remember to place an (R) next to rectal readings or an (Ax) next to axillary readings.
10. Without touching the sheath or probe cover, remove it from the probe (see figure 14-15B). Many thermometers have a button you push to remove the sheath. Discard the sheath in an infectious waste container.
11. Reposition the patient. Observe all safety checkpoints before leaving the patient.
12. Return the probe to the correct storage position in the thermometer unit. Turn off the

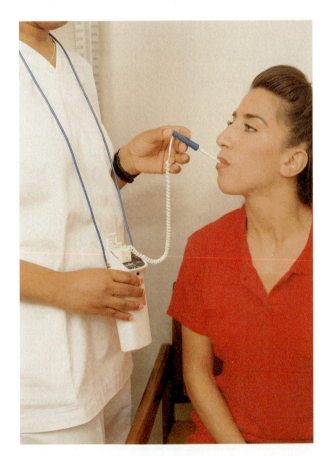

FIGURE 14-15A While taking a temperature, hold the probe of the electronic thermometer in place.

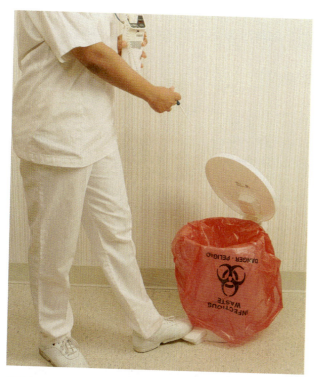

FIGURE 14-15B Discard the probe cover in an infectious waste container without touching the cover.

unit if this is necessary. Place the unit in the charging stand if the model has a charging unit.

13. Replace all equipment.

14. Remove gloves and discard in an infectious waste container. Wash hands.

15. **C** Record required information on the patient's chart or agency form, for example, date and time, T 98⁸, your signature and title. Report any abnormal reading immediately to your supervisor.

Practice *Go to the workbook and use the evaluation sheet for 14:2F, Measuring Temperature with an Electronic Thermometer, to practice this procedure. When you feel you have mastered this skill, sign the sheet and give it to your instructor for further action.*

Final Checkpoint Using the criteria listed on the evaluation sheet, your instructor will grade your performance.

14:3 INFORMATION
Measuring and Recording Pulse

OBRA Pulse is a vital sign that you will be required to take. There are certain facts you must know when you take this measurement. This section provides the main information.

 Pulse is defined as "the pressure of the blood pushing against the wall of an artery as the heart beats and rests." In other words, it is a throbbing of the arteries that is caused by the contractions of the heart. The pulse is more easily felt in arteries that lie fairly close to the skin and can be pressed against a bone by the fingers.

The pulse can be felt at different arterial sites on the body. Some of the major sites are shown in figure 14-16 and include:

◆ temporal—at the side of the forehead

◆ carotid—at the neck

◆ brachial—inner aspect of forearm at the antecubital space (crease of the elbow)

◆ radial—at the inner aspect of the wrist, above the thumb

◆ femoral—at the inner aspect of the upper thigh

◆ popliteal—behind the knee

◆ dorsalis pedis—at the top of the foot arch

NOTE: Pulse is usually taken over the radial artery.

Pulse rate is measured as the number of beats per minute. Pulse rates vary among individuals, depending on age, sex, and body size:

◆ Adults have a general range of 60 to 90 beats per minute.

◆ Adult men: 60 to 70 beats per minute.

◆ Adult women: 65 to 80 beats per minute.

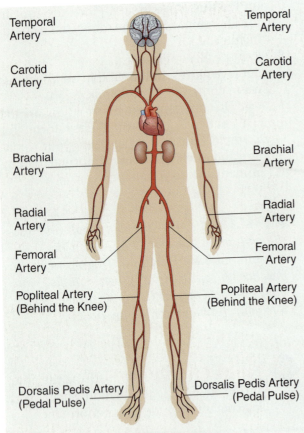

Temporal Artery
Temporal Artery
Carotid Artery
Carotid Artery
Brachial Artery
Brachial Artery
Radial Artery
Radial Artery
Femoral Artery
Femoral Artery
Popliteal Artery (Behind the Knee)
Popliteal Artery (Behind the Knee)
Dorsalis Pedis Artery (Pedal Pulse)
Dorsalis Pedis Artery (Pedal Pulse)

FIGURE 14-16 Major pulse sites.

◆ Children aged over 7: 70 to 90 beats per minute.

◆ Children aged from 1 to 7: range of 80 to 110 beats per minute.

◆ Infants: 100 to 160 beats per minute.

◆ **Bradycardia** is a pulse rate under 60 beats per minute.

◆ **Tachycardia** is a pulse rate over 100 beats per minute (except in children).

NOTE: Any variations or extremes in pulse rates should be reported immediately.

Rhythm of the pulse is also noted. Rhythm refers to the regularity of the pulse, or the spacing of the beats. It is described as *regular* or *irregular*. An **arrhythmia** is an irregular or abnormal rhythm, usually caused by a defect in the electrical conduction pattern of the heart.

Volume, or the strength or intensity of the pulse, is also noted. It is described by words such as *strong, weak, thready,* or *bounding.*

Various factors will change pulse rate. Increased, or accelerated, rates can be caused by exercise, stimulant drugs, excitement, fever, shock, nervous tension, and other similar factors. Decreased, or slower, rates can be caused by sleep, depressant drugs, heart disease, coma, physical training, and other similar factors.

STUDENT: *Go to the workbook and complete the assignment sheet for 14:3, Measuring and Recording Pulse. Then return and continue with the procedure.*

PROCEDURE 14:3

OBRA

Measuring and Recording Radial Pulse

Equipment and Supplies

Watch with second hand, paper, pencil/pen

Procedure

1. Assemble equipment.
2. Wash hands.
3. Introduce yourself. Identify the patient. Explain the procedure.

4. Place the patient in a comfortable position, with the arm supported and the palm of the hand turned downward.
   NOTE: If the forearm rests on the chest, it will be easier to count respirations after taking the pulse.

5. With the tips of your first two or three fingers, locate the pulse on the thumb side of the patient's wrist (see figure 14-17).

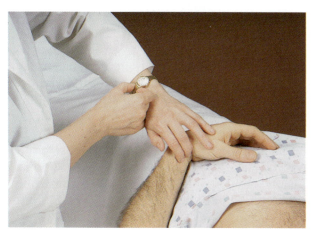

FIGURE 14-17 To count a radial pulse, put the tips of two or three fingers on the thumb side of the patient's wrist.

NOTE: Do not use your thumb; use your fingers. The thumb contains a pulse that you may confuse with the patient's pulse.

6. When the pulse is felt, exert slight pressure and start counting. Use the second hand of the watch and count for 1 full minute.

    NOTE: In some agencies, the pulse is counted for 30 seconds and the final number multiplied by 2. To detect irregularities, it is better to count for 1 full minute.

7. While counting the pulse, also note the volume (character or strength) and the rhythm (regularity).
8. Record the following information: date, time, rate, rhythm, and volume. Follow your agency's policy for recording.
9. Check the patient before leaving. Observe all safety precautions to protect the patient.
10. Replace all equipment used.
11. Wash hands.
12. **C** Record all required information on the patient's chart or agency form, for example, date, time, P 82 strong and regular, your signature and title. Report any unusual observations immediately to your supervisor.

Practice *Go to the workbook and use the evaluation sheet for 14:3, Measuring and Recording Radial Pulse, to practice this procedure. When you feel you have mastered this skill, sign the sheet and give it to your instructor for further action.*

Final Checkpoint Using the criteria listed on the evaluation sheet, your instructor will grade your performance.

INFORMATION

14:4 Measuring and Recording Respirations

OBRA Respirations are another vital sign that you must observe, count, and record correctly. This section provides the main points you must note when counting and recording the quality of respirations.

Respiration is the process of taking in oxygen (O_2) and expelling carbon dioxide (CO_2) from the lungs and respiratory tract. One respiration consists of one inspiration (breathing in) and one expiration (breathing out).

The normal rate for respirations in adults is 14 to 18 breaths per minute, although wider ranges may be observed (12 to 20 breaths per minute). In children, respirations are slightly faster than those for adults and average 16 to 25 per minute. In infants, the rate may be 30 to 50 per minute.

In addition to rate, the character and rhythm of respirations should be noted. **Character** refers to the depth and quality of respirations. Words used to describe character include *deep, shallow, labored, difficult, stertorous* (abnormal sounds like snoring), and *moist.* Rhythm refers to the regularity of respirations, or equal spacing between breaths. It is described as *regular* or *irregular.*

The following terminology is used to describe abnormal respirations:

◆ **dyspnea**—difficult or labored breathing.
◆ **apnea**—absence of respirations, usually temporary.

◆ **tachypnea**—respiratory rate above 25 respirations per minute.

◆ **bradypnea**—slow respiratory rate, usually below 10 respirations per minute.

◆ **orthopnea**—severe dyspnea in which breathing is very difficult in any position other than sitting erect or standing.

◆ **Cheyne–Stokes** respirations—periods of dyspnea followed by periods of apnea; frequently noted in the dying patient.

◆ **rales**—bubbling or noisy sounds caused by fluids or mucus in the air passages.

◆ **wheezing**—difficult breathing with a high-pitched whistling or sighing sound during expiration; caused by a narrowing of bronchioles (as seen in asthma) and/or an obstruction or mucus accumulation in the bronchi.

◆ **cyanosis**—a dusky, bluish discoloration of the skin, lips, and/or nail beds as a result of decreased oxygen and increased carbon dioxide in the bloodstream.

Respirations must be counted in such a way that the patient is unaware of the procedure. Because respirations are partially under voluntary control, patients may breathe more quickly or more slowly when they become aware of the fact that respirations are being counted. Do not tell the patient you are counting respirations. Also, leave your hand on the pulse site while counting respirations. The patient will think you are still counting pulse and will not be likely to alter the respiratory rate.

STUDENT: *Go to the workbook and complete the assignment sheet for 14:4, Measuring and Recording Respirations. Then return and continue with the procedure.*

PROCEDURE 14:4

OBRA

Measuring and Recording Respirations

Equipment and Supplies

Watch with second hand, paper, pen/pencil

Procedure

1. Assemble equipment.
2. Wash hands.
3. Introduce yourself. Identify the patient.
4. After the pulse rate has been counted, leave your hand in position on the pulse site and count the number of times the chest rises and falls during one minute (see figure 14-18).

   NOTE: This is done so the patient is not aware that respirations are being counted. If patients are aware, they can alter their rate of breathing.
5. Count each expiration and inspiration as one respiration.
6. Note the depth (character) and rhythm (regularity) of the respirations.

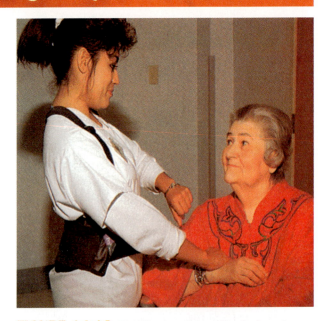

FIGURE 14-18 Positioning the patient's hand on his or her chest makes it easier to count pulse and respiration.

7. Record the following information: date, time, rate, character, and rhythm.
8. Check the patient before leaving the area. Observe all safety precautions to protect the patient.
9. Replace all equipment.
10. Wash hands.
11. **C** Record all required information on the patient's chart or agency form, for example, date, time, R 16 deep and regular (or even), your signature and title. Report any unusual observations immediately to your supervisor.

Practice *Go to the workbook and use the evaluation sheet for 14:4, Measuring and Recording Respirations, to practice this procedure. When you feel you have mastered this skill, sign the sheet and give it to your instructor for further action.*

✔ Final Checkpoint Using the criteria listed on the evaluation sheet, your instructor will grade your performance.

14:5 INFORMATION
Graphing TPR

C In some agencies, you may be required to chart temperature, pulse, and respirations (TPR) on graphic records. This section provides basic information about these records.

Graphic sheets are special records used for recording temperature, pulse, and respirations. The forms vary in different health care facilities, but all contain the same basic information. The graphic chart presents a visual diagram of variations in a patient's vital signs. The progress is easier to follow than a list of numbers that give the same information. Graphic charts are used most often in hospitals and long-term-care facilities. However, similar records may be kept in medical offices or other health care facilities. Patients are sometimes taught how to maintain these records.

Some charts make use of color coding. For example, temperature is recorded in blue ink, pulse is recorded in red ink, and respirations are recorded in green ink. Other agencies use blue ink for 7 AM to 7 PM (days) and red ink for 7 PM to 7 AM (nights). Follow the policy of your institution.

Factors that affect vital signs are often included on the graph. Examples include surgery, medications that lower temperature (such as aspirin), and antibiotics.

 The graph is a medical record, so it must be neat, legible, and accurate. Double check all information recorded on the graph. If an error occurs, it should be crossed out carefully with red ink and initialed. Correct information should then be inserted on the graph.

STUDENT: *Read the complete procedure for 14:5, Graphing TPR. Then go back and start doing the procedure. Your assignment will follow the procedure.*

PROCEDURE 14:5
Graphing TPR

Equipment and Supplies
Blank TPR graphic sheets in the workbook, TPR sample graph, assignment sheets on graphing in the workbook, pen, ruler

Procedure
1. Assemble equipment.
2. Examine the sample graphic sheet (see figure 14-19). This will vary, depending on the

GRAPHIC CHART

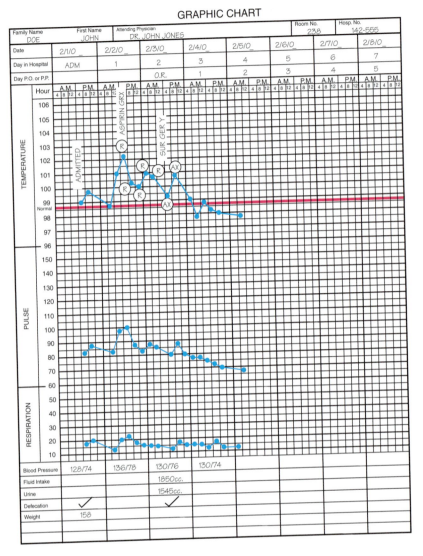

FIGURE 14-19 A sample graphic sheet.

agency. However, most graphic sheets contain time blocks across the top and number blocks for TPRs on the side. Note areas for recording temperature, pulse, and respirations. Refer to the example while completing the procedure steps.

3. Using a blank graphic sheet, fill in patient information in the spaces provided at the top. Write last name first in most cases. Be sure patient identification, hospital, and room number are accurate.

   NOTE: Forms vary. Follow directions as they apply to your form.

4. Fill in the dates in the spaces provided after DATE.

   NOTE: A graphic chart provides a day-to-day visual representation of the variations in a patient's TPRs.

5. If your chart calls for DAY IN HOSPITAL below the dates, enter *Adm.* under the first date. This stands for day of admission. The second date would then be day *1*, or first full day in the hospital. The third date would be day *2*, and so forth.

6. Some graphs contain a third line, DAYS P.O. or PP, which means days post-op (after surgery) or postpartum (after delivery of a baby). The day of surgery would be shown as O.R. or *Surgery*. The next day would be day *1*, or first day after surgery. The day of delivery of a baby is shown as *Del.*, with the next day as day *1*, or first day after delivery. Numbers continue in sequence for each following day.

7. Go to the Assignment Sheet #1. Note the TPRs. On the graphic sheet, find the correct

Date and Time column. Move down the column until the correct temperature number is found on the side of the chart. Mark this with a dot (•) in the box. Do the same for the pulse and respirations.

> ⚠ **CAUTION:** Double check your notations. Be sure they are accurate.

> ✔ **CHECKPOINT:** Your instructor will check your notations.

8. Repeat step 7 for the next TPR. Check to be sure you are in the correct time column. Mark the dots clearly under the time column and at the correct temperature measurement, pulse rate, or respiration rate.

9. Use a straight paper edge or ruler to connect the dots for temperature. Do the same with the dots for pulse and, finally, with the dots for respiration.

   NOTE: A ruler makes the line straight and neat, and the readings are more legible.

10. Continue to graph the remaining TPRs from Assignment Sheet #1. Double check all entries for accuracy. Use a ruler to connect all dots for each of the vital signs.

11. Any drug that might alter or change temperature or other vital signs is usually noted on the graph in the time column closest to the time when the drug was first given. Turn the paper sideways and write the name of the drug in the correct time column. Aspirin is often recorded in this column because it lowers temperature. A rapid drop in body temperature would be readily explained by the word *aspirin* in the time column. Antibiotics and medications that alter heart rate are also noted in many cases.

12. Other events in a patient's hospitalization are also recorded in the time column. Examples include surgery and discharge. In some hospitals, if the patient is placed in isolation, this is also noted on the graph.

13. Blood pressure, weight, height, defecation (bowel movements), and other similar kinds of information are often recorded in special areas at the bottom of the graphic record. Record any information required in the correct areas on your form.

14. Recheck your graph for neatness, accuracy, and completeness of information.

> **Practice** *Go to the workbook and complete Assignment Sheet #1 for Graphing TPR. Give it to your instructor for grading. Note all changes. Then complete Assignment Sheet #2 for graphing TPR in the workbook. Repeat this process by completing Graphing TPR assignments #3 to #5 until you have mastered graphic records.*

 Final Checkpoint Your instructor will grade your performance on this skill according to the accuracy of the completed assignments.

14:6   INFORMATION
Measuring and Recording Apical Pulse

At times, you will be required to take an apical pulse. This section provides basic information on this topic.

An **apical pulse** is a pulse count taken with a **stethoscope** at the apex of the heart. The actual heartbeat is heard and counted. A stethoscope is an instrument used to listen to internal body sounds. The stethoscope amplifies the sounds so they are easier to hear. Parts of the stethoscope include the earpieces, tubing, and bell or thin, flexible disk called a *diaphragm* (see figure 14-20). The tips of the earpieces should be bent forward when they are placed in the ears. The earpieces should fit snugly but should not cause pain or discomfort. To prevent the spread of microorganisms, the earpieces and bell/diaphragm of the stethoscope should be cleaned with a disinfectant such as alcohol before and after every use.

Usually, a physician orders an apical pulse. It is frequently ordered for patients with irregular heartbeats, hardening of the arteries, or weak or

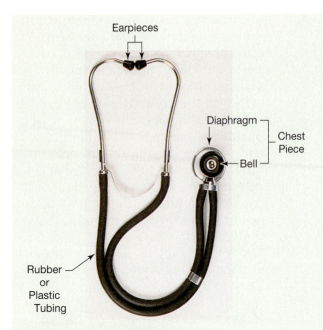

Earpieces

Diaphragm

Chest Piece

Bell

Rubber or Plastic Tubing

FIGURE 14-20 Parts of a stethoscope.

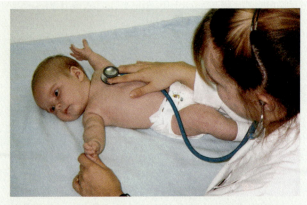

FIGURE 14-21 An apical pulse is frequently taken on infants and small children because their pulses are more rapid.

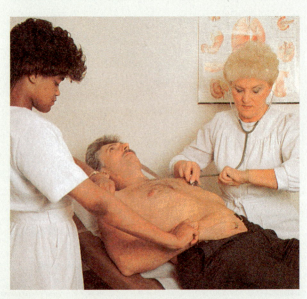

FIGURE 14-22 To determine a pulse deficit, one person should count an apical pulse while another person is counting a radial pulse.

rapid radial pulses. Because children and infants have very rapid radial pulse counts, apical pulse counts are usually taken (see figure 14-21). It is generally easier to count a rapid pulse while listening to it (through a stethoscope) than by feeling it with your fingers.

It is important that you protect the patient's privacy when counting an apical pulse. Avoid exposing the patient during this procedure.

Two separate heart sounds are heard while listening to the heartbeat. The sounds resemble a "lubb-dupp." Each lubb-dupp counts as one heartbeat. The sounds are caused by the closing of the heart valves as blood flows through the chambers of the heart. Any abnormal sounds or beats should be reported immediately to your supervisor.

A **pulse deficit** is a condition that occurs with some heart conditions. In some cases, the heart is weak and does not pump enough blood to produce a pulse. In other cases, the heart beats too fast (tachycardia), and there is not enough time for the heart to fill with blood; therefore, the heart does not produce a pulse during each beat. In such cases, the apical pulse rate is higher than the pulse rate at other pulse sites on the body. For the most accurate determination of a pulse deficit, one person should check the apical pulse while a second person checks another pulse site, usually the radial

pulse (see figure 14-22). If this is not possible, one person should first check the apical pulse and then immediately check the radial pulse. Then, subtract the rate of the radial pulse from the rate of the apical pulse. The difference is the pulse deficit. For example, if the apical pulse is 130 and the radial pulse is 92, the pulse deficit would be 38 (130 − 92 = 38).

STUDENT: *Go to the workbook and complete the assignment sheet for 14:6, Measuring and Recording Apical Pulse. Then return and continue with the procedure.*

PROCEDURE 14:6

Measuring and Recording Apical Pulse

Equipment and Supplies

Stethoscope, watch with second hand, paper, pencil/pen, alcohol or disinfectant swab

Procedure

1. Assemble equipment. Use alcohol or a disinfectant to wipe the earpieces and the bell/diaphragm of the stethoscope.
2. Wash hands.
3. Introduce yourself. Identify the patient and explain the procedure. If the patient is an infant or child, explain the procedure to the parent(s).

   NOTE: It is usually best to say, "I am going to listen to your heartbeat." Some patients do not know what an apical pulse is.
4. Close the door to the room. Screen the unit or draw curtains around the bed to provide privacy.
5. Uncover the left side of the patient's chest. The stethoscope must be placed directly against the skin.
6. Place the stethoscope tips in your ears. Locate the apex of the heart, 2 to 3 inches to the left of the breastbone. Use your index finger to locate the fifth intercostal (between the ribs) space at the midclavicular (collarbone) line (see figure 14-23). Place the bell/diaphragm over the apical region and listen for heart sounds.

   ! CAUTION: Be sure the tips of the stethoscope are facing forward before placing them in your ears.
7. Count the apical pulse for 1 full minute. Note the rate, rhythm, and volume.

   NOTE: Remember to count each lubb-dupp as one beat.
8. If you doubt your count, recheck your count for another minute.
9. Record your reading. Note date, time, rate, rhythm, and volume. Chart according to the agency policy. Some use an *A* and others use an *AP* to denote apical pulse.

   NOTE: If both a radial and apical pulse are taken, it may be recorded as A82/R82. If a pulse deficit exists, it should be noted. For example, with A80/R64, there

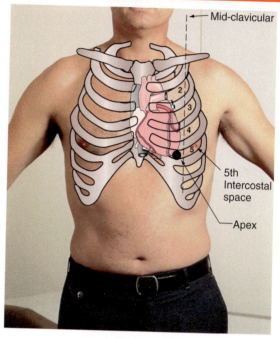

FIGURE 14-23 Locate the apex of the heart at the fifth intercostal (between the ribs) space by the midclavicular (middle of the collarbone) line.

is a pulse deficit of 16 (that is, 80 − 64 = 16). This would be recorded as A80/R64 Pulse deficit: 16.

10. Check all safety and comfort points before leaving the patient.
11. Use an alcohol or disinfectant swab to clean the earpieces and the bell/diaphragm of the stethoscope. Replace all equipment.
12. Wash hands.
13. **C** Record all required information on the patient's chart or agency form. For example: date, time, AP 86 strong and regular, your signature and title. If any abnormalities or changes were observed, note and report these immediately.

Practice *Go to the workbook and use the evaluation sheet for 14:6, Measuring and Recording Apical Pulse, to practice this procedure. When you feel you have mastered this skill, sign the sheet and give it to your instructor for further action.*

✔ **Final Checkpoint**   Using the criteria listed on the evaluation sheet, your instructor will grade your performance.

14:7 INFORMATION Measuring and Recording Blood Pressure

OBRA   Blood pressure (BP) is one of the vital signs you will be required to take. It is important that your recording be accurate and that you understand what the blood pressure reading means. This section provides basic information on this topic.

Blood pressure (BP) is a measurement of the pressure that the blood exerts on the walls of the arteries during the various stages of heart activity. Blood pressure is read in millimeters (mm) of mercury (Hg) on an instrument known as a **sphygmomanometer.**

There are two types of blood pressure measurements: systolic and diastolic. **Systolic** pressure occurs in the walls of the arteries when the left ventricle of the heart is contracting and pushing blood into the arteries.

◆ A normal systolic reading is 120 millimeters mercury (120 mm Hg).

◆ Normal range for systolic readings is from 100 to 140 mm Hg.

Diastolic pressure is the constant pressure in the walls of the arteries when the left ventricle of the heart is at rest, or between contractions. Blood has moved forward into the capillaries and veins, so the volume of blood in the arteries has decreased.

◆ A normal diastolic reading is 80 mm Hg.

◆ Normal range for diastolic readings is from 60 to 90 mm Hg.

Pulse pressure is the difference between systolic and diastolic pressure. The pulse pressure is an important indicator of the health and tone of arterial walls. A normal range for pulse pressure in adults is 30 to 50 mm Hg. For example, if the systolic pressure is 120 mm Hg and the diastolic pressure is 80 mm Hg, the pulse pressure is 40 mm Hg (120 minus 80 = 40).

Hypertension, or high blood pressure, is indicated when pressures are greater than 140 mm Hg systolic and 90 mm Hg diastolic. Common causes include stress, anxiety, obesity, high-salt intake, aging, kidney disease, thyroid deficiency, and vascular conditions such as arteriosclerosis. If hypertension is not treated, it can lead to stroke, kidney disease, and/or heart disease.

Hypotension, or low blood pressure, is indicated when pressures are less than 100 mm Hg systolic and 60 mm Hg diastolic. Hypotension may occur with heart failure, dehydration, depression, severe burns, hemorrhage, and shock. *Orthostatic*, or postural, hypotension occurs when there is a sudden drop in both systolic and diastolic pressure when an individual moves from a lying to a sitting or standing position. It is caused by the inability of blood vessels to compensate quickly to the change in position. The individual becomes lightheaded and dizzy and may experience blurred vision. The symptoms last a few seconds until the blood vessels compensate and more blood is pushed to the brain.

Various factors can influence blood pressure readings. Some of these factors are:

◆ force of the heartbeat

◆ resistance of the arterial system

◆ elasticity of the arteries

◆ volume of the blood in the arteries

Many other factors can also influence blood pressure readings. These factors can cause blood pressure to be high or low. Some examples are as follows:

◆ factors that may increase blood pressure:
   (1) excitement, anxiety, nervous tension
   (2) stimulant drugs

(3) exercise and eating

(4) smoking

♦ factors that may decrease blood pressure:

(1) rest or sleep

(2) depressant drugs

(3) shock

(4) excessive loss of blood

(5) fasting (not eating)

♦ factors that may cause changes in readings:

(1) lying down

(2) sitting position

(3) standing position

Blood pressure is recorded as a fraction. The systolic reading is the top number, or numerator. The diastolic reading is the bottom number, or denominator. For example, a systolic reading of 120 and a diastolic reading of 80 is recorded as 120/80.

Two main types of sphygmomanometers are used to obtain blood pressure readings. The mercury sphygmomanometer has a long column of mercury (see figure 14-24). Each mark on the gauge represents 2 mm Hg. The mercury sphygmomanometer must always be placed on a flat, level surface or mounted on a wall. If it is calibrated correctly, the level of mercury should be at zero when viewed at eye level. The Occupational Health and Safety Administration (OSHA) discourages the use of mercury sphygmomanometers because of the possibility of a mercury spill and contamination. The aneroid sphygmomanometer does not have a mercury column (see figure 14-25). However, it is calibrated in mm Hg. Each line represents 2 mm Hg pressure. When the cuff is deflated, the needle must be on zero. If the needle is not on zero, the sphygmomanometer should not be used until it is recalibrated. Electronic sphygmomanometers are used in some health care facilities (see figure 14-26). Blood pressure and pulse readings are shown on a digital display after a cuff is placed on the patient.

In order to obtain accurate blood pressure readings, it is important to observe several factors. The American Heart Association (AHA) recommends that the patient sit quietly for at least 5 minutes before blood pressure is taken. The AHA also recommends that two separate readings be taken and averaged, with a minimum wait of 30 seconds between readings.

The size and placement of the sphygmomanometer cuff is also important (see figure 14-27). The cuff contains a rubber bladder that fills with air to apply pressure to the arteries. Cuffs that are too wide or too narrow give inaccurate readings. A cuff that is too small will give an artificially high reading; if it is too large it will give an artificially low reading. To ensure the greatest degree of accuracy, the width of the cuff should be approximately 20 percent wider than the diameter (or width) of the patient's upper arm. The patient should be seated or lying comfortably and have the forearm supported on a flat surface. The area of the arm covered by the cuff should be at heart level. The arm must be

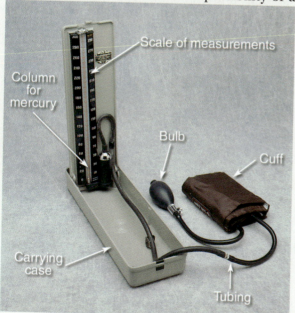

FIGURE 14-24 The gauge on a mercury sphygmomanometer has a column of mercury.

Scale of measurements

Column for mercury

Bulb

Cuff

Carrying case

Tubing

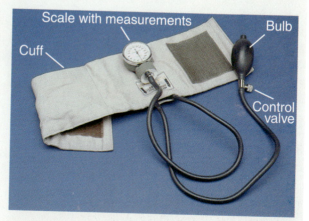

FIGURE 14-25 The gauge on an aneroid sphygmomanometer does not contain a column of mercury.

Scale with measurements

Bulb

Cuff

Control valve

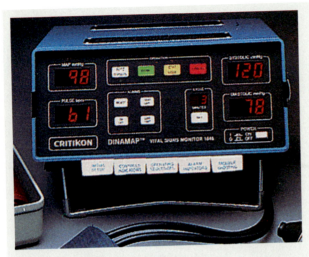

FIGURE 14-26 Electronic sphygmomanometers provide a digital display of blood pressure and pulse readings.

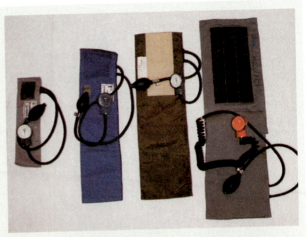

FIGURE 14-27 It is important to use the correct size cuff because cuffs that are too wide or too narrow will result in inaccurate readings.

free of any constrictive clothing. The deflated cuff should be placed on the arm with the center of the bladder in the cuff directly over the brachial artery, and the lower edge of the cuff 1 to 1½ inches above the antecubital area (bend of the elbow).

A final point relating to accuracy is placement of the stethoscope bell/diaphragm. The bell/diaphragm should be placed directly over the brachial artery at the antecubital area and held securely but with as little pressure as possible.

C For a health care worker, a major responsibility is accuracy in taking and recording

blood pressure. You should *not* discuss the reading with the patient. This is the responsibility of the physician because the information may cause a personal reaction that can affect the treatment. Only the physician should determine whether an abnormal blood pressure is indication for treatment.

STUDENT: *Go to the workbook and complete the assignment sheets for 14:7, Measuring and Recording Blood Pressure, Reading a Mercury Sphygmomanometer, and Reading an Aneroid Sphygmomanometer. Then return and continue with the procedure.*

PROCEDURE 14:7   OBRA

Measuring and Recording Blood Pressure

Equipment and Supplies

Stethoscope, sphygmomanometer, alcohol swab or disinfectant, paper, pencil/pen

Procedure

1. Assemble equipment. Use an alcohol swab or disinfectant to clean the earpieces and bell/diaphragm of the stethoscope.
2. Wash hands.
3. Introduce yourself. Identify the patient. Explain the procedure.
   NOTE: If possible, allow the patient to sit quietly for 5 minutes before taking the blood pressure.
   NOTE: Reassure the patient as needed. Nervous tension and excitement can alter or elevate blood pressure.
4. Roll up the patient's sleeve to approximately 5 inches above the elbow. Position the arm so that it is supported, comfortable, and

close to the level of the heart. The palm should be up.

NOTE: If the sleeve constricts the arm, remove the garment. The arm must be bare and unconstricted for an accurate reading.

5. Wrap the deflated cuff around the upper arm 1 to 1½ inches above the elbow and over the brachial artery. The center of the bladder inside the cuff should be over the brachial artery.

   ⚠ **CAUTION:** Do not pull the cuff too tight. The cuff should be smooth and even.

6. Determine the palpatory systolic pressure (see figure 14-28A). To do this, find the radial pulse and keep your fingers on it. Inflate the cuff until the radial pulse disappears. Inflate the cuff 30 mm Hg above this point. Slowly release the pressure on the cuff while watching the gauge. When the pulse is felt again, note the reading on the gauge. This is the palpatory systolic pressure.

7. Deflate the cuff completely. Ask the patient to raise the arm and flex the fingers to promote blood flow. Wait 30 to 60 seconds to allow blood flow to resume completely.

8. Use your fingertips to locate the brachial artery (see figure 14-28B). The brachial artery is located on the inner part of the arm at the antecubital space (area where the elbow bends). Place the stethoscope over the artery (see figure 14-28C). Put the earpieces in your ears.

NOTE: Earpieces should be pointed forward.

9. Check to make sure the tubings are separate and not tangled together.

10. Gently close the valve on the rubber bulb by turning it in a clockwise direction. Inflate the cuff to 30 mm Hg above the palpatory systolic pressure.

    NOTE: Make sure the sphygmomanometer gauge is at eye level.

11. Open the bulb valve slowly and let the air escape gradually.

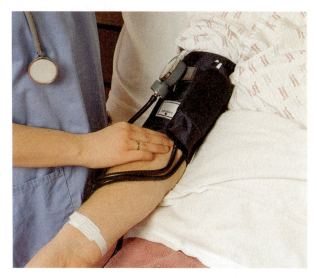

FIGURE 14-28B Locate the brachial artery on the inner part of the arm at the antecubital space.

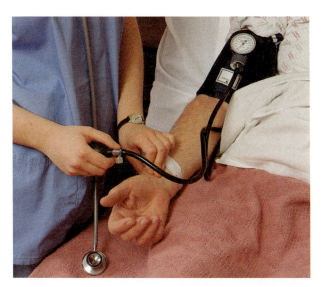

FIGURE 14-28A Determine the palpatory systolic pressure by checking the radial pulse as you inflate the cuff.

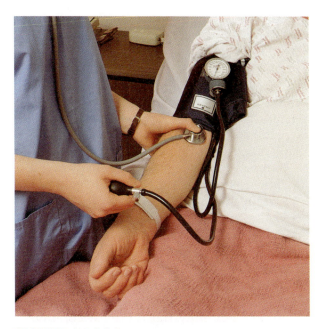

FIGURE 14-28C Place the stethoscope over the brachial artery as you listen for the blood pressure sounds.

12. When the first sound is heard, note the reading on the manometer. This is the systolic pressure.

13. Continue to release the air until there is an abrupt change of the sound, usually soft or muffled. Note the reading on the manometer. Continue to release the air until the sound changes again, becoming first faint and then no longer heard. Note the reading on the manometer. The point at which the first change in sound occurs is the diastolic pressure in children. The diastolic pressure in adults is the point at which the sound becomes very faint or stops.

    NOTE: If you still hear sound, continue to the zero mark. Record both readings (the change of sound and the zero reading). For a systolic of 122 and a continued diastolic of 78, this can be written as 122/78/0.

14. When the sound ceases, rapidly deflate the cuff.

15. If you need to repeat the procedure to recheck your reading, completely deflate the cuff, wait 1 minute, and repeat the procedure. Ask the patient to raise the arm and flex the fingers to promote blood flow.

    ! CAUTION: If you cannot obtain a reading, report to your supervisor promptly.

16. Record the time and your reading. The reading is written as a fraction, with systolic over diastolic. For example, BP 124/72 (or 124/80/72 if the change in sound is noted).

17. Remove the cuff. Expel any remaining air by squeezing the cuff. Use alcohol or a disinfectant to clean the stethoscope earpieces and diaphragm/bell. Replace all equipment.

18. Check patient for safety and comfort before leaving.

19. Wash hands.

20. **C** Record all required information on the patient's chart or agency form, for example, date, time, B. P. 126/74, your signature and title. Report any abnormal readings immediately to your supervisor.

Practice *Go to the workbook and use the evaluation sheet for 14:7, Measuring and Recording Blood Pressure, to practice this procedure. When you feel you have mastered this skill, sign the sheet and give it to your instructor for further action.*

 Final Checkpoint Using the criteria listed on the evaluation sheet, your instructor will grade your performance.

UNIT 14 SUMMARY

Vital signs are important indicators of health states of the body. The four main vital signs are temperature, pulse, respiration, and blood pressure.

Temperature is a measurement of the balance between heat lost and heat produced by the body. It can be measured orally, rectally, aurally (by way of the ear), and between folds of skin. An abnormal body temperature can indicate disease.

Pulse is the pressure of the blood felt against the wall of an artery as the heart contracts or beats. Pulse can be measured at various body sites, but the most common site is the radial pulse, which is at the wrist. The rate, rhythm, and volume (strength) should be noted each time a pulse is taken. An apical pulse is taken with a stethoscope at the apex of the heart. The stethoscope is used to listen to the heart beat. Apical pulse is frequently taken on infants and small children with rapid pulse rates.

Respiration refers to the breathing process. Each respiration consists of an inspiration (breathing in) and an expiration (breathing out). The rate, rhythm, and character, or type, of respirations should always be noted.

Blood pressure is the force exerted by the blood against the arterial walls when the heart contracts or relaxes. Two measurements are noted: systolic and diastolic. An abnormal blood pressure can indicate disease.

Vital signs are major indications of body function. The health care worker must use precise methods to measure vital signs so results are as accurate as possible. A thorough understanding of vital signs and what they indicate will allow the health care worker to be alert to any abnormalities so they can be immediately reported to the correct individual.

INTERNET SEARCHES

Use the suggested search engines in Unit 11:4 of this textbook to search the Internet for additional information on the following topics:

1. *Organization:* find the American Heart Association web site to obtain information on the heart, pulse, arrhythmias, and blood pressure.

2. *Vital signs:* research body temperature, pulse, respiration, blood pressure, and apical pulse.

3. *Temperature scales:* research Celcius (Centigrade) versus Fahrenheit temperatures. Try to locate conversion charts which can be used to compare the two scales.

4. *Diseases:* research hypothermia, fever or pyrexia, hypertension, hypotension, and heart arrhythmias.

REVIEW QUESTIONS

1. List the four (4) main vital signs.

2. State the normal value or range for an adult for each of the following:
   a. oral temperature
   b. rectal temperature
   c. axillary or groin temperature
   d. pulse
   e. respiration

3. What three (3) factors must be noted about every pulse?

4. Why is an apical pulse taken?

5. What is the pulse deficit if an apical pulse is 112 and the radial pulse is 88?

6. Differentiate between hypertension and hypotension and list the basic causes of each.

7. How does systolic pressure differ from diastolic pressure? What are the normal ranges for each?

8. Define each of the following:
   a. bradycardia
   b. arrhythmia
   c. dyspnea
   d. tachypnea
   e. rales

UNIT 14

SUGGESTED REFERENCES

American Heart Association. *Hypertension Primer.* 2nd ed. Dallas, TX: American Heart Association, 1999.

American Heart Association. *Recommendations for Human Blood Pressure Determination by Sphygmomanometers.* Dallas, TX: American Heart Association, n.d.

Cohen, Barbara, and Dena Wood. *Memmler's Structure and Function of the Human Body.* 7th ed. Philadelphia, PA: Lippincott, Williams, & Wilkins, 2000.

Hegner, Barbara, Esther Caldwell, and Joan Needham. *Nursing Assistant: A Nursing Process Approach.* 8th ed. Clifton Park, NY: Delmar Learning, 1999.

Huber, Helen, and Audree Spatz. *Homemaker–Home Health Aide.* 5th ed. Clifton Park, NY: Delmar Learning, 1998.

Keir, Lucille, Connie Krebs, and Barbara A. Wise. *Medical Assisting: Clinical and Administrative Competencies.* 5th ed. Clifton Park, NY: Delmar Learning, 2003.

Phipps, Wilma, Judith Sands, and Jane Marek. *Medical Surgical Nursing: Concepts and Clinical Practice.* St. Louis, MO: C. V. Mosby, 1998.

Simmers, Louise. *Practical Problems in Mathematics for Health Occupations.* Clifton Park, NY: Delmar Learning, 1996.

Zakus, Sharron. *Clinical Skills for Medical Assistants.* 4th ed. St. Louis, MO: C. V. Mosby, 2001.

UNIT 15

First Aid

Unit Objectives

After completing this unit of study, you should be able to:

◆ Demonstrate cardiopulmonary resuscitation for one-person rescue, two-person rescue, infants, children, and obstructed-airway victims

◆ Describe first aid for
  — bleeding and wounds
  — shock
  — poisoning
  — burns
  — heat exposure
  — cold exposure
  — bone and joint injuries, including fractures
  — specific injuries to the eyes, head, nose, ears, chest, abdomen, and genital organs
  — sudden illness including heart attack, stroke, fainting, convulsions, and diabetic reactions

◆ Apply dressings and bandages, observing all safety precautions and using the circular, spiral, figure-eight, and recurrent, or finger wrap

◆ Define, pronounce, and spell all the key terms

 Observe Standard Precautions

 Safety—Proceed with Caution

 Math Skill

 Science Skill

 C Communications Skill

 Instructors Check—Call Instructor at This Point

 OBRA OBRA Requirement— Based on Federal Law

 Legal Responsibility

 Career Information

 Technology

378

KEY TERMS

abrasion
(ah″-bray′-shun)

amputation

avulsion
(ay′-vul′-shun)

bandages

burn

cardiopulmonary resuscitation
(car′-dee-oh-pull′-meh-nah-
ree ree″-suh-sih-tay′-shun)

cerebrovascular accident
(seh-ree′-bro-vass″-ku-lehr
ax′-ih-dent)

convulsion

diabetic coma

diaphoresis
(dy″-ah-feh-ree′-sis)

dislocation

dressing

fainting

first aid

fracture

frostbite

heart attack

heat cramps

heat exhaustion

heat stroke

hemorrhage

hypothermia

incision

infection

insulin shock

laceration

poisoning

puncture

shock

sprain

strain

triage
(tree′-ahj)

wound

15:1 INFORMATION
Providing First Aid

In every health care career you may have experiences that require a knowledge of first aid. This section provides basic guidelines for all the first aid topics discussed in the remaining sections of this unit. All students are strongly encouraged to take the First Aid Certification Course through their local Red Cross divisions to become proficient in providing first aid.

First aid is not full and complete treatment. Rather, **first aid** is best defined as "immediate care that is given to the victim of an injury or illness to minimize the effect of the injury or illness until experts can take over." Application of correct first aid can often mean the difference between life and death, or recovery versus permanent disability. In addition, by knowing the proper first aid measures, you can help yourself and others in a time of emergency.

C In any situation where first aid treatment is necessary, it is essential that you remain calm. Avoid panic. Evaluate the situation thoroughly. Always have a reason for anything you do. The treatment you provide will vary depending on the type of injury or illness, the environment, others present, equipment or supplies on hand, and the availability of medical help. Therefore, it is important for you to think about all these factors and determine what action is necessary.

The first step of first aid is to recognize that an emergency exists. Many senses can alert you to an emergency. Listen for unusual sounds such as screams, calls for help, breaking glass, screeching tires, or changes in machinery or equipment noises. Look for unusual sights such as an empty medicine container, damaged electrical wires, a stalled car, smoke or fire, a person lying motionless, blood, or spilled chemicals. Note any unusual, unfamiliar, or strange odors such as those of chemicals, natural gas, or pungent fumes. Watch for unusual appearances or behaviors in others such as difficulty in breathing, clutching of the chest or throat, abnormal skin colors, slurred or confused speech, unexplained confusion or drowsiness, excessive perspiration, signs of pain, and any symptoms of distress. Sometimes, signs of an emergency are clearly evident. An example is an automobile accident with victims in cars or on the street. Other times, signs are less obvious and require an alert individual to note that something is different or wrong. An empty medicine container and a small child with slurred speech, for example, are less obvious signs.

After determining that an emergency exists, the next step is to take appropriate action to help the victim or victims. Check the scene and make sure it is safe to approach. A quick glance at the area can provide information on what has occurred, dangers present, number of people involved, and other important factors. If live electrical wires are lying on the ground around an accident victim, for example, a rescuer could be electrocuted while trying to assist the victim. An infant thrown from a car during an automobile accident may be overlooked. A rescuer who pauses briefly to assess the situation will avoid such dangerous pitfalls and provide more efficient care. If the scene is not safe, call for medical help. Do not endanger your own life or the lives of other bystanders. Allow professionals to handle fires, dangerous chemicals, damaged electrical wires, and other life-threatening situations. If the scene appears safe, approach the victim. Determine whether the victim is conscious (see figure 15-1). If the victim shows no sign of consciousness, tap him gently and call to him. If the victim shows signs of consciousness, try to find out what happened and what is wrong. Never move an injured victim unless the victim is in a dangerous area such as an area filled with fire and/or smoke, flood waters, or carbon monoxide or poisonous fumes, or one with dangerous traffic, where vehicles cannot be stopped. If it is necessary to move the victim, do so as quickly and carefully as possible. Victims have been injured more severely by improper movement at the scenes of accidents, so avoid any unnecessary movement.

In an emergency, it is essential to call the emergency medical services (EMS) as soon as possible (see figure 15-2). The time factor is critical. Early access to the EMS system and advanced medical care increases the victim's chance of survival. Use a telephone, cellular phone, or CB radio to contact the police, ambulance or rescue squad, fire department, utility company, or other resources. In many areas of the country, the emergency number 911 can be used to contact any of the emergency medical services. Sometimes, it may be necessary to instruct others to contact authorities while you are giving first aid. Make sure that complete, accurate information is given to the correct authority. Describe the situation, actions taken, exact location, telephone number from which you are calling, assistance required, number of people involved, and the condition of the victim(s). Do not hang up the receiver or end the CB radio call until the other party has all the necessary information. If you are alone, call EMS immediately before providing any care to:

◆ an unconscious adult

◆ an unconscious child 8 years old or older

◆ an unconscious infant or child with a high risk for heart problems

If you are alone, shout for help and start cardiopulmonary resuscitation (CPR) if needed for:

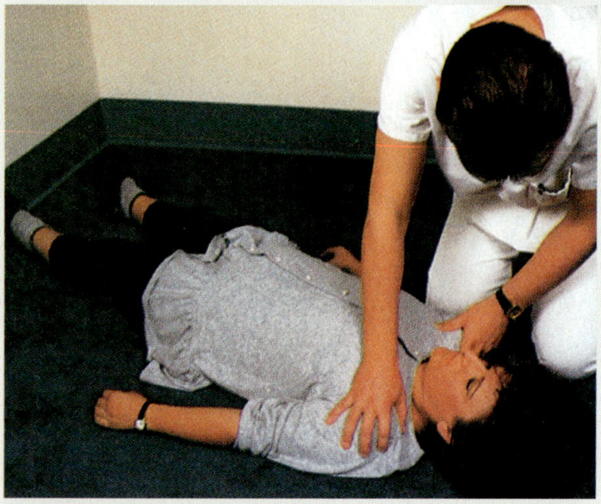

FIGURE 15-1 Determine whether the victim is conscious by gently tapping and by calling to him or her.

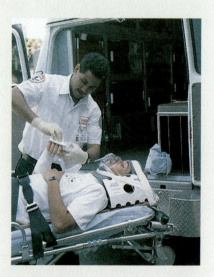

FIGURE 15-2 Call for emergency medical services (EMS) as soon as possible.

- an unconscious infant or child less than 8 years old

- any victim of submersion or near drowning

- any victim with cardiac arrest caused by trauma

- any victim with cardiac arrest caused by a drug overdose

If no one arrives to call EMS, continue providing care for approximately 1 minute, and then go to the nearest telephone, call for EMS, and return immediately to the victim.

After calling for help, provide care to the victim. If possible, obtain the victim's permission before providing any care. Introduce yourself and ask if you can help. If the victim can respond, he or she should give you permission before you provide care. If the victim is a child or minor, and a parent is present, obtain permission from the parent. If the victim is unconscious, confused, or seriously ill and unable to consent to care, and no other relative is available to give permission, you can assume that you have permission. It is important to remember that every individual has the right to refuse care. If a person refuses to give consent for care, do not proceed. If possible, have someone witness the refusal of care. If a life-threatening emergency exists, call EMS, alert them to the situation, and allow the professionals to take over.

At times it may be necessary to **triage** the situation. Triage is a method of prioritizing treatment. If two or more people are involved, triage also determines which person is treated first. Always attend to life-threatening emergencies first. Examples include no breathing or difficulty in breathing; no pulse; severe bleeding; persistent pain in the chest or abdomen; vomiting or passing blood; poisoning; head, neck, or spine injuries; open chest or abdominal wounds; shock; and severe second- and third-degree burns. Proper care for these emergencies is described in the sections that follow. If the victim is conscious, breathing, and able to talk, reassure the victim and try to determine what has happened. Ask the victim about pain or discomfort.

Check the victim for other types of injuries. Examples include fractures (broken bones), burns, shock, specific injuries, and other similar conditions. Always have a sound reason for anything you do. Examine the victim thoroughly and note any abnormal signs or symptoms. Check vital signs. Note the temperature, color, and moistness of the skin. Check and compare the pupils of the eyes. Look for fluids or blood draining from the mouth, nose, or ears. Gently examine the body for cuts, bruises, swelling, and painful areas. Report any abnormalities noted to emergency medical services when they arrive at the scene.

Obtain as much information regarding the accident, injury, or illness as possible. This information can then be given to the correct authorities. Information can be obtained from the victim, other persons present, or by examination of items present at the scene. Emergency medical identification contained in a bracelet, necklace, medical card, or Vial-of-Life is an important source of information. Empty medicine containers, bottles of chemicals or solutions, or similar items also can reveal important information. Be alert to all such sources of information. Use this information to determine how you may help the victim.

Some general principles of care should be observed whenever first aid is necessary. Some of these principles are:

- Obtain qualified assistance as soon as possible. Report all information obtained, observations noted, treatment given, and other important facts to the correct authorities. It may sometimes be necessary to send someone at the scene to obtain help.

- Avoid any unnecessary movement of the victim. Keep the victim in a position that will allow for providing the best care for the type of injury or illness.

- Reassure the victim. A confident, calm attitude will help relieve the victim's anxiety.

- If the victim is unconscious or vomiting, do not give him or her anything to eat or drink. It is best to avoid giving a victim anything to eat or drink while providing first aid treatment, unless the specific treatment requires that fluids or food be given.

- Protect the victim from cold or chilling, but avoid overheating the victim.

- Work quickly, but in an organized and efficient manner.

- Do not make a diagnosis or discuss the victim's condition with observers at the scene. It is essential to maintain confidentiality and protect the victim's right to privacy while providing treatment.

◆ Make every attempt to avoid further injury.

 CAUTION: Provide only the treatment that you are qualified to provide.

STUDENT: *Go to the workbook and complete the assignment sheet for 15:1, Providing First Aid.*

15:2 INFORMATION Performing Cardiopulmonary Resuscitation

At some time in your life, you may find an unconscious victim who is not breathing. This is an emergency situation. Correct action can save a life. Certification courses in cardiopulmonary resuscitation (CPR) are offered by the American Red Cross and American Heart Association. This section provides the basic facts about cardiopulmonary resuscitation.

The word parts of **cardiopulmonary resuscitation** provide a fairly clear description of the procedure: cardio (the heart) plus pulmonary (the lungs) plus resuscitation (to remove from apparent death or unconsciousness). When you administer CPR, you breathe for the person *and* circulate the blood. The purpose is to keep oxygenated blood flowing to the brain and other vital body organs until the heart and lungs start working again, or until medical help is available.

Clinical death occurs when the heart stops beating and the victim stops breathing. *Biological death* refers to the death of the body cells. Biological death occurs 4 to 6 minutes after clinical death and can result in permanent brain damage as well as damage to other vital organs. If CPR can be started immediately after clinical death occurs, the victim may be revived.

Cardiopulmonary resuscitation is as simple as ABCD. In fact, the *ABCD*s serve as guides to lifesaving techniques for persons who have stopped breathing and have no pulse.

◆ *A stands for airway.* To open the victim's airway, use the *head-tilt/chin-lift* method (see figure 15-3). Put one hand on the victim's forehead and put the fingertips of the other hand under the bony part of the jaw, near the chin. Tilt the head back without closing the victim's mouth. This action prevents the tongue from falling back and blocking the air passage. If the victim has a suspected neck or upper spinal cord injury, try to open the airway by lifting the chin without tilting the head back. If it is difficult to keep the jaw lifted with one hand, use a *jaw-thrust maneuver* to open the airway. Grasp the angles of the victim's lower jaw by positioning one hand on each side. Lift with both hands to move the lower jaw forward, making every attempt to avoid excessive backward tilting or side-to-side movement of the head.

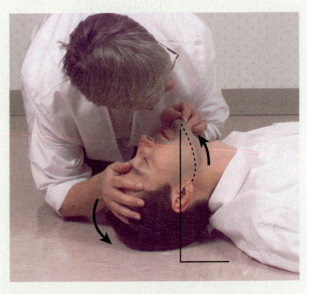

FIGURE 15-3 Open the airway by using the head-tilt/chin-lift method.

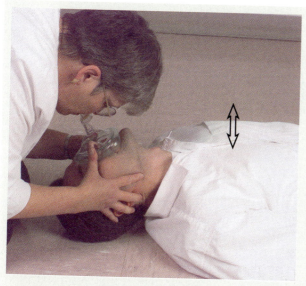

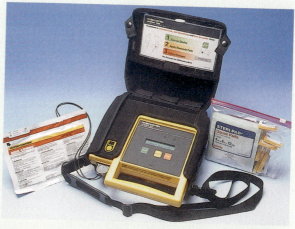

FIGURE 15-4 Whenever possible, use a CPR barrier mask to prevent transmission of disease while giving respirations.

FIGURE 15-5 When cardiac arrest occurs, an automated external defibrillator (AED) can be used to analyze the electrical rhythm of the heart and to apply a shock to try to restore the normal heart rhythm.

◆ *B stands for breathing.* Breathing means that you breathe into the victim's mouth or nose to supply needed oxygen or provide ventilations. To avoid loss of air when providing mouth-to-mouth breathing, it is important to pinch the victim's nose shut and make a tight seal around the victim's mouth with your mouth.

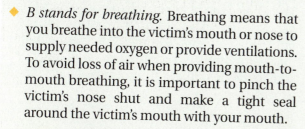 **CAUTION:** Follow standard precautions. If possible, use a CPR pocket face mask with a one-way valve to provide a barrier and prevent the transmission of disease (see figure 15-4). Special training is required for the use of this mask. Other protective barrier face shields are also available.

◆ *C stands for circulation.* By applying pressure to a certain area of the breastbone (sternum), the heart is compressed between the sternum and vertebral column. Blood is squeezed out of the heart and into the blood vessels. In this way, oxygen is supplied to body cells.

◆ *D stands for defibrillation.* One of the most common causes of cardiac arrest is ventricular fibrillation, an arrhythmia, or abnormal electrical conduction pattern in the heart. When the heart is fibrillating, it does not pump blood effectively. A defibrillator is a machine that delivers an electric shock to the heart to try to restore the normal electrical pattern and rhythm. Automated external

defibrillators (AEDs) are now available for use by trained first responders, emergency medical technicians, and even citizens (see figure 15-5). After electrode pads are positioned on the victim's chest, the AED determines the heart rhythm, recognizes abnormal rhythms that may respond to defibrillation, and sounds an audible or visual warning telling the operator to push a "shock" button. Some AEDs are fully automatic and even administer the shock. Studies have shown that the sooner defibrillation is provided, the greater the chances of survival are from a cardiac arrest caused by an arrhythmia. However, it is essential to remember that CPR is used until an AED is available. CPR will circulate the blood and prevent biological death. In addition, the use of AEDs is not recommended for an infant or child less than 8 years old, or for anyone who weighs less than 55 pounds.

Following the ABCDs in proper sequence is an essential part of CPR. Extreme care must be taken to evaluate the victim's condition before CPR is started. The first step is to determine whether the victim is conscious. Tap the victim gently and ask, "Are you OK?" If you know the victim, call the victim by name and speak loudly. If there is no response and the victim is unconscious, call for help. The American Heart Association and the American Red Cross recommend a "*call first, call fast*" priority. If you are alone, *call first* before providing any care to:

◆ an unconscious adult

◆ an unconscious child 8 years old or older

◆ an unconscious infant or child with a high risk for heart problems

If you are alone, shout for help, and start cardiopulmonary resuscitation (CPR) if needed for:

◆ an unconscious infant or child less than 8 years old

◆ any victim of submersion or near drowning

◆ any victim with cardiac arrest caused by trauma

◆ any victim with cardiac arrest caused by a drug overdose

If no help arrives to call EMS, provide care for approximately 1 minute, and then *call fast* for EMS. Return to the victim immediately to continue providing care until EMS arrives.

After determining that a victim is unconscious, the second step is to check for breathing. Try not to move the victim while you check breathing. If the victim is breathing, leave the victim in the same position and proceed with other needed care. If the victim is not breathing, or you are unable to determine whether the victim is breathing, position the victim on his or her back. If you must turn the victim, support the victim's head and neck and keep the victim's body in as straight a line as possible while turning. Then, open the airway by using the head-tilt/chin-lift or jaw-thrust maneuver. This step will sometimes start the victim breathing. To check for breathing, use a three-point evaluation for approximately 5 but not more than 10 seconds. *Look* for chest movement. *Listen* for breathing through the nose or mouth. *Feel* for movement of air from the nose or mouth. If the victim is not breathing, give two slow, gentle breaths, each breath lasting approximately 2 seconds. Watch for the victim's chest to rise slowly. Pause between breaths to allow air flow back out of the lungs. In addition, take a breath between the two breaths to increase the oxygen content of the rescue breath. After giving two breaths, check the carotid pulse in the neck to determine whether cardiac compression is needed. Take no more than 10 seconds to determine whether the pulse is absent before starting compressions.

! **CAUTION:** Cardiac compressions are not given if the pulse can be felt. If a person has stopped breathing but still has a pulse, it may be necessary to give only pulmonary respiration.

Correct hand placement is essential before performing chest compressions. For adults, the hand is placed on the lower half of the sternum. While kneeling alongside the victim, find the correct position by using the middle finger of your hand that is closest to the victim's feet to follow the ribs up to where the ribs meet the sternum, at the substernal notch. Keep the middle finger on the notch and position the index finger above it so two fingers are on the sternum. Then place the heel of your opposite hand (the hand closest to the victim's head) on the sternum, next to the index finger. Measuring in this manner minimizes the danger of applying pressure to the tip of the sternum, called the xiphoid process.

! **CAUTION:** The xiphoid process can be broken off quite easily and therefore should not be pressed.

Cardiopulmonary resuscitation can be performed on adults, children, and infants. In addition, it can be done by one person or two persons. Rates of ventilations and compressions vary according to the number of persons giving CPR and the age of the victim.

◆ *One-person rescue:* For adults, the person performing the rescue should provide 15 compressions followed by 2 ventilations, for a cycle ratio of 15:2. If 15 compressions are given at the rate of approximately 100 per minute, this will allow time for the rescuer to stop for 2 ventilations and still complete a 15:2 cycle in approximately 15 seconds. Four 15:2 cycles should be completed every minute. The hands should be positioned correctly on the sternum. The two hands should be interlaced and only the heel of the palm should rest on the sternum. Pressure should be applied straight down to compress the sternum approximately 1½ to 2 inches, or 3.8 to 5.0 centimeters.

♦ *Two-person rescue:* Two people performing a rescue on an adult victim allows one person to give breaths while the second person provides compressions. During the rescue, the person giving breaths can check the effectiveness of the compressions by feeling for a carotid pulse while chest compressions are administered. One rescuer applies the compressions at the rate of 100 per minute. After every 15 compressions, the rescuer applying compressions pauses, and the second rescuer provides 2 ventilations. Thus, there is a 15:2 ratio.

♦ *Infants:* Cardiopulmonary resuscitation for an infant is different than that for an adult because of the infant's size. Ventilations are given by covering both the infant's nose and mouth; a seal is made by the mouth of the rescuer. Breaths are given slowly until the infant's chest rises gently. Extreme care must be taken to avoid overinflating the lungs and/or forcing air into the stomach. The brachial pulse site in the arm is used to check pulse (see figure 15-6). Compressions are given by placing two fingers on the sternum one finger's width below an imaginary line drawn between the nipples. The sternum should be compressed ½ to 1 inch (approximately 1.3 to 2.5 centimeters). Compressions are given at a rate of at least 100 per minute. Even with a one-person rescue, one respiration is given after every five compressions, for a 5:1 ratio. The infant's back must be supported at all times when giving compressions. In addition, the infant's head should not be tilted as far back as an adult's because this can obstruct the infant's airway. If two rescuers are available to perform CPR on an infant, a two-thumb technique can be used by one rescuer to perform compressions while the second rescuer gives breaths. The rescuer providing compressions stands at the infant's feet and places his or her thumbs next to each other on the lower half of the

sternum about one finger's width below the nipple line. The rescuer then wraps his or her hands around the infant to support the infant's back with the fingers. The same ratio of 5 compressions to 1 ventilation is used by the two rescuers.

♦ *Children:* Cardiopulmonary resuscitation for children depends on the size of the child. The CPR method for an adult is usually used if the child is relatively large or is older than 8. The initial steps of CPR for a child are the same steps used in adult CPR, except that the head is not tilted as far back when the airway is opened. The main differences relate to compressions. The heel of one hand is placed on the sternum one finger's width above the substernal-notch, that is, in the same position used for adult compressions. The other hand remains on the forehead to keep the airway open. The sternum is compressed 1 to 1½ inches (approximately 2.5 to 3.8 centimeters). Compressions are given at a rate of 100 per minute. After each five compressions, one slow breath is given until the chest rises gently. This provides a 5:1 ratio. Each cycle of 5 compressions and 1 ventilation should take

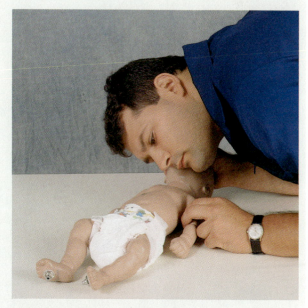

FIGURE 15-6 Use the brachial pulse site in the arm to check for a pulse in an infant.

approximately 5 seconds, and ten to twelve cycles should be completed every minute.

OBRA There are times when a victim has an obstructed airway (an object blocking the airway). Special measures must be taken to clear this obstruction.

◆ If the victim is conscious, coughing, talking or making noise, and/or able to breathe, the airway is not completely obstructed. Remain calm and encourage the victim to remain calm. Encourage the victim to cough hard. Coughing is the most effective method of expelling the object from the airway.

◆ If the victim is conscious but not able to talk, make noise, breathe, or cough, the airway is completely obstructed. The victim usually grasps his or her throat and appears cyanotic (blue discoloration of the skin), see figure 15-7. Immediate action must be taken to clear the airway. Abdominal thrusts, as described in Procedure 15:2E, are given to provide a force of air to push the object out of the airway.

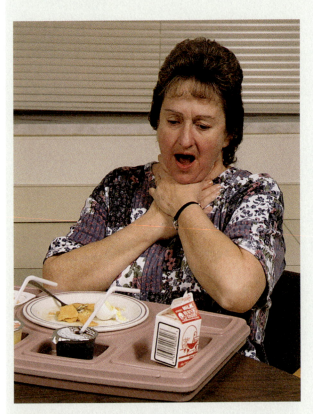

FIGURE 15-7 A choking victim usually grasps her throat and appears cyanotic.

◆ If the victim is unconscious and has an obstructed airway, a sequence of steps is performed to remove the obstruction. The sequence includes giving five abdominal thrusts, performing a mouth sweep, opening the airway, and attempting to ventilate (give breaths). The sequence, described in detail in Procedure 15:2F, is repeated until the object is expelled, ventilations are successful, or other qualified medical help arrives.

◆ If an infant (birth to 1 year old) has an obstructed airway, a different sequence of steps is used to remove the obstruction. The sequence includes five back blows; five chest thrusts; a check of the mouth; a finger sweep, if the object is seen; and an attempt to ventilate. The sequence, described in detail in Procedure 15:2F, is repeated until the object is expelled, ventilations are successful, or other qualified medical help arrives.

◆ If a child aged 1 to 8 has an obstructed airway, the same sequence of steps used for an adult is followed. However, a finger sweep of the mouth is *not* performed unless the object can be seen in the mouth.

◆ Until the airway is cleared, chest compressions have no value. Compressions circulate oxygen to the body cells. Unless the airway is cleared and oxygen is supplied to the lungs, however, there is no oxygen to circulate.

Once CPR is started, it must be continued unless one of the following situations occur:

◆ The victim recovers and starts to breathe.

◆ Other qualified help arrives and takes over.

◆ A doctor or other legally qualified person orders you to discontinue the attempt.

◆ The rescuer is so physically exhausted, CPR can no longer be continued.

◆ The scene suddenly becomes unsafe.

◆ You are given a legally valid do not resuscitate (DNR) order.

STUDENT: *Go to the workbook and complete the assignment sheet for 15:2, Performing Cardiopulmonary Resuscitation. Then return and continue with the procedures.*

PROCEDURE 15:2A
Performing CPR—One-Person Rescue

Equipment and Supplies

CPR manikin, alcohol or disinfecting solution, gauze sponges

Procedure

⚠ CAUTION: Only a CPR training manikin (see figure 15-8) should be used to practice this procedure. *Never* practice CPR on another person.

1. Assemble equipment. Position the manikin on a firm surface, usually the floor.
2. Check for consciousness. Shake the "victim" by tapping the shoulder. Ask, "Are you OK?" If the victim does not respond, activate EMS immediately. Follow the "call first, call fast" priority.
3. Open the airway. Use the head-tilt/chin-lift method. Place one hand on the victim's forehead. Place the fingertips of the other hand under the bony part of the victim's jaw, near the chin. Tilt the head without closing the victim's mouth.

    NOTE: This action moves the tongue away from the back of the throat and prevents the tongue from blocking the airway.

⚠ CAUTION: If the victim has a suspected neck or upper spinal cord injury, use a jaw-thrust maneuver to open the airway. Grasp the angles of the victim's lower jaw by positioning one hand on each side. Lift with both hands to move the lower jaw forward, making every attempt to avoid excessive backward tilting or side-to-side movement of the head.

4. Check for breathing. Put your ear close to the victim's nose and mouth while looking at the chest. Look, listen, and feel for respirations for about 5 but not more than 10 seconds.
5. *If the victim is breathing,* keep the airway open and obtain medical help. *If the victim is not breathing,* administer mouth-to-mouth resuscitation as follows:
    a. Keep the airway open.
    b. Resting your hand on the victim's forehead, use your thumb and forefinger to pinch the victim's nose shut.
    c. Seal the victim's mouth with your mouth.
    d. Give two slow breaths, each lasting approximately 2 seconds until the chest rises gently (see figure 15-9A). Pause slightly between breaths. This allows air to flow out and provides you with a chance to

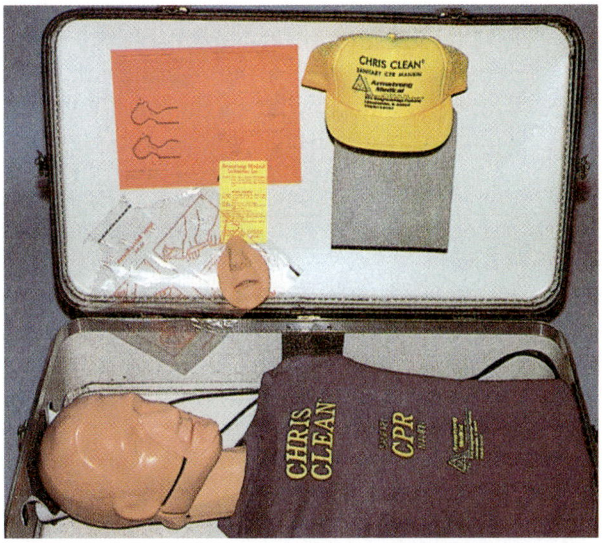

FIGURE 15-8 Use only training manikins while practicing CPR.

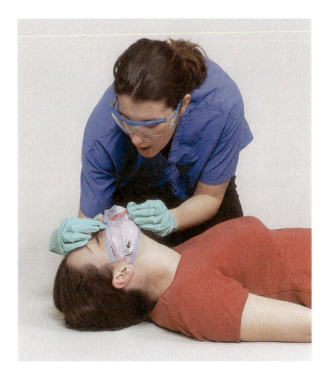

FIGURE 15-9A If the victim is not breathing, open the airway and give two slow, gentle breaths.

take a breath and increase the oxygen level for the second rescue breath.

e. Watch the chest for movement to be sure the air is entering the victim's lungs. Avoid overinflating the lungs and/or forcing air into the stomach.

CAUTION: Follow standard precautions. If possible, use a CPR pocket face mask with a one-way valve to provide a barrier and prevent the transmission of disease.

6. Palpate the carotid pulse: kneeling at the victim's side, place the fingertips of your hand on the victim's voice box. Then slide the fingers toward you and into the groove at the side of the victim's neck, where you should find the carotid pulse. Take at least 5 seconds but not more than 10 seconds to feel for the pulse (see figure 15-9B). At the same time, watch for breathing, signs of circulation, and/or movement.

NOTE: The pulse may be weak, so check carefully.

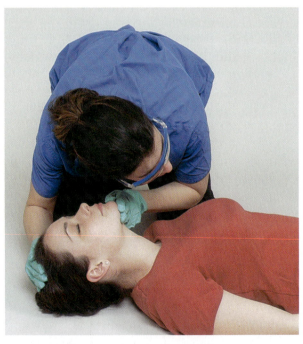

FIGURE 15-9B Palpate the carotid pulse for at least 5 but not more than 10 seconds to determine whether the heart is beating.

7. *If the victim has a pulse,* continue providing mouth-to-mouth resuscitation. Give one slow, gentle breath every 5 seconds. Count, "One, one thousand; two, one thousand; three, one thousand; four, one thousand; and breathe," to obtain the correct timing. After 1 minute of rescue breathing (approximately twelve breaths), recheck the pulse to make sure the heart is still beating.

8. *If the victim does not have a pulse,* administer chest compressions as follows:

a. Locate the correct place on the sternum: while kneeling alongside the victim, use the middle finger of your hand that is closest to the victim's feet to follow the ribs up to where the ribs meet the sternum, at the substernal notch. Keep the middle finger on the notch and position the index finger above it so two fingers are on the sternum. Then, place the heel of the opposite hand (the one closest to the victim's head) on the sternum, next to the index finger.

CAUTION: The heel of your hand should be approximately 1 to 1½ inches above the end of the sternum.

b. Place your other hand on top of the hand that is correctly positioned. Keep your fingers off the victim's chest. It may help to interlock your fingers.

c. Rise up on your knees so that your shoulders are directly over the victim's sternum. Lock your elbows and keep your arms straight.

NOTE: This position will allow you to push straight down on the sternum and compress the heart, which lies between the sternum and vertebral column.

d. Push straight down to compress the chest approximately 1½ to 2 inches, or 3.8 to 5.0 centimeters (see figure 15-9C). Use a smooth, even motion.

e. Administer 15 compressions at the rate of 100 per minute. Count, "One and, two and, three and," and so forth, to obtain the correct rate.

f. Allow the chest to relax completely after each compression. Keep your hands on

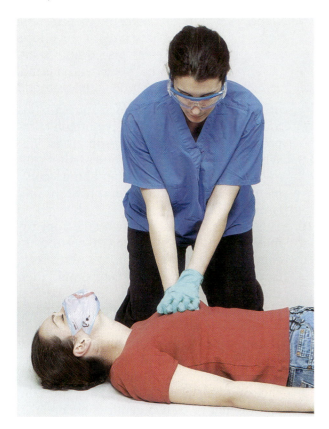

FIGURE 15-9C Use smooth, even motions to compress the chest straight down while giving 15 compressions.

the sternum during the upstroke (chest relaxation period).

   g. The 15 compressions should be completed in approximately 10 seconds.

9. After administering 15 compressions, give the victim 2 ventilations, or respirations. Avoid excessive body movement while giving the ventilations. Keep your knees in the same position and swing your body upward to give the respirations. Respirations should be completed in approximately 5 seconds.

10. Repeat the cycle of 15 compressions followed by 2 ventilations. After four cycles of a 15:2 ratio, take 5 seconds to check the victim for breathing and the presence of a carotid pulse. If no pulse is felt, continue providing 15 compressions followed by 2 respirations.

NOTE: Remember, cardiac compressions are applied only if the victim has no pulse.

11. After you begin CPR, do not stop unless
   a. The victim recovers.
   b. Help arrives to take over and give CPR and/or apply an AED.
   c. A physician or other legally qualified person orders you to discontinue the attempt.
   d. You are so physically exhausted, you cannot continue.
   e. The scene suddenly becomes unsafe.
   f. You are given a legally valid do not resuscitate (DNR) order.

12. After the practice session, use a gauze pad saturated with 70-percent alcohol or a 10-percent bleach disinfecting solution to clean the manikin. Wipe the face and clean inside the mouth thoroughly. Saturate a clean gauze pad with the solution and lay it on the mouth area for at least 30 seconds. Use another gauze pad to wipe the area dry. Follow manufacturer's instructions for any additional cleaning required.

   NOTE: A 10-percent bleach solution is more effective than alcohol. Some manikins have disposable mouthpieces that are discarded after use. If the mouthpiece is discarded, the remainder of the face should still be disinfected.

13. Replace all equipment used. Wash hands.

Practice *Go to the workbook and use the evaluation sheet for 15:2A, Performing CPR—One-Person Rescue, to practice this procedure. When you feel you have mastered this skill, sign the sheet and give it to your instructor for further action.*

 Final Checkpoint Using the criteria listed on the evaluation sheet, your instructor will grade your performance.

PROCEDURE 15:2B

Performing CPR—Two-Person Rescue

Equipment and Supplies

CPR manikin, alcohol or disinfecting solution, gauze sponges

Procedure

! **CAUTION:** Only a CPR training manikin should be used to practice this procedure. *Never* practice CPR on another person.

1. Assemble equipment. Position the manikin on a firm surface, usually the floor.
2. Shake the victim to check for consciousness. Ask, "Are you OK?"
3. If the victim is unconscious, one rescuer checks for breathing and begins CPR. The second rescuer contacts emergency medical services.
4. Use the head-tilt/chin-lift method to open the victim's airway. Place one hand on the victim's forehead. Place the fingertips of the other hand under the bony part of the victim's jaw, near the chin. Tilt the victim's head back without closing the victim's mouth.
5. Check for breathing. Look, listen, and feel for breathing for 5 but not more than 10 seconds.
6. *If the victim is not breathing,* give two slow, gentle breaths, each lasting approximately 2 seconds. Watch the chest for movement to be sure air is entering the victim's lungs. Avoid overinflating the lungs and/or forcing air into the stomach.

☣ **CAUTION:** Follow standard precautions. If possible, use a CPR pocket face mask with a one-way valve to provide a barrier and prevent the transmission of disease.

7. Feel for the carotid pulse for at least 5 seconds and not more than 10 seconds. Watch for signs of breathing, circulation, and/or movement.
8. *If there is no pulse,* give chest compressions. Locate the correct hand position on the sternum. Until the second rescuer returns, provide compressions and respirations as for a one-person rescue. Give fifteen compressions followed by two respirations.
9. When the second rescuer returns after calling for help, the first rescuer should complete the cycle of fifteen compressions and two respirations.
10. The first rescuer should then take approximately 5 but not more than 10 seconds to check for breathing and the presence of a carotid pulse. The first rescuer should then state, "No pulse. Continue CPR." The first rescuer then gives two gentle, slow breaths for approximately 2 seconds each.
11. The second rescuer should get into position for compressions and locate the correct hand placement while the first rescuer is checking for pulse and breathing. After the first rescuer gives two gentle, slow breaths, the second rescuer should begin compressions at the rate of 100 per minute, or 15 compressions in approximately 10 seconds (see figure 15-10A). The second rescuer should count out loud, "One and, two and, three and, four and, five and . . . ." After

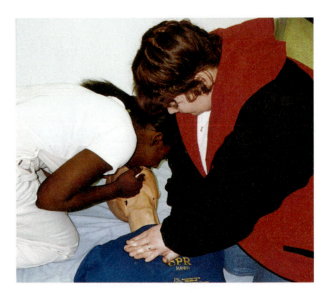

FIGURE 15-10A In a two-person rescue, two breaths are given after every 15 compressions.

each 15 compressions, the second rescuer should pause slightly to allow the first rescuer to give two slow breaths. Rescue then continues with two breaths after each 15 compressions.

12. Continue with the cycle of 15 compressions and two ventilations. The rescuer giving breaths should recheck pulse and breathing every few minutes by asking the rescuer giving compressions to pause for approximately 5 but not more than 10 seconds. In addition, the rescuer giving breaths can monitor the carotid pulse during compressions to assess the effectiveness of the compressions.

13. If one rescuer gets tired, the rescuers can change positions. The person giving compressions should provide a clear signal to change positions, such as, "Change, and two, and three, and four, and. . . ." The compressor should complete a cycle of 15 compressions. The ventilator should give two breaths at the end of the 15 compressions. The ventilator should then move to the chest and locate the correct hand placement for compressions (see figure 15-10B).

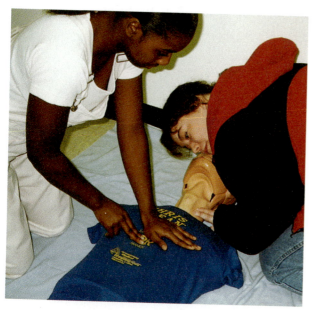

FIGURE 15-10B When the person doing compressions gets tired, the rescuers can change positions.

The compressor should move to the head, open the airway, and check the pulse and breathing for approximately 5 but not more than 10 seconds. After checking for pulse and breathing, the person should then give two gentle slow breaths and state, "No pulse. Continue CPR." The new compressor should then give 15 compressions at the rate of 100 per minute. The rescue should continue with two ventilations after each 15 compressions.

14. The rescuers should continue CPR until qualified medical help arrives, the victim recovers, a doctor or other legally qualified person orders CPR discontinued, the scene suddenly becomes unsafe, or they are presented with a legally valid do not resuscitate (DNR) order.

15. After the practice session, use a gauze pad saturated with 70-percent alcohol or a 10-percent bleach disinfecting solution to clean the manikin. Wipe the face and clean inside the mouth thoroughly. Saturate a clean gauze pad with the solution and lay it on the mouth area for at least 30 seconds. Use another gauze pad to wipe the area dry. Follow manufacturer's instructions for any additional cleaning required.
    NOTE: A 10-percent bleach solution is more effective than alcohol. Some manikins have disposable mouthpieces that are discarded after use. If the mouthpiece is discarded, the remainder of the face should still be disinfected.

16. Replace all equipment used. Wash hands.

Practice Go to the workbook and use the evaluation sheet for 15:2B, Performing CPR—Two-Person Rescue, to practice this procedure. When you feel you have mastered this skill, sign the sheet and give it to your instructor for further action.

 Final Checkpoint Using the criteria listed on the evaluation sheet, your instructor will grade your performance.

PROCEDURE 15:2C & D

Performing CPR on Infants and Children

Equipment and Supplies

CPR infant and child manikins, alcohol or disinfecting solution, gauze pads

Procedure

⚠️ **CAUTION:** Only CPR training manikins should be used to practice these procedures. *Never* practice CPR on a human infant or child.

1. Assemble equipment.

2. Gently shake the infant or child or tap the infant's foot (for reflex action) to determine consciousness. Call to the infant or child.

3. If the infant or child is unconscious, call aloud for help, and begin the steps of CPR. If no one arrives to call EMS, stop CPR after one minute to telephone for medical assistance. Resume CPR as quickly as possible.

   NOTE: If the infant or child is known to have a high risk for heart problems, call first and then begin CPR.

4. Use the head-tilt/chin-lift method to open the infant's or child's airway. Tip the head back gently, taking care not to tip it as far back as you would an adult's head.

⚠️ **CAUTION:** Tipping the head too far will cause an obstruction of the infant's airway.

   NOTE: For CPR techniques, infants are usually considered to be under 1 year old; children are ages 1 to 8 years. Children over 8 years old usually require the same techniques as do adults. Use your judgment for this age group, depending on the size of the child.

5. Look, listen, and feel for breathing. Check for at least 5 but not more than 10 seconds.

6. *If there is no breathing,* give two slow, gentle breaths, each breath lasting approximately 1½ seconds. For an infant, cover the infant's nose and mouth with your mouth (see figure 15-11). For a child, cover the child's nose and mouth with your mouth, or pinch the child's nose and cover the child's mouth with your mouth. Breathe until the chest rises gently during each ventilation and allow for chest deflation after each breath.

7. Check the pulse. For an infant, check the pulse over the brachial artery: place your fingertips on the inside of the upper arm and halfway between the elbow and shoulder (refer to figure 15-6). Put your thumb on the posterior (outside) of the arm. Squeeze your fingers gently toward your thumb. Feel for the pulse for 5 but not more than 10 seconds. For a child, check the pulse at the carotid pulse site. Feel for the pulse for 5 but not more than 10 seconds.

8. *If a pulse is present,* continue providing ventilations by giving the infant or child one ventilation every 3 seconds. After 1 minute (approximately 20 breaths), recheck the pulse and breathing for approximately 5 but not more than 10 seconds.

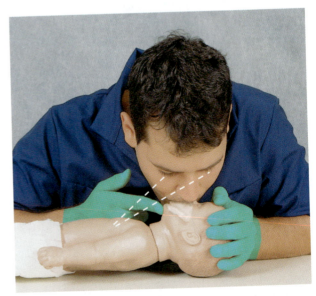

FIGURE 15-11 If an infant is not breathing, cover the infant's mouth and nose with your mouth and give two slow, gentle breaths.

9. *If no pulse is present,* administer cardiac compressions. For an infant, locate the correct position for compressions by drawing an imaginary line between the nipples. Place two fingers on the sternum and one finger's width below this imaginary line. Give compressions at the rate of 100 per minute. For a child, place the heel of one hand one finger's width above the substernal notch of the breastbone. Keep the other hand on the child's forehead (see figure 15-12). Give compressions at the rate of 100 per minute. Make sure the infant or child is on a firm surface, or use one hand to support the infant's or child's back while administering compressions. Press hard enough to compress the infant's chest ½ to 1 inch, or 1.3 to 2.5 centimeters, or the child's chest 1 to 1½

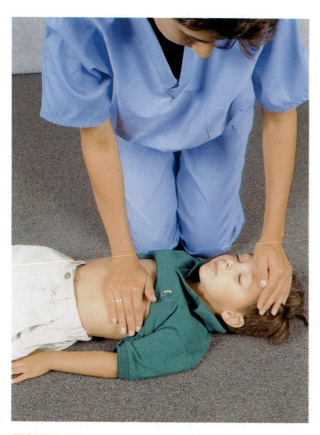

FIGURE 15-12 Use one hand to give chest compressions to a child. Keep the other hand on the child's forehead.

inches, or 2.5 to 3.8 centimeters. Give 5 compressions in approximately 3 seconds.

10. After every five compressions, give one slow, gentle breath until the chest rises gently.

11. Continue the cycle of five compressions followed by one ventilation. To establish the correct rate, count, "One, two, three, four, five, breathe."

12. After one minute (about 12 cycles), check for breathing and pulse for approximately 5 but not more than 10 seconds. Continue CPR if no breathing or pulse is noted. Recheck the pulse and breathing every few minutes.

13. After the practice session, use a gauze pad saturated with 70-percent alcohol or a 10-percent bleach disinfecting solution to clean the manikin. Wipe the face and clean inside the mouth thoroughly. Saturate a clean gauze pad with the solution and lay it on the mouth area for at least 30 seconds. Use another gauze pad to wipe the area dry. Follow manufacturer's instructions for specific cleaning.

   NOTE: The 10-percent bleach solution is more effective than alcohol. Some manikins have disposable mouthpieces that are discarded after use. If the mouthpiece is discarded, the remainder of the face should still be disinfected.

14. Replace all equipment used. Wash hands.

Practice *Go to the workbook and use the evaluation sheets for 15:2C, Performing CPR on Infants and 15:2D, Performing CPR on Children, to practice these procedures. When you feel you have mastered these skills, sign the sheets and give them to your instructor for further action.*

 Final Checkpoint Using the criteria listed on the evaluation sheet, your instructor will grade your performance.

PROCEDURE 15:2E

Performing CPR—Obstructed Airway on Conscious Adult Victim

Equipment and Supplies

CPR manikin or choking manikin

Procedure

⚠ **CAUTION:** Only a manikin should be used to practice this procedure. Do not practice on another person. Hand placement can be tried on another person, but the actual abdominal thrust should *never* be performed unless the person is choking.

1. Assemble equipment. Position the manikin in an upright position sitting on a chair.
2. Determine whether the victim has an airway obstruction. Ask, "Are you choking?" Check to see whether the victim can cough or speak.

⚠ **CAUTION:** If the victim is coughing, the airway is not completely obstructed. Encourage the victim to remain calm and cough hard. Coughing is usually very effective for removing an obstruction.

3. If the victim cannot cough, talk, make noise, or breathe, call for help.
4. Perform abdominal thrusts to try to remove the obstruction. Follow these steps:
   a. Stand behind the victim.
   b. Wrap both arms around the victim's waist.
   c. Make a fist of one hand (see figure 15-13A). Place the thumb side of the victim's fist in the middle of the victim's abdomen, slightly above the navel (umbilicus) but well below the xiphoid process at the end of the sternum.

d. Grasp the fist with your other hand (see figure 15-13B).
e. Use quick, upward thrusts to press into the victim's abdomen (see figure 15-13C).

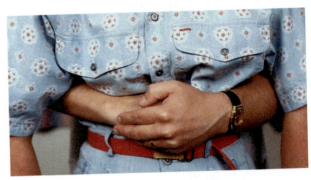

FIGURE 15-13B Place the thumb side of the fist above the umbilicus but well below the xiphoid process at the end of the sternum. Grasp the fist with your other hand.

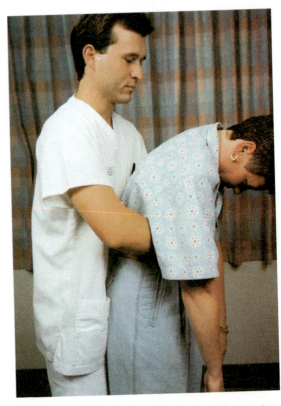

FIGURE 15-13C Use quick, upward thrusts to press into the victim's abdomen.

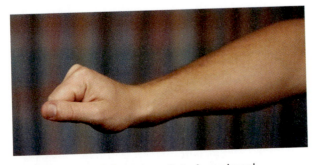

FIGURE 15-13A Make a fist of one hand.

NOTE: The thrusts should be delivered hard enough to cause a force of air to push the obstruction out of the airway.

 CAUTION: Make sure that your forearms do not press against the victim's rib cage while the thrusts are being performed.

f. If you cannot reach around the victim to give abdominal thrusts (the victim is very obese), or if a victim is in the later stages of pregnancy, give chest thrusts. Stand behind the victim. Wrap your arms under the victim's axilla (armpits) and around to the center of the chest. Make a fist with one hand and place the thumb side of the fist against the center of the sternum but well above the xiphoid process. Grab your fist with your other hand and thrust inward.

g. Repeat the thrusts until the object is expelled or until the victim becomes unconscious. If the victim loses consciousness, follow Procedure 15:2F, Performing CPR—Obstructed Airway on Unconscious Victim. Start with a mouth sweep, try to give two breaths, reposition the head and try to give two more breaths if the first breaths do not go in, and then give five abdominal thrusts if you are unable to ventilate the victim.

5. Make every effort to obtain medical help for the victim as soon as possible. Send someone to call for help. If no one is present, yell for help. If no one answers your calls, you may have to stop your efforts for a short period of time to call EMS.

6. After the practice session, replace all equipment used. Wash hands.

Practice *Go to the workbook and use the evaluation sheet for 15:2E, Performing CPR—Obstructed Airway on Conscious, Adult Victim, to practice these procedure. When you feel you have mastered this skill, sign the sheet and give it to your instructor for further action.*

✔ **Final Checkpoint** Using the criteria listed on the evaluation sheet, your instructor will grade your performance.

PROCEDURE 15:2F

Performing CPR—Obstructed Airway on Unconscious Victim

Equipment and Supplies

CPR manikin, alcohol or disinfecting solution, gauze sponges

Procedure

 CAUTION: Only a manikin should be used to practice this procedure. Do *not* practice on another person.

1. Assemble equipment. Place the manikin on a firm surface, usually the floor.
2. Shake the victim gently. Ask, "Are you OK?"
3. If the victim is unconscious, yell for help. If no one arrives to help, call EMS. If the victim is an infant or child, yell for help, and perform the steps for an unconscious choking victim for approximately one minute. If no one arrives to call EMS, stop after one minute to call EMS. Resume the steps for an unconscious choking victim as quickly as possible.
4. Use the head-tilt/chin-lift method to open the airway.
5. Look, listen, and feel for breathing for approximately 5 but not more than 10 seconds.
6. If the victim is not breathing, give two slow, gentle breaths. If air does not go into the lungs, reposition the victim's head and try to

breathe again. If the chest still does not rise, the airway is probably obstructed.

CAUTION: Follow standard precautions. If possible, use a CPR pocket face mask with a one-way valve to provide a barrier and prevent the transmission of disease.

7. Perform five abdominal thrusts. Position the victim on his or her back. Place one of your legs on either side of the hips and thighs and "straddle" the victim (see figure 15-14A). Place the heel of one hand on the victim's abdomen, making sure the heel is positioned well below the tip of the xiphoid process, at the end of the sternum, but slightly above the navel (umbilicus). Place your other hand on top of the first hand. Give five quick, upward thrusts into the abdomen.

   NOTE: This action provides a force of air to help free the object obstructing the airway.

   NOTE: If the victim is pregnant or very obese, it may be necessary to give chest thrusts instead of abdominal thrusts. Position your hands in the same position used for chest compressions. Push straight down five times.

8. Check the mouth for the object. Open the victim's mouth by grasping the lower jaw between your thumb and fingers and lifting it. This pushes the tongue out of the airway and away from the object that may be lodged there. Use the index finger of your opposite hand to sweep along the inside of the mouth. With a C-shape or hooking motion, bring the finger along one cheek and sweep across the throat from the side and toward the opposite cheek (see figure 15-14B). Remove the object if it is seen.

   CAUTION: Take care not to push straight into the throat because this may force the object to lodge deeper in the airway.

9. Open the airway and try to give two slow, gentle breaths. If the chest rises, check the pulse and continue with ventilations or CPR as needed.

10. *If the chest does not rise,* reposition the head, and try to breathe again. If the chest still does not rise, repeat the sequence. Give five thrusts, check the mouth, and attempt to ventilate. Continue repeating the sequence until you are able to get air into the chest during ventilation.

    NOTE: Unless you are able to get oxygen into the lungs of the victim, chest compressions

have no value. The purpose of chest compressions is to circulate the oxygen.

NOTE: After a period of time without oxygen, the muscles of the throat will relax and you may be able to remove the object using the previous methods.

11. To care for an infant who has an obstructed airway, follow these steps:
    a. Gently shake the infant to determine consciousness. Call to the infant. Call for help if there is no response.
    b. Use the head-tilt/chin-lift method to open the airway.
    c. Look, listen, and feel for breathing for 5 but not more than 10 seconds.
    d. If there is no breathing, cover the infant's nose and mouth with your mouth and

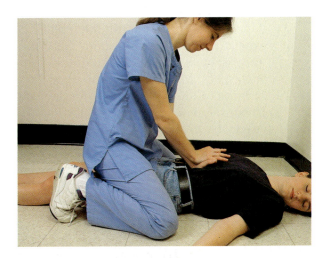

FIGURE 15-14A Straddle the unconscious victim to give five abdominal thrusts.

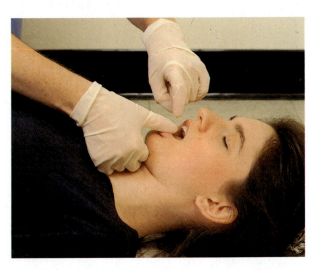

FIGURE 15-14B Use a C-shaped, or hooking, motion to check the mouth for the object.

attempt to ventilate. If the breaths do not go in, reposition the infant's head and try to breathe a second time. If the breaths still do not go in, assume that the infant has an obstructed airway.

e. Give five back blows. Hold the infant face down, with your arm supporting the infant's body and your hand supporting the infant's head and jaw. Position the head lower than the chest (see figure 15-15A). Use the heel of your other hand to give five firm back blows between the infant's shoulder blades.

⚠ **CAUTION:** When performing back blows on an infant, do not use excessive force.

f. Give five chest thrusts. Turn the infant face up, holding the head lower than the chest. Position two to three fingers on the sternum one finger's width below an imaginary line drawn between the nipples. Gently press straight down five times (see figure 15-15B), to compress the sternum ½ to 1 inch.

g. Check the mouth for the object. If you see the object, remove it by using a finger to sweep the mouth.

⚠ **CAUTION:** If you do *not* see the object, do not sweep the mouth with a finger.

h. Attempt to ventilate by giving two slow breaths. If the infant's chest rises, check for pulse and then continue with pulmonary

resuscitation or cardiac compressions, as needed. If the chest does not rise, keep repeating the sequence of five back blows, five chest thrusts, checking the mouth, and ventilating until the object can be removed.

12. To care for a child who has an obstructed airway, follow the same procedure used for adult victims *except* look in the mouth during the mouth check. Do *not* perform a finger sweep unless the object can be seen in the mouth. Therefore the sequence of steps is to give five abdominal thrusts, look in the mouth, sweep the mouth if the object is seen, and attempt to ventilate.

13. After the practice session, use a gauze pad saturated with 70-percent alcohol or a 10-percent bleach disinfecting solution to clean the manikin. Wipe the face and clean inside the mouth thoroughly. Saturate a clean gauze pad with the solution and lay it on the mouth area for at least 30 seconds. Use another gauze pad to wipe the area dry. Follow manufacturer's recommendations for specific cleaning or care.

NOTE: A 10-percent bleach solution is more effective than alcohol. Some manikins have disposable mouthpieces that are discarded after use. If the mouthpiece is discarded, the remainder of the face should still be disinfected.

14. Replace all equipment used. Wash hands.

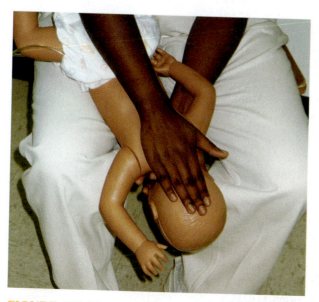

FIGURE 15-15A To give an infant five back blows, position the infant face down, with the head lower than the chest.

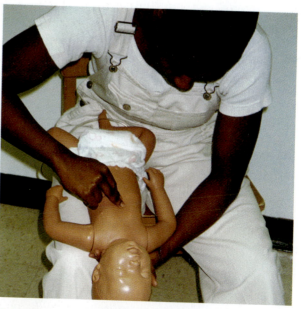

FIGURE 15-15B Give the infant five chest thrusts, keeping the head lower than the chest.

Practice *Go to the workbook and use the evaluation sheet for 15:2F, Performing CPR—Obstructed Airway on Unconscious Victim, to practice these procedure. When you feel you have mastered this skill, sign the sheet and give it to your instructor for further action.*

 Final Checkpoint Using the criteria listed on the evaluation sheet, your instructor will grade your performance.

15:3 INFORMATION Providing First Aid for Bleeding and Wounds

In any health career as well as in your personal life, you may need to provide first aid to control bleeding or care for wounds. This section provides basic information on the principles to observe when providing such first aid.

A **wound** involves injury to the soft tissues. Wounds are usually classified as open or closed. With an open wound, there is a break in the skin or mucous membrane. With a closed wound, there is no break in the skin or mucous membrane but injury occurs to the underlying tissues. Wounds can result in bleeding, infection, and/or tetanus (lockjaw, a serious infection caused by bacteria). First aid care must be directed toward controlling bleeding before the bleeding leads to death, and toward preventing or obtaining treatment for infection.

Open wounds are classified into types according to the injuries that occur. Some main types are abrasions, incisions, lacerations, punctures, avulsions, and amputations.

◆ **Abrasion:** With this type of wound the skin is scraped off. Bleeding is usually limited, but infection must be prevented because dirt and contaminants often enter the wound.

◆ **Incision:** This is a cut or injury caused by a sharp object such as a knife, scissors, or razor blade. The edges of the wound are smooth and regular. If the cut is deep, bleeding can be heavy and can lead to excessive blood loss. In addition, damage to muscles, nerves, and other tissues can occur (see figure 15-16).

◆ **Laceration:** This type of wound involves tearing of the tissues by way of excessive force. The wound often has jagged, irregular edges. Bleeding may be heavy. If the wound is deep, contamination may lead to infection.

◆ **Puncture:** This type of wound is caused by a sharp object such as a pin, nail, or pointed instrument. External bleeding is usually limited, but internal bleeding can occur. In addition, the chance for infection is increased and tetanus may develop if tetanus bacteria enter the wound.

◆ **Avulsion:** This type of wound occurs when tissue is torn or separated from the victim's body. It can result in a piece of torn tissue hanging from the ear, nose, hand, or other body part. Bleeding is heavy and usually extensive. It is important to preserve the

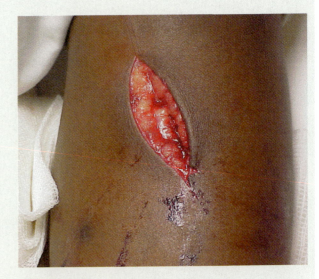

FIGURE 15-16 An incision, caused by a sharp object such as a knife or razor blade, can cause heavy bleeding and/or damage to muscles, nerves, and other tissues. *(Courtesy of Ron Stram, MD, Albany Medical Center, Albany, NY).*

body part while caring for this type of wound, because a surgeon may be able to reattach it.

◆ **Amputation:** This type of injury occurs when a body part is cut off and separated from the body. Loss of a finger, toe, hand, or other body part can occur. Bleeding can be heavy and extensive. Care must be taken to preserve the amputated part because a surgeon may be able to reattach it. The part should be wrapped in a cool, moist dressing (use sterile water or normal saline, if possible), and placed in a plastic bag. The plastic bag should be kept cool or placed in ice water and transported with the victim. The body part should never be placed directly on ice.

Controlling bleeding is the first priority in caring for wounds, because it is possible for a victim to bleed to death in a short period of time. Bleeding can come from arteries, veins, and capillaries. Arterial blood usually spurts from a wound, results in heavy blood loss, and is bright red in color. Arterial bleeding is life-threatening and must be controlled quickly. Venous blood is slower, steadier, and dark red or maroon in color. Venous bleeding is easier to control. Capillary blood "oozes" from the wound slowly, is less red than arterial blood, and clots easily. The four main methods for controlling bleeding are listed in the order in which they should be used: direct pressure, elevation, pressure bandage, and pressure points.

CAUTION: If possible, use some type of protective barrier, such as gloves or plastic wrap, while controlling bleeding, see figure 15-17. If this is not possible in an emergency, use thick layers of dressings and try to avoid contact of blood with your skin. Wash your hands thoroughly and as soon as possible after giving first aid to a bleeding victim.

◆ *Direct pressure:* Using your gloved hand over a thick dressing or sterile gauze, apply pressure directly to the wound. If no dressing is available, use a clean cloth or linen-type towel. In an emergency when no materials are available, it may even be necessary to use a bare hand. Continue to apply pressure for 5 to 10 minutes or until the bleeding stops. If blood soaks through the dressing, apply a second dressing over the first and continue to apply direct pressure. Do *not* disturb blood clots once they have formed. Direct pressure will usually stop most bleeding.

◆ *Elevation:* Raise the injured part above the level of the victim's heart to allow gravity to aid in stopping the blood flow from the wound. Continue applying direct pressure while elevating the injured part.

CAUTION: If fractures (broken bones) are present or suspected, the part should *not* be elevated.

◆ *Pressure bandage:* Apply a pressure bandage to hold the dressings in place. Maintain direct pressure and elevation while applying the pressure bandage. The procedure for applying a pressure bandage is described in step 4 of Procedure Sheet 15:3.

◆ *Pressure points:* If direct pressure, elevation, and the pressure bandage do not stop severe bleeding, it may be necessary to apply pressure to pressure points. By applying pressure to a main artery and pressing it against an underlying bone, the main blood supply to the injured area can be cut off. However, because this technique also stops circulation to other parts of the limb, it should *not* be used any longer than

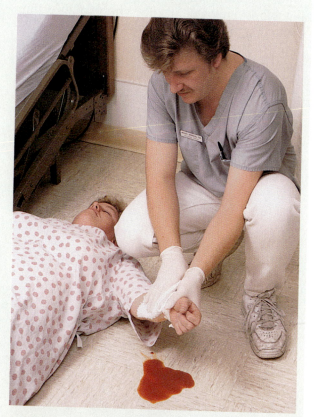

FIGURE 15-17 If possible, use some type of protective barrier, such as gloves or plastic wrap, while controlling bleeding.

is absolutely necessary. Direct pressure and elevation should also be continued while pressure is being applied to the pressure point.

The main pressure point for the arm is the brachial artery. It is located on the inside of the arm, approximately halfway between the armpit and the elbow (see figure 15-18A). The main pressure point for the leg is the femoral artery. The pulsation can be felt at the groin (the front middle point of the upper leg, in the crease where the thigh joins the body), see figure 15-18B. When bleeding stops, slowly release pressure on the pressure point. Continue using direct pressure and elevation. If bleeding starts again, be ready to reapply pressure to the correct pressure point.

After severe bleeding has been controlled, obtain medical help for the victim. Do not disturb any blood clots or remove the dressings that were used to control the bleeding, because this may result in additional bleeding. Make no attempt to clean the wound, because this too is likely to result in additional bleeding.

In treating minor wounds that do not involve severe bleeding, prevention of infection is the first priority. Wash your hands thoroughly before treating the wound. Put on gloves to avoid contamination from blood or fluid draining from the wound. Use soap and water and sterile gauze, if possible, to wash the wound. Wipe in an outward direction, away from the wound. Discard the wipe after each use. Rinse the wound thoroughly with cool water. Use sterile gauze to gently blot the wound dry. Apply a sterile dressing or bandage. Watch for any signs of infection. Be sure to tell the victim to obtain medical help if any signs of infection appear.

Infection can develop in any wound. It is important to recognize the signs of infection and to seek medical help if they appear. Some signs and symptoms are swelling, heat, redness, pain, fever, pus, and red streaks leading from the wound. Prompt medical care is needed if any of these symptoms occur.

Tetanus bacteria can enter an open wound and lead to serious illness and death. Tetanus infection is most common in puncture wounds and wounds that involve damage to tissue underneath the skin. When this type of wound occurs, it is important to obtain information from the patient regarding his or her last tetanus shot and to get medical advice regarding protection in the form of a tetanus shot or booster.

With some wounds, objects can remain in the tissues or become embedded in the wound. Examples of such objects include splinters, small pieces of glass, small stones, and other similar objects. If the object is at the surface of the skin, remove it gently with sterile tweezers or tweezers wiped clean with alcohol or a disinfectant. Any objects embedded in the tissues should be left in the skin and removed by a physician.

Closed wounds (those not involving breaks in the skin) can occur anywhere in the body as a result of injury. If the wound is a bruise, cold applications can be applied to reduce swelling.

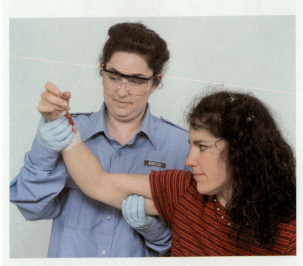

FIGURE 15-18A The main pressure point for the arm is the brachial artery. Pressure is applied to the artery only until the bleeding stops.

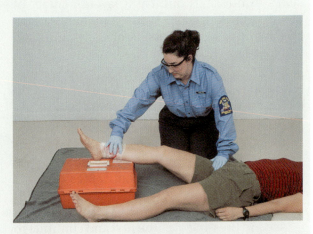

FIGURE 15-18B The main pressure point in the leg is the femoral artery. Pressure is applied while maintaining direct pressure to and elevation of the injured part.

Other closed wounds can be extremely serious and cause internal bleeding that may lead to death. Signs and symptoms may include pain, tenderness, swelling, deformity, cold and clammy skin, rapid and weak pulse, a drop in blood pressure, uncontrolled restlessness, excessive thirst, vomited blood, or blood in the urine or feces. Get medical help for the victim as soon as possible. Check breathing, treat for shock, avoid unnecessary movement, and avoid giving any fluids or food to the victim.

While caring for any victim with severe bleeding or wounds, always be alert for the signs of shock. Be prepared to treat shock while providing care to control bleeding and prevent infection in the wound.

C At all times, remain calm while providing first aid. Reassure the victim. Obtain appropriate assistance or medical care as soon as possible in every case requiring additional care.

STUDENT: *Go to the workbook and complete the assignment sheet for 15:3, Providing First Aid for Bleeding and Wounds. Then return and continue with the procedure.*

PROCEDURE 15:3
Providing First Aid for Bleeding and Wounds

Equipment and Supplies

Sterile dressings and bandages, disposable gloves

Procedure
Severe Wounds

1. Follow the steps of priority care, if indicated.
   a. Check the scene. Move the victim only if absolutely necessary.
   b. Check the victim for consciousness and breathing.
   c. Call emergency medical services (EMS).
   d. Provide care to the victim.
2. To control severe bleeding, proceed as follows:
    a. If possible, put on gloves or wrap your hands in plastic wrap to provide a protective barrier while controlling bleeding. If this is not possible in an emergency, use thick layers of dressings and try to avoid contact of blood with your skin.
   b. Using your hand over a thick dressing or sterile gauze, apply pressure directly to the wound.
   c. Continue to apply pressure to the wound for approximately 5 to 10 minutes. Do *not* release the pressure to check whether the bleeding has stopped.
   d. If blood soaks through the first dressing, apply a second dressing on top of the first dressing, and continue to apply direct pressure.
   NOTE: If sterile gauze is *not* available, use clean material or a bare hand.

   ! CAUTION: Do *not* disturb blood clots once they have formed. This will cause the bleeding to start again.
3. Elevate the injured part above the level of the victim's heart unless a fracture or broken bone is suspected.
   NOTE: This allows gravity to help stop the blood flow to the area.
   NOTE: Direct pressure and elevation are used together. Do *not* stop direct pressure while elevating the part.
4. To hold the dressings in place, apply a pressure bandage. Maintain direct pressure and elevation while applying the pressure bandage. To apply a pressure bandage, proceed as follows:
   a. Apply additional dressings over the dressings already on the wound.
   b. Use a roller bandage to hold the dressings in place by wrapping the roller bandage around the dressings. Use overlapping turns to cover the dressings and to hold them securely in place.
   c. Tie off the ends of the bandage by placing the tie directly over the dressings (see figure 15-19).
   d. Make sure the pressure bandage is secure. Check a pulse site below the pressure

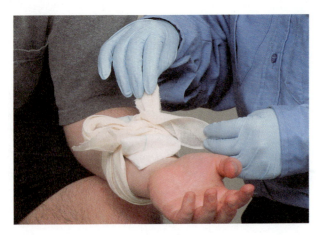

FIGURE 15-19 Tie the ends of the bandage directly over the dressings to secure a pressure bandage.

bandage to make sure the bandage is not too tight. A pulse should be present and there should be no discoloration of the skin to indicate impaired circulation. If any signs of impaired circulation are present, loosen and replace the pressure bandage.

5. If the bleeding continues, it may be necessary to apply pressure to the appropriate pressure point. Continue using direct pressure and elevation, and apply pressure to the pressure point as follows:

   a. If the wound is on the arm or hand, apply pressure to the brachial artery. Place the flat surface of your fingers (not your fingertips) against the inside of the victim's upper arm, approximately halfway between the elbow and axilla area. Position your thumb on the outside of the arm. Press your fingers toward your thumb to compress the brachial artery and decrease the supply of blood to the arm.

   b. If the wound is on the leg, place the flat surfaces of your fingers or the heel of one hand directly over the femoral artery where it passes over the pelvic bone. The position is on the front, middle part of the upper thigh (groin) where the leg joins the body. Straighten your arm and apply pressure to compress the femoral artery and to decrease the blood supply to the leg.

6. When the bleeding stops, slowly release the pressure on the pressure point while continuing to use direct pressure and elevation.

If the bleeding starts again, be ready to reapply pressure to the pressure point.

7. Obtain medical help for the victim as soon as possible. Severe bleeding is a life-threatening emergency.

8. While caring for any victim experiencing severe bleeding, be alert for the signs and symptoms of shock. Treat the victim for shock if any signs or symptoms are noted.

9. **C** During treatment, constantly reassure the victim. Encourage the victim to remain calm by remaining calm yourself.

10. After controlling the bleeding, wash your hands as thoroughly and quickly as possible to avoid possible contamination from the blood. Wear gloves and use a disinfectant solution to wipe up any blood spills. Always wash your hands thoroughly after removing gloves.

Procedure
Minor Wounds

1. Wash hands thoroughly with soap and water. Put on gloves.

2. Use sterile gauze, soap, and water to wash the wound. Start at the center and wash in an outward direction. Discard the gauze after each pass.

3. Rinse the wound thoroughly with cool water to remove all of the soap.

4. Use sterile gauze to dry the wound. Blot it gently.

5. Apply a sterile dressing to the wound.

6. Caution the victim to look for signs of infection. Tell the victim to obtain medical care if any signs of infection appear.

7. If tetanus infection is possible (for example, in cases involving puncture wounds), tell the victim to contact a doctor regarding a tetanus shot.

   ! CAUTION: Do *not* use any antiseptic solutions to clean the wound and do *not* apply any substances to the wound unless specifically instructed to do so by your immediate supervisor.

8. Obtain medical help as soon as possible for any victim requiring additional care. Any victim who has particles embedded in a wound, risk of tetanus, severe bleeding, or other complications must be referred for medical care.

9. When care is complete, remove gloves and wash hands thoroughly.

Practice *Go to the workbook and use the evaluation sheet for 15:3, Providing First Aid for Bleeding and Wounds, to practice these procedures. When you feel you have mastered these skills, sign the sheet and give it to your instructor for further action.*

 Final Checkpoint Using the criteria listed on the evaluation sheet, your instructor will grade your performance.

15:4 INFORMATION Providing First Aid for Shock

Shock is a state that can exist with any injury or illness requiring first aid. It is important that you are able to recognize it and provide treatment.

Shock, also called *hypoperfusion,* can be defined as "a clinical set of signs and symptoms associated with an inadequate supply of blood to body organs, especially the brain and heart." If it is not treated, shock can lead to death, even when a victim's injuries or illness might not themselves be fatal.

Many different things can cause the victim to experience shock: **hemorrhage** (excessive loss of blood); excessive pain; infection; heart attack; stroke; poisoning by chemicals, drugs, or gases; lack of oxygen; psychological trauma; and dehydration (loss of body fluids) from burns, vomiting, or diarrhea. The eight main types of shock are shown in Table 15-1. All types of shock impair circulation and decrease the supply of oxygen to body cells, tissues, and organs.

When shock occurs, the body attempts to increase blood flow to the brain, heart, and vital organs by reducing blood flow to other body parts. This can lead to the following signs and symptoms that indicate shock:

◆ Skin is pale or bluish gray in color. Check the nail beds and the mucous membrane around the mouth.

◆ Skin is cool to the touch.

◆ **Diaphoresis,** or excessive perspiration, may result in a wet, clammy feeling when the skin is touched.

◆ Pulse is rapid, weak, and difficult to feel. Check the pulse at one of the carotid arteries in the neck.

◆ Respirations are rapid, shallow, and may be irregular.

◆ Blood pressure is very low or below normal, and may not be obtainable.

◆ Victim experiences general weakness. As shock progresses, the victim becomes listless and confused. Eventually, the victim loses consciousness.

◆ Victim experiences anxiety and extreme restlessness.

◆ Victim may experience excessive thirst, nausea, and/or vomiting.

◆ Victim may complain of blurred vision. As shock progresses, the victim's eyes may appear sunken and have a vacant or confused expression. The pupils may dilate or become large.

It is essential to get medical help for the victim as soon as possible because shock is a life-threatening condition. Treatment for shock is directed toward (1) eliminating the cause of shock; (2) improving circulation, especially to the brain and heart; (3) providing an adequate oxygen supply; and (4) maintaining body temperature. Some of the basic principles for treatment are as follows:

◆ Reduce the effects of or eliminate the cause of shock: control bleeding, provide oxygen if available, ease pain through position change, and/or provide emotional support.

◆ The position for treating shock must be based on the victim's injuries.

! **CAUTION:** If neck or spine injuries are suspected, the victim should not be moved

TABLE 15-1 Types of Shock

TYPE OF SHOCK	CAUSE	DESCRIPTION
Anaphylactic	Hypersensitive or allergic reaction to a substance such as food, medications, insect stings or bites, or snake bites	Body releases histamine causing vasodilation (blood vessels get larger); blood pressure drops and less blood goes to body cells; urticaria (hives) and respiratory distress may occur
Cardiogenic	Damage to heart muscle from heart attack or cardiac arrest	Heart cannot effectively pump blood to body cells
Hemorrhagic	Severe bleeding or loss of blood plasma	Decrease in blood volume causes blood pressure to drop; decreased blood flow to body cells
Metabolic	Loss of body fluid from severe vomiting, diarrhea, or a heat illness; disruption in acid–base balance as occurs in diabetes	Decreased amount of fluid causes dehydration and disruption in normal acid–base balance of body; blood pressure drops and less blood circulates to body cells
Neurogenic	Injury and trauma to brain and/or spinal cord	Nervous system loses ability to control the size of blood vessels; blood vessels dilate and blood pressure drops; decreased blood flow to body cells
Psychogenic	Emotional distress such as anger, fear, or grief	Emotional response causes sudden dilation of blood vessels; blood pools in areas away from the brain; some individuals faint
Respiratory	Trauma to respiratory tract; respiratory distress or arrest (chronic disease, choking)	Interferes with exchange of oxygen and carbon dioxide between lungs and blood stream; insufficient oxygen supply for body cells
Septic	Acute infection (toxic shock syndrome)	Poisons or toxins in blood cause vasodilation; blood pressure drops; less oxygen to body cells

unless it is necessary to remove him or her from danger.

The best position for treating shock is usually to keep the victim lying flat on the back, because this improves circulation. Raising the feet and legs 12 inches can also provide additional blood for the heart and brain. However, if the victim is vomiting or has bleeding and injuries of the jaw or mouth, the victim should be positioned on the side to prevent him or her from choking on blood and/or vomitus. If a victim is experiencing breathing problems, it may be necessary to raise the victim's head and shoulders to make breathing easier. If the victim has a *head* (not neck) injury and has difficulty breathing, the victim should be positioned lying flat or with the head raised slightly. It is important to position the victim based on the injury or illness involved.

◆ Cover the patient with blankets or additional clothing to prevent chilling or exposure to the cold. Blankets may also be placed between the ground and the victim. However, it is important to avoid overheating the victim. If the skin is very warm to the touch and perspiration is noted, remove some of the blankets or coverings.

◆ Avoid giving the victim anything to eat or drink. If the victim complains of excessive thirst, a wet cloth can be used to provide some comfort by moistening the lips and mouth.

Remember that it is important to look for signs of shock while providing first aid for any injury or illness. Provide care that will reduce the effect of shock. Obtain medical help for the victim as soon as possible.

STUDENT: *Go to the workbook and complete the assignment sheet for 15:4, Providing First Aid for Shock. Then return and continue with the procedure.*

PROCEDURE 15:4
Providing First Aid for Shock

Equipment and Supplies

Blankets, watch with second hand (optional), disposable gloves

Procedure

1. Follow the steps of priority care, if indicated.
   a. Check the scene. Move the victim only if absolutely necessary.
   b. Check the victim for consciousness and breathing.
   c. Call emergency medical services (EMS).
   d. Provide care to the victim.
   e. Control severe bleeding.
      CAUTION: If possible, wear gloves or use a protective barrier while controlling bleeding.

2. Obtain medical help for the victim as soon as possible. Call or send someone to obtain help.

3. Observe the victim for any signs of shock. Look for a pale or bluish color to the skin. Touch the skin and note if it is cool, moist, or clammy to the touch. Note diaphoresis, or excessive perspiration. Check the pulse to see if it is rapid, weak, or irregular. If you are unable to feel a radial pulse, check the carotid pulse. Check the respirations to see if they are rapid, weak, irregular, shallow, or labored. If equipment is available, check blood pressure to see if it is low. Observe the victim for signs of weakness, apathy, confusion, or consciousness. Note if the victim is nauseated or vomiting, complaining of excessive thirst, restless or anxious, or complaining of blurred vision. Examine the eyes for a sunken, vacant, or confused appearance, and dilated pupils.

4. Try to reduce the effects or eliminate the cause of shock: control bleeding by applying pressure at the site; provide oxygen, if possible; attempt to ease pain through position changes and comfort measures; give emotional support.

5. Position the victim based on the injuries or illness present.
   a. If an injury of the neck or spine is present or suspect, do not move the victim.
   b. If the victim has bleeding and injuries to the jaw or mouth, or is vomiting, position the victim's body on either side. This allows fluids, vomitus, and/or blood to drain and prevents the airway from becoming blocked by these fluids.
   c. If the victim is having difficulty breathing, position the victim on the back, but raise the head and shoulders slightly to aid breathing.
   d. If the victim has a head injury, position the victim lying flat or with the head raised slightly.
      NOTE: Never allow the head to be positioned lower than the rest of the body.
   e. If none of these conditions exist, position the victim lying flat on the back. To improve circulation, raise the feet and legs 12 inches (see figure 15-20). If raising the legs causes pain or leads to difficult breathing, however, lower the legs to the flat position.
      CAUTION: Do not raise the legs if the victim has head, neck, or back injuries, or if there are possible fractures of the hips or legs.
   f. If in doubt on how to position a victim according to the injuries involved, keep the victim lying down flat or in the position in which you found him or her. Avoid any unnecessary movement.

6. Place enough blankets or coverings on the victim to prevent chilling. Sometimes, a

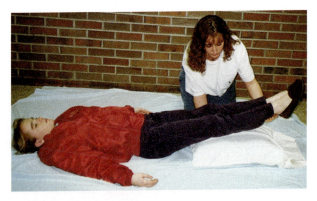

FIGURE 15-20 Position a shock victim flat on the back and elevate the feet and legs 12 inches. Do *not* use this position if the victim has a neck, spinal, head, or jaw injury, or if the victim is having difficulty breathing.

blanket can be placed between the victim and the ground. Avoid overheating the victim.

7. Do not give the victim anything to eat or drink. If the victim complains of excessive thirst, use a moist cloth to wet the lips, tongue, and inside of the mouth.

8. **C** Constantly reassure the victim. Encourage the victim to remain calm by remaining calm yourself.

9. Observe and provide care to the victim until medical help is obtained.

10. Replace all equipment used. Wash hands.

Practice *Go to the workbook and use the evaluation sheet for 15:4, Providing First Aid for Shock, to practice this procedure. When you feel you have mastered this skill, sign the sheet and give it to your instructor for further action.*

Final Checkpoint Using the criteria listed on the evaluation sheet, your instructor will grade your performance.

15:5 INFORMATION Providing First Aid for Poisoning

Poisoning can occur anywhere, anytime—not only in health care settings, but also in your personal life. **Poisoning** can happen to any individual, regardless of age. It can be caused by swallowing various substances, inhaling poisonous gases, injecting substances, or contacting the skin with poison. Any substance that causes a harmful reaction when applied or ingested can be called a poison. Immediate action is necessary for any poisoning victim. Treatment varies depending on the type of poison, the injury involved, and the method of contact.

If the poisoning victim is unconscious, check for breathing. Provide artificial respiration if the victim is not breathing. Obtain medical help as soon as possible. If the unconscious victim is breathing, position the victim on his or her side so fluids can drain from the mouth. Obtain medical help quickly.

 If a poison has been swallowed, immediate care must be provided before the poison can be absorbed into the body. Call a poison control center (PCC) or a physician immediately. If you cannot contact a PCC, call emergency medical services (EMS). Most areas have poison control centers that provide information on specific antidotes and treatment. Save the label or container of the substance taken so this information can be given to the PCC or physician. It is also helpful to know or estimate how much was taken and the time at which the poisoning occurred. If the victim vomits, save a sample of the vomited material.

If the poison control center tells you to induce vomiting, get the victim to vomit. When inducing vomiting, place the victim on one side with the head slightly downward. Syrup of ipecac followed by a glass of water can be given to induce vomiting. (Follow dosage recommended on bottle.) Syrup of ipecac is available in most drug stores and can be kept in a first aid kit for poisoning victims. If syrup of ipecac is not available, tickle the back of the victim's throat or administer warm salt water.

⚠️ **CAUTION:** Vomiting must *not* be induced in unconscious victims, victims who swallowed an acid or alkali, victims who swallowed petroleum products, victims who are convulsing, or victims who have burns on the lips and mouth.

Because vomiting removes only about one-half of the poison, the PCC may recommend using activated charcoal to counteract the remaining poison. Activated charcoal is available in most drug stores and helps absorb any remaining poison. Follow the directions on the bottle to determine the correct dosage.

If poisoning is caused by inhalation of dangerous gases, the victim must be removed immediately from the area before being treated. A commonly inhaled poison is carbon monoxide. It is odorless, colorless, and very difficult to detect. Before entering the danger area, take a deep breath of fresh air and do *not* breathe the gas while you are removing the victim from the area. After rescuing the victim, immediately check for breathing. Provide artificial respiration if needed. Obtain medical help immediately; death may occur very quickly with this type of poisoning.

If poisoning is caused by chemicals or poisons coming in contact with the victim's skin, use large amounts of water to wash the skin for at least 15 to 20 minutes, diluting the substance and removing it from the skin. Remove any clothing and jewelry that contain the substance. Call a PCC or physician for additional information. Obtain medical help as soon as possible for burns or injuries that may result from contact with the poison.

Contact with a poisonous plant such as poison ivy, oak, or sumac can cause a serious skin reaction if not treated immediately. If such contact occurs, wash the area thoroughly with soap and water. If a rash or weeping sores develop after two to three days, lotions such as Calamine or Caladryl, or a paste made from baking soda and water may help relieve the discomfort. If the condition is severe and affects large areas of the body or face, obtain medical help.

If poisoning is caused by injection from an insect bite or sting or a snakebite, and an arm or leg is affected, position the affected area below the level of the heart. For an insect bite, remove any embedded stinger by scraping the stinger away from the skin with the edge of a rigid card, such as a credit card, or a tongue depressor. Do not use tweezers because tweezers can puncture the venom sac attached to the stinger, injecting more poison into body tissues. Then wash the area well with soap and water. Apply a sterile dressing and a cold pack to reduce swelling. If a tick is embedded in the skin, use tweezers to slowly pull the tick out of the skin. Wash the area thoroughly with soap and water and apply an antiseptic. Watch for signs of infection and obtain medical help if needed. Ticks can cause Rocky Mountain spotted fever or Lyme disease, dangerous diseases if untreated. For a snakebite, wash the wound and immobilize the injured area, positioning it lower than the heart, if possible. Do *not* cut the wound or apply a tourniquet. Monitor the breathing of the victim and give artificial respiration if necessary. Obtain medical help for the victim as soon as possible. Watch for allergic reaction in all victims (see figure 15-21). Signs and symptoms of allergic reaction include redness and swelling at the site, itching, hives, pain, swelling of the throat, difficult or labored breathing, dizziness, and a change in the level of consciousness. Maintain respirations and obtain medical help as quickly as possible for the victim who experiences an allergic reaction.

C In all poisoning victims, observe for signs of anaphylactic shock. Treat the victim for shock, if necessary. Try to remain calm and confident while providing first aid for poisoning victims. Reassure the victim as needed. Act quickly and in an organized, efficient manner.

STUDENT: *Go to the workbook and complete the assignment sheet for 15:5, Providing First Aid for Poisoning. Then return and continue with the procedure.*

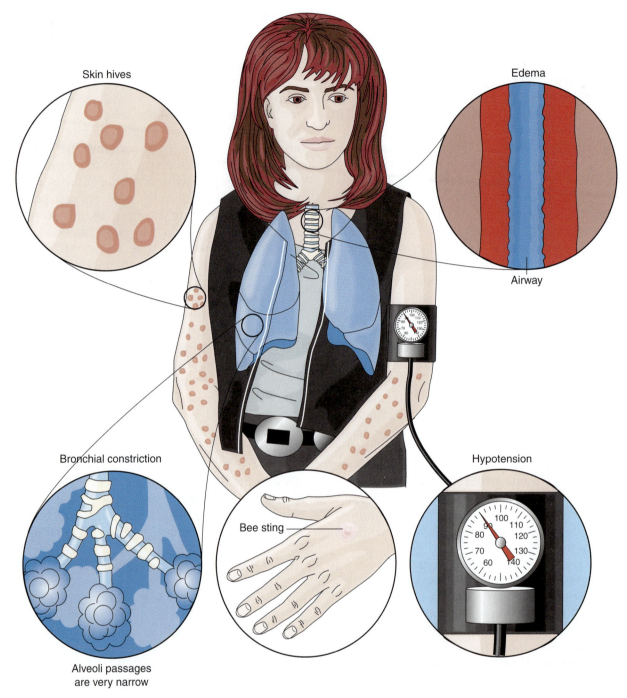

Skin hives

Edema

Airway

Bronchial constriction

Bee sting

Hypotension

Alveoli passages
are very narrow

FIGURE 15-21 Watch for allergic reactions in all poisoning victims.

PROCEDURE 15:5

Providing First Aid for Poisoning

Equipment and Supplies

Telephone, disposable gloves

Procedure

1. Follow the steps of priority care, if indicated:
   a. Check the scene. Move the victim only if absolutely necessary.
   b. Check the victim for consciousness and breathing.
   c. Call emergency medical services.
   d. Provide care to the victim.
   e. Control severe bleeding.

   CAUTION: If possible, wear gloves or use a protective barrier while controlling bleeding.

2. Check the victim for signs of poisoning. Signs may include burns on the lips or mouth, odor, a container of poison, or presence of the poisonous substance on the victim or in the victim's mouth. Information may also be obtained from the victim or from an observer.

3. If the victim is conscious, not convulsing, and has swallowed a poison:
   a. Try to determine the type of poison, how much was taken, and when the poison was taken. Look for the container near the victim.
   b. Call a poison control center (PCC) or physician immediately for specific information on how to treat the poisoning victim. Provide as much information as possible.
   c. Follow the instructions received from the PCC. Obtain medical help if needed.
   d. If the victim vomits, save a sample of the vomited material.

4. If the PCC tells you to get the victim to vomit, induce vomiting. Give the victim syrup of ipecac or warm salt water, or tickle the back of the victim's throat.

   CAUTION: Do *not* induce vomiting if the victim is unconscious or convulsing, has burns on the lips or mouth, or has swallowed an acid, alkali, or petroleum product.

5. If the victim is unconscious:
   a. Check for breathing. If the victim is not breathing, give artificial respiration.
   b. If the victim is breathing, position the victim on his or her side to allow fluids to drain from the mouth.
   c. Call a PCC or physician for specific treatment. Obtain medical help immediately.
   d. If possible, save the poison container and a sample of any vomited material. Check with any observers to find out what was taken, how much was taken, and when the poison was taken.

6. If chemicals or poisons have splashed on the victim's skin, wash the area thoroughly with large amounts of water. Remove any clothing and jewelry containing the substance. If a large area of the body is affected, a shower, tub, or garden hose may be used to rinse the skin. Obtain medical help immediately for burns or injuries caused by the poison.

7. If the victim has come in contact with a poisonous plant such as poison ivy, oak, or sumac, wash the area of contact thoroughly with soap and water. Remove any contaminated clothing. If a rash or weeping sores develop in the next few days after exposure, lotions such as Calamine or Caladryl, or a paste made from baking soda and water, may help relieve the discomfort. If the condition is severe and affects large areas of the body or face, obtain medical help.

8. If the victim has inhaled poisonous gas, do not endanger your life by trying to treat the victim in the area of the gas. Take a deep breath of fresh air before entering the area and hold your breath while you remove the victim from the area. When the victim is in a safe area, check for breathing. Provide artificial respiration, if necessary. Obtain medical help immediately.

9. If poisoning is caused by injection from an insect bite or sting or a snakebite, proceed as follows:
   a. If an arm or leg is affected, position the affected area below the level of the heart.

b. For an insect bite, remove any embedded stinger by scraping it off with an object like a credit card. Wash the area well with soap and water. Apply a sterile dressing and a cold pack to reduce swelling.

c. If a tick is embedded in the skin, use tweezers to gently pull the tick out of the skin. Wash the area thoroughly with soap and water and apply an antiseptic. Obtain medical help if needed.

d. For a snakebite, wash the wound. Immobilize the injured area, positioning it lower than the heart, if possible. Monitor the breathing of the victim and give artificial respiration if necessary. Obtain medical help for the victim as soon as possible.

e. Watch for the signs and symptoms of allergic reaction in all victims. Signs and symptoms of allergic reaction include redness and swelling at the site, itching, hives, pain, swelling of the throat, difficult or labored breathing, dizziness, and a change in the level of consciousness. Maintain respirations and obtain medical help as quickly as possible for the victim experiencing an allergic reaction.

10. Observe for signs of anaphylactic shock while treating any poisoning victim. Treat for shock as necessary.

11. Remain calm while treating the victim. Reassure the victim.

12. **C** Always obtain medical help for any poisoning victim. Some poisons may have delayed reactions. Always keep the telephone numbers of a PCC and other sources of medical assistance in a convenient location so you will be prepared to provide first aid for poisoning.

Practice *Go to the workbook and use the evaluation sheet for 15:5, Providing First Aid for Poisoning, to practice this procedure. When you feel you have mastered this skill, sign the sheet and give it to your instructor for further action.*

✔ **Final Checkpoint** Using the criteria listed on the evaluation sheet, your instructor will grade your performance.

15:6 INFORMATION Providing First Aid for Burns

A **burn** is an injury that can be caused by fire, heat, chemical agents, radiation, and/or electricity. Burns are classified as either first, second, or third degree (see figure 15-22). Characteristics of each type of burn are as follows:

◆ *First-degree, or superficial, burn:* This is the least severe type of burn. It involves only the top layer of skin, the epidermis, and usually heals in 5 to 6 days without permanent scarring. The skin is usually reddened or discolored. There may be some mild swelling, and the victim feels pain. Three common causes are overexposure to the sun (sunburn), brief contact with hot objects or steam, and exposure of the skin to a weak acid or alkali.

◆ *Second-degree, or partial-thickness, burn:* This type of burn involves injury to the top layers of skin, including both the epidermis and dermis. A blister or vesicle forms. The skin is red or has a mottled appearance. Swelling usually occurs, and the surface of the skin frequently appears to be wet. This is a painful burn and may take 3 to 4 weeks to heal. Frequent causes include excessive exposure to the sun, a sunlamp, or artificial radiation; contact with hot or boiling liquids; and contact with fire.

◆ *Third-degree, or full-thickness, burn:* This is the most severe type of burn and involves injury to all layers of the skin plus the underlying tissue. The area involved has a white or charred appearance. This type of burn can be either extremely painful or, if nerve endings are destroyed, relatively painless. Third-degree burns can be life-threatening because of fluid loss, infection, and shock.

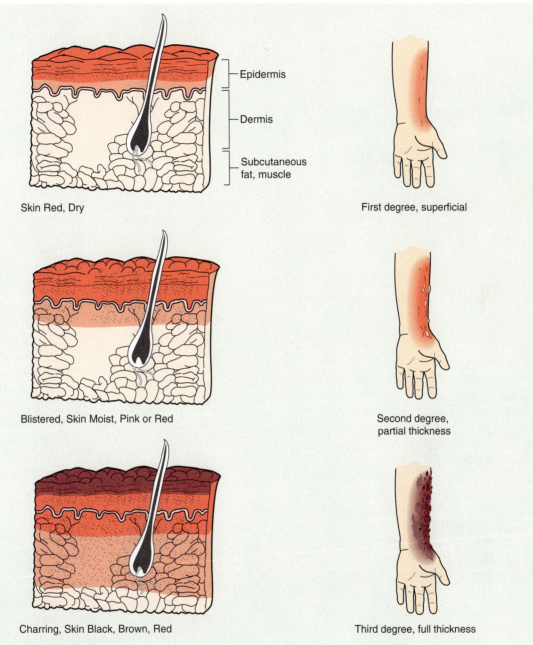

Skin Red, Dry

First degree, superficial

Blistered, Skin Moist, Pink or Red

Second degree, partial thickness

Charring, Skin Black, Brown, Red

Third degree, full thickness

FIGURE 15-22 Types of burns.

Frequent causes include exposure to fire or flames, prolonged contact with hot objects, contact with electricity, and immersion in hot or boiling liquids.

First aid treatment for burns is directed toward removing the source of heat, cooling the affected skin area, covering the burn, relieving pain, observing and treating for shock, and preventing infection. Medical treatment is not usually required for first-degree and mild second-degree burns. However, medical care should be obtained if more than 15 percent of the surface of an adult's body is burned (10 percent in a child). The rule of nines is used to calculate the percentage of body surface burned (see figure 15-23). Medical care should also be obtained if the burns affect the face or respiratory tract, if the victim has difficulty breathing, if burns cover more than one body part, if the victim has a partial-thickness burn and is under 5 or over 60 years of age, or if the burns resulted from chemicals, explosions, or electricity. All victims with third-degree burns should receive medical care.

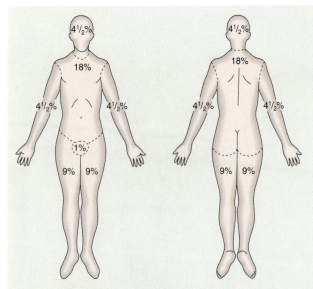

FIGURE 15-23 The *rule of nines* is used to calculate the percentage of body surface burned.

The main treatment for first-degree and mild second-degree burns is to cool the area by flushing it with large amounts of cool water. Do *not* use ice or ice water on burns because doing so causes the body to lose heat. After the pain subsides, use dry, sterile gauze to blot the area dry. Apply a dry, sterile dressing to prevent infection. If nonadhesive dressings are available, it is best to use them because they will not stick to the injured area. If possible, elevate the affected part to reduce swelling caused by inflammation. If necessary, obtain medical help.

CAUTION: Do *not* apply cotton, tissues, ointment, powders, oils, grease, butter, or any other substances to the burned area unless you are instructed to do so by a physician or your immediate supervisor. Do *not* break or open any blisters that form on burns because doing so will just cause an open wound that is prone to infection.

Call for medical help immediately if the victim has severe second-degree or third-degree burns. Cover the burned areas with thick, sterile dressings. Elevate the hands or feet if they are burned. If the feet or legs are burned, do *not* allow the victim to walk. If particles of clothing are attached to the burned areas, do *not* attempt to remove these particles. Watch the victim closely for signs of respiratory distress and/or shock. Provide artificial respiration and treatment for shock, as necessary. Watch the victim closely until medical help arrives.

For burns caused by chemicals splashing on the skin, use large amounts of water to flush the affected areas for 15 to 30 minutes or until medical help arrives. Gently remove any clothing, socks and shoes, or jewelry that contains the chemical to minimize the area injured. Continue flushing the skin with cool water and watch the victim for signs of shock until medical help can be obtained.

If the eyes have been burned by chemicals or irritating gases, flush the eyes with large amounts of water for at least 15 to 30 minutes or until medical help arrives. If only one eye is injured, be sure to tilt the victim's head in the direction of the injury so the injured eye can be properly flushed. Start at the inner corner of the eye and allow the water to run over the surface of the eye and to the outside. Continue flushing the eye with cool water and watch the victim for signs of shock until medical help can be obtained.

CAUTION: Make sure that the water (or remaining chemical) does not enter the *uninjured* eye.

Loss of body fluids (dehydration) can occur very quickly with severe burns, so shock is frequently noted in burn victims. Be alert for any signs of shock and treat the burn victim for shock immediately.

C Remain calm while treating the burn victim. Reassure the victim. Obtain medical help as quickly as possible for any burn victim requiring medical assistance.

STUDENT: *Go to the workbook and complete the assignment sheet for 15:6, Providing First Aid for Burns. Then return and continue with the procedure.*

PROCEDURE 15:6

Providing First Aid for Burns

Equipment and Supplies

Water, sterile dressings, disposable gloves

Procedure

1. Follow the priorities of care, if indicated:
   a. Check the scene. Move the victim only if absolutely necessary.
   b. Check the victim for consciousness and breathing.
   c. Call emergency medical services (EMS) if necessary.
   d. Provide care to the victim.
   e. Check for bleeding. Control severe bleeding.

      CAUTION: If possible, wear gloves or use a protective barrier while controlling bleeding.
2. Check the burned area carefully to determine the type of burn. A reddened or discolored area is usually a superficial, or first-degree, burn. If the skin is wet, red, swollen, painful, and blistered, the burn is usually a partial-thickness, or second-degree, burn (see figure 15-24A). If the skin is white or charred and there is destruction of tissue, the burn is a full-thickness, or third-degree, burn (see figure 15-24B).

   NOTE: Victims can have more than one type of burn at one time. Treat for the most severe type of burn present.
3. For a first-degree or mild second-degree burn:
   a. Cool the burn by flushing it with large amounts of cool water. If this is not possible, apply clean or sterile cloths that are cold and wet. Continue applying cold water until the pain subsides.
   b. Use sterile gauze to gently blot the injured area dry.
   c. Apply dry, sterile dressings to the burned area. If possible, use nonadhesive (nonstick) dressings, because they will not stick to the burn.
   d. If blisters are present, do *not* break or open them.
   e. If possible, elevate the burned area to reduce swelling caused by inflammation.
   f. Obtain medical help for burns to the face, or if burns cover more than 15 percent of the surface of an adult's body or 10 percent of the surface of a child's body. If the

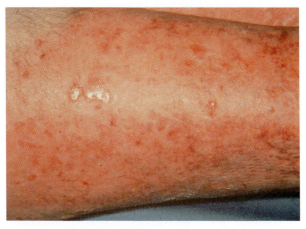

FIGURE 15-24A The skin is wet, red, swollen, painful, and blistered when a second-degree or partial-thickness burn is present. *(Courtesy of the Phoenix Society of Burn Survivors, Inc.)*

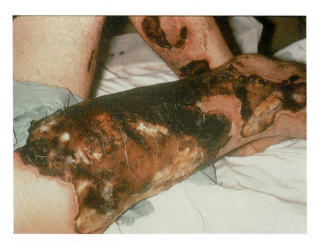

FIGURE 15-24B A third-degree or full thickness burn destroys or affects all layers of the skin plus fat, muscle, bone, and nerve tissue. The skin is white or charred in appearance. *(Courtesy of the Phoenix Society of Burn Survivors, Inc.)*

victim is having difficulty breathing, or any other distress is noted, obtain medical help.

   g. Do *not* apply any cotton, ointment, powders, grease, butter, or similar substances to the burned area.

   NOTE: These substances may increase the possibility of infection.

4. For a severe second-degree or any third-degree burn:

   a. Call for medical help immediately.

   b. Use thick, sterile dressings to cover the injured areas.

   c. Do *not* attempt to remove any particles of clothing that have stuck to the burned areas.

   d. If the hands and arms or legs and feet are affected, elevate these areas.

   e. If the victim has burns on the face or is experiencing difficulty in breathing, elevate the head.

   f. Watch the victim closely for signs of shock and provide care if necessary.

5. For a burn caused by a chemical splashing on the skin:

   a. Using large amounts of water, immediately flush the area for 15 to 30 minutes or until medical help arrives.

   b. Remove any articles of clothing, socks and shoes, or jewelry contaminated by the substance.

   c. Continue flushing the area with large amounts of cool water.

   d. Obtain medical help immediately.

6. If the eye has been burned by chemicals or irritating gases:

   a. If the victim is wearing contact lenses or glasses, ask him or her to remove them quickly.

   b. Tilt the victim's head toward the injured side.

   c. Hold the eyelid of the injured eye open. Pour cool water from the inner part of the eye (the part closest to the nose) toward the outer part (see figure 15-25).

   d. Use cool water to irrigate the eye for 15 to 30 minutes or until medical help arrives.

   ⚠ **CAUTION:** Take care that the water or chemicals do not enter the uninjured eye.

   e. Obtain medical help immediately.

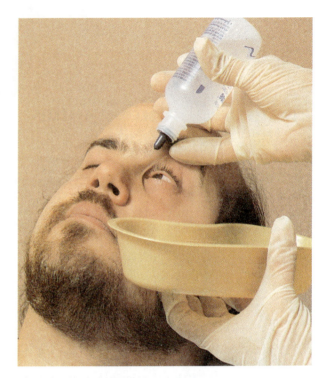

FIGURE 15-25 To irrigate an eye, hold the eyelid open and irrigate from the inner part of the eye toward the outer part.

7. Observe for the signs of shock in all burn victims. Treat for shock as necessary.

8. Ⓒ Reassure the victim as you are providing treatment. Remain calm and encourage the victim to remain calm.

9. Obtain medical help immediately for any burn victim with extensive burns, third-degree burns, burns to the face, signs of shock, respiratory distress, eye burns, and/or chemical burns to the skin.

Practice *Go to the workbook and use the evaluation sheet for 15:6, Providing First Aid for Burns, to practice this procedure. When you feel you have mastered this skill, sign the sheet and give it to your instructor for further action.*

 Final Checkpoint Using the criteria listed on the evaluation sheet, your instructor will grade your performance.

15:7 INFORMATION Providing First Aid for Heat Exposure

Excessive exposure to heat or high external temperatures can lead to a life-threatening emergency (see figure 15-26). Overexposure to heat can cause a chemical imbalance in the body that can eventually lead to death. Harmful reactions can occur when water or salt are lost through perspiration or when the body cannot eliminate excess heat.

Heat cramps are caused by exposure to heat. They are muscle pains and spasms that result from the loss of water and salt through perspiration. Firm pressure applied to the cramped muscle will provide relief from the discomfort. The victim should rest and move to a cooler area. In addition, small sips of water or an electrolyte solution, such as sport drinks, can be given to the victim.

Heat exhaustion occurs when a victim is exposed to heat and experiences a loss of fluids through sweating. Signs and symptoms include pale and clammy skin, profuse perspiration (diaphoresis), fatigue or tiredness, weakness, headache, muscle cramps, nausea and/or vomiting, and dizziness and/or fainting. Body temperature is about normal or just slightly elevated. Treatment methods include moving the victim to a cooler area whenever possible; loosening or removing excessive clothing; applying cool, wet cloths; laying the victim down and elevating the victim's feet 12 inches; and giving the victim small sips of cool water, approximately 4 ounces every 15 minutes if the victim is alert and conscious. If the victim vomits, develops shock, or experiences respiratory distress, obtain medical help immediately.

Heat stroke is caused by prolonged exposure to high temperatures. It is a medical emergency. The body is unable to eliminate the excess heat, and internal body temperature rises to 105°F (40.6°C) or higher. Normal body defenses such as the sweating mechanism no longer function. Signs and symptoms in addition to the high body temperature include red, hot, and dry skin. The pulse is usually rapid, but may remain strong. The victim may lose consciousness. Treatment is geared primarily toward ways of cooling the body quickly, because a high body temperature can cause convulsions and/or death in a very short period of time. The victim can be placed in a tub of cool water, or the skin can be sponged with cool water. Ice or cold packs can be placed on the victim's wrists, ankles, in each axillary (armpit) area, and in the groin. Be alert for signs of shock at all times. Obtain medical help immediately.

C After victims have recovered from any condition caused by heat exposure, they must be warned to avoid abnormally warm or hot temperatures for several days. They should also be encouraged to drink sufficient amounts of water and to consume adequate amounts of salt.

STUDENT: *Go to the workbook and complete the assignment sheet for 15:7, Providing First Aid for Heat Exposure. Then return and continue with the procedure.*

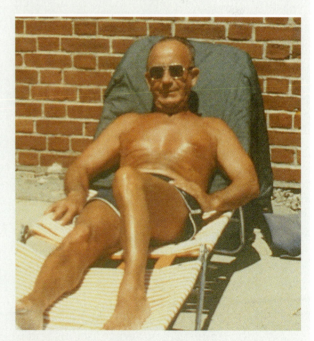

FIGURE 15-26 Excessive exposure to heat or high external temperatures can lead to a life-threatening emergency. *(Courtesy of the Phoenix Society of Burn Survivors, Inc.)*

PROCEDURE 15:7
Providing First Aid for Heat Exposure

Equipment and Supplies

Water, wash cloths or small towels

Procedure

1. Follow the priorities of care, if indicated:
   a. Check the scene. Move the victim only if absolutely necessary.
   b. Check the victim for consciousness and breathing.
   c. Call emergency medical services (EMS) if necessary.
   d. Provide care to the victim.
   e. Check for bleeding. Control severe bleeding.

   CAUTION: If possible, wear gloves or use a protective barrier while controlling bleeding.

2. Observe the victim closely for signs and symptoms of heat exposure. Information may also be obtained directly from the victim or from observers. If the victim has been exposed to heat or has been exercising strenuously, and is complaining of muscular pain or spasm, he or she is probably experiencing heat cramps. If the victim has close-to-normal body temperature but has pale and clammy skin, is perspirating excessively, and complains of nausea, headache, weakness, dizziness, or fatigue, he or she is probably experiencing heat exhaustion. If body temperature is high (105°F, or 40.6°C, or higher); skin is red, dry, and hot; and the victim is weak or unconscious, he or she is experiencing heat stroke.

3. If the victim has heat cramps:
   a. Use your hand to apply firm pressure to the cramped muscle(s). This helps relieve the spasms.
   b. Encourage relaxation. Allow the victim to lie down in a cool area, if possible.
   c. If the victim is alert and conscious and is not nauseated or vomiting, give him or her small sips of cool water, approximately 4 ounces every 15 minutes.
   d. If the heat cramps continue or get worse, obtain medical help.

4. If the victim has heat exhaustion:
   a. Move the victim to a cool area, if possible. An air-conditioned room is ideal, but a fan can also help circulate air and cool the victim.
   b. Help the victim lie down flat on the back. Elevate the victim's feet and legs 12 inches.
   c. Loosen any tight clothing. Remove excessive clothing such as jackets and sweaters.
   d. Apply cool, wet cloths to the victim's face.
   e. If the victim is conscious and is not nauseated or vomiting, give him or her small sips of cool water, approximately 4 ounces every 15 minutes.
   f. If the victim complains of nausea and/or vomits, discontinue water. Obtain medical help.

5. If the victim has heat stroke:
   a. Immediately move the victim to a cool area, if at all possible.
   b. Remove excessive clothing.
   c. Sponge the bare skin with cool water, or place ice or cold packs on the victim's wrists, ankles, and in the axillary and groin areas. The victim can also be placed in a tub of cool water to lower body temperature.

   CAUTION: Watch that the victim's head is not submerged in water. If the victim is unconscious, you may need assistance to place him or her in the tub.

   d. If vomiting occurs, position the victim on his or her side. Watch for signs of difficulty in breathing and provide care as indicated.
   e. Obtain medical help immediately. This is a life-threatening emergency.

6. Shock can develop quickly in all victims of heat exposure. Be alert for the signs of shock and treat as necessary.

CAUTION: Obtain medical help for heat cramps that do not subside, heat exhaustion with signs of shock or vomiting, and *all* heat stroke victims as soon as possible.

7. **C** Reassure the victim as you are providing treatment. Remain calm.

Practice *Go to the workbook and use the evaluation sheet for 15:7, Providing First Aid for Heat Exposure, to practice this procedure. When you feel you have mastered this skill, sign the sheet and give it to your instructor for further action.*

 Final Checkpoint Using the criteria listed on the evaluation sheet, your instructor will grade your performance.

15:8   INFORMATION   Providing First Aid for Cold Exposure

Exposure to cold external temperatures can cause body tissues to freeze and body processes to slow. If treatment is not provided immediately, the victim can die. Factors such as wind velocity, amount of humidity, and length of exposure all affect the degree of injury.

Prolonged exposure to the cold can result in **hypothermia,** a condition in which the body temperature is less than 95°F (35°C). Elderly individuals are more susceptible to hypothermia than are younger individuals (see figure 15-27). Signs and symptoms include shivering, numbness, weakness or drowsiness, low body temperature, poor coordination, confusion, and loss of consciousness. If prolonged exposure continues, body processes will slow down and death can occur. Treatment consists of getting the victim to a warm area, removing wet clothing, slowly warming the victim by wrapping in blankets or putting on dry clothing, and, if the victim is fully conscious, giving warm nonalcoholic, noncaffeinated liquids by mouth. Avoid warming the victim too quickly, because rapid warming can cause dangerous heart arrhythmias.

Frostbite is actual freezing of tissue fluids accompanied by damage to the skin and underlying tissues (see figure 15-28). It is caused by exposure to freezing or below-freezing temperatures. Early signs and symptoms include redness and tingling. As frostbite progresses, signs and symptoms include pale, glossy skin, white or grayish-yellow in color; in some cases, blisters; skin that is cold to the touch; numbness; and, sometimes, pain that gradually subsides until the victim does not feel any pain. If exposure continues, the victim may become confused, lethargic, and incoherent. Shock may develop followed by unconsciousness and death. First aid for frostbite is directed at maintaining respirations, treating for shock, warming the affected parts, and preventing further injury. Frequently, small areas of the body are affected by frostbite. Common sites include the fingers, toes, ears, nose, and cheeks. Extreme care must be taken to avoid further injury to areas damaged by frostbite. Because the victim usually does not feel pain, the part must be warmed

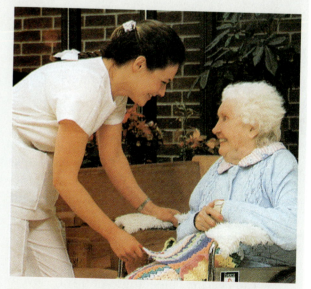

FIGURE 15-27 Elderly individuals are more susceptible to hypothermia than are younger individuals.

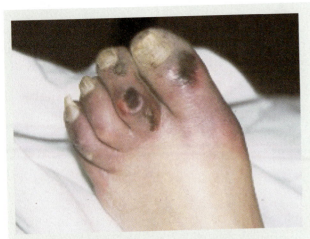

FIGURE 15-28 Frostbite is actual freezing of tissue fluids accompanied by damage to skin and underlying tissues. *(Courtesy of Deborah Funk, MD, Albany Medical Center, Albany, NY)*

! CAUTION: Heat lamps, hot water above 104°F (40°C), or heat from a stove or oven should *not* be used. Furthermore, the parts should *not* be rubbed or massaged, because this may cause gangrene (death of the tissue). Avoid opening or breaking any blisters that form, because doing so will create an open wound. Do *not* allow the victim to walk or stand if the feet, legs, or toes are affected. Dry, sterile dressings can be placed between toes or fingers to prevent them from rubbing and causing further injury. Medical help should be obtained as quickly as possible.

Shock is frequently noted in victims exposed to the cold. Be alert for all signs of shock and treat for shock as necessary.

carefully, taking care not to burn the injured tissue. The parts affected may be immersed in warm water at 100°F to 104°F (37.8°C to 40°C).

STUDENT: *Go to the workbook and complete the assignment sheet for 15:8, Providing First Aid for Cold Exposure. Then return and continue with the procedure.*

PROCEDURE 15:8

Providing First Aid for Cold Exposure

Equipment and Supplies

Blankets, bath water and thermometer, sterile gauze sponges

Procedure

1. Follow the priorities of care, if indicated:
   a. Check the scene. Move the victim only if absolutely necessary.
   b. Check the victim for consciousness and breathing.
   c. Call emergency medical services (EMS) if necessary.
   d. Provide care to the victim.
   e. Check for bleeding. Control severe bleeding.

   CAUTION: If possible, wear gloves or use a protective barrier while controlling bleeding.

2. Observe the victim closely for signs and symptoms of cold exposure. Information may also be obtained directly from the victim or observers. Note shivering, numbness, weakness or drowsiness, confusion, low body temperature, and lethargy. Check the skin, particularly on the toes, fingers, ears, nose, and cheeks. Suspect frostbite if any areas are pale, glossy, white or grayish-yellow, and cold to the touch, and if the victim complains of any part of the body feeling numb or painless.

3. Move the victim to a warm area as soon as possible.

4. Immediately remove any wet or frozen clothing. Loosen any tight clothing that decreases circulation.

5. Slowly warm the victim by wrapping the victim in blankets or dressing the victim in dry, warm clothing. If a body part is affected by frostbite, immerse the part in warm water measuring 100°F to 104°F (37.8°C to 40°C).

   ! CAUTION: Warm a victim of hypothermia slowly. Rapid warming can cause heart problems or increase circulation to the surface of the body, which causes additional cooling of vital organs.

⚠ CAUTION: Do *not* use heat lamps, hot water above the stated temperatures, or heat from stoves or ovens. Excessive heat can burn the victim.

6. After the body part affected by frostbite has been thawed and the skin becomes flushed, discontinue warming the area because swelling may develop rapidly. Dry the part by blotting gently with a towel or soft cloth. Gently wrap the part in clean or sterile cloths. Use sterile gauze to separate the fingers and/or toes to prevent them from rubbing together.

⚠ CAUTION: *Never* rub or massage the frostbitten area, because doing so can cause gangrene.

7. Help the victim lie down. Do not allow the victim to walk or stand if the legs, feet, or toes are injured. Elevate any injured areas.

8. Observe the victim for signs of shock. Treat for shock as necessary.

9. If the victim is conscious and is not nauseated or vomiting, give warm liquids to drink.

⚠ CAUTION: Do *not* give beverages containing alcohol or caffeine. Give the victim warm broth, water, or milk.

10. **C** Reassure the victim while providing treatment. Remain calm and encourage the victim to remain calm.

11. Obtain medical help as soon as possible.

> **Practice** *Go to the workbook and use the evaluation sheet for 15:8, Providing First Aid for Cold Exposure, to practice this procedure. When you feel you have mastered this skill, sign the sheet and give it to your instructor for further action.*

✔ Final Checkpoint Using the criteria listed on the evaluation sheet, your instructor will grade your performance.

15:9 INFORMATION Providing First Aid for Bone and Joint Injuries

Injuries to bones and joints are common in accidents and falls. A variety of injuries can occur to bones and joints. Such injuries sometimes occur together; other times, these injuries occur by themselves. Examples of injuries to bones and joints are fractures, dislocations, sprains, and strains.

A **fracture** is a break in a bone. A closed, or simple, fracture is a bone break that is not accompanied by an external or open wound on the skin. A compound, or open, fracture is a bone break that is accompanied by an open wound on the skin. Main facts regarding fractures are as follows:

◆ Signs and symptoms of fractures can vary. Not all signs and symptoms will be present in every victim. Common signs and symptoms include deformity, limited motion or loss of motion, pain and tenderness at the fracture site, swelling and discoloration, and the protrusion of bone ends through the skin. Additional information obtained from the victim may include hearing a bone break or snap, feeling a grating sensation (crepitation), and abnormal movements within a part of the body.

◆ Treatment for fractures is directed toward maintaining respirations, treating for shock, keeping the broken bone from moving, and preventing further injury. Devices such as splints and slings can be utilized to prevent movement of the injured part. Whenever a fracture is evident or suspected, medical help must be obtained.

A **dislocation** is when the end of a bone is either displaced from a joint or moved out of its normal position within a joint. This injury is frequently accompanied by a tearing or stretching of ligaments, muscles, and other soft tissue.

◆ Signs and symptoms that may occur include deformity, limited or abnormal movement, swelling, discoloration, pain, tenderness, and a shortening or lengthening of the affected arm or leg.

◆ First aid for dislocations is basically the same as that for fractures. No attempt should be made to reduce the dislocation (that is, replace the bone in the joint). The affected part must be immobilized in the position in which it was found. Immobilization is accomplished by using splints and/or slings. Movement of the injured part can lead to additional injury to nerves, blood vessels, and other tissue in the area. Obtain medical help immediately.

A **sprain** is an injury to the tissues surrounding a joint; it usually occurs when the part is forced beyond its normal range of movement. Ligaments, tendons, and other tissues are stretched or torn. Common sites for sprains include the ankles and wrists.

◆ Signs and symptoms of a sprain include swelling, pain, discoloration and, sometimes, impaired motion. Frequently, sprains resemble fractures or dislocations. If in doubt, treat the injury as a fracture.

◆ First aid for a sprain includes application of cold to decrease swelling and pain, elevation of the affected part, and rest. In addition, an elastic bandage can be used to provide support for the affected area. If swelling is severe or if there is any question of a fracture, medical help should be obtained.

A **strain** is the overstretching of a muscle; it is caused by overexertion or lifting. A frequent site for strains is the back.

◆ Signs and symptoms of a strain include sudden pain, swelling, and/or bruising.

◆ Treatment for a strain is directed toward resting the affected muscle while providing support. Bedrest with a backboard under the mattress is recommended for a strained back. Cold applications can be used initially to reduce the swelling. However, warm, wet applications are the main treatment later, because warmth relaxes the muscles. Different types of cold and heat packs are available (see figure 15-29). Medical help should be

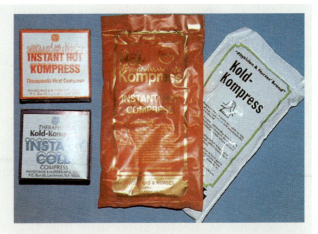

FIGURE 15-29 Disposable heat and cold packs contain chemicals that must be activated before using.

obtained for severe strains and all back injuries.

Splints are devices that can be used to immobilize injured parts when fractures, dislocations, and other similar injuries are present or suspected. Many commercial splints are available, including inflatable, or air, splints, padded boards, and traction splints. Splints can also be made from cardboard, newspapers, blankets, pillows, boards, and other similar materials. Some basic principles regarding the use of splints are:

◆ Splints should be long enough to immobilize the joint above and below the injured area (see figure 15-30). By preventing movement in these joints, the injured bone or area is held in position and further injury is prevented.

◆ Splints should be padded, especially at bony areas and over the site of injury. Cloths, thick dressings, towels, and similar materials can be used as padding.

◆ Strips of cloth, roller gauze, triangular bandages folded into bands or strips, and similar materials can be used to tie splints in place.

◆ Splints must be applied so that they do not put pressure directly over the site of injury.

◆ If an open wound is present, use a sterile dressing to apply pressure and control bleeding.

CAUTION: Wear gloves or use a protective barrier while controlling bleeding to avoid contamination from the blood.

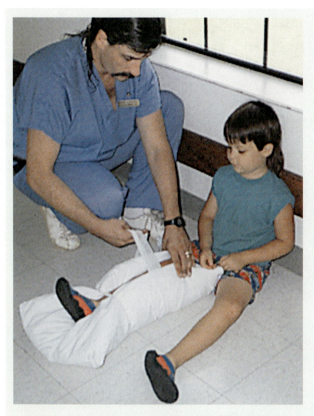

FIGURE 15-30 Splints should be long enough to immobilize the joint above and below the injured area.

> ⚠ **CAUTION:** Leave the dressing in place, and apply the splint in such a way that it does *not* put pressure on the wound.

◆ *Never* make any attempt to replace broken bones or reduce a fracture or dislocation; and do *not* move the victim. Splint wherever you find the victim.

◆ *Pneumatic* splints are available in various sizes and shapes for different parts of the arms and legs. Care must be taken to avoid any unnecessary movement while the splint is being positioned. There are two main types of pneumatic splints: air (inflatable) and vacuum (deflatable). If an air splint is positioned over a fracture site, air pressure is used to inflate the splint (see figure 15-31A). Some air splints have nozzles; these splints are inflated by blowing into the nozzles. Other air splints require the use of pressurized material in cans, while still others are inflated with cool air from a refrigerant solution. The coldness reduces swelling. Care must be taken to avoid overinflating air splints. To test whether the splint is properly inflated, use a thumb to apply slight

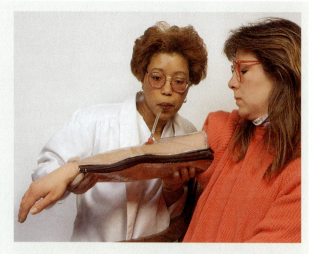

FIGURE 15-31A Some air splints are inflated by blowing into a nozzle. Care must be taken to avoid overinflating this type of splint.

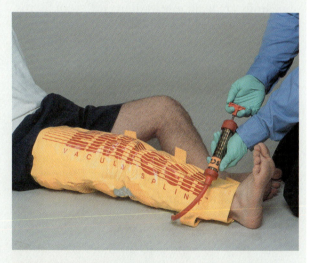

FIGURE 15-31B Vacuum pneumatic splints are deflated until the splint molds to the fracture site to provide support.

pressure to the splint; an indentation mark should result. Vacuum pneumatic splints are deflated after being positioned over a fracture site. Air is removed from the splint with a hand pump or suction pump until the splint molds to the fracture site to provide support (see figure 15-31B). Care must be taken to avoid overdeflation of the splint. A pulse site below the splint should be checked to make sure the splint is not applying too much pressure and cutting off circulation.

◆ Traction splints are special devices that provide a pulling or traction effect on the injured bone. They are frequently used for fractures of the femur, or thigh bone.

⚖ **CAUTION:** Only persons specifically trained in the application of traction splints should apply them.

◆ After a splint is applied, it is essential to note the circulation and the effects on the nerve endings of the skin below the splint to make sure the splint is not too tight. Check skin temperature (it should be warm to the touch), skin color (pale or blue indicates poor circulation), swelling or edema, numbness or tingling, and pulse, if possible.

🛑 **CAUTION:** If any signs of impaired circulation or impaired neurological status are present, immediately loosen the ties holding the splint.

Slings are available in many different forms. Commercial slings usually have a series of straps that extend around the neck and/or thoracic (chest) region, see figure 15-32. A common type of sling used for first aid is the triangular bandage. Slings are usually used to support the arm, hand, forearm, and shoulder. They may be used when casts are in place. In addition, they are also used to provide immobility if a fracture of the arm or shoulder is suspected. Basic principles to observe with slings include:

◆ When a sling is applied to an arm, the sling should be positioned in such a way that the hand is higher than the elbow. The purpose of elevating the hand is to promote circulation, prevent swelling (edema), and decrease pain.

◆ Circulation in the limb and nerve supply to the limb must be checked frequently. Specifically, check for skin temperature (should be warm if circulation is good), skin color (blue or very pale indicates poor circulation), swelling (edema), amount of pain, and tingling or numbness. Nail beds can also be used to check circulation. When the nail beds are pressed slightly, they blanch (turn white). If circulation is good, the pink color should return to the nail beds immediately after the pressure is released.

◆ If a sling is being applied because of a suspected fracture to the bone, extreme care must be taken to move the injured limb as little as possible while the sling is being applied. The victim can sometimes help by

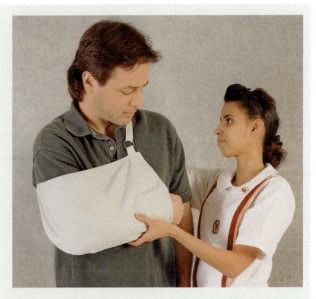

FIGURE 15-32 Commercial slings usually have a series of straps that extend around the neck and/or thoracic region.

holding the injured limb in position while the sling is slipped into place.

◆ If a triangular bandage is used, care must be taken so that the knot tied at the neck does not press against a bone. The knot should be tied to either side of the spinal column. Place gauze or padding under the knot of the sling to protect the skin.

◆ When shoulder injuries are suspected, it may be necessary to keep the arm next to the body. After a sling has been applied, another bandage can be placed around the thoracic region to hold the arm against the body.

Injuries to the neck or spine are the most dangerous types of injuries to bones and joints.

🛑 **CAUTION:** If a victim who has such injuries is moved, permanent damage resulting in paralysis can occur. If at all possible, avoid any movement of a victim with neck or spinal injuries. Wait until a backboard and adequate help for transfer is available.

Many victims with injuries to bones and/or joints also experience shock. Always be alert for signs of shock and treat as needed.

C Injuries of this type usually involve a great deal of anxiety, pain, and discomfort, so constantly reassure the victim. Encourage the victim to relax, and position the victim as comfortably as possible. Advise the victim that medical help is on the way. First aid measures are directed toward relieving the pain as much as possible.

Obtain medical help for all victims of bone or joint injuries. The only definite diagnosis of a closed fracture is an X-ray of the area. Whenever a fracture and/or dislocation is suspected, treat the victim as though one of these injuries has occurred.

STUDENT: *Go to the workbook and complete the assignment sheet for 15:9, Providing First Aid for Bone and Joint Injuries. Then return and continue with the procedure.*

PROCEDURE 15:9
Providing First Aid for Bone and Joint Injuries

Equipment and Supplies

Blankets, splints of various sizes, air or inflatable splints, triangular bandages, strips of cloth or roller gauze, disposable gloves

Procedure

1. Follow the priorities of care, if indicated:
   a. Check the scene. Move the victim only if absolutely necessary. If the victim must be moved from a dangerous area, pull in the direction of the long axis of the body (that is, from the head or feet). If at all possible, tie an injured leg to the other leg or secure an injured arm to the body before movement.

      CAUTION: If neck or spinal injuries are suspected, avoid any movement of the victim unless movement is necessary to save the victim's life.
   b. Check the victim for consciousness and breathing.
   c. Call emergency medical services (EMS) if necessary.
   d. Provide care to the victim.
   e. Control severe bleeding. If an open wound accompanies a fracture, take care not to push broken bone ends into the wound.

      CAUTION: If possible, wear gloves or use a protective barrier while controlling bleeding.
2. Observe for signs and symptoms of a fracture, dislocation, or joint injury. Note deformities (such as a shortening or lengthening of an extremity), limited motion or loss of motion, pain, tenderness, swelling, discoloration, and bone fragments protruding through the skin. Also, the victim may state that he or she heard a bone snap or crack, or may complain of a grating sensation.
3. Immobilize the injured part to prevent movement.

   CAUTION: Do *not* attempt to straighten a deformity, replace broken bone ends, or reduce a dislocation. Avoid any unnecessary movement of the injured part. If a bone injury is suspected, treat the victim as though a fracture or dislocation has occurred. Use splints or slings to immobilize the injury.
4. *To apply splints:*
   a. Obtain commercial splints or improvise splints by using blankets, pillows, newspapers, boards, cardboard, or similar supportive materials.
   b. Make sure that the splints are long enough to immobilize the joint both above and below the injury.
   c. Position the splints, making sure that they do *not* apply pressure directly at the site of injury. Two splints are usually used. However, if a pillow, blanket, or similar item is used, one such item can be rolled around the area to provide support on all sides.
   d. Use thick dressings, cloths, towels, or other similar materials to pad the splints. Make sure bony areas are protected. Avoid direct contact between the splint material and the skin.

      NOTE: Many commercial splints are already padded. However, additional padding is often needed to protect the bony areas.

e. Use strips of cloth, triangular bandages folded into strips, roller gauze, or other similar material to tie or anchor the splints in place. The use of elastic bandage is discouraged because the bandages may cut off or interfere with circulation. If splints are long, three to five ties may be required. Tie the strips above and below the upper joint and above and below the lower joint. An additional tie should be placed in the center region of the splint.

f. Avoid any unnecessary movement of the injured area while splints are being applied. If possible, have another individual support the area while you are applying the splints.

5. *To apply air (inflatable) splints:*
   a. Obtain the correct splint for the injured part.
   NOTE: Most air splints are available for full arm, lower arm, wrist, full leg, lower leg, and ankle/foot.
   b. Some air splints have zippers for easier application, but others must be slipped into position on the victim. If the splint has a zipper, position the open splint on the injured area, taking care to avoid any movement of the affected part. Use your hand to support the injured area. Close the zipper. If the splint must be slipped into position, slide the splint onto your arm first. Then hold the injured leg or arm and slide the splint from your arm to the victim's injured extremity. This technique prevents unnecessary movement.
   c. Inflate the splint. Many splints are inflated by blowing into the nozzle. Others require the use of a pressure solution in a can. Follow instructions provided by the manufacturer of the splint.
   d. Check to make sure that the splint is not overinflated. Use your thumb to press a section of the splint. Your thumb should leave a slight indentation if the splint is inflated correctly.

6. *To apply a sling,* follow the manufacturer's instructions for commercial slings. To use a triangular bandage for a sling (see figure 15-33), proceed as follows:
   a. If possible, obtain the help of another individual to support the injured arm while the sling is being applied. Sometimes, the victim can hold the injured arm in place.

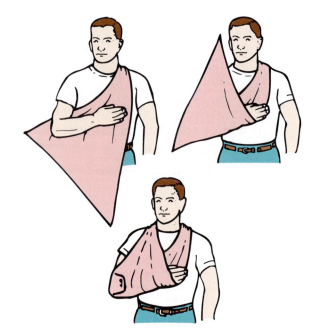

FIGURE 15-33 Steps for applying a triangular bandage as a sling.

b. Place the long straight edge of the triangular bandage on the uninjured side. Allow one end to extend over the shoulder of the uninjured arm. The other end should hang down in front of the victim's chest. The short edge of the triangle should extend back and under the elbow of the injured arm.
   ! CAUTION: Avoid excessive movement of the injured limb while positioning the sling.

c. Bring the long end of the bandage up and over the shoulder of the injured arm.

d. Use a square knot to tie the two ends together near the neck. Make sure the knot is not over a bone. Tie it to either side of the spinal column. Place gauze or padding between the knot and the skin. Make sure the hand is elevated 5 to 6 inches above the elbow.

e. The point of the bandage is now near the elbow. Bring the point forward, fold it, and pin it to the front of the sling. If no pin is available, coil the end and tie it in a knot.
   ! CAUTION: If you use a pin, put your hand between the pin and the victim's skin while inserting the pin.

f. Check the position of the sling. The fingers of the injured hand should extend beyond the edge of the triangular bandage. In addition, the hand should be slightly elevated to prevent swelling (edema).

7. After splints and/or slings have been applied, check for signs of impaired circulation. Skin color should be pink. A pale or bluish color is a sign of poor circulation. The skin should be warm to the touch. Swelling can indicate poor circulation. If the victim complains of pain or pressure from the splints and/or slings, or of numbness or tingling in the area below the splints/sling, circulation may be impaired. Slightly press the nail beds on the foot or hand so they temporarily turn white. If circulation is good, the pink color will return to the nail beds immediately after pressure is released. If you note any signs of impaired circulation, loosen the splints and/or sling immediately.

8. Watch for signs of shock in any victim with a bone and/or joint injury. Remember, inadequate blood flow is the main cause of shock. Watch for signs of impaired circulation, such as a bluish tinge around the lips or nail beds. Treat for shock, as necessary.

9. If medical help is delayed, cold applications such as cold compresses or an ice bag can be used on the injured area to decrease swelling.

⓵ CAUTION: To prevent injury to the skin, make sure that the ice bag is covered with a towel or other material.

10. Place the victim in a comfortable position, but avoid any unnecessary movement.

⓵ CAUTION: Avoid *any* movement if a neck or spinal injury is suspected.

11. **Ⓒ** Reassure the victim while providing first aid. Try to relieve the pain by carefully positioning the injured part, avoiding unnecessary movement, and applying cold.

12. Obtain medical help as quickly as possible.

Practice *Go to the workbook and use the evaluation sheet for 15:9, Providing First Aid for Bone and Joint Injuries, to practice this procedure. When you feel you have mastered this skill, sign the sheet and give it to your instructor for further action.*

✔ **Final Checkpoint** Using the criteria listed on the evaluation sheet, your instructor will grade your performance.

15:10 INFORMATION Providing First Aid for Specific Injuries

Although treatment for burns, bleeding, wounds, poisoning, and fractures is basically the same for all regions of the body, injuries to specific body parts require special care. Examples of these parts are the eyes, ears, nose, brain, chest, abdomen, and genital organs.

Eye Injuries

Any *eye* injury always involves the danger of vision loss, especially if treated incorrectly. In most cases involving serious injury to the eyes, it is best *not* to provide major treatment.

Obtaining medical help, preferably from an eye specialist, is a top priority of first aid care.

◆ Foreign objects such as dust, dirt, and similar small particles frequently enter the eye. These objects cause irritation and can scratch the eye or become embedded in the eye tissue. Signs and symptoms include redness, a burning sensation, pain, watering or tearing of the eye, and/or the presence of visible objects in the eye. If the foreign body is floating freely, prevent the victim from rubbing the eye, wash your hands thoroughly, and gently draw the upper lid down over the lower lid. This stimulates the formation of tears. The proximity of the lids also creates a wiping action, which may remove the particle. If this does not remove the foreign body, use your thumb and forefinger to grasp the eyelashes and gently raise the upper eyelid. Tell the victim to look down and tilt his or her head toward the injured side. Use water to gently flush the eye or use the corner of a piece of sterile gauze to gently remove the object.

CAUTION: If this does not remove the object or if the object is embedded, make *no* attempt to remove it.

Apply a dry, sterile dressing and obtain medical help for the victim. Serious injury can occur if any attempt is made to remove an object embedded in the eye tissue.

◆ Blows to the eye from a fist, accident, or explosion may cause contusions or black eyes as a result of internal bleeding and torn tissues inside the eye. Because this can lead to loss of vision, the victim should be examined as soon as possible by an eye specialist. Apply sterile dressings or an eye shield, keep the victim lying flat, and obtain medical help. It is sometimes best to cover both eyes to prevent involuntary movement of the injured eye.

◆ Penetrating injuries that cut the eye tissue are extremely dangerous.

CAUTION: If an object is protruding from the eye, make *no* attempt to remove the object. Rather, support it by *loosely* applying dressings. A paper cup with a hole cut in the bottom can also be used to stabilize the object and prevent it from moving (see figure 15-34).

Apply dressings to both eyes to prevent involuntary movement of the injured eye.

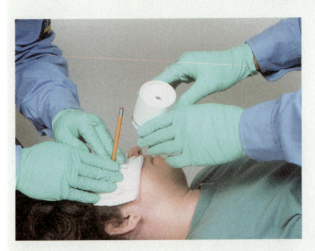

FIGURE 15-34 A cup can be used to stabilize an object impaled in the eye and to prevent it from moving.

Avoid applying pressure to the eye while applying the dressings. Keep the victim lying flat on his or her back to prevent fluids from draining out of the eye. Obtain medical help immediately.

Ear Injuries

Injuries to the *ear* can result in rupture or perforation of the eardrum. These injuries also require medical care. Treatment for specific types of ear injuries is as follows:

◆ Wounds of the ear frequently result in torn or detached tissue. Apply sterile dressings with light pressure to control bleeding.

CAUTION: If possible, wear gloves or use a protective barrier while controlling bleeding.

Save any torn tissue and use sterile water or sterile normal saline solution to keep it cool and moist. Send the torn tissue to the medical facility along with the victim.

NOTE: If sterile water is not available, use cool, clean water.

Keep the victim lying flat, but raise his or her head (if no other conditions prohibit raising the head).

◆ If the eardrum is ruptured or perforated, place sterile gauze loosely in the outer ear canal. Do *not* allow the victim to hit the side of the head in an attempt to restore hearing and do *not* put any liquids into the ear. Obtain medical help for the victim.

◆ Clear or blood-tinged fluid draining from the ear can be a sign of skull or brain injury. Allow the fluid to flow from the ear. Keep the victim lying down. If possible, turn the victim on his or her injured side and slightly elevate the head and shoulders to allow the fluid to drain. Obtain medical help immediately and report the presence and description of the fluid.

CAUTION: Wear gloves or use a protective barrier to avoid skin contact with fluid draining from the ear.

Head or Skull Injuries

Wounds or blows to the *head* or *skull* can result in injury to the brain. Again, it is important to obtain medical help as quickly as possible for the victim.

◆ Signs and symptoms of brain injury include clear or blood-tinged cerebrospinal fluid draining from the nose or ears, loss of consciousness, headache, visual disturbances, pupils unequal in size, muscle paralysis, speech disturbances, convulsions, and nausea and vomiting.

◆ Keep the victim lying flat and treat for shock. If there is no evidence of neck or spinal injury, raise the victim's head slightly by supporting the head and shoulders on a small pillow or a rolled blanket or coat.

◆ Watch closely for signs of respiratory distress and provide artificial respiration as needed.

◆ Make *no* attempt to stop the flow of fluid. Loose dressings can be positioned to absorb the flow.

> **CAUTION:** Wear gloves or use a protective barrier to avoid contamination from the cerebrospinal fluid.

◆ Do *not* give the victim any liquids. If the victim complains of excessive thirst, use a clean, cool, wet cloth to moisten the lips, tongue, and inside of the mouth.

◆ Note how long the victim is unconscious and report this to the emergency rescue personnel.

Nose Injuries

Injuries to the *nose* frequently cause a nosebleed, also called an epistaxis. Nosebleeds are usually more frightening than they are serious. Nosebleeds can also be caused by change in altitude, strenuous activity, high blood pressure, and rupture of small blood vessels after a cold. Treatment for a nosebleed includes:

◆ Keep the victim quiet and remain calm.

◆ If possible, place the victim in a sitting position with the head leaning slightly forward.

◆ Apply pressure to control bleeding by pressing the bleeding nostril toward the midline. If both nostrils are bleeding, press both nostrils toward the midline.
NOTE: If both nostrils are blocked, tell the victim to breathe through the mouth.

> **CAUTION:** Wear gloves or use a protective barrier to avoid contamination from blood.

◆ If application of pressure against the midline or septum does not stop the bleeding, insert a small piece of gauze in the nostril and then apply pressure on the outer surface of the nostril.

> **CAUTION:** Do not use cotton balls because the fibers will shed and stick.

Be sure to leave a portion of the gauze extending out of the nostril so that the packing can be removed later.

◆ Apply a cold compress to the bridge of the nose. A covered ice pack or a cold, wet cloth can be used.

◆ If the bleeding does not stop or a fracture of the nose is suspected, obtain medical assistance. If a person has repeated nosebleeds, a referral for medical attention should be made. Nosebleeds can indicate an underlying condition that requires medical care and treatment, such as high blood pressure.

Chest Injuries

Injuries to the *chest* are usually medical emergencies because the heart, lungs, and major blood vessels may be involved. Chest injuries include sucking chest wounds, penetrating wounds, and crushing injuries. In all cases, obtain medical help immediately.

◆ *Sucking chest wound:* a deep, open chest wound that allows air to flow directly in and out with breathing. The partial vacuum that is usually present in the pleura (sacs surrounding the lungs) is destroyed, causing the lung on the injured side to collapse. Immediate medical help must be obtained. An airtight dressing must be placed over the wound to prevent air flow into the wound. Aluminum foil, plastic wrap, or other nonporous material should be used to cover the wound. Tape or a bandage can be used to hold the nonporous material in place on three sides. The fourth side should be left loose to allow air to escape when the victim exhales. Maintain an open airway (through the nose or mouth) and provide artificial respiration as needed. If possible, position the victim on his or her injured side and elevate the head and chest slightly. This allows the uninjured lung to expand more freely and prevents pressure

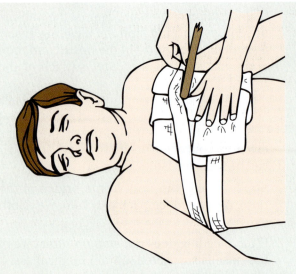

FIGURE 15-35 Immobilize an object protruding from the chest by placing dressings around the object and taping the dressings in place.

on the uninjured lung from blood and damaged tissue.

◆ *Penetrating injuries to the chest:* can result in sucking chest wounds or damage to the heart and blood vessels. If an object (for example, a knife) is protruding from the chest, do *not* attempt to remove the object. If possible, immobilize the object by placing dressings around it and taping the dressings in position (see figure 15-35). Place the victim in a comfortable position, maintain respirations, and obtain medical help immediately.

◆ *Crushing chest injuries:* caused in vehicular accidents or when heavy objects strike the chest. Fractured ribs and damage to the lungs and/or heart can occur. Place the victim in a comfortable position and, if possible, elevate the head and shoulders to aid breathing. If an injury to the neck or spine is suspected, avoid moving the victim. Obtain medical help immediately.

Abdominal Injuries

Abdominal injuries can damage internal organs and cause bleeding in major blood vessels. The intestines and other abdominal organs may protrude from an open wound. Medical help must be obtained immediately; bleeding, shock, and organ damage can lead to death in a short period of time.

◆ Signs and symptoms include severe abdominal pain or tenderness, protruding organs, open wounds, nausea and vomiting (particularly of blood), abdominal muscle rigidity, and symptoms of shock.

◆ Position the victim flat on his or her back. Place a pillow or rolled blanket under the knees to bend the knees slightly. This helps relax the abdominal muscles. Elevate the head and shoulders slightly to aid breathing.

◆ Remove clothing from around the wound or protruding organs. Use a large sterile dressing moistened with sterile water or normal saline solution to cover the area. If sterile water or normal saline is not available, use warm tap water to moisten the dressings. Cover the dressings with plastic wrap, if available, to keep the dressings moist. Then cover the dressings with aluminum foil or a folded towel to keep the area warm.

⚠ **CAUTION:** Make no attempt to reposition protruding organs.

◆ Avoid giving the victim any fluids or food. If the victim complains of excessive thirst, use a cool, wet cloth to moisten the lips, tongue, and inside of the mouth.

Injuries to Genital Organs

Injuries to *genital organs* can result from falls, blows, or explosions. Zippers catching on genitals and other accidents sometimes bruise the genitals. Because injuries to the genitals may cause severe pain, bleeding, and shock, medical help is required. Basic principles of first aid include the following:

◆ Control severe bleeding by using a sterile (or clean) dressing to apply direct pressure to the area.

☣ **CAUTION:** Wear gloves or use a protective barrier to avoid contamination from blood.

◆ Treat the victim for shock.

◆ Do not remove any penetrating or inserted objects.

◆ Save any torn tissue and use sterile water or sterile normal saline to keep it cool and moist. Send the torn tissue to the medical facility along with the victim.

◆ Use a covered ice pack or other cold applications to decrease bleeding and relieve pain.

◆ Obtain medical help.

Shock frequently occurs in victims with specific injuries to the eyes, ears, chest, abdomen, or other vital organs. Be alert for the signs of shock and immediately treat all victims.

C Most of the specific injuries discussed in this section result in extreme pain for the victim. It is essential that you reassure the victim constantly and encourage the victim to relax as much as possible. Direct first aid care toward providing as much relief from pain as possible.

STUDENT: *Go to the workbook and complete the assignment sheet for 15:10, Providing First Aid for Specific Injuries. Then return and continue with the procedure.*

PROCEDURE 15:10
Providing First Aid for Specific Injuries

Equipment and Supplies

Blankets, pillows, dressings, bandages, tape, aluminum foil or plastic wrap, eye shields or sterile dressings, sterile water, disposable gloves

Procedure

1. Follow the priorities of care, if indicated:
   a. Check the scene. Move the victim only if absolutely necessary.
   b. Check the victim for consciousness and breathing.
   c. Call emergency medical services (EMS), if necessary.
   d. Provide care to the victim.
   e. Check for bleeding. Control severe bleeding.

      CAUTION: If possible, wear gloves or use a protective barrier while controlling bleeding.

2. **C** Observe the victim closely for signs and symptoms of specific injuries. Do a systematic examination of the victim. Always have a reason for everything you do. Explain what you are doing to the victim and/or observers.

3. If the victim has an eye injury, proceed as follows:
   a. If the victim has a free-floating particle or foreign body in the eye, warn the victim *not* to rub the eye. Wash your hands thoroughly to prevent infection. Gently grasp the upper eyelid and draw it down over the lower eyelid. If this does not remove the object, use your thumb and forefinger to grasp the eyelashes and gently raise the upper eyelid. Tell the victim to look down and tilt his or her head slightly to the injured side. Use water to gently flush the eye or use the corner of a piece of sterile gauze to gently remove the object. If this does not remove the object or if the object is embedded, proceed to step b.
   b. If an object is embedded in the eye, make *no* attempt to remove it. Rather, apply a dry, sterile dressing to loosely cover the eye. Obtain medical help.
   c. If an eye injury has caused a contusion, a black eye, internal bleeding, and/or torn tissue in the eye, apply sterile dressings or eye shields to both eyes. Keep the victim lying flat. Obtain medical help.

      NOTE: Both eyes are covered to prevent involuntary movement of the injured eye.
   d. If an object is protruding from the eye, make *no* attempt to remove the object. If possible, support the object in position by loosely placing dressings around it. A paper cup with the bottom removed can also be used to surround and prevent any movement of the object. Apply dressings to the uninjured eye to prevent movement of the injured eye. Keep the victim lying flat. Obtain medical help immediately.

4. If the victim has an ear injury:
   a. Control severe bleeding from an ear wound by using a sterile dressing to apply light pressure.

   CAUTION: Wear gloves or use a protective barrier to prevent contamination from the blood.

   b. If any tissue has been torn from the ear, preserve the tissue by placing it in cool, sterile water or normal saline solution. The tissue may also be put in sterile gauze that has been moistened with sterile water. Send the torn tissue to the medical facility along with the victim.

   NOTE: If sterile water is not available, use cool, clean water.

   c. If a rupture or perforation of the eardrum is suspected or evident, place sterile gauze loosely in the outer ear canal. Caution the victim against hitting the side of the head to restore hearing. Obtain medical help.

   d. If cerebrospinal fluid is draining from the ear, make no attempt to stop the flow of the fluid. If no neck or spinal injury is suspected, turn the victim on his or her injured side and slightly elevate the head and shoulders to allow the fluid to drain. A dressing may be positioned to absorb the flow. Obtain medical help immediately.

   CAUTION: Wear gloves or use a protective barrier to prevent contamination from the cerebrospinal fluid.

5. If the victim has a brain injury:
   a. Keep the victim lying flat. Treat for shock. If there is no evidence of a neck or spinal injury, place a small pillow or a rolled blanket or coat under the victim's head and shoulders to elevate the head slightly.

   CAUTION: Never position the victim's head lower than the rest of the body.

   b. Watch closely for signs of respiratory distress. Provide artificial respiration if needed.

   NOTE: Remove the pillow if artificial respiration is given.

   c. If cerebrospinal fluid is draining from the ears, nose, and/or mouth, make *no* attempt to stop the flow. Position dressings to absorb the flow.

   CAUTION: Wear gloves or use a protective barrier to prevent contamination from the cerebrospinal fluid.

d. Avoid giving the victim any fluids by mouth. If the victim complains of excessive thirst, use a cool, wet cloth to moisten the lips, tongue, and inside of the mouth.

e. If the victim is unconscious, note for how long and report this information to the emergency rescue personnel.

f. Obtain medical help as quickly as possible.

6. If the victim has a nosebleed:
   a. Try to keep the victim calm. Remain calm yourself.

   b. Position the victim in a sitting position, if possible. Lean the head forward slightly. If the victim cannot sit up, slightly elevate the head.

   c. Apply pressure by pressing the nostril(s) toward the midline. Continue applying pressure for at least 5 minutes and longer if necessary to control the bleeding.

   NOTE: If both nostrils are bleeding and must be pressed toward the midline, tell the victim to breathe through the mouth.

   CAUTION: Wear gloves or use a protective barrier to prevent contamination from the blood.

   d. If application of pressure does not control the bleeding, insert gauze into the bleeding nostril, taking care to allow some of the gauze to hang out. Then apply pressure again by pushing the nostril toward the midline.

   e. Apply cold compresses to the bridge of the nose. Use cold, wet cloths or a covered ice bag.

   f. If the bleeding does not stop, a fracture is suspected, or the victim has repeated nosebleeds, obtain medical help.

   NOTE: Nosebleeds can indicate a serious underlying condition that requires medical attention, such as high blood pressure.

7. If the victim has a chest injury:
   a. If the wound is a sucking chest wound, apply a nonporous dressing. Use plastic wrap or aluminum foil to create an airtight seal. Use tape on three sides to hold the dressing in place. Leave the fourth side loose to allow excess air to escape when the victim exhales (see figure 15-36).

   b. Maintain an open airway. Constantly be alert for signs of respiratory distress. Provide artificial respiration as needed.

   c. If there is no evidence of a neck or spinal injury, position the victim with his or her injured side down. Slightly elevate the

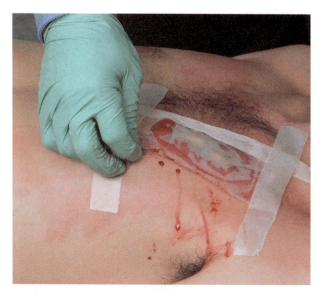

FIGURE 15-36 An airtight dressing is used to cover a sucking chest wound. It is taped on three sides. The fourth side is left open to allow excess air to escape when the victim exhales.

head and chest by placing small pillows or blankets under the victim.

d. If an object is protruding from the chest, make *no* attempt to remove it. If possible, immobilize the object with dressings, and tape around it.

e. Obtain medical help immediately for all chest injuries.

8. If the victim has an abdominal injury:

a. Position the victim flat on the back. Place a small pillow or a rolled blanket or coat under the victim's knees to flex them slightly. Elevate the head and shoulders to aid breathing. If movement of the legs causes pain, leave the victim lying flat.

b. If abdominal organs are protruding from the wound, make *no* attempt to reposition the organs. Remove clothing from around the wound or protruding organs. Use a sterile dressing that has been moistened with sterile water or normal saline solution to cover the area. If sterile water or normal saline is not available, use warm tap water to moisten the dressings.

c. Cover the dressing with plastic wrap, if available, to keep the dressing moist. Then apply a folded towel or aluminum foil to keep the area warm.

d. Avoid giving the victim any fluids or food. If the victim complains of excessive thirst, use a cool, wet cloth to moisten the lips, tongue, and inside of the mouth.

e. Obtain medical help immediately.

9. If the victim has an injury to the genital organs:

a. Control severe bleeding by using a sterile dressing to apply direct pressure.

   CAUTION: Wear gloves or use a protective barrier to prevent contamination from the blood.

b. Position the victim flat on the back. Separate the legs to prevent pressure on the genital area.

c. If any tissue is torn from the area, preserve the tissue by placing it in cool, sterile water or normal saline solution or in gauze moistened with sterile water. Put the tissue on ice and send it to the medical facility along with the victim.

d. Apply cold compresses such as covered ice bags to the area to relieve pain and reduce swelling.

e. Obtain medical help for the victim.

10. Be alert for the signs of shock in all victims. Treat for shock immediately.

11. **C** Constantly reassure all victims while providing care. Remain calm. Encourage the victim to relax as much as possible.

12. Always obtain medical help as quickly as possible. Shock, pain, and injuries to vital organs can cause death in a very short period of time.

Practice *Go to the workbook and use the evaluation sheet for 15:10, Providing First Aid for Specific Injuries, to practice this procedure. When you feel you have mastered this skill, sign the sheet and give it to your instructor for further action.*

 Final Checkpoint Using the criteria listed on the evaluation sheet, your instructor will grade your performance.

15:11 INFORMATION Providing First Aid for Sudden Illness

The victim of a sudden illness requires first aid until medical help can be obtained. Sudden illness can occur in any individual. At times, it is difficult to determine the exact illness being experienced by the victim. However, by knowing the signs and symptoms of some major disorders, you should be able to provide appropriate first aid care. Information regarding a specific condition or illness may also be obtained from the victim, medical alert bracelets or necklaces, or medical information cards. Be alert to all of these factors while caring for the victim of a sudden illness.

Heart Attack

A **heart attack** is also called a *coronary thrombosis, coronary occlusion,* or *myocardial infarction.* It may occur when one of the coronary arteries supplying blood to the heart is blocked. If the attack is severe, the victim may die. If the heart stops beating, cardiopulmonary resuscitation (CPR) must be started. Main facts regarding heart attacks are as follows:

◆ Signs and symptoms of a heart attack may vary depending on the amount of heart damage. Severe, painful pressure under the breastbone (sternum) with pain radiating to the shoulders, arms, neck, and jaw is a common symptom (see figure 15-37). The victim usually experiences intense shortness of breath. The skin, especially near the lips and nail beds, becomes pale or bluish in color. The victim feels very weak but is also anxious and apprehensive. Nausea, vomiting, diaphoresis (excessive perspiration), and loss of consciousness may occur.

◆ First aid for a heart attack is directed toward encouraging the victim to relax, placing the victim in a comfortable position to relieve pain and assist breathing, and obtaining medical help. Shock frequently occurs, so provide treatment for shock. Prevent any

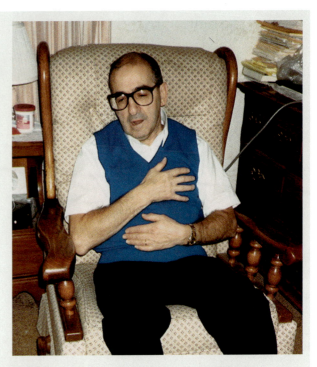

FIGURE 15-37 Severe pressure under the sternum with pain radiating to the shoulders, arms, neck, and jaw is a common symptom of a heart attack.

unnecessary stress and avoid excessive movement because any activity places additional strain on the heart. Reassure the victim constantly, and obtain appropriate medical assistance as soon as possible.

Cerebrovascular Accident or Stroke

A *stroke* is also called a **cerebrovascular accident** (CVA), *apoplexy,* or *cerebral thrombosis.* It is caused by either the presence of a clot in a cerebral artery that provides blood to the brain or hemorrhage from a blood vessel in the brain.

◆ Signs and symptoms of a stroke vary depending on the part of the brain affected. Some common signs and symptoms are numbness, paralysis, eye pupils unequal in size, mental confusion, slurred speech, nausea, vomiting, difficult breathing and swallowing, and loss of consciousness.

◆ First aid for a stroke victim is directed toward maintaining respirations, laying the victim flat on the back with the head slightly elevated or on the side to allow secretions to drain from the mouth, and avoiding any fluids by mouth. Reassure the victim, prevent any unnecessary stress, and avoid any unnecessary movement.

C **NOTE:** Always remember that although the victim may be unable to speak or may appear to be unconscious, he or she may be able to hear and understand what is going on.

◆ Obtain medical help as quickly as possible. Immediate care during the first three hours can help prevent brain damage. If the CVA is caused by a blood clot, treatment with thrombolytic or "clot busting" drugs such as TPA (tissue plasminogen activator) or angioplasty of the cerebral arteries can dissolve a blood clot and restore blood flow to the brain.

Fainting

Fainting occurs when there is a temporary reduction in the supply of blood to the brain. It may result in partial or complete loss of consciousness. The victim usually regains consciousness after being in a supine position (that is, lying flat on the back).

◆ Early signs of fainting include dizziness, extreme pallor, diaphoresis, coldness of the skin, nausea, and a numbness and tingling of the hands and feet.

◆ If early symptoms are noted, help the victim to lie down or to sit in a chair and position his or her head at the level of the knees.

◆ If the victim loses consciousness, try to prevent injury. Provide first aid by keeping the victim in a supine position. If no neck or spine injuries are suspected, use a pillow or blankets to elevate the victim's legs and feet 12 inches. Loosen any tight clothing and maintain an open airway. Use cool water to gently bathe the victim's face. Check for any injuries that may have been caused by the fall. Permit the victim to remain flat and quiet until color improves and the victim has recovered. Then allow the victim to get up gradually. If recovery is not prompt, if other injuries occur or are suspected, or if fainting occurs again, obtain medical help. Fainting can be a sign of a serious illness or condition that requires medical attention.

Convulsion

A **convulsion,** which is a type of *seizure*, is a strong, involuntary contraction of muscles. Convulsions may occur in conjunction with high body temperatures, head injuries, brain disease, and brain disorders such as epilepsy.

◆ Convulsions cause a rigidity of body muscles followed by jerking movements. During a convulsion, a person may stop breathing, bite the tongue, lose bladder and bowel control, and injure body parts. The face and lips may develop a bluish color. The victim may lose consciousness. After regaining consciousness at the end of the convulsion, the victim may be confused and disoriented, and complain of a headache.

◆ First aid is directed toward preventing self-injury. Removing dangerous objects from the area, providing a pillow or cushion under the victim's head, and providing artificial respiration, as necessary, are all ways to assist the victim.

◆ Do *not* try to place anything between the victim's teeth. This can cause severe injury to your fingers, and/or damage to the victim's teeth or gums.

◆ Do *not* use force to restrain or stop the muscle movements; this only causes the contractions to become more severe.

◆ When the convulsion is over, watch the victim closely. If fluid, such as saliva or vomit, is in the victim's mouth, position the victim on his or her side to allow the fluid to drain from the mouth. Allow the victim to sleep or rest. Obtain medical help if the seizure lasts more than a few minutes, if the victim has repeated seizures, if other severe injuries are apparent, if the victim does not have a history of seizures, or if the victim does not regain consciousness.

Diabetic Reactions

Diabetes mellitus is a metabolic disorder caused by a lack or insufficient production of insulin (a hormone produced by the pancreas). Insulin helps the body transport glucose, a form of sugar, from the bloodstream into body cells where the glucose is used to produce energy.

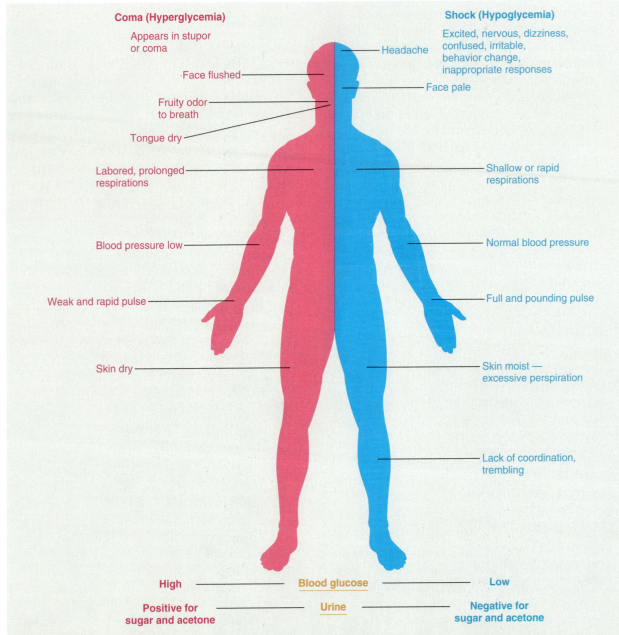

Coma (Hyperglycemia)

Appears in stupor or coma

Face flushed

Fruity odor to breath

Tongue dry

Labored, prolonged respirations

Blood pressure low

Weak and rapid pulse

Skin dry

Shock (Hypoglycemia)

Excited, nervous, dizziness, confused, irritable, behavior change, inappropriate responses

Headache

Face pale

Shallow or rapid respirations

Normal blood pressure

Full and pounding pulse

Skin moist — excessive perspiration

Lack of coordination, trembling

High ——— Blood glucose ——— Low

Positive for sugar and acetone ——— Urine ——— Negative for sugar and acetone

FIGURE 15-38 Diabetic coma (hyperglycemia) versus insulin shock (hypoglycemia).

When there is a lack of insulin, sugar builds up in the bloodstream. Insulin injections can reduce and control the level of sugar in the blood. Individuals with diabetes are in danger of developing two conditions that require first aid: diabetic coma and insulin shock (see figure 15-38).

◆ **Diabetic coma** is caused by an increase in the level of glucose in the bloodstream. The condition may result from an excess intake of sugar, failure to take insulin, or insufficient production of insulin. Signs and symptoms include confusion; weakness or dizziness;

nausea and/or vomiting; rapid, deep respirations; dry, flushed skin; and a sweet or fruity odor to the breath. The victim will eventually lose consciousness and die unless the condition is treated. Medical assistance must be obtained as quickly as possible.

◆ **Insulin shock** is caused by an excess amount of insulin (and a low level of glucose) in the bloodstream. It may result from failure to eat the recommended amounts, vomiting after taking insulin, or taking excessive amounts of insulin. Signs and symptoms include muscle weakness; mental confusion; restlessness or anxiety; diaphoresis; pale, moist skin; hunger pangs; and/or palpitations (rapid, irregular heartbeats). The victim may lapse into a coma and develop convulsions. The onset of insulin shock is sudden, and the victim's condition can deteriorate quickly; therefore, immediate first aid care is required. If the victim is conscious, give him or her a drink containing sugar, such as sweetened orange juice. A cube or teaspoon of granulated sugar can also be placed in the victim's mouth. If the victim is confused, avoid giving hard candy.

NOTE: Unconsciousness could occur, and the victim could choke on the hard candy.

The intake of sugar should quickly control the reaction. If the victim loses consciousness or convulsions start, provide care for the convulsions and obtain medical assistance immediately.

◆ By observing symptoms carefully and obtaining as much information as possible from the victim, you can usually determine whether the condition is diabetic coma or insulin shock. Ask the victim, "Have you eaten today?" and "Have you taken your insulin?" If the victim has taken insulin but has not eaten, insulin shock is developing because there is too much insulin in the body. If the victim has eaten but has not

taken insulin, diabetic coma is developing. In cases when you know that the victim is diabetic but the victim is unconscious and there are no definite symptoms of either condition, you may not be able to determine whether the condition is diabetic coma or insulin shock. In such cases, the recommendation is to put granulated sugar under the victim's tongue before calling for an ambulance. This is the lesser of two evils. If the patient is in diabetic coma, the blood-sugar level can be lowered as needed when the victim is transported for medical care. If the victim is in insulin shock, however, brain damage can occur if the blood-sugar level is not raised immediately. Medical care cannot correct brain damage.

C In all cases of sudden illness, constantly reassure the victim and make every attempt to encourage the victim to relax and avoid further stress. Be alert for the signs of shock and provide treatment for shock to all victims. The pain, anxiety, and fear associated with sudden illness can contribute to shock.

STUDENT: *Go to the workbook and complete the assignment sheet for 15:11, Providing First Aid for Sudden Illness. Then return and continue with the procedure.*

PROCEDURE 15:11

Providing First Aid for Sudden Illness

Equipment and Supplies

Blankets, pillows, sugar, clean cloth, cool water, disposable gloves

Procedure

1. Follow the priorities of care, if indicated.
   a. Check the scene. Move the victim only if absolutely necessary.
   b. Check the victim for consciousness and breathing.
   c. Call emergency medical services (EMS), if necessary.
   d. Provide care to the victim.
   e. Check for bleeding. Control severe bleeding.

   CAUTION: If possible, wear gloves or use a protective barrier while controlling bleeding.

2. Closely observe the victim for specific signs and symptoms. If the victim is conscious, obtain information about the history of the illness, type and amount of pain, and other pertinent details. If the victim is unconscious, check for a medical bracelet or necklace or a medical information card. Always

have a reason for everything you do. Explain your actions to any observers, especially if it is necessary to check the victim's wallet for a medical card.

3. If you suspect the victim is having a *heart attack,* provide first aid as follows:
   a. Place the victim in the most comfortable position possible but avoid unnecessary movement. Some victims will want to lie flat, but others will want to be in a partial or complete sitting position. If the victim is having difficulty breathing, use pillows or rolled blankets to elevate the head and shoulders.
   b. Obtain medical help for the victim immediately. Advise EMS that oxygen may be necessary.
   c. Encourage the victim to relax. Reassure the victim. Remain calm and encourage others to remain calm.
   d. Watch for signs of shock and treat for shock as necessary. Avoid overheating the victim.
   e. If the victim complains of excessive thirst, use a wet cloth to moisten the lips, tongue, and inside of the mouth. Small sips of water can also be given to the victim, but avoid giving large amounts of fluid.

      ⚠ CAUTION: Do *not* give the victim ice water or very cold water because the cold can intensify shock.

4. If you suspect that the victim has had a *stroke:*
   a. Place the victim in a comfortable position. Keep the victim lying flat or slightly elevate the victim's head and shoulders to aid breathing. If the victim has difficulty swallowing, turn the victim on his or her side to allow secretions to drain from the mouth and prevent choking on the secretions.
   b. Reassure the victim. Encourage the victim to relax.
   c. Avoid giving the victim any fluids or food by mouth. If the victim complains of excessive thirst, use a cool, wet cloth to moisten the lips, tongue, and inside of the mouth.
   d. Obtain medical help for the victim as quickly as possible.

5. If the victim has *fainted:*
   a. Keep the victim in a supine position (that is, lying flat on the back). Raise the legs and feet 12 inches.
   b. Check for breathing. Provide artificial respiration, if necessary.
   c. Loosen any tight clothing.
   d. Use cool water to gently bathe the face.
   e. Check for any other injuries.
   f. Encourage the victim to continue lying down until his or her skin color improves.
   g. If no other injuries are suspected, allow the victim to get up slowly. First, elevate the head and shoulders. Then place the victim in a sitting position. Allow the victim to stand slowly. If any signs of dizziness, weakness, or pallor are noted, return the victim to the supine position.
   h. If the victim does not recover quickly, or if any other injuries occur, obtain medical care. If fainting has occurred frequently, refer the victim for medical care.
      NOTE: Fainting can be a sign of a serious illness or condition.

6. If the victim is having a *convulsion:*
   a. Remove any dangerous objects from the area. If the victim is near heavy furniture or machinery that cannot be moved, move the victim to a safe area.
   b. Place soft material such as a blanket, small pillow, rolled jacket, or other similar material under the victim's head to prevent injury.
   c. Closely observe respirations at all times. During the convulsion, there will be short periods of apnea (cessation of breathing).
      NOTE: If breathing does not resume quickly, artificial respiration may be necessary.
   d. Do *not* try to place anything between the victim's teeth. This can cause injury to the teeth and/or gums.
   e. Do *not* attempt to restrain the muscle contractions.
   f. **C** Note how long the convulsion lasts and what parts of the body are involved. Be sure to report this information to the EMS personnel.
   g. After the convulsion ends, closely watch the victim. Encourage the victim to rest.

h. Obtain medical assistance if the seizure lasts more than a few minutes, if the victim has repeated seizures, if other severe injuries are apparent, if the victim does not have a history of seizures, or if the victim does not regain consciousness.

7. If the victim is in *diabetic coma:*

a. Place the victim in a comfortable position. If the victim is unconscious, position him or her on either side to allow secretions to drain from the mouth.

b. Frequently check respirations. Provide artificial respiration as needed.

c. Obtain medical help immediately so the victim can be transported to a medical facility.

8. If the victim is in *insulin shock:*

a. If the victim is conscious and can swallow, offer a drink containing sugar.

b. If the victim is unconscious, place a small amount of granulated sugar under the victim's tongue.

c. Place the victim in a comfortable position. Position an unconscious victim on either side to allow secretions to drain from the mouth.

d. If recovery is not prompt, obtain medical help immediately.

9. Observe all victims of sudden illness for signs of shock. Treat for shock as necessary.

10. Constantly reassure any victim of sudden illness. Encourage relaxation to decrease stress.

Practice *Go to the workbook and use the evaluation sheet for 15:11, Providing First Aid for Sudden Illness, to practice this procedure. When you feel you have mastered this skill, sign the sheet and give it to your instructor for further action.*

Final Checkpoint Using the criteria listed on the evaluation sheet, your instructor will grade your performance.

15:12 INFORMATION Applying Dressings and Bandages

In many cases requiring first aid, it will be necessary for you to apply dressings and bandages. This section provides basic information on types of bandages and dressings and on application methods.

A **dressing** is a sterile covering placed over a wound or an injured part. It is used to control bleeding, absorb blood and secretions, prevent infection, and ease pain. Materials that may be used as dressings include gauze pads in a variety of sizes, and compresses of thick, absorbent material (see figure 15-39). Fluff cotton should *not* be used as a dressing because the loose cotton fibers may contaminate the wound. In an emergency when no dressings are available, a clean handkerchief or pillowcase may be used.

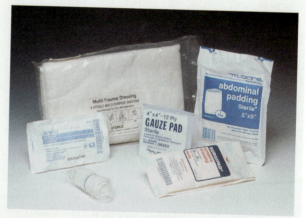

FIGURE 15-39 Dressings to cover a wound are available in many different sizes.

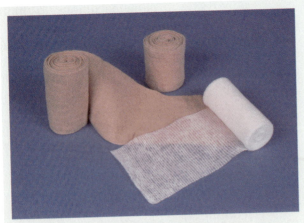

FIGURE 15-40 Roller gauze and elastic bandages can be used to hold dressings in place.

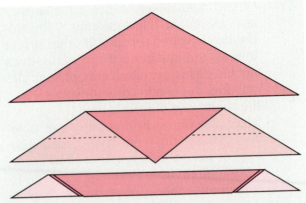

FIGURE 15-41 Folding a cravat bandage from a triangular bandage.

The dressing is held in place with tape or a bandage.

Bandages are materials used to hold dressings in place, to secure splints, and to support and protect body parts. Bandages should be applied snugly enough to control bleeding and prevent movement of the dressing, but not so tightly that they interfere with circulation. Types of bandages include roller gauze bandages, triangular bandages, and elastic bandages (see figure 15-40).

◆ Roller gauze bandages come in a variety of widths, most commonly 1-, 2-, and 3-inch widths. They can be used to hold dressings in place on almost any part of the body.

◆ Triangular bandages can be used to secure dressings on the head/scalp or as slings. A triangular bandage is sometimes used as a covering for a large body part such as a hand, foot, or shoulder. By folding the triangular bandage into a band of cloth called a cravat (see figure 15-41), the bandage can be used to secure splints or dressings on body parts.

◆ Elastic bandages are easy to apply because they readily conform, or mold, to the injured part. However, they can be quite hazardous; if they are applied too tightly or are stretched during application, they can cut off or constrict circulation. Elastic bandages are sometimes used to provide support and stimulate circulation.

Several methods are used to wrap bandages. The method used depends on the body part involved. Some common wraps include the spiral wrap, the figure-eight wrap for joints, and the finger, or recurrent, wrap. The wraps are described in Procedure 15:12, immediately following this information section.

After any bandage has been applied, it is important to check the body part below the bandage to make sure the bandage is not so tight as to interfere with blood circulation. Signs that indicate poor circulation include swelling, a pale or blue (cyanotic) color to the skin, coldness to the touch, and numbness or tingling. If the bandage has been applied to the hand, arm, leg, or foot, press lightly on the nail beds to blanch them (that is, make them turn white). The pink color should return to the nail beds immediately after pressure is released. If the pink color does not return or returns slowly, this is an indication of poor or impaired circulation. If any signs of impaired circulation are noted, loosen the bandages immediately.

STUDENT: *Go to the workbook and complete the assignment sheet for 15:12, Applying Dressings and Bandages. Then return and continue with the procedure.*

PROCEDURE 15:12
Applying Dressings and Bandages

Equipment and Supplies

Sterile gauze pads, triangular bandage, roller gauze bandage, elastic bandage, tape, disposable gloves

Procedure

1. Assemble equipment.
2. 🔶 Wash hands. Put on gloves if there is any chance of contact with blood or body fluids.
3. Apply a dressing to a wound as follows:
   a. Obtain the correct size dressing. The dressing should be large enough to extend at least 1 inch beyond the edges of the wound.
   b. Open the sterile dressing package, taking care not to touch or handle the sterile dressing with your fingers.
   c. Use a pinching action to pick up the sterile dressing so you handle only one part of the outside of the dressing. (The ideal situation would involve the use of sterile transfer forceps or sterile gloves to handle the dressing. However, these items are usually not available in emergency situations.)
   d. Place the dressing on the wound. The untouched (sterile) side of the dressing should be placed on the wound. Do *not* slide the dressing into position. Instead, hold the dressing directly over the wound and then lower the dressing onto the wound.
   e. Secure the dressing in place with tape or with one of the bandage wraps.
      🛑 **CAUTION:** If tape is used, do not wrap it completely around the part. This can lead to impaired circulation.
4. Apply a triangular bandage to the head or scalp (see figure 15-42):
   a. Fold a 2-inch hem on the base (longest side) of the triangular bandage.
   b. Position and secure a sterile dressing in place over the wound.
   c. Keeping the hem on the outside, position the middle of the base of bandage on the forehead, just above the eyebrows.
   d. Bring the point of the bandage down over the back of the head.
   e. Bring the two ends of the base of the bandage around the head and above the ears. Cross the ends when they meet at the back of head. Bring them around to the forehead.
   f. Use a square knot to tie the ends in the center of the forehead.
   g. Use one hand to support the head. Use the other hand to gently but firmly pull

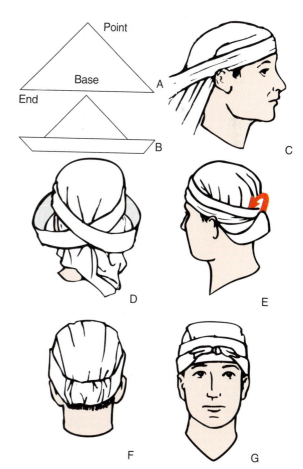

FIGURE 15-42 Steps for applying a triangular bandage to the head or scalp.

down on the point of the bandage at the back of the head until the bandage is snug against the head.

  h. Bring the point up and tuck it into the bandage where the bandage crosses at the back of the head.

5. Make a cravat bandage from a triangular bandage (review figure 15-41):

  a. Bring the point of the triangular bandage down to the middle of the base (the long end of the bandage).

  b. Continue folding the bandage lengthwise until the desired width is obtained.

6. Apply a circular bandage with the cravat bandage (see figure 15-43):

  a. Place a sterile dressing on the wound.

  b. Place the center of the cravat bandage over the sterile dressing.

  c. Bring the ends of the cravat around the body part and cross them when they meet.

  d. Bring the ends back to the starting point.

  e. Use a square knot to tie the ends of the cravat over the dressing.

    CAUTION: Avoid tying or wrapping the bandage too tightly. This could impair circulation.

    NOTE: Roller gauze bandage can also be used.

    CAUTION: This type of wrap is *never* used around the neck because it could strangle the victim.

7. Apply a spiral wrap using roller gauze bandage or elastic bandage:

  a. Place a sterile dressing over the wound.

  b. Hold the roller gauze or elastic bandage so that the loose end is hanging off the bottom of the roll.

  c. Start at the farthest end (the bottom of the limb) and move in an upward direction.

  d. Anchor the bandage by placing it on an angle at the starting point. To do this, encircle the limb once, leaving a corner of the bandage uncovered. Turn down this free corner and then encircle the part again with the bandage (see figure 15-44A).

  e. Continue encircling the limb. Use a spiral type motion to move up the limb. Overlap each new turn approximately one-half the width of the bandage.

  f. Use one or two circular turns to finish the wrap at the end point.

g. Secure the end by taping, pinning, or tying. To avoid injury when pins are used, place your hand under the double layer of bandage and between the pin and the skin before inserting the pin (see figure 15-44B). The end of the bandage can also be cut in half and the two halves brought around opposite sides and tied into place.

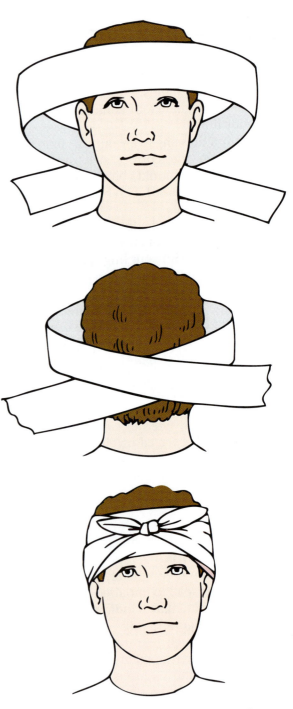

FIGURE 15-43 Steps for applying a circular bandage with a cravat bandage.

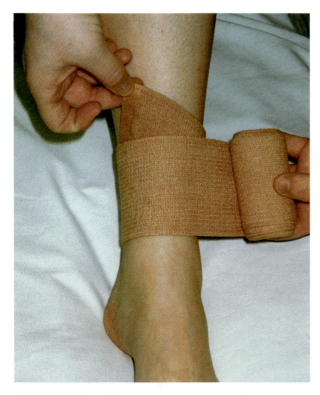

FIGURE 15-44A Anchor the bandage by leaving a corner exposed. This corner is then folded down and covered when the bandage is circled around the limb.

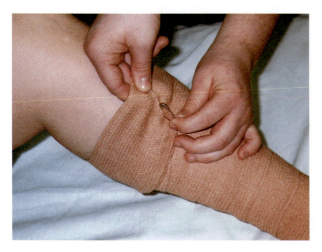

FIGURE 15-44B Place your hand between the bandage and the victim's skin while inserting a pin.

8. Use roller gauze bandage or elastic bandage to apply a figure-eight ankle wrap:
   a. Position a dressing over the wound.
   b. Anchor the bandage at the instep of the foot.
   c. Make one or two circular turns around the instep and foot (see figure 15-45A).

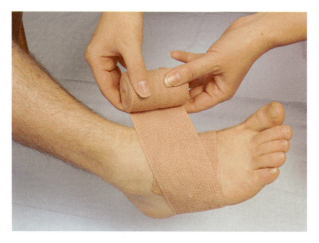

FIGURE 15-45A Bring the bandage over the foot in a diagonal direction for the start of the figure-eight pattern.

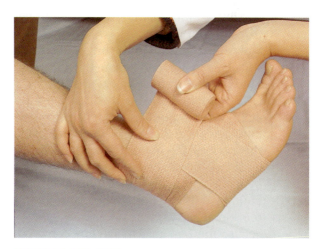

FIGURE 15-45B Keep repeating the figure-eight pattern by moving downward and backward toward the heel with each turn.

   d. Bring the bandage up over the foot in a diagonal direction. Bring it around the back of the ankle and then down over the top of the foot. Circle it under the instep. This creates the figure-eight pattern.
   e. Repeat the figure-eight pattern. With each successive turn, move downward and backward toward the heel (see figure 15-45B). Overlap the previous turn by one-half to two-thirds the width of the bandage.
   NOTE: Hold the bandage firmly but do not pull it too tightly. If you are using elastic bandage, avoid stretching the material during the application.
   f. Near completion, use one or two final circular wraps to circle the ankle.

g. Secure the bandage in place by taping, pinning, or tying the ends, as described in 7g, preceding.

 CAUTION: To avoid injury to the victim when pins are used, place your hand between the bandage and the victim's skin.

9. Use roller gauze bandage to apply a recurrent wrap to the fingers (see figure 15-46).

   a. Place a sterile dressing over the wound.

   b. Hold the roller gauze bandage so that the loose end is hanging off the bottom of the roll.

   c. Place the end of the bandage on the bottom of the finger. Then bring the bandage up to the tip of the finger and down to the bottom of the opposite side of the finger. With overlapping wraps, fold the bandage backward and forward over the finger three or four times.

   d. Start at the bottom of the finger and use a spiral wrap up and down the finger to hold the recurrent wraps in position.

   e. Complete the bandage by using a figure-eight wrap around the wrist. Bring the bandage in a diagonal direction across the back of the hand. Circle the wrist at least two times. Bring the bandage back over the top of the hand and circle the bandaged finger. Repeat this figure-eight motion at least twice.

   f. Secure the bandage by circling the wrist once or twice. Tie the bandage at the wrist.

10. After any bandage has been applied, check the circulation below the bandage at frequent intervals. Note any signs of impaired circulation, including swelling, coldness, numbness or tingling, pallor or cyanosis, and poor return of pink color after nail beds are blanched by lightly pressing on them. If any signs of poor circulation are noted, loosen the bandages immediately.

11. Obtain medical help for any victim who may need additional care.

12. Remove gloves and wash hands.

Practice *Go to the workbook and use the evaluation sheet for 15:12, Applying Dressings and Bandages, to practice this procedure. When you feel you have mastered this skill, sign the sheet and give it to your instructor for further action.*

✔ **Final Checkpoint**   Using the criteria listed on the evaluation sheet, your instructor will grade your performance.

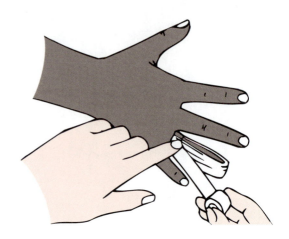

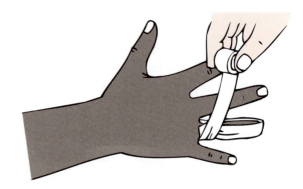

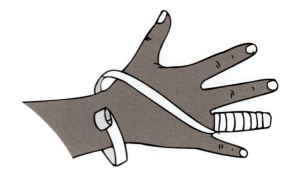

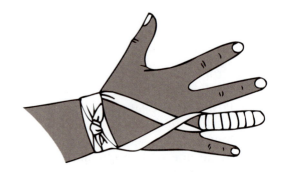

FIGURE 15-46 Recurrent wrap for the finger.

UNIT 15 SUMMARY

First aid is defined as "the immediate care given to the victim of an injury or illness to minimize the effect of the injury or illness until experts can take over." Nearly everyone at some time experiences situations for which a proper knowledge of first aid is essential. It is important to follow correct techniques while administering first aid and to provide only the treatment you are qualified to provide.

The basic principles of first aid were presented in this unit. Methods of cardiopulmonary resuscitation (CPR) for infants, children, adults, and choking victims were described. Proper first aid for bleeding, shock, poisoning, burns, heat and cold exposure, bone and joint injuries, specific injuries, and sudden illness were covered. Instructions were given for the application of common dressings and bandages. By learning and following the suggested methods, the health care worker can provide correct first aid treatment in emergency situations until the help of experts can be obtained.

INTERNET SEARCHES

Use the suggested search engines in Unit 11:4 of this textbook to search the Internet for additional information on the following topics:

1. *Organizations:* find web sites for the American Red Cross, the American Heart Association, Emergency Medical Services, and Poison Control Centers to learn services offered.

2. *CPR:* look for sites that discuss the principles of cardiopulmonary resuscitation, abdominal thrusts or the Heimlich maneuver, and cardiac emergencies.

3. *Automated External Defibrillators:* search for manufacturers of AEDs and compare different models.

4. *First aid treatments:* find information on recommended treatment for bleeding, wounds, shock, poisoning, snakebites, insect stings, ticks, burns, heat exposure, heat stroke, hypothermia, frostbite, fractures, dislocations, sprains, strains, eye injuries, nose injuries, head and skull injuries, spine injuries, chest injuries, abdominal injuries, myocardial infarction, cerebrovascular accident, fainting, convulsions or seizures, diabetic coma, and insulin shock.

REVIEW QUESTIONS

Review the following case histories. List the correct first aid care, in proper order of use, that should be used to treat each victim.

1. You are slicing carrots and cut off the end of your finger.

2. You find your 2-year-old brother in the bathroom. An empty bottle of aspirin tablets is on the floor. His mouth is covered with a white powdery residue.

3. You are watching television with your parents. Suddenly your father complains of severe pain in his chest and left arm. He is very short of breath and his lips appear blue in color.

4. You are working in chemistry lab. Suddenly an experiment boils over and concentrated hydrochloric acid splashes into your lab partner's face and eyes. She starts screaming with pain.

5. You are driving and the car ahead of you loses control, goes off the road, and hits a tree. When you get to the car, the driver is slumped over the wheel. His arm is twisted at an odd angle. You notice a small fire at the rear of the car. A small child is crying in a car seat in the back seat.

6. You are playing tennis on a hot summer day with a friend. Suddenly your friend collapses on the tennis court. When you get to her, her skin is hot, red, and dry. She is breathing but she is unconscious.

UNIT 15

SUGGESTED REFERENCES

American National Red Cross. *Community First Aid and Safety.* Boston, MA: Staywell, 2001.
American National Red Cross. *CPR for the Professional Rescuer.* Boston, MA: Staywell, 2002.
American National Red Cross. *Emergency Response.* Boston, MA: Staywell, 2001.

American National Red Cross. *First Aid/CPR/AED.* Boston, MA: Staywell, 2001.

Beebe, Richard. *Functional Anatomy for Emergency Medical Services.* Clifton Park, NY: Delmar Learning, 2002.

Beebe, Richard, and Deborah Funk. *Fundamentals of Emergency Care.* Clifton Park, NY: Delmar Learning, 2001.

Buttarovoli, Philip, and Thomas Stair. *Minor Emergencies: Splinters to Fractures.* St. Louis, MO: Mosby, 1999.

Chernega, Janet. *Emergency Guide for Dental Auxiliaries.* 3rd ed. Clifton Park, NY: Delmar Learning, 2002.

Des Jardins, Terry. *Cardiopulmonary Anatomy and Physiology: Essentials for Respiratory Care.* 4th ed. Clifton Park, NY: Delmar Learning, 2002.

Heckman, James (Ed.). *Emergency Care and Transportation of the Sick and Injured.* 6th ed. Park Ridge, IL: American Academy of Orthopaedic Surgeons, 1995.

Hernandez, Lisa de. *Emergencia: Emergency Translation Manual.* Clifton Park, NY: Delmar Learning, 2002.

Instructional Materials Laboratory. *Emergency Victim Care.* Columbus, OH: Ohio State University, n.d.

Myers, Jeffrey, Marianne Neighbors, Ruth Tannehill-Jones. *Principles of Pathophysiology and Emergency Medical Care.* Clifton Park, NY: Delmar Learning, 2002.

Scott, Ann Sensi, and Elizabeth Fong. *Functional Anatomy for EMS Providers.* Clifton Park, NY: Delmar Learning, 2002.

Shea, Donna, and Adrienne Carter-Ward. *Telephone Triage Card Deck.* Clifton Park, NY: Delmar Learning, 1996.

Tuttle-Yoder, Jeryll, and Susan Fraser-Nobbe. *Stat! Medical Office Emergency Manual.* Clifton Park, NY: Delmar Learning, 1996.

Walz, Bruce J. *Introduction to EMS Systems.* Clifton Park, NY: Delmar Learning, 2002.

Wertz, Elizabeth. *Emergency Care for Children.* Clifton Park, NY: Delmar Learning, 2002.

Whittle, James. *911 Responding for Life: Case Studies in Emergency Care.* Clifton Park, NY: Delmar Learning, 2001.

For additional information on first aid and emergency care, write to:

◆ American Red Cross—contact your local chapter for First Aid and CPR courses and certification, or check the web site at *www.redcross.org.*

◆ U.S. Department of Transportation Emergency Medical Services Branch N-42-13 Washington, D.C. 20540

Preparing for the World of Work

Unit Objectives

After completing this unit of study, you should be able to:

- ◆ Identify at least five job-keeping skills and explain why employers consider them to be essential skills
- ◆ Write a letter of application containing all required information and using correct form for letters
- ◆ Prepare a resumé containing all necessary information and meeting standards for neatness and correctness
- ◆ Complete a job application form that meets standards of neatness and accuracy
- ◆ Demonstrate how to participate in a job interview, including wearing correct dress and meeting standards established in this unit
- ◆ Determine gross and net income
- ◆ Calculate an accurate budget for a one-month period, accounting for fixed expenses and variable expenses without exceeding net monthly income
- ◆ Define, pronounce, and spell all the key terms

  Observe Standard Precautions

 Instructors Check—Call Instructor at This Point

 Safety—Proceed with Caution

 **OBRA** OBRA Requirement— Based on Federal Law

 Math Skill

 Legal Responsibility

 Science Skill

Career Information

 C Communications Skill

 Technology

KEY TERMS

application forms	gross income	net income
budget	income	resumé
deductions	job interview	*(rez'-ah-may)*
fixed expenses	letter of application	variable expenses

16:1 INFORMATION Developing Job-Keeping Skills

In order to obtain and keep a job, there are certain characteristics that you must develop to be a good employee. A recent survey of employers asked for information on the deficiencies of high school graduates. The most frequent complaints included poor written grammar, spelling, speech, and math skills. Other complaints included lack of respect for work, lack of self-initiative, poor personal appearance, not accepting responsibility, excessive tardiness and poor attendance, and inability to accept criticism. Any of these defects would be detrimental in a health care worker.

In order to be successful in a health care career, it is essential that you develop good job-keeping skills. Being aware of and striving to achieve the qualities needed for employment are as important as acquiring the knowledge and skills required in your chosen health care profession.

Job-keeping skills include:

◆ **C** *Use correct grammar at all times:* This includes both the written and spoken word. Patients often judge ability on how well a person speaks or writes information. Use of words like *ain't* indicates a lack of education and does not create a favorable or professional impression. You must constantly strive to use correct grammar. Listen to how other health care professionals speak and review basic concepts of correct grammar. It

may even be necessary to take a communications course to learn to speak correctly. Because you will be completing legal written records for health care, the use of correct spelling, punctuation, and sentence structure is also essential. Use a dictionary to check spelling, or use the spell check on a computer system. Refer to standard English books or secretarial manuals for information on sentence structure and punctuation. Constantly strive to improve both oral and written communication skills.

◆ *Report to work on time and when scheduled:* Because many health care facilities provide care seven days a week, 365 days per year, and often 24-hours per day, an employee who is frequently late or absent can cause a major disruption in schedule and contribute to an insufficiency of personnel to provide patient care. Most health care facilities have strict rules regarding absenteeism, and a series of absences can result in job loss.

◆ *Be prepared to work when you arrive at work:* An employer does not pay workers to socialize, make personal telephone calls, consult others about personal or family problems, bring their children to work, or work in a sloppy and inefficient manner. Develop a good work ethic. Observe all legal and ethical responsibilities. Follow the policies and procedures of your health care facility. Recognize your limitations and seek help when you need it. Be willing to learn new procedures and techniques. Watch efficient and knowledgeable staff members and learn by their examples. Constantly strive to do the best job possible. A worker who has self-initiative, who sees a job that needs to be done and does it, is a valuable employee who is likely to be recognized and rewarded.

◆ *Practice teamwork:* Because health care typically involves a team of different professionals working together to provide patient care, it is important to be willing to work with others. If you are willing to help others when they need help, they will likely be willing to help you. Two or three people working together can lift a heavy patient much more readily than can one.

◆ *Promote a positive attitude:* By being positive, you create a good impression and encourage the same attitude in others. Too often, employees concentrate only on the negative aspects of their jobs. Every job has some bad points; and it is easy to criticize these points. It is also easy to criticize the bad points in others with whom you work. However, this leads to a negative attitude and helps create poor morale in everyone. By concentrating on the good aspects of a job and the rewards it can provide, work will seem much more pleasant, and employees will obtain more satisfaction from their efforts.

◆ *Accept responsibility for your actions:* Most individuals are more than willing to take credit for the good things they have done. In the same manner, it is essential to take responsibility for mistakes. If you make a mistake, report it to your supervisor and make every effort to correct the error. Every human being will do something wrong at some time. Recognizing an error, taking responsibility for it, and making every effort to correct it or prevent it from happening again is a sign of a competent worker. Honesty is essential in health care. Not accepting responsibility for your actions is dishonest. It is often a reason for dismissal and can prevent you from obtaining another position.

◆ *Be willing to learn:* Health care changes constantly because of advances in technology and research. Every health care worker must

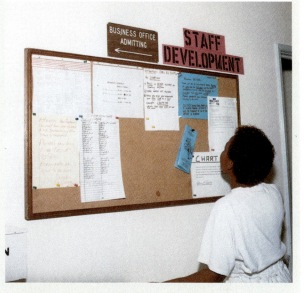

FIGURE 16-1 Participating in staff development programs is one way to improve your own knowledge and skills.

be willing to learn new things and adapt to change. Participating in staff development programs (see figure 16-1), taking courses at technical schools or colleges, attending special seminars or meetings, reading professional journals, and asking questions of other qualified individuals are all ways to improve your knowledge and skills. Employers recognize these efforts. Ambition is often rewarded with a higher salary and/or job advancement.

Without good job-keeping skills, no amount of knowledge will help you keep a job. Therefore, it is essential for you to strive to develop the qualities that employers need in workers. Be courteous, responsible, enthusiastic, cooperative, reliable, punctual, and efficient. Strive hard to be the best you can be. If you do this, you will not only be likely to retain your job, but you will probably be rewarded with job advancement, increased salary, and personal satisfaction.

STUDENT: *Go to the workbook and complete the assignment sheet for 16:1, Developing Job-Keeping Skills.*

16:2 INFORMATION Writing a Letter of Application and Preparing a Resumé

In your search for a job, you will often respond in writing to advertisements or sources. This usually involves sending a resumé, which should be accompanied by a letter of application, or cover letter.

Letter of Application

The purpose of a **letter of application** is to obtain an interview. You must create a good impression in the letter so that the employer will be interested in possibly obtaining you as an employee. In most cases, you will be responding to a job advertised either in the newspaper or through other sources. However a resumé may be sent to potential employers even though they have not advertised a job opportunity. A cover letter should accompany all resumés.

The letter should be computer printed or typewritten on good quality paper. It must be neat, complete, and done according to correct form for letters. Care must be taken to ensure that spelling and punctuation are correct. Remember, this letter is the employer's first impression of you.

C If possible, the letter should be addressed to the correct individual. If you know the name of the agency or company, call to obtain this information. Be sure you obtain the correct spelling of the person's name as well as the person's correct title. If you are responding to a box number, follow the instructions in the advertisement. Another possibility is to address the letter to the personnel director or the head of a particular department.

The letter usually contains three to four paragraphs. The contents of each paragraph are described as follows:

◆ Paragraph one: state your purpose for writing and express interest in the position for which you are applying. If you are responding to an advertisement, state the name and date of the publication. If you were referred by another individual, give this person's name and title.

◆ Paragraph two: state why you feel you are qualified for the position. It may also state why you want to work for this particular employer. Information should be brief because most of the information will be included on your resumé.

◆ Paragraph three: state that a resumé is included. You may also want to draw the employer's attention to one or two important features on your resumé. If you are not including a resumé, state that one is available on request. Whenever possible, it is best to enclose a resumé.

◆ Paragraph four: closes the letter with a request for an interview. Be sure you clearly state how the employer can contact you for additional information. Include a telephone number and the times you will be available to respond to a telephone call. Finally, include a thank you to the potential employer for considering your application.

Figure 16-2 is a sample letter of application to serve as a guide to writing a good letter. However, remember this is only one guide. Letters must be varied to suit each circumstance.

Resumé

A **resumé** is a record of information about an individual. It is a thorough yet concise summary of an individual's education, experience, and abilities. It is used to provide an employer with basic information that makes you appear qualified as an employee.

A resumé should be computer printed or typed and attractive in appearance. Like a letter of application, a resumé creates an impression on the employer. Information should be presented in an organized fashion. At the same time, the resumé should be concise and pertinent. Good-quality paper; correct spelling and punctuation; straight, even margins; and an attractive style are essential. If you are sending out a series of resumés, professional copies are permitted. However, be sure the copies are clear, on good-quality paper, and appealing in appearance.

```
18 Hireme Lane
Job City, Ohio 44444
June 3, 20--


Mr. Prospective Employer
Personnel Director
Health Care Facility
12 Nursing Lane
Dental City, Ohio 44833

Dear Mr. Employer:

In response to your advertisement in the _____
on _____, 20 _____, I would like to apply for
the position of _____.

I recently graduated from _____. I majored in
_____ and feel I am well qualified for this
position. I enjoy working with people and have a sincere
interest in additional training in _____.

My resume is enclosed. I have also enclosed a specific list of
skills which I mastered during my school experience. I feel
that previous positions noted on the resume have provided me
with a good basis for meeting your job requirements.

Thank you for considering my application. I would appreciate
a personal interview at your earliest convenience to discuss
my qualifications. Please contact me at the above address or
by telephone at 589-1111 after 2:00 PM any day.


Sincerely,


Iamjob Hunting
```

FIGURE 16-2 A sample letter of application.

Resumé format can vary. Review sample sources and find a style that you feel best presents your information. A one-page resumé is usually sufficient.

Parts of a resumé can also vary. Some of the most important parts that should be included are shown in figures 16-3A and 16-3B and are described as follows:

◆ *Personal identification:* This includes your name, address, and telephone number. Be sure to include the area code.

FLORENCE NURSE
22 SOUTH MAIN STREET
NURSING, OHIO 33303
(419) 589-1111

EMPLOYMENT OBJECTIVE: NURSING ASSISTANT

SKILLS

RECORDING VITAL SIGNS
OBSERVING INFECTION CONTROL
ADMINISTERING CPR AND FIRST AID
UNDERSTANDING MEDICAL TERMINOLOGY
ASSISTING WITH ADMISSIONS/DISCHARGES

MOVING/TRANSFERRING PATIENTS
PROVIDING PERSONAL HYGIENE
MAKING BEDS
APPLYING HEAT/COLD APPLICATIONS
COLLECTING SPECIMENS

EDUCATION

CAREER HIGH SCHOOL
5 DIAMOND STREET
NURSING, OHIO 33302

GRADUATION: JUNE 5, 2002
MAJOR: HEALTH OCCUPATIONS
GRADE AVERAGE: A'S AND B'S

WORK EXPERIENCE

SUMMER 2002 TO PRESENT

COUNTRY KING FRIED CHICKEN
5 SOUTHERN LANE
MANSFIELD, OHIO 33302

FAST FOOD WORKER

DUTIES: OPERATE REGISTER,
RECORD ORDERS, PROMOTE SALES

SUMMER OF 2000 AND 2001

MADISON RAM HOSPITAL
602 ESLEY LANE
MANSFIELD, OHIO 33301

CANDY STRIPER

VOLUNTEER DUTIES: DELIVER MAIL
AND FLOWERS, ASSISTED NURSES

EXTRACURRICULAR ACTIVITIES

SCHOOL MARCHING BAND
VOCATIONAL INDUSTRIAL CLUBS OF AMERICA (VICA)
RED CROSS CLUB MEMBER
RED CROSS BLOOD MOBILE
MARCH OF DIMES WALKATHON
CHURCH YOUTH GROUP

THREE YEARS
CLASS TREASURER - TWO YEARS
THREE YEARS
VOLUNTEER WORKER - TWO YEARS
WALKER FOR FIVE YEARS
MEMBER FOR SEVEN YEARS

REFERENCES

JANE SMARTO, R.N.
TEACHER
CAREER HIGH SCHOOL

55 EDUCATION LANE
NURSING, OHIO 33303
(419) 589-2134

JEAN SMITH, L.P.N.
GERIATRIC NURSE
HAPPY FOLKS HOME

432 GERIATRIC PATH
OLDVILLE, OHIO 33300
(419) 529-9865

JERRY BROWN
PERSONNEL DIRECTOR
MADISON HEALTH CARE PROVIDERS

556 EXECUTIVE ROAD
MANSFIELD, OHIO 33300
(419)747-2993

FIGURE 16-3A A sample resumé with information centered.

```
                        THOMAS  J.  TOOTH

   340 DENTAL LANE          FLOSS,  OHIO  44598          (524)  333-2435


   CAREER GOAL:    POSITION AS A DENTAL ASSISTANT IN GENERAL PRACTICE WITH A
                   GOAL OF BECOMING A CERTIFIED DENTAL ASSISTANT

   EDUCATION:      OHIO JOINT VOCATIONAL SCHOOL, OPPORTUNITY, OHIO 44597
                   GRADUATED IN JUNE 2002
                   MAJORED IN DENTAL ASSISTANT PROGRAM FOR TWO YEARS

   SKILLS:         IDENTIFICATION OF TEETH, CHARTING CONDITIONS OF THE
                   TEETH, MIXING DENTAL CEMENTS AND BASES, POURING MODELS
                   AND CUSTOM TRAYS, PREPARING ANESTHETIC SYRINGE, SETTING
                   UP BASIC DENTAL TRAYS, STERILIZING OF INSTRUMENTS,
                   DEVELOPING AND MOUNTING X RAYS, TYPING BUSINESS LETTERS,
                   COMPLETING INSURANCE FORMS

   WORK            DENTAL LAB PRODUCTS, 55 MODEL STREET, FLOSS, OHIO 44598
   EXPERIENCE:     EMPLOYED SEPTEMBER 2001 TO PRESENT AS DENTAL LAB ASSISTANT
                   PROFICIENT IN MODELS, CUSTOM TRAYS, PROSTHETIC DEVICES

                   DRUGGIST STORES, 890 PHARMACY LANE, OPPORTUNITY, OHIO 44597
                   EMPLOYED JUNE 2000 TO AUGUST 2001 AS SALESPERSON
                   EXPERIENCE IN CUSTOMER RELATIONS, INVENTORY, REGISTER, AND
                   SALES PROMOTION

   ACTIVITIES:     HEALTH OCCUPATIONS STUDENTS OF AMERICA (HOSA) TREASURER
                   FIRST PLACE STATE AWARD IN HOSA DENTAL ASSISTANT CONTEST
                   VOLUNTEER WORKER DURING DENTAL HEALTH WEEK
                   MEMBER OF SCHOOL PEP CLUB
                   HOBBIES INCLUDE FOOTBALL, SWIMMING, BASKETBALL, READING
                   VOLUNTEER FOR MEALS-ON-WHEELS

   PERSONAL        DEPENDABLE, CONSIDERATE OF OTHERS, WILLING TO LEARN,
   TRAITS:         ADAPTABLE TO NEW SITUATIONS, RESPECTFUL AND HONEST,
                   ADEPT AT DENTAL TERMINOLOGY, ABLE TO PERFORM A VARIETY
                   OF DENTAL SKILLS

   REFERENCES:     REFERENCES WILL BE FURNISHED ON REQUEST
```

FIGURE 16-3B A sample resumé with left margin highlights.

◆ *Employment objective,* job desired, or career goal: Briefly state the title of the position for which you are applying.

◆ *Educational background:* List the name and address of your high school. Be sure to include special courses or majors if they relate to the job position. If you have taken additional courses or special training, list them also. If you have completed college or technical school, this information should be placed first.

◆ *Work or employment experience:* This includes previous positions of employment. Always start with the most recent position and work backward. Each entry should include the name and address of the employer, dates employed, your job title, and a brief description of duties. Avoid use of the word *I.* For example, instead of stating, "I sterilized supplies," state, "sterilized supplies," using action verbs to describe duties.

◆ *Skills:* List special knowledge, computer, and work skills you have that can be used in the job you are seeking. The list of skills should be specific and indicate your qualifications and ability to perform the job duties. When work experience is limited, a list of skills is important to show an employer that you are qualified for the position.

◆ *Other activities:* These can include organizations of which you are a member, offices held, community activities, special awards received, volunteer work, hobbies, special interests, and other similar facts. Keep this information brief, but do not hesitate to include facts that indicate school, church, and community involvement. This section can show an employer that you are a well-rounded person who participates in activities, assumes leadership roles, strives to achieve, and practices good citizenship. Write out the full names of organizations rather than the identifying letters. For example, write *Vocational Industrial Clubs of America* rather than *V.I.C.A.* and *Health Occupations Students of America* rather than *H.O.S.A.*

◆ *References:* Most sources recommend stating that "references will be furnished on request." For a high school student with limited experience, however, references can provide valuable additional information. Always be sure you have an individual's permission before using that person as a reference. List the full name, title, address, and telephone number of the reference. It is best not to use relatives or high school friends as references. Select professionals in your field, clergy, teachers, or other individuals with responsible positions.

Honesty is always the best policy, and this is particularly true regarding resumés. Never give information that you think will look good but is exaggerated or only partly true. Inaccurate or false information can cost you a job. If you have an A to B average in school, include this information. If your average is lower than an A to B, do *not* include this information.

Before preparing your resumé, it is important to list all of the information you wish to include. Then select the format that best presents this information. The two sample resumés shown in figures 16-3A and 16-3B are meant to serve as guidelines only. Do not hesitate to evaluate other formats and present your information in the best possible way.

The envelope should be the correct size for your letter of application and resumé. Do *not* fold the letter into small sections and put it in an undersized envelope. This creates a sloppy impression. When possible, it is best to buy standard business envelopes that match your paper. A 9 × 12 envelope eliminates the need to fold the cover letter and resumé and helps create a more professional appearance. Be sure the envelope is addressed correctly and neatly. It should also be computer printed or typewritten.

Career Passport or Portfolio

A *career passport* or *portfolio* is a professional way to highlight your knowledge, abilities, and skills as you prepare for employment or extended education. It allows you to present yourself in an organized and efficient manner when you interview for schools or employment. Most career passports or portfolios contain the following types of information:

◆ *Introductory letter:* provides a brief synopsis of yourself including your background, education, and future goals

◆ *Resumé:* provides an organized record of information on education, employment experience, special skills, and activities

◆ *Skill list and competency level:* provides a list of skills you have mastered and the level of competency for each skill; some health occupation programs provide summaries of competency evaluations that can be used; if your program does not provide this, a list of skills and final competency grades can be compiled by using the evaluation sheets in the *Diversified Health Occupations Workbook*

◆ *Letter(s) of recommendation:* include letters of recommendation from your instructors, guidance counselors, supervisors at clinical areas or agencies where you perform volunteer work, respected members of the community, advisors of activities in which you participate, and presidents of organizations of which you are a member

◆ *Copies of work evaluations:* include copies of evaluations you receive at job-training sites, volunteer activities, and/or paid work experiences

◆ *Documentation of mastering job-keeping skills:* the federal government has created SCANS, or the Secretaries Commission on Acquiring Necessary Skills, to designate skills employers desire in employees. SCANS lists three foundation skills that employers desire: *basic skills* (able to read, write, solve math problems, speak, and listen), *thinking skills* (able to learn, reason, think creatively, make decisions, and solve problems), and *personal qualities* (display responsibility, self-initiative, sociability, honesty, and integrity). In addition, SCANS lists five workplace competencies: *manage resources* (demonstrate ability to allocate time, money, materials, and space), *display interpersonal skills* (demonstrate ability to work in a team, lead, negotiate, compromise, teach others, and work with individuals from diverse backgrounds), *utilize information* (acquire and evaluate data, file information, interpret information, and communicate with others), *comprehend systems* (understand social, organizational, and technical systems), and *use technologies* (use computers, apply technology to specific tasks, and maintain equipment). Write brief paragraphs to document how you have mastered skills such as teamwork, self-motivation, leadership, a willingness to learn, responsibility, organization, and other SCANS qualities

◆ *Leadership and organization abilities:* include information that demonstrates leadership and organization abilities you have mastered; participation in Health Occupations Students of America (HOSA) or Vocational Industrial Clubs of America (VICA) should be included

Organize the above information in a neat binder or portfolio. Use tab dividers to separate it into organized sections. Make sure that you use correct grammar and punctuation on all written information. The effort you put into creating a professional portfolio or passport will be beneficial when you have this document ready to present during a school or job interview.

STUDENT: *Go to the workbook and complete the assignment sheet for 16:2, Writing a Letter of Application and Resumé. Then return and continue with the procedure.*

PROCEDURE 16:2   Ⓒ

Writing a Letter of Application and Preparing a Resumé

Equipment and Supplies

Good-quality paper, inventory sheet for resumés (see workbook), computer with word processing software and a printer, or typewriter

Procedure

1. Assemble equipment.

2. Re-read the preceding information section on letters of application and resumés.

3. Review the sample letters of application and resumés.

4. Go to the workbook and complete the inventory sheet for resumés. Check dates for accuracy. Be sure that names are spelled correctly. Use the telephone book or other sources to check addresses and zip codes.

5. Carefully evaluate all your information. Determine the best method of presenting your information. Try different ways of writing your material. Do not hesitate to show several different versions to your instructor or others and get their opinions on which way seems most effective.

6. Type a rough draft of a letter of application. Follow the correct form for letters. Use correct spacing and margins. Check for correct spelling and punctuation.

7. Type a final letter of application. Be sure it contains the required information. Proofread the letter for spelling errors and other mistakes. If possible, ask someone else to proofread your letter and evaluate it.

8. Type a rough draft of your resumé. Position the information in an attractive manner. Be sure that spacing is standard throughout the resumé and margins are even on all sides.

9. Review your sample resumé. Reword any information, if necessary. Be sure all information is pertinent and concise. Ask your instructor or others for opinions regarding suggested changes.

10. Type your final resumé. Take care to avoid errors. If you are not a good typist, it might be wise to have someone else complete the final draft. Proofread the final copy, checking carefully for errors. If possible, ask someone else to proofread your resumé and evaluate it.

NOTE: Resumés can be copies of the original; but be sure the copies are of good quality. Letters of application must be originals; they are individually tailored for each potential job, and, therefore, are not copied.

11. Replace all equipment.

Practice *Go to the workbook and use the evaluation sheet for 16:2, Writing a Letter of Application and Resumé, to practice this procedure. When you feel you have mastered this skill, sign the sheet and give it to your instructor for further action. Also give your instructor your letter of application and resumé along with the evaluation sheet.*

 Final Checkpoint Using the criteria listed on the evaluation sheet, your instructor will grade your letter of application and resumé.

16:3 INFORMATION Completing Job Application Forms

Even though you provide each potential employer with a resumé, most employers still require you to complete an application form. **Application forms** are used by employers to collect specific information. Forms vary from employer to employer, but most request similar information.

Before completing any application form, it is essential that you first read the entire form. Note areas where certain information is to be placed. Read instructions that state how the form is to be completed. Some forms request that the applicant type or print all answers. Others request that the form be completed in the person's handwriting. If a scanner is available, an application form can be scanned into a computer so information can be keyed onto the application. The application can then be printed. Some health care facilities are using on-line applications. A computer is used to key information into the appropriate spaces. The application form is then printed and mailed or sent electronically by e-mail to the employer.

Be sure you have all the required information with you when you go for a job interview. Many employers will ask you to complete the application form at that time. Others will allow you to take the form home. Still others will even send the form to you prior to the interview. The latter two options allow you more time to obtain complete information and print or type the form (unless otherwise requested).

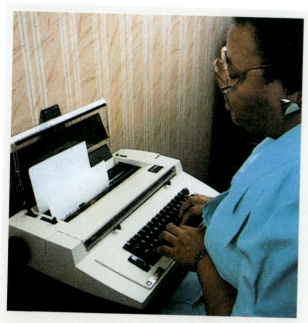

FIGURE 16-4 To complete a job application form, type the information or use black ink.

C Fill out each item neatly and completely. Do *not* leave any areas blank. Put "none" or "NA" (meaning "not applicable") when the item requested does not apply to you. Be sure addresses include zip codes and all other required information. Watch spelling and punctuation. Errors will not impress the potential employer. If the application does not state otherwise, it is best to type or to print neatly (see figure 16-4). Use a black pen if printing. Be sure you take your time and that all information is legible. Take care *not* to write in spaces that state "office use only" or "do not write below this line." Employers often judge how well you follow directions by your reaction to these sections.

Be sure all information is correct and truthful. Remember, material can be checked and verified. A simple half-truth can cost you a job.

Always proofread your completed application. Check for completeness, spelling, proper answers to questions, and any errors.

If references are requested, be sure to include all information requested. Before using anyone's name as a reference, it is best to obtain that person's permission. Be prepared to provide reference information when you go for a job interview.

Even though questions vary on different forms, some basic information is usually requested on all of them. In order to be sure you have this information, it is useful to take a "wallet card" with you. A sample card is included in the workbook (as Assignment 1). Employers will not be impressed if you have to ask for a telephone book in order to find requested information; you may appear to be unprepared. Of course, if you are allowed to take the application home or if it is mailed or sent electronically (e-mail) to you, looking for information would not be a problem.

Remember that employers use application forms as a screening method. In order to avoid being eliminated from consideration for a position of employment, be sure your application creates a favorable impression.

STUDENT: *Go to the workbook and complete the assignment sheets for 16:3, Completing Job Application Forms and Wallet Card. Then return and continue with the procedure.*

PROCEDURE 16:3 **C**
Completing Job Application Forms

Equipment and Supplies
Typewriter or computer and scanner or pen, wallet card (sample in workbook), sample application forms (sample in workbook)

Procedure
1. Assemble equipment. If a typewriter is used, be sure the ribbon is of good quality. If a scanner is available, scan the application

form into the word processing program of a computer. The application form can then be completed with the computer and printed on a printer.

2. Complete all information on the wallet card. A sample is included in the workbook (as Assignment 2). Check dates and be sure information is accurate. List full addresses, zip codes, and names.

3. Review the preceding information section on completing job application forms. Read additional references, as needed.

4. Read the entire sample application form (Assignment 3) in the workbook. Be sure you understand the information requested for each part. Read all directions completely.

5. Unless otherwise directed, type all information requested. If a typewriter is not available, use a black ink pen to print all information.

6. Complete all areas of the form. Use "none" or "NA" as a reply to items that do not apply to you.

7. Take care not to write in spaces labeled "office use only" or "do not write below this line." Leave these areas blank.

8. In the space labeled "*signature*," sign your name. Note any statement that may be printed by the signature line. Be sure you are aware of what you are signing and the permission you may be giving. Most employers request permission to contact previous employers and/or references, and a verification that information is accurate.

9. Recheck the entire application. Be sure information is correct and complete. Note and correct any spelling errors. Be sure you have answered all of the questions.

10. Replace all equipment.

Practice *Go to the workbook and use the evaluation sheet for 16:3, Completing Job Application Forms, to practice this procedure. Obtain sample job application forms from your instructor or other sources. When you feel you have mastered this skill, sign the sheet and give it to your instructor for further action.*

 Final Checkpoint   Using the criteria listed on the evaluation sheet, your instructor will grade your job application form.

16:4 INFORMATION
Participating in a Job Interview

A job interview is what you are seeking when you send a letter of application and a resumé. You must prepare for an interview just as hard as you did when composing your resumé. A poor interview can mean a lost job.

A **job interview** is usually the last step before getting or being denied a particular position of employment. Usually, you have been screened by the potential employer and have been selected for an interview as a result of your resumé and application form. To the employer, the interview serves at least two main purposes: (1) it provides the opportunity to evaluate you in person, obtain additional information, and ascertain whether you meet the job qualifications; and (2) it allows the employer to tell you about the position in more detail.

Careful preparation is needed before going to an interview. Be sure you have all required information. Your "wallet card," resumé, and completed application form (if you have done one) must be ready. If you have completed a career passport or portfolio, be sure to take it to the interview. If possible, find out about the position and the agency offering the job. In this way, you will be more aware of the agency's needs.

Be sure of the scheduled date and time of the interview. Know the name of the individual you must contact and the exact place of the interview. Write this information down and take it with you.

Dress carefully. It is best to dress conservatively. Coats and ties are still best for men. Although pantsuits are sometimes acceptable for women, employers still generally prefer dresses or skirts. Even though it shouldn't be the case, first impressions can affect the employer. All clothes should fit well and be clean and pressed, if needed. Avoid bright, flashy colors and very faddish styles.

Check your entire appearance. Hair should be neat, clean, and styled attractively. Nails should be clean. Women should avoid wearing bright nail polish, too much makeup, and perfume. Men should be clean shaven. Be sure that your teeth are clean and your breath is fresh. Jewelry should not be excessive. And last but not least, use a good antiperspirant. When you are nervous, you perspire.

It is best to arrive 5 to 10 minutes early for your interview. Late arrival could mean a lost job. Allow for traffic, trains blocking the road, and other complications that might interfere with your arriving on time.

During the interview, observe all of the following points:

◆ Greet the interviewer by name when you are introduced. Introduce yourself. Shake hands firmly and smile (see figure 16-5).

◆ Remain standing until the interviewer asks you to sit. Be aware of your posture and sit straight. Keep both feet flat on the floor or cross your legs at the ankles only.

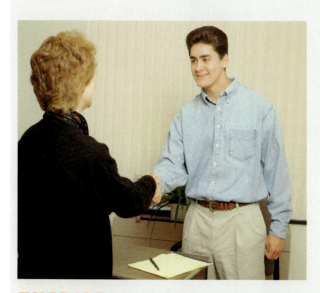

FIGURE 16-5 Shake hands firmly and smile when you greet an interviewer.

◆ Use correct grammar. Avoid using slang words.

◆ Speak slowly and clearly. Don't mumble.

◆ Be polite. Practice good manners.

◆ **C** Maintain eye contact. Avoid looking at the floor, ceiling, or away from the interviewer. Looking at the middle of the interviewer's forehead or at the tip of the interviewer's nose can sometimes help when you are nervous and experiencing difficulty with direct eye contact.

◆ Answer all questions thoroughly, but don't go into long, drawn-out explanations.

◆ Do *not* smoke, chew gum, or eat candy during the interview.

◆ Smile but avoid excessive laughter or giggling.

◆ Be yourself. Do not try to assume a different personality or different mannerisms; doing so will only increase your nervousness.

◆ Be enthusiastic. Display your positive attitude.

◆ Listen closely to the interviewer. Do not interrupt in the middle of a sentence. Allow the interviewer to take the lead.

◆ Avoid awkward habits such as swinging your legs, jingling change in your pocket, waving your hands or arms, or patting at your hair.

◆ Never discuss personal problems, finances, or other situations in an effort to get the job. This usually has a negative effect on the interviewer.

◆ Do not criticize former employers or degrade them in any way.

◆ Answer all questions truthfully to the best of your ability.

◆ Think before you respond. Try to organize the information you present.

◆ Be proud of yourself, to a degree. You have skills and are trained. Make sure the interviewer is aware of this. However, be sure to show a willingness to learn and to gain additional knowledge.

◆ Do not immediately question the employer about salary, fringe benefits, insurance, and other similar items. This information is usually mentioned before the end of the interview. If the employer asks whether you have any questions, ask about the job description or responsibilities, type of uniform required, potential for career growth, continuing education or in-service programs, and job orientation. These types of questions indicate a sincere interest in the job rather than a "What's in it for me?" attitude.

◆ Do not expect a definite answer at the end of the interview. The interviewer will usually tell you that he or she will contact you.

◆ Thank the interviewer for the interview as you leave. If the interviewer extends a hand, shake hands firmly. Smile, be polite, and exit with confidence.

◆ Never try to extend the interview if the interviewer indicates that he or she is ready to end it.

After the interview, it is best to send a follow-up note or letter to thank the employer for the interview (see figure 16-6). You may indicate that you are still interested in the position. You may also state that you are available for further questioning. When an employer is evaluating several applicants, a thank-you note is sometimes the deciding factor in who gets the job.

C Because you may be asked many different questions during an interview, it is impossible to prepare all answers ahead of time. However, it is wise to think about some potential questions and your responses to them. The following is a suggested list of questions to review. Additional questions may be found in any book on job interviews.

◆ *Tell me a little about yourself.* (Note: Stick to job-related information.)

◆ *What are your strong points/weak points?* (Note: Be sure to turn a weakness into a positive point. For example, say, "One of my weaknesses is poor spelling, but I use a dictionary to check spelling and try to learn to spell ten new words each week.")

◆ *Why do you feel you are qualified for this position?*

◆ *What jobs have you held in the past? Why did you leave these jobs?* (Note: Avoid criticizing former employers.)

◆ *What school activities are you involved in?*

◆ *What kind of work interests you?*

◆ *Why do you want to work here?*

◆ *What skills do you have that would be of value?*

◆ *What is your attitude toward work?*

◆ *What do you want to know about this job opening?*

◆ *What were your favorite subjects in school and why?*

◆ *What does success mean to you?*

◆ *How do you manage your time?*

◆ *What is your image of the ideal job?*

◆ *How skilled are you with computers?*

◆ *What are the three most important things to you in a job?*

◆ *Do you prefer to work alone or with others? Why?*

◆ *How many days of school did you miss last year?*

◆ *What do you do in your spare time?*

◆ *Do you have any plans for further education?*

Any questions that may reflect discrimination or bias do *not* have to be answered during a job interview. Federal law prohibits discrimination with regard to age, cultural or ethnic background, marital status, parenthood, religion, race, and gender. Employers are aware

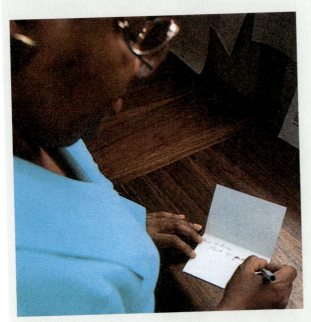

FIGURE 16-6 After a job interview, send a thank-you note or letter to the employer.

that it is illegal to ask questions of this nature, and the large majority will not ask such questions. If an employer does ask a question of this nature, however, you have the right to refuse to answer. An example of this type of question might be, "I see you married recently. Do you plan to start having children in the next year or two?" Be polite but firm in your refusal. A statement such as "I prefer not to answer that question" or "Can I ask you how this would affect the job we are discussing?" is usually sufficient.

At the end of the interview, you may be asked to provide proof of your eligibility to work. Under the Bureau of Immigration Reform Act of 1986, employers are now required by federal law to ask you to complete an Employment Eligibility Verification Form I-9. This form helps the employer verify that you are legally entitled to work in the United States. To complete this form, you must provide documents that indicate your identity. A birth certificate, passport, and/or immigration card can be used for this purpose. You must also have a photo identification, such as a driver's license, and a social security card. The employer must make copies of these documents and include them in your file. Having these forms readily available shows that you are prepared for a job.

STUDENT: *Go to the workbook and complete the assignment sheet for 16:4, Participating in a Job Interview. Then return and continue with the procedure.*

PROCEDURE 16:4   C
Participating in a Job Interview

Equipment and Supplies

Desk, two chairs, evaluation sheets, lists of questions

Procedure

1. Assemble equipment. Role play a mock interview with four persons. Arrange for two people to evaluate the interview, one person to be the interviewer, and you to be the interviewee.

2. Position the two evaluators in such a way that they can observe both the interviewer and you, the person being interviewed. Make sure they will not interfere with the interview.

3. The interviewer should be seated at the desk and have a list of possible questions to ask during the interview.

4. Play the role of the person being interviewed. Prepare for this role by doing the following:

   ◆ Be sure you have all necessary information. Prepare your wallet card, resumé, job application form, and/or career passport or portfolio.

   ◆ Dress appropriately for the interview (as outlined in the preceding information section).

   ◆ Arrive at least 5 to 10 minutes early for the interview.

5. When you are called for the interview, introduce yourself. Be sure to refer to the interviewer by name.

6. Sit in the chair indicated. Be aware of your posture, making sure to sit straight. Keep your feet flat on the floor or cross your legs at the ankles only.

7. Listen closely to the employer. Answer all questions thoroughly and completely. Think before you speak. Organize your information.

8. Maintain eye contact. Avoid distracting mannerisms.

9. Use correct grammar. Avoid slang expressions. Speak in complete sentences. Practice good manners.

10. When you are asked whether you have any questions, ask questions pertaining to the job responsibilities. Avoid a series of questions on salary, fringe benefits, vacations, time off, and so forth.

11. At the end of the interview, thank the interviewer for his or her time. Shake hands as you leave.

12. Check your performance by looking at the evaluation sheets completed by the two observers. Study suggested changes.

13. Replace all equipment.

Practice *Go to the workbook and use the evaluation sheet for 16:4, Participating in a Job Interview, to practice this procedure. When you feel you have mastered this skill, sign the sheet and give it to your instructor for further action.*

✔ **Final Checkpoint** Using the criteria listed on the evaluation sheet, your instructor will grade your performance.

16:5 INFORMATION Determining Net Income

 Obtaining a job means, in part, that you will be earning your own money. This often means that you will be responsible for your own living expenses. To avoid debt and financial crisis, it is important that you learn about managing your money effectively, including understanding how to determine net income.

The term **income** usually means money that you earn or that is available to you. However, the amount you actually earn and the amount you receive to spend may vary. The following two terms explain the difference.

◆ **Gross Income:** This is the total amount of money you earn for hours worked. It is the amount determined before any deductions have been taken out of your pay.

◆ **Net Income:** This is commonly referred to as "take home pay." It is the amount of money available to you after all payroll **deductions** have been taken out of your salary. Some common deductions are Social Security tax, federal and state taxes, and city taxes. Other deductions may include payroll deductions such as those for United Appeal, medical or life insurance, union dues, and other similar items.

To determine gross income, simply multiply your wage per hour times the number of hours worked. For example, if you earn $7.00 per hour and work a 40 hour week, 7 × 40 = $280.00. In this example, then, $280.00 would be your gross income.

To determine net income, you must first determine the amounts of the various deductions that will be taken out of your gross pay. Deduction percentages usually vary depending on your income level. You can usually determine approximate deduction percentages and, therefore, your approximate net income by referring to tax charts. Never hesitate to ask about deduction percentages. It is your responsibility to check your own paycheck for accuracy. Starting with the example of gross pay of $280.00, the following shows how net pay may be determined.

Gross Pay $280.00

◆ Deduction for federal tax in this income range is usually approximately 15 percent. Check tax tables for accuracy.

15%, or 0.15, × 280 = $42.00   − 42.00
                                                    238.00

◆ Deduction for state tax is approximately 2 percent.

2%, or 0.02, × 280 = $5.60   − 5.60
                                                    232.40

◆ Deduction for city tax is approximately 1 percent.

1%, or 0.01, × 280 = 2.80

$$- 2.80 \over 229.60$$

◆ Deduction for F.I.C.A., or Social Security tax, includes 6.2 percent of the first $84,900 in income and a Medicare deduction of 1.45 percent of the total in income, for a total deduction of 7.65 percent.

7.65%, or 0.0765, × 280 = 21.42

$$- 21.42 \over 208.18$$

◆ Net income after taxes, then, would be $208.18. Therefore, before you even receive your paycheck, $71.82 will be deducted from it. Additional deductions for insurance, union dues, contributions to charity, and other items may also be taken out of your gross pay.

In order to manage your money effectively, it is essential that you be able to calculate your net income. Because this is the amount of money you will have to spend, it will to some extent determine your lifestyle.

STUDENT: *Read and complete Procedure 16:5, Determining Net Income.*

PROCEDURE 16:5
Determining Net Income

Equipment and Supplies

Assignment sheet for 16:5, Determining Net Income; pen or pencil

Procedure

1. Assemble equipment. If a calculator is available, you may use it to complete this assignment.
2. Read the instructions on the assignment sheet in the workbook for 16:5, Determining Net Income. Use the assignment sheet with this procedure.
3. Determine your wage per hour by using your salary in a current job or an amount assigned by your instructor. Multiply this amount by the number of hours you work per week. This is your gross weekly pay.
4. If your instructor has tax tables, read the tax tables to determine the percentage, or amount of money, that will be withheld for federal tax. If tax tables are not available, check with your employer to obtain this information.
   NOTE: The average withholding tax for an initial income bracket is usually approximately 15 percent. If you cannot find the exact amount or percentage, use this amount (0.15) for an approximate determination.
5. Multiply the percentage for federal tax times your gross weekly pay to determine the amount deducted for federal tax.
6. Determine the deduction for state tax by reading your state tax tables or by consulting your employer.
   NOTE: An average state tax is 2 percent. If you cannot find the exact amount or percentage, use this amount (0.02) for an approximate determination.
7. Multiply the percentage for state tax by your gross weekly pay to determine the amount deducted for state tax.
8. Determine the deduction for any city or corporation tax by reading the city/corporation tax tables or consulting your employer.
   NOTE: An average city/corporation tax is 1 percent. If you cannot find the exact amount or percentage, use this amount (0.01) for an approximate determination.
9. Multiply the percentage for city/corporation tax by your gross weekly pay to determine the amount deducted for city/corporation tax.
10. Check the current deduction for F.I.C.A., or Social Security and Medicare, by checking

the tax tables or asking your employer for this information. Determine the deduction for F.I.C.A. by multiplying your gross weekly pay by this percentage.

NOTE: In 2002, the F.I.C.A. rate was 6.2 percent of the first $84,900 in income and 1.45 percent of total income for Medicare. Use this total of 7.65 percent, or 0.0765, if you cannot obtain another percentage.

11. List the amounts for any other deductions. Examples include insurance, charitable donations, union dues, and similar items.

12. Add the amounts determined for federal tax, state tax, city/corporation tax, social security, and other deductions together.

13. Subtract the total amount for deductions from your gross weekly pay. The amount left is your net, or take home, pay.

14. Recheck any figures, as needed.

15. Replace all equipment.

Practice Go to the workbook and use the evaluation sheet for 16:5, Determining Net Income. Practice determining net income according to the criteria listed on the evaluation sheet. When you feel you have mastered this skill, sign the sheet and give it to your instructor for further action.

✔ **Final Checkpoint** Using the criteria listed on the evaluation sheet, your instructor will grade your performance.

16:6   INFORMATION   Calculating a Budget

 In order to use your net income wisely, it is best to prepare a budget. This section provides basic information on this topic.

A **budget** is an itemized list of living expenses. It must be realistic to be effective.

A budget usually consists of two main types of expenses: fixed expenses and variable expenses. **Fixed expenses** include items such as rent or house payments, utilities, food, car payments, and insurance payments. **Variable expenses** include items such as entertainment, clothing purchases, and donations.

The easiest way to prepare a budget is to simply list all anticipated expenses for a one-month period. Then, determine your net monthly pay. Allow a fair percentage of the net monthly pay for each of the budget items listed.

Savings should be incorporated into every budget. If saving money is regarded as an obligation, it is easier to set aside money for this purpose. When an emergency occurs, money is then available to cover the unexpected expenditure.

Some payments are due once or twice a year. An example is insurance payments. To be realistic, a monthly amount should be budgeted for this purpose. To determine a monthly amount, divide the total yearly cost for the insurance by twelve. Then, budget this amount each month. In this way, when insurance payments are due, the money is available for payment, and one month's budget will not have to bear the full amount of the insurance payment.

It is important that budgeted expenses do *not* exceed net monthly income. It may sometimes be necessary to limit expenses that are not fixed. Entertainment, clothing purchases, and similar items are examples of expenses that can be limited.

The final step is to live by your budget and avoid any spending over the allotted amounts. This is one way to prevent financial problems and excessive debt. If your fixed expenses or net income increases, you will have to revise your budget. Remember, creating a budget leads to careful management of hard-earned money.

STUDENT: *Read Procedure 16:6, Calculating a Budget. Then go to the workbook and complete the corresponding assignment sheet.*

PROCEDURE 16:6

Calculating a Budget

Equipment and Supplies

Assignment sheet for 16:6, Calculating a Budget; pen or pencil

Procedure

1. Assemble equipment. If a calculator is available, you may use it to complete this procedure.
2. Go to the workbook and read the instructions on the assignment sheet for 16:6, Calculating a Budget.
3. Determine your fixed expenses for a one-month period. This includes amounts you must pay for rent, utilities, loans, charge accounts, insurance, and similar items. List these expenses.
4. Determine your variable expenses for a one-month period. This includes amounts for clothing purchases, personal items, donations, entertainment, and similar items. List these expenses.
5. List any other items that must be included in your monthly budget. Be sure to list a reasonable amount for each item.
6. Determine a reasonable amount for savings. Many people prefer to set aside a certain percentage of their net monthly pay as savings.
7. Determine your net monthly pay. Double-check all figures for accuracy.
8. Add all of your monthly budget expenses together. The sum represents your total expenditures per month.

9. Compare your expense total to your net monthly income. If your expense total is higher than your net income, you will have to revise your budget and reduce any expenses that are not fixed. If your expense total is lower than your net income, you may increase the dollar amounts of your budget items. If the other figures in your budget are realistic, it may be wise to increase the dollar amount of savings.
10. When the expense total in your budget equals your monthly net income, you have a balanced budget. Live by this budget and avoid any expenditures not listed on the budget.
11. Replace all equipment.

Practice *Go to the workbook and use the evaluation sheet for 16:6, Calculating a Budget, to practice this procedure. When you feel you have mastered this skill, sign the sheet and give it to your instructor for further action. Give your instructor a completed budget along with the evaluation sheet.*

 Final Checkpoint Using the criteria listed on the evaluation sheet, your instructor will grade your budget.

UNIT 16 SUMMARY

Even if an individual is proficient in many skills, it does not necessarily follow that the individual will obtain the "ideal" job. Just as it is important to learn the skills needed in your chosen health care career, it is important to learn the skills necessary to obtain a job.

Job-keeping skills important to an employer include using correct grammar in both oral and written communications, reporting to work on time and when scheduled, being prepared to work, following correct policies and procedures, having a positive attitude, working well with others, taking responsibility for your actions, and being willing to learn. Without good job-keeping skills, no amount of knowledge will help you keep a job.

One of the first aspects of obtaining a job involves preparing a letter of application and a resumé. These are the "press releases" that tell a potential employer about your skills and abilities. A properly prepared resumé will help you obtain an interview.

It is important to prepare for an interview. Careful consideration should be given to dress and appearance. Answers should be prepared for common interview questions. The applicant should also try to learn as much as possible about the potential employer; this way, the applicant will be able to match his or her skills and abilities to the needs of the employer. Finally, practice completing job application forms. A neat, correct, and thorough application form will also help you get a job.

Certain other skills become essential when a person has a job. Everyone should be able to calculate gross and net income. In addition, everyone should be able to develop a budget based on needs and income. Having and following a budget makes it more likely that money earned will be spent wisely and minimizes the chance of debt. Learn the job-seeking and job-keeping skills well. They will benefit you throughout your life as you seek new positions of employment and advance in your chosen health career.

INTERNET SEARCHES

Use the suggested search engines in Unit 11:4 of this textbook to search the Internet for additional information on the following topics:

1. *Components of a job search:* find information on letters of application or cover letters, resumes, job interviews, and job application forms.

2. *Requirements of employers:* locate information on skills and qualities that employers desire.

3. *Job search:* look for sites that provide information on employment opportunities. For specific health care careers, look for opportunities under organizations for the specific career. Also check general sites such as *monster.com, job-listing.com, jobsleuth.com,* and *joblocator.com.*

4. *Salary and wages:* check sites such as the Internal Revenue Service (IRS), state and local tax departments, and Social Security Administration for information on taxes and tax rates. Also locate sites on money management, budgeting, and fiscal or financial management for information on how to manage money.

REVIEW QUESTIONS

1. Choose four (4) job-keeping skills that you feel you have mastered. Write a paragraph describing why you feel you have mastered these skills.

2. What is the main purpose of a letter of application or cover letter? When is it used?

3. List the main sections of a resumé and briefly describe the information that should be included in each section.

4. State six (6) basic principles that must be followed while completing a job application form.

5. Create answers for the following interview questions.
   a. Why do you feel you are qualified for this job?
   b. Why do you want to leave your current job?
   c. Tell me about two or three of your major accomplishments and why you feel they are important.

6. You have obtained a job and will receive a salary of $7.20 per hour. Calculate the following:
   a. Gross pay for a 40-hour week
   b. Federal tax deduction of 15%
   c. State tax deduction of 3%
   d. City tax deduction of 0.5%
   e. FICA or social security deduction of 7.65%
   f. Net pay after above deductibles

UNIT 16

SUGGESTED REFERENCES

Anderson, Shirley, and Jody Smith. *Delmar's Handbook for Health Information Careers.* Clifton Park, NY: Delmar Learning, 1998.

Baily, M. *Career Success for the 21st Century.* 3rd ed. Cincinnati, OH: South-Western, 2003.

Colbert, Bruce. *Workplace Readiness for Health Occupations.* Clifton Park, NY: Delmar Learning, 2000.

Field, Ben, and Paul Wright. *Better Job Search in 3 Easy Steps.* Clifton Park, NY: Delmar Learning, 2000.

Field, Ben, Dan Strakal, and Paul Wright. *Better Job Skills in 3 Easy Steps.* Clifton Park, NY: Delmar Learning, 2000.

Field, Ben, and Paul Wright. *Better Resumes in 3 Easy Steps.* Clifton Park, NY: Delmar Learning, 2000.

Krantman, Stan. *The Resumé Writer's Workbook.* 2nd ed. Clifton Park, NY: Delmar Learning, 2001.

Kushner, John. *How to Find and Apply for a Job.* 6th ed. Cincinnati, OH: South-Western, 1996.

O'Donnell, Michael. *Health Promotion in the Workplace.* 3rd ed. Clifton Park, NY: Delmar Learning, 2002.

Pigford, Lois. *The Successful Interview and Beyond.* Clifton Park, NY: Delmar Learning, 2001.

Ryan, Joan S. *Managing Your Personal Finances.* 4th ed. Cincinnati, OH: South-Western, 2002.

Simmers, Louise. *Practical Problems in Mathematics for Health Occupations.* Clifton Park, NY: Delmar Learning, 1996.

Villemarie, Doreen, and Lorraine Villemarie. *Grammar and Writing Skills for the Health Professional.* Clifton Park, NY: Delmar Learning, 2001.

Wallace, B., and J. Masters. *Personal Development for Life and Work.* Cincinnati, OH: South-Western, 2001.

Wray, J., L. Luft, and M. Highland. *Fundamentals of Human Relations: Applications for Life and Work.* Cincinnati, OH: South-Western, 1996.

Zedlitz, T. *Getting a Job: Process Kit.* 4th ed. Cincinnati, OH: South-Western, 1998.

Part 2

Special Health Care Skills

Introduction

This part is divided into six major units. The topics are designed to provide you with the basic knowledge and skills required to perform a wide variety of procedures used in specific health careers. Before you start a unit, read the unit objectives so you will know exactly what is expected of you. The objectives identify the competencies you should have mastered upon completing the unit.

For each procedure discussed in this part, you will find information and procedure sections in the textbook. In the workbook, you will find two types of sheets: assignment sheets and evaluation sheets. Following are brief explanations of these main components of the textbook and workbook.

1. *Information Sections (Textbook):* The information sections are designed to provide the basic knowledge you must have to perform the procedures. The sections explain why things are done, give necessary facts, and stress key points that should be observed. Each information section refers you to a specific assignment sheet in the workbook.

2. *Assignment Sheets (Workbook):* The assignment sheets provide review of the main facts and related information about the procedures. After you have read each information section in the text, try to answer the questions on the assignment sheet. Then refer back to the information section to see whether your answers are correct. Let your instructor grade your completed assignment sheet. Note and learn from any points that were incorrect. Be sure you understand all information before performing the procedure.

3. *Procedure Sections (Textbook):* The procedure sections provide step-by-step instructions on how to perform the procedures. Follow the steps while you practice the procedures. Each procedure lists the equipment and supplies you will need. Be sure you have all the necessary equipment and supplies before you begin.

At times you will see one of three words within the procedure sections: **Note, Caution**, and **Checkpoint. Note** means to carefully read the comment following. These comments usually stress points of knowledge or explain why certain techniques are used. **Caution** means that a safety factor is involved and that you should proceed carefully while doing this step in order to avoid injury to yourself or the patient. **Checkpoint** means to ask your instructor to check you at this point in the procedure. Checkpoints are usually located at critical points in the procedures. Each procedure section in this part of the text refers you to a specific evaluation sheet in the workbook.

4. *Evaluation Sheets (Workbook):* Each evaluation sheet contains a list of the criteria on which you will be tested when you have demonstrated that you have mastered a particular procedure. Use these sheets as you practice the procedures. Make sure that your performance meets the established standards. When you feel you have mastered a particular procedure, sign the evaluation sheet and give it to your instructor. Your instructor will grade you by using the listed criteria and checking each step against your performance.

You will find a list of suggested references at the end of each unit in this part. If you want additional information about any of the procedures discussed in the unit, refer to these references.

As was the case in Part 1, you will notice icons throughout this part of the textbook. The purpose of these icons is to accentuate particular factors or denote specific types of knowledge. The icons and their meanings are as follows:

 Observe Standard Precautions

 Safety—Proceed with Caution

 Math Skill

 Science Skill

 Communications Skill

 Instructors Check—Call Instructor at This Point

 OBRA Requirement— Based on Federal Law

 Legal Responsibility

 Career Information

 Technology

UNIT 17

Dental Assistant Skills

Unit Objectives

After completing this unit of study, you should be able to:

- Locate and name all the structures and tissues of a tooth
- Identify deciduous and permanent teeth by their full proper names
- Identify teeth by the Universal Numbering System and the Federation Dentaire International System
- Identify surfaces of the teeth
- Chart conditions of teeth
- Operate and maintain dental equipment according to general guidelines and principles
- Identify the main dental instruments and set up dental trays for each of the following: oral examination, amalgam restoration, composite restoration, and surgical extraction
- Position a patient in a dental chair, observing all safety precautions
- Demonstrate the Bass method of brushing
- Demonstrate flossing technique
- Prepare alginate and take an impression from dentures
- Prepare rubber base impression material and load a syringe
- Pour plaster and stone models that meet required standards
- Make a custom tray
- Describe proper maintenance of anesthetic carpules and an aspirating syringe
- Load an anesthetic aspirating syringe without contaminating it
- Mix cements and bases for dental use
- Mix amalgam and load the amalgam carrier
- Mix composite for restorations
- Develop dental X-rays that meet required standards
- Mount full-mouth and bitewing X-rays
- Define, pronounce, and spell all the key terms

Observe Standard Precautions

  Instructors Check—Call Instructor at This Point

 Safety—Proceed with Caution

 OBRA Requirement— Based on Federal Law

 Math Skill

 Legal Responsibility

 Science Skill

 Career Information

 Communications Skill

Technology

KEY TERMS

air compressor

alginate
  (ahl'-jih-nate")

alveolar process
  (al-vee'-o-lar)

amalgam
  (ah-mahl'-gam)

anesthesia
  (an-es-thee'-sha) Note: th as
  in "thin"

anterior

apex

apical foramen

aspirating syringe

assistant's cart

base

bicuspids

bitewings

buccal
  (buck'-kal)

burs

carious lesions (caries)
  (care'-ee"-us lee'-shunz)

carpules

cavity

cement

cementum

cervix

composite
  (kom-poz'-it)

contra angle

crown

cuspids

cuspidor

custom trays

dental chair

dental light

dentin

dentitions

distal

doctor's cart

enamel

Federation Dentaire
  International System

gingiva
  (jin'-jih"-vah)

halitosis
  (hal"-ih-toe'-sis)

high-speed handpiece

high-velocity oral evacuator

impression

incisal

incisors

labial
  (lab'-ee"-ahl)

line angles

liner

lingual
  (lynn'-gwal)

low-speed handpiece

mandibular

maxillary

mesial
  (me'-ze-ahl)

model

molars

occlusal
  (oh-klew'-sal)

occlusal films

odontology

oral-evacuation system

panoramic

pedodontic (child) films
  (pee-doe-don'-tick)

periapical films
  (per-ree-ape'-ih-kal)

permanent (succedaneous)
  teeth

periodontal ligament
  (pear"-e-o-don'-till)

periodontium

plaque
  (plak')

plaster

point angles

posterior

primary (deciduous) teeth

prophylaxis angle
  (proh"-fill-ax'-sis an'-gull)

pulp

quadrant

radiographs

radiolucent
  (ray"-dee-oh-lew'-sent)

radiopaque
  (ray"-dee-oh-payk')

restoration

rheostats
  (ree'-oh-stats")

root

rubber base

saliva ejector

stone

temporary

tri-flow (air–water) syringe

Universal Numbering System

CAREER HIGHLIGHTS

Dental assistants work under the supervision of doctors, called dentists, and they are important members of the dental health care team. Educational requirements vary from state to state, but can include on-the-job training, one- or two-year health occupations education programs, and/or an associate's degree.

Certification is available through the Dental Assisting National Board. Graduation from an accredited program of dental assisting or two years of full-time employment as a dental assistant is required before an individual can take the certification examination. The duties of dental assistants vary depending on the size and type of practice, and on the dental practice laws of the state in which they work. In addition to the knowledge and skills presented in this unit, dental assistants must also learn and master skills such as:

◆ Presenting a professional appearance and attitude

◆ Obtaining knowledge regarding health care delivery systems, organizational structure, and teamwork

◆ Meeting all legal responsibilities

◆ Communicating effectively

◆ Being sensitive to and respecting cultural diversity

◆ Comprehending human anatomy, physiology, and pathophysiology with an emphasis on oral anatomy and physiology

◆ Learning dental terminology

◆ Observing all safety precautions

◆ Practicing all principles of infection control

◆ Taking and recording vital signs

◆ Administering first aid and cardiopulmonary resuscitation

◆ Promoting good nutrition and a healthy life-style to maintain dental health

◆ Utilizing computer skills

◆ Performing administrative duties such as answering the telephone, scheduling appointments, preparing correspondence, completing insurance forms, maintaining accounts, recording dental histories, and maintaining patient records

◆ Ordering and maintaining supplies and materials

INFORMATION
17:1 Identifying the Structures and Tissues of a Tooth

An understanding of the basic structures and tissues of a tooth is essential for a dental assistant. **Odontology** is the study of the anatomy, growth, and diseases of the teeth. Teeth are accessory organs of the digestive tract that aid in the *mastication*, or chewing, of food. Individuals have two **dentitions**, or sets, of teeth: a primary, or deciduous, dentition, and a permanent, or succedaneous, dentition (see figure 17-1). At birth, a newborn has approximately forty-four teeth buds at various stages of development. When a child is approximately 6 months old, these teeth buds begin to erupt into the mouth to form the primary dentition. When a child is approximately 2 years old, all of the twenty primary teeth will have erupted. These teeth maintain proper spacing for the permanent, or succedaneous, teeth and are used for mastication and speech. Between the ages of 6

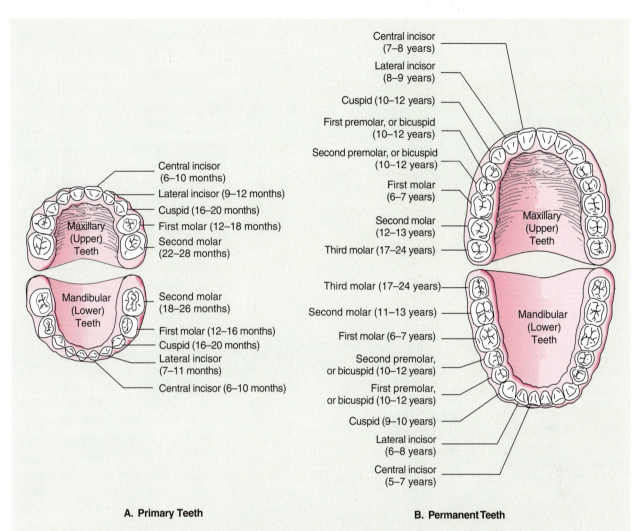

A. Primary Teeth

Central incisor (6–10 months)
Lateral incisor (9–12 months)
Cuspid (16–20 months)
First molar (12–18 months)
Second molar (22–28 months)

Maxillary (Upper) Teeth

Mandibular (Lower) Teeth

Second molar (18–26 months)
First molar (12–16 months)
Cuspid (16–20 months)
Lateral incisor (7–11 months)
Central incisor (6–10 months)

B. Permanent Teeth

Central incisor (7–8 years)
Lateral incisor (8–9 years)
Cuspid (10–12 years)
First premolar, or bicuspid (10–12 years)
Second premolar, or bicuspid (10–12 years)
First molar (6–7 years)
Second molar (12–13 years)
Third molar (17–24 years)

Maxillary (Upper) Teeth

Third molar (17–24 years)
Second molar (11–13 years)
First molar (6–7 years)
Second premolar, or bicuspid (10–12 years)
First premolar, or bicuspid (10–12 years)
Cuspid (9–10 years)
Lateral incisor (6–8 years)
Central incisor (5–7 years)

Mandibular (Lower) Teeth

FIGURE 17-1 Eruption times of (A) primary (deciduous) and (B) permanent (succedaneous) teeth.

and 12 years, all of the primary teeth are lost and are replaced by the permanent dentition. These permanent teeth begin to erupt when a child is approximately 5 years old. They continue erupting and replacing primary teeth until the individual reaches approximately 17 to 20 years of age, when the third molars, or wisdom teeth, erupt. Most of the thirty-two teeth in the permanent dentition are in place by 12 years of age. A child 5 to 12 years old who has both primary and permanent teeth erupted in the mouth has a *mixed dentition.*

Every tooth in both the primary and permanent dentitions has four main sections, or divisions: the crown, the root, the cervix, and the apex (see figure 17-2):

◆ **Crown**: This is the section of the tooth that is visible in the mouth. It is protected on the outside by the tissue called *enamel.*

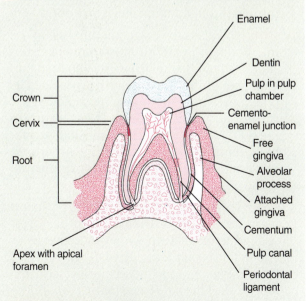

Enamel
Dentin
Pulp in pulp chamber
Cemento-enamel junction
Free gingiva
Alveolar process
Attached gingiva
Cementum
Pulp canal
Periodontal ligament

Crown
Cervix
Root

Apex with apical foramen

FIGURE 17-2 The structures and tissues of a tooth.

◆ **Root**: This is the section of the tooth below the gingiva, or gums. It is covered on the outside by the tissue called *cementum*. The root is normally not visible in the mouth; it helps anchor, or hold, the tooth in the bony socket of the jaw. A tooth may have a single root or multiple roots. If it has two roots, it is called *bifurcated*; if it has three roots, it is called *trifurcated*.

◆ **Cervix**: This is also called the *neck*, or *cemento-enamel junction*, because it is the area where the enamel covering the crown meets the cementum covering the root. It is the narrow section where the crown joins with the root.

◆ **Apex**: This is the tip of the root of the tooth. It contains an opening called the **apical foramen**, through which nerves and blood vessels enter the tooth.

Each tooth is made of four main tissues: enamel, cementum, dentin, and pulp (see figure 17-2):

◆ **Enamel**: This is the hardest tissue in the body and covers the outside of the crown. It is made up mainly of calcium and phosphorus and forms a protective layer for the tooth. Once a tooth is fully developed, the enamel cannot grow or repair itself.

◆ **Cementum**: This is the hard, bonelike tissue that covers the outside of the root. In addition to providing a thin layer of protection, it also helps hold the tooth in place. Cementum is formed throughout the life of the tooth.

◆ **Dentin**: This is the tissue that makes up the main bulk of the tooth. It is a bonelike substance that is softer than the enamel but harder than the cementum that provides its outer coverings. Although it has no nerves, it carries sensations of pain and temperature to the pulp. Dentin is a living tissue that is capable of limited repair and continued growth. The internal surface of dentin forms the wall of the pulp chamber.

◆ **Pulp**: This is the soft tissue located in the innermost area of the tooth. It is made up of blood vessels and nerves held in place by connective tissue. The section of pulp located in the crown is called the *pulp chamber*, and the section located in the root is called the *pulp canal* (or *root canal*). The pulp chamber and the pulp canal create a space in the center of the tooth known as the *pulp cavity*. The pulp provides sensation and nourishment for the tooth and helps produce dentin.

The **periodontium** consists of those structures that surround and support the teeth and includes the alveolar process, the periodontal ligament, and the gingiva:

◆ **Alveolar process** or ridge: This is the bone tissue of the maxilla (upper jawbone) and mandible (lower jawbone) that surrounds the roots of the teeth. It contains a series of sockets, or *alveoli*—one for each tooth. Although the tooth sits in the alveolus and is supported by it, the tooth does not touch the bone.

◆ **Periodontal ligament**: This consists of dense fibers of connective tissue that attach to the cementum of the tooth and to the alveolus. The periodontal ligament supports or suspends the tooth in the socket. It acts as a shock absorber and prevents the tooth from resting on or rubbing against the bone during chewing. The periodontal ligament also contains nerves and blood vessels that provide nourishment, aid in the production of cementum, and produce sensation when pressure is applied to the tooth.

◆ **Gingiva**, or gums: These are made of epithelial tissue covered with mucous membrane. They cover the alveolar bone and surround the teeth. The gingiva that surrounds the cervix of a tooth and fills the interproximal spaces (spaces between the teeth) is called *free gingiva* because it is not attached to the tooth. The space between the free gingiva and the tooth is the *gingival sulcus*. Dental floss is used to clean this area of the tooth. Gingiva attached to the alveolar bone is called *attached gingiva*.

The supporting structures and tissues of the teeth are meant to last a lifetime. However, disease can affect the teeth and supporting structures just as it can affect other organs of the body. Dental care is directed toward preventing and treating dental disease and preserving and prolonging the life of the teeth. The information and procedures presented in this unit are all methods of preventing and treating dental disease.

STUDENT: *Go to the workbook and complete the assignment sheet for 17:1, Identifying the Structures and Tissues of a Tooth. Then return and continue with the procedure.*

PROCEDURE 17:1

Identifying the Structures and Tissues of a Tooth

Equipment and Supplies

Anatomical model or chart of the structures and tissues of a tooth, paper, and pen or pencil

Procedure

1. Assemble equipment.
2. Wash hands.
3. Review Information Section 17:1 and then answer the following questions by writing the answers or discussing the information with a lab partner:
   a. Differentiate between primary (deciduous) and permanent (succedaneous) dentitions.
   b. State the ages when primary teeth begin to erupt in the mouth and when they finish erupting.
   c. What is the first primary tooth to erupt?
   d. State the age when permanent teeth begin to erupt to replace the primary teeth.
   e. What is the first permanent tooth to erupt?
   f. What is the total number of primary teeth? Of permanent teeth?
   g. What does the term *mixed dentition* mean? At what ages does it usually occur?
4. Use an anatomical model or chart of a tooth to identify and locate each of the following sections or divisions of a tooth:
   a. crown
   b. root
   c. cervix
   d. apex and apical foramen
5. Use an anatomical model or chart of a tooth to identify and describe the function of each of the following tissues of a tooth:
   a. enamel
   b. cementum
   c. dentin
   d. pulp
6. Use an anatomical model or chart of a tooth to identify and state the function of each of the following structures of the periodontium:
   a. alveolar process
   b. periodontal ligament
   c. gingiva
7. Without looking at the model or chart, draw a tooth and label all of the divisions, tissues, and supporting structures. Then compare your drawing to the model or chart. Check it for accuracy and correct any errors.
   NOTE: If you make any errors, return to Information Section 17:1 to review the material. Then correct your drawing.
8. Replace all equipment.
9. Wash hands.

> **Practice** *Go to the workbook and use the evaluation sheet for 17:1, Identifying the Structures and Tissues of a Tooth, to practice this procedure. When you feel you have mastered this skill, sign the sheet and give it to your instructor for further action.*

 Final Checkpoint Using the criteria listed on the evaluation sheet, your instructor will grade your performance.

17:2 INFORMATION
Identifying the Teeth

 The four main types of teeth and their locations and characteristics are:

◆ **Incisors**
Located in the front and center of the mouth
Broad, sharp edge
Used to cut or bite food
Central incisors are in the center
Lateral incisors are on the sides of the centrals

◆ **Cuspids**
Also called *canines,* or *eyeteeth*
Located at angles of lips
Used to tear food
Longest teeth in the mouth

◆ **Bicuspids**
Also called *premolars*
Located before the molars, from front to back
Used to pulverize or grind food

◆ **Molars**
Teeth in the back of the mouth
Largest and strongest teeth
Used to chew and grind food

Primary, or **deciduous, teeth**: This is the first set of teeth. Although they are also called "baby" teeth, this is an inappropriate term because it implies that the primary teeth have no permanent value and are unimportant. In reality, they serve the important function of maintaining correct spacing for permanent teeth. There are twenty primary teeth:

Ten maxillary (upper):
Two central incisors
Two lateral incisors
Two cuspids
Two 1st molars
Two 2nd molars
Ten mandibular (lower):
Two central incisors
Two lateral incisors
Two cuspids
Two 1st molars
Two 2nd molars

NOTE: There are no bicuspids in primary dentition.

To name the primary teeth, the mouth is divided into **quadrants** or four sections: maxillary right, maxillary left, mandibular right, and mandibular left. A *transverse,* or horizontal, plane separates the mouth into an upper, or *maxillary,* and lower, or *mandibular,* arch or jaw. Each tooth is then labeled as either **maxillary** or **mandibular**. Teeth in the sockets, or alveoli, of the maxilla, or upper jawbone, are called *maxillary.* Teeth in the alveoli of the mandible, or lower jawbone, are called *mandibular.* A *midsagittal* plane divides the mouth into a right and left half. Each tooth is then identified as *right* or *left,* depending on its location in the mouth. In figure 17-3, positions of the teeth are shown as though you were facing another person and looking into the mouth. This creates a mirror image and right and left are reversed.

NOTE: Your left is the patient's right; your right is the patient's left.

Each primary tooth has a specific name. For example, the central incisor in the maxillary right quadrant or arch is called the *maxillary right central incisor.* The central incisor in the maxillary left quadrant is called the *maxillary left central incisor.* The central incisor in the mandibular left quadrant is called the *mandibular left central incisor.* The central incisor in the mandibular right quadrant is called the *mandibular right central incisor.* The same pattern applies to all of the lateral incisors, cuspids, 1st molars, and 2nd molars.

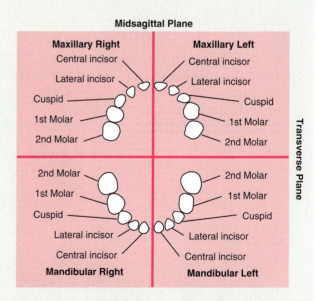

FIGURE 17-3 Primary (deciduous) teeth.

Permanent, or **succedaneous, teeth**: This is the second set of teeth (see figure 17-4). There are thirty-two permanent teeth:

Sixteen maxillary (upper):

Two central incisors

Two lateral incisors

Two cuspids

Two 1st bicuspids

Two 2nd bicuspids

Two 1st molars

Two 2nd molars

Two 3rd molars (wisdom teeth)

Sixteen mandibular (lower):

Two central incisors

Two lateral incisors

Two cuspids

Two 1st bicuspids

Two 2nd bicuspids

Two 1st molars

Two 2nd molars

Two 3rd molars (wisdom teeth)

NOTE: Each permanent tooth in figure 17-4 has its own name, depending on the quadrant it is in. Each is labeled as *maxillary* or *mandibular*

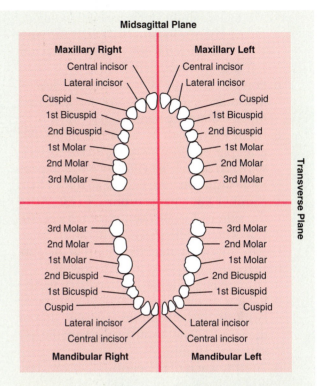

FIGURE 17-4 Permanent (succedaneous) teeth.

and *right* or *left,* following the same pattern used to name each primary tooth.

STUDENT: *Go to the workbook and complete the assignment sheet for 17:2, Identifying the Teeth. Then return and continue with the procedure.*

PROCEDURE 17:2

Identifying the Teeth

Equipment and Supplies

Model or unlabeled chart of primary or deciduous teeth, model or unlabeled chart of permanent or succedaneous teeth, paper, and pen or pencil

Procedure

1. Assemble equipment.
2. Wash hands.
3. Use the model or unlabeled chart of primary teeth to practice the following:

   a. Point to all of the upper teeth and state the name *maxillary.* Write the word *maxillary* on paper. Check for correct spelling.
   b. Point to all of the lower teeth and state the name *mandibular.* Write the word *mandibular* on paper. Check for correct spelling.
   c. Imagine a line in the midsagittal plane that divides the mouth into right and left sides. Point to all the teeth on the right side of the mouth. Point to all the teeth on the left side of the mouth.

NOTE: Remember, you are on the outside of the mouth looking in. Teeth on your right side are *left* teeth, and teeth on your left side are *right* teeth.

d. Point to all four central incisors, lateral incisors, cuspids, 1st molars, and 2nd molars. State the names out loud.

e. Name each tooth by its correct name. For example, say *maxillary right central incisor, maxillary right lateral incisor,* and continue until you have named all the teeth.

f. Number your paper from 1 to 20. Write the names for all twenty primary teeth. Check the spelling of each name.

4. Use the model or unlabeled chart of the permanent teeth to practice the following:

a. Point to all the upper, or maxillary, teeth.

b. Point to all the lower, or mandibular, teeth.

c. Point to all the teeth on the right side of the mouth. Point to all the teeth on the left side of the mouth.

d. Point to each of the central incisors, lateral incisors, cuspids, 1st bicuspids, 2nd bicuspids, 1st molars, 2nd molars, and 3rd molars.

e. Name each tooth by its correct name. For example, state *maxillary right 3rd molar, maxillary right 2nd molar,* and continue until you have named all the teeth.

f. Number your paper from 1 to 32. Write the names for all thirty-two permanent teeth. Check the spelling of each name.

5. Replace all equipment.

6. Wash hands.

Practice *Go to the workbook and use the evaluation sheet for 17:2, Identifying the Teeth, to practice this procedure. When you feel you have mastered this skill, sign the sheet and give it to your instructor for further action.*

 Final Checkpoint Using the criteria listed on the evaluation sheet, your instructor will grade your performance.

INFORMATION
Identifying Teeth Using the Universal Numbering System and the Federation Dentaire International System

17:3

Several charting methods are used to identify the teeth. The most common method used in the United States is the Universal Numbering System. It was adopted by the American Dental Association in 1968 and is used on most dental insurance forms and dental charts.

The **Universal Numbering System** is an abbreviated form for identifying the teeth. Each tooth has a number or letter by which it is identified. It is much easier to call a permanent tooth *number 8* rather than to call it the *maxillary right central incisor.*

Primary, or deciduous, teeth:

◆ Are identified by letters from *A* to *T.*

◆ Labeling takes place in a circular pattern.

◆ Starting at the maxillary right 2nd molar, which is *A,* and moving to the left side of the maxillary arch, each tooth is assigned a different letter. The maxillary left 2nd molar is *J.*

◆ Dropping down to the mandibular left 2nd molar, which is *K,* and moving from the left to the mandibular right teeth, continue lettering each mandibular tooth. The mandibular right 2nd molar is *T.*

◆ Figure 17-5 demonstrates how deciduous teeth are identified by the Universal Numbering System. Remember, this is a mirror image. The teeth on *your* right are the patient's left teeth, and teeth on *your* left are the patient's right teeth.

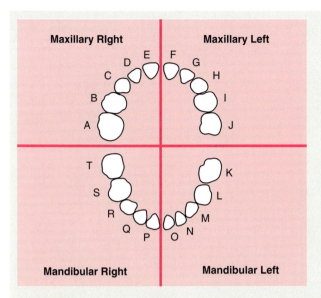

FIGURE 17-5 Coding by the Universal Numbering System for primary or deciduous teeth.

Permanent, or succedaneous, teeth:

♦ Are identified by numbers from *1* to *32*.

♦ The mouth is encircled as each tooth is labeled.

♦ Starting at the maxillary right 3rd molar, which is *1*, and moving around the arch to the left side of the maxillary arch, each tooth is assigned a number. The maxillary left 3rd molar is number *16*.

♦ Dropping down to the mandibular left 3rd molar, which is number *17*, and moving from the left to the mandibular right teeth, continue numbering each tooth in the mandibular arch. The mandibular right 3rd molar is number *32*.

♦ Figure 17-6 demonstrates how permanent teeth are identified by the Universal Numbering System.

The **Federation Dentaire International System** is another method for numbering the teeth. It is used in some dental offices in the United States, and is the most widely used system in Canada and European countries. It uses a two-digit code that identifies the quadrant and the tooth. This makes it easy to use on a computerized system. To identify primary teeth:

♦ The mouth is divided into 4 quadrants.

♦ Code numbers are assigned to each quadrant: maxillary right is *5*, maxillary left is *6*, mandibular left is *7*, and mandibular right is *8*.

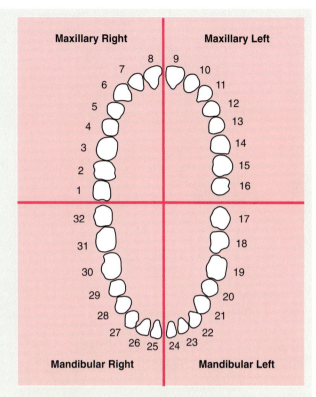

FIGURE 17-6 Coding by the Universal Numbering System for permanent or succedaneous teeth.

♦ Teeth in each quadrant are numbered from *1* to *5*, starting with the central incisor and ending with the second molar.

♦ The number of the quadrant and the number of the tooth are combined to code the tooth. For example, the maxillary right first molar is tooth number *54*. The *5* represents maxillary right and the *4* represents first molar.

♦ Figure 17-7 demonstrates how primary teeth are identified by the Federation Dentaire International System.

To identify permanent teeth:

♦ The mouth is divided into 4 quadrants.

♦ Code numbers are assigned to each quadrant: maxillary right is *1*, maxillary left is *2*, mandibular left is *3*, and mandibular right is *4*.

♦ Teeth in each quadrant are numbered from *1* to *8*, starting with the central incisor and ending with the third molar.

♦ The number of the quadrant and the number of the tooth are combined to code the tooth. For example, the mandibular left lateral incisor is tooth number *32*. The *3* represents

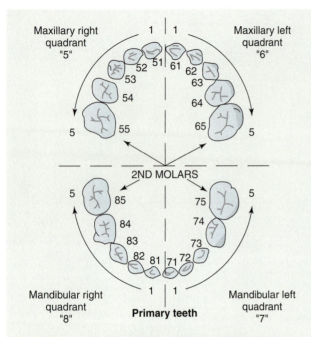

FIGURE 17-7 The Federation Dentaire International System of coding for primary teeth.

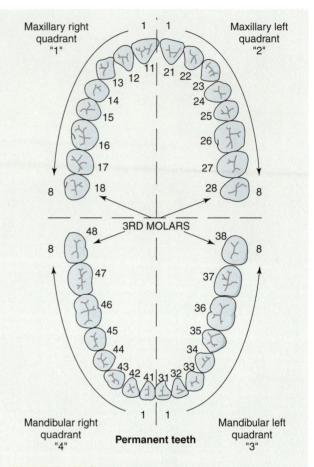

FIGURE 17-8 The Federation Dentaire International System of coding for permanent teeth.

mandibular left and the *2* represents lateral incisor.

◆ Figure 17-8 demonstrates how permanent teeth are identified by the Federation Dentaire International System.

The Federation Dentaire International System can also be used to describe the oral cavity and/or the maxillary or mandibular arches:

◆ *00* refers to the entire oral cavity. For example: *panoramic X-ray 00*

◆ *01* refers to the entire maxillary arch. For example: *fluoride treatment 01*

◆ *02* refers to the entire mandibular arch. For example: *denture 02*

Dental assistants must use the method of numbering the dentist prefers. It is important to become familiar with the various systems to assist with charting conditions and completing insurance forms.

STUDENT: *Go to the workbook and complete the assignment sheet for 17:3, Identifying Teeth Using the Universal Numbering System and Federation Dentaire International System. Then return and continue with the procedure.*

PROCEDURE 17:3A

Identifying Teeth Using the Universal Numbering System

Equipment and Supplies

Model or chart of primary or deciduous teeth, model or chart of permanent or succedaneous teeth, paper, and pen or pencil

Procedure

1. Assemble equipment.
2. Wash hands.
3. Use the model or chart of primary teeth to practice the following:
   a. Draw a sketch of the twenty primary teeth. Label each tooth in your sketch using the letters of the Universal Numbering System. Start by labeling the maxillary right 2nd molar as *A*. Continue labeling all maxillary teeth from *A* to *J*, moving from the maxillary right teeth to the maxillary left teeth. Then, label the mandibular teeth from *K* to *T*, moving from the mandibular left teeth to the mandibular right teeth.
   b. Look at the model or chart of primary teeth. Name teeth at random using the full names, such as *maxillary right central incisor*. Then, determine the correct letter for each tooth. In the previous example, the letter would be *E*. Refer to your sketch as needed.
   c. Call out letters from *A* to *T* at random. Name the tooth that corresponds with each letter.
   d. Repeat the previous two steps until you feel confident about using the Universal Numbering System to identify primary teeth.
4. Use the model or chart of permanent teeth to practice the following:
   a. Draw a sketch of the thirty-two permanent teeth. Label each tooth in your sketch using the numbers of the Universal Numbering System. Start by labeling the maxillary right 3rd molar as number *1*. Continue labeling all maxillary teeth from *1* to *16*, moving from the maxillary right teeth to the maxillary left teeth. Then, label the mandibular teeth from *17* to *32*, moving from the mandibular left teeth to the mandibular right teeth.
   b. Look at the model or chart of permanent teeth. Name teeth at random using the full names, such as *mandibular left 2nd molar*. Then, determine the correct number for each tooth. In the previous example, the number would be *18*. Refer to your sketch as needed.
   c. Call out numbers from *1* to *32* at random. Name the tooth that corresponds with each number.
   d. Repeat the previous two steps until you feel confident about using the Universal Numbering System to identify permanent teeth.
5. Replace all equipment.
6. Wash hands.

Practice *Go to the workbook and use the evaluation sheet for 17:3A, Identifying Teeth Using the Universal Numbering System, to practice this procedure. When you feel you have mastered this skill, sign the sheet and give it to your instructor for further action.*

 Final Checkpoint Using the criteria listed on the evaluation sheet, your instructor will grade your performance.

PROCEDURE 17:3B

Identifying Teeth Using the Federation Dentaire International System

Equipment and Supplies

Model or chart of primary teeth, model or chart of permanent teeth, paper, and pen or pencil

Procedure

1. Assemble equipment.
2. Wash hands.
3. Use the model or chart of primary teeth to practice the following:
   a. Draw a sketch of the twenty primary teeth. Divide the mouth into four quadrants. Draw a transverse line to separate the teeth into maxillary or upper and mandibular or lower teeth. Draw a midsagittal line to separate the mouth into right and left sides.
   b. Label the maxillary right quadrant as *5*, the maxillary left quadrant as *6*, the mandibular left quadrant as *7*, and the mandibular right quadrant as *8*.
   c. Label the teeth in each quadrant from *1* to *5*. Begin with the central incisor as *1*, and end with the second molar as *5*.
   d. Examine the model of primary teeth. Name teeth at random using correct names, such as *maxillary left central incisor*. Then, combine the number of the quadrant with the number of the tooth to determine the correct code for the tooth. In the previous example, the correct code for the tooth is number *61*. The *6* represents maxillary left and the *1* represents central incisor.
   e. Call out number codes at random. Name the tooth that corresponds with each number.
   f. Repeat the previous two steps until you feel confident about using the Federation Dentaire International System to identify primary teeth.
4. Use the model or chart of permanent teeth to practice the following:
   a. Draw a sketch of the thirty-two permanent teeth. Divide the mouth into four quadrants. Draw a transverse line to separate the teeth into maxillary or upper and mandibular or lower teeth. Draw a midsagittal line to separate the mouth into right and left sides.
   b. Label the maxillary right quadrant as *1*, the maxillary left quadrant as *2*, the mandibular left quadrant as *3*, and the mandibular right quadrant as *4*.
   c. Label the teeth in each quadrant from *1* to *8*. Begin with the central incisor as *1*, and end with the third molar as *8*.
   d. Examine the model of permanent teeth. Name teeth at random using correct names, such as *mandibular left first bicuspid*. Then, combine the number of the quadrant with the number of the tooth to determine the correct code for the tooth. In the previous example, the correct code for the tooth is number *34*. The *3* represents mandibular left and the *4* represents first bicuspid.
   e. Call out number codes at random. Name the tooth that corresponds with each number.
   f. Repeat the previous two steps until you feel confident about using the Federation Dentaire International System to identify permanent teeth.
5. Replace all equipment.
6. Wash hands.

Practice *Go to the workbook and use the evaluation sheet for 17:3B, Identifying Teeth Using the Federation Dentaire International System, to practice this procedure. When you feel you have mastered this skill, sign the sheet and give it to your instructor for further action.*

 Final Checkpoint Using the criteria listed on the evaluation sheet, your instructor will grade your performance.

17:4 INFORMATION
Identifying the Surfaces of the Teeth

To chart conditions of the teeth, the dental assistant must be familiar with the crown surfaces of the teeth.

The first step is to differentiate between anterior or posterior teeth (see figure 17-9).

◆ **Anterior** means "toward the front." The central and lateral incisors and cuspids are anterior teeth.

◆ **Posterior** means "toward the back." The bicuspids and molars are posterior teeth.

Each tooth then is divided into two main sections: the crown and the root. The crown is the part that is visible in the mouth, or oral cavity. The root is the section that is located below the gingiva, or gums. The crown is divided into five sections, or surfaces.

Crown surfaces of the anterior teeth (see figure 17-10) are as follows:

◆ **Labial:** crown surface next to the lips; *facial* surface

◆ **Lingual:** crown surface next to the tongue

◆ **Incisal:** cutting edge of the tooth

◆ **Mesial:** side surface closest to the midline (the imaginary line dividing mouth into a right half and a left half)

◆ **Distal:** side surface away from the midline (that is, the side surface facing toward the back of the mouth)

Crown surfaces of the posterior teeth (see figure 17-11) are as follows:

◆ **Buccal:** crown surface next to face or cheek; *facial* surface

◆ **Lingual:** crown surface next to the tongue

◆ **Occlusal:** chewing or grinding surface of the tooth

◆ **Mesial:** side surface toward the midline of the mouth

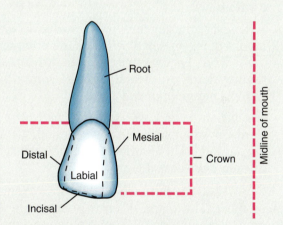

FIGURE 17-10 Crown surfaces on an anterior tooth. The lingual (tongue) surface is not seen on this diagram.

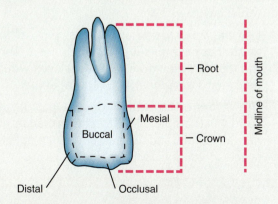

FIGURE 17-11 Crown surfaces on a posterior tooth. The lingual (tongue) surface is not seen on this diagram.

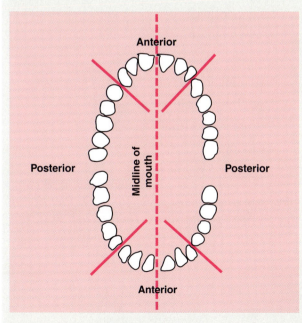

FIGURE 17-9 Anterior and posterior teeth.

◆ **Distal:** side surface away from the midline of the mouth

A suggested list of abbreviations for the crown surfaces follows:

Mesial	*M*
Distal	*D*
Labial	*La*
Lingual	*L* or *Li* or *Lin*
Incisal	*I*
Occlusal	*O*
Buccal	*B*

Line angles form where two crown surfaces meet. The name of each angle is formed by combining the names of the surfaces involved. Use the following guidelines when naming line angles:

◆ Drop the suffix *al* of the *first* word and replace it with *o.*

◆ Whenever mesial or distal surfaces are involved, use *mesial* or *distal* as the first part of the word. For example, a line angle formed by the mesial and labial surfaces would be called a *mesiolabial* line angle.

◆ Use *incisal* or *occlusal* as the last part of the word. For example, a line angle formed by the lingual and occlusal surfaces would be called a *linguoocclusal* line angle.

Point angles form where three crown surfaces meet. The name of each point angle is formed by combining the names of the surfaces involved. Use the following guidelines when naming point angles:

◆ Drop the suffix *al* of the first *two* words and replace with *o.*

◆ Use *mesial* or *distal* as the first part of the word. For example, a point angle formed by the distal, labial, and incisal surfaces would be called a *distolabioincisal* point angle.

◆ Use *incisal* or *occlusal* as the last part of the word. For example, a point angle formed by the mesial, lingual, and occlusal surfaces would be called a *mesiolinguoocclusal* point angle.

A suggested list of abbreviations for anterior teeth line angles and point angles follows:

Line Angles

Linguoincisal	*LiI*
Labioincisal	*LaI*
Mesiolabial	*MLa*
Mesioincisal	*MI*
Mesiolingual	*MLi*
Distolingual	*DLi*
Distoincisal	*DI*
Distolabial	*DLa*

Point Angles

Mesiolinguoincisal	*MLiI*
Mesiolabioincisal	*MLaI*
Distolabioincisal	*DLaI*
Distolinguoincisal	*DLiI*

A suggested list of abbreviations for posterior teeth line angles and point angles follows:

Line Angles

Mesioocclusal	*MO*
Mesiolingual	*MLi*
Mesiobuccal	*MB*
Distoocclusal	*DO*
Distolingual	*DLi*
Distobuccal	*DB*
Linguoocclusal	*LiO*
Buccoocclusal	*BO*

Point Angles

Mesiolinguoocclusal	*MLiO*
Mesiobuccoocclusal	*MBO*
Distobuccoocclusal	*DBO*
Distolinguoocclusal	*DLiO*

STUDENT: *Go to the workbook and complete the assignment sheet for 17:4, Identifying the Surfaces of the Teeth. Then return and continue with the procedure.*

PROCEDURE 17:4

Identifying the Surfaces of the Teeth

Equipment and Supplies

Model of the teeth, paper, pen or pencil

Procedure

1. Assemble equipment.
2. Wash hands.
3. Use the model of the teeth to point out and identify the teeth and surfaces.
4. Identify the anterior teeth. Identify the posterior teeth.
5. Locate the following crown surfaces on the anterior teeth:
   a. Labial
   b. Incisal edge
   c. Lingual
   d. Mesial (draw an imaginary line to separate the mouth into a right and left side)
   e. Distal
6. Locate the following crown surfaces on the posterior teeth:
   a. Buccal
   b. Occlusal
   c. Lingual
   d. Mesial
   e. Distal
7. Locate the line angles on the anterior teeth. Write the correct names on paper. Remember, a line angle forms where two crown surfaces meet. There are a total of eight line angles.
8. Locate the line angles on the posterior teeth. Write the correct names on paper. There are a total of eight line angles.
9. Locate the point angles on the anterior teeth. Write the correct names on the paper. Remember, a point angle forms where three crown surfaces meet. There are a total of four point angles.
10. Locate the point angles on the posterior teeth. Write the correct names on the paper. There are a total of four point angles.
11. Practice steps 4 to 10 until you feel confident about identifying the surfaces on the teeth.
12. Replace all equipment.
13. Wash hands.

Practice *Go to the workbook and use the evaluation sheet for 17:4, Identifying the Surfaces of the Teeth, to practice this procedure. When you feel you have mastered this skill, sign the sheet and give it to your instructor for further action.*

 Final Checkpoint Using the criteria listed on the evaluation sheet, your instructor will grade your performance.

INFORMATION
17:5 Charting Conditions of the Teeth

A dental assistant may be required to chart conditions of the teeth on dental charts or insurance forms. Forms, symbols, and abbreviations vary from office to office.

Dental charts are legal records. They must be complete, neat, and correct. Information must be current and should be updated each time a patient visits the office. The dental charts must be stored in a locked file cabinet to maintain confidentiality and to prevent loss. A dental chart may contain the following sections:

◆ Personal patient information: full name of patient, birthdate or age, address, telephone number, place of employment, physician's name and address, and insurance information

◆ Medical history: diseases or medical conditions patient has, special medical precautions, allergies, and other pertinent medical information (Unit 22:4 in this textbook discusses a medical history in detail.)

◆ Charting area: anatomical or geometric diagrams of the teeth

◆ Treatment section: written record of treatment, services performed, and in some cases, fees and amounts paid

◆ Radiographic history: record of date and type of dental radiographs or X-rays

◆ Remarks: area for written notations by dentist or dental hygienist

In figure 17-12A, permanent, or succedaneous, teeth are represented by the anatomic diagrams. The teeth are numbered according to the Universal Numbering System. Maxillary teeth are above the transverse line and mandibular teeth are below the line. In figure 17-12B, both primary and permanent teeth are represented by the geometric diagrams. Primary teeth are labeled with letters according to the Universal Numbering System. Permanent teeth are labeled with numbers.

Surfaces of the teeth are also shown in figures 17-12A and 17-12B. The surfaces have been shaded to help familiarize you with chart representations. Note the examples for the following surfaces, the numbers of which refer to the Universal Numbering System:

◆ Occlusal: numbers 1 and 32

◆ Incisal: numbers 8 and 25

◆ Buccal: numbers 3 and 30

◆ Labial: numbers 9 and 24

◆ Lingual: numbers 5, 10, 23, and 28

◆ Mesial: numbers 6 and 27; not actually shown on the anatomic diagram but noted along the mesial edges of other surfaces

◆ Distal: numbers 12 and 21; not actually shown on the anatomic diagram but noted along the distal edges of other surfaces

NOTE: Figures 17-12A and 17-12B are sample charts. Dental charts vary slightly. Never hesitate to ask questions about which surfaces are represented by different diagrams.

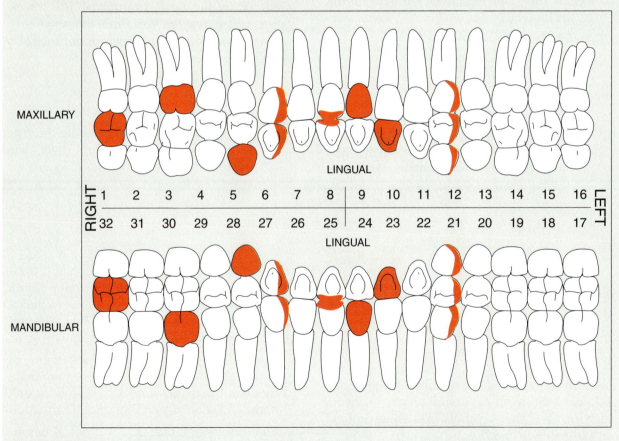

FIGURE 17-12A A sample anatomical diagram dental chart of permanent dentition with different crown surfaces shaded.

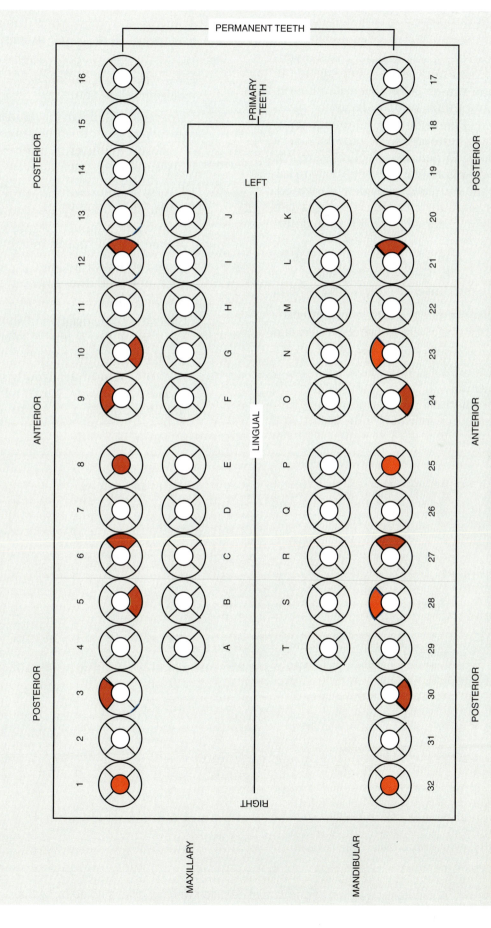

FIGURE 17-12B A sample geometric diagram dental chart with different crown surfaces shaded on permanent dentition.

Notation methods for dental charting vary. In some cases, a pencil is used so that if errors occur, they can be erased. In other cases, a pencil is initially used but charting is completed in ink. In still other cases, colored pencils are used. Red indicates carious lesions (decay) or treatment needed. Blue indicates treatment completed, such as restorations or crowns. Check with the doctor to determine which system is used and learn this system. Never hesitate to ask questions while you learn the preferred method.

Symbols used for anatomic diagrams can also vary. Again, check with the doctor to determine which symbols you should use.

Samples of symbols are shown on figures 17-13A and 17-13B. The numbers used in this figure refer to the Universal Numbering System:

○ Circle or outline any area involving a carious *lesion* or *decay*. In figures 17-13A and 17-13B, carious lesions are shown on the following teeth and surfaces:

1 Occlusal	6 Distal
2 Distoocclusal	7 Incisal
3 Mesioocclusodistal	8 Lingual

4 Buccal	9 Labial
5 Lingual	10 Mesiolingual

● Use a circle filled in solid to indicate *amalgam restoration* (number 12, occlusal amalgam restoration)

⊙ Use a circle with dot in the middle to indicate *esthetic restoration* such as composite or silicates (number 11, composite on labial surface)

X Draw an X over the entire diagram of a *missing tooth* (number 13)

/ Draw one line through the entire diagram of a tooth *to be extracted* (number 14)

// Draw two lines through the entire diagram of a tooth that *has been extracted* (number 15)

○ Circle the entire diagram of an *impacted tooth* (tooth that is unable to erupt into its proper position) (number 16)

RCT or ENDO Write under a tooth that *needs endodontic* (root canal) *treatment* (number 17)

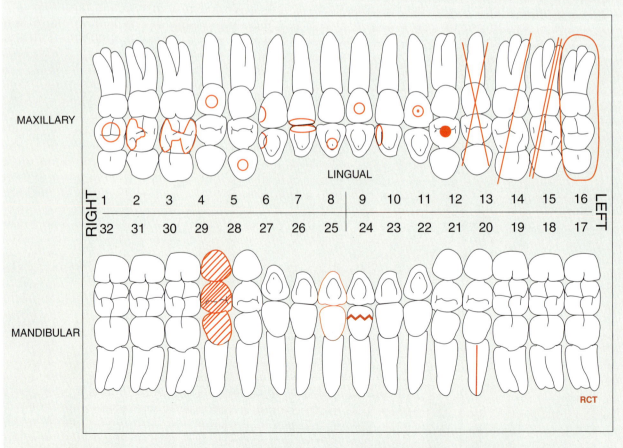

FIGURE 17-13A An anatomic diagram of permanent dentition with conditions noted by symbols.

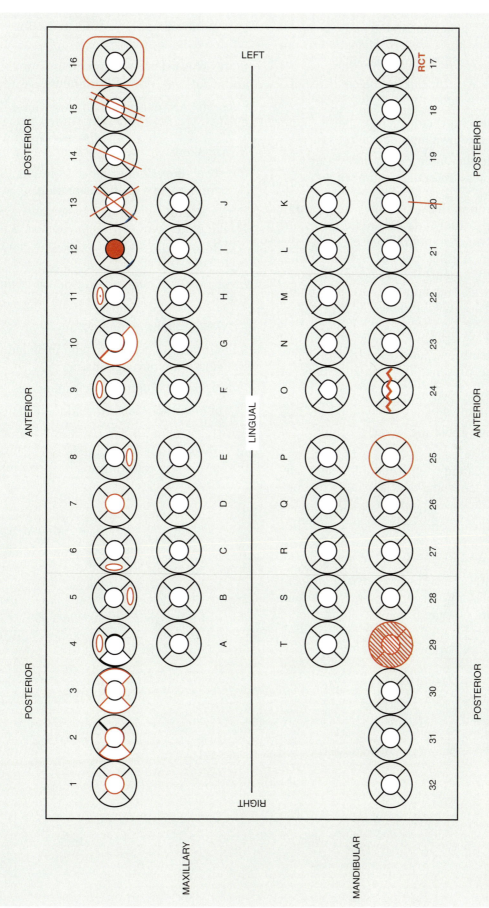

| Draw a heavy line in the pulp canal of a tooth with *completed endodontic* (root canal) *treatment* (number 20)

∧∧ Draw a saw line in the affected area of a *fractured tooth* (number 24)

○ Circle entire crown for a *porcelain* or *esthetic* crown (number 25)

⊖ Circle the entire crown and fill in with lines for a *gold crown* (number 29)

NOTE: Remember, these are only one group of symbols. Many other symbols are in use. Learn the symbols you are required to use.

In addition to using symbols in the anatomic diagram, all treatments or services rendered to the patient are also recorded on the dental chart. The following points should be noted:

◆ Only services performed are recorded in this section. Treatment performed by a previous dentist, the presence of carious lesions, or missing teeth are *not* noted here.

◆ Information must be recorded in ink.

◆ Information must be neat, correct, and complete.

◆ Abbreviations are used to denote teeth, surfaces, treatment completed, and base cements.

◆ Information recorded usually includes date, number of teeth, and services performed (for example, exam, X-rays, restorations, crowns, impressions).

◆ If treatment was not done to a *particular tooth* (for example, only full-mouth X-rays and exam were performed), the number column should be left blank.

Common abbreviations used for services rendered are as follows:

NOTE: This list varies from area to area. Use the abbreviations your doctor prefers.

AM or *Amal.:* Amalgam restoration, silver filling

Anes: Anesthetic

BWXR: Bitewing X-rays

Com or *Ant:* Composite restoration, anterior restoration, or esthetic restoration

Cr or *CR:* Crown; type may be included (*FGCr* for full gold crown, *PFMCr* for porcelain fused to metal crown, and *PJCr* for porcelain jacket crown)

Ex. or *Clin. Ex.:* Examination or clinical examination

Ext.: Extraction

FMXR: Full-mouth series of X-rays

Imp.: Impression; type may be included (*Alg* for Alginate, *RB* for rubber base)

Pro or *Prophy:* Prophylaxis, cleaning teeth

RCT or *Endo:* Root canal, or endodontic, treatment

Check your understanding of what treatment was completed in the following examples of charting by referring to the previous list of abbreviations.

2/10/—		Ex., Pro, FMXR
3/1/—	30	AM to MOD, Anes
5/6/—	8	Ant to MLa

STUDENT: *Read Procedure 17:5, Charting Conditions of the Teeth. Then go to the workbook and complete assignment sheet 17:5, Charting Conditions of the Teeth.*

PROCEDURE 17:5

Charting Conditions of the Teeth

Equipment and Supplies

Dental cards or charts; charting assignments; pen, pencil, or colored pencils

Procedure

1. Assemble equipment.
2. Wash hands.
3. Use the dental card or chart to complete Charting Assignment 1.
4. Use a pen, pencil, or colored pencils to complete all information. Your instructor will specify which to use.
5. Fill in the patient information area. Put name, address, and telephone number. You may place your name, address, and telephone number on the practice chart.
6. Chart each condition noted on the assignment. Check to be sure you are using the correct anatomic diagram. Refer to Information section 17:5 to determine correct symbols.
7. On the anatomic diagrams of the teeth and in the services rendered area, chart all treatment completed. Use appropriate abbreviations for treatment completed. Refer to Information section 17:5 to determine common abbreviations for services rendered.
8. Double-check all notations on the chart for accuracy. Make sure all notations are neat and legible.
9. When you have completed Charting Assignment 1, give it to your instructor. Your instructor will grade the assignment according to the criteria listed on the evaluation sheet.
10. Note all corrections on your graded assignment. Question your instructor if you do not understand the corrections. Then, complete Assignment 2 and give it to your instructor. Repeat the entire process for Assignment 3.
11. Replace all equipment.
12. Wash hands.

✔ **Final Checkpoint** Using the criteria listed on the evaluation sheet, your instructor will grade the three charting assignments.

INFORMATION

17:6 Operating and Maintaining Dental Equipment

Correct use and maintenance of dental equipment may be one of the responsibilities of the dental assistant. Remember always to check the manufacturer's recommendations prior to using or maintaining any equipment. This section provides some basic facts about the various pieces of dental equipment. Note that the equipment discussed is used for four-handed dentistry. The term *four-handed dentistry* describes the dentist and dental assistant working together as a team while seated on either side of a patient who is lying in a supine position in the dental chair.

 Infection control is essential while operating and maintaining any piece of dental equipment. During dental procedures, equipment can be contaminated with blood, saliva, and body fluids. Standard precautions, described in Unit 13:3, must be observed at all times. After any dental procedure, any contaminated equipment must be disinfected or sterilized before it is used on another patient. Gloves must be worn while cleaning any contaminated areas. In addition, protective barriers must be placed on many parts of the equipment prior to use (see figure 17-14). Special covers can be purchased for the dental chair, for handles and switches on the dental light, and to cover the X-ray tube head. Plastic wrap or aluminum foil can also be used to cover surfaces such as the

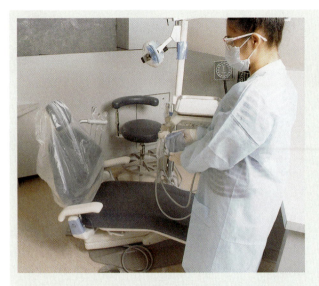

FIGURE 17-14 Protective barriers, such as plastic wrap or commercial covers, must be placed on many parts of the dental equipment prior to use.

handles and switches on the dental light. Clear plastic wrap can be used on the X-ray tube head. Plastic-backed paper or plastic wrap can be used on the headrest, armrest, and other parts of the dental chair, and to cover the tops of the dental carts. Protective barriers are put in place prior to a dental procedure. When the procedure is complete, the assistant must wear gloves to remove the contaminated barriers. The areas must then be disinfected. All surfaces are sprayed with a disinfectant and wiped to remove any particles or debris. The areas are then sprayed a second time, and the solution is left in place for the period of time recommended by the manufacturer, usually 10 minutes (see figure 17-15A and B). All surfaces are then wiped again, and the contaminated gloves removed. After the hands are washed thoroughly, clean protective barriers must be put in place before the next dental procedure. By observing standard precautions and proper disinfection/sterilization procedures, the transmission of disease by dental equipment can be prevented.

Dental light: Most dental lights are mounted on the ceiling of the dental unit. The light is used to illuminate the oral cavity, or mouth, while the doctor works. The light is positioned 30 to 50 inches from the oral cavity. Most lights contain dimmer switches to adjust the intensity of the light. Prior to a procedure, protective barriers such as plastic wrap, aluminum

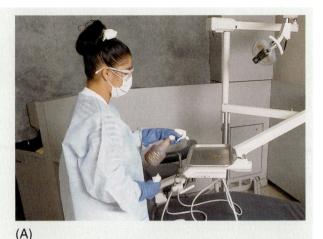

(A)

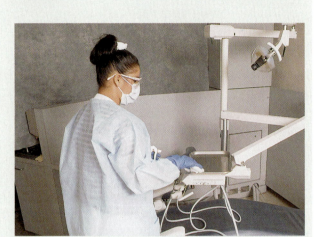

(B)

FIGURE 17-15 After a dental procedure is complete, contaminated surfaces are (A) sprayed with a disinfectant and then (B) wiped and sprayed a second time with a disinfectant.

foil, or commercial covers are placed on the handles and switches of the light. These must be removed and replaced with clean barriers after each patient. In addition, all parts that are touched must be disinfected after each patient. Most manufacturers recommend the use of a mild detergent and a soft cloth to clean the light shield. The soft cloth prevents the formation of scratches on the light shield. At least once a week, all moving parts on the light should be lubricated with a general, all-purpose oil.

Dental chair: The dental chair (see figure 17-16) is designed to position the patient comfortably while providing the doctor and the dental assistant with easy access to the oral cavity. Most chairs have thin, narrow headrests so the doctor and the dental assistant can position each patient. Most manufacturers recommend frequent, thorough cleaning with special upholstery cleaners or mild soap solutions.

Air compressor: The air compressor provides air pressure to operate the handpieces and air syringes on the dental units. It is usually located in a storage area or basement, and air lines are installed to carry the air pressure to the dental units. The compressor is usually set to provide 100 pounds of pressure. The pressure gauge on the air compressor should be checked frequently. If pressure goes above 120 pounds, the doctor should be notified. Careful maintenance of the air compressor is essential.

Manufacturer's recommendations must be read and followed. Some air compressors are sealed units and require no lubrication. In units that require oil to operate, the oil level should be checked frequently, usually weekly. Most air compressors have oil reservoirs covered by a cap or plug. Remove the cap or plug to check the oil level. If the oil level is low, the doctor should be notified immediately. In addition, water from the compression of moist air accumulates in the main tank of the compressor. This water should be drained daily. The pressure should be at zero before the drain faucet or valve is opened to release the accumulated water. Most air compressors contain special drain faucets or valves on their tanks.

Oral-evacuation system: This system, also called a *central vacuum system,* uses water to provide the dental units with a suction action. It aids in removing particles, debris, and liquids from the oral cavity. Its action is similar to that of a vacuum cleaner. The system consists of a main pump with vacuum lines to the dental unit and is usually located in a storage area or utility closet. Electrical control switches to turn the pump on and off are usually located on or near the dental unit. Wastes and liquids drawn into the system are discharged into a sanitary sewer line. A solids collector trap is located on the oral evacuation unit or in the dental unit. This trap catches large particles and must be cleaned daily. The particles should be emptied into a paper towel and placed in the correct waste container. The trap should be washed with a mild detergent, rinsed thoroughly, and dried. Some manufacturers recommend using a germicide spray or liquid daily to prevent the growth of organisms and the development of unpleasant odors. Again, it is important to read and follow

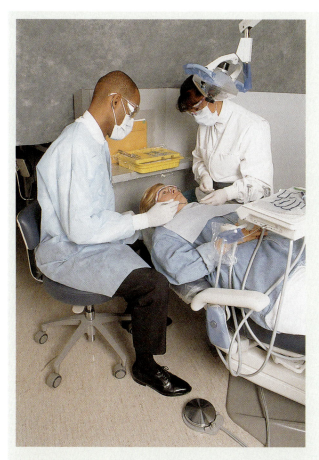

FIGURE 17-16 The dental chair allows the patient to be positioned comfortably while providing the doctor and the dental assistant easy access to the oral cavity.

themselves close to the patient. The chair reclines to place the patient in a supine, or lying down, position. Most chairs contain controls on both sides and/or on the floor so they can be operated by the doctor or the dental assistant. The control to raise and lower the height of the chair is usually located on the chair base and is operated by foot. The control to recline or raise the chair is usually located on the side of the chair and near the headrest; it is operated by hand. Many chairs also have foot controls to lock the chairs in position. This prevents movement of the chair while the patient is getting in or out of it. Cleaning the chair between patients is mandatory for infection control. The headrest, armrest, and any other contaminated area must be wiped clean with a disinfectant, then resprayed, left in place for the required time, and wiped again. The headrest is usually covered with a plastic disposable cover, which is discarded and replaced with a clean one after

the manufacturer's instructions on specific care and maintenance of the oral-evacuation system.

Assistant's cart: Carts for assistants vary from office to office, but most carts contain the same basic equipment (see figure 17-17). Drawers or areas for instrument storage are found on some carts. Other carts have sliding tops with storage areas under the tops. In addition, the following equipment is usually located on the cart:

◆ **Tri-flow**, or **air–water, syringe:** This is also called a *three-way syringe* (see figure 17-18). It provides air, water, or a combination of air and water for various dental procedures. After each use, the air-water syringe should be run for at least 30 seconds to flush out the unit. Plastic disposable tips are used in some offices. Other offices use a metal tip that is removable for sterilization in an autoclave. It must be changed and replaced with a sterile

tip after each patient. The syringe and tubing must be wiped with a disinfectant after each patient.

◆ **Saliva ejector:** This provides constant, low-volume suction to remove saliva from the mouth. Most ejectors contain screw-type knobs that are used to turn the suction on and off. The tips are disposable (see figure 17-19). They must be changed after each patient. The tip holder is covered with a protective barrier during use. The barrier is removed after each patient, the holder and tubing are disinfected and a new barrier is put in place. At least once daily, the inside of the tip holder must be cleaned thoroughly with a brush. A germicide solution or spray can also be used to clean the inside of the tip holder. The tubing can be sanitized by turning the saliva ejector on and drawing a disinfecting and deodorizing solution into it.

◆ **High-velocity oral evacuator:** This is also called a *high-volume* or *high-vacuum evacuator* (see figure 17-20). It is used to remove particles, debris, and large amounts of liquid from the oral cavity. Various tips can be used

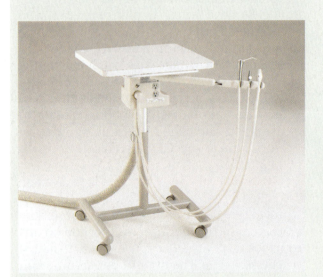

FIGURE 17-17 A sample assistant's cart. *(Courtesy of A-dec, Inc., Newberg, OR, USA)*

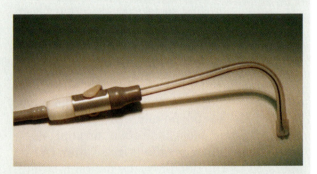

FIGURE 17-19 A saliva ejector with a disposable tip in position.

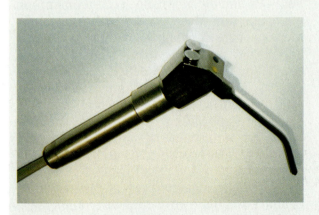

FIGURE 17-18 An air–water, or tri-flow, syringe.

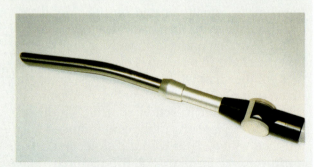

FIGURE 17-20 A high-velocity oral evacuator removes particles, debris, and large amounts of liquid from the oral cavity.

in the evacuator. Plastic disposable tips are discarded. Metal tips and nondisposable, heavy plastic tips are cleaned and sterilized in an autoclave. The evacuator holder is covered with a protective barrier during the procedure. The barrier is removed after each patient, the holder and tubing are disinfected, and a new barrier is put in place. A disinfecting and deodorizing solution can be suctioned into the tubing to sanitize the interior of the unit. Most units contain filter screens to trap larger particles drawn into the evacuator. These screens must be changed or emptied and cleaned daily. In addition, a slide valve is usually attached to the unit. This is used to turn the unit on and off with ease. The valve should be removed daily for thorough cleaning. It should be lubricated with a silicone-type lubricant to prevent sticking.

CAUTION: Because of possible contamination from saliva, blood, or body fluids, standard precautions must be observed while operating the saliva ejector and/or the oral-evacuation systems. Gloves, masks, and protective eyewear must be worn at all times. Gloves and masks are discarded after each patient. In addition, masks must be changed any time they become wet or are worn for longer than 30 minutes. Protective eyewear must be disinfected, rinsed to remove the disinfectant, and dried before being used for another patient.

◆ **Cuspidor:** This is a bowl or cup that can be used to allow the patient to expectorate (spit out) particles and water. Some cuspidors are installed on dental units; others are portable units. Most cuspidors are automatically flushed with running water. After each patient, the cuspidor must be cleaned and disinfected. Portable units are frequently sterilized.

Doctor's cart: Style and type of doctors' carts also vary from office to office (see figure 17-21). Many contain air-water syringes in addition to a variety of handpieces. Most carts also have **rheostats**, or foot controls used to operate the handpieces. Basic handpieces found on a doctor's cart are as follows:

◆ **Low-speed handpiece:** This is also called a *conventional-speed handpiece.* It is used for dental caries (decay) removal and fine-finishing work. The lower speed of this handpiece allows the doctor maximum control.

Different attachments can be used on this handpiece. Two of the most common are the contra angle and the prophylaxis angle.

(1) **Contra angle:** This is used for cutting and polishing during various dental procedures (see figure 17-22). Instruments called **burs** are inserted into the contra angle. Burs are rotary instruments used to cut, shape, finish, and polish teeth, restorations, and dental appliances. Burs have three parts: the *head* or cutting portion, the *shank* or part inserted in the handpiece, and the *neck,* which joins the head to the shank. Some contra angles use latch-type burs, which contain a groove at the shank. Others use friction-grip, or FG, burs, which have a smooth shank. Friction-grip burs are held

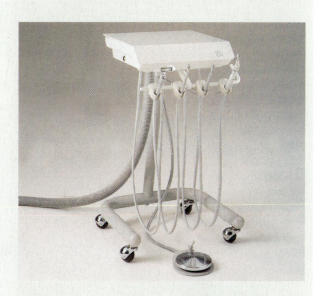

FIGURE 17-21 A sample doctor's cart. *(Courtesy of A-dec, Inc., Newberg, OR, USA)*

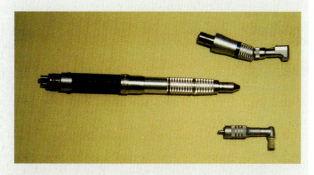

FIGURE 17-22 A low-speed handpiece with a contra-angle attachment (top) and a prophylaxis-angle attachment (bottom).

in place by a friction chuck in the head of the contra angle (see figure 17-23).

(2) **Prophylaxis angle:** This attachment holds polishing cups, disks, and brushes that are used to clean the teeth or to polish restorations (see figure 17-22).

◆ **High-speed handpiece:** This is sometimes called *an ultraspeed handpiece* (see figure 17-24). It is used to do most of the cutting and preparation of the tooth during dental procedures. This handpiece contains a friction-grip chuck; therefore, only friction-grip, or FG, burs can be used. A bur tool/wrench or a button release lever on the handpiece is used to insert and remove the burs. When this handpiece is used, intense heat is generated by the friction action of the bur. This requires the handpiece to be water-cooled with a fine mist of water when it is used. A high velocity oral evacuator or saliva ejector is used to suction the water that accumulates in the patient's mouth.

After each patient, handpieces must be scrubbed thoroughly to remove debris, rinsed, dried, and sterilized. If a handpiece cannot be sterilized according to manufacturer's instructions, it must be flushed with water, cleaned thoroughly, and disinfected with a chemical germicide. All tubings must be wiped with a disinfectant. The burs should be cleaned well with a bur brush and then sterilized. Manufacturer's recommendations must be followed when sterilizing burs because different types of materials used in burs require different methods of sterilization. Both low-speed and high-speed handpieces require lubrication. It is important to follow the manufacturer's instructions regarding the type of lubrication and method of application.

☣ **CAUTION:** Because of possible contamination from saliva, blood, or body fluids, standard precautions must be observed while handpieces are in use. Gloves, masks, and protective eyewear must be worn at all times. Gloves and masks are discarded after each patient. In addition, masks must be changed any time they become wet or are worn for longer than 30 minutes. Protective eyewear must be disinfected, rinsed to remove the disinfectant, and dried before being used for another patient.

The dental assistant's responsibilities for the use and maintenance of dental equipment vary. It is your responsibility to learn exactly what maintenance is expected. Read specific manufacturer's instructions for the equipment you handle.

STUDENT: *Go to the workbook and complete the assignment sheet for 17:6, Operating and Maintaining Dental Equipment. Then return and continue with the procedure.*

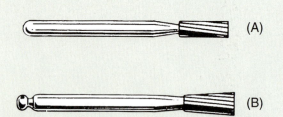

FIGURE 17-23 (A) A friction grip (FG) bur has a smooth shank. (B) A latch-type bur has a groove.

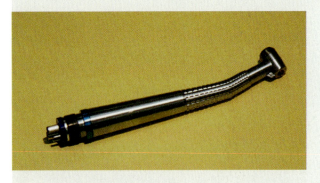

FIGURE 17-24 A high-speed handpiece is used to do most of the cutting and preparation of the tooth during dental procedures.

PROCEDURE 17:6

Operating and Maintaining Dental Equipment

Equipment and Supplies

Dental light, dental chair, air compressor, oral-evacuation system, assistant's cart with equipment, doctor's cart with equipment, latch-type bur, friction-grip (FG) bur, bur tool, lubricants, cleaning brush, soft cloths, disinfecting solution, protective barriers, disposable gloves

Procedure

1. Assemble equipment.
2. Wash hands. Put on gloves. If the equipment will be operated, a mask and protective eyewear must also be used.

   CAUTION: Dry hands thoroughly. You will be working with electrical equipment.
3. Practice operating the dental light:

   a. Locate the on–off switch. Turn the light on.

   b. Position the light so that it is above the dental chair. From a seated position, practice moving the light.

   NOTE: You will be sitting on a chair while assisting the doctor and will frequently reposition the light.

   c. Locate the dimmer switch. Turn the switch to adjust the intensity of the light.

   d. Practice applying protective barriers to the handles and/or switches of the light. Use commercial covers, plastic wrap, or aluminum foil to cover and protect the areas of the light that may be touched during a dental procedure.

   CAUTION: Remember to wear gloves while removing contaminated protective barriers. After the covers are discarded, wipe the areas with a disinfectant. Then respray the areas and leave the disinfectant in place for the amount of time recommended by the manufacturer. Then rewipe all areas. Remove the gloves, and wash your hands. Then, apply clean protective barriers.

   e. Use a mild detergent and a soft cloth to clean the shield of the light.

   f. Locate all moving parts on the light fixture. Use a general, all-purpose oil to lubricate these parts, if lubrication is needed.

4. Practice operating the dental chair:

   a. Locate the chair lock. It is usually on the base of the chair. Lock and unlock the chair.

   CAUTION: The chair must be locked when a patient is getting in or out of it.

   b. Locate the elevation control, which raises and lowers the height of the chair. It is usually a foot control on the base of the chair. Raise and lower the chair.

   CAUTION: The chair must be in its lowest position when a patient is getting in or out of the chair.

   NOTE: At least once each week, the chair should be elevated to its highest position and then lowered to its lowest position. This lubricates the hydraulic system.

   c. Locate the forward-backward control, which reclines or raises the back of the chair. It is usually located on the side of the chair and near the headrest or on a foot control. Put the chair in a reclining position. Raise the chair to a sitting position.

   NOTE: The chair must be in an upright position when a patient is getting in or out of it.

   d. Locate the reset button, found on many chairs. It is usually located near the forward-backward control. Operate the button. It automatically raises the back of the chair to an upright position and lowers the chair to its lowest position from the floor.

   e. Place a clean, disposable cover on the headrest of the chair. Some offices also drape the armrests and other parts of the chair with plastic-backed paper or plastic wrap. Wear gloves to remove contaminated protective barriers, wipe the areas with a disinfectant, respray the area and leave the solution in place for the correct amount of time, and then rewipe. Remove the gloves, and wash your hands before putting clean protective barriers in place.

   f. Use a mild detergent and a soft cloth to wash the chair. Rinse and dry the chair.

   NOTE: Some manufacturers recommend special upholstery cleaners.

5. Practice operating and maintaining the air compressor:
   a. Read the manufacturer's instructions.
   b. Turn the compressor on. Before inserting the plug into an electrical socket, always check the electrical cord for breaks or tears, and the plug for the third prong. Some air compressors operate immediately after being plugged into an electric wall socket; others have on-off switches.
   c. Watch the pressure gauge on the compressor. If the pressure goes above 120 pounds, turn the compressor off, and notify your doctor immediately.
      NOTE: Most air compressors are set to provide 100 pounds of pressure.
   d. Turn the compressor off.
   e. Locate the oil reservoir, if the air compressor has one. Remove the cap or plug. Check the level of oil. If the oil level is low, notify your doctor immediately.
      NOTE: Some air compressors are sealed units and require no lubrication.
   f. Locate the drain faucet or valve on the bottom of the main tank. Check the pressure gauge to be sure it is at zero. Open the faucet or valve to allow the water that has accumulated in the tank to drain.
      ⚠ CAUTION: Do *not* open this valve unless the pressure is at zero.
      NOTE: A pan can be placed under the tank to catch the draining water.

6. Practice operating and maintaining the oral-evacuation system:
   a. Read the manufacturer's instructions.
   b. Turn the system on. Some systems have on-off switches in the dental units; other, smaller systems have switches on the evacuation units themselves.
   c. Turn the system off.
   d. Locate the solids collector trap. Empty any particles in the trap onto a paper towel. Place the towel and particles in the proper waste container. Wash the trap with a mild detergent, rinse, and dry. Replace the trap on the system.
      ☣ CAUTION: Always wear gloves when emptying the solids collector trap.
      NOTE: Many manufacturers recommend using a germicide spray or solution in the trap to prevent the growth of organisms and the development of unpleasant odors.

NOTE: Systems vary, so follow individual instructions on removing and replacing the trap.

7. Practice operating the tri-flow, or air-water, syringe. It is located on the assistant's cart and/or the doctor's cart.
   a. Push the button to release air. It is usually marked with an *A* (for air).
   b. Direct the tip of the syringe into a cup or sink. Push the button to release water. It is usually marked with a *W* (for water).
   c. Continue to hold the tip over a cup or sink. Push both the air and water buttons. Water under air pressure will spray out of the syringe.
   d. Remove and replace the syringe tip. The tip must be sterilized after each patient. Some plastic tips are disposable and are discarded in an infectious-waste container.
   e. Use a disinfectant solution to clean the tip holder and tubing.

8. Practice operating the saliva ejector:
   a. Insert a tip into the ejector.
   b. Locate the screw knob or control and turn the ejector on.
      NOTE: The oral-evacuation system must be on before the ejector will work.
   c. Turn the ejector off.
   d. Remove the tip. The tips are disposable and are placed in an infectious-waste can after being used on a patient.
   e. Use a brush to clean inside the ejector tip holder. Use a disinfectant solution to clean the tip holder and tubing.
   f. Turn the saliva ejector on. Place the end into a disinfecting and deodorizing solution to draw the solution into the ejector unit to sanitize it.

9. Practice operating the high-velocity oral evacuator:
   a. Insert a tip into the evacuator. Tips can be plastic or metal.
   b. Locate the slide valve. Move the valve to turn the evacuator on. Move it in the opposite direction to turn the evacuator off.
   c. Remove the slide valve from the evacuator. Scrub it with a brush. Rinse it thoroughly. Dry the valve. Place a silicone lubricant on the valve. Replace the valve in the evacuator unit.
      NOTE: The lubricant prevents the slide valve from sticking.

d. Locate the filter screen on the evacuator unit. It is usually located under the cart or on the tubing. Empty the particles in the screen onto a paper towel. Place the towel and particles in an infectious-waste can. Scrub the screen gently with a brush. Rinse the screen and replace it in the evacuator unit. Some screens are disposable. These are discarded in an infectious-waste container and replaced with a new screen.

NOTE: Follow specific instructions on removing and replacing the screen.

e. Remove the tip. Place a disposable tip in an infectious-waste bag. Scrub a metal tip, using a brush to clean the inside. Rinse the tip. Sterilize it correctly.

f. Use a disinfectant solution to clean the tip holder and tubing.

g. Turn the evacuator on. Place the tip into a disinfecting and deodorizing solution to draw the solution into the tubing to sanitize it.

10. Practice maintaining the low-speed handpiece. It is located on the doctor's cart.

a. Read the manufacturer's instructions.

b. Insert a contra-angle head or attachment on the handpiece. Tighten the handpiece to hold the head in place.

NOTE: The handpiece should be kept open when an attachment or head is not in place. If the handpiece is closed while empty, the units that hold the heads in place are destroyed.

c. Check the contra angle to determine which type of bur is required. If a small latch is present on the back, latch-type burs are required. Obtain a bur that has a groove at the end and insert it in the contra angle. Close the latch to hold the bur in place. If no latch is present on the contra angle, friction-grip, or FG, burs are required. Obtain an FG bur. Use a bur tool to push the bur into position on the contra angle.

NOTE: Some new handpieces have levers that are pushed to insert and remove burs. Bur tools are not used with these handpieces.

d. Remove the bur from the contra angle by releasing the latch, pushing the bur out with the bur tool, or using the lever on the handpiece, if a lever is present.

e. Remove the contra angle from the handpiece by loosening the top of the handpiece. Use a low-speed lubricant to lubricate the contra angle. Spray the lubricant into the hole at the end, where the contra angle attaches to the handpiece.

f. Insert and remove a prophylaxis angle on the handpiece. Use a low-speed lubricant to moisten the hole at the end of the prophylaxis angle, where the angle attaches to the handpiece.

g. Remove the handpiece from the unit. Scrub it thoroughly to remove debris, rinse and dry it, and then sterilize it. Use a disinfectant to clean the outside of the tubing. Follow manufacturer's instructions to sterilize the burs and the contra angle or prophylaxis angle.

h. Follow manufacturer's instructions to lubricate the handpiece. Most handpieces unclip in the center. Spray low-speed lubricant into the lower end of the top section; the tubing looks like two *V*s in this area. Then, unscrew the handpiece from the base. The lower end of this section has four holes. Spray low-speed lubricant into the second largest hole only. Reassemble the handpiece. Push the rheostat, or foot control, on the cart to operate the handpiece and to remove excess oil. Turn it off and use a paper towel to wipe the handpiece dry. Then, clean the handpiece again with a disinfectant.

NOTE: Most manufacturers recommend daily lubrication.

11. Practice maintaining the high-speed handpiece:

a. Use a bur tool to insert and remove a friction-grip bur on the handpiece.

NOTE: Only friction-grip burs are used in this handpiece.

NOTE: Some new handpieces have levers that are pushed to insert and remove burs. Bur tools are not used with these handpieces.

b. Remove the handpiece from the unit. Scrub it thoroughly to remove debris, rinse and dry it, and then sterilize it. Use a disinfectant to clean the outside of the tubing.

c. Follow manufacturer's instructions to lubricate the handpiece. Most handpieces are unscrewed at the base. Spray high-speed lubricant into the large hole only. Reassemble the handpiece. Operate the handpiece to remove excess lubricant. Wipe the handpiece dry with a paper towel and then clean the handpiece again with a disinfectant.

12. Clean and replace all equipment.
13. Wash hands.

Final Checkpoint Using the criteria listed on the evaluation sheet, your instructor will grade your performance.

INFORMATION
17:7 Identifying Dental Instruments and Preparing Dental Trays

Assisting with a variety of dental procedures may be one of the responsibilities of the dental assistant. Correct preparation includes setting up trays of instruments and supplies used in specific procedures. Therefore, a dental assistant must be familiar with dental instruments.

Various methods are used for setting up trays for specific dental procedures. In some settings, the trays are set up immediately before use. The dental assistant prepares the room, seats the patient, and then sets up a tray with supplies and sterilized instruments. The instruments and supplies are determined by the procedure that will be performed on the patient. In other settings, preset sterilized trays are used. Tray contents are determined by the doctor. Trays are set up for oral examinations, amalgam restorations, composite restorations, surgical extractions, and other similar procedures. During an oral examination, the patient's teeth are cleaned and examined. Dental radiographs or X rays may be taken. Amalgam and composite are the two main restorative materials used to repair carious lesions or tooth decay. The doctor removes the damaged tooth structure and creates an opening called a cavity preparation. Amalgam, the silver restorative material, or composite, an esthetic restorative material is then placed in the cavity preparation. A surgical extraction is removal of a damaged tooth. After determining the procedure that is to be performed, the dental assistant seats the patient and positions the correct tray containing the sterilized instruments. Additional instruments or supplies can be added if needed. In many settings, preset trays are color coded (for example, red for amalgam, blue for composite) and are sterilized as a unit.

Items on the trays should be organized and placed in proper sequence. Instruments are usually arranged in the order of use. After an instrument is used, it is returned to the same place on the tray, in case it is needed again. This makes it easier for the dental assistant to locate instruments and increases overall efficiency (see figure 17-25).

The main parts of a dental hand instrument are:

◆ *Blade or nib or point:* A blade is the cutting portion of an instrument; a nib is the blunt, serrated, or smooth working end of a condensing (packing) instrument; a point is the sharp end used to explore and detect.

◆ *Shank:* The portion that connects the shaft, or handle, to the blade, nib, or point.

◆ *Shaft:* The handle of the instrument, usually hexagonal (six sides) to provide a better grip.

Instruments used vary from office to office. However, some instruments are standard and are used in all dental offices. The following briefly describes some of the main instruments.

◆ *Mouth mirror:* Used to view areas of the oral cavity, reflect light on dark surfaces, and retract the lips for better visibility. It is used in

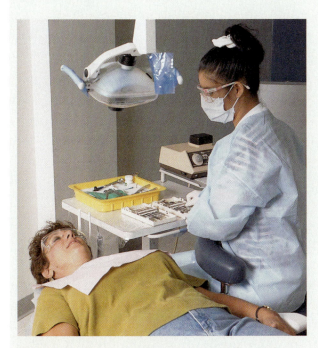

FIGURE 17-25 Instruments are arranged in order of use to make it easier for the dental assistant to locate them.

every basic tray set-up. Mirrors are available in various sizes and with plain or magnifying ends (see figure 17-26).

◆ *Explorer:* Used to examine the teeth, detect carious lesions, and note other oral conditions. Explorers are available in many shapes and sizes. They may be single or double ended (see figure 17-27).

◆ *Cotton pliers:* Used to carry objects such as cotton pellets or rolls to and from the mouth. Some lock, some do not. They are also called *operating pliers* or *college pliers* (see figure 17-28).

◆ *Scalers:* Used to remove calculus (tartar) and debris from the teeth and subgingival pockets. Scalers are used mainly for prophylactic (cleaning) or periodontal (gum, or gingiva) treatments. They are available in many shapes (see figure 17-29).

◆ *Periodontal probes:* Used to measure the depth of the gingival sulcus (the space between the tooth and the free gingiva). It has a round, tapered blade with a blunt tip that is marked in millimeters (mm) (see figure 17-30).

◆ *Excavators:* Used mainly for removal of caries and refinement of the internal opening in a cavity preparation (see figure 17-31).

(1) *Spoon:* Used to remove soft decay from a cavity. It is a cutting instrument with a small curve or scoop at the working end.

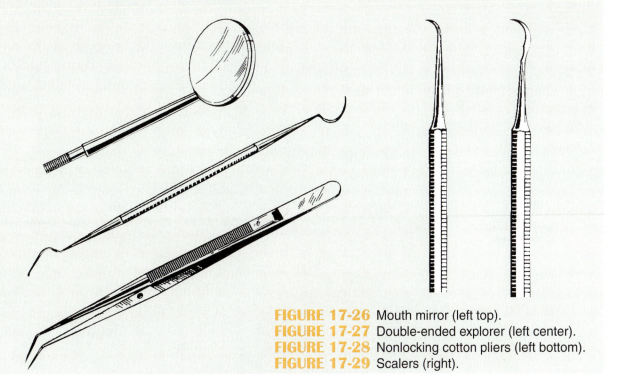

FIGURE 17-26 Mouth mirror (left top).
FIGURE 17-27 Double-ended explorer (left center).
FIGURE 17-28 Nonlocking cotton pliers (left bottom).
FIGURE 17-29 Scalers (right).

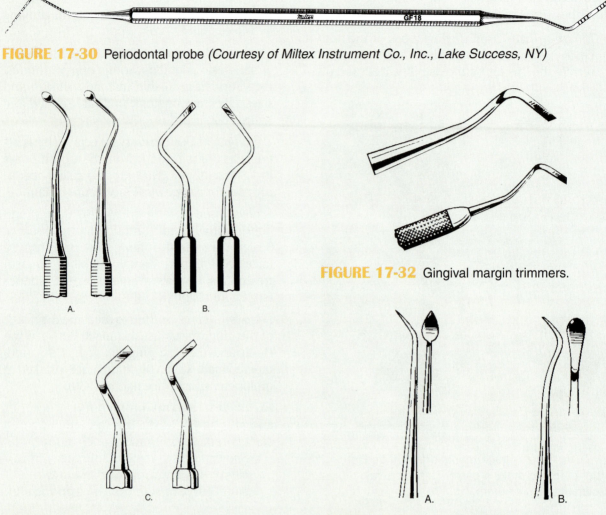

FIGURE 17-30 Periodontal probe *(Courtesy of Miltex Instrument Co., Inc., Lake Success, NY)*

FIGURE 17-32 Gingival margin trimmers.

FIGURE 17-31 Excavators: (A) spoons, (B) hoes, and (C) hatchets.

FIGURE 17-33 Carvers: (A) cleoid and (B) discoid.

(2) *Hoe:* Used primarily on anterior teeth to remove caries, smooth and shape a cavity preparation, and/or form line angles. A hoe has one or more angles to the shaft, with the last length forming the blade. It is also used in scraping, planing, and direct-thrust cutting.

(3) *Hatchet:* Used to refine internal line angles, smooth and shape the sides of a cavity preparation, and remove hard-type caries.

◆ *Chisels:* Used for cutting and shaping enamel. Instruments in this group include:

(1) *Enamel hatchet:* Similar to other hatchets but the blade is larger, heavier, and beveled on only one side.

(2) *Gingival margin trimmer:* Special chisel for placing bevels on gingival enamel margins of proximoocclusal cavity preparations. It has the chisel blade placed at an angle to the shaft, not straight across like a hatchet. In addition, the blade is curved, not flat like a hatchet (see figure 17-32).

◆ *Cleoid-discoid carver:* A double-ended instrument. It is also available as a cleoid or discoid single-ended instrument. The cleoid has a claw-shaped cutting end, and the cutting edge surrounds the entire end. The discoid is disc shaped and also has the cutting edge around the blade. It is used as a carver for amalgam, but can also be used as an excavator (see figure 17-33).

◆ *Plastic filling instrument (PFI):* Used to shape and condense restorative material that is still malleable (capable of being shaped or

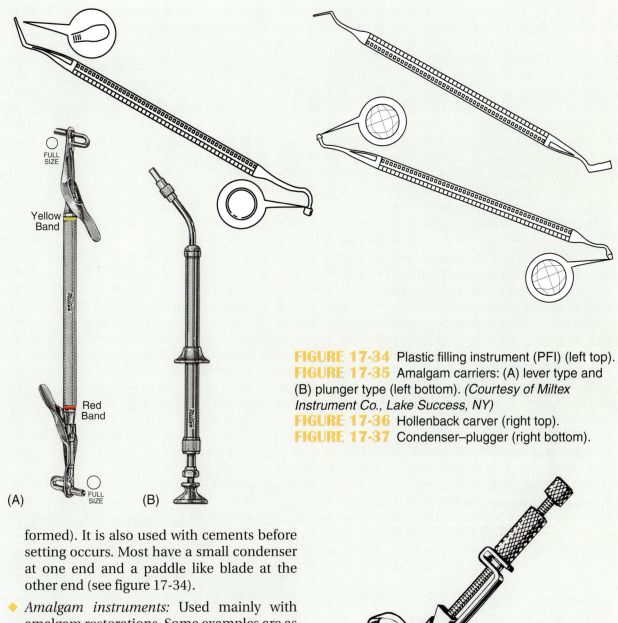

FULL
SIZE

Yellow
Band

Red
Band

FULL
SIZE

(A)   (B)

FIGURE 17-38 Matrix retainer and band.

formed). It is also used with cements before setting occurs. Most have a small condenser at one end and a paddle like blade at the other end (see figure 17-34).

♦ *Amalgam instruments:* Used mainly with amalgam restorations. Some examples are as follows:

(1) *Amalgam carrier:* Used to carry small masses of freshly mixed amalgam to the cavity preparation (see figure 17-35).

(2) *Amalgam carvers:* Used to carve or shape freshly placed amalgam and restore the tooth to natural anatomy. One example is the Hollenback carver (see figure 17-36).

(3) *Condenser–plugger:* Used for condensing and packing amalgam into the prepared cavity. The ends may be serrated or plain (see figure 17-37).

(4) *Matrix retainer* and *matrix band:* The matrix retainer is used to hold the matrix band in place (see figure 17-38). A matrix band is a short strip of steel or other metal that is not affected by mercury. It is used to form a wall around a cavity so amalgam can be packed into place.

NOTE: Plastic matrix strips are used with composite restorative material.

♦ *Burnisher:* Contains working points in the shapes of balls or "beavertails." Burnishers are used primarily to burnish (adapt) the margins of gold restorations to a better fit.

Burnishers are also used to polish other metals (see figure 17-39).

♦ *Plastic composite instruments:* A set of plastic instruments used with composite restorations. Because metal instruments can discolor composite, doctors use plastic instruments.

♦ *Surgical instruments:* Instruments used depend on the type of oral surgery being performed. The main instruments used in extraction procedures are listed. Other specific instruments and supplies such as chisels, hemostats, needle holders, and suture materials might also be used.

(1) *Surgical forceps:* Also called *extracting forceps.* These are used for extracting teeth. There are many different types, one for each type of tooth to be extracted (see figure 17-40).

(2) *Periosteal elevators:* Used for lifting the mucous membrane and tissue covering the bone. It is a double-ended instrument with a blade at each end (see figure 17-41).

(3) *Root elevator:* Used to loosen the tooth out of its socket prior to being removed with forceps. There are various types, shapes, and sizes (see figure 17-42).

(4) *Root-tip pick:* Used to remove small tips from a socket such as a root tip or piece of bone. There are straight and contra-angled versions (see figure 17-43).

(5) *Rongeur forceps:* Used to trim or cut bone tissue. The tips of the forcep may

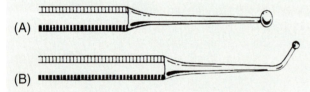

(A)

(B)

FIGURE 17-39 (A) Oval burnisher; (B) Ball burnisher.

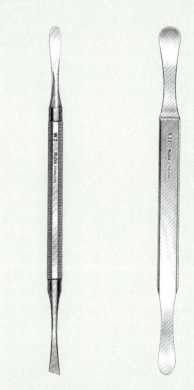

FIGURE 17-41 Periosteal elevators. *(Courtesy of Miltex Instrument Co., Lake Success, NY)*

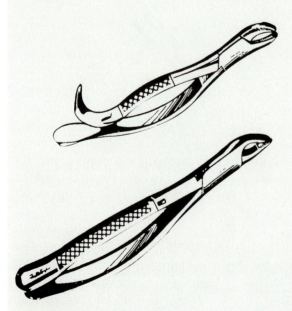

FIGURE 17-40 Surgical forceps.

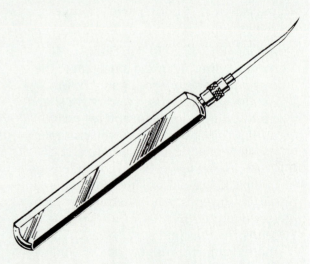

FIGURE 17-42 Root elevator.

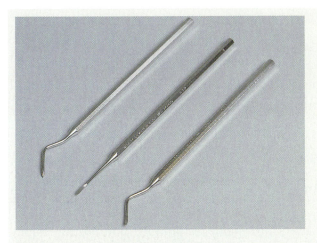

FIGURE 17-43 Root-tip picks.

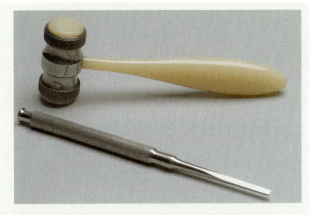

FIGURE 17-45 Bone or surgical chisel and mallet.

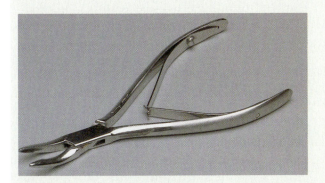

FIGURE 17-44 Rongeur forceps.

be round or square with a tough sharp blade that extends around both sides and the end of the tips (see figure 17-44).

(6) *Lancet:* Used to lance and incise tissue. A lancet is similar to a scalpel and blade.

(7) *Bone or surgical chisels:* Used for cutting bone structure in oral surgery. Some are used by hand, others require the use of a surgical mallet (see figure 17-45).

When setting up trays for various procedures, it is important to remember to place only items that are usually needed. Setting the tray with instruments and supplies that are needed only occasionally can decrease efficiency and crowd all the items. Items usually kept in the cart include the drape and clips, dental bases and cements, restorative materials, extra cotton products or dressings, and instruments used for specific problems or procedures. Some instruments and supplies are placed on almost all trays. Examples include the mouth mirror,

cotton pliers, explorer, cotton pellets, cotton rolls, and gauze sponges.

Trays can be set up for a variety of dental procedures. Four examples of tray set-ups include:

♦ *Prophylactic, or general examination, tray:* This type of tray is used for basic examination and cleaning of the teeth. Supplies and instruments placed on the tray include scalers; a periodontal probe for an adult; prophylactic cups, paste, and brushes; and fluoride-treatment supplies.

♦ *Amalgam restoration tray:* This type of tray is used for an amalgam restoration procedure. Instruments placed on the tray include amalgam carriers, condenser-pluggers, and carvers.

♦ *Composite, or esthetic, restoration tray:* This type of tray is used for the placement of a composite restoration. Special composite instruments such as a fine brush and plastic instruments are placed on this tray.

♦ *Surgical extraction tray:* This type of tray is used for extraction, or removal, of teeth. Instruments and supplies vary depending on the type of extraction. In most cases, however, surgical instruments such as extracting forceps, root elevators, root-tip picks, periosteal elevators, Rongeur forceps, lancets, bone chisels, and a needle holder with suture materials are placed on the tray.

STUDENT: *Go to the workbook and complete the assignment sheet for 17:7, Identifying Dental Instruments and Preparing Dental Trays. Then return and continue with the procedure.*

PROCEDURE 17:7

Identifying Dental Instruments and Preparing Dental Trays

Equipment and Supplies

Patient records, X-rays, variety of instruments, cotton pellets and rolls, tray for supplies and instruments, cements, mixing pads, drape and clips, carts with handpieces, assorted supplies and equipment for specific procedures, personal protective equipment (PPE) including gloves, gown, mask, and eye shield

Procedure

1. Assemble equipment.
2. Wash hands. Put on required personal protective equipment including gloves, a gown, mask, and eye shield.
3. Read the Information sections on dental instruments, amalgam, composite, cements, and anesthesia.
4. Place the dental tray in a convenient location. Make sure the tray is clean.
5. Examine each of the following instruments until you are able to identify them and state why they are used. Refer to the information on Identifying Dental Instruments to complete this task.
   a. Mouth mirror
   b. Explorers
   c. Cotton pliers
   d. Scalers
   e. Periodontal probe
   f. Spoons
   g. Hoes
   h. Hatchet
   i. Enamel hatchet
   j. Gingival margin trimmer
   k. Cleoid-discoid carver
   l. Plastic filling instrument
   m. Amalgam carrier
   n. Amalgam carvers
   o. Condenser–plugger
   p. Matrix retainer and band
   q. Burnisher
   r. Plastic composite instruments
   s. Surgical forceps
   t. Periosteal elevator
   u. Root elevator
   v. Root-tip pick
   w. Rongeur forcep
   x. Lancet
   y. Bone or surgical chisel and mallet
6. Set up trays for the following procedures: prophylactic cleaning and oral examination, amalgam restoration, composite restoration, and surgical extraction. Perform the following steps for each procedure and tray.
   a. Lay out the general patient equipment, including records, X-rays, drape, clips, and other similar items.
   b. Review the parts of the carts. Think about which handpieces will be used. Make sure all are in good working condition.
   c. Set the tray with the main instruments to be used. Place these instruments in the order of use. Refer to references and Information sections to be sure you include all required instruments. Make sure that the basic instruments (mirror, explorer, cotton pliers) are on the tray.
   d. Have the correct dental cements or bases available for any procedure that might involve the use of these materials. Do not forget to have mixing pads and instruments ready for use.
   e. Think about additional equipment that might be used. Add these to the tray. Such items might include prophy paste, fluoride trays, matrix bands, wooden wedges, finishing strips, and articulation paper.
   f. Add additional equipment that might be necessary. Examples might include the amalgamator and special handpieces.
   g. Add needed supplies. These might include cotton pellets, rolls, gauze, and other similar items.
7. Review all of the equipment and supplies you have prepared for each of the four procedures. Read the steps of each procedure and make sure that you have the equipment and materials the doctor will require for each.
8. If your doctor uses a rubber dam (a device to keep the oral cavity dry during a procedure) or special types of anesthesia, be sure that you have prepared these materials.

9. Remember that equipment, supplies, and instruments used vary from doctor to doctor. It is the dental assistant's responsibility to know the doctor's preferences and to prepare these things for use.
10. Replace all equipment.
11. Remove personal protective equipment. Wash hands.

Practice *Go to the workbook and use the evaluation sheet for 17:7, Identifying Dental Instruments and Preparing Dental Trays, to practice this procedure. When you feel you have mastered this skill, sign the sheet and give it to your instructor for further action.*

 Final Checkpoint Using the criteria listed on the evaluation sheet, your instructor will grade your performance.

INFORMATION

17:8 Positioning a Patient in the Dental Chair

Positioning a patient in the dental chair is one of the responsibilities of a dental assistant. Correct positioning of a patient in the dental chair allows the doctor to complete dental procedures efficiently. In four-handed dentistry, the patient is placed in a supine, or lying-down, position.

Before a patient gets in or out of the chair, the chair must be locked in the upright position. The patient could be injured if the chair moves. Always check the chair to be sure it is in a locked position before seating a patient or before assisting a patient out of the chair.

The patient's head rests on the upper, narrow headrest of the chair. Positioning the patient's head in this narrow section of the chair allows the doctor and the dental assistant closer access to the oral cavity. Short adults and children must be positioned in the chair starting with correct placement of the head first.

The chair must be elevated from the floor to the height that will allow both the doctor to be seated comfortably near the chair and the patient's head to be above the doctor's lap.

After a patient has been seated in the chair, it is best to recline the chair slowly. Lowering a patient to a supine position quickly can cause dizziness, discomfort, and fear in some patients. It is best to lower the chair part way, pause to allow the patient time to adjust to the change in position, and then finish lowering the chair. The chair should recline until the patient is lying almost flat. An imaginary line from the patient's chin to the patient's ankles should be parallel to the floor. The legs and head should be at the same level.

C Explain all chair movements to the patient. Inform the patient before elevating or lowering the chair, before reclining the back of the chair, and before returning the patient to a sitting position. Unexpected movements can frighten the patient.

Before any dental procedure is performed, a protective drape is placed over the patient's chest. This protects the patient's clothing during the procedure. Most drapes have a paper side and a plastic side. The plastic side is placed against the patient's clothing; the paper side is placed facing up. In this way, the paper absorbs moisture and the plastic keeps moisture from soaking through to the patient's clothing.

After the patient is in the correct position, the light should be positioned 30 to 50 inches from the oral cavity, or mouth. Care must be taken to ensure that the light illuminates the mouth but does not shine in the patient's eyes.

C When positioning a patient in the dental chair, it is important to show a friendly and pleasant attitude toward the patient. Make the patient feel welcome and allow the patient to talk about his or her interests. Knowledge about the patient allows the dental assistant to ask questions such as, "How was your vacation?" or "How did your basketball team do in the last game?" Displaying an interest in patients makes them more at ease and less apprehensive. When a procedure is complete, a comment such as, "It was good to see you again, Mrs. Brown" or, "I hope you enjoy your first year at college" is much better than, "You're done for today."

STUDENT: *Go to the workbook and complete the assignment sheet for 17:8, Positioning a Patient in the Dental Chair. Then return and continue with the procedure.*

PROCEDURE 17:8

Positioning a Patient in the Dental Chair

Equipment and Supplies

Dental chair and light, headrest cover, drape, alligator clips, protective barriers for dental light, gloves, mask, protective eyewear, disinfectant solution, gauze sponges

Procedure

1. Wash hands.
2. Assemble equipment. Use a disposable plastic cover to cover the headrest. Use protective barriers, such as commercial covers, plastic wrap, or aluminum foil to cover the handles and/or switches of the dental light. Use plastic cloths to cover the tops of dental carts.
3. Introduce yourself. Identify the patient. Explain the procedure.
   C
   NOTE: Patients are often apprehensive.
4. Lock the chair to prevent movement of the chair.
   ⚠ CAUTION: Double-check the lock to prevent injury to the patient.
5. Assist the patient into the chair.
6. Adjust the headrest for comfort and correct position.
7. Use the alligator clips to secure the drape around the patient's neck and shoulders (see figure 17-46). Place the plastic side of the drape against the patient's clothing.
   NOTE: The drape can also be applied later, when the patient is in a reclining position.
   NOTE: In some offices, the patient's health history is updated at this time.
8. Use the elevation control to raise the chair to the height desired by the doctor.
   NOTE: Tell the patient you are raising the chair before doing so.

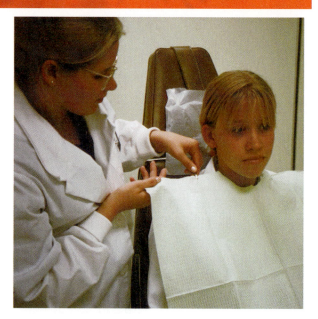

FIGURE 17-46 A protective drape is used to protect the patient's clothing during dental procedures.

9. Use the backward control to place the patient in the correct reclining position. Pause after reclining the patient halfway to allow the patient to adjust to the change in position.
   NOTE: Inform the patient. Observe the patient closely for signs of respiratory distress.
10. Position the light 30 to 50 inches from the oral cavity. Leave the light off until the doctor is ready to work on the patient.
    NOTE: Make sure the light does *not* shine in the patient's eyes.
11. Put on gloves, a mask, and protective eyewear before assisting the doctor with any dental procedure that may result in the splashing of saliva, blood, or body fluids.

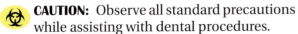

CAUTION: Observe all standard precautions while assisting with dental procedures.

12. When the doctor is done, lock the chair. Check to be sure it does not move. Position the dental light out of the patient's way.
13. Warn the patient *not* to get out of the chair until it has stopped moving.
14. Use the reset button to lower the chair and to return it to an upright position. Remove the drape and place it in an infectious-waste container.
15. Help the patient out of the chair.
16. After the patient has left the area, remove the protective barriers from the light, dental chair, and carts. Put the barriers in an infectious-waste container. Use a disinfectant solution to wipe all contaminated areas. Then respray all areas, leave the disinfectant in place for the required amount of time, and rewipe the areas.

17. Clean and prepare all instruments and handpieces for sterilization. Replace all equipment.
18. Remove and discard gloves. Wash hands thoroughly.

Practice *Go to the workbook and use the evaluation sheet for 17:8, Positioning a Patient in the Dental Chair, to practice this procedure. When you feel you have mastered this skill, sign the sheet and give it to your instructor for further action.*

✔ **Final Checkpoint** Using the criteria listed on the evaluation sheet, your instructor will grade your performance.

17:9 INFORMATION Demonstrating Brushing and Flossing Techniques

Using correct brushing and flossing techniques is essential to prevent dental disease. Teaching the patient the correct methods to use is part of the responsibility of a dental assistant.

Correct brushing and flossing are important parts of prophylactic (preventive) care. Purposes include:

◆ Prevention of decay, or **carious lesions (caries)**.

◆ Removal of plaque. **Plaque** is a thin, tenacious, filmlike deposit that adheres to the teeth and can lead to decay. It contains microorganisms and a protein substance.

◆ Prevention of **halitosis** (bad breath).

C The importance of proper brushing and flossing techniques must be stressed to the patient. Demonstrations should be given to all patients. Talk slowly and clearly. Repeat and stress important points.

The brushing technique taught will depend on the preference of the doctor. A common technique is the Bass method. The brush is placed at a 45° angle to the gumline and then a vibrating motion is used.

Five surfaces on each tooth must be cleaned:

◆ *Chewing, or biting, surface*

◆ *Facial surface:* the tooth side that faces the inside of the lips and cheeks; facial surfaces are seen from the front, as in a smile

◆ *Lingual surface:* the tooth side nearest the tongue

◆ *Side, or interproximal, surfaces:* the surfaces located between the teeth; there are two on each tooth; floss is used to clean these surfaces because a brush cannot get between the teeth, and the bristles do not provide enough coverage

Toothbrushes vary in size, shape, and texture of the bristles. A soft-bristled brush is usually recommended. It will not injure the gum, or gingival tissue. The head of the brush should be the correct size and fit easily into the mouth. Brushes should be discarded when the bristles are frayed or worn. Many kinds of electric toothbrushes are also available and are effective in cleaning the teeth if used correctly. They can be very beneficial for people with limited function of the hands and arms, such as people with arthritis.

Toothpastes or dentrifices are used to clean the teeth and provide a pleasant taste. Many doctors recommend toothpaste with fluoride. The American Dental Association supports the use of fluoride as an aid in preventing decay. Toothpastes with tartar control help prevent the hard deposits that accumulate on the teeth. Toothpastes with whitening agents help remove stains from teeth. The type of toothpaste recom-

mended to the patient depends on the needs of the patient and the doctor's preference.

Dental floss is used to remove plaque and bacteria from the side surfaces of the teeth. Floss is available in waxed and unwaxed types. The type suggested to the patient depends on the doctor's preference. Both types are effective if used correctly.

STUDENT: *Go the workbook and complete the assignment sheet for 17:9, Demonstrating Brushing and Flossing Techniques. Then return and continue with the procedures.*

PROCEDURE 17:9A

Demonstrating Brushing Technique

Equipment and Supplies

Soft-textured toothbrush, demonstration model of teeth

Procedure

1. Assemble equipment.
2. Wash hands.
3. Introduce yourself. Identify the patient.
4. **C** Explain the importance of correctly brushing the teeth. Stress that proper brushing helps prevent decay and removes plaque, a soft deposit leading to decay. Also stress that teeth should be brushed immediately after eating.
5. Suggest the use of a soft-textured brush to prevent gum damage.
   NOTE: If the doctor has recommended another type of toothbrush, follow the doctor's preference.
6. Use a toothbrush and demonstration model of teeth to show the patient how to brush the teeth.
7. Tell the patient to begin brushing in one area of the mouth and then to systematically brush each tooth. Suggest starting on the facial surfaces of the right, rear teeth.
8. Place the brush at a 45° angle to the gumline (see figure 17-47A).

9. Rotate the brush slightly and gently push the bristles between the teeth.
10. Use a very short, back-and-forth, vibrating movement to clean the teeth.
11. Move the brush to the next group of teeth. Repeat steps 8 to 10. Continue until the facial surfaces of all the teeth are clean.
12. Repeat steps 8 to 10 on the lingual, or tongue, surfaces of the teeth. To brush the lingual surfaces of the front, or anterior, teeth, place the brush in a vertical position (see figure 17-47B).
13. Brush the biting surfaces of all teeth. Place the brush on the surfaces. Use a very short, vibrating motion (see figure 17-47C). Move the brush to the next area. Repeat until all biting surfaces are clean.
14. Stress to the patient that the areas between the teeth must be cleaned with floss.
15. Ask whether the patient has any questions. Make sure the patient understands the technique to use.
    C **NOTE:** Asking the patient to demonstrate the technique is a good method of determining whether the main points have been understood.
16. Clean and replace all equipment.
17. Wash hands.

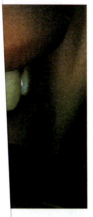

a 45° angle

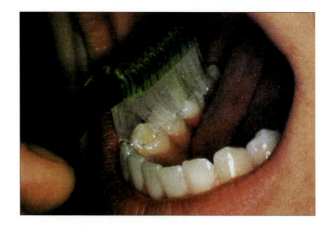

FIGURE 17-47C Use a short, vibrating motion to clean the biting surfaces of the teeth.

> ***Practice*** *Go to the workbook and use the evaluation sheet for 17:9A, Demonstrating Brushing Technique, to practice this procedure. When you feel you have mastered this skill, sign the sheet and give it to your instructor for further action.*

✔ **Final Checkpoint**   Using the criteria listed on the evaluation sheet, your instructor will grade your performance.

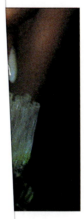

position to clean the lingual, or tongue, surfaces of the anterior teeth.

PROCEDURE 17:9B

Demonstrating Flossing Techniques

Equipment and Supplies

Dental floss, demonstration model of teeth

Procedure

1. Assemble equipment.
2. Wash hands.
3. Introduce yourself. Identify the patient.
4. Explain the importance of flossing. Stress that flossing is the way to remove food and plaque from between the teeth. Mention that this is an area where decay often begins because brushing is not enough.
5. Use dental floss and a demonstration model of the teeth to show the patient how to floss the teeth.
6. Remove 12 to 18 inches of floss from the spool. **NOTE:** Floss is waxed or unwaxed. The type recommended depends on the doctor's preference.
7. Wrap the floss around the middle fingers of both hands. This anchors the floss. As floss is used, unroll new floss from the middle finger

of one hand and wrap used floss around the middle finger of the opposite hand.

8. To clean the upper (maxillary) teeth, wrap the floss around the index finger of one hand and the thumb of the other hand or the two thumbs. To clean the lower (mandibular) teeth, use the index fingers of both hands.
   NOTE: Floss still remains anchored on middle fingers.

9. Keep the fingers and thumb approximately 1 to 2 inches apart. This is the length of floss to be used.

10. Gently insert the floss between the teeth. Do not snap the floss into the gums.
    CAUTION: Snapping the floss into the gums can injure the gum tissue.

11. Gently slide the floss into the space between the gum and tooth. Stop when you feel resistance. Curve the floss into a C-shape around the side of the tooth (see figure 17-48).

12. Hold the floss tightly against the tooth and move the floss away from the gum by scraping the floss up and down against the side of the tooth.
    CAUTION: A side-to-side or front-to-back motion could cut the gums.

13. Repeat steps 10 to 12 until both sides of every tooth in the mouth have been flossed. Move the floss on the fingers as it becomes soiled. Use fresh floss at all times.

14. Warn the patient that some bleeding and soreness may occur the first few times teeth are flossed. If bleeding or soreness continues, flossing should be stopped and the doctor notified.

15. Make sure the patient understands the procedure.
    C **NOTE:** Asking the patient to demonstrate the technique is a good way to determine whether the main points have been understood.

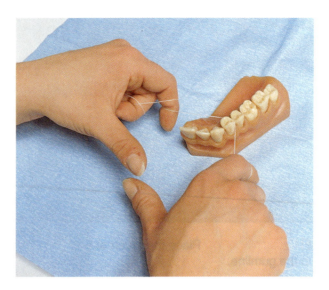

FIGURE 17-48 After curving the floss into a C-shape around the side of the tooth, use an up-and-down motion to clean the side.

16. Clean and replace all equipment.
17. Wash hands.

Practice *Go to the workbook and use the evaluation sheet for 17:9B, Demonstrating Flossing Technique, to practice this procedure. When you feel you have mastered this skill, sign the sheet and give it to your instructor for further action.*

 Final Checkpoint Using the criteria listed on the evaluation sheet, your instructor will grade your performance.

17:10 INFORMATION Taking Impressions and Pouring Models

The dental assistant may prepare a wide variety of impression and model materials for the doctor. This section provides basic facts about the purposes and types of some of these materials.

An **impression** is a negative reproduction of a tooth, several teeth, or the dental arch (see figure 17-49). It is taken to form a model of the area for restorative treatment that will take place outside of the mouth. Common materials used to take impressions are alginate, rubber base, and polysiloxane or polyvinylsiloxane.

A **model**, also called a *cast,* is a positive reproduction of the arches or teeth that is created from the negative impression (see figure 17-50). Common materials used for models are plaster

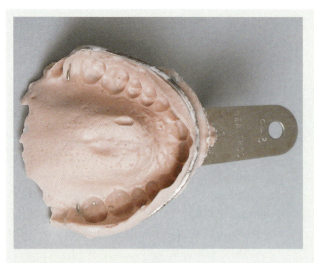

FIGURE 17-49 An impression is a negative reproduction of a tooth, several teeth, or a dental arch.

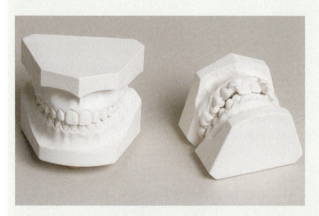

FIGURE 17-50 A model is a positive reproduction of the teeth that is used for the construction of dentures, partials, or other prosthetics.

or stone. A model serves as the basis for construction of dentures, partials, or other prosthetics for the mouth.

Alginate is an *irreversible,* hydrocolloid impression material. It cannot be returned from a gel to its original state. Advantages include:

◆ it is simple and economical to use

◆ setting time can be controlled by the water temperature

◆ it has adequate strength for an accurate impression

◆ it yields an adequate basic reproduction of detail

◆ it is easily removed from tissues and instruments during cleaning

Disadvantages include:

◆ it is not good for final impressions of cavity preparations or small areas requiring fine detail, such as final impressions for crowns or bridges

◆ it changes in dimension by shrinking as it loses water content and must be poured immediately for an accurate duplication

◆ it tears or breaks easily when set

Alginate powder is supplied as a fast set (type I) or regular set (type II), flavored or unflavored, and/or regular or heavy-bodied material. Some alginates have an antimicrobial agent added to prevent the growth of microorganisms in the impression. Some are powder-free to reduce inhalation of the dry material. Proper measuring techniques are essential to obtain the correct set. Always follow the manufacturer's directions. Alginate material should be stored in a cool, dry place to avoid deterioration. To prevent moisture contamination, the lid should be replaced immediately after the material is used.

Rubber base or polysulfide is an elastomeric impression material that is elastic and rubbery in nature. Three types are produced. One is a light-bodied material for use in a syringe. The second is a heavy-bodied material for use in trays. The third is a regular- or medium-bodied material for use in both syringes and trays. Frequently, two types are used together. A syringe is used to place light-bodied material into the area of the impression. Then, a custom tray filled with heavy-bodied material is placed into the mouth and over the light-bodied material to complete the impression. Rubber-base materials can be used for any dental procedure that requires an impression. They are particularly good for use in cavity preparations that require fine detail, such as an impression taken prior to the construction of a crown. Rubber-base materials are not subject to dimension changes as much as are alginates. However, rubber-base materials should be poured promptly if possible, preferably within 1 to 2 hours after they are made. Disadvantages of rubber-base or polysulfide materials are the sulfur-like odor, taste, long setting-time (approximately 10 minutes), and the fact that it causes permanent stains on cloth and other materials.

Polysiloxane or polyvinylsiloxane impression materials are silicone materials. They are available in light-bodied, regular- (medium-) bodied, and heavy-bodied versions. They are supplied in two tubes, which are placed in a special mixing

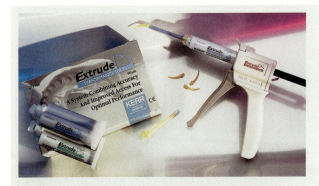

FIGURE 17-51 An extruder gun automatically mixes the cartridges of catalyst and base of polysiloxane or polyvinylsiloxane impression materials. *(Courtesy of Kerr Corporation)*

device called an *extruder,* or *automix gun* (see figure 17-51). A disposable mixing tip is placed on the end of this gun, and as the pastes are expelled into the mixing tip, the catalyst and base are automatically mixed. Syringe-tipped mixing tubes can also be used, and the material can be placed directly on the area of the impression as it is expelled from the gun. This provides for easy cleanup after use. Polysiloxane or polyvinylsiloxane materials are not affected by fluids in the oral cavity. This allows these materials to spread evenly over the impression area, creating a highly accurate impression. This impression retains its shape and size for a long period of time. Another important advantage is that these materials are odor-free and have a pleasant taste. One disadvantage is that latex gloves may inhibit the setting of these materials; thus, vinyl gloves must be worn while taking impressions. A second disadvantage is that they are more expensive than rubber-base or polysulfide impression materials.

There are two main gypsum products used to form models: plaster and stone. **Plaster** is the weaker of the two. It is used mainly where strength is not a critical factor, such as for study models and preliminary models. It is also a less expensive material. **Stone** is a more refined gypsum product than is plaster. It produces a stronger, more regular and uniform model. However, it is more expensive than plaster. Stone is used for making diagnostic models or casts, and for any work requiring a high degree of strength and accuracy.

Basic principles for the use of plaster and stone include:

◆ Both products must be stored in a tightly closed container and in a cool, dry area.

Moisture contamination of gypsum products leads to defective models or casts.

◆ Correct amounts of water and powder must be used. Usually, 45 to 50 cubic centimeters of water is used for 100 grams of plaster; 30 cubic centimeters of water is used for 100 grams of stone. If an insufficient amount of water is used, the mixture will be too thick and crumbly to flow into the impression. If too much water is used, the model will be weak, set slowly, and develop air bubbles that destroy the effectiveness of the model.

◆ Impressions should be clean and dry before the models or casts are poured. Drying by blotting is preferred. Drying with an air blast can cause dehydration or shrinkage of the impression material, especially of alginate.

◆ The use of cold water when mixing plaster provides the greatest amount of working time. When you are learning how to prepare the plaster mix, use the coldest water available to provide more time.

◆ Air bubbles in the mix can ruin a model. Stir and spatulate the mix in such a way that as little air as possible enters the mix. To remove as many air bubbles as possible, always place the bowl on a vibrator before pouring.

Because contact with saliva and/or blood is very possible while taking impressions and pouring models, the Centers for Disease Control and Prevention (CDC) has established guidelines for infection control. Gloves, a gown, face mask, and eye protection must be worn at all times. Hands must be washed immediately after removing gloves at the end of the procedure. All completed impressions must be rinsed gently for at least 30 seconds with room-temperature tap water to remove any mouth debris. The impression must then be disinfected with a solution such as 10-percent sodium hypochlorite (household bleach), iodophor, glutaraldehyde, or phenylphenol. All mixing containers, spatulas, and impression trays must be disinfected or sterilized prior to being used for another patient. Standard precautions must be followed at all times while taking impressions and pouring models.

STUDENT: *Go to the workbook and complete the assignment sheet for 17:10, Taking Impressions and Pouring Models. Then return and continue with the procedures.*

PROCEDURE 17:10A

Preparing Alginate

Equipment and Supplies

Alginate powder; large, rubber mixing bowl; spatula; powder scoop and water-measuring cup provided by the manufacturer; room-temperature water, denture; impression trays; disinfectant solution or spray; disposable gloves; gown; face mask; eye protection

Procedure

1. Assemble equipment. Select an impression tray to fit the denture.
   NOTE: If an impression is being made of the patient's mouth, the doctor usually measures and selects the impression tray to be used.

2. Wash hands. Put on disposable gloves, a gown, face mask, and eye protection.

   CAUTION: The denture or the mouth will contain saliva and even blood at times. Standard precautions must be observed while taking an impression of the mouth.

3. Make sure all equipment, especially the bowl and spatula, are clean.

4. Measure out the correct amount of room-temperature (70°F or 21°C) water.
   NOTE: Follow the manufacturer's directions for the correct amount of water. Usually, one measure of water is used with one scoop or envelope of powder.

5. Place the water in the mixing bowl.

6. Fluff the powder in the container by rolling the container from side to side several times. Open the lid cautiously to avoid inhaling the powder, which can be hazardous if inhaled. Wearing a face mask reduces this risk.

7. Measure out the correct amount of powder. Fill the scoop with powder. Tap the top of the scoop lightly with the spatula to fill air voids. With the spatula, level the powder at the top of the scoop (see figure 17-52A).
   NOTE: Follow the manufacturer's instructions for the correct amount of powder. A basic guide is as follows:
   three scoops: large upper (maxillary) impression
   two scoops: medium maxillary or any mandibular impression
   one scoop: partial impression

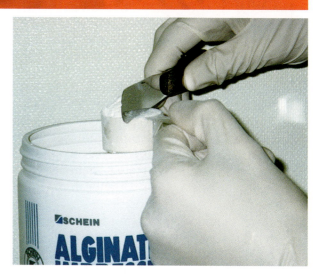

FIGURE 17-52A Use the spatula to level the scoop of alginate powder.

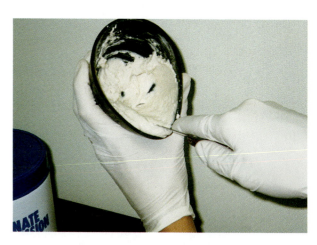

FIGURE 17-52B Use a stropping action to press the mix against the side of the bowl.

8. Add the measured powder to the water in the bowl.

9. Use a circular motion to press the spatula against the side of the bowl and to mix all of the powder with the water.

10. Use a stropping (beating or pressing) action with the spatula to press the mix against the side of the bowl (see figure 17-52B). Rotate the bowl as you mix. This makes the mix creamy and smooth and removes air bubbles.

11. Mixing should be completed within 1 minute for regular-set and 30 to 45 seconds for fast-set alginate.

12. Fill the impression tray with the mix. Smooth the surface with a wet finger or wet spatula. Remove any excess material from the back of the tray.

> **CAUTION:** Regular-set alginate mix sets in 2 to 4 minutes, and fast-set alginate sets in 1 to 2 minutes, so work quickly.

> **NOTE:** Make sure the impression tray is the correct size.

> **NOTE:** The impression tray can be sprayed with a special lubricant spray before being filled. This makes it easier to remove the alginate at the end of the procedure (see figure 17-52C). Some impression trays require the use of an adhesive. Follow manufacturer's instructions provided with the impression trays.

13. Hand the filled impression tray to the doctor. Pass the tray handle first.

> **NOTE:** In some states, a dental assistant may be allowed to take a preliminary impression of a patient's dentition. Check the legal requirements for your state.

14. To take an impression from a denture, soak the denture in water first.

> **NOTE:** This allows the denture to more readily come out of the alginate.

> **CAUTION:** Gloves should be worn while handling any denture to avoid contamination from saliva or fluids from the mouth.

15. Shake the excess water from the denture. Place it in position on the alginate. Press the anterior teeth of the denture into place. Then press the back of the denture into position.

> **CAUTION:** Do not press too hard or the denture will go completely through the alginate.

16. Use steady pressure with the index finger and the middle finger to hold the denture in place (see figure 17-52D). Hold for at least 1 minute.

17. After the alginate has set completely (usually in 2 to 4 minutes), check it for smoothness. If it is smooth and does *not* stick to your fingers, it is ready.

18. Gently remove the denture from the alginate.

> **NOTE:** A very slight side-to-side motion often releases the denture.

19. Use room-temperature tap water to gently rinse the impression for at least 30 seconds. Spray the impression with a disinfecting solution to prevent contamination from saliva, blood, or mouth fluids that may be present on the impression.

20. Pour the model as quickly as possible, preferably within 20 minutes. If you are unable to immediately pour the model, wrap the alginate impression in a wet paper towel. Place the towel-wrapped impression in a plastic bag or covered air-tight container to maintain 100 percent humidity. Soaking an impression in a bowl of water is not recommended. Label the bag or container with the patient's name and date.

> **CAUTION:** The alginate will shrink almost immediately if left to air dry, and this shrinkage leads to an inaccurate model.

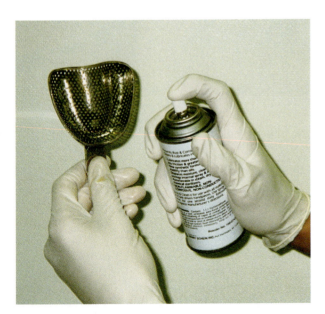

FIGURE 17-52C Before using the impression tray, spray it with lubricant to make it easier to remove the alginate material from the tray when the procedure is complete.

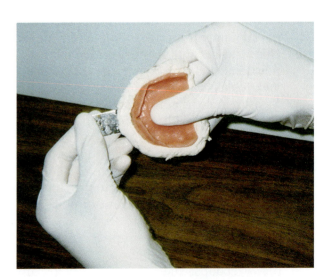

FIGURE 17-52D Use steady pressure to hold the denture in the alginate.

21. Clean the bowl and spatula. Place all excess alginate in a trash container. *Never* pour alginate into the sink because it will clog the drain. The bowl and spatula must be disinfected or sterilized. Some offices use disposable bowls and spatulas. These are discarded in an infectious-waste container.

22. To clean the impression tray, remove the alginate. Discard all alginate in a trash container. Use pipe cleaners to clean out the holes in the tray. Scrub the tray with a brush and place it in the ultrasonic unit for cleaning. Sterilize the tray according to manufacturer's instructions prior to using it on another patient.

23. Replace all equipment.

24. Remove all personal protective equipment. Wash hands thoroughly.

Practice *Go to the workbook and use the evaluation sheet for 17:10A, Preparing Alginate, to practice this procedure. When you feel you have mastered this skill, sign the sheet and give it to your instructor for further action.*

 Final Checkpoint Using the criteria listed on the evaluation sheet, your instructor will grade your performance.

PROCEDURE 17:10B

Preparing Rubber Base (Polysulfide)

Equipment and Supplies

Tubes of accelerator and base rubber-base materials, paper mixing pad (coated), metal spatula, impression tray, adhesive, syringe, tip, paper to make funnel, cleaning brush, disinfecting solution or spray, disposable gloves, gown, face mask, eye protection

Procedure

1. Assemble equipment.

2. Wash hands. Put on disposable gloves, a gown, face mask, and eye protection.

   CAUTION: The mouth will contain saliva and even blood at times. Standard precautions must be observed while taking an impression of the mouth.

3. Prepare tray and/or syringe, depending on which will be used. Use heavy-bodied rubber-base material for a tray, light-bodied rubber-base material for a syringe.

   a. To prepare the impression tray, apply adhesive over the entire surface of the tray. Allow the adhesive to dry.

   b. To prepare the syringe, put a plastic tip on the end of the syringe (see figure 17-53A). Make a paper funnel to load the syringe: fold the paper in half; then, fold a bias fold with one end ¼ inch and one end 1 inch (see figure 17-53B).

4. Mark the mixing pad with the length of strip desired (see figure 17-53C). The amount is determined by the impression to be taken.

5. Dispense an even line of accelerator material.
   NOTE: Strip of accelerator must be smooth and even for correct proportions.

6. Dispense a strip of base material that is the same length as the accelerator.
   NOTE: Strip will be wider in diameter, but it is the same weight.

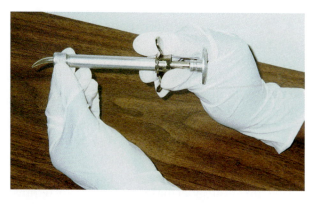

FIGURE 17-53A Put a plastic tip on the syringe before mixing the rubber base material.

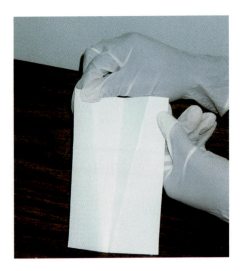

FIGURE 17-53B Fold a sheet of mixing-pad paper to make a paper funnel to load the rubber-base syringe.

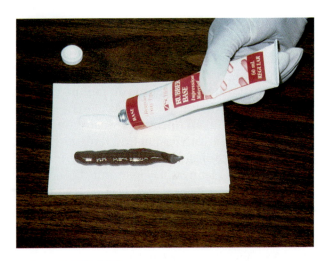

FIGURE 17-53D Keep the materials separate while dispensing equal strips of the accelerator and base.

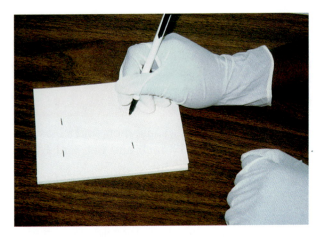

FIGURE 17-53C Mark the mixing pad with the length of strip desired.

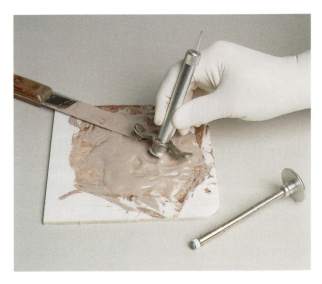

FIGURE 17-53E The syringe can also be filled by pushing the end of the barrel into the rubber base material.

NOTE: Keep the materials separate (see figure 17-53D).

7. Use accelerator material to coat both sides of the metal spatula.

8. Mix the accelerator and the base. Use smooth strokes and broad sweeps. Mix well until no strips or streaks of color are evident.
   NOTE: Mixing should be complete in 45 to 60 seconds.

9. Place the rubber-base mix in the prepared impression tray. If a syringe is to be used, first place the material in the paper funnel. Then, roll the funnel and squeeze the material into the syringe. Another way to fill the syringe with the rubber-base material is to remove the plastic tip and plunger. Use a repetitive stroking motion to push the end of the barrel

into the material so that the material fills the inside of the syringe (see figure 17-53E). Replace the plastic tip and plunger so the syringe is ready to use.

10. If a syringe is used, pass this to the doctor first. The doctor uses the syringe to place the impression material directly in the area of the impression. The filled impression tray is then passed to the doctor for insertion into the patient's mouth.

 CAUTION: In many states, a dental assistant is *not* permitted to take a rubber-base impression of a patient's dentition. The assistant's role is to prepare the material for the doctor.

NOTE: Work quickly before the impression sets. Curing time is usually 5 to 10 minutes.

11. After the impression tray is removed from the mouth, rinse it in room-temperature tap water for 30 seconds. Spray it with a disinfectant or soak it in a disinfecting solution.

☣ **CAUTION:** The impression may be contaminated with saliva, blood, and mouth fluids. Observe standard precautions.

12. A model can now be poured. It is best to pour a model as quickly as possible for the greatest degree of accuracy.

13. To clean the syringe, first squeeze out excess material. Then, soak the syringe in warm water for approximately 15 minutes. Soak the impression tray after the impression has been removed.

NOTE: Soaking allows the material to set and makes it easy to peel off the tray, spatula, or syringe.

14. Use a brush to remove any material left on the spatula or tray or in the syringe. Clean the syringe, spatula, and tray in an ultrasonic unit. Follow manufacturer's instructions to sterilize the syringe, spatula, and tray.

NOTE: The syringe tips are disposable and discarded after use. Disposable impression trays are sometimes used for rubber-base impressions.

15. Discard all excess rubber-base material and the mixing sheet in an infectious-waste container. Replace all equipment. Close caps tightly on both tubes of material.

16. Remove all personal protective equipment. Wash hands thoroughly.

Practice *Go to the workbook and use the evaluation sheet for 17:10B, Preparing Rubber Base (Polysulfide), to practice this procedure. When you feel you have mastered this skill, sign the sheet and give it to your instructor for further action.*

✔ **Final Checkpoint** Using the criteria listed on the evaluation sheet, your instructor will grade your performance.

PROCEDURE 17:10C
Pouring a Plaster Model

Equipment and Supplies

Alginate or rubber-base impression, mixing bowl, hard spatula, plaster, metric graduate and scale, vibrator, glass slab or tile square, water, personal protective equipment (gloves, gown, face mask, and eye protection)

Procedure

1. Assemble equipment.
2. Wash hands. Put on all personal protective equipment (gloves, gown, face mask, and eye protection).

☣ **CAUTION:** Observe standard precautions while working with an impression.

3. Prepare an alginate impression or use a rubber-base impression a doctor has prepared. Blot excess disinfecting solution from the impression.

4. Measure the water. Use 45 to 50 cubic centimeters. The water should be room temperature (70°F or 21°C) or cooler.

NOTE: Colder water allows more working time for beginners.

5. Pour the water into the bowl.
6. Measure the plaster powder. Use 100 grams.
7. Sift the powder into the bowl, allowing it to drop to the bottom of the bowl (see figure17-54A). Allow the powder to absorb all of the water.
8. With the spatula, use a wiping and scraping motion to mix the powder and water.

 CAUTION: Avoid using a whipping motion because this creates air bubbles.

9. Scrape the mix against the side of the bowl to remove any lumps.
10. Place the bowl on the vibrator platform. Hold the bowl in place to remove air bubbles from the mix (see figure 17-54B).

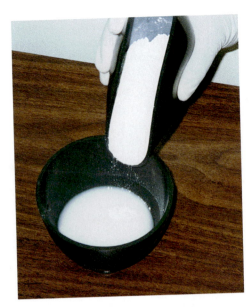

FIGURE 17-54A Allow the plaster to drop to the bottom of the bowl and absorb the water.

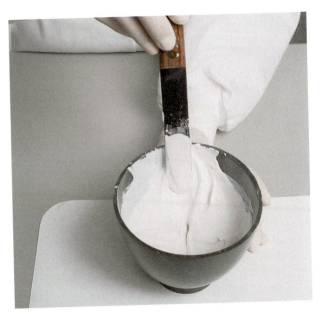

FIGURE 17-54C The consistency of the plaster mix is correct if the mix does not run back together after being cut with a spatula.

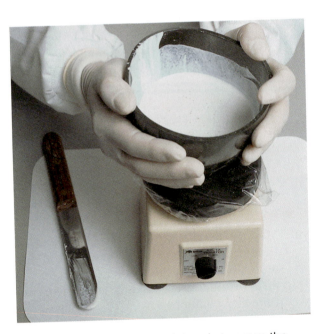

FIGURE 17-54B Use both hands to grasp the bowl of mix firmly on the vibrator platform to remove air bubbles from the plaster.

11. Test the mix by holding the bowl upside down. The mixture should not flow out of the bowl. Cut through the mixture with the spatula. The mix is the correct consistency if it does not run back together (see figure 17-54C).

12. Place a plastic bag over the vibrator. Place the impression on the covered vibrator platform.
    NOTE: The plastic cover protects the vibrator.

13. Use the spatula to place a small amount of plaster on the back, or heel, of the impression (see figure 17-54D). Vibrate the tray lightly so the mix flows into the impression, filling the "teeth."
    CAUTION: Use only a small amount of plaster at a time to ensure even filling and prevent air bubble formation.

14. Repeat step 13. Add the mix to the same area each time. Try to keep the flow as even as possible. Repeat until the impression is completely filled.

15. Form the base of the model by placing the remaining mix on a glass slab or tile. The mix should be approximately 1 inch thick.

16. Very carefully invert the entire impression and place it on the base. Do not push down on the model.
    NOTE: Use a damp paper towel to create an arch on the mandibular model to keep the plaster mix out of this area.
    NOTE: In some dental settings, the remaining mix is simply placed on top of the model and built up to the correct thickness. In other settings, a base former is used. It is filled with plaster to form the base; the impression is then inverted on top.

17. Smooth the mix on the sides of the impression and base so the two areas join. The model should be kept as level as possible.

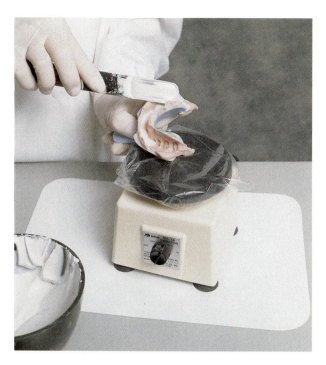

FIGURE 17-54D While holding the impression tray on the vibrator platform, place a small amount of plaster mix on the back, or heel, of the impression.

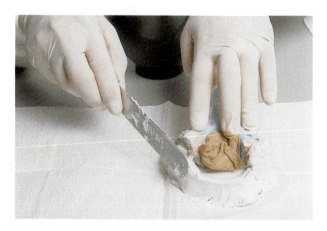

FIGURE 17-54E Remove excess amounts of plaster from the sides of the model to create a smooth edge.

18. Remove excess amounts of mix from the sides and top of the model. Keep the model basically smooth, (see figure 17-54E).
19. Put the model in a safe place. Allow it to set. Do not disturb it for at least 1 hour.
    NOTE: Setting time varies from 1 to 3 hours.
    NOTE: The model will get hot. As heat is produced, the water evaporates, and the model sets (becomes solid). This is called an *exothermic* reaction.

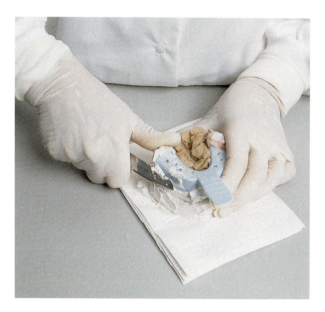

FIGURE 17-54F Use a laboratory knife or spatula to remove dry plaster from the impression tray before lifting the tray off the model.

20. When the model is completely dry, remove it from the impression tray. Use a laboratory knife or spatula to gently scrape away any plaster material on the impression tray (see figure 17-54F). Use firm but steady pressure to lift the tray away from the model. Do *not* pull because this may break the model or separate it from the base. Avoid breaking the teeth.
21. Clean and replace all equipment. Place all waste plaster in a trash container. Use large amounts of water to flush the sink. Scrub the bowls and other equipment thoroughly. If the impression tray is not disposable, it must be cleaned and sterilized prior to being used for another patient. Clean the counter top immediately.
22. Remove all personal protective equipment. Wash hands.

Practice *Go to the workbook and use the evaluation sheet for 17:10C, Pouring a Plaster Model, to practice this procedure. When you feel you have mastered this skill, sign the sheet and give it to your instructor for further action.*

 Final Checkpoint Using the criteria listed on the evaluation sheet, your instructor will grade your performance.

PROCEDURE 17:10D

Pouring a Stone Model

Equipment and Supplies

Alginate or rubber-base impression, mixing bowl, hard spatula, stone powder, metric graduate and scale, vibrator, glass slab or tile, water, personal protective equipment (gloves, gown, face mask, and eye protection)

Procedure

1. Assemble equipment.
2. Wash hands. Put on personal protective equipment.

   CAUTION: Observe standard precautions while working with an impression.
3. Prepare an alginate impression or use a rubber-base impression a doctor has prepared. Blot excess disinfecting solution from the impression.
4. Measure the water. Use 30 cubic centimeters (following manufacturer's instructions). The water should be room temperature (70°F or 21°C) or slightly cooler.
5. Pour the water into the bowl.
6. Measure the stone. Use 100 grams or follow the manufacturer's instructions (see figure 17-55).
7. Sift the powder into the bowl. Allow the powder to absorb the water.

   NOTE: Place the bowl on the vibrator platform for 5 to 10 seconds to aid mixing.
8. Use a wiping and scraping motion to mix the stone powder and water until a uniform, creamy mixture is obtained.

   CAUTION: Avoid using a whipping motion, because this causes air bubbles.
9. Place the bowl on the vibrator platform. Hold the bowl firmly in place to remove air bubbles from the mix.
10. To pour the model, follow steps 11 to 20 of Procedure 17:10C, Pouring a Plaster Model.
11. Clean and replace all equipment. Place excess stone in a trash container. Do *not* wash stone material down the sink drain because it will clog the plumbing. Scrub the bowl, spatula, and countertop thoroughly. Disinfect or sterilize the bowl and spatula. If they are disposable, place them in an infectious-waste container.
12. Remove personal protective equipment. Wash hands.

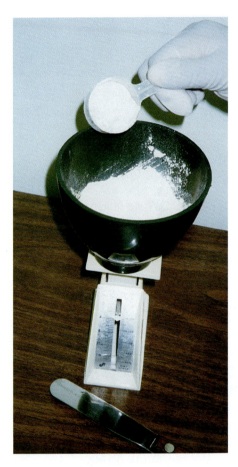

FIGURE 17-55 A small scale is used to weigh the correct amount of stone material, usually 100 grams.

Practice *Go to the workbook and use the evaluation sheet for 17:10D, Pouring a Stone Model, to practice this procedure. When you feel you have mastered this skill, sign the sheet and give it to your instructor for further action.*

 Final Checkpoint Using the criteria listed on the evaluation sheet, your instructor will grade your performance.

PROCEDURE 17:10E

Trimming a Model

Equipment and Supplies

Prepared model, model trimmer, bowl of water, safety glasses

Procedure

1. Assemble equipment.
2. Wash hands.
3. Soak the model in a bowl of water for 5 minutes.
   NOTE: A wet model is easier to trim and less likely to break.
4. Put on safety glasses.
5. Turn on the water supply to the model trimmer. Turn on the model trimmer. Allow water to moisten the wheel.
6. Use light, even pressure to hold the model and trim the base so it is smooth and even (see figure 17-56.) The base should be parallel to the biting surfaces. It should be at least ½ inch thick and ⅓ the entire height of the model.
   CAUTION: Keep fingers away from the wheel at all times (see figure 17-57). Use steady pressure to hold the model.
7. Trim the back, or heel, of the model. Approximately ¼ inch should remain behind the third molars. The heel should be perpendicular to the base.
   NOTE: If working on a set of models, first trim the mandibular model. Then, hold the two models together so they are in occlusion and fit together. Trim the maxillary model parallel to the base of the mandibular model.
8. Trim the sides of the model. On the maxillary model, form a 63° angle with the heel. Cut to within ¼ to ⅜ inch of the bicuspids (see figure 17-56). On the mandibular model, form a 55° angle with the heel. Cut to within ¼ to ⅜ inch of the bicuspids.
9. Trim the heel points to approximately ½ inch in length and to form a 125° angle with the heel.
10. On the maxillary model, mark the cuspids and the center of the central incisors. Make two cuts, one on each side, to form a point between the two central incisors. On the

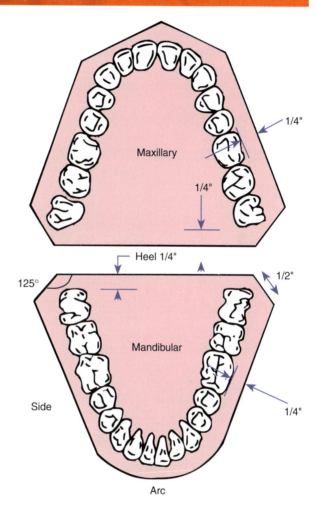

FIGURE 17-56 Measurements for trimming a model.

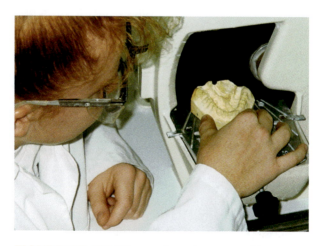

FIGURE 17-57 Wear safety glasses and keep fingers away from the wheel at all times while using a model trimmer.

mandibular model, mark the cuspids and make an arc cut.

11. Label the model(s) with the patient's name and the date. Recheck both the maxillary and mandibular model to make sure they are trimmed correctly (refer to figure 17-50).

12. Clean the trimmer thoroughly. Use a brush to clean the wheel. Remove the platform to wash and dry the inside of the trimmer.

13. Use large amounts of water to rinse the sink drain.

14. Replace all equipment.

15. Wash hands.

Practice *Go to the workbook and use the evaluation sheet for 17:10E, Trimming a Model, to practice this procedure. When you feel you have mastered this skill, sign the sheet and give it to your instructor for further action.*

Final Checkpoint   Using the criteria listed on the evaluation sheet, your instructor will grade your performance.

17:11 INFORMATION Making Custom Trays

Making custom trays for impressions may be one of the responsibilities of the dental assistant. **Custom trays** are impression trays made to fit a particular patient's mouth. To obtain exact impressions, a tray must be exactly fitted to the patient's mouth. Thus, a custom tray is produced.

Quick-curing acrylic resins or shellac-based materials are used to produce custom trays. The acrylic resins are more popular because they produce a stronger tray and one that can be used with all types of impression materials.

To make a custom tray, first a model or cast of the patient's mouth is made from a standard impression tray. An impression is taken, and a stone or plaster model is poured. This is often referred to as a *preliminary impression*. The stone or plaster model of the patient's mouth is then used as a base to form the custom tray. In this way, the tray is fitted perfectly for the individual. The tray can then be used with a variety of impression materials to get an exact impression of the patient's mouth.

Because acrylic resins are difficult to remove from mixing jars or containers, a plastic-or wax-lined disposable paper cup and tongue blades are used to mix the material. Coating the fingers lightly with petroleum jelly helps prevent the material from sticking to the hands.

STUDENT: *Go to the workbook and complete the assignment sheet for 17:11, Making Custom Trays. Then return and continue with the procedure.*

PROCEDURE 17:11

Making Custom Trays

Equipment and Supplies

Powder and liquid tray materials, measuring devices, paper cups and tongue blades, petroleum jelly, glass slab, baseplate wax, alcohol lamp or bunsen burner, wax knife, acrylic bur or stone, plaster or stone model, safety glasses

Procedure

1. Assemble equipment.
2. Wash hands.
3. Use a single layer of baseplate wax to cover the teeth and other specified areas of the model. This serves as a spacer for the tray.

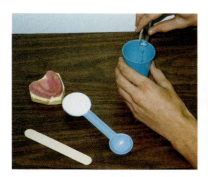

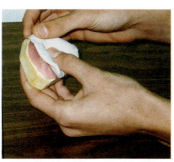

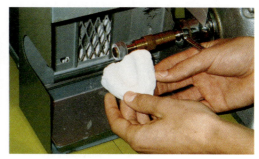

FIGURE 17-58A Pour the required amount of liquid into a paper cup.

FIGURE 17-58B Start at the palate area to adapt the wafer of custom tray material to the model.

FIGURE 17-58C A lathe can be used to trim and smooth the edges of a custom tray.

NOTE: Use warm water to warm the wax to make it more pliable.

NOTE: Special rolls of liner material are also available to cover the teeth. The liner material is cut to size, moistened, and then placed over the teeth.

4. Pour the required amount of liquid (follow manufacturer's instructions) into a paper cup (see figure 17-58A). A wax- or plastic-lined paper cup is preferred. Measure the correct amount of powder and add it to the liquid in the cup.

⚠ CAUTION: Never use a rubber bowl for mixing. Paper cups provide for easier cleanup because they can be discarded.

5. Use a tongue blade for mixing. Mix thoroughly for approximately 1 minute until the mix is uniform.

6. Allow the mixture to stand until it is not sticky to the touch and is stringy when pulled, approximately 2 to 3 minutes.

7. Coat the model, glass slab, and your hands with petroleum jelly to prevent the material from sticking.

8. Place the material on the glass slab. Roll or form it into a wafer with a uniform thickness of approximately ¹⁄₁₆ to ⅛ inch.

9. Remove the wafer from the tray. Slowly adapt it to the model. Start at the palate area and extend to the sides (see figure 17-58B).

10. Form a handle on the tray. Extra material can be applied by using a small amount of the resin liquid at the point of attachment.

11. Use a knife to remove excess material from the sides.

12. Allow the tray to cure for 7 to 10 minutes. Then, gently remove the tray from the model.

13. Remove the wax spacer, unless the doctor wants it left in place. Label the tray with patient's name.

14. Use special acrylic burs or an arbor band on a lathe to trim and smooth the tray (see figure 17-58C).

⚠ CAUTION: Wear safety glasses while trimming the tray.

15. Clean and replace all equipment. The resin liquid can be used to remove mix from surfaces, but it should be used sparingly.

16. Wash hands.

Practice *Go to the workbook and use the evaluation sheet for 17:11, Making Custom Trays, to practice this procedure. When you feel you have mastered this skill, sign the sheet and give it to your instructor for further action.*

 Final Checkpoint Using the criteria listed on the evaluation sheet, your instructor will grade your performance.

17:12 INFORMATION Maintaining and Loading an Anesthetic Aspirating Syringe

Anesthesia is used in many dental procedures to decrease pain or discomfort. Some responsibilities of the dental assistant with regard to anesthesia are discussed in this section. It is important to note, however, that the degree of responsibility may vary from state to state.

Pain control is an important part of any dental procedure. **Anesthesia**, which means "absence of feeling," is the term used to describe the condition that exists when the sensation of feeling pain has been decreased or eliminated. The type of anesthesia used depends on the needs of the patient. Different types of anesthesia include:

◆ *General anesthesia:* This type renders the patient unconscious. It is usually used in a hospital and administered by an anesthesiologist. It is seldom used in dental offices.

◆ *Analgesia or sedation:* This type causes loss of ability to feel pain but not loss of consciousness. In dental offices, analgesia is usually given by having the patient inhale a mixture of nitrous oxide and oxygen gases. This causes the patient to feel pleasantly relaxed but remain awake and able to cooperate. The effects wear off very quickly after the administration is stopped. Other forms of sedation are also used. These include oral doses or injections of mild sedatives, or tranquilizers.

◆ *Local anesthesia:* This is the form of anesthesia used most frequently in dental offices. An anesthetic is injected into the area where loss of sensation is desired. This decreases or eliminates the sensation of pain in the specific area but has no effect on the patient's level of consciousness.

◆ *Topical anesthesia:* Topical anesthetics are frequently used to reduce the pain or discomfort caused by the injection for local anesthesia. These anesthetics are applied to the mucous membrane to desensitize the area where another anesthetic is to be injected. Topical anesthetics are available as liquids, sprays, gels, and ointments.

There are two main kinds of injections used to produce local anesthesia in the oral cavity (see figure 17-59):

◆ *Block:* The anesthetic is injected near a main nerve trunk. This kind of injection is used primarily for mandibular teeth. Several teeth are anesthetized.

◆ *Infiltration, or field:* The anesthetic is injected around the terminal nerve branches of the teeth. This kind of injection is used mainly for maxillary teeth, but it can be used for anterior mandibular teeth. Each tooth usually requires a separate injection.

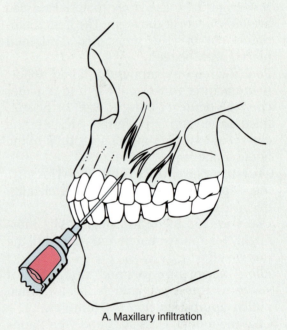

A. Maxillary infiltration

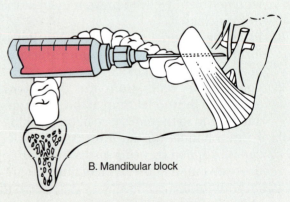

B. Mandibular block

FIGURE 17-59 Types of injections for dental anesthesia: (A) maxillary infiltration and (B) mandibular block.

A variety of medications are used to produce local anesthesia. The main local-anesthetic medication is lidocaine (Xylocaine). It decreases nerve sensation. Other anesthetics that may be used include mepivacaine, or Carbocaine, and prilocaine, or Citanest. Procaine, or Novocain, is used infrequently. Vasoconstrictors are often added to anesthetics. Vasoconstrictors decrease the size of the blood vessels in the area and, thus, keep the blood from rapidly carrying away the anesthetic. In this way, the anesthesia effect is prolonged. Vasoconstrictors also help reduce bleeding at the site. Epinephrine is a common vasoconstrictor.

CAUTION: Vasoconstrictors can be dangerous for patients with heart disease, hyperthyroidism, and hypertension (high blood pressure). It is important to review the patient's health history and follow the doctor's directions before epinephrine is used.

Carpules are glass cartridges that contain premeasured amounts of anesthetic solutions (see figure 17-60). The carpule fits into the barrel of a syringe. This is the most common delivery system for local-anesthetic injection. The following points must be observed when using carpules:

♦ Check the glass: Do not use if cracks or chips are present.

♦ Check the solution: It should be clear in color. If it is yellow or straw colored, this may mean that the epinephrine has broken down. Do *not* use a carpule containing discolored solution.

♦ Check the rubber plunger: It should be level with or just slightly below the top of the cartridge.
  (1) An extruded (pushed-out) plunger with a large air bubble usually means that the cartridge was frozen. Do *not* use.
  (2) An extruded plunger with no air bubble usually means that the cartridge was left in a disinfecting solution too long. The solution passes through the rubber diaphragm and enters the carpule. Do *not* use.

♦ Check the bubble: Small bubbles (1 mm to 2 mm) are normal. Large bubbles are usually caused by freezing. Return a carpule containing large bubbles to the supplier for replacement.

♦ Check the aluminum cap: Rust from the container can contaminate the caps. It is best *not* to use a carpule having rust on the cap.

♦ Care of carpules: Do *not* autoclave carpules. They are sterile on the inside. It is best *not* to soak any carpule for a long time because the disinfecting solution can pass into the rubber diaphragm and contaminate the solution inside. Prior to using any carpule, use a sterile pad moistened with 70-percent ethyl alcohol or 91-percent isopropyl alcohol to rub the aluminum cap end and rubber-plunger end. Cartridge dispensers are available for conveniently storing carpules (see figure 17-61).

Aspirating syringes are commonly used to inject local anesthetic (see figure 17-62). Each syringe contains an open area for insertion of the carpule. In most cases, a disposable needle is placed on the end just before the syringe is to be used.

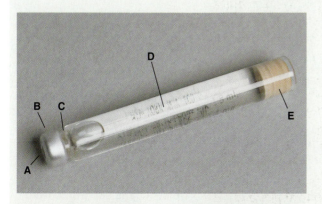

FIGURE 17-60 Parts of an anesthetic carpule: (A) Rubber diaphragm, (B) aluminum cap, (C) neck, (D) glass cylinder, and (E) rubber plunger.

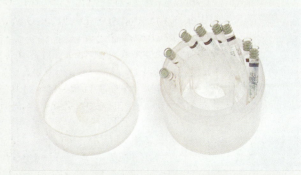

FIGURE 17-61 Cartridge dispensers are used to store the carpules conveniently.

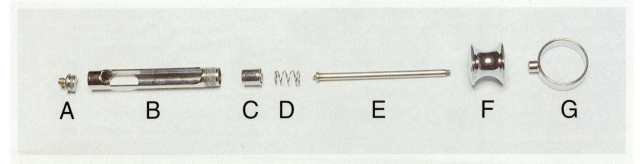

FIGURE 17-62 Parts of the aspirating syringe: (A) needle adaptor, (B) barrel, (C) guide bearing, (D) spring, (E) piston with harpoon, (F) finger grip, and (G) thumb ring.

◆ *Aspiration* means "drawing back by suction." After penetrating the mucous membrane with the syringe, the doctor draws back on the syringe to be sure the needle has not penetrated a blood vessel and to be sure it is properly inserted in the tissues before injecting the medication.

◆ After each use, the syringe must be washed thoroughly and rinsed. It must then be autoclaved.

◆ After each five uses, the syringe should be dismantled, or taken apart. All parts should be checked carefully. Worn or defective parts should be replaced. Threaded areas should be lubricated.

◆ Standard precautions must be followed while handling the disposable needle after an injection has been given. Handle the needle carefully to avoid needle sticks. The needle must be removed from the syringe and placed in a leakproof puncture-resistant sharps box. It must *not* be bent, broken, or recapped. If the needle

must be recapped during the procedure, a one-handed scoop technique must be used. The needle guard or cover must be placed on a tray or in a special recap device designed to hold the guard in position (see figure 17-63A to C). The used needle should then be inserted into the guard or cap. Fingers must be kept off of the guard until the end of the needle is covered. Once the needle

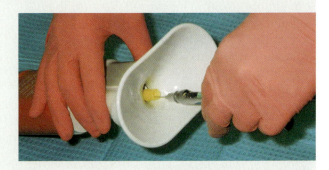

FIGURE 17-63B The needle guard is clamped into the recap device. The used needle is then placed in the needle guard. *(Courtesy of Patrick Reineck, DDS)*

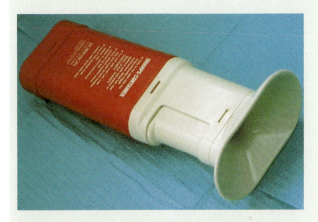

FIGURE 17-63A This recap device has its own sharps container to dispose of the used needle and guard. *(Courtesy of Patrick Reineck, DDS)*

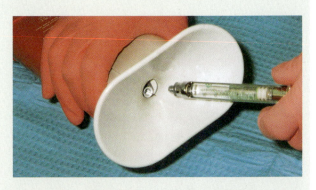

FIGURE 17-63C The syringe is separated from the needle. Then the clamp on the recap device is released to allow the used needle and guard to drop into the sharps container. *(Courtesy of Patrick Reineck, DDS)*

end is covered by the guard or cap, it is safe to pick up the guard and slip it firmly into position over the needle.

Correct care of carpules and syringes and correct loading of syringes are part of the responsibilities of a dental assistant. Procedures 17:12A and 17:12B provide additional information.

STUDENT: *Go to the workbook and complete the assignment sheet for 17:12, Maintaining and Loading an Anesthetic Aspirating Syringe. Then return and continue with the procedures.*

PROCEDURE 17:12A
Maintaining an Anesthetic Aspirating Syringe

Equipment and Supplies

Soap, water, aspirating syringe, pliers, lubrication, personal protective equipment (gloves, gown, face mask, and eye protection)

Procedure

1. Assemble equipment.
2. Wash hands. Put on personal protective equipment.

   CAUTION: Observe standard precautions while working with a contaminated aspirating syringe.

3. Use pliers and gentle pressure to unscrew the parts of the syringe.
4. Use the manufacturer's instructions to identify all of the following parts:

   NOTE: Parts may vary slightly depending on the manufacturer.

   ◆ Thumb ring

   ◆ Finger grip

   ◆ Spring

   ◆ Guide bearing

   ◆ Piston with harpoon

   ◆ Barrel

   ◆ Needle adaptor

5. Use soap and water to clean all parts thoroughly. Rinse all parts.
6. Inspect the piston and harpoon. Make sure the harpoon is sharp and *not* damaged.
7. Check the needle adaptor. Make sure the hole is open and *not* plugged.
8. Check all other parts. Make sure they are *not* damaged or defective.

NOTE: Parts can be replaced. This is more economical than replacing the entire syringe.

9. Lubricate all of the threaded joints: thumb ring, piston top, barrel, and adaptor.
10. Put the syringe back together. First, put the needle adaptor on the barrel. Then, place the guide bearing narrow end down on the piston. Next, place the spring on top. Screw on the finger grip and thumb ring. Finally, place on the barrel and secure.
11. Check the syringe to make sure it is secure and correctly assembled.
12. After each use, wash the syringe thoroughly. Rinse and dry the syringe. Sterilize it in the autoclave.
13. After each five uses, repeat steps 1 to 11 of this procedure to check the anesthetic aspirating syringe and keep it in good condition. Replace any defective parts. Then, sterilize by autoclaving prior to use.
14. Replace all equipment.
15. Remove personal protective equipment. Wash hands thoroughly.

Practice *Go to the workbook and use the evaluation sheet for 17:12A, Maintaining an Anesthetic Aspirating Syringe, to practice this procedure. When you feel you have mastered this skill, sign the sheet and give it to your instructor for further action.*

 Final Checkpoint Using the criteria listed on the evaluation sheet, your instructor will grade your performance.

PROCEDURE 17:12B
Loading an Anesthetic Aspirating Syringe

Equipment and Supplies

Aspirating syringe, needles, carpules, cartridge dispenser, gauze with disinfectant solution, sharps container, personal protective equipment (gloves, gown, face mask, and eye protection)

Procedure

1. Assemble equipment. Check with the doctor to determine the type of cartridge and needle length and gauge to use.

   ⚠ CAUTION: The doctor will determine the type of medication after checking the patient's medical history. If the patient has allergies, hyperthyroidism, heart disease, or hypertension, epinephrine (a vasoconstrictor) is usually *not* used.

2. Wash hands. Put on personal protective equipment.

   ☣ CAUTION: Observe standard precautions while working with an aspirating syringe.

3. Check the carpule. Note color of solution, location of plunger, condition of aluminum cap, presence of bubbles, and condition of glass. Use gauze containing 70-percent ethyl alcohol or 91-percent isopropyl alcohol to wipe the rubber-diaphragm on the aluminum cap end and the plunger end of the carpule.

   ⚠ CAUTION: Never use a defective carpule. Discard or return it to the supplier.

4. Check the syringe. Note condition of the harpoon and other parts.

5. Place fingers and thumb on the thumb ring and finger grip. Retract the piston all the way back.

6. Place the carpule in the syringe, with the plunger end going into the harpoon end first (see figure 17-64A). The aluminum-cap end will then fall into place.

   ⚠ CAUTION: Never force the carpule into place; it will break.

7. Engage the harpoon into the rubber plunger. Use moderate pressure to push the piston forward until the harpoon is firmly engaged in the plunger. Make sure not to push too far.

8. Attach the needle to the needle adaptor by screwing it in place (see figure 17-64B).

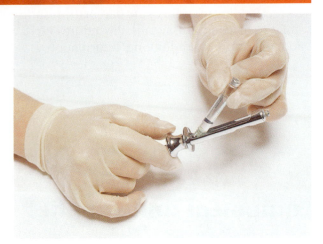

FIGURE 17-64A Place the plunger end of the cartridge into the barrel first, and the aluminum cap end will then fall into place.

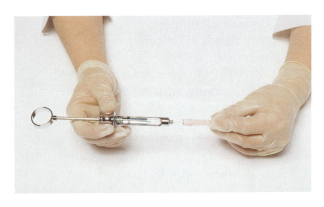

FIGURE 17-64B Attach the needle to the needle adaptor by screwing it in place.

Make sure the needle is engaged in the center of the rubber diaphragm on the cap of the carpule.

NOTE: Size (gauge and length) of the needle used will be determined by the doctor.

NOTE: The needle can be attached before the harpoon is engaged in the rubber plunger.

⚠ CAUTION: Always leave the cover on the needle end to prevent contamination and accidental needle stick injuries.

9. Prior to administration of the injection, remove the protective cap from the needle. Expel a few drops of the solution to make sure the eye of the needle is open.

10. Expel all air bubbles from the carpule. Using extreme caution, replace the protective cap on the needle loosely so it can be easily removed.

11. When the doctor is ready for the anesthesic, first pass a gauze sponge to dry the injection area. Then, pass topical anesthetic as needed. Position the needle with the beveled side toward the patient's teeth. Direct the entire syringe toward the path of insertion. Use a palm-grasp position to place the syringe in the doctor's hand. As the doctor grasps the syringe, carefully remove the protective cap from the needle. Some doctors prefer to remove the cap with a recap device. **NOTE:** Keep the syringe out of the patient's sight by passing it at the patient's chin level or below.

12. To unload the syringe, carefully unscrew the needle and place it in a sharps container. Then, use one hand to hold the carpule in position and use the other hand to disengage the harpoon. Invert the syringe so that the carpule falls out. Keep the piston retracted.

CAUTION: Never recap the needle by hand after use. If it must be recapped to protect the doctor or the dental assistant, use a one-handed scoop technique. Put the needle cap, cover, or guard on a tray or in a special re-cap device that holds the cover securely. Insert the needle into the cap without touching the cap. When the needle end is covered by the cap, push the cap firmly in place over the needle. At the end of the procedure, remove the needle with the cap in place from the syringe and discard the needle and cap in a sharps container.

13. Record the type and amount of local anesthetic used on the patient's chart.

14. Care for the syringe as instructed in Procedure 17:12A. Place the empty carpule in a sharps container.

15. Replace all equipment.

16. Remove personal protective equipment. Wash hands thoroughly.

Practice *Go to the workbook and use the evaluation sheet for 17:12B, Loading an Anesthetic Aspirating Syringe, to practice this procedure. When you feel you have mastered this skill, sign the sheet and give it to your instructor for further action.*

 Final Checkpoint Using the criteria listed on the evaluation sheet, your instructor will grade your performance.

INFORMATION
17:13 Mixing Dental Cements and Bases

Cements and bases are used in a variety of dental procedures. They are used to line or prepare a tooth for a restoration and/or as *luting* agents to cause materials to stick together. Important terminology includes the following:

◆ **Liner:** Material used to cover, line, or seal exposed tooth tissue, such as dentin. It is usually in the form of a varnish.

◆ **Base:** Protective material that is placed over the pulpal area of a tooth to reduce irritation and thermal (heat) shock. Used under large restorations.

◆ **Cement:** Material used to permanently seal inlays, orthodontic appliances, crowns, and bridges in place. It is sometimes used as a temporary filling or as a base for restorations when sedation is necessary.

◆ **Temporary:** Material used as a restorative material for a short time and only until permanent restoration can be done.

A large variety of products are available. Some products have several uses and can act as a base, cement, or temporary, depending on the need. Always read manufacturer's directions for mixing and use. Some of the types available are as follows:

◆ *Varnish* acts as a liner to protect exposed surfaces of dentin from thermal shock and irritation. It is placed under a restoration. Many brands of varnish are available, including Copal, Copalite, Varnal, and Handi-Liner.

- ◆ *Zinc oxide eugenol (ZOE)* has a sedative effect when placed under a restoration. When it is reinforced with other substances, ZOE is also used as a base under metallic restorations or as a temporary cement or restoration. It is not recommended as a base material for resins or composites (anterior restorations) because it interferes with the setting reaction of these materials. Brand names for zinc oxide eugenol are I.R.M., Cavitec, Wonder Pak, and Interval.

- ◆ *Calcium hydroxide* is used as a base in larger restorations and for pulp capping. It stimulates the formation of secondary dentin to protect the pulp. Because it is water soluble, calcium hydroxide is not used for temporary restorations. Brand names include Dycal, Preline, Hypocal, and Dropsin.

- ◆ *Zinc phosphate* is used as a thermally protective base under metallic fillings and as a cement to retain gold restorations such as inlays, crowns, and bridges. Tenacin and Fleck's are brand names.

- ◆ *Carboxylate* is also called *zinc polyacrylate* or *polycarboxylate.* It is used as a cement for orthodontic bands and brackets, crowns, and bridges, and as a base under some restorations. Brand names include Durelon, Hybond, and Tylock-Plus.

Correct mixing techniques must be followed when using bases or cements. Amounts must be measured carefully. Mixing times and proper manipulation techniques must be followed. Improper mixing techniques can lead to a poor base or cement and shorten the life of the restoration that is placed on top. Read the instructions carefully for each type.

Cements and bases are available in many different forms. Sometimes, a liquid and paste are used. Other times liquids and powders, or two pastes are used. In most cases, care must be taken to avoid mixing the substances in their containers because a small amount of liquid added to a powder in a container can ruin or destroy the entire contents of the container. Therefore, it is important to follow precautions that prevent mixing the containers of material together and to use clean measuring devices.

Some brands of cements and bases require light curing. A visible light source is held close to the preparation for a brief time, usually about 20 seconds for each 1 millimeter layer. This causes the material to "cure" or set and become hard. Light shields must be used by the dentist and assistant to prevent eye irritation from the visible light source.

Procedures for mixing some types of cements and bases are described on the following pages. These procedures provide a basic introduction.

STUDENT: *Go to the workbook and complete the assignment sheet for 17:13, Mixing Dental Cements and Bases. Then return and continue with the procedures.*

PROCEDURE 17:13A

Preparing Varnish

Equipment and Supplies

Cavity varnish, varnish solvent or thinner, cotton pliers, cotton pellets, special applicators (with some products), air syringe, personal protective equipment (gloves, gown, face mask, and eye protection)

NOTE: Copal, Copalite, Varnal, and Handi-Liner are brand names of varnish.

Procedure

1. Assemble equipment. Read and follow the manufacturer's instructions for the specific varnish being used.

2. Wash hands. Put on personal protective equipment.

☣ **CAUTION:** Observe standard precautions while assisting with any dental procedure.

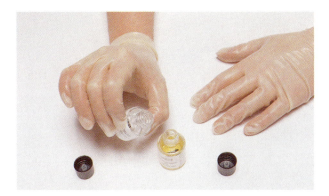

FIGURE 17-65A Some types of varnish must be thinned with a thinner solution when they become thick.

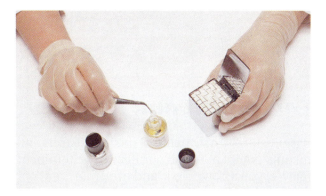

FIGURE 17-65B Cotton pliers can be used to hold the cotton pellet while saturating the pellet with varnish.

3. Check the bottle of varnish. If the contents are too thick, add thinner (see figure 17-65A). Loosen caps slightly, but leave in place until ready for use.
    NOTE: Evaporation occurs if caps are left off bottles.

4. When the doctor has completed the cavity preparation, pass the air-water, or tri-flow, syringe to the doctor. The cavity preparation must be dry before varnish is applied.

5. Put two cotton pellets in the cotton pliers. Dip the pellets into the varnish to saturate them (see figure 17-65B). Remove the excess varnish by placing both pellets on a 2 × 2 gauze pad. Pick up one saturated cotton pellet with the cotton pliers and pass it to the doctor.
    NOTE: Two pellets are saturated at the same time to avoid contamination of the varnish with the cotton pliers. To prepare the pellets one at a time, two pairs of cotton pliers must be used.
    NOTE: Special applicators are sometimes used. Cotton fibers are placed on the end of the applicator, and the applicator is then dipped in the varnish. A second applicator must be used for the second pellet.

6. The doctor paints the dentin surface with the varnish. The dental assistant should be ready to receive the pliers.

7. Pass the air syringe to the doctor. The area is dried with warm air for approximately 15 to 30 seconds.

8. Discard the used cotton pellet. Pick up the second saturated cotton pellet with the cotton pliers. Pass the pliers to the doctor.

9. The doctor will apply a second coat of varnish. Very porous teeth sometimes require three applications. If a third coat is necessary, use clean, uncontaminated cotton pliers to saturate a new cotton pellet with varnish.
    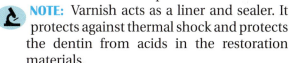
    NOTE: Varnish acts as a liner and sealer. It protects against thermal shock and protects the dentin from acids in the restoration materials.

10. When you receive the pliers, discard the pellet. Close the lid on the varnish bottle immediately to avoid evaporation.
    NOTE: The thinner can be used to clean the screw threads on the top of the varnish bottle. This helps prevent the lid from sticking on the varnish bottle.

11. Thinner can be used as a solvent to clean varnish from instruments. It can also be used to clean varnish from the enamel of the tooth being prepared.

12. Clean and replace all equipment. Scrub and sterilize all instruments.

13. Remove personal protective equipment. Wash hands thoroughly.

Practice *Go to the workbook and use the evaluation sheet for 17:13A, Preparing Varnish, to practice this procedure. When you feel you have mastered this skill, sign the sheet and give it to your instructor for further action.*

 Final Checkpoint Using the criteria listed on the evaluation sheet, your instructor will grade your performance.

PROCEDURE 17:13B

Preparing Calcium Hydroxide

Equipment and Supplies

Base, catalyst, ball-pointed mixing instrument, mixing pad, personal protective equipment (gloves, gown, face mask, and eye protection)

NOTE: Brand names for calcium hydroxide include Dycal, Preline, Hypocal, and Dropsin. This procedure is for Dycal.

Procedure

1. Assemble equipment. Read and follow the manufacturer's instructions for the brand being used.
2. Wash hands. Put on personal protective equipment.

   CAUTION: Observe standard precautions while assisting with any dental procedure.
3. Place equal small dots of the base and the catalyst on the mixing pad side by side.

   CAUTION: Take care that neither substance contaminates the tube of the other substance. If the catalyst mix enters the base tube, it can destroy the base material.
4. When the doctor is ready for the base, use the ball-pointed mixing instrument to mix the two pastes together (see figure 17-66). The mix should be uniform in color. Mixing should be completed in 10 seconds.
5. Immediately place a small amount of the mix on the end of the mixing instrument. Pass the mixing instrument to the doctor.

   NOTE: Calcium hydroxide is used as a base under restorations. It serves as a protective barrier between the dentin and pulp and between cements and restorative materials. Because it is water soluble, it cannot be used as a temporary filling material.
6. Reapply the mix to the mixing instrument until the doctor has used the required amount of base. The mixing pad of material can also be held near the patient's chin so that the doctor can obtain mix as needed.

   NOTE: Calcium hydroxide sets in approximately 2½ to 3 minutes. In the mouth, it sets faster because of moisture and mouth temperature. Therefore, it is important to work quickly and efficiently.

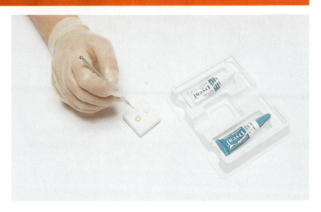

FIGURE 17-66 A ball-pointed instrument can be used to mix the base and catalyst together.

NOTE: Some brands of calcium hydroxide are light-cured. A visible light source is used to cure or set these materials.

7. Hand instruments to the doctor to remove excess material.
8. Clean and replace all equipment. A 10-percent sodium hydroxide solution or orange solvent can be used to remove the calcium hydroxide from instruments. Instruments must then be scrubbed and sterilized. Check to be sure the caps are secure on both tubes. Clean the outsides of the tubes, if necessary. Tear the used sheet off of the mixing pad and discard the sheet in a waste container.
9. Remove personal protective equipment. Wash hands thoroughly.

Practice *Go to the workbook and use the evaluation sheet for 17:13B, Preparing Calcium Hydroxide, to practice this procedure. When you feel you have mastered this skill, sign the sheet and give it to your instructor for further action.*

 Final Checkpoint Using the criteria listed on the evaluation sheet, your instructor will grade your performance.

PROCEDURE 17:13C

Preparing Carboxylate

Equipment and Supplies

Powder, scoop, liquid, mixing pad or glass slab, flexible stainless steel or plastic spatula, personal protective equipment (gloves, gown, face mask, and eye protection)

NOTE: Durelon, Hybond, and Tylock-Plus are brands of carboxylate. They are used as a cement and as a base under restorations. This procedure is written for Durelon.

Procedure

1. Assemble equipment. Read and follow the manufacturer's instructions for the brand being used.
2. Wash hands. Put on personal protective equipment.

   CAUTION: Observe standard precautions while assisting with any dental procedure.

3. Press the measuring scoop down into the powder. Use firm pressure to fill the scoop. Withdraw the scoop. Use the spatula to remove excess powder from the outside of the scoop. Use the spatula to level the powder.
4. Invert the scoop over the mixing pad (or glass slab). Tap the side with the spatula to release all of the powder.

   NOTE: If a glass slab is used, first cool it by placing it under cold, running water. Dry it thoroughly.

5. Hold the bottle of liquid in a vertical position. Squeeze the required number of drops of liquid onto the pad and beside the powder. Follow the manufacturer's recommendations for amount. Sample measurements are as follows:

   a. Cement: Use three drops of liquid for one scoop of powder.

   b. Base: Use two drops of liquid for one scoop of powder.

   NOTE: Some manufacturers provide calibrated, syringe-type liquid dispensers. Follow instructions to use this type of dispenser. Usually, the plunger is moved from one full calibration to the next calibration to obtain each drop of liquid required. If two drops of liquid are needed, the plunger would be moved through two calibrations on the syringe.

6. Use the spatula to add all of the powder to the liquid at one time. Mix vigorously. The mix should be completed in 30 seconds. The final mix should appear glossy.

   CAUTION: Do not start mixing until the doctor is ready. Dispense the liquid only when you are ready to use it.

7. The final mix should be used while it is glossy. The doctor has approximately 2 to 3 minutes of manipulation time, so it is important to work quickly and efficiently.
8. Close the lid on the bottles of liquid and powder immediately after use. The opening of the dropper bottle must be kept clean.
9. Use water to wipe the mixing spatula and instruments clean immediately after use. If the material has set, a 10-percent sodium hydroxide solution or orange solvent can be used to clean the instruments.
10. Clean and replace all equipment. Wash all instruments thoroughly and then sterilize them correctly. Tear the used sheet off of the mixing pad and discard the sheet in a waste container.
11. Remove personal protective equipment. Wash hands thoroughly.

Practice *Go to the workbook and use the evaluation sheet for 17:13C, Preparing Carboxylate, to practice this procedure. When you feel you have mastered this skill, sign the sheet and give it to your instructor for further action.*

 Final Checkpoint Using the criteria listed on the evaluation sheet, your instructor will grade your performance.

PROCEDURE 17:13D

Preparing Zinc Oxide Eugenol (ZOE)

Equipment and Supplies

Containers of powder and liquid, mixing pad, small spatula, measuring devices, personal protective equipment (gloves, gown, face mask, and eye protection)

NOTE: I.R.M. is a brand of a reinforced zinc oxide eugenol. Other brands include Cavitec, Wonder Pak, and Interval. This procedure is written for I.R.M. It is used as a base under amalgam restorations and as a temporary cement or restoration. It *cannot* be used under resin or composite restorations.

Procedure

1. Assemble equipment. Read and follow the manufacturer's instructions for the brand being used.
2. Wash hands. Put on personal protective equipment.
   CAUTION: Observe standard precautions while assisting with any dental procedure.
3. Fluff the powder by gently shaking the container. This ensures uniform bulk density of the contents. Open the lid carefully to avoid inhaling the powder.
4. Fill the powder scoop to excess without packing. Use the spatula to level the scoop (see figure 17-67A). Place the powder on the mixing pad.

5. Dispense one drop of liquid for each scoop of powder used or follow manufacturer's instructions. Dispense the drop of liquid on the pad next to the powder (see figure 17-67B).
   CAUTION: Do not drop the liquid *into* the powder.
6. Return the empty dropper into the holder on the bottle. Close the cap of the bottle containing the liquid immediately.
   NOTE: Prolonged contact between the dropper and the liquid eugenol will cause deterioration of the dropper. If the cap is left off the bottle, evaporation of the liquid will occur.
7. Use the spatula to mix half of the powder and all of the liquid (see figure 17-67C). Use a stropping action with the spatula to thoroughly combine this powder with the liquid.
8. Add the rest of the powder to the mix in two or three increments. Spatulate thoroughly to mix.
9. When all of the powder has been added, whip the mix vigorously for 5 to 10 seconds. The final mix should be smooth and adaptable.
   NOTE: Total mixing should be complete in 1 to 1½ minutes.
10. Pass the mix and the preferred instrument to the doctor. The initial set occurs approximately 3 to 5 minutes from the start of mixing, so work quickly and efficiently.

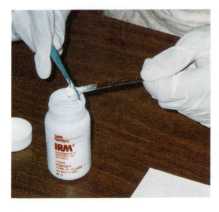

FIGURE 17-67A Use a spatula to level the powder in the scoop.

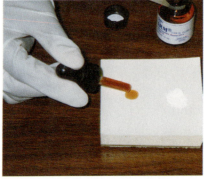

FIGURE 17-67B Dispense the liquid onto the pad next to the powder.

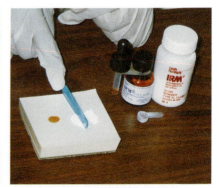

FIGURE 17-67C To begin mixing the powder and liquid, use the spatula to add half the powder to the liquid and mix thoroughly.

11. Clean and replace all equipment. Check to be sure the lids on the bottles of powder and liquid are secure. Tear the sheet off of the mixing pad and discard the sheet in a waste container. Use orange solvent or alcohol to clean the spatula and other instruments. Scrub and sterilize all instruments.

12. Remove personal protective equipment. Wash hands thoroughly.

Practice *Go to the workbook and use the evaluation sheet for 17:13D, Preparing Zinc Oxide Eugenol (ZOE), to practice this procedure. When you feel you have mastered this skill, sign the sheet and give it to your instructor for further action.*

✔ **Final Checkpoint** Using the criteria listed on the evaluation sheet, your instructor will grade your performance.

INFORMATION
17:14 Preparing Restorative Materials—Amalgam and Composite

A main method of treating dental caries is restoration by the placement of filling materials. **Restoration** is defined as "the process of replacing a diseased portion of a tooth or a lost tooth by artificial means." This may include filling material, a crown, bridge, denture, partial denture, or implant.

Dental caries, or decay, is a disease process that attacks the hard tissues of the teeth, demineralizing and eventually destroying these tissues. When the enamel, dentin, and/or cementum are destroyed, a hollow space called a **cavity** is created in the tooth. To repair the damage caused by a carious lesion, the doctor removes the decayed and damaged tissue and fills the cavity preparation with a restorative material, or filling. Two of the most commonly used restorative materials are amalgam and composite.

Dental **amalgam** is a restorative material used primarily on posterior teeth.

◆ Dental amalgam is a mixture of metals (an alloy) combined with the metal mercury.

◆ Amalgam alloy contains four main metals. Each metal has certain properties that help form a durable restoration. To ensure a uniform product, the American Dental Association has established percentages by weight for each of these metals. The metals and their properties are as follows:

(1) *Silver* is the main component. It provides high strength, low flow (resistance to change in shape under biting forces), high expansion, rapid setting, and silver color.

(2) *Tin* is added to counterbalance the silver. It reduces expansion, slows setting time, reduces strength, increases the ability of the alloy to combine with mercury, and allows the restoration to be carved.

(3) *Copper* is added in small amounts to provide increased strength, hardness, and low flow, to increase expansion, and to stabilize the other metals. It should make up 13 to 30 percent of a high-copper alloy. An amalgam containing less than 6 percent copper is called a *low-copper alloy,* a type used less frequently.

(4) *Zinc* is used in very small amounts to remove oxides and other impurities. It is sometimes referred to as a *scavenger metal.* It is not used in all alloys.

◆ *Mercury* is a metal that is a liquid at room temperature. It is added to other metals to form amalgam. It must be handled with care because it is highly toxic. It can vaporize (evaporate and float freely in the air) and be absorbed into the body through inhalation or skin pores. Mercury vapor has no odor, color, or taste, and is extremely difficult to detect.

Many sources can produce a vapor. Examples include a leaking capsule, a mercury spill, air exposure while preparing and dispensing amalgam, particle release while polishing a restoration or removing old amalgam restorations, and/or improper storage of amalgam scraps. Even carpeting in a treatment room can retain amalgam particles; vacuuming can cause the mercury to vaporize into the air. Personal protective equipment (PPE), including disposable gloves, a gown, a face mask, and eye protection (glasses or a face shield) should be worn while working with dental amalgam. If skin is accidentally exposed to mercury, the skin should be scrubbed with soap and water and rinsed thoroughly. Mercury must be stored in well-sealed, unbreakable containers. Mercury spills should be cleaned up immediately. Spill kits, containing gloves, a mercury-vapor respirator (to prevent inhalation of the mercury), a sulfur solution (to coat the droplets), a syringe with a large needle (to draw in the mercury), and polyethylene bags are used to clean up spills (see figure 17-68). In addition, proper cleanup is essential after working with dental amalgam. Mercury-contaminated items, such as gloves, masks, or used capsules should be discarded in a labeled and sealed polyethylene bag. Scrap amalgam should be submerged in a tightly sealed, unbreakable jar containing sulfur water, glycerin, or mineral oil. Most dental offices have a program of mercury hygiene to control mercury hazards. The dental assistant must become familiar with this program and follow established regulations.

- *Amalgamation* is the process that occurs when amalgam alloy is mixed with mercury. A new alloy is formed, which becomes the restorative (filling) material, called *dental amalgam.*

- *Trituration* is the mixing process used to combine mercury with the amalgam alloy. It is done with a mechanical amalgamator (a mixing machine). It is important to follow the manufacturer's instructions regarding mixing (trituration) time.

- Amalgam alloy is available in pellets or powder and as low-copper or high-copper alloys. Low-copper alloys, used less frequently, are composed of comminuted (lathe-cut filings) or spherical particles. High-copper alloys are available as comminuted, spherical, or admixed (combination of particles). Alloys with smaller particles will usually produce a stronger amalgam restoration with a smoother surface. The type of alloy used depends on the doctor's preference.

- Dental amalgam alloy is purchased in disposable capsules containing premeasured amounts of amalgam alloy powder and mercury (see figure 17-69). The American Dental

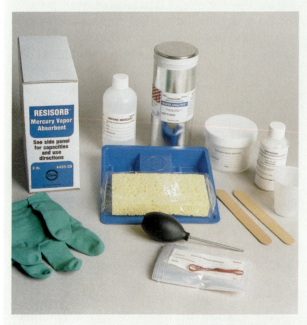

FIGURE 17-68 A mercury spill kit should be used to clean up mercury to prevent mercuric poisoning.

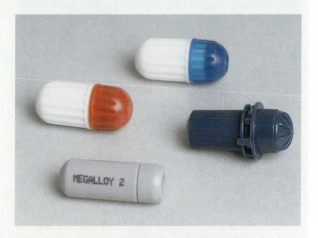

FIGURE 17-69 Dental amalgam alloy is purchased in disposable capsules containing premeasured amount of amalgam alloy and mercury.

Association (ADA) encourages the use of these premeasured capsules because they eliminate mercury dispensers and decrease the possibility of a mercury spill, accidental inhalation of mercury vapor, or skin contact with the mercury. A membrane inside the capsule separates the amalgam alloy powder and mercury until the capsule is used. Usually, the capsule must be twisted or pressed to break the membrane and combine the alloy powder and mercury before the capsule is placed in the amalgamator for trituration.

◆ After amalgam has been triturated, it must be used immediately to produce a good restoration. The doctor uses an amalgam carrier to place the amalgam in the prepared cavity. The amalgam is then condensed, or packed, into the cavity preparation, after which the restoration is carved to correct occlusion (alignment between maxillary and mandibular teeth) and tooth contour.

◆ Amalgam bonding agents are used for many restorations. These agents help the amalgam adhere to the tooth surfaces and increase the retention of the restoration. It is important to follow the manufacturer's recommendations while using any bonding agents.

Composite is the restorative material used most frequently in the repair of anterior teeth, but it can also be used to restore posterior teeth. In comparison to other, older resins, composite offers improved appearance, increased strength, and the ability to withstand chemical actions caused by mouth fluids. It has an organic polymer matrix, such as dimethacrylate, and inorganic filler particles such as quartz and/or lithium aluminum silicate. *Self-curing,* or *chemical-curing, composite* is supplied as two pastes that are mixed together to cause a chemical reaction. One paste is a *base*, and the other is an *accelerator* (catalyst). When the composite base and accelerator are mixed together, substances present in the base and accelerator cause the reaction called *polymerization*, which results in a hardening of the material. *Light-cured composite* is sensitive to light, and polymerization does not occur until the composite is exposed to a curing light (see figure 17-70). Light-cured composite is available in a premixed,

syringe form. It is available in various shades to blend with the teeth. The amount needed is dispensed from the syringe and then placed in the tooth cavity. When the restoration is in place, a curing light is used on the composite, and the material sets (polymerizes). Both the doctor and the dental assistant must wear light-filtering glasses or use light-screening paddles while using the curing light to prevent eye damage. Ask the patient to close his or her eyes when the curing light is used. Before the composite is placed in the prepared cavity, the cavity is etched, and a bonding agent, or resin, is applied. The etching solution roughens the surface so that the composite will adhere (stick) and bond more securely to the tooth tissue. The bonding agent is then applied to help the composite material adhere to the tooth. Before using any composite, etching, or bonding materials, read and follow the manufacturer's instructions.

STUDENT: *Go to the workbook and complete the assignment sheet for 17:14, Preparing Restorative Materials—Amalgam and Composite. Then return and continue with the procedures.*

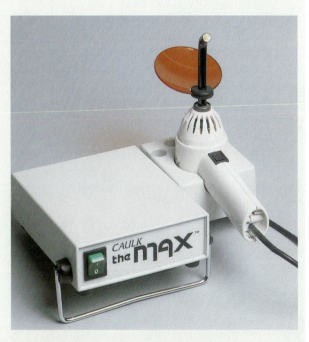

FIGURE 17-70 A curing light is used on light-cured composite to cause polymerization or hardening. *(Courtesy of Lasermed, Inc., Salt Lake City, Utah)*

PROCEDURE 17:14A

Preparing Amalgam

Equipment and Supplies

Premeasured amalgam capsule, amalgamator, amalgam carrier, amalgam well or dappen dish, amalgam instruments, articulating paper, personal protective equipment (gloves, gown, face mask, and eye protection)

Procedure

1. Wash hands. Put on personal protective equipment.

   CAUTION: Observe standard precautions while assisting with any dental procedure.

2. Assemble equipment.

3. Assist the doctor as required for preparation of the cavity.

4. If a bonding agent is used, read and follow the manufacturer's instructions to prepare the materials for the doctor. The bonding agent helps the amalgam adhere to the exposed tooth surfaces.

5. Prepare the amalgam capsule according to manufacturer's instructions. Some capsules are activated by twisting the cap to break a seal and combine the amalgam alloy with the mercury. Other capsules are activated by pressing the capsule together (see figure 17-71A).

   CAUTION: Avoid skin contact with the mercury. Also, avoid inhalation of mercury vapors. Both may lead to mercury poisoning.

6. Place the capsule in the amalgamator (see figure 17-71B). Close the cover of the amalgamator to enclose the capsule. Set the timer for the correct time. Follow the manufacturer's instructions for trituration time.

   NOTE: Time is usually 7 to 10 seconds.

7. When the doctor has completed the cavity preparation, push the start button on the amalgamator to start trituration.

8. When trituration is complete, unscrew the capsule. Tap both ends into an amalgam well or dappen dish to empty the container.

9. Fill the amalgam carrier. The carrier should be packed tightly, smoothly, and quickly (see figure 17-71C).

10. Pass the filled carrier to the doctor. Be ready to pass a condensing instrument, because the amalgam must be condensed into the tooth.

11. Repeat steps 9 and 10 until the cavity preparation is filled. It may be necessary to prepare a new mix of amalgam for large cavities.

    NOTE: Setting time is usually 3 to 4 minutes, so work quickly.

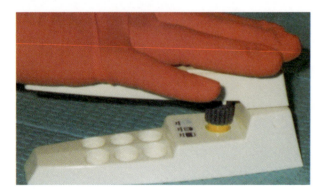

FIGURE 17-71A Some disposable amalgam capsules are activated by pressing the two ends of the capsule together to break the membrane and combine the alloy powder and mercury. Some brands of capsules must be twisted. Follow manufacturer's instructions. *(Courtesy of Patrick Reineck, DDS)*

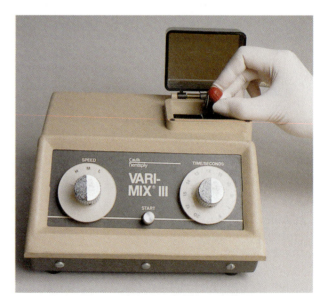

FIGURE 17-71B Place the capsule in the amalgamator. Read the manufacturer's instructions for correct trituration time.

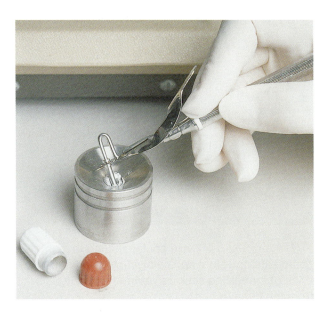

FIGURE 17-71C The amalgam carrier should be packed tightly, smoothly, and quickly.

sure on the new restoration for one to two hours. Some doctors recommend a soft diet or suggest that the patient not use the area for chewing for one to eight hours. Some doctors request a follow-up appointment to check and polish the restoration.

NOTE: Before the restoration can be polished properly, it usually must set for 24 hours. Polishing helps prolong the life of the restoration.

16. Clean and replace all equipment. Scrub and sterilize all instruments. Place any disposable items contaminated with mercury in a sealed polyethylene bag. Submerge any unused, mixed amalgam in a tightly-sealed, unbreakable jar containing sulfur water, glycerin, or mineral oil. Many offices save this amalgam and return a large amount of it to manufacturers who reclaim the silver.

17. Remove personal protective equipment. Wash hands thoroughly.

12. After the amalgam has been condensed, pass the carving instruments. The restoration must be carved so that correct occlusion and contour is achieved.

13. At all times, have the tri-flow syringe and oral evacuator ready to rinse the patient's mouth and remove excess amalgam particles and liquids.

14. Pass articulating paper when the doctor is ready to check occlusion.

15. **C** When the restoration is complete, make sure the patient receives correct instructions. Most patients are told *not* to put pres-

Practice *Go to the workbook and use the evaluation sheet for 17:14A, Preparing Amalgam, to practice this procedure. When you feel you have mastered this skill, sign the sheet and give it to your instructor for further action.*

✔ **Final Checkpoint** Using the criteria listed on the evaluation sheet, your instructor will grade your performance.

PROCEDURE 17:14B

Preparing Composite

Equipment and Supplies

Etching liquid, resin (universal and catalyst), composite (universal and catalyst) or light-cured composite syringe, cotton pellets, cotton pliers, mixing pads, mixing stick, plastic composite instruments, personal protective equipment (gloves, gown, face mask, and eye protection)

Procedure

1. Assemble equipment.
2. Wash hands. Put on personal protective equipment.
    CAUTION: Observe standard precautions while assisting with any dental procedure.
3. Assist doctor as required for the cavity preparation.

4. Open the bottle of etching liquid. Dispense one to two drops on a mixing pad. Moisten a cotton pellet in the liquid. Pass cotton pliers and the moistened pellet to the doctor.

   NOTE: Etching liquid can also be dispensed into a disposable, plastic well and placed on a disposable brush for placement in the cavity. Wells and brushes are supplied with certain brands of etching liquid.

   NOTE: The doctor etches the surface for approximately 1 minute. This roughens the tooth surface to increase bond strength.

   NOTE: If dentin is exposed, a calcium hydroxide base may be placed on the area prior to etching.

5. Pass the tri-flow syringe. The restorative area must be washed thoroughly with oil-free water and then dried after etching.

6. Prepare the resin material. Place equal amounts (one to two drops) of universal and catalyst on a mixing pad or in a disposable, plastic well. Mix thoroughly for 5 to 10 seconds with a fine brush or plastic placement instrument. The doctor will apply this to the tooth surface.

   NOTE: The resin helps the composite material adhere to the tooth.

   ⚠ CAUTION: Take care to avoid contaminating the contents of the universal container with those of the catalyst container. Such contamination may cause a reaction that destroys the contents of both containers.

7. Prepare the composite. Place an amount of universal paste equal to approximately one-half the size of the cavity on the mixing pad; use one end of the mixing stick (usually marked *U*). Use the opposite end of the mixing stick (usually curved and marked *C*) to place an equal amount of catalyst on the mixing pad. Mix the two pastes together for approximately 20 seconds and until the mix is smooth and well blended.

   ⚠ CAUTION: Again, take care to avoid contaminating the contents of the universal jar with those of the catalyst jar (see figure 17-72A). Such contamination may cause a reaction that destroys the contents of both jars.

   NOTE: If a premixed, light-cured composite is used, dispense the amount required from the syringe (see figure 17-72B). This type of composite material does not have to be mixed.

8. Use plastic composite instruments to pass the prepared composite paste to the doctor.

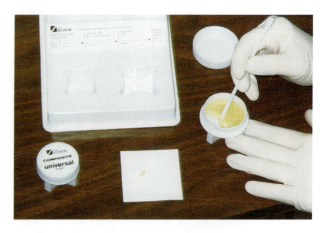

FIGURE 17-72A Avoid contaminating the jars of composite universal and catalyst by using opposite ends of the mixing stick as you remove materials from the jars.

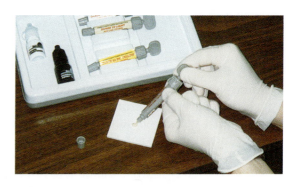

FIGURE 17-72B If a premixed, light-cured composite is used, dispense the amount required from the syringe.

NOTE: Plastic instruments will not discolor the mix. They also reduce the tendency of the composite to stick to the instruments.

9. Refill the instruments with composite mix as needed. Work quickly but efficiently.

   NOTE: Setting usually occurs 4 minutes after mixing. This allows approximately 1 to 2 minutes for placement.

   NOTE: If light-sensitive composite resin is used, the curing light is given to the doctor when the restoration is in place. The material will not harden, or set, until it is exposed to this light.

   ⚠ CAUTION: The doctor and the dental assistant must wear light-filtering glasses or use light-screening paddles while using the curing light. Ask the patient to close his or her eyes.

10. Have composite finishing and polishing strips ready for use.

11. Clean materials from instruments immediately. The mixing sticks are usually disposable. Discard these immediately to avoid contaminating the jars. Scrub and sterilize all instruments.

12. Replace all equipment. Check to make sure the lids on all containers are securely in place.

13. Remove personal protective equipment. Wash hands.

Practice *Go to the workbook and use the evaluation sheet for 17:14B, Preparing Composite, to practice this procedure. When you feel you have mastered this skill, sign the sheet and give it to your instructor for further action.*

Final Checkpoint Using the criteria listed on the evaluation sheet, your instructor will grade your performance.

17:15 INFORMATION Developing and Mounting Dental X-Rays

The dental assistant develops and mounts dental X-rays or radiographs. Dental **radiographs** are negatives taken of the teeth, similar to the negatives received when photographs are taken. X-ray beams are passed through the teeth and tissues. A series of shadows are then produced on film. Images on the developed film are described as radiolucent or radiopaque:

◆ **Radiolucent:** These areas appear dark on X-rays. This means that the X-rays penetrate through the structures. Examples of these areas are the pulp and caries.

◆ **Radiopaque:** These areas appear light or white on X-rays. This means that the structures stop the X-rays, or that the X-rays are unable to penetrate the structures. Most tooth structures, including enamel and dentin, are radiopaque. Metallic restorations also appear very white, or radiopaque, on X-rays.

There are several different types of dental radiographs:

◆ **Bitewings** (BWXR): These show only the crowns of the maxillary and mandibular teeth (see figure 17-73). They are called cavity-detecting X-rays because they are primarily used to detect interproximal (between the teeth) decay and recurring decay under restorations. They do not show root-end

infection or abscess. Usually, two to four bitewings are taken of the posterior teeth. Sometimes two to four bitewings are taken of anterior teeth in adults. Two common sizes of bitewing film include: size *1* used for anterior teeth, and size *3* used for posterior teeth.

◆ **Periapical films** (PA): These show the tooth and the surrounding area, and can show root-end infection. They are also used to determine the number and shape of roots, the condition of supporting structures of the teeth, and the relationship of a tooth to other teeth. Usually, fourteen periapical X-rays are taken for a full-mouth series. This shows the complete dentition (see figure 17-74). Size *2* film is usually used for periapical films, but a size *1* film can be used for adults with small mouths or children over six years of age.

◆ **Pedodontic (child) films:** These are smaller films, usually size *0*, used on children to show disease or other conditions of the teeth. Both bitewings (BWs) and periapicals (PAs) are taken.

◆ **Occlusal films:** These films, size *4*, are approximately twice the size of a number *2*

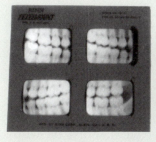
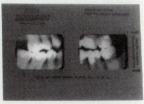

FIGURE 17-73 Bitewing (BW) X-rays show only the crowns of the maxillary and mandibular teeth.

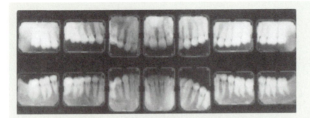

FIGURE 17-74 A full-mouth series of periapical (PA) X-rays shows the crowns and roots of all the teeth.

film. They are used to view the occlusal (chewing) planes of the maxilla or mandible.

◆ **Panoramic:** This is a special type of film that shows the entire dental arch, or all of the teeth, on one film. The film is placed in a film cassette in a panoramic X-ray unit that rotates around the patient's head (see figure 17-75A). One developed film shows complete dentition, bone structure, and surrounding tissues (see figure 17-75B).

Care must be taken while developing films. Developing involves a series of chemical reactions. The following points should be noted:

◆ Dental film is specially prepared and wrapped in a packet containing moisture-proof paper. The film is between two sheets of protective black paper. It is backed with lead foil. The lead foil stops the X-ray beams once they have passed through the teeth structures to the film (see figure 17-76).

◆ Exposure of the film to light will destroy the image on the film. Film must be opened and exposed in a dark room. Only safety dark room lights should be used. No outside light can enter the room during this procedure.

◆ Dental film contains a film emulsion, with a layer of silver halide suspended in a gelatin. The gelatin keeps the silver from settling and keeps it suspended on the surface of the film. The X-ray beams reduce, or expose, some of the silver salts. When the film is later exposed to chemicals, the chemicals act on the exposed silver to create the shadows seen on the X-ray.

◆ Care must be taken while the film is being unwrapped. Hands must be clean and dry. Personal protective equipment, including gloves and eye protection, must be worn.

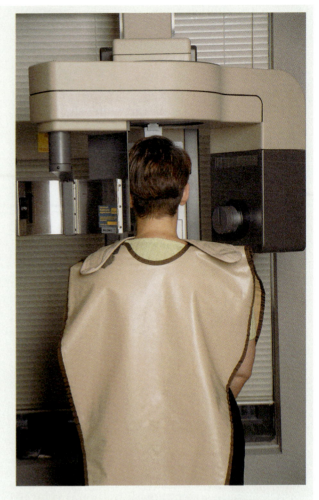

FIGURE 17-75A After a patient is positioned in a panoramic X-ray machine, the unit rotates around the patient's head.

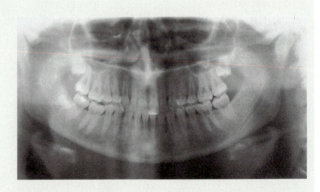

FIGURE 17-75B A panoramic X-ray shows complete dentition, bone structure, and surrounding tissue.

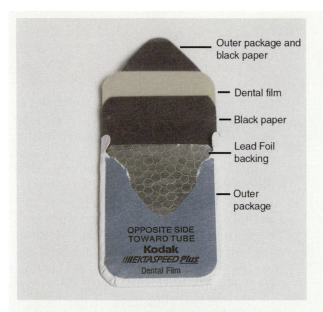

Outer package and black paper

Dental film

Black paper

Lead Foil backing

Outer package

OPPOSITE SIDE TOWARD TUBE
Kodak
EKTASPEED Plus
Dental Film

FIGURE 17-76 The lead foil in the packet of X-ray film stops the X-ray beams after they have passed through the teeth structures.

Fingerprints and marks can damage the film. Handle the film by the edges only.

◆ Developing solution is used to break down the exposed silver. This fluid is a chemical mixture that is alkaline in nature. It must be mixed according to the manufacturer's directions. Developing fluid must be replaced periodically when it is diluted, outdated, or causing poor quality images on the film.

◆ Fixing solution is used to stop the developing process. Fixing solution is a chemical solution that is acidic in nature. It must be mixed according to the manufacturer's instructions. Fixing solution must be replaced when it is diluted, outdated, or causing poor quality images on the film.

◆ The developing and fixing solutions must be monitored daily for temperature, amount, cleanliness, and quality. Read and follow the manufacturer's instructions provided with the solutions. The solutions must be handled with care because they are toxic to the skin and eyes. Personal protective equipment must be worn when handling, mixing, replenishing, or disposing of solutions.

◆ Temperature of the developer, fixer, and water used should be 68°F, or 20°C. All solutions should be mixed well before using.

◆ Most offices have automatic developing machines. Manufacturer's instructions should be followed.

X-rays are placed in special mounts for viewing. They must be mounted correctly.

◆ Each film contains a dimple. This dimple points toward the X-ray machine. One side of the film shows a concave (pointing inward) dimple. The other side shows a convex (pointing outward) dimple.

◆ In one mount, all dimples must be facing the same direction.

◆ When all the dimples are convex (pointing outward), you are viewing the facial surface (buccal or labial). When the films are placed in the mount in this manner, the films on your left are the patient's right teeth, and the films on your right are the patient's left teeth. This is the most widely used method for mounting X-rays because most dental charts use this facial view of the teeth.

◆ When all the dimples are concave (pointing inward), you are viewing the lingual (tongue) surface. Thus, the films on your right are the patient's right teeth, and the films on your left are the patient's left teeth.

◆ The doctor determines the manner in which films should be mounted.

STUDENT: *Go to the workbook and complete the assignment sheet for 17:15, Developing and Mounting Dental X-Rays. Then return and continue with the procedures.*

PROCEDURE 17:15A

Developing Dental X-Rays

Equipment and Supplies

Exposed dental X-ray film, dark room, developing tanks, film clip rack, pen, personal protective equipment (gloves, gown, face mask, and protective eyewear)

NOTE: This procedure would *not* be used with an automatic processor or developer. Follow manufacturer's instructions on the automatic units.

Procedure

1. Assemble equipment.
2. Wash hands. Put on personal protective equipment.
   NOTE: The exposed X-ray film may be contaminated with saliva or mouth fluids.
3. Stir the developing and fixing solutions thoroughly.
4. Turn on the rinse water. Regulate the temperature at 68°F, or 20°C. The water bath should be running constantly.
   NOTE: This ensures a clean supply of water for rinsing.
5. Secure the darkroom. Close all doors tightly. Turn on the outside warning light. Turn off the main lights. Turn on the safe lights.
   CAUTION: Any beam of light will destroy the X-ray film. Double-check for any light beams.
6. Unwrap the film. Turn the tab toward you. Pull open the tab. Pull the black paper out approximately one-half its length. Fold back the lead shield and the moisture-proof paper to expose the film.
7. Use a gloved thumb and forefinger to grasp the sides of the film. Gently remove the film from the pack.
   CAUTION: Avoid getting fingerprints or marks on the film.
8. Clip the film on the film rack. Tug gently to be sure the film is securely in place.
   NOTE: If the film is loose, it may fall off the rack and into the solutions.
9. When all films from one patient have been placed on the film rack, use a pen to label one plastic, waterproof wrap with the patient's name. Place this name wrap on the clip above the patient's films.
   NOTE: This identifies films when more than one set are processed.
10. Smoothly immerse the film into the developer (see figure 17-77A and B). Gently agitate the hanger up and down several times to make sure the film is coated with developer. Hook the hanger over the side of the tank, making sure all of the films are below the level of solution in the tank. Set the timer for 5 minutes or the developing time specified by the manufacturer of the film and solution. Cover the tank.
    CAUTION: Avoid jerking motions while putting the film in the developer. Jerking motions will cause streaking of the film.
    NOTE: Check the time charts provided with solutions and film speeds to determine the correct developing time. Correct time and temperature are essential for diagnostically acceptable X-rays. Many ultraspeed films develop in 2 minutes or less.
    NOTE: Tanks should be kept covered to prevent evaporation of solutions.
11. At the end of the developing time, lift the film rack out of the developing solution. Gently shake off excess solution.
12. Place the rack in the running-water bath. Agitate the rack up and down several times so that the film surfaces are thoroughly rinsed for at least 30 seconds.
    NOTE: This helps remove the developer from the films. In this way, developing solution will *not* contaminate the fixing solution.
13. Hold the rack above the water bath and gently shake off excess water.
14. Place the rack in the fixing solution. Agitate the rack up and down to cover all surfaces of the film. Set the timer for 10 minutes or the time specified by the film and solution manufacturers. Cover the tanks.
    NOTE: Film is usually left in the fixer twice as long as it is left in the developer.
    NOTE: This stops the developing process. The fixer clears the film and hardens it.

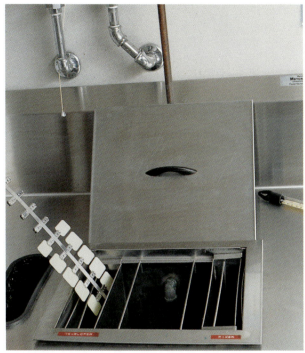

(A)

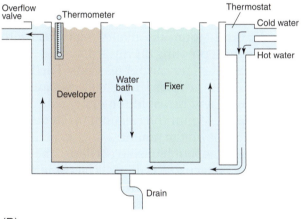

Overflow valve | Thermometer | Thermostat | Cold water | Hot water

Developer | Water bath | Fixer

Drain

(B)

FIGURE 17-77 (A) Smoothly immerse the film in the developing solution. (B) The developing solution is on the left and separated from the fix solution on the right by the water bath.

15. When the fixing time is complete, remove the film rack from the fixing solution. Shake off excess solution.

16. Rinse the rack in the water bath. Agitate the rack to cover the films with water. Rinse the films for at least 20 minutes. Cover the tanks.

    NOTE: Films can be left in the final rinse for longer periods.

17. At the end of the rinse period, put the film rack on a drying rack. Make sure the films are not in contact with any surface (for example, a wall) while they are drying.

    NOTE: Films should be thoroughly dried before being removed from the film rack. They should not be handled or mounted until dry.

18. Clean all solutions off the countertops or sink immediately. Replace all supplies. Make sure the tanks are covered prior to leaving the darkroom area.

19. If no further films are to be developed, turn off the running-water bath. In a dental office, this bath is always turned off at the end of the day.

20. Remove personal protective equipment. Wash hands.

Practice *Go to the workbook and use the evaluation sheet for 17:15A, Developing Dental X-Rays, to practice this procedure. When you feel you have mastered this skill, sign the sheet and give it to your instructor for further action.*

 Final Checkpoint Using the criteria listed on the evaluation sheet, your instructor will grade your performance.

PROCEDURE 17:15B

Mounting Dental X-Rays

Equipment and Supplies

Developed, full-mouth series of X-rays; X-ray mounts; view box

Procedure

1. Assemble equipment. Label the X-ray mount with the patient's name and the date the films were taken.
2. Wash hands.
3. Turn on view box. Make sure surface is dry and clean.
4. Lay out the series of X-rays. Make sure each dimple is pointing in the same direction, that is, either concave (inward) or convex (outward).

   NOTE: Convex is the facial-surface view; concave is the lingual-surface view.

   NOTE: A full-mouth series of X-rays usually consists of fourteen periapical films plus two or four bitewings.
5. Review the following facts about dentition. They are essential for mounting films:
   a. Bitewing X-rays show only the crowns of maxillary and mandibular teeth.
   b. Periapical films show the crowns and roots of teeth.
   c. Maxillary films often each have a hazy or swirly area, which is the maxillary sinus.
   d. Maxillary central incisors are larger than mandibular central incisors.
   e. Maxillary lateral incisors are larger than mandibular lateral incisors.
   f. Mandibular lateral incisors are wider than mandibular central incisors.
   g. Maxillary cuspids are the longest teeth in the mouth.
   h. Maxillary molars each have three blurred roots.
   i. Mandibular molars each have two distinct roots.
6. Locate the four (or two) bitewings (BW). Mount these in the correct areas on the mount (see figure 17-78). The bicuspid views should be placed closer to the center of the mount.
7. Locate the two central incisor (CI) and lateral incisor (LI) films. Look at the size of the teeth to determine which are maxillary films and which are mandibular films. Mount the maxillary films with the roots pointing upward. Mount the mandibular films with the roots pointing downward.

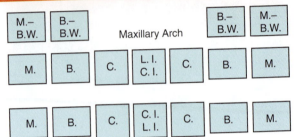

Abbreviations:
B.W. Bite wings
C.I. Central incisors
L.I. Lateral incisors
C. Cuspids
B. Bicuspids
M. Molars

FIGURE 17-78 Correct placement for a full-mouth series of X-rays.

8. Locate the four cuspid (C) films. The larger or longer cuspids are maxillary. Note the incisors and bicuspids on either side of the cuspids. Mount the cuspid films in the correct areas on the mount.
9. Locate the four bicuspid (B) films. The maxillary 1st bicuspid is the only bicuspid that is bifurcated (having two roots). Note the two maxillary films. Place them in the mount by noting cuspids and molars on either side. Do the same for the mandibular bicuspids.
10. Locate the four molar (M) films. Note the blurred, trifurcated (three) roots of the maxillary molars. Look for hazy or swirly areas that indicate the maxillary sinuses. Note the arch curvature in the back of the mouth. Place these films in the correct mount positions. Note the bifurcated (two) roots of the mandibular molars. Use the arch and bicuspid locations to place these films in the correct mount positions.

    NOTE: Some people find it easier to mount all maxillary films and then all mandibular films. Either way is satisfactory.
11. Check whether there are restorations on the films, for purposes of comparison and verification of placement accuracy. Restorations

can also serve as clues to placement when the quality of one film is poor or the film has been taken incorrectly.

NOTE: If the films do not fit, always check the dimples to be sure they are pointing in the same direction. One reversed dimple can cause a great deal of difficulty.

12. Recheck the entire mount for accuracy, noting the facts listed in Step 5. Make sure all maxillary roots are pointing upward and all mandibular roots are pointing downward.

13. Clean and replace all equipment. Turn off view box.

14. Wash hands.

Practice *Go to the workbook and use the evaluation sheet for 17:15B, Mounting Dental X-Rays, to practice this procedure. When you feel you have mastered this skill, sign the sheet and give it to your instructor for further action.*

Final Checkpoint Using the criteria listed on the evaluation sheet, your instructor will grade your performance.

UNIT 17 SUMMARY

Many different skills are performed by the dental assistant. Some of the more common skills were discussed in this unit.

A knowledge of the structure, names, and surfaces, and of the Universal Numbering System and the Federation Dentaire International System for identifying teeth is essential. This knowledge allows the dental assistant to help with charting dental conditions and provides a better understanding of the procedures performed by the doctor. This knowledge is also necessary in order to develop and mount dental X-rays.

Taking impressions and pouring models of the teeth are tasks frequently performed when dental restorative or orthodontic treatment is necessary. In addition, custom trays are made to obtain more exact models of patients' mouths.

A knowledge of basic dental instruments allows the dental assistant to assist the doctor when basic dental restorative procedures are performed. The use of amalgam or composite as restorative or filling material for teeth with carious lesions or decay is one of the most common procedures. The dental assistant helps by preparing dental anesthetic materials, mixing bases and cements, and preparing restorative materials. After procedures are complete, the dental assistant is often responsible for the maintenance and care of the equipment and instruments used.

By mastering the basic skills, the dental assistant can become a valuable member of the dental team and help provide quality dental care to the patient.

INTERNET SEARCHES

Use the suggested search engine in Unit 11:4 of this textbook to search the Internet for additional information on the following topics:

1. *Organization:* search the web sites for the American Dental Association, American Dental Hygienists' Association, and the American Dental Assistants' Association to obtain information on dental careers.

2. *Dental anatomy:* research information on the tissues of a tooth (enamel, dentin, pulp, and cementum), periodontium (alveolar process, periodontal ligament, and gingiva), and eruption of teeth.

3. *Restorative treatments:* research amalgam, composite, prophylactic treatments (e.g., fluoride), orthdontic treatment, and periodontic treatment.

4. *Dental supply companies:* search for suppliers of dental instruments, equipment, and materials to compare and contrast the products available.

REVIEW QUESTIONS

1. Draw a diagram of a tooth. Label the three (3) sections or divisions of the tooth, the four (4) tissues of the tooth, and the structures of the periodontium.

2. Name the five (5) surfaces, eight (8) line angles, and four (4) point angles for both anterior and posterior teeth.

3. Identify both the Universal Numbering System and the Federation Dentaire International System code for each of the following permanent teeth:
   a. maxillary right central incisor
   b. maxillary left 2nd molar
   c. mandibular left cuspid
   d. mandibular right 1st bicuspid

4. Explain the maintenance and disinfection requirements for each of the following types of dental equipment:
   a. dental chair
   b. dental light
   c. tri-flow or air–water syringe
   d. low speed handpiece

5. List the main dental instruments that would be placed on the tray for each of the following procedures:
   a. prophylactic and oral examination
   b. amalgam restoration
   c. composite restoration
   d. surgical extraction

6. If teeth are brushed correctly, why must they be flossed?

7. Differentiate between general anesthesia, analgesia or sedation, local anesthesia, and topical anesthesia.

8. State the main function of a dental varnish, base, cement, and temporary.

9. Why is mercury dangerous? List four (4) safety precautions that must be observed while working with mercury and dental amalgam.

10. Draw a diagram of the 14 periapical films for a full-mouth series of X-rays. Identify the teeth that are shown in each film.

UNIT 17

SUGGESTED REFERENCES

American Dental Association, *Dental Letters with Impact.* Chicago, IL: American Dental Association, 2001.

Bird, Doni, Debbie Robinson, and Audrey Behrans. *Modern Dental Assisting.* 6th ed. Philadelphia, PA: W. B. Saunders, 2001.

Bird, William, Carol Hatrick, and W. Stephen Eakle. *Dental Materials: Clinical Applications for Dental Assistants and Dental Hygienists.* Philadelphia, PA: W. B. Saunders, 2002.

Chernega, Janet. *Emergency Guide for Dental Auxiliaries.* 3rd ed. Clifton Park, NY: Delmar Learning, 2002.

Colwell Systems. *Dental Appointment Forms Kit.* Champaign, IL: Colwell Systems, n.d.

Craig, Robert, Joan Powers, and John Wataha. *Dental Materials: Properties and Manipulation.* 7th ed. St. Louis, MO: Mosby, 1999.

Davidson, Judith Ann. *Legal and Ethical Considerations for Dental Hygienists and Assistants.* St. Louis, MO: Mosby, 1999.

Dietz, Ellen. *Dental Office Managment.* Clifton Park, NY: Delmar Learning, 2000.

Dietz, Ellen. *Safety Standards and Infection Control for Dental Assistants.* Clifton Park, NY: Delmar Learning, 2002.

Dofka, Charline. *Dental Terminology.* Clifton Park, NY: Delmar Learning, 2000.

Ferracane, Jack. *Materials in Dentistry.* Philadelphia, PA: Lippincott, Williams, & Wikins, 2001.

Finkbeiner, Betty, and Charles Allan Finkbeiner. *Practice Management for the Dental Team.* 5th ed. St. Louis, MO: Mosby, 2001.

Frommer, Herbert. *Radiology for Dental Auxiliaries.* 7th ed. St. Louis, MO: Mosby, 2000.

Graf, Jill. *Dental Charting: A Standard Approach.* Clifton Park, NY: Delmar Learning, 2000.

Miyasaki-Ching, Cara. *Chasteen's Essentials of Clinical Dental Assisting.* St. Louis, MO: Mosby, 2001.

Novak, Darlene. *Contemporary Dental Assisting.* St. Louis, MO: Mosby, 2000.

Pendleton, Alice, and Pauline Anderson. *The Dental Assistant.* 7th ed. Clifton Park, NY: Delmar Learning, 2001.

Phinney, Donna, and Judy Halstead. *Delmar's Dental Assisting: A Comprehensive Approach.* Clifton Park, NY: Delmar Learning, 2000.

Phinney, Donna, and Judy Halstead. *Delmar's Handbook of Essential Skills and Procedures for Chairside Dental Assisting.* Clifton Park, NY: Delmar Learning, 2002.

Schuster, Greg, Greg Wetterhus, and Phyllis Dryden. *Handbook of Clinical Dental Assisting.* Philadelphia, PA: W. B. Saunders, 1999.

Scott, Ann Senisi, and Elizabeth Fong. *Body Structures and Functions.* 9th ed. Clifton Park, NY: Delmar Learning, 1998.

Short, Marjorie J. *Head, Neck & Dental Anatomy.* 3rd ed. Clifton Park, NY: Delmar Learning, 2002.

Thibodeaus, Melissa. *Delmar's Dental Exam Review.* Clifton Park, NY: Delmar Learning, 2000.

Woelfel, Julian, and Rickne Scheid. *Dental Anatomy.* Philadelphia, PA: Lippincott, Williams, & Wilkins, 2001.

For additional information on dental careers, contact the following associations:

◆ American Dental Assistants' Association
203 N. Lasalle, Suite 1320
Chicago, Illinois 60611
Internet address: *www.dentalassistant.org*

◆ American Dental Association
211 E. Chicago Avenue
Chicago, Illinois 60611
Internet address: *www.ada.org*

◆ American Dental Hygienists' Association
444 N. Michigan Avenue, Suite 3400
Chicago, Illinois 60611
Internet address: *www.adha.org*

◆ National Association of Dental Laboratories
1530 Metropolitan Boulevard
Tallahassee, FL 32308
Internet address: *www.nadl.org*

UNIT 18

Laboratory Assistant Skills

Unit Objectives

After completing this unit of study, you should be able to:

- ◆ Operate the microscope and identify its parts
- ◆ Obtain a culture specimen without contaminating it
- ◆ Streak an agar plate or slide
- ◆ Stain a bacterial slide using the Gram's stain technique
- ◆ Puncture the skin to obtain blood, observing all safety factors
- ◆ Perform a microhematocrit
- ◆ Perform a hemoglobin test with a hemoglobinometer and a photometer
- ◆ Count white blood cells and red blood cells using a hemacytometer counting chamber
- ◆ Prepare and stain a blood smear using Wright's stain
- ◆ Test blood for type and Rh factors using anti-serums
- ◆ Perform an erythrocyte sedimentation rate (ESR)
- ◆ Measure blood-sugar (glucose) level
- ◆ Test urine using a reagent strip
- ◆ Measure specific gravity of urine
- ◆ Prepare urine for sedimentation examination
- ◆ Define, pronounce, and spell all the key terms

 Observe Standard Precautions

 Safety—Proceed with Caution

 Math Skill

 Science Skill

 C Communications Skill

 Instructors Check—Call Instructor at This Point

 OBRA OBRA Requirement— Based on Federal Law

 Legal Responsibility

 Career Information

 Technology

550

KEY TERMS

agar plate

antibody screen

anticoagulant
   (an"-tie-coh-ag'-you-lant)

antigen
   (an'-tih-jen")

anuria
   (ah-nur'-ree"-ah)

blood smear

culture specimen

differential count

direct smear

erythrocyte counts
   (eh-rith'-row-site")

erythrocyte sedimentation rate

fasting blood sugar

glucose

glycosuria
   (gly"-coh-shur'-ee-ah)

Gram's stain

hemacytometer
   (hee"-ma-sy-tom'-et-er)

hematocrit
   (hih"-mat'-oh-krit)

hematuria
   (hee"-mah-tyour'-ee-ah)

hemoglobin
   (hee'-mow-glow"-bin)

hemolysis
   (hih"-mall'-ah-sis)

hyperglycemia
   (high"-purr-gly-see'-me-ah)

hypoglycemia
   (high"-poh-gly-see'-me-ah)

leukocyte counts

microscope

oliguria
   (oh"-lih-goo'-ree-ah)

polyuria

reagent strips

refractometer
   (ree-frack-tum'-ee-ter)

resistant

sensitive

skin puncture

specific gravity

typing and crossmatch

urinalysis
   (your'-in-al'-ee-sis)

urinary sediment

urinometer

venipuncture

CAREER HIGHLIGHTS

Medical, or clinical, laboratory personnel work under the supervision of doctors, usually pathologists. They are important members of the health care team. They perform laboratory tests on body tissues, fluids, and cells to aid in the detection, diagnosis, and treatment of disease. Levels of personnel are the technologist, technician, and laboratory assistant. Medical laboratory technologists perform more complex tests and usually have a bachelor's or master's degree. Medical laboratory technicians perform less complex tests and usually have an associate's degree. Medical laboratory assistants perform basic laboratory tests and usually have specialized health occupation education training. Some states require laboratory personnel to be licensed or registered. Certification can be obtained from the American Society for Clinical Laboratory Science or the American Medical Technologists Association, each of which has specific requirements.

Any medical laboratory or medical office that performs tests on human specimens is regulated by a federal amendment called the Clinical Laboratory Improvement Amendment (CLIA) of 1998. CLIA established standards, regulations, and performance requirements based on the complexity of a test and the risk factors associated with incorrect results. Levels of complexity include waived tests (including provider-performed microscopy tests or PPM), moderately complex tests, and highly complex tests. Each of these levels has different requirements for personnel and quality control. Laboratories are certified by the United States Department of Health and Human Services (USDHHS) based on these levels. Therefore, *medical laboratory assistants/medical assistants must follow all legal requirements before performing any laboratory test.* Some examples of waived tests, or tests that can be performed by assistants if the agency where they are working has a CLIA waiver certificate, include:

◆ Most urinary reagent strip or reagent tablet tests

◆ Spun microhematocrit

◆ Erythrocyte sedimentation rate (nonautomated)

◆ Hemoglobin: copper sulfate (nonautomated) or automated by instruments with self-contained components to perform specimen-reagent interaction and provide direct measurement and readout

◆ Blood glucose by glucose testing devices cleared by the Federal Drug Administration

◆ Ovulation and pregnancy tests by visual color comparison

◆ Fecal occult blood

◆ Cholesterol monitoring by specific kits

◆ Rapid streptococcal identification by specific kits

◆ Gastric occult blood

Many of the waived tests are discussed in this unit. In addition to the knowledge and skills presented in this unit, medical laboratory assistants must also learn and master skills such as:

◆ Presenting a professional appearance and attitude

◆ Obtaining knowledge regarding health care delivery systems, organizational structure, and teamwork

◆ Meeting all legal responsibilities

◆ Communicating effectively

◆ Being sensitive to and respecting cultural diversity

◆ Comprehending human anatomy, physiology, and pathophysiology with an emphasis on cells, tissues, and body fluids, especially blood and urine

◆ Learning medical terminology

◆ Observing all safety precautions

◆ Practicing all principles of infection control

◆ Performing other duties such as answering the telephone, scheduling appointments, preparing correspondence, completing insurance forms, maintaining accounts, and maintaining patient records

◆ Utilizing computer skills

◆ Cleaning and maintaining laboratory equipment

◆ Ordering and maintaining supplies and materials

18:1 INFORMATION *Operating the Microscope*

The **microscope** is a valuable tool used in many health professions. In order to obtain the desired results when working with the microscope, it is important that you first become familiar with its parts and how to use them correctly.

Many different models of microscopes are available. A *monocular microscope* has one eyepiece, and a *binocular microscope* has two eyepieces. The quality of microscopes also varies, according to the type of lenses, attachments, and magnification ability. The compound, bright-field microscope, described in this unit, is one of the most commonly used microscopes. An epifluorescence microscope is used to detect antibodies and specific organisms by using a fluorescent dye stain. An electron microscope, which is extremely expensive and requires special expertise to operate, uses electron beams instead of a light source to view objects. Electron microscopes are used to view extremely small objects such as cell organelles and viruses. However, all microscopes have one basic purpose. They are designed to magnify or enlarge objects so the objects become more visible.

Most microscopes contain the same basic parts. A list and a brief description of the function of each part follows. Parts are shown in figure 18-1.

◆ *Base:* The solid stand on which the microscope rests.

◆ *Arm:* The long, back stem of the microscope. In most cases the arm is used to carry the microscope.

◆ *Eyepiece(s):* The part(s) of the microscope through which the eye views the object or slide. The eyepiece usually has a magnification power of 10X (ten times). This means

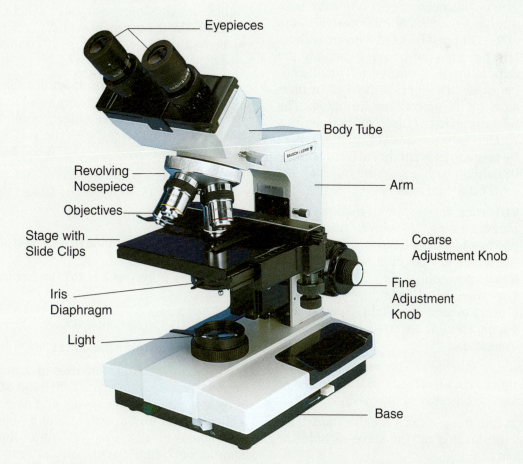

Eyepieces

Body Tube

Revolving Nosepiece

Arm

Objectives

Stage with Slide Clips

Coarse Adjustment Knob

Iris Diaphragm

Fine Adjustment Knob

Light

Base

FIGURE 18-1 Parts of a microscope.

that it makes the object on the slide appear ten times larger than normal. Some microscopes have zoom lenses. On these, the magnification can range from 10X to 20X, depending on how the eyepiece is positioned. Special lens paper should be used to clean the eyepiece to avoid scratching the lenses. The eyepiece is also called the *ocular viewpiece.*

◆ *Objectives:* The parts of the microscope that magnify the object being viewed. They work with the eyepiece. A microscope may have three or four objectives, and they can vary. Some of the more common objectives are:

(1) The low-power objective is the shortest in length. It magnifies the object being viewed four times (4X).

(2) Another low-power objective magnifies the object ten times (10X).

(3) The high-power objectives magnify the object forty or forty-five times (40X or 45X).

(4) The oil-immersion (OI) objective usually has a magnification power of 95X to 100X. Oil must be used with this objective because the image is usually too dark to be seen otherwise. The oil concentrates the light. A drop of immersion oil is placed on the slide. The oil-immersion objective is carefully rotated into the drop of oil. Care must be taken to prevent the oil from coming in contact with any of the other objectives on the microscope.

NOTE: Smaller specimens require greater magnification. However, the high-power objectives have small openings. Therefore, to view small specimens, use a high-power objective and more light. For large specimens, use low-power objectives and less light. Special lens paper should be used to clean the objectives.

◆ *Revolving nosepiece:* The section to which the objectives are attached. It is turned to change the objective being used.

◆ *Stage:* The flat platform for the slide. Slide clips are located on the stage to hold the slide in place.

◆ *Coarse adjustment:* The larger knob on the arm. It moves the objectives up and down and also brings the slide into rough focus. The coarse adjustment should be used only on the low power (10X) objective. It is important to watch the stage while moving the objectives to avoid breaking the slide and/or objectives.

◆ *Fine adjustment:* The smaller knob on the arm. It moves the objectives slowly for a precise and clear image. The fine adjustment is used on the low-power (10X), high-power (40–45X), and oil immersion (95–100X) objectives.

◆ *Iris diaphragm:* A circular structure directly underneath the stage. The diaphragm controls the amount of light that enters the microscope through the bottom of the stage. To increase or decrease the amount of light, turn the diaphragm to a larger or smaller hole.

◆ *Illuminating light:* Located under the stage, the illuminating light provides the necessary light for viewing; the amount of light is controlled by the iris diaphragm.

◆ *Body Tube:* The section that connects the eyepiece and the objectives.

To determine total magnification of an object (how many times you are magnifying or enlarging the object) multiply the power of the eyepiece times the power of the objective in use.

◆ *Example 1:* If the eyepiece is 10X and the objective is 4X, multiply the 10 and the 4.

$$10 \times 4 = 40$$

The object is magnified or enlarged 40 times its original size.

◆ *Example 2:* Eyepiece is 20X, and objective is 40X.

$$20 \times 40 = 800$$

You are enlarging the object 800 times.

Proper care and cleaning of any microscope is important because dirt and dust can interfere with proper viewing and damage the delicate glass on the eyepiece and objectives. The glass in the eyepiece and objectives should be cleaned with special lens paper.

Paper towels, tissues, and cloths can scratch the delicate glass. The rest of the microscope should be wiped clean with a damp, soft cloth after use. When oil is used with an oil-immersion objective, the oil should be wiped off immediately after use because it can seep into the lens case. Before storing the microscope, the low-power objective should be in place and the nosepiece should be moved to its lowest position. When the microscope is not in use, it should be covered with a dust cover or stored in a dust-free cabinet. It is also important to avoid jarring or bumping the microscope because it is a delicate instrument. To carry or move a microscope, place one hand firmly on the arm and the other hand under the base (see figure 18-2). Always put the microscope down gently when placing it on a desk or counter. Before using any microscope, read and follow the specific operating instructions provided by the manufacturer.

STUDENT: *Go to the workbook and complete the assignment sheet for 18:1, Operating the Microscope. Then return and continue with the procedure.*

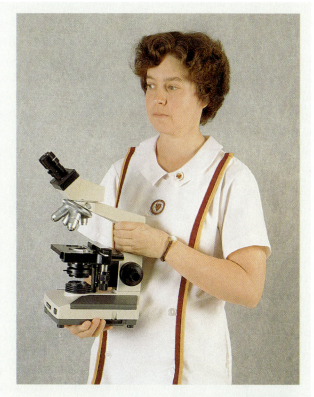

FIGURE 18-2 To carry a microscope, place one hand firmly on the arm and your other hand under the base.

PROCEDURE 18:1

Operating the Microscope

Equipment and Supplies

Microscope; lens paper; slide and cover slip; hair, paper, or other small object; drop of water; immersion oil

Procedure

1. Assemble equipment.
2. Wash hands.

    CAUTION: Wear gloves and observe standard precautions while handling any specimen contaminated by blood or body fluids, or while examining pathogenic organisms.

3. Use a prepared slide or get a clean slide. Place a human hair, shred of paper, or other small object on the slide. Add a drop of water or normal saline. Cover with a clean cover slip by holding the cover slip at an angle and allowing it to drop on the specimen.

    NOTE: Make sure there are no air bubbles between the slide and cover slip. If air bubbles are present, remove the cover slip and position it again.

4. Use lens paper to clean the eyepiece (ocular viewpiece) and the objectives.

     CAUTION: Do not use any other material to clean these surfaces. Towels, rags, and tissues can scratch these surfaces.

5. Turn on the illuminating light. Open the iris diaphragm so that the largest hole is located directly under the hole in the stage platform.

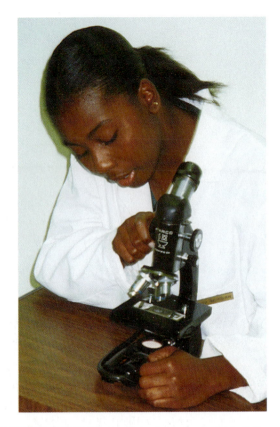

FIGURE 18-3 Watch the stage and slide while using the coarse adjustment to move the objective downward.

6. Turn the revolving nosepiece until the low-power objective clicks into place.

7. Place the slide on the stage. Fasten it with the slide clips.
   NOTE: Avoid getting fingerprints or smudges on the slide.

8. Watch the stage and slide (see figure 18-3). Turn the coarse adjustment so that the objective moves down close to the slide.
   CAUTION: Do *not* look into the eyepiece while moving the objective down. The objective could crack the slide and/or be damaged.

9. Now, look through the eyepiece. Slowly turn the body tube upward until the object comes into focus.

10. Change to the fine adjustment. Turn the knob slowly until the object comes into its sharpest focus.

11. Do the following while still using low power:
    a. Move the slide to the right while looking through the eyepiece. In which direction does the image move?
    b. Move the slide to the left. In which direction does the image move?

c. Open and close the iris diaphragm. How does this affect the image?

12. Without moving the body tube, turn the revolving nosepiece until the high-power objective is in place. Focus with the fine adjustment only.
    CAUTION: Watch the slide while turning the objectives to avoid breaking the slide or objectives.

13. Under high power, make the following observations:
    a. How does the amount of light compare with that needed under low power? (You may need to adjust the diaphragm for better viewing.)
    b. Do you see a larger or a smaller area of the object than was seen under low power?

14. If the microscope has an oil-immersion objective, do the following:
    a. Turn the revolving nosepiece until the oil-immersion objective is in position. Focus with fine adjustment only.
       CAUTION: Watch the slide while turning the objectives to avoid breaking the slide or objectives.
    b. Move the oil-immersion objective slightly to either side so that no objective is in position.
    c. Place a small drop of immersion oil on the part of the slide that will be directly under the objective.
       CAUTION: Use the oil sparingly.
    d. Move the oil-immersion objective back into position, taking care that no other objective comes in contact with the oil. Make sure that the oil-immersion objective is touching the drop of oil.
    e. Look through the eyepiece and use the fine adjustment to bring the slide into focus.
    f. Move the diaphragm as necessary to adjust the amount of light for viewing the slide.
    g. When you are done viewing the slide, turn the revolving nosepiece until the low-power objective is in position.
       CAUTION: Make sure no other objective comes in contact with the oil on the slide.
    h. Use lens paper to carefully remove all the oil from the oil-immersion objective.

15. When you are done viewing the slide, remove the slide and the coverslip. Wash and dry both items.

⚠ **CAUTION:** Handle both with care. They break easily.

16. Use the special lens paper to clean the eyepiece and the objectives.

⚠ **CAUTION:** Do *not* use any other material to clean these parts. Towels, rags, and tissues can scratch these surfaces.

17. Use a damp, soft cloth to wipe the other parts of the microscope.

18. Using the coarse adjustment, move the low-power objective so that it is in its lowest position, down close to the stage.

19. Turn off the illuminating light.

20. Place the cover back on the microscope. This protects it from dust in the room. The microscope can also be stored in a dust-free cabinet.

⚠ **CAUTION:** Remember to place one hand on the arm and the other hand under the base while moving the microscope.

21. Make sure that the microscope is kept away from the counter's edge. This prevents the microscope from being knocked to the floor.

22. Clean and replace all equipment.

23. Remove gloves. Wash hands.

Practice *Go to the workbook and use the evaluation sheet for 18:1, Operating the Microscope, to practice this procedure. When you feel you have mastered this skill, sign the sheet and give it to your instructor for further action.*

✔ **Final Checkpoint** Using the criteria listed on the evaluation sheet, your instructor will grade your performance.

18:2 INFORMATION Obtaining and Handling Cultures

 In some health careers, it may be necessary for you to obtain a specimen of microorganisms, grow them on a culture medium, and stain a small sample.

A **culture specimen** is obtained when a doctor wants to identify the causative agent of a disease. The sample specimen is then either examined promptly or grown and examined for identification. Specimens may be obtained from a variety of sites, including lesions on the skin or from the eyes, ears, nose, throat, or other body openings. Care must be taken while obtaining a specimen. A sterile applicator swab should be used to prevent contamination from other sources. The specimen must be kept moist and free from contact with other things once it has been obtained.

Sometimes, the specimen is placed immediately on a slide. This is called a **direct smear,** or bacteriological smear. The swab containing the culture specimen is rolled across the surface of the slide to place a thin film of culture material on the slide. The smear is air dried and heat-fixed, or passed through a flame, so the organisms will adhere, or stick, to the slide. After the direct smear is stained so that organisms are visible, it is examined by a qualified individual, and the organism causing the disease is tentatively identified.

Other times, the specimen is placed or streaked on an **agar plate,** also called a *culture plate* or *petri dish,* or in a culture media tube (see figure 18-4). Agar is a special solid medium

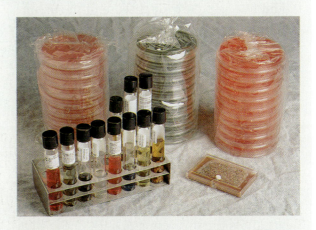

FIGURE 18-4 There are many different types of agar plates and media tubes.

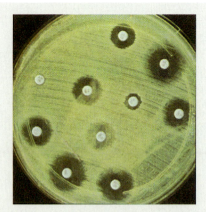

FIGURE 18-5 An agar plate prepared for a sensitivity study with small antibiotic disks positioned on the plate.

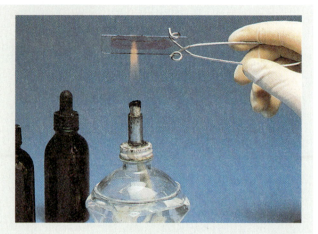

FIGURE 18-6 The slide is fixed with heat so organisms will adhere (stick) to the slide.

that provides both nourishment and moisture for the organism. The agar plate is placed in an incubator at 35° to 37°C for 24 to 36 hours, and the organism is grown. This is called *culturing an organism*. A small sample of the cultured organism (called a *colony*) is placed on a slide, stained, and then examined for identification. Exact identification sometimes requires growing a sample of the cultured organism (the colony) on another special medium, which helps differentiate the microorganisms. In this manner, the organism can be isolated.

In some instances, a culture and sensitivity study is done. Small, sterile disks containing different antibiotics are placed on the agar plate after the organism has been applied (see figure 18-5). If the organisms grow up to the edge of a particular disk, this means the organism is **resistant** to that antibiotic. The antibiotic would *not* work against the organism and would not help cure the disease. If the organisms do not grow close to the disk, this means the organisms are **sensitive** to the antibiotic on the disk. This antibiotic would work against the organism and aid in the curing of the disease. In this manner, a doctor is better able to determine which drug to give a patient for the disease or infection.

Before a slide that has been smeared with microorganisms can be stained, the slide must be fixed. To fix a slide, it must be held over a source of heat, such as a bunsen burner or alcohol lamp, for a very brief period of time. The heat causes the organisms to stick to the slide

(see figure 18-6). As a result, the organisms will not wash off of the slide when various solutions or stains are applied to the slide.

A common technique for staining cultures is the **Gram's stain.** This staining technique not only colors the organisms so that they are visible, but also provides another method of identifying organisms. The Gram's stain technique involves the following four steps:

1. Gentian violet or crystal violet stain is applied to the slide for approximately 1 minute. This is called the *primary dye*. It is purple in color. Any organism that keeps the purple color at the end of the procedure is a gram-positive organism.

2. Iodine is applied to the slide for approximately 1 minute. This solution sets the gentian violet or crystal violet stain, or makes the primary dye adhere to the organisms on the slide.

3. A 95-percent solution of ethyl alcohol or an acetone–alcohol decolorizer is applied to the slide until the solution running off the slide is no longer purple in color. This alcohol solution removes the purple color of the gentian violet or crystal violet stain from gram-negative organisms. Only gram-positive organisms retain the purple color after this step.

4. Safranin solution is applied to the slide for approximately 30 to 60 seconds. This solution is a counterstain. It stains the gram-negative organisms red so that they can be seen under a microscope.

NOTE: Times may vary depending on the type of stain used. Read and follow the manufacturer's instructions.

After the slide is stained, organisms on the slide are identified as *gram positive* if they retain the purple color of the gentian violet or crystal violet stain, and *gram negative* if they retain the red color of the safranin solution. A qualified lab technologist or physician examines the slide. By noting the shape of the organism and whether it is gram positive or negative, a preliminary identification of the type of organism can be made.

Because any culture may contain pathogenic (disease-producing) organisms or be contaminated with blood and body fluids, standard precautions (see Unit 13:3) must be observed at all times while handling cultures. Hands must be washed frequently and thoroughly, and gloves must be worn. Protective clothing such as lab coats or lab aprons must be worn. If splashing of specimens is possible, a mask and protective eyewear must be worn. All culture specimens and disposable equipment contaminated with the culture are placed in an infectious-waste bag for disposal according to legal requirements for infectious waste. Any lab counter or contaminated area must be wiped immediately with a disinfectant solution.

STUDENT: *Go to the workbook and complete the assignment sheet for 18:2, Obtaining and Handling Cultures. Then return and continue with the procedures.*

PROCEDURE 18:2A

Obtaining a Culture Specimen

Equipment and Supplies

Sterile cotton applicator swabs, culture medium (some prepacked with sterile swabs), sterile test tube with medium (if no prepacked medium), label, pen or pencil for marking, disposable gloves, infectious-waste bag

Procedure

1. Check physician's written order or obtain an order from your immediate supervisor.
2. Assemble equipment.
3. Wash hands. Put on gloves.

    CAUTION: Observe standard precautions while obtaining and handling the culture specimen. If splashing of specimens is possible, a gown, mask, and eye protection must be worn.

4. **C** Introduce yourself. Greet and identify the patient. Explain the procedure to the patient. Obtain the patient's consent.
5. Check the body area where the specimen is to be obtained. The order should state the site for taking the specimen.

    NOTE: Specimens can be taken from the nose, throat, or other body areas, or from open wounds.

6. Remove the sterile applicator from its package. Pick it up by the wooden end only. Make sure you do not touch the sterile cotton tip to any surface or contaminate it in any way (see figure 18-7A).

    CAUTION: If the tip does not remain sterile, the test will be inaccurate.

7. Place the sterile tip on the area to be cultured. Use a gentle yet firm rotating motion to cover the tip of the applicator with a sample specimen (see figure 18-7B).
8. Remove the applicator from the culture site. Be careful not to contaminate the tip.
9. Place the applicator into the sterile tube or culture-medium container.

    CAUTION: Take care not to touch the sides of the container, because the specimen will smear against the sides of the container instead of being placed in the medium.

    NOTE: Brace your arms against your body to keep your hands steady while inserting the applicator swab.

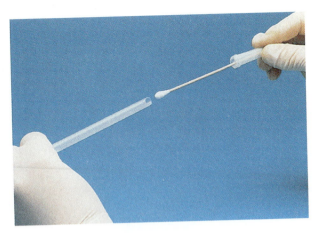

FIGURE 18-7A Take care not to contaminate the sterile tip as you remove the sterile applicator from its package.

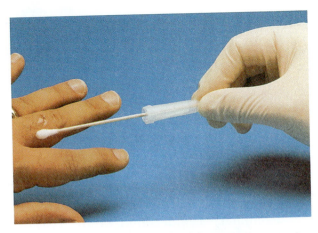

FIGURE 18-7B Rotate the applicator tip to obtain a specimen from the site.

10. Check to be sure the tip is in the medium.
    NOTE: This keeps the specimen sterile and moist for examination.
    NOTE: Some culture-medium tubes contain a liquid culture medium separated from a gauze layer by a thin layer of glass or other material. In order to saturate the gauze layer with the liquid medium, it is necessary to squeeze the container gently to break the glass or other material (see figure 18-7C). Read and follow the manufacturer's instructions when using any culture-medium container.

11. Label the specimen with the patient's name, address, identification number, doctor's name, the date, the type of test ordered, and the site from which the specimen was obtained.

12. Take or send the specimen to the laboratory. If you will be transferring the specimen to a slide or an agar plate, place the specimen in a safe location until you are ready to use it. Keep it away from direct sunlight and sources of heat.

13. Clean and replace all equipment. Place all contaminated disposable materials in the infectious-waste bag. Use a disinfectant to wipe the counter and any contaminated areas.

14. Remove gloves. Wash hands thoroughly.

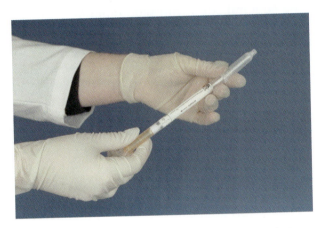

FIGURE 18-7C Squeeze the container gently to crush the glass and release the culture medium.

Practice *Go to the workbook and use the evaluation sheet for 18:2A, Obtaining a Culture Specimen, to practice this procedure. When you feel you have mastered this skill, sign the sheet and give it to your instructor for further action.*

 Final Checkpoint Using the criteria listed on the evaluation sheet, your instructor will grade your performance.

PROCEDURE 18:2B

Preparing a Direct Smear

Equipment and Supplies

Culture specimen for direct smear, clean glass slide, bunsen burner or alcohol lamp, staining rack, rubber-tipped hemostats or slide clamps, disposable gloves, infectious-waste bag

Procedure

1. Assemble equipment.
2. Wash hands. Put on gloves.
   CAUTION: Observe standard precautions while handling any culture specimen.
3. Clean the slide thoroughly. Avoid touching the top of the slide once it has been cleaned.
4. Carefully remove the specimen from the medium tube. Handle the applicator by the wooden end only.
   CAUTION: Avoid contaminating the applicator tip.
5. Use the thumb and forefinger of one hand to pick up the clean slide. Hold it securely. The slide can also be placed on a table or counter and held securely.
6. Place the tip of the applicator swab containing the culture on the slide approximately 1/2 inch away from the thumb holding the slide.
7. Hold the applicator tip firmly on the slide and roll it toward the opposite end of the slide. Use firm, even pressure to allow for the transfer of the organisms to the slide (see figure 18-8). Stop ½ inch from the end of the slide.
8. Allow the slide to dry at room temperature.
   CAUTION: If the slide does not dry prior to being fixed, the heat from fixing the slide will drive the moisture out of the organisms, and distort their shape.
9. Dispose of the contaminated applicator swab by placing it in an infectious-waste bag.
   CAUTION: Handle the swab carefully to avoid infecting yourself or contaminating other surfaces.
10. When the slide is dry, place it in a set of rubber-tipped hemostats or slide clamps. Make sure the smear side is facing upward.
11. Turn on the bunsen burner or alcohol lamp.
    CAUTION: If a match is used to turn on the flame, extinguish the match and then hold it under water before putting it in a trash container.
12. Hold the clamped slide 1 to 2 inches above the flame for 1 to 2 seconds. Do this three to four times. Do *not* get the slide too hot. Check the temperature by touching the bottom of the slide lightly on your hand. It should feel warm but not too hot.
    NOTE: This is called *fixing*. The heat causes the organisms to stick to the slide.
    CAUTION: Excess heat will shrink the organisms, and they will no longer be identifiable.
13. Place the slide on the staining rack; the slide must be stained prior to being viewed.
14. Label the slide with the patient's name, doctor's name, address, identification number, and any other necessary information.
15. Clean and replace all equipment. Place all contaminated disposable materials in the infectious-waste bag. Use a disinfectant to wipe the counter and any contaminated areas.

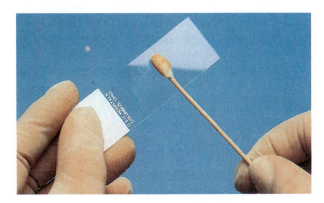

FIGURE 18-8 Roll the applicator tip across the slide to transfer the organisms to the slide.

16. Make sure the bunsen burner or alcohol lamp is extinguished.
17. Remove gloves. Wash hands thoroughly.

> **Practice** *Go to the workbook and use the evaluation sheet for 18:2B, Preparing a Direct Smear, to practice this procedure. When you feel you have mastered this skill, sign the sheet and give it to your instructor for further action.*

 Final Checkpoint Using the criteria listed on the evaluation sheet, your instructor will grade your performance.

PROCEDURE 18:2C
Streaking an Agar Plate

Equipment and Supplies

Agar plate with correct medium, specimen for direct smear, label, pen or marker, incubator, disposable gloves, infectious-waste bag

Procedure

1. Assemble equipment.
2. Wash hands. Put on gloves.

    CAUTION: Observe standard precautions while handling any culture specimen.

3. Remove the applicator containing the culture specimen from its tube. Hold it by the wooden end. Take care to avoid contaminating the applicator tip. Look at the tip to be sure it is still moist.

    NOTE: If the specimen is dry, the organisms have probably died, and the results will not be accurate.

4. The agar plate is made up of two parts: the lower disk, which contains the agar, and the upper lid. Open the agar plate. Take care not to touch the inside of the plate. Invert the lid: that is, place the lid with the top against the counter. In this way, the inside of the lid stays clean.

    NOTE: The agar plate can also be placed upside down, with the agar on top. The agar plate should then be lifted. The lid will remain on the table, with the inside facing up.

5. Hold the plate firmly in one hand (see figure 18-9A) or place it on a flat surface.
6. Starting at the top of the agar, gently place the applicator tip in one corner. Using a rotary motion, turning the top of the tip so that all sides of the tip touch the agar, go from side to side approximately one-quarter of the way down the plate. To cover the second quadrant of the plate, turn the plate one-quarter turn and repeat the side-to-side motion of the applicator tip, crossing the first quadrant two to three times. Turn the

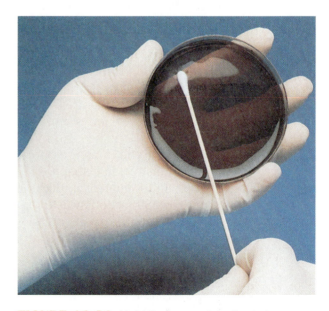

FIGURE 18-9A Hold the agar plate firmly in one hand while streaking it with the specimen.

plate one-quarter turn and use the same motion to cover the third quadrant. To cover the fourth quadrant, turn the plate one-quarter turn, and cross into the third quadrant one or two times. Note the sample streaking pattern in figure 18-9B. This streaking method helps isolate the colonies of organisms in the fourth quadrant (see figure 18-9C).

NOTE: This is only one type of streaking pattern.

⚠ **CAUTION:** Be gentle. Do not break into the agar.

NOTE: An innoculating loop can also be used to streak the agar. After each quadrant is streaked, the loop is placed in a flame and cooled. Use the method the laboratory or physician prefers.

NOTE: Cover the agar only one time in each area. Do *not* go back over areas already covered.

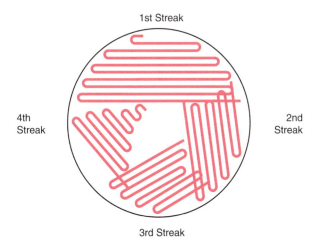

FIGURE 18-9B A sample streaking pattern.

7. Check to be sure all areas of the agar have been streaked. Different streaking methods can be used. Use the one the laboratory or physician prefers.

8. Discard the applicator swab in the infectious-waste bag or a biohazard container. Some laboratories require the swab to be placed in a container of disinfectant prior to disposal in an infectious-waste bag.

9. If a sensitivity study is to be done, place antibiotic disks on the agar. You can use an automatic dispenser of medicated disks to do so. If an automatic dispenser is not available, use sterile thumb forceps. Place the disks around the agar. Leave spaces between the disks. Make sure that the disks are not too close to the edge of the agar plate (refer to figure 18-5).

    NOTE: The agar plate must be streaked heavily and completely for a sensitivity study.

10. Pick up the agar plate lid by the side edges. Take care not to touch the inside. Place the lid on top of the agar plate.

    NOTE: The agar plate can be placed into the lid instead, but be careful not to contaminate the insides.

11. Label the bottom of the agar plate with the patient's name, doctor's name, address, identification number, date, time, site of specimen, and other required information.

12. Invert the agar plate and place it in the incubator at 35° to 37°C for 24 to 36 hours (see figure 18-9D). Be sure the plate is upside down with the agar on top. This prevents moisture from settling on the agar.

    NOTE: The incubator provides darkness and warmth for growth of the organism. The

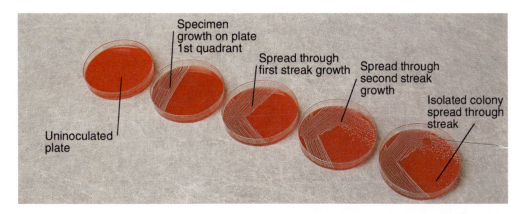

FIGURE 18-9C Note the isolated colonies of organisms in the fourth quadrant after the culture has grown in the incubator.

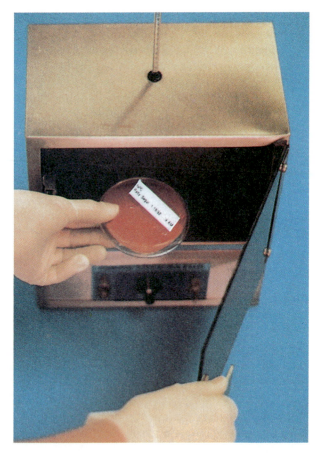

FIGURE 18-9D Invert the agar plate and place it in the incubator for 24 to 36 hours at 35° to 37°C.

agar provides food and moisture to stimulate growth.

13. Check the temperature of the incubator. It is usually set at 35° to 37° Celsius (95° to 99° Fahrenheit).

14. Clean and replace all equipment. Place all contaminated disposable equipment in the infectious-waste bag. Use a disinfectant to wipe the counter and any contaminated areas.

15. Remove gloves. Wash hands thoroughly to prevent infection and spread of the disease.

Practice *Go to the workbook and use the evaluation sheet for 18:2C, Streaking an Agar Plate, to practice this procedure. When you feel you have mastered this skill, sign the sheet and give it to your instructor for further action.*

 Final Checkpoint Using the criteria listed on the evaluation sheet, your instructor will grade your performance.

PROCEDURE 18:2D

Transferring Culture from Agar Plate to Slide

Equipment and Supplies

Agar plate with growth, innoculating loop, bunsen burner or alcohol lamp, rubber-tipped hemostat or slide clamps, slide, normal saline solution, staining rack, disposable gloves, infectious-waste bag, pen or pencil

Procedure

1. Assemble equipment.
2. Wash hands. Put on gloves.

    CAUTION: Observe standard precautions while handling any culture specimen.

3. Light the bunsen burner or alcohol lamp.

    CAUTION: Wet the match before discarding it in a trash can.

4. Open the agar plate. Handle the outside of the plate only. To prevent contamination, place the lid with the top against the counter (that is, with the inside facing up).

    NOTE: The agar plate can also be placed upside down, with the agar on top. The agar plate should then be lifted. The lid will remain on the table, with the inside facing up.

5. Place the innoculating loop in the flame until the loop end gets red hot.

    NOTE: This kills organisms that might be present on the loop.

6. Cool the loop by dipping it into an area of agar that has no organisms present.

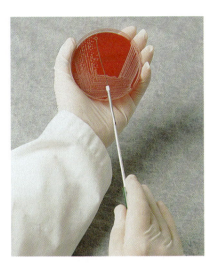

FIGURE 18-10 Dip the loop into a small portion of an isolated growth of the cultured organism.

> **NOTE:** A hot loop will destroy the shape of the organisms, making them unidentifiable.

7. Dip the loop into a small portion of the colony growth (see figure 18-10). Skim the top of the growth to get some organisms on the loop.

> **NOTE:** Only a small sample is needed. If too large a mass is obtained, the slide will be too concentrated.

8. Immediately place the lid on the agar plate to prevent contamination to yourself or the environment from the organism.

9. Place a small drop of normal saline on a clean glass slide.

> **NOTE:** Normal saline provides a liquid medium for the organisms.

10. Mix the specimen (on the loop) and the saline on the slide. This loosens the organisms and suspends them in liquid.

 CAUTION: Do not rub the mixture against the slide, because doing so could damage the shape of the organisms.

11. Starting at one end of the slide, spread the solution thinly over the slide. Cover the entire width with the culture.

12. Place the slide on the staining rack to air dry. Fix as previously taught.

13. Place the loop in the flame until red hot. This destroys all organisms.

14. Label the slide with the patient's name, doctor's name, address, identification number, and other required information.

15. Clean and replace all equipment. Place all contaminated disposable equipment in the infectious-waste bag. Use a disinfectant to wipe the counter and any contaminated areas.

16. Remove gloves. Wash hands thoroughly.

> **Practice** *Go to the workbook and use the evaluation sheet for 18:2D, Transferring Culture from Agar Plate to Slide, to practice this procedure. When you feel you have mastered this skill, sign the sheet and give it to your instructor for further action.*

✔ **Final Checkpoint** Using the criteria listed on the evaluation sheet, your instructor will grade your performance.

PROCEDURE 18:2E

Staining with Gram's Stain

Equipment and Supplies

Slide with fixed smear, staining rack, gentian violet or crystal violet stain, Gram's iodine, 95-percent ethyl alcohol or acetone–alcohol decolorizer, safranin solution, distilled water, asepto syringe or plastic squeeze bottle, disposable gloves, infectious-waste bag

> **NOTE:** Timing may vary with types of solutions used. Read the instructions provided with the solutions or follow agency policy.

Procedure

1. Assemble equipment.
2. Wash hands. Put on gloves.

CAUTION: Observe standard precautions while handling any culture specimen.

3. Use your thumb and forefinger to pick up the fixed slide. Place the slide on the staining rack. Check to be sure the smear side is facing up.

   CAUTION: Avoid touching the top of the slide with your fingers.

4. Cover the slide with gentian violet or crystal violet stain (see figure 18-11). Leave the stain in place for the recommended time, usually 1 minute. Stain only the smeared side of the slide. This is the primary dye.

   NOTE: To avoid staining the sink, it is best to let water run during the entire procedure.

   NOTE: The primary stain is purple and will dye all gram-positive organisms. Thus, any organisms that remain purple in color at the end of this procedure are gram-positive organisms.

5. Rinse the slide thoroughly with distilled water. Use an asepto syringe or plastic squeeze bottle to rinse gently.

6. Use Gram's iodine solution to cover the slide. Tilt the slide to allow the iodine and remaining water to run off. Then, cover the slide again with iodine. Leave in place for the recommended time, usually 1 minute. This sets the primary dye.

NOTE: The first application of iodine is allowed to run off the slide so that the second application will result in a full-strength iodine covering.

NOTE: Any gram-positive organisms will now have the purple primary dye set into them. After this step, gram-negative organisms will also be dyed purple. This dye must be removed.

7. Use an asepto syringe or plastic squeeze bottle to rinse the slide thoroughly with distilled water.

8. Use 95-percent ethyl alcohol or acetone–alcohol to decolorize the slide. Apply the alcohol to the slide. Immediately tilt the slide to allow the decolorizer to run off. Reapply the alcohol and again tilt the slide to allow the alcohol to run off. After each application, check the color of the alcohol as it runs off the slide. Stop immediately when the decolorizer is no longer purple. This usually occurs in 3 to 5 seconds.

   NOTE: This step removes the primary dye from the gram-negative organisms. Only the gram-positive organisms remain purple.

   CAUTION: This is a crucial step. Too many applications of alcohol can also decolorize gram-positive organisms. Stop as soon as the alcohol is no longer purple in color.

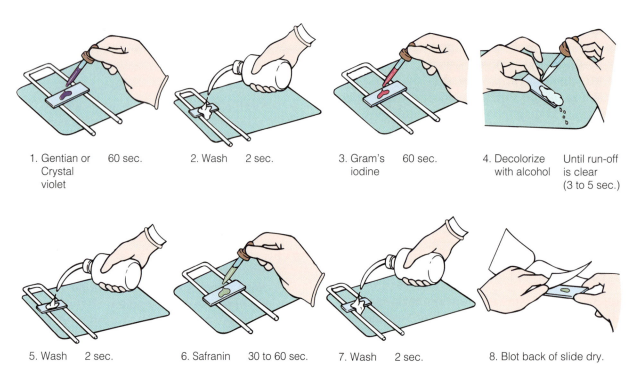

1. Gentian or   60 sec.
   Crystal
   violet

2. Wash   2 sec.

3. Gram's   60 sec.
   iodine

4. Decolorize   Until run-off
   with alcohol   is clear
                   (3 to 5 sec.)

5. Wash   2 sec.

6. Safranin   30 to 60 sec.

7. Wash   2 sec.

8. Blot back of slide dry.

FIGURE 18-11 The Gram's stain technique.

9. Rinse the slide well with distilled water to remove any remaining decolorizer.

10. Use safranin solution to counterstain the slide. Apply the safranin, tilt the slide to allow the safranin and remaining water to run off, and then reapply the safranin. This stain should remain on the slide for the recommended time, usually 30 to 60 seconds.
    NOTE: Safranin stains gram-negative organisms red so that they can be seen and identified under a microscope.

11. Use distilled water to rinse the slide.

12. Use a paper towel to dry the *back* of the slide. Do *not* dry the front, or smear, side because rubbing it can remove the smear from the slide. Allow the front of the slide to air dry.

13. Once dry, the slide is fairly permanent and is ready for microscopic examination. A laboratory technologist or doctor can examine the slide and identify the type of organism present by noting the shape and color. If purple, the organism is gram-positive; if red, it is gram-negative.

14. Clean the area thoroughly. Replace all equipment.
    NOTE: The dyes can permanently stain the counter if not removed immediately.

15. Remove gloves. Wash hands.

> **Practice** *Go to the workbook and use the evaluation sheet for 18:2E, Staining with Gram's Stain, to practice this procedure. When you feel you have mastered this skill, sign the sheet and give it to your instructor for further action.*

✔ **Final Checkpoint** Using the criteria listed on the evaluation sheet, your instructor will grade your performance.

18:3 INFORMATION Puncturing the Skin to Obtain Capillary Blood

Blood tests are often done to assist a physician in making a diagnosis. Depending on your chosen health career, you may be responsible for performing some basic blood tests. In order to do these tests, blood must be obtained. This section provides basic facts on performing a skin puncture to obtain blood. *No* procedures should be attempted without classroom instruction and supervision.

Blood for testing can be obtained in various ways. For many routine tests, a simple **skin puncture** provides a sufficient amount of blood. Skin punctures are used only for tests requiring small quantities of blood. This blood is obtained from the capillaries and is often called *peripheral blood.* For other tests requiring larger quantities of blood, a **venipuncture** is performed. In a venipuncture, the blood is taken from a vein. For still other tests, blood is taken from an artery. Arterial blood is used for specific tests such as those which measure the amount of blood gases (oxygen and carbon dioxide) or determine acid–base balance.

 Responsibility for obtaining blood for various blood tests varies. Liability should be checked for individual states. *In some states, health occupations students are not permitted to perform any procedure involving obtaining blood. It is vital that you determine what you are legally permitted to do.*

The procedure that follows discusses only the skin puncture. If you are required to do a venipuncture or to draw arterial blood, you need specific training in these procedures. Only legally qualified individuals should perform venipunctures and arterial punctures.

Careful aseptic technique must be followed while performing a skin puncture. The skin must be cleaned thoroughly with 70-percent isopropyl alcohol or a similar antiseptic. The lancet used to puncture the skin must be sterile. Finally, the puncture site should be covered with sterile gauze after the skin puncture is complete.

Common puncture sites used to obtain capillary blood include the fingers, heels, and ear lobes (see figure 18-12A). The heel is frequently used for infants until they learn to walk. A finger is usually used for children and adults. When a finger puncture is performed, care must be taken in the selection of the finger. The thumb, index finger, or pinkie finger should not be used because they have arteries close to the surface. In addition, they are used most frequently, and the chance for infection is greater. The finger to be used must be examined closely. Avoid fingers with edema (swelling), callouses, scars, rashes, or sores. Make sure the skin is warm and pink. If the finger is cyanotic (blue), do not use it. Cyanosis indicates poor circulation.

The skin puncture should be 2 to 4 millimeters deep in order to reach the capillary beds under the skin. The puncture should be made across the grain of lines in the finger, or at right angles to the fingerprint striations (see figure 18-12B). This type of puncture heals more rapidly in most cases.

The first drop of blood obtained is always removed. It is contaminated with alcohol, perspiration, excess tissue fluid, and other substances on the skin. The second or succeeding drops of blood can be used for the various blood tests.

After performing a skin puncture, the health care worker must remain with the patient until the blood stops flowing. When sufficient blood has been obtained, sterile gauze should be held firmly against the puncture to help stop the bleeding.

Standard precautions (Unit 13:3) must be observed at all times while obtaining and handling blood. Many diseases, including hepatitis B (HBV), hepatitis C (HCV), and acquired immune deficiency syndrome (AIDS), can be transmitted by blood. Hands must be washed thoroughly and gloves must be worn at all times. If splashing of the blood is possible, masks, protective eyewear, and gowns must also be worn. Any blood spills must be wiped up immediately with a disinfectant solution.

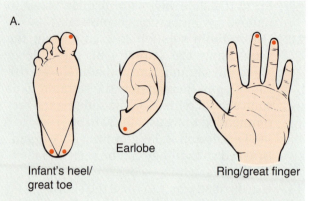

A.

Infant's heel/ great toe

Earlobe

Ring/great finger

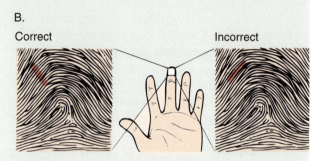

B.

Correct

Incorrect

FIGURE 18-12A & B (A) Common skin puncture sites for obtaining capillary blood. (B) Skin punctures should be made across the grain of lines in the finger.

All contaminated disposable materials or supplies and any remaining blood samples are placed in an infectious-waste bag prior to being disposed of as infectious-waste according to legal requirements. Any sharps, such as lancets or needles, must be placed in a leakproof puncture-resistant sharps box. They should *not* be bent, broken, or recapped. It is important for the health care worker to observe all precautions established by his or her agency for workers who handle blood samples. All blood must be regarded as hazardous, because many illnesses can be transmitted through improper handling of blood samples.

STUDENT: *Go to the workbook and complete the assignment sheet for 18:3, Puncturing the Skin to Obtain Capillary Blood. Then return and continue with the procedure.*

PROCEDURE 18:3

Puncturing the Skin to Obtain Capillary Blood

Equipment and Supplies

Sterile lancet, 70-percent isopropyl alcohol, sterile gauze pads, disposable gloves, sharps box, infectious-waste bag

Procedure

1. Assemble equipment.
2. Wash hands. Put on gloves.

   CAUTION: Observe all standard precautions while obtaining and testing blood. If splashing of blood is possible, put on a gown, face mask, and protective eyewear.

3. **C** Introduce yourself. Identify the patient. Explain the procedure. Obtain the patient's consent.

   NOTE: It is usually best to seat the patient in a comfortable position.

4. Select a finger. Make sure it is free from edema, cyanosis, scars, sores, and callouses. Do *not* use the thumb, index finger, or pinkie finger. If the hand and fingers are cold to the touch, wrap them in a warm cloth or hold them under warm water for a few minutes to stimulate circulation.

   NOTE: Check the circulation in the finger. The finger should be warm and pink for good blood supply. Check the color of the nail bed.

   NOTE: Although this procedure describes a finger puncture, the same principles should be observed when using any skin site to obtain capillary blood.

5. Cleanse the finger thoroughly with a sterile alcohol swab or a sterile gauze pad saturated with 70-percent isopropyl alcohol. Allow the area to air dry.

   NOTE: Do *not* allow the finger to touch anything.

6. Grasp the finger firmly with your thumb and forefinger. Hold the sterile lancet in the other hand. Use a quick, clean, stabbing stroke to puncture the finger with the sterile

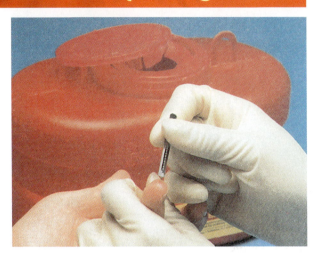

FIGURE 18-13 A sterile lancet is used to puncture the skin 2 to 4 millimeters deep.

lancet (see figure 18-13). Make the cut at right angles to the fingerprint striations, near the top of the finger but not too close to the fingernail.

NOTE: The puncture should be 2 to 4 millimeters deep.

NOTE: Many agencies use automatic lancet devices. The lancet is positioned over the skin site and activated to allow the lancet to puncture the skin (see figure 18-14). Read and follow manufacturer's instructions when using an automatic device.

CAUTION: Do *not* squeeze or milk the finger because doing so will cause tissue fluid to mix with the blood. If necessary, use gentle pressure at a distance from the puncture site to start the blood flow.

CHECKPOINT: Your instructor will check the puncture to be sure it is at a correct angle and is free flowing.

7. Immediately place the lancet in a puncture-resistant sharps container. Do *not* bend or break the lancet before discarding it.

8. Use sterile gauze to remove the first drop of blood. This blood is contaminated with alcohol, perspiration, and other substances

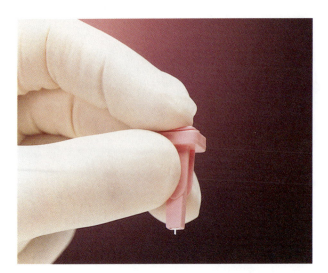

FIGURE 18-14 To use an automatic lancet device, position the lancet over the skin and depress the plunger to make the puncture. *(Courtesy of Becton Dickinson VACUTAINER Systems)*

from the skin. Discard the gauze in the infectious-waste bag.

9. Use the second and succeeding drops of blood to perform the blood tests ordered (for example, hemoglobin). Work quickly to avoid cessation of bleeding.

10. When sufficient blood has been obtained, instruct the patient to hold sterile gauze firmly against the puncture.

 CAUTION: Remain with the patient until the bleeding stops. You must be certain that bleeding has stopped before you leave the area.

11. Clean and replace all equipment. Put all contaminated disposable supplies in the infectious-waste bag. Use a disinfectant to wipe the counter and any contaminated equipment.

12. Remove gloves. Wash hands thoroughly.

Practice *Go to the workbook and use the evaluation sheet for 18:3, Puncturing the Skin to Obtain Capillary Blood, to practice this procedure. When you feel you have mastered this skill, sign the sheet and give it to your instructor for further action.*

Final Checkpoint Using the criteria listed on the evaluation sheet, your instructor will grade your performance.

18:4 INFORMATION *Performing a Microhematocrit*

One of the basic blood tests you may be required to perform is the microhematocrit. A **hematocrit** (HCT), or "crit," is a blood test that measures the volume of packed red blood cells (RBCs), or erythrocytes, in the blood. It is often described as a measurement of the percentage of RBCs per volume of blood. Red blood cells carry oxygen from the lungs to the body cells. They also carry carbon dioxide from the body cells to the lungs, where it is eliminated from the body.

Several different methods can be used to perform a hematocrit. A popular method is the microhematocrit. This test requires less blood and can be done in a shorter period of time compared to other methods. A special centrifuge is used for the microhematocrit. This machine spins the blood tubes at approximately 10,000 revolutions per minute with a centrifugal (driving away from the center) force. The force separates the blood into three main layers: RBCs, a buffy coat, and plasma (see figure 18-15). The buffy coat is a very thin, whitish layer consisting of white blood cells (WBCs) and platelets. By using the graphic reading device on the microhematocrit centrifuge, the percentage of RBCs can be measured (see figure 18-16).

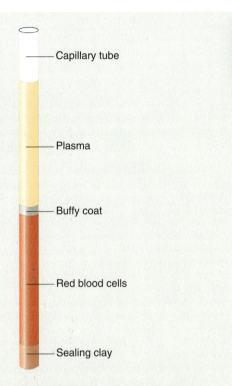

FIGURE 18-15 The microhematocrit centrifuge separates the blood into three main layers: red blood cells, a buffy coat, and plasma.

Special capillary tubes are used in the microhematocrit centrifuge. The tubes are usually lined with an anticoagulant such as heparin. An **anticoagulant** is a substance that prevents the blood from clotting. The tubes are filled to the indicated level with blood from a free-flowing skin puncture. The empty (that is, without blood) ends of the tubes are sealed with special plastic sealing clay (see figure 18-17). This clay keeps the blood from running out of the tube during centrifuging. Extreme care must be taken to avoid contaminating the clay block with the blood. Self-sealing tubes are available for use. These tubes contain a plug with a small air channel to allow air to escape when blood is drawn into the tube. When the blood touches the plug, the air channel seals automatically.

In some agencies, two tubes are filled for the test and the readings of the two tubes are averaged to determine the specific hematocrit of a patient. For example, if one tube registers at 41 percent and the second tube registers at 44 percent, the two numbers are added together:

$$41 + 44 = 85$$

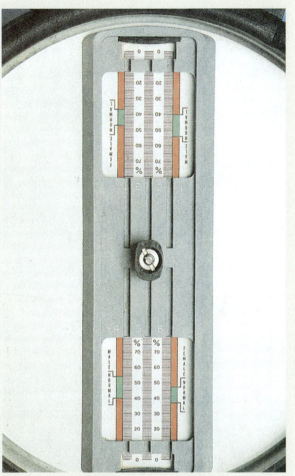

FIGURE 18-16 By using the graphic reading device on the microhematocrit centrifuge, the percentage of red blood cells can be measured.

The total is divided by 2 to obtain the average:

$$
\begin{array}{r}
42.5 \\
2\,\overline{)85.0} \\
\underline{-\ 8\ \ \ \ } \\
05 \\
\underline{-\ 4\ } \\
10 \\
\underline{-\ 10} \\
0
\end{array}
$$

The hematocrit reading for the two tubes would be recorded as 42.5 percent. In other agencies, one tube is used to obtain the hematocrit reading for a patient. The reading obtained from the single tube is recorded as the hematocrit percentage.

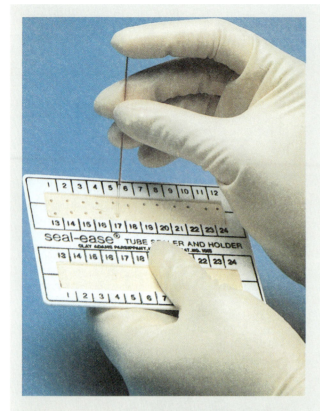

FIGURE 18-17 The empty end of the capillary tube is sealed with clay to prevent the blood from running out of the tube during centrifuging.

Normal values for the test vary slightly depending on the types of microhematocrit centrifuge and capillary tube used. An average value for adults is 35 to 45 percent for women and 40 to 55 percent for men. In other words, 35 to 45 percent of the total blood volume is RBCs in females, and 40 to 55 percent of the total blood volume in men is RBCs. Newborns have a value of 51 to 61 percent, children 1 year old average 32 to 38 percent, and children 6 years old average 34 to 42 percent.

A low hematocrit often indicates *anemia*. A high hematocrit reading can indicate *polycythemia*. Anemia is a low number of RBCs, and polycythemia is a high number of RBCs. Because there are several different types of each of these conditions, the physician usually conducts other, more extensive blood tests to evaluate the condition. Patients with burns or dehydration can also have a high hematocrit, but their red blood cell counts will be normal. Patients with severe bleeding may have a low hematocrit.

Accuracy is essential while performing this test because the test is used to diagnose disease. False results can lead to improper diagnosis and care.

⬡**CAUTION:** If any results are questionable, *do not hesitate* to repeat the test.

Careful recording of the test is also essential. Hematocrit is often abbreviated *hct*. The recording of a test might look like this: *hct.* 35%. Double-check all readings to make sure they are accurate.

⚖ It is the physician's responsibility to report the results of this test to the patient.

STUDENT: *Go to the workbook and complete the assignment sheet for 18:4, Performing a Microhematocrit. Then return and continue with the procedure.*

PROCEDURE 18:4

Performing a Microhematocrit

Equipment and Supplies

Sterile lancet, alcohol swabs, microhematocrit capillary tubes, microhematocrit centrifuge, capillary tube, sealing clay (if the tube is not self-sealing), sterile gauze, disposable gloves, sharps container, infectious-waste bag, paper, pen or pencil

NOTE: The following procedure is for the Readacrit centrifuge. Follow specific manufacturer's instructions when using other equipment.

Procedure

1. Assemble equipment.
2. Wash hands. Put on gloves.

CAUTION: Observe standard precautions while obtaining and testing blood.

3. **C** Introduce yourself. Identify the patient. Explain the procedure. Obtain the patient's consent.

   NOTE: It is best to seat the patient in a comfortable position.

4. Perform the procedure for a skin puncture. Put the used lancet in the sharps container immediately.

5. Use sterile gauze to remove the first drop of blood. Discard the gauze in the infectious-waste bag.

6. Use the second drop of blood. Hold the capillary tube at a slight angle to the skin. Place the end without the indicator mark into the drop of blood (see figure 18-18A). Do *not* touch the skin. Allow the blood to flow into the tube until it reaches the indicator mark. Check to make sure there are no air bubbles in the tube.

   NOTE: If the tube does not have an indicator mark, fill it to within 2 millimeters of the end, or approximately three-quarters full.

   CAUTION: Do *not* use blood that has started to clot.

7. Hold a gloved finger over the end of the tube to prevent the blood from flowing out. Seal the opposite end (the one without blood) by tapping the tube into a tray of sealing clay (refer to figure 18-17). Check the seal to be sure there are no openings. If a self-sealing tube is used, check to make sure that the plug has expanded to close the air channel and seal the tube.

   CAUTION: Avoid applying pressure while sealing the tube because the tube may break.

8. If your agency requires two capillary tubes for the test, fill and seal the second tube.

9. When sufficient blood has been obtained, instruct the patient to hold sterile gauze firmly against the puncture.

   CAUTION: Remain with the patient until the bleeding stops.

10. Place the tube into the microhematocrit centrifuge. Make sure the tube end with the clay seal is against the rubber buffer (see figure 18-18B). The open end of the tube should face the center of the centrifuge. If slots are designated for male or female, place the tube in the correct slot. If one tube is used, many manufacturers recommend placing an empty tube in the opposite slot to balance the centrifuge. If two tubes are used, they can be placed on opposite sides.

    NOTE: Read specific manufacturer's instructions regarding loading the centrifuge.

    CAUTION: Handle tubes carefully to avoid breakage.

    NOTE: Check to be sure the tube is in the correct slot.

11. Lock the centrifuge cover by turning it to the marked angle. Be sure the outside lid is also securely closed. Set the timer to the recommended time (usually 3 to 5 minutes) and turn the machine on.

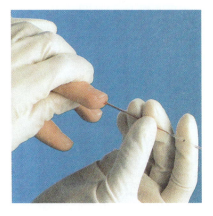

FIGURE 18-18A Hold the capillary tube at a slight angle to the skin to fill the tube with blood to the indicator mark.

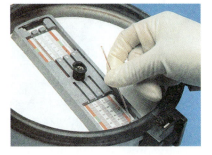

FIGURE 18-18B Place the sealed end of the capillary tube against the rubber buffer on the outer edge of the micro-hematocrit centrifuge.

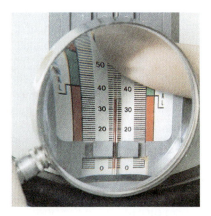

FIGURE 18-18C After positioning the tube so the top of the clay line is at zero, read the percentage number at the top of the red blood cell layer.

⬡ **CAUTION:** Recheck the lids. If they are not secure, the tube could fly out.

12. When spinning stops completely, open the lid. Push the tube upward so the top of the clay line is at zero. Read the number at the top of the RBC layer (see figure 18-18C).

NOTE: Remember that three layers are present in the tube. The lower layer is RBCs, the middle layer is a thin, buffy coat of WBCs and platelets, and the top, clear layer is plasma (refer to figure 18-15).

13. ◯ Double-check the accuracy of your reading. If two tubes are used, obtain a reading for each of the tubes. Add the two readings together. Divide the sum by 2. This number is the hematocrit reading.

NOTE: The final reading for two tubes is an average reading of both tubes.

14. Record your reading.

15. Check the patient to be sure bleeding from the puncture has stopped.

16. Clean and replace all equipment. Put the capillary tube in the sharps container. Place any contaminated disposable supplies in the infectious-waste bag. Use a disinfectant to wipe the centrifuge, the counter, and any contaminated areas.

17. Remove gloves. Wash hands thoroughly.

18. ◯**C** Record required information on the patient's chart or the agency form, for example: date; time; Hct: 45%; and your signature and title. Report any abnormal readings immediately.

Practice *Go to the workbook and use the evaluation sheet for 18:4, Performing a Microhematocrit, to practice this procedure. When you feel you have mastered this skill, sign the sheet and give it to your instructor for further action.*

✔ **Final Checkpoint** Using the criteria listed on the evaluation sheet, your instructor will grade your performance.

18:5 INFORMATION *Measuring Hemoglobin*

Another blood test you may be required to perform is the hemoglobin test. Various methods are used to perform this test. Using a hemoglobinometer is one method.

 The **hemoglobin** (Hgb) test is used to determine the oxygen-carrying capacity of the blood. Hemoglobin is a substance found in red blood cells (RBCs). It is composed of two parts: (1) heme, an iron-containing portion, and (2) globin, a protein. The hemoglobin combines with oxygen and transports it to the body cells. Hemoglobin also assists in carrying carbon dioxide from the body cells to the lungs.

Before hemoglobin concentration can be determined, the blood must be hemolyzed. **Hemolysis** is the destruction of RBCs. When RBCs are destroyed, the hemoglobin is released into the solution that surrounds the cells. Whole blood is normally red and cloudy in appearance. When the cells rupture during hemolysis and hemoglobin is released, however, the blood becomes clear, or transparent. Hemolysis solutions contain special chemicals that cause this reaction outside the body.

The hemoglobinometer is a special instrument used to measure the hemoglobin concentration in blood (see figure 18-19). The hemoglobinometer is used with an offset chamber and hemolysis stick. Blood is placed on the chamber, and the hemolytic stick is applied; a cover clip is lowered over the hemolyzed blood specimen, and the chamber is inserted into the hemoglobinometer for a reading. By using a color comparison, an approximate reading for an individual patient can be obtained. This test is not as accurate as other types of hemoglobin tests because it relies on the ability of the human eye to perform a color match.

An automated photometer can also be used to check the level of hemoglobin. A disposable cuvette, or microcuvette, filled with a

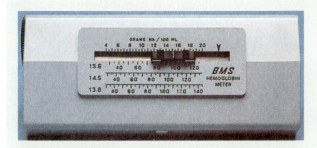

FIGURE 18-19 The hemoglobinometer is a special instrument used to measure the hemoglobin concentration in blood.

hemolyzing solution, is used to obtain a blood sample. The hemolyzing solution in the cuvette hemolyzes the blood and releases the hemoglobin. The cuvette with the hemolyzed blood sample is then placed in the photometer, which automatically measures the color intensity. This test is more accurate because it does not depend on an individual's ability to compare color intensities. For accurate readings, it is important to read and follow the instructions provided by the manufacturer of the photometer.

Normal values for hemoglobin vary with the type of test. An average range is 12 to 18 grams of hemoglobin per 100 milliliters of blood. Males average 13 to 18 grams, females average 12 to 16 grams, newborns average 16 to 23 grams, and children from 1 to 10 years of age average 10 to 14 grams of hemoglobin per 100 milliliters of blood.

A low hemoglobin level can indicate anemia. A high level can indicate polycythemia, which is characterized by high hemoglobin concentration and number of RBCs.

Accuracy is essential while performing this test. Care must be taken to follow the procedure exactly. The reading should be double-checked. If any results are questionable, the test should be repeated.

 It is the physician's responsibility to report the results of this test to the patient.

STUDENT: *Go to the workbook and complete the assignment sheet for 18:5, Measuring Hemoglobin. Then return and continue with the procedure.*

PROCEDURE 18:5A

Measuring Hemoglobin with a Hemoglobinometer

Equipment and Supplies

Sterile lancet, alcohol swab, sterile gauze pads, hemoglobinometer, blood chamber, hemolysis applicator sticks, lens paper, disposable gloves, sharps container, infectious-waste bag, paper, pencil or pen

Procedure

1. Assemble equipment.
2. Wash hands. Put on gloves.
   CAUTION: Observe standard precautions while obtaining and testing blood.
3. Use lens paper to clean the blood chamber.
   NOTE: Lens paper prevents scratches on the chamber.

4. **C** Introduce yourself. Identify the patient. Explain the procedure to the patient. Obtain the patient's consent.
5. Perform a skin puncture. Put the used lancet in the sharps container immediately.
6. Wipe off the first drop of blood. Use the second drop. Place a large drop of blood on the clean chamber (see figure 18-20A). Avoid touching the chamber with the patient's skin.
   CAUTION: The first drop of blood is not used because it is diluted and contaminated.
7. When sufficient blood has been obtained, instruct the patient to hold sterile gauze firmly against the puncture.
   CAUTION: Remain with the patient until the bleeding stops.

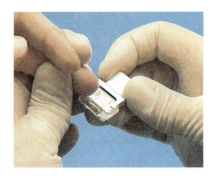

FIGURE 18-20A Place a large drop of blood on the glass chamber, taking care not to touch the chamber with the patient's skin.

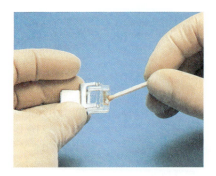

FIGURE 18-20B Use the hemolysis applicator stick to hemolyze the blood until it is clear or transparent.

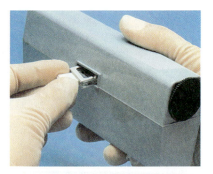

FIGURE 18-20C Slide the loaded chamber into the slot on the side of the hemoglobinometer.

8. Use the hemolysis applicator stick to hemolyze the blood (see figure 18-20B). Use a rotating motion to agitate the blood. Use the end of the stick that has the hemolysis solution (the end shiny in appearance). This usually takes 30 to 45 seconds, but it is best to observe the appearance of the blood rather than depend on the time factor. The blood will look red and cloudy at the start and then become clear, or transparent, when it is hemolyzed.

NOTE: This procedure ruptures the walls of the blood cells. The hemoglobin goes into a uniform solution, which is transparent.

CAUTION: Make sure the entire sample of blood is completely hemolyzed.

9. Use the cover glass to cover the chamber; push the chamber and coverglass into the clip. The chamber is now ready to use.

10. Look into the hemoglobinometer. Check the lighting to make sure it is equal in the entire field. If one side is darker, inform your instructor.

CAUTION: An exact color match is essential to be sure the hemoglobinometer is calibrated correctly. An incorrect calibration will result in inaccurate readings. Follow manufacturer's instructions to calibrate the device.

NOTE: Many agencies use a quality control test chamber with a predetermined hemoglobin reading. The chamber is placed into the hemoglobinometer, the technician performs a color match, and the reading is checked. If the reading is not the same as the predetermined reading for the test chamber,

the hemoglobinometer should not be used. In some cases, the technician needs additional training in order to perform a correct color match.

11. Slide the loaded chamber into the hemoglobinometer (see figure 18-20C).

CAUTION: Avoid applying force when loading the chamber because the chamber may break.

12. Look into the eyepiece. Use your thumb to turn on the light. Slide the slide button until the two halves of the field are equally light and appear as a single field of the same color.

CHECKPOINT: Your instructor will check the color match.

13. Read the scale to determine the number of grams per 100 milliliters of blood. The reading will be 12, 12.5, 13, or a similar number.

NOTE: Normal values for hemoglobin are 12 to 18 grams per 100 milliliters of blood.

14. Record your reading as in the following example: *Hgb 12 gm.*

15. Recheck your reading to be sure it is accurate.

16. Check the patient to be sure the skin puncture has stopped bleeding.

17. Clean and replace all equipment. Wash the chamber and coverglass and then wipe with a disinfectant solution. Some agencies require that the glass be soaked in a disinfectant. Dry it with lens paper to prevent scratches. Use a disinfectant solution to wipe off the outside of the hemoglobinometer. Place all contaminated disposable materials in the infectious-waste bag. Use a disinfectant to wipe the counter and any contaminated areas.

18. Remove gloves. Wash hands thoroughly.
19. **C** Record the required information on the patient's chart or the agency form, for example, date; time; Hgb: 14.5 gm; and your signature and title. Report any abnormal readings immediately.

> **Practice** *Go to the workbook and use the evaluation sheet for 18:5A, Measuring Hemoglobin with a Hemoglobinometer, to practice this procedure. When you feel you have mastered this skill, sign the sheet and give it to your instructor for further action.*

 Final Checkpoint Using the criteria listed on the evaluation sheet, your instructor will grade your performance.

PROCEDURE 18:5B
Measuring Hemoglobin with a Photometer

Equipment and Supplies

Sterile lancet, alcohol swab, sterile gauze pads, hemoglobin photometer, control cuvette, disposable cuvette, tissue or lens paper, disposable gloves, sharps container, infectious-waste bag, paper, pencil or pen

NOTE: This procedure describes the use of the HemoCue Hemoglobin Photometer.

Procedure

1. Assemble equipment. Read manufacturer's instructions provided with the photometer.
2. Wash hands. Put on gloves

    CAUTION: Observe all standard precautions while obtaining and testing blood.
3. Check the photometer to make sure it is calibrated correctly:
    a. Press on the power button to turn the photometer on.
    b. Pull out the cuvette holder to the load position. The display will show the letters *Hb*.
    c. When the indicator displays ready, insert the red control cuvette into the cuvette holder. Gently push the holder into the unit. When the holder is inserted correctly, the photometer will display *Measuring* followed by three dashes.
    d. In 10 to 15 seconds, the photometer will display a value for the control cuvette. Compare this value with the assigned value on the control cuvette card provided with the unit. The value displayed should not be more then ± 0.3g/dl from the value on the control cuvette card. If the value is within this range, the photometer is calibrated correctly.

        ! CAUTION: If the photometer is *not* calibrated correctly, notify your instructor or refer to the troubleshooting guide in the manual provided with the photometer. *Do not use the photometer if the calibration is not correct.* Inaccurate test results would be obtained.
4. **C** Introduce yourself. Identify the patient. Explain the procedure to the patient. Obtain the patient's consent.
5. Perform a skin puncture. Put the used lancet in the sharps container immediately.
6. Wipe off the first and/or second drop of blood. Use the second or third drop. Use your gloved index finger and thumb to hold the cuvette at the square end (see figure 18-21A). Place the angled tip end into the middle of the drop of blood (see figure 18-21B). Hold the cuvette steady to allow capillary action to completely fill the cavity at the tip end

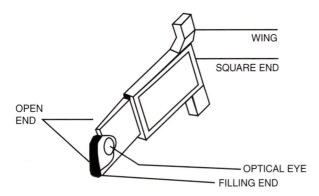

FIGURE 18-21A Always hold the disposable cuvette at the square end to prevent fingerprints or smudges from contaminating the optical eye at the filling end. *(Courtesy of HemoCue, Mission Viejo, CA)*

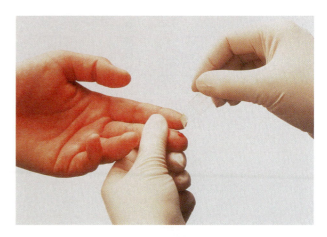

FIGURE 18-21B Place the tip end of the cuvette in the middle of the drop of blood. *(Courtesy of HemoCue, Mission Viejo, CA)*

with blood. Check the filled cuvette to make sure no air bubbles are present in the optical eye. If air bubbles are present, discard the cuvette in the sharps container. Obtain a new cuvette and repeat the filling process with another drop of blood.

CAUTION: Never touch or handle the angled filling tip end of the cuvette. Finger marks or smudges will cause an inaccurate reading.

NOTE: The reagent inside the cavity of the cuvette will hemolyze the erythrocytes and release the hemoglobin.

7. When sufficient blood has been obtained, instruct the patient to hold sterile gauze firmly against the puncture.

8. Use clean lint-free tissue or lens paper to wipe off the excess blood on the outside of the cuvette. Make sure you do *not* draw blood out of the cuvette tip while you are cleaning the outside surface.

9. Check to make sure the photometer is displaying *ready*. Immediately place the filled cuvette into the cuvette holder (see figure 18-21C). Gently push the holder into the unit. If the holder is inserted correctly, *Measuring* followed by three dashes will appear on the display.

    NOTE: Obtain the hemoglobin measurement as quickly as possible after filling the cuvette. *Never* wait more than 10 minutes or test results will be inaccurate.

10. Within 60 seconds, the unit will display the hemoglobin reading in grams per deciliter (g/dl) of blood (see figure 18-21D). Record the reading on the display.

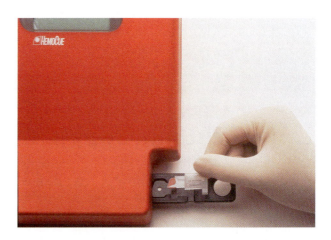

FIGURE 18-21C Place the filled cuvette into the cuvette holder and gently push the holder into the photometer unit. *(Courtesy of HemoCue, Mission Viejo, CA)*

NOTE: Normal values for hemoglobin are 12 to 18 grams per deciliter of blood.

11. Record your reading as in the following example: *Hgb 12.8 gm.*

12. Recheck the reading to be sure it is accurate. Pull the cuvette holder out to the load position, wait until flashing dashes and *Ready* appear on the display, and then gently push the cuvette holder back into the unit. Within 60 seconds, the reading will appear.

13. Remove the cuvette from the photometer unit. Immediately place the used cuvette in the sharps container. Turn the photometer off.

14. Check the patient to be sure the skin puncture has stopped bleeding.

15. Clean and replace all equipment. Use a disinfecting solution to wipe off the outside of

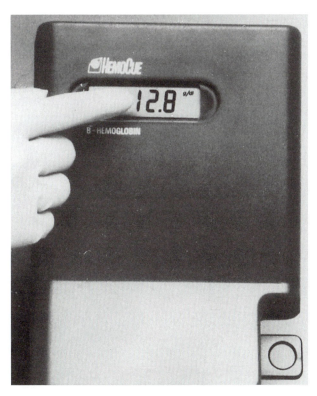

FIGURE 18-21D The photometer unit displays the hemoglobin reading in grams per deciliter (g/dl) of blood. *(Courtesy of HemoCue, Mission Viejo, CA)*

the photometer or follow manufacturer's recommendations for cleaning. Place all contaminated disposable materials in the infectious-waste bag. Use a disinfectant to wipe the counter and any contaminated areas.

16. Remove gloves. Wash hands thoroughly.
17. **C** Record the required information on the patient's chart or agency form, for example, date; time; Hgb: 12.8 gm; and your signature and title. Report any abnormal readings immediately.

> **Practice** *Go to the workbook and use the evaluation sheet for 18:5B, Measuring Hemoglobin with a Photometer, to practice this procedure. When you feel you have mastered this skill, sign the sheet and give it to your instructor for further action.*

✔ **Final Checkpoint** Using the criteria listed on the evaluation sheet, your instructor will grade your performance.

18:6 INFORMATION Counting Blood Cells

Counting blood cells may be one of your responsibilities in an office or laboratory. To be able to do this, you must understand the equipment used.

Erythrocyte and leukocyte counts are done to determine the number of blood cells in the blood. **Erythrocyte counts** are done for red blood cells, or RBCs, and **leukocyte counts** are done for white blood cells, or WBCs. Because RBC counts are more complicated and the number of RBCs can be determined in part by hemoglobin and hematocrit tests, leukocyte counts are more common.

Various methods are used. Most large laboratories use automated cell counters especially designed for this purpose. In smaller offices or agencies, however, counts are performed using a counting chamber. The procedures that follow involve the use of the counting chamber.

The **hemacytometer** counting chamber is a carefully calibrated slide with a measured and lined area for counting cells. A solution containing cells is placed on the slide; then certain areas of the slide or chamber are counted. Study figure 18-22A and note the following information:

◆ Each side of the hemacytometer slide contains a counting chamber

◆ Nine large, distinct squares can be located on the counting chamber when it is placed under a microscope. These are called *primary squares.*

◆ The primary squares on the corners (outer-corner squares) are used to count WBCs. Each of these four corner squares contains sixteen smaller squares. This provides a specifically measured area for counting, shown as *W* in the figure.

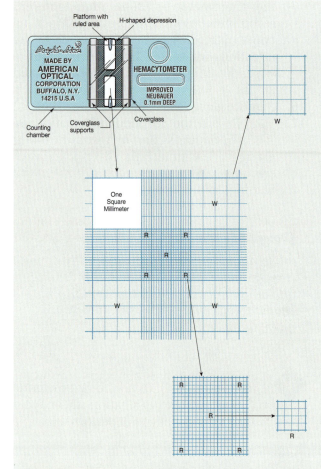

FIGURE 18-22A A hemacytometer counting chamber. Areas marked *W* are used to count white blood cells, or leukocytes. Areas marked *R* are used to count red blood cells, or erythrocytes.

◆ The center square is used for RBC counts. This center square is divided into twenty-five smaller secondary squares; each of these smaller squares contains sixteen squares. Only the four corner squares and the center squares of the twenty-five squares in the large center square are counted. Thus, five areas are counted for RBCs, shown as *R* in the figure.

◆ Only the cells that touch the left line or the top line of each of the large squares (the nine primary squares) are counted. Cells touching the right line or the bottom line are not counted (see figure 18-22B).

◆ Formulas used to determine final counts are as follows:

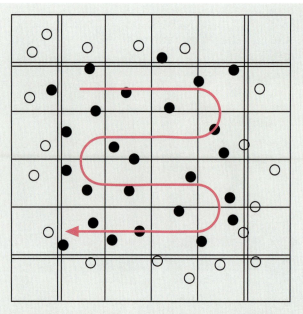

FIGURE 18-22B A sample counting chamber showing cells to count: ● = cells counted, ○ = cells not counted. The arrow indicates a counting pattern that should be followed.

Leukocytes or WBCs:
Count the four primary squares on one side of the slide and add the 4 numbers together:

$$43 + 38 + 40 + 37 = 158$$

Count the four primary squares on the opposite side of the slide and add the 4 numbers together:

$$40 + 36 + 39 + 41 = 156$$

Add the two totals together:

$$158 + 156 = 314$$

Divide the sum by 2 to obtain the average reading for the two sides of the slide:

$$314 \div 2 = 157$$

Multiply the average by 50 (if dilution is 1:20)

$$157 \times 50 = 7,850$$

The leukocyte or WBC count is 7,850.

Erythrocytes or RBCs:
Count the five secondary squares on one side of the slide and add the 5 numbers together:

$$103 + 98 + 100 + 104 + 99 = 504$$

Count the five secondary squares on the other side of the slide and add the 5 numbers together:

$$96 + 101 + 98 + 93 + 95 = 483$$

Add the two totals together:

$$504 + 483 = 987$$

Divide the sum by 2 to obtain the average reading for the two sides of the slide:

$$987 \div 2 = 493.5$$

Multiply the average by 10,000 (*Hint:* Add zeros and move the decimal point 4 places to the right)

$$493.5 \times 10,000 = 4,935,000$$

The erythrocyte or RBC count is 4,935,000.

Blood must be diluted before it is placed on the hemacytometer counting chamber. The formulas are based on this fact, and dilution of the blood is required for the formulas to work accurately. Disposable, self-filling, blood-diluting pipette units are used to dilute the blood correctly (see figure 18-23). A common type is the Unopette system. These units consist of a capillary pipette, pipette shield, and a sealed, plastic reservoir containing a premeasured volume of diluting fluid. Different diluting fluids are used for RBC counts and WBC counts. The diluting fluid for WBC counts will hemolyze, or destroy, the RBCs so that the WBCs are visible. Therefore, it is extremely important to select the correct pipette unit with the proper diluting fluid before doing any blood cell count. It is important to follow the manufacturer's instructions for proper filling and use of the pipette unit. The blood sample is usually collected in the capillary pipette, drawn into the reservoir containing the diluting fluid, mixed correctly, and then dispensed from the reservoir. The units automatically dilute the blood 20 times for a WBC count and 200 times for an RBC count. These dilution ratios are part of the formula for counting blood cells. Some Unopettes dilute the blood for a WBC count 100 times. This alters the formula for calculating WBC counts. If this type of Unopette is used, the total count is multiplied by 250 instead of 50.

White blood cell counts are usually done under the low-power objective (the 10X power) of the microscope. Red blood cell counts are done under high-power because only a small section of the chamber is counted. Lab counters are used in most cases. The procedures that follow list the step-by-step methods of completing these tasks.

The normal count for WBCs is 5,000 to 10,000 cells per cubic millimeter of blood. A low count, below 5,000, is called *leukopenia.*

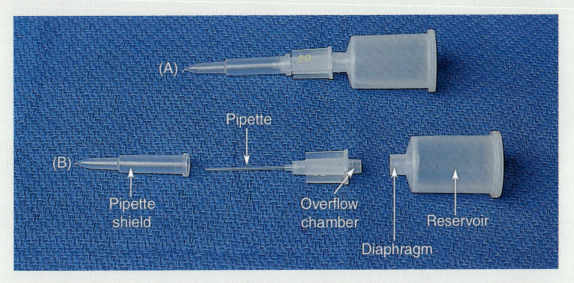

FIGURE 18-23A & B Parts of a disposable Unopette blood-diluting pipette: (A) assembled unit and (B) unassembled unit.

Leukopenia can occur after X-ray therapy, after administration of certain drugs, and with pernicious anemia. A high count, above 10,000, is called *leukocytosis*. Leukocytosis can occur with many acute infections, leukemia, and other conditions.

The normal count for RBCs is 4 to 6 million per cubic millimeter of blood. Males usually have a relatively high erythrocyte count of 4.5 to 6.0 million, while females have a relatively low count of 4.0 to 5.5 million per cubic millimeter of blood. A low erythrocyte count can indicate anemia. A high erythrocyte count can indicate polycythemia.

As with all blood tests, accuracy is essential when counting blood cells. Double-check all calculations and counts. Note the principles and follow all steps of the procedures. Repeat the test if there are any questionable results.

STUDENT: *Go to the workbook and complete the assignment sheet for 18:6, Counting Blood Cells. Then return and continue with the procedures.*

PROCEDURE 18:6A
Counting Erythrocytes

Equipment and Supplies

Sterile lancet; alcohol swab; sterile gauze; alcohol; disposable, self-filling diluting pipette with erythrocyte-diluting fluid; hemacytometer counting chamber and coverglass; microscope; disposable gloves; sharps container; infectious-waste bag; paper; pencil or pen

Procedure

1. Assemble equipment. Use lens paper to clean the hemacytometer and coverglass.
2. Wash hands. Put on gloves. If splashing of blood is possible, put on a gown, face mask, and eye protection.

    CAUTION: Observe standard precautions while obtaining and testing blood.
3. **C** Introduce yourself. Identify the patient. Explain the procedure. Obtain the patient's consent.
4. Do a skin puncture. Put the used lancet in the sharps container immediately.
5. Wipe off the first drop of blood. To fill a Unopette pipette, do the following:
    a. Place the reservoir on a flat surface and hold it firmly with one hand. With the pipette shield attached to the pipette, puncture the diaphragm in the neck of the reservoir by using your other hand to push the tip of the pipette shield through the diaphragm (see figure 18-24, step 1a).
    b. Remove the shield from the reservoir. Then, use a twisting motion to remove the shield from the pipette (see figure 18-24, step 1b).
    c. While holding the pipette in an almost horizontal position, place the tip of the pipette in the second drop of blood (see figure 18-24, step 2a). The pipette will fill by capillary action and will stop automatically when the blood reaches the top of the tube. Use a gauze pad to wipe any excess blood from the outside of the capillary pipette, taking care not to remove any blood from the pipette.

    CAUTION: Do *not* wipe the hole at the tip because blood will be drawn out of the pipette.

    NOTE: To use a different type of disposable, self-filling, diluting pipette, read and follow the manufacturer's instructions.
6. When sufficient blood has been obtained, instruct the patient to hold sterile gauze firmly against the puncture.

    CAUTION: Remain with the patient until the bleeding stops.
7. To mix the blood and the diluting fluid in the reservoir of the Unopette, do the following:
    a. Use the thumb and forefinger of one hand to squeeze the reservoir slightly and expel

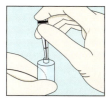

1. Puncture diaphragm

Using the protective shield on the capillary pipette, puncture the diaphragm of the reservoir as follows:

a. Place reservoir on a flat surface. Grasping reservoir in one hand, take pipette assembly in other hand. Push tip of pipette shield firmly through diaphragm in neck of reservoir, then remove.

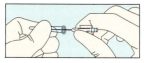

b. Remove shield from pipette assembly with a twist.

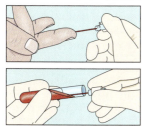

2. Add sample

Fill capillary with sample and transfer to reservoir as follows:

a. Holding pipette almost horizontally, touch tip of pipette to sample. (See alternate methods in illustrations above.) Pipette will fill by capillary action. Filling is complete and will stop automatically when sample reaches end of capillary bore in neck of pipette.

b. Wipe excess sample from outside of capillary pipette, making certain that no sample is removed from capillary bore.

c. Squeeze reservoir slightly to force out some air. Do not expel any liquid. Maintain pressure on reservoir.

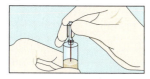

d. Cover opening of overflow chamber with index finger and seat pipette securely in reservoir neck.

e. Release pressure on reservoir. Then remove finger from pipette opening. Negative pressure will draw blood into diluent.

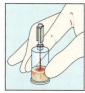

f. Squeeze reservoir gently two or three times to rinse capillary bore, forcing diluent into, but not out of, overflow chamber, releasing pressure each time to return mixture to reservoir.

CAUTION: If reservoir is squeezed too hard, some of the specimen may be expelled through the top of the overflow chamber.

some air, taking care not to expel any liquid (see figure 18-24, step 2c). While maintaining the pressure on the reservoir, use the index finger of your other hand to cover the opening of the overflow chamber on the capillary pipette. Place the pipette securely in the reservoir neck.

b. Release the pressure on the reservoir and then remove your other finger from the pipette opening. Negative pressure will draw the blood in the capillary pipette into the diluting fluid in the reservoir. Squeeze the reservoir gently two or three times to rinse the capillary pipette, taking care not to force the diluting solution out of the overflow chamber on the pipette (see figure 18-24, step 2f).

c. Place an index finger over the opening and invert the reservoir several times to mix the blood and the diluting fluid (see figure 18-24, step 2g).

   NOTE: The blood is now diluted to a 1:200 ratio, or 200 times.

8. To transfer the diluted blood from the reservoir, do the following:

a. Place your finger over the opening and invert the reservoir several times to resuspend the cells.

b. Remove the capillary pipette from the reservoir. Turn it upside down and attach the opposite end of it to the reservoir. This action turns the reservoir and pipette into a dropper.

c. Invert the reservoir and squeeze the sides gently to discard the first three or four drops onto a gauze pad.

   CAUTION: Immediately place the contaminated gauze pad in the infectious-waste bag.

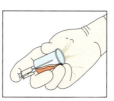

g. Place index finger over upper opening and gently invert several times to thoroughly mix sample with diluent.

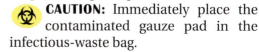

FIGURE 18-24 Procedure for using the Unopette system to prepare blood for cytology counts. *(Courtesy of Becton Dickinson VACUTAINER Systems)*

d. The unit is now ready to be used to charge the hemacytometer counting chamber.

9. Check the coverglass to be sure it is centered on the counting chamber. Place a drop of the diluted blood mixture on the chamber platform so that the drop contacts the edge of the coverglass. Capillary action will draw the drop under the coverglass and over the ruled area. This is called *charging the chamber.*
   NOTE: Use only one drop of the blood mixture.
   NOTE: No air bubbles should be present.
   NOTE: The drop must be large enough to cover the area but should not spill into the moats on either side. If this occurs, the chamber must be cleaned and recharged.

10. Charge the opposite side of the chamber in the same manner.

11. Allow 2 minutes for the cells to settle in one place on the chamber.

12. Carefully place the chamber on the microscope stage. Make sure you hold the chamber level at all times.

13. To focus the chamber, move the 10X objective in place on the microscope. Find the moat and bring it into focus. Next, move the slide to the side until the indicator arrow appears as a whiter area. Focus the arrow so that the tip is clearly seen through the microscope. Slowly move the slide toward you until the chamber counting area comes into view. Bring it into clear focus with the fine-adjustment knob.
   ! **CAUTION:** Do *not* move the coarse adjustment downward unless you are watching the stage. The counting chamber and coverglass are likely to break.

14. Scan the area. Make sure that the cells are evenly distributed. If not, the chamber must be recharged.
   ✔ CHECKPOINT: Your instructor will check the distribution before the count is performed.

15. Locate the center primary square of the ruled area. Move the chamber to center the upper left secondary square. Switch to high power. Adjust lighting and focus (see figure 18-25). Count all of the RBCs in the four corner secondary squares and the central square. The difference between any two squares should not be more than fifteen cells. Recheck counts, if necessary.

16. Add the five totals together. For example, if the counts are 103, 98, 100, 104, and 99, the total would be 504 red

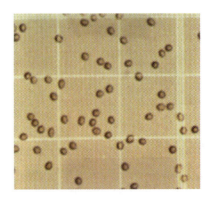

FIGURE 18-25 Use high power to count erythrocytes on the hemacytometer slide.

blood cells counted on the first side of the hemacytometer counting chamber.

17. Repeat the process on the other side of the chamber. Count the five designated areas and add the totals together. For example, if the counts are 96, 101, 98, 93, and 95, the total would be 483 red blood cells counted on the second side of the hemacytometer counting chamber. The two RBC counts should be similar.

18. Calculate the average red blood cell count. Add the two totals together and divide the sum by 2. For example, adding 504 to 483 equals 987. Dividing the sum of 987 by 2 equals 493.5. The average red blood cell count is 493.5

19. Multiply the average red blood cell count by 10,000 to obtain the actual red blood cell count. For example, 493.5 multiplied by 10,000 equals 4,935,000 red blood cells. (*Hint:* to multiply by 10,000, simply add zeros and move the decimal point four places to the right). The actual red blood cell count that is recorded is 4,935,000. Double-check all math for accuracy to be sure you have calculated the correct red blood cell count.

20. Clean and replace all equipment. Place the disposable diluting pipette unit in a sharps container. Put any other contaminated disposable materials in the infectious-waste bag. Use a disinfectant to wipe the counter and any other contaminated areas.

21. Use lens paper saturated with a disinfectant solution to clean the hemacytometer chamber and coverglass. Some agencies require that the chamber and coverglass be soaked in a disinfecting solution. Use lens paper to dry the chamber and coverglass. Store the

chamber and coverglass in a protective container to prevent scratches.

22. Remove gloves, face mask, and eye protection. Discard the gloves and mask in an infectious-waste container. Clean and disinfect the eye protection. Wash hands thoroughly.

23. **C** Record required information on the patient's chart or the agency form, for example: date; time; RBC count: 4,935,000; and your signature and title. Report any abnormal counts immediately.

 Practice *Go to the workbook and use the evaluation sheet for 18:6A, Counting Erythrocytes, to practice this procedure. When you feel you have mastered this skill, sign the sheet and give it to your instructor for further action.*

 Final Checkpoint Using the criteria listed on the evaluation sheet, your instructor will grade your performance.

PROCEDURE 18:6B

Counting Leukocytes

Equipment and Supplies

Sterile lancet; alcohol swab; disposable, self-filling diluting pipette with leukocyte-diluting fluid; sterile gauze; hemacytometer counting chamber and coverglass; microscope; disposable gloves; sharps container; infectious-waste bag; paper; pen or pencil

NOTE: Check the diluting pipette to determine if the dilution ratio is 1:20 or 1:100. This procedure determines calculations based on a dilution of 1:20. If the dilution of the pipette is 1:100, the average WBC count would be multiplied by 250, not 50 as shown in this procedure.

Procedure

1. Assemble equipment. Use lens paper to clean the hemacytometer and coverglass.
2. Wash hands. Put on gloves. If splashing of blood is possible, put on a gown, face mask, and eye protection.
   CAUTION: Observe standard precautions while obtaining and testing blood.
3. **C** Introduce yourself. Identify the patient. Explain the procedure. Obtain the patient's consent.
4. Do a skin puncture. Put the used lancet in the sharps container immediately.
5. Wipe off the first drop of blood. Fill a Unopette pipette following the procedure

described in step 5 of Procedure 18:6A, Counting Erythrocytes, and figure 18-24.

6. When sufficient blood has been obtained, instruct the patient to hold sterile gauze firmly against the puncture.
   CAUTION: Remain with the patient until the bleeding stops.
7. To mix the blood and the diluting fluid in the reservoir of the Unopette, follow the procedure described in step 7 of Procedure 18:6A, Counting Erythrocytes.
   NOTE: The white blood cell diluting fluid hemolyzes, or destroys, the red blood cells. After the blood is mixed with the diluting fluid, *wait 5 to 10 minutes* before using the diluted blood. This allows the RBCs to hemolyze so that the WBCs are visible.
   NOTE: The blood is now diluted to a 1:20 ratio, or 20 times.
8. To transfer the diluted blood from the reservoir, follow the procedure described in step 8 of Procedure 18:6A, Counting Erythrocytes.
9. Check the coverglass to be sure it is centered on the counting chamber. Place a drop of diluted blood on the chamber platform so that the drop contacts the edge of the coverglass (see figure 18-26). Capillary action will draw the drop of diluted blood under the coverglass and over the ruled area. This is called charging the chamber.
   NOTE: Use only one drop of diluted blood.

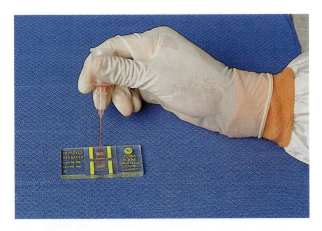

FIGURE 18-26 Place a drop of diluted blood at the edge of the cover slip on the chamber platform.

FIGURE 18-27 The low power objective of a microscope is used to count leukocytes.

NOTE: No air bubbles should be present.

NOTE: The drop should be large enough to cover the area but should not spill into the moats on either side. If this occurs, the chamber must be cleaned and recharged.

10. Charge the other side of the chamber.

11. Allow approximately 2 minutes for the cells to settle in one place.

12. Carefully place the chamber on the microscope stage. Hold the chamber level at all times.

13. Move the 10X objective into place on the microscope. Find the moat on the bottom edge of the slide and bring it into focus. Move the slide sideways until the clearer, white arrow indicator comes into focus. Next, pull the slide toward you until the ruled chamber area is in view. Use fine adjustment to focus the area.

⚠ **CAUTION:** Do *not* move the coarse adjustment downward while looking through the eyepiece. The slide and coverglass are likely to break.

14. Scan the area to be sure the cells are evenly distributed. If not, the chamber must be recharged.

✔ **CHECKPOINT:** Your instructor will check the distribution before the count is performed.

15. Center the upper-left primary square. Under low power (10X), count the cells in the sixteen small squares of this square (see figure 18-27). Count all cells touching the top line or the left line. Do *not* count any cells touching the right line or the bottom line.

16. Obtain counts for the other three primary squares on the outer corners.

17. Total the counts from the four squares. For example, if the counts are 43, 38, 40, and 37, the total would be 158 white blood cells counted on the first side of the hemacytometer counting chamber.

NOTE: The difference between any two primary squares should not be more than ten cells.

18. Count the four primary squares on the other side of the chamber. Find the sum of the counts from these four squares. For example, if the counts are 40, 36, 39, and 41, the total would be 156 white blood cells counted on the second side of the chamber.

19. Calculate the average white blood cell count. Add the two totals together and divide the sum by 2. For example, adding 158 to 156 equals 314. Dividing the sum of 314 by 2 equals 157. The average white blood cell count is 157.

20. Multiply the average white blood cell count by 50 (if the dilution ratio is 1:20) to obtain the actual white blood cell count. For example, 157 multiplied by 50 equals 7,850. The actual white blood cell count that is recorded is 7,850. Double-check all math for accuracy to be sure you have calculated the correct white blood cell count.

21. Clean and replace all equipment. Place the disposable diluting pipette unit in a sharps container. Put any other contaminated disposable materials in the infectious-waste bag. Use a disinfectant to wipe the counter and any other contaminated areas.

22. Use lens paper saturated with a disinfectant solution to clean the hemacytometer chamber and coverglass. Some agencies require

that the chamber and coverglass be soaked in a disinfecting solution. Use lens paper to dry the chamber and coverglass. Store the chamber and coverglass in a protective container to prevent scratches.

23. Remove gloves, face mask, and eye protection. Discard the gloves and mask in an infectious-waste container. Clean and disinfect the eye protection. Wash hands thoroughly.

24. **C** Record the required information on the patient's chart or the agency form, for example, date, time, WBC count: 7,850; and your signature and title. Report any abnormal counts immediately.

Practice *Go to the workbook and use the evaluation sheet for 18:6B, Counting Leukocytes, to practice this procedure. When you feel you have mastered this skill, sign the sheet and give it to your instructor for further action.*

✔ **Final Checkpoint** Using the criteria listed on the evaluation sheet, your instructor will grade your performance.

18:7 INFORMATION
Preparing and Staining a Blood Film or Smear

 A blood film or smear is used for a variety of blood tests. A **blood smear** or film is prepared by placing a small drop of blood on a slide. Another slide, coverslip, or special spreader is then used to spread the blood in a thin layer across the slide. An important test that uses the blood film or smear is the **differential count** of white blood cells (WBCs). There are five different types of WBCs, or leukocytes, each with its own characteristic appearance. In a differential count, 100 WBCs are counted. As the count is performed, a total is kept of each type of leukocyte seen by using a differential counter or calculator. The percentage of each type is then calculated. For example, if 33 lymphocytes are counted, the blood is said to contain 33 percent lymphocytes. Because certain types of WBCs increase after specific infections, the differential count aids in making diagnoses. For example, after certain viral illnesses, an increase in lymphocytes (a specific type of leukocyte) is often

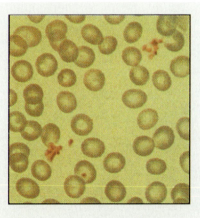

FIGURE 18-28 A photomicrograph of a slide stained with Wright's stain and showing erythrocytes and platelets (1,000X).

noted. Likewise, an infection involving certain parasites can lead to an increase in the number of eosinophils, another type of leukocyte.

The blood film or smear is also used to examine the form, structure, and relative number of erythrocytes (red blood cells, or RBCs), leukocytes, and platelets (see figure 18-28). In addition to abnormal blood counts, abnormal shapes can also be signs of diseases. For example, a sickle-shaped RBC can indicate the presence of sickle cell anemia. Abnormal shapes and an increase in leukocytes are seen in certain types of leukemia.

All the equipment used for preparing the blood smear or film must be extremely clean. Fingerprints, smears, stains, and other similar contaminants will interfere with, and in some cases even distort, the appearance of the cells. Wiping the slide and spreader with alcohol is one way to remove contaminants.

Before the slide can be viewed under a microscope, the cells must be stained so that they are visible. A common stain is Wright's stain. The stain fixes the smear, or makes the cells in the blood adhere to the slide. When a buffer is then added, the stain colors or dyes the blood cells so that they become visible under the microscope.

Another common stain is a quick stain, or three-step method. The blood smear slide is dipped into a fixative solution for about 1 second. It is then dipped into two separate staining solutions for approximately 1 second each (see figure 18-29). This three-step procedure is repeated four to five times following manufacturer's instructions. Then the slide is gently rinsed with water and allowed to air dry before it is examined. This method is faster and requires less than one minute to complete. It is important to read and follow manufacturer's

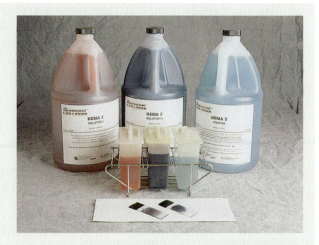

FIGURE 18-29 A quick stain, or three-step method, is another way of staining blood smear slides.

instructions in order to obtain a properly stained blood smear.

STUDENT: *Go to the workbook and complete the assignment sheet for 18:7, Preparing and Staining a Blood Film or Smear. Then return and continue with the procedures.*

PROCEDURE 18:7A

Preparing a Blood Film or Smear

Equipment and Supplies

Lancet, alcohol swab, sterile gauze, alcohol, slide, coverslip or spreader slide, disposable gloves, sharps container, infectious-waste bag

Procedure

1. Assemble equipment.
2. Wash hands. Put on gloves.

   CAUTION: Observe standard precautions while obtaining and testing blood.

3. Use an alcohol swab to clean the slide and coverslip (spreader slide). Check both for defects or chips. Any defects could interfere with the smear pattern.
4. Introduce yourself. Identify the patient. Explain the procedure. Obtain the patient's consent.
5. Perform a skin puncture. Wipe off the first drop of blood. Put the used lancet in the sharps container immediately.
6. Place a small drop of blood on the slide by touching the slide to the blood. The drop of blood should be placed approximately ¼ to ½

inch from the end of the slide and centered on the slide.

> ❗ **CAUTION:** Do *not* touch the slide to the skin because doing so will cause the blood to smear.

NOTE: The blood drop should be approximately 2 millimeters in diameter, or the size of a matchhead.

7. When sufficient blood has been obtained, instruct the patient to hold sterile gauze firmly against the puncture.

> ❗ **CAUTION:** Remain with the patient until the bleeding stops.

8. Place the edge of the coverslip or spreader slide in front of the blood on the slide (see figure 18-30A).

9. Hold the spreader slide at a 30 to 45° angle. Pull the spreader back until it touches the blood. Hold it steady while the blood spreads evenly to the edges of the spreader slide (see figure 18-30B).

10. Using a firm, steady movement, push the spreader to the opposite end of the slide (see figure 18-30C). Use a smooth, continuous motion. Keep the spreader in contact with the slide at all times. Finish by raising the spreader in a smooth low arc. If the coverslip or spreader slide is disposable, put it in the sharps container. If it is not disposable, wash it thoroughly and clean or soak it in a disinfecting solution.

11. Allow the slide to air dry. It is now ready for staining.

NOTE: The smear should be approximately 1½ inches long, smooth, thin, and have an even margin on all sides.

NOTE: If the slide cannot be stained immediately, immerse the dried smear in methanol for 30 to 60 seconds to fix the slide and preserve the smear. Remove the slide from the methanol solution and allow it to air dry.

12. Check the patient to be sure that the skin puncture has stopped bleeding.

13. Clean and replace all equipment. Put all contaminated disposable supplies in the infectious-waste bag. Use a disinfectant to wipe the counter and any contaminated areas.

14. Remove gloves. Wash hands.

> **Practice** *Go to the workbook and use the evaluation sheet for 18:7A, Preparing a Blood Film or Smear, to practice this procedure. When you feel you have mastered this skill, sign the sheet and give it to your instructor for further action.*

✔ **Final Checkpoint** Using the criteria listed on the evaluation sheet, your instructor will grade your performance.

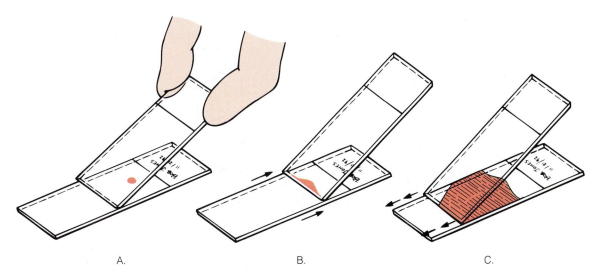

FIGURE 18-30A, B, & C To prepare a blood smear: (A) place the edge of the spreader slide in front of the drop of blood on the slide; (B) hold the slide at a 30 to 45° angle and pull it back until it touches the drop of blood; (C) use a firm, steady movement to push the spreader slide to the opposite end of the slide.

PROCEDURE 18:7B

Staining a Blood Film or Smear

Equipment and Supplies

Blood smear film slide, staining rack, Wright's stain with distilled water/buffer solution or quick stain kit, timer, disposable gloves, infectious-waste bag

Procedure

1. Assemble equipment.
2. Wash hands. Put on gloves.

   CAUTION: Observe standard precautions while obtaining and testing blood.
3. Prepare a blood smear film if you have not already done so.

   NOTE: The slide should be smooth and have an even margin on all sides. There should be no streaks, hesitation marks, or holes.
4. Place the slide with the smear side up on a staining rack. Make sure the rack is level.
5. To stain the slide with Wright's stain:

   a. Use Wright's stain to completely cover the dry smear (see figure 18-31A). Count the number of drops of the stain as you apply it. Leave the stain in place for 1 to 3 minutes.

   NOTE: The time and number of drops may vary with different stains; read and follow manufacturer's instructions.

   b. Add an equal amount of distilled water or buffer (see figure 18-31B). Place it on the slide one drop at a time. Between drops, blow gently along the length of the slide to mix the stain and water. Allow it to stand 2 to 4 minutes.

   NOTE: The solutions are well mixed when an oily, greenish sheen appears.

   CAUTION: Make sure none of the mixture runs off of the slide.

   c. Wash the slide by flooding it gently with distilled water. Allow the stain mixture to flow off of the slide.
6. To stain the slide with a quick stain kit:

   a. Read the manufacturer's instructions.

   b. Dip the slide into the fix solution for about 1 second.

   c. Quickly dip the slide into each of the two staining solutions for about 1 second each.

   NOTE: Touch the end of the slide on a paper towel between solutions to remove excess solution. Do *not* allow the slide to dry between solutions.

   d. Repeat the three-step dip process approximately four to five times, following manufacturer's instructions.

   e. Rinse the slide gently with water (if required by the manufacturer).

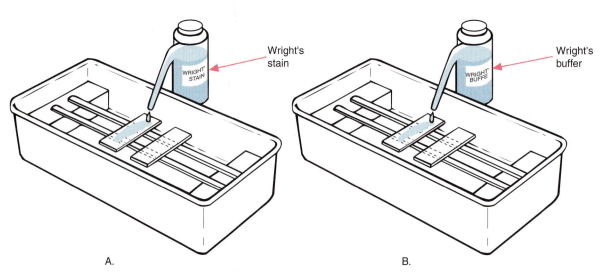

Wright's stain

Wright's buffer

A.

B.

FIGURE 18-31A & B (A) Use Wright's stain to cover the dry smear. (B) After waiting 1 to 3 minutes, add an equal amount of distilled water or buffer solution.

7. Wipe the dye from the back of the slide. Observe which part of the slide has the heaviest concentration of blood smear. Stand the slide on its end (vertically) to dry. Place the part with the heaviest concentration downward and allow the dye to flow down from the less concentrated (thinner) area. In an emergency, the front of the slide can be blotted dry, but this is not recommended. It is best to allow the slide to air dry at room temperature.

8. The finished smear should have a lavender-pink color. If it appears too purple, hold the slide under gently running cold water until the desired color is obtained. Let the water strike the slide above the thick portion of the smear and flow downward.

   NOTE: The slide is now ready to be examined. A differential count of leukocytes is usually done with this type of stain. Examinations of erythrocytes and platelets can also be done.

9. Clean and replace all equipment. Put all contaminated disposable supplies in the infectious-waste bag. Use a disinfectant to wipe the counter and any contaminated areas.

10. Remove gloves. Wash hands.

> **Practice** *Go to the workbook and use the evaluation sheet for 18:7B, Staining a Blood Film or Smear, to practice this procedure. When you feel you have mastered this skill, sign the sheet and give it to your instructor for further action.*

✔ **Final Checkpoint** Using the criteria listed on the evaluation sheet, your instructor will grade your performance.

18:8 INFORMATION
Testing for Blood Types

 Human beings inherit a certain blood type from their parents. The type of blood is determined by the presence of certain factors, called *antigens,* on red blood cells (RBCs) or erythrocytes. An **antigen** is a substance, usually a protein, that causes the body to produce a protein, called an *antibody,* that reacts against the antigen. An antigen may be introduced into the body, such as the antigens that enter the body as viruses, or an antigen may be formed within the body, such as the RBCs that contain antigens. The variety of antigens that may be present on the RBCs serve as the basis for blood group systems and blood types. Two of the major systems are called the ABO blood type system and the Rh system.

In the ABO blood type system, two specific antigens can be present: antigen A and antigen B. There are four main blood types: A, B, AB, and O. The letters refer to the kind of antigen present in the RBCs of an individual. Red blood cells are not the only body cells with the A and B antigens. Most other cells also have them. Thus, in forensic (legal) medicine, a piece of skin or other tissue found at a crime scene can be typed. In this way, the blood type of the victim and/or criminal can be determined.

◆ *Type A* contains antigen A on the RBCs.

◆ *Type B* contains antigen B on the RBCs.

◆ *Type AB* contains both antigen A and antigen B on the RBCs.

◆ *Type O* contains neither antigen A nor antigen B on the RBCs.

In addition to an ABO blood type, every individual has an Rh type. Rh stands for *rhesis monkey,* in which it was first found. In the Rh blood type system, only one factor, the D antigen, is involved. If the Rh factor, or D antigen, is present on the RBCs, the blood type is called *Rh positive.* If the Rh factor is *not* present, the blood type is called *Rh negative.*

If an antigen not present in a person's RBCs is introduced into the blood, the individual will produce antibodies to destroy the foreign antigen. These antibodies remain in the individual's blood plasma or serum. They are specific for a particular antigen, or act against only the antigen they were produced to act against. These antibodies destroy the RBCs having the foreign antigen in one of two main ways. They cause the RBCs to either hemolyze (dissolve and go into solution, releasing hemoglobin) or to agglutinate (clump together). Because RBCs carry oxygen and carbon dioxide to maintain vital body functions, their destruction can lead to death.

Before anyone can receive a transfusion (transfer of blood from one individual to another), a **typing and crossmatch** must be performed on the blood. The blood typing reveals the ABO, Rh factors, and other, rarer blood type systems. *Crossmatching* consists of a series of tests performed on the blood of the donor (the person giving blood) and on the blood of the recipient (the person receiving blood). The purpose is to detect any possible incompatibility (difference that would make the blood unsuitable for transfusion) between the recipient's serum and the cells of the donor. Most blood banks also do an **antibody screen** of blood prior to a transfusion being performed. This screening is performed to check for unexpected antibodies that may be present in the blood and that could lead to an incompatibility reaction. Only when the two types of blood are compatible, or identical in antigens and antibodies present, can the blood from one individual be given to another individual.

Blood typing is also performed on pregnant women. An Rh incompatibility between a pregnant woman and the fetus (developing infant) can cause hemolytic disease of the newborn (HDN). The problem occurs when the woman is Rh negative and the fetus is Rh positive. The Rh antigen, or D antigen, enters the mother's bloodstream through the placenta. The mother's bloodstream then produces anti-D antibodies against the D antigen. When these antibodies enter the developing infant's bloodstream through the placenta, the antibodies can hemolyze or destroy the infant's red blood cells. Fortunately, a medicine called RhoGAM can be given to the pregnant woman to prevent the formation of the anti-D antibodies. The RhoGAM injection is usually given to the woman once or twice during the pregnancy and within 72 hours after delivery if the infant is Rh positive.

The procedure that follows demonstrates blood typing using an anti-A serum and an anti-B serum; the Rh factor is checked using an anti-Rh, or anti-D, serum. The three serums are designed to cause an agglutination reaction if the antigens are present in the blood. Thus, if the blood reacts to the anti-A serum by agglutinating, but does not react to the anti-B serum, only antigen A is present, and the blood type is type A (see figure 18-32). Conversely, if the blood reacts to the anti-B serum but does not react to the anti-A serum, only antigen B is present, and the blood type is B. If the blood reacts to both the anti-A serum and anti-B serum, both antigen A and antigen B are present, and the blood type is AB. If the blood reacts to neither the anti-A serum nor the anti-B serum, neither antigen is present, and the blood type is O. If the blood reacts to the anti-Rh serum, the Rh factor is present, and the blood is Rh positive. If the blood does not react to the anti-RH serum, the Rh factor is not present, and the blood type is Rh negative. This test is used for screening purposes. Additional and more extensive laboratory tests are performed on blood before a transfusion is given.

STUDENT: *Go to the workbook and complete the assignment sheet for 18:8, Testing for Blood Types. Then return and continue with the procedure.*

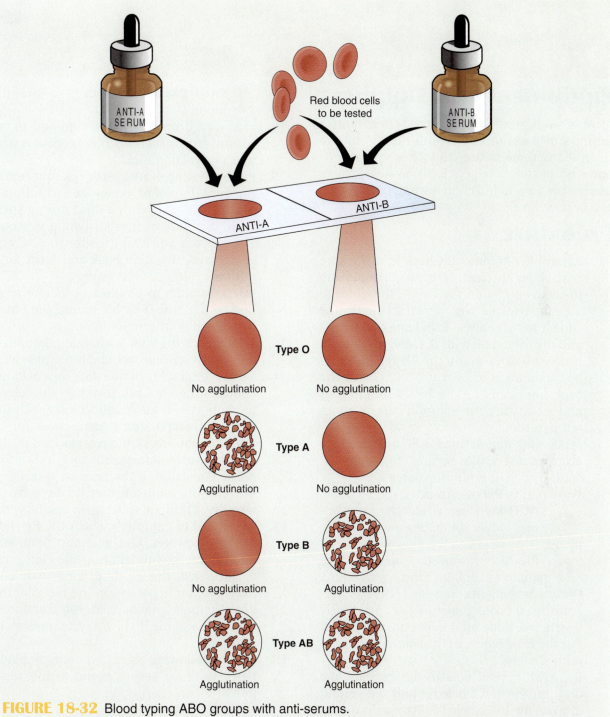

FIGURE 18-32 Blood typing ABO groups with anti-serums.

PROCEDURE 18:8

Testing for Blood Types

Equipment and Supplies

Alcohol swab, sterile lancet, sterile gauze, anti-A serum, anti-B serum, anti-D (anti-Rh) serum, two clean slides, three mixing sticks, Rh-typing viewbox with heater, wax pencil, disposable gloves, sharps container, infectious-waste bag, paper, pen or pencil

Procedure

1. Assemble equipment. Check to make sure both slides are clean or use an alcohol swab to clean each slide, then allow the slides to air dry. Use the wax pencil to mark one slide into two halves. Label one half with *A* and the other half with *B*. Label the second slide with *Rh*. Turn on the Rh-typing viewbox to allow it to heat to 37°C. Check the expiration dates on the anti-serum bottles and make sure the solutions are at room temperature.

   NOTE: Old anti-serums will not produce accurate test results. Serums should be discarded on their expiration dates.

2. Wash hands. Put on gloves.

   CAUTION: Observe standard precautions while obtaining and testing blood.

3. **C** Introduce yourself. Identify the patient. Explain the procedure. Obtain the patient's consent.

4. Perform a skin puncture as previously instructed. Wipe off the first drop of blood. Put the used lancet in the sharps container immediately.

5. Place two drops of blood on the first slide, one drop on the half labeled *A* and the second drop on the half labeled *B*. Place a third drop of blood on the second slide, labeled *Rh*.

   CAUTION: Take care *not* to touch the skin to the slide.

6. When sufficient blood has been obtained, instruct the patient to hold sterile gauze firmly against the puncture.

   CAUTION: Remain with the patient until the bleeding stops.

7. Place one drop of anti-A serum next to the first drop of blood. Immediately mix the blood and serum with a mixing stick.

   CAUTION: Work quickly, before the blood clots.

8. Place one drop of anti-B serum next to the second drop of blood. Mix immediately with a second mixing stick.

9. Place one drop of anti-Rh or D serum next to the third drop of blood on the second slide. Mix immediately with a third mixing stick. Place the slide on the Rh-typing viewbox. The viewbox will heat the slide to 37°C and gently rock the slide back and forth for 2 minutes.

   NOTE: In order to obtain an accurate reaction to the anti-D or Rh serum, the blood must be at body temperature.

10. Gently rock the slide containing the anti-A and anti-B serums back and forth for at least 1 to 2 minutes. Make sure the drops of blood and serum do not mix together. This allows the antigens in the blood to react with the serums. Using a strong light, check for an agglutination, or clumping, reaction in the two drops of blood. Agglutination indicates a positive reaction. If the reaction is positive, the cells will clump together. If the reaction is negative, the blood will remain unchanged.

11. At the end of 2 minutes, check the Rh slide on the viewbox. Use a strong light and observe for agglutination. If the cells have agglutinated, the reaction is positive, and the Rh factor is present in the blood. If the blood remains unchanged, the reaction is negative, and the Rh factor is not present in the blood.

12. Use the following chart to determine blood type based on serum agglutination reactions.

TYPE OF BLOOD	ANTI-A	ANTI-B	ANTI-RH OR ANTI-D
O	Negative	Negative	
A	Positive	Negative	
B	Negative	Positive	
AB	Positive	Positive	
Rh positive			Positive
Rh negative			Negative

13. Recheck any questionable results. Correctly record the information.

NOTE: Blood type is noted as A positive (A+), AB negative (AB−), and so forth for the various blood types.

14. Check the patient to make sure the skin puncture has stopped bleeding.

15. Clean and replace all equipment. If the slides are disposable, put them in the sharps container. If the slides are not disposable, wash them thoroughly and then clean or soak them in a disinfecting solution. Put all contaminated disposable supplies in the infectious-waste bag. Use a disinfectant to wipe the counter, viewbox, and other contaminated areas.

16. Remove gloves. Wash hands.

17. **C** Record all required information on the patient's chart or the agency form,

for example, date, time, Blood Type AB+, and your signature and title. Report any abnormal readings immediately.

Practice *Go to the workbook and use the evaluation sheet for 18:8, Testing for Blood Types, to practice this procedure. When you feel you have mastered this skill, sign the sheet and give it to your instructor for further action.*

Final Checkpoint Using the criteria listed on the evaluation sheet, your instructor will grade your performance.

18:9 INFORMATION
Performing an Erythrocyte Sedimentation Rate

 An erythrocyte sedimentation rate is another blood test for red blood cells (RBCs). An **erythrocyte sedimentation rate** (ESR) measures the distance that RBCs fall and settle in a glass test tube in a specific period of time. The test is also called a *sedimentation rate*, or *sed rate*. Venous blood is used for this test. An anticoagulant, such as oxalate or sequestrene, is added to the blood to prevent clotting. The blood is then placed in a special tube. The RBCs fall and settle in the tube. The distance is measured in millimeters by using graduated marks on the tube or rack. The measurement is taken at the point where the clear plasma line is noted above the settled RBCs (see figure 18-33).

In order for the RBCs to fall and settle correctly, the tube containing the blood must be placed in a special rack. The rack is designed to hold the tube in an exact vertical position. Many sedimentation racks contain a level indicator. This indicator must be adjusted so that the rack is 100 percent level with it.

Measurements of ESR are usually taken at specific time periods. Some laboratories check the distance at 15-minute intervals; other laboratories check the distance at 20-minute intervals. A measurement is always taken at the 1-hour period. The various readings and times are then placed on a graphic chart. By reading the chart, the physician can determine both the rate and distance of fall for the RBCs.

Normal values for ESR can vary slightly. The normal range depends to some extent on the method used. Most normal values are from 0 to 15 millimeters per hour for adult females and 0 to 10 millimeters per hour for adult males.

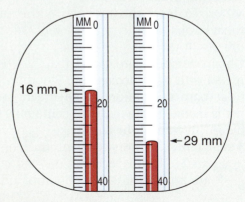

FIGURE 18-33 Read the level at the marked line between the cells and the plasma of the blood.

A faster-than-normal sedimentation rate signifies that inflammation and/or cell destruction has taken place. This may occur in conjunction with many medical conditions, including infections, cancers (such as certain carcinomas and leukemia), inflammatory processes (such as rheumatic fever and rheumatoid arthritis), and acute viral hepatitis. Pregnant or menstruating females may also have an increased sedimentation rate. A slower-than-normal sedimentation rate can occur in conjunction with polycythemia (a high number of RBCs), sickle-cell anemia, certain types of heart disease (such as congestive heart failure), and severe liver disease.

STUDENT: *Go to the workbook and complete the assignment sheet for 18:9, Performing an Erythrocyte Sedimentation Rate. Then return and continue with the procedure.*

PROCEDURE 18:9

Performing an Erythrocyte Sedimentation Rate

Equipment and Supplies

Venous blood with oxalate or sequestrene (anticoagulant), sedimentation rack, sedimentation-rate tubes, transfer pipette, timer, disposable gloves, infectious-waste bag, paper, pen or pencil

NOTE: The following procedure is for the Wintrobe method. Other methods vary slightly.

Procedure

1. Assemble equipment.
2. Wash hands. Put on gloves.

    CAUTION: Observe standard precautions while obtaining and testing blood.
3. Check the sedimentation rack. Make sure the rack is level. Check the bubble or level indicator for the level mark.

    NOTE: To level the rack, turn the platform knobs located near the feet (see figure 18-34A).
4. Obtain venipuncture blood that has been mixed with an anticoagulant. Blood should be at room temperature. Make sure the stopper is secure on the test tube containing the blood. Invert the tube and shake it gently for 3 to 5 minutes to thoroughly mix the blood.

    NOTE: Health occupation students are *not* permitted to obtain blood by venipuncture unless they receive special training.
5. Place the sedimentation tube in the rack. Make sure the black line on the tube is at the zero on the rack.

    NOTE: The tube must be clean and dry for an accurate measurement.

    NOTE: The tube can also be filled with the proper amount of blood first and then placed in the rack.

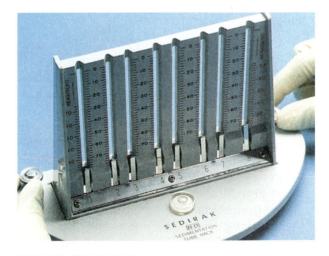

FIGURE 18-34A Turn the platform knobs to center the bubble in the indicator and to level the sedimentation rack.

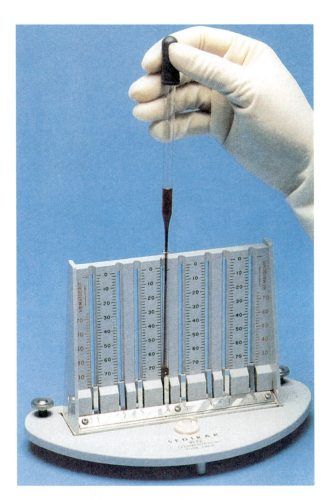

FIGURE 18-34B Transfer the blood from the pipette to the sedimentation-rate tube, taking care to keep the pipette below the level of the blood at all times to prevent air bubble formation.

6. With a transfer pipette, withdraw blood from the blood tube into the pipette and place the filled pipette in the bottom of the sedimentation-rate tube (see figure 18-34B). Gradually withdraw the pipette while expelling the blood to prevent air bubble formation. Fill the tube to the zero mark.
   NOTE: Before placing the pipette in the sedimentation-rate tube, use a gentle, even motion to expel all air from the bottom of the pipette.
   NOTE: If air bubbles are present, start over.
7. Recheck the level of the rack.

8. The RBCs will fall and settle. At specific time intervals, read the level to which the RBCs have fallen. Most tests are done at 20-, 40- and 60-minute intervals, but some laboratories and agencies take readings at 15-, 30-, 45- and 60-minute intervals, and others record only a 60-minute reading.
   NOTE: Read at eye level. Take the reading at the marked line between the cells and plasma of the blood (refer to figure 18-33).
9. Record the readings in millimeters. Note the times of the readings. Make sure all readings are recorded.
   NOTE: Normal readings vary. With the Wintrobe method, the reading is usually 0 to 15 millimeters per hour for females and 0 to 10 millimeters per hour for males.
10. Clean and replace all equipment. Most tubes are disposable. Place disposable tubes in a sharps container. Put other contaminated disposable supplies in the infectious-waste bag. Use a disinfectant to wipe the rack, counter, and any other contaminated areas.
11. Remove gloves. Wash hands thoroughly.
12. Record required information on the patient's chart or the agency form, for example, date; time; ESR 6 mm-20 min, 9 mm-40 min, or 12 mm-60 min; and your signature and title. Report any abnormal readings immediately.

Practice *Go to the workbook and use the evaluation sheet for 18:9, Performing an Erythrocyte Sedimentation Rate, to practice this procedure. When you feel you have mastered this skill, sign the sheet and give it to your instructor for further action.*

✔ **Final Checkpoint** Using the criteria listed on the evaluation sheet, your instructor will grade your performance.

INFORMATION

18:10 Measuring Blood-Sugar (Glucose) Level

Many health care careers involve measuring blood-sugar (glucose) level. **Glucose** is a form of sugar found in the bloodstream. Insulin, which is produced by the islets of Langerhans in the pancreas, normally allows glucose to cross cell membranes so that it can be metabolized. In a disease known as diabetes mellitus, however, there is an insufficient amount of insulin. Diabetics therefore cannot metabolize glucose, or convert it into energy. Glucose builds up in the bloodstream. Excess amounts are filtered out by the kidneys and eliminated from the body in the urine. **Hyperglycemia,** or high blood-sugar, and **glycosuria,** or sugar in the urine, are two main signs of diabetes.

Diabetics control their disease by following calculated diets that meet nutritional needs while controlling blood-sugar levels. In some cases, diet control can regulate blood-sugar level. However, many diabetics must also take insulin injections to control blood-sugar levels. Correct insulin dosage and proper diet can maintain normal blood-sugar level. However, the dosage of insulin required can vary depending on body metabolism, food intake, amount of exercise, other illness, and stress. For this reason, many diabetics are taught to check blood-sugar levels and regulate insulin dosages based on glucose levels. Because too much insulin can lead to severe **hypoglycemia,** or low blood sugar, and a condition called *insulin shock,* proper insulin dosage is essential.

A variety of blood tests can be used to check the level of glucose. One method of checking blood-sugar level is a **fasting blood sugar** (FBS). This test is usually performed in medical laboratories. The patient does not eat or drink anything (fasts) for 8 to 12 hours before the test. A venipuncture is done to obtain a sample of blood, and the amount of glucose is checked. Normal fasting blood sugar is 70 to 110 milligrams per deciliter of blood.

Another test called the *glucose tolerance test (GTT)* evaluates how well a person metabolizes a calculated amount of glucose. The GTT is frequently used to diagnose diabetes. The patient fasts for 8 to 12 hours before the GTT. A blood and urine specimen are obtained and tested for fasting levels. The patient then drinks a calibrated amount of glucose. Blood and urine specimens are usually obtained and tested at 30 minutes, one hour, two hours, and three hours, but test times vary. Normally, the glucose ingested would be metabolized by the end of the GTT and blood and urine levels of glucose would be in normal ranges. In a person with diabetes mellitus, the levels would remain elevated.

Another blood test that is performed on diabetics is the *glycohemoglobin test* (HbA1C or HbA1). This test measures the amount of glucose that attaches to the hemoglobin on red blood cells (RBCs). Because RBCs live approximately 120 days or four months, this test provides information on the average blood-sugar levels for the previous two to three months. Although normal values depend on the test used, a common normal range is 4.0 to 6.0 percent. A person with well-controlled diabetes averages 6 to 7 percent. A person with untreated or uncontrolled diabetes might have levels of 10 to 12 percent or even higher. If the glycohemoglobin level rises, it indicates that the patient's diabetic management plan must be improved. This can be accomplished by more frequent evaluations of daily glucose levels, changes in the type or dosage of insulin, and/or stricter dietary control. The American Diabetes Association recommends that diabetics with good glucose control be tested for glycohemoglobin levels once or twice a year. Diabetics with poor control should have the test four times a year.

In past years, most diabetics checked the level of glucose in the urine. A high level of glucose in the urine can indicate a high blood-sugar level, because excess glucose is filtered out of the blood by the kidneys. However, urine tests do *not always* accurately indicate a current blood-sugar level because the urine may show glucose that was excreted several hours earlier. Therefore, diabetics are now encouraged to check blood-glucose levels rather than urine-glucose levels. Advantages of checking blood glucose include increased accuracy compared to urine tests, unlimited flexibility with regard to timing of the test, ability to detect both low and high glucose levels, better regulation of insulin dosage, and improved control of diabetes.

It is now possible to use reagent strips to test blood-sugar level. These are plastic strips with a chemical-reagent pad or pads. A drop of blood from a skin puncture is placed on the pad. When glucose in the blood reacts with the chemicals on the pad, color changes occur. The amount of glucose present can be determined by comparing the color on the chemical-reagent pad to a color chart usually located on the bottle of reagent strips. This method is not as accurate because it relies on the operator performing a color match. Usually the strips are placed in a special photometer or glucose meter. The glucose meter provides a more accurate reading of the reagent strip and shows the amount of glucose in milligrams by way of numbers that light up on the screen.

In order to obtain the most accurate results, the following should be done:

◆ Store all reagent strips properly. Reagent strips are very sensitive to heat, light, and moisture. They should be stored in a dark, dry, cool area, but should not be refrigerated. The bottle containing the strips is usually made of dark or light-resistant glass. To prevent contamination from moisture in the air, the bottle should be closed immediately after use.

◆ Handle the reagent strips carefully. Never touch the chemical-reagent pad(s). Chemicals and moisture on the skin can cause inaccurate results. In addition, the chemicals on the strips can burn or injure the skin.

◆ Read all instructions carefully. Times and procedure methods vary with different strips. A few require rinsing before a reading is taken. Others must be blotted at a set time interval. If a glucose meter is used, it is important to use the strip designed for that particular brand of meter.

◆ Read all instructions provided with the glucose meter. To ensure accuracy, meters have to be calibrated before use. Test strips or solutions are used to calibrate the meter. Different time intervals and procedures are used for different meters.

◆ Some new glucose meters do not require the use of reagent strips. An example is the Hemo-Cue glucose meter (see figure 18-35). A disposable cuvette is filled with a drop of blood and the cuvette is inserted into the holder on the side of the unit. When the cuvette holder is pushed into the unit, the photometer measures the glucose level in 15 to 240 seconds and displays the reading on the monitor. The cuvette is then discarded in a sharps container. It is important to measure the sample of blood within 40 seconds to obtain the most accurate results.

◆ Glucose meters must be cleaned carefully after each use. Accumulation of dirt, dust, or other residue can lead to inaccurate readings. Most manufacturers recommend specific cleaning procedures. Lens paper is frequently recommended to prevent scratching the screen. Water is usually the only solution used for cleaning because alcohol can damage many meters. If possible, disinfect the meter.

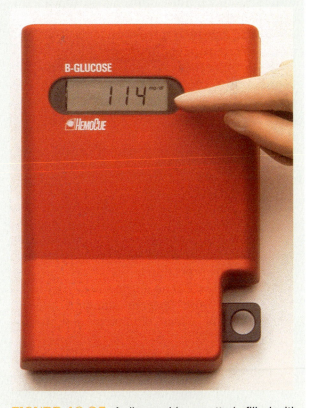

FIGURE 18-35 A disposable cuvette is filled with blood and inserted into the HemoCue glucose meter. The glucose level is displayed on the screen in 15 to 240 seconds. Reagent strips are *not* used with this type of glucose meter. *(Courtesy of HemoCue, Mission Viejo, CA)*

C Most patients check their own blood-glucose levels. Even children can be taught to monitor their own blood sugar levels. Patients must be given complete instructions on the correct procedure to use. Correct skin puncture techniques must be taught. Asepsis must be stressed. Proper use and storage of reagent strips and operation and cleaning of the glucose meter must be demonstrated.

Patients frequently are taught to determine insulin dosages based on glucose levels, so their determinations of glucose levels must be as accurate as possible.

STUDENT: *Go to the workbook and complete the assignment sheet for 18:10, Measuring Blood-Sugar (Glucose) Level. Then return and continue with the procedure.*

PROCEDURE 18:10

Measuring Blood-Sugar (Glucose) Level

Equipment and Supplies

Sterile lancet, alcohol swabs, sterile gauze, glucose reagent strips or disposable cuvette (depending on which glucose meter is used), glucose meter, lens paper, tissues or blotter paper, watch or timer with second hand, disposable gloves, sharps container, infectious-waste bag, paper, and pen or pencil

NOTE: The method used varies slightly depending on the type of reagent strip and/or glucose meter used. Follow specific manufacturer's instructions.

Procedure

1. Assemble equipment. Carefully read instructions provided with the glucose reagent strips and the glucose meter. Note times that must be observed during each step of the procedure.
2. Wash hands. Put on gloves.

   CAUTION: Observe standard precautions while obtaining and testing blood.
3. Calibrate the glucose meter for accuracy. Follow the manufacturer's instructions. Most meters have test reagent strips or solutions that are placed on a reagent strip to check calibration.
4. C Introduce yourself. Identify the patient. Explain the procedure. Obtain the patient's consent.

NOTE: It is best to seat the patient in a comfortable position.

5. Perform the procedure for a skin puncture. Place the used lancet in the sharps container immediately.
6. Use sterile gauze to remove the first drop of blood.
7. Remove one reagent strip from the bottle, being careful not to touch the chemical-reagent pad on the strip. Immediately close the lid of the bottle.

   CAUTION: If the chemical reagent pad touches the skin, injury or burns can occur, as can inaccurate readings.
8. Press the start button on the glucose meter. A beep or light usually indicates the correct time for placing a large drop of blood on the reagent strip. Make sure the drop of blood completely covers the chemical-reagent pad. Hold the strip level to avoid spilling the blood. Do not allow the chemical-reagent pad to touch the skin while applying the drop of blood.

NOTE: If the glucose meter uses a disposable cuvette instead of a reagent strip, place the tip end of the cuvette into the middle of the drop of blood. Hold the cuvette steady to allow the chamber to fill completely through capillary action. Use a lint-free tissue or lens paper to wipe off excess blood on the outside of the cuvette. Immediately place the cuvette into the holder on the side of the glucose meter (refer to figure 18-35). Gently push the cuvette holder into the glucose meter. Within 15 to 240 seconds, the glucose reading will be displayed on the screen. Steps 10 and 11 of this procedure are not used with this type of glucose meter.

9. When sufficient blood has been obtained, instruct the patient to hold sterile gauze firmly against the skin puncture.

   ⬡! CAUTION: Remain with the patient until the bleeding stops.

10. The glucose meter signals with a beep or light when the blood has been on the strip for the required period of time. If necessary, blot the strip gently by placing it between a fold of tissue or blotter paper. Some glucose meters do not require blotting of the reagent strip, so it is important to follow manufacturer's instructions.

    NOTE: Blood usually remains on the strip for 10 to 60 seconds. It is important to follow the time period established by the manufacturer, because this is a crucial step.

    ⬡! CAUTION: Never wipe the strip while blotting it. Wiping removes too much of the blood and causes inaccurate results.

11. Immediately insert the strip into the correct position in the meter (see figure 18-36). Most manufacturers require that the reagent pad faces the window on the meter. Check to be sure the strip is in the correct position. Follow manufacturer's instructions to obtain an accurate reading.

12. Record your reading in milligrams (mg), for example, *102 mg*. Be sure to include the date, time, glucose test, your name or initials, and other required information. Double-check your reading for accuracy.

13. Check the patient to make sure that bleeding from the skin puncture has stopped.

14. Clean and replace all equipment. Place the reagent strip and any contaminated disposable equipment in the infectious-waste bag. If a disposable cuvette was used, place the cuvette in the sharps container. Use a disinfectant to wipe the counter and any contaminated areas. Follow the manufacturer's instructions for proper cleaning of the glucose meter.

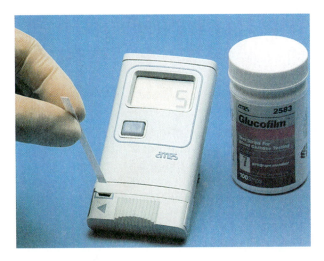

FIGURE 18-36 Insert the reagent strip into the correct position in the glucose meter to obtain an accurate blood-glucose level.

NOTE: Most manufacturers recommend using lens paper and water to clean the window, strip slot, and other areas on the meter. A disinfectant solution should then be put on these areas unless prohibited by the manufacturer.

15. Remove gloves. Wash hands thoroughly.

16. **C** Record all required information on the patient's chart or the agency form, for example, date; time; Blood Glucose: 102 mg; and your signature and title. Report any abnormal readings immediately.

Practice *Go to the workbook and use the evaluation sheet for 18:10, Measuring Blood-Sugar (Glucose) Level, to practice this procedure. When you feel you have mastered this skill, sign the sheet and give it to your instructor for further action.*

 Final Checkpoint Using the criteria listed on the evaluation sheet, your instructor will grade your performance.

18:11 INFORMATION Testing Urine

Urine tests are often done to determine the physical condition of a patient. Abnormal urine tests are often the first indications of a disease process. Table 18-1 provides the main facts regarding urine, specifically normal and abnormal characteristics of urine. Refer to this table as you perform the basic urine tests.

A **urinalysis** is an examination of urine and consists of three main areas of testing: *physical, chemical,* and *microscopic.*

Physical testing of urine is usually done first and consists of observing and recording color, odor, transparency, and specific gravity. The urine specimen should be fresh and mixed gently prior to being checked for physical characteristics. The normal and abnormal physical characteristics are listed in Table 18-1.

Chemical testing of urine is performed to check pH, protein, glucose, ketone, bilirubin, urobilinogen, and blood. Reagent strips, described in detail in Information section 18:12, are usually used for chemical testing. Diseases indicated by the presence of abnormal chemicals in the urine are listed in Table 18-1.

Microscopic testing of the urine is done to examine formed elements in the urine, such as cells, casts, crystals, and amorphous deposits. To do a microscopic examination, the urine is centrifuged to spin out the solid particles and form urinary sediment. This procedure is described in detail in Information Section 18:14. The sediment is then examined under a microscope and checked for the presence of blood cells, bacteria, casts (formed in the kidney tubules and expelled during kidney damage), and other elements.

For the most accurate results, a urinalysis should be performed on fresh, warm urine. If possible, a urine specimen should be examined within 1 hour after it is collected. If this is not possible, the specimen can be refrigerated. After refrigeration, it should be returned to room temperature before being examined.

Urine is a body fluid, so standard precautions (Unit 13:3) must be observed while collecting and handling urine. Hands must be washed frequently, and gloves must be worn at all times. If splashing of the urine is possible, a mask, protective eyewear, and protective clothing must be worn. Urine should be discarded in a toilet, but is sometimes poured down a sink. If this is done, the sink must be flushed with water and wiped with a disinfectant. Any areas contaminated by the urine must be wiped with a disinfectant. The specimen containers and other contaminated disposable supplies must be discarded in the infectious-waste bag prior to being discarded as infectious-waste according to legal requirements.

STUDENT: *Go to the workbook and complete the assignment sheet for 18:11, Testing Urine.*

18:12 INFORMATION Using Reagent Strips to Test Urine

This section describes the urine reagent strip test, which is frequently used as a screening test for urine. Many different types of reagent strips are available, and all work according to the same basic principles. Read the label of the reagent strip container for directions.

Excess amounts of many substances in the blood are eliminated from the body by the kidneys as part of urine. By testing the urine for the presence of these substances, certain diseases in the body can be detected. The most common method of testing for the presence or absence of these substances is the use of the urine reagent strip, or dipstic.

Urine **reagent strips** are firm, plastic strips. Small pads containing chemical reactants are attached to the strip. Each pad reacts to a specific substance. If the substance is present in the urine, it reacts with the chemical

TABLE 18-1 Characteristics of Urine

CHARACTERISTIC	NORMAL	ABNORMAL
Volume or amount	1,000 to 2,000 cc daily	**Polyuria**—increased amount, over 2,000 cc in 24 hours **Oliguria**—decreased amount, less than 500 cc in 24 hours **Anuria**—no formation
Color	Some shade of yellow; straw-yellow to amber	Pale or colorless—diluted Dark-yellow, orange, or brown—concentrated Yellow or beer-brown—bilirubin or bile pigment, can precede jaundice and indicate hepatitis Cloudy-red—caused by presence of RBCs (hematuria) Clear-red—hemoglobin, due to increased RBC destruction
Transparency	Clear	Cloudy because of pus, mucus, WBCs, and/or old specimen Milky because of fats or lipids
Odor	Faintly aromatic	Ammonia—old specimen Foul/putrid—bacteria or infection Fruity or sweet—acetone or ketones, diabetes mellitus
pH reaction	Range 5.5 to 8.0, Average 6 (Mildly Acidic)	Alkaline—infection, chronic renal failure, or old specimen High acidity—diarrhea, starvation, and ketones (diabetes mellitus)
Specific gravity	1.005 to 1.030	Increased—diabetes mellitus, concentrated urine, low fluid intake, dehydration Decreased-renal disease, diluted urine, high fluid intake, diuretic medications (water pills)
Glucose	None	Presence, glycosuria, may mean diabetes mellitus
Albumin, protein	None to trace	Presence, proteinuria or albuminuria, can indicate kidney disease
Acetones–ketones	None	Presence, ketonuria, can indicate starvation, diabetes mellitus, or a high-fat diet
Blood	None	Presence, hematuria, indicates kidney, ureter, or bladder disease or infection
Pus	None	Presence, pyuria, indicates infection in urinary system
Bacteria	None in catheter specimen Small amount in routine specimen is normal	Large amount may indicate infection
Red blood cells (Erythrocytes)	None	Presence may indicate disease of kidneys, bleeding in the urinary tract
White blood cells (Leukocytes)	Few normal	Large number indicates infection
Bilirubin	None	Presence, bilirubinuria, can indicate liver disease, hepatitis, or bile duct obstruction
Urobilinogen	0.1 to 1.0 E.U./dl (Ehrlich units per deciliter)	Presence can indicate liver disease, destruction of red blood cells (hemolytic diseases)

reactant on the strip and produces a color change. In addition to showing the presence of the substance, most of the chemical reactants will also measure the amount of the substance present by producing different color changes according to the amount of substance present.

⚠️ Most urine reagent strips are very sensitive to light, heat, and moisture. They must be stored in a dry, cool, dark area. The bottle containing the strips is usually made of dark or light-resistant glass. A moisture-absorbent pad or pack is usually present in the bottle. The bottle must be closed immediately after use. Care must be taken not to touch or handle any of the chemical-reactant pads on the strip. Chemicals and moisture on the skin can lead to an inaccurate test. In addition, many of the chemicals on the strip are poisonous and can burn or injure the skin. Many patients use reagent strips in their homes for specific urine tests, so it is important to make sure that the patient understands the importance of correct storage and handling of reagent strips. The patient should be cautioned against storing the strips in a bathroom, on windowsills, or close to sources of heat. The strips must also be stored out of the reach of children.

Chemical reactants on the pads of the strips are only effective for a certain period of time. An expiration date is printed on every bottle of strips. Never use reagent strips after the expiration date, because inaccurate test results will occur. In an agency where many bottles of strips are kept in stock, it is important to rotate the strips so that the bottle with the closest expiration date is used first.

Reagent strips can be used to test for a variety of substances present in the urine. Some of the more common ones include the following:

◆ *pH* is a measure of the acidity or alkalinity of urine. pH is measured on a scale of 1 to 14. A neutral pH is 7. A pH below 7 indicates acidic urine, and a pH above 7 indicates alkaline urine. Urine is usually slightly acidic, with a pH range of 5.5 to 8.0. Diet, medications, kidney disease, starvation, and diabetes can each change pH.

◆ *Protein* should be retained in the blood and it is not normally found in the urine. Its presence (proteinuria), usually in the form of albumin (albuminuria), may indicate kidney disease.

◆ *Glucose* is usually metabolized to produce energy and is not normally found in the urine. If the level of glucose in the blood is high, glucose will be eliminated in the urine, a condition called glycosuria. The presence of glucose can indicate diabetes mellitus.

◆ *Ketones* and *acetones* are the end products of the metabolism of fat in the body. They are not normally found in the urine. Their presence (ketonuria) can indicate diabetes mellitus, starvation, fasting, dieting, a high-fat diet, and metabolic disorders.

◆ *Blood* is not normally found in the urine. A test sometimes shows positive for blood when the patient is menstruating. If blood is detected in the urine, a microscopic examination of the urine should be performed. Blood in the urine is called **hematuria.** Its presence can indicate injury, infection, or disease in the kidneys and/or urinary tract.

◆ *Bilirubin* is not usually present in the urine. It is a breakdown product of the hemoglobin on red blood cells (RBCs) and is usually eliminated through the intestines. Its presence (bilirubinuria) in the urine can indicate liver disease such as hepatitis or bile duct obstruction.

◆ *Urobilinogen* is bilirubin that has been converted by intestinal bacteria. It is usually excreted by the intestines. Small amounts of 0.1 to 1.0 Ehrlich units (EU) per deciliter of urine are normal. The presence of larger amounts usually indicates heart, spleen, liver, or hemolytic (destruction of blood cells) disease.

Many different types of reagent strips are available. Some of the more common types and the substances they test for include:

◆ Albustix: protein

◆ Bili-Labstix: pH, protein, glucose, ketone, bilirubin, and blood

◆ Chemstrip-GK: glucose and ketone

◆ Chemstrip-GP: glucose and protein

- Clinistix: glucose

- Combistix: pH, glucose, and protein

- Diastix: glucose

- Hemastix: blood

- Keto-Diastix: glucose and ketone

- Ketostix: ketone

- Labstix: pH, glucose, protein, ketone, and blood

- Multistix: pH, specific gravity, glucose, protein, ketone, blood, bilirubin, urobilinogen, and nitrite

- Uristix: protein, glucose, nitrites, and leukocytes

It is important to read the instructions carefully when using any type of reagent strip. A color comparison chart is usually located on the bottle of reagent strips or on a paper enclosed in the box. This chart lists the substances to be tested and the correct time interval for reading each reaction. The exact time for reading each chemical reaction must be followed for the most accurate results. Adequate lighting is essential to correctly match colors.

Most laboratories and offices perform quality control checks on reagent strips to make sure the strips produce accurate results. A urine control solution, with predetermined results, is tested with a reagent strip. If the results do not meet the predetermined range, the strips must not be used. Quality control checks should be run at least once a day, whenever a new container of strips is opened, and any time test results seem questionable.

Automated strip readers or analyzers are available (see figure 18-37). The strip readers, or spectophotometers, analyze the color change and intensity for each reagent on the strip. The results are displayed on a lighted screen and/or printed. The automated strip readers are more accurate than the human eye, but they are expensive.

To obtain the greatest degree of accuracy with a reagent strip, fresh urine specimens should be used. Urine should be tested within 1 hour of collection. If this is not possible, the urine specimen should be refrigerated.

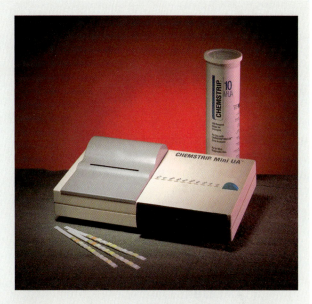

FIGURE 18-37 The Chemstrip Mini UA urine analyzer is one example of an automated strip reader that analyzes the reagent strip more accurately than the human eye. *(Courtesy of Boehringer Mannheim)*

However, refrigerated specimens should be allowed to return to room temperature prior to being tested. Results are most accurate if testing can be done immediately after collecting the specimen, while the specimen is still warm.

C When results of the test are recorded, the type of test used must be specified, for example, *Labstix* or *Multistix*. All substances tested must be listed along with the results for each. The date and time of the test should also be noted. Put your name or initials near the recording. A sample charting is as follows:

1/30/–9:00 A.M. Miss Smith
Labstix Test: pH: 6
　　　　　　 Protein: neg.
　　　　　　 Glucose: 1%
　　　　　　 Ketone: mod.
　　　　　　 Blood: neg.

STUDENT: *Go to the workbook and complete the assignment sheet for 18:12, Using Reagent Strips to Test Urine. Then return and continue with the procedure.*

PROCEDURE 18:12

Using Reagent Strips to Test Urine

Equipment and Supplies

Fresh, early morning urine specimen, if possible; urine-specimen container; reagent strips and color comparison chart; disposable gloves; infectious-waste bag; paper; pen or pencil; watch with second hand or timer

Procedure

1. Assemble equipment. Read instructions for the reagent strip.
2. Wash hands. Put on gloves.

   CAUTION: Observe standard precautions while obtaining and testing urine.
3. **C** Introduce yourself. Identify the patient. Explain the procedure. Obtain the patient's consent.
4. Obtain a fresh urine specimen and pour it into the specimen container.
5. Gently rotate the container between your hands to mix the urine specimen.
6. Hold a reagent strip by the clear end (see figure 18-38A). Immerse the strip in the urine specimen, making sure all reagent areas are submersed.
7. Remove the strip immediately. Tap the edge of the strip against the side of the specimen container to remove excess urine (see figure 18-38B).

NOTE: This will prevent urine from dropping on the color comparison chart during color matching.

8. Turn the strip so that the reagent areas are facing you. Hold the strip horizontally near the color comparison charts on the bottle (see figure 18-38C).
9. Note the time. A watch or clock with a second hand is essential because many readings are done in a period of seconds.

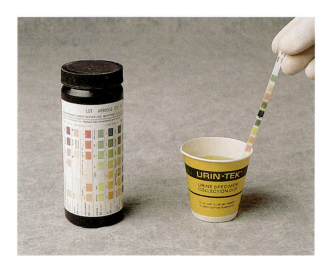

FIGURE 18-38B Tap the edge of the strip against the side of the specimen container to remove excess urine.

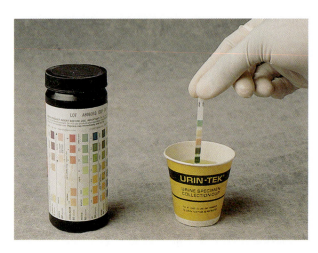

FIGURE 18-38A Hold the reagent strip by the clear end to immerse the strip in the urine specimen.

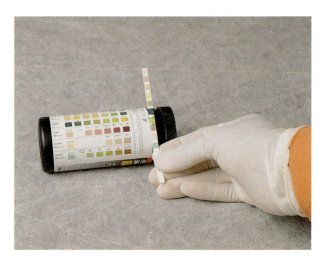

FIGURE 18-38C Under good lighting, compare the strip to the color charts to determine correct readings.

10. Start at the center of the strip. Read any reagent areas that require immediate readings. Record these readings.

11. Watch the time and read additional reagent areas at the correct time intervals. Some are read at 10 seconds, 15 seconds, 30 seconds, or 60 seconds. Record all readings.

    NOTE: The time lapses between readings are usually sufficient to allow you to read readily down the strip.

12. Recheck all readings. Using a second reagent strip to check accuracy of results is sometimes required.

13. Discard the strip and any contaminated disposable supplies in the infectious-waste bag. Pour the urine into a toilet or down a sink. If a sink is used, flush the sink with water and wipe with a disinfectant. Use a disinfectant to wipe the counter and any contaminated areas. Clean and replace all equipment.

14. Remove gloves. Wash hands.

15. **C** Record all required information on the patient's chart or the agency form, for example: date, time; Labstix: pH: 6, Protein: neg., Glucose: 1%, Ketones: Tr., Blood: Neg; and your signature and title. Report any abnormal readings to your supervisor immediately.

Practice *Go to the workbook and use the evaluation sheet for 18:12, Using Reagent Strips to Test Urine, to practice this procedure. When you feel you have mastered this skill, sign the sheet and give it to your instructor for further action.*

✔ **Final Checkpoint** Using the criteria listed on the evaluation sheet, your instructor will grade your performance.

18:13 INFORMATION *Measuring Specific Gravity*

Specific gravity is defined as the weight of a substance compared to the weight of distilled water, in equal volumes. Specific gravity of urine, then, is the weight of urine compared to the weight of an equal amount of distilled water. The weight of distilled water is 1.000. Its specific gravity is expressed as: *Sp. Gr. 1.000.*

The normal range for specific gravity of urine is 1.005 to 1.030 with most specimens ranging between 1.010 to 1.025. Variations occur as follows:

◆ *Low specific gravity,* below 1.005, is usually caused by diluted urine possibly resulting from excessive fluid intake, kidney disease in which the kidneys cannot concentrate urine, diuretic medications, or diabetes insipidus.

◆ *High specific gravity,* above 1.030, is usually caused by concentrated urine possibly resulting from low fluid intake, dehydration, excessive fluid loss through other body parts, kidney disease in which too many substances are excreted, and/or diabetes mellitus, in which sugar is present in the urine.

 One way to determine specific gravity is to measure it with a **urinometer.** Urine is poured into a urinometer jar or cylinder. The urinometer, which is a float with a calibrated stem, is placed in the urine with a spinning motion. The urine collects at a line at a curved angle on the urinometer float. This line is known as the *meniscus.* The reading for specific gravity is taken at the lower part of the meniscus. It must be read at eye level to be accurate. Each calibration on the urinometer float is in thousandths. The top line represents 1.000, the specific gravity of distilled water, and each small line below it represents .001. The calibrations read 1.000, 1.001, 1.002, 1.003, 1.004, and so forth. It is important that the urinometer be free floating and away from the sides and bottom of the jar or cylinder when the reading for specific gravity is taken.

Another way to determine specific gravity is with a **refractometer** (see figure 18-39). One drop of well-mixed urine is placed on the refractometer. Specific gravity is read by looking through an ocular, or eyepiece. It is important to follow manufacturer's instructions and to calibrate the refractometer with distilled water when it is used.

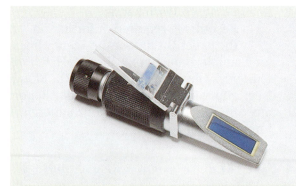

STUDENT: *Go to the workbook and complete the assignment sheet for 18:13, Measuring Specific Gravity. Then return and continue with the procedure.*

FIGURE 18-39 A refractometer can be used to calculate specific gravity of urine.

PROCEDURE 18:13
Measuring Specific Gravity

Equipment and Supplies

Urine specimen in a container, urinometer float, urinometer jar or cylinder, refractometer, transfer pipette or eye dropper, disposable gloves, infectious-waste bag, paper towels or gauze, paper, pencil or pen

Procedure

1. Assemble equipment.
2. To use a urinometer, clean the urinometer float and cylinder or jar thoroughly and make sure they are dry. To use a refractometer, place one drop of distilled water on the glass plate and close the lid gently. Look through the eyepiece and read the specific gravity to make sure it is 1.000. If it is not, the refractometer must be calibrated according to manufacturer's instructions. Use lens paper to dry and clean the glass plate.
   NOTE: Dirty equipment will interfere with the reading.
3. Wash hands. Put on gloves.
   CAUTION: Observe standard precautions while obtaining and testing urine.
4. **C** Introduce yourself. Identify the patient. Explain the procedure. Obtain the patient's consent.
5. Obtain a fresh urine specimen. Do *not* refrigerate the specimen because this can alter the test results. It is best to perform the test as soon as possible after obtaining the urine. The most accurate results are obtained when the urine is at room temperature.
   NOTE: An early-morning, first-voided specimen is the most concentrated and is therefore preferred.
6. To check specific gravity using a urinometer, proceed as follows:
   a. Fill the urinometer jar or cylinder with urine to within 1 inch from the top.
      NOTE: Make sure the urine is mixed well.
   b. Using paper or a piece of gauze, remove any bubbles from the top of the urine.
   c. Grasp the urinometer stem at the top and slowly insert it into the jar or cylinder containing the urine. Avoid wetting the top of the stem. As you insert the urinometer float, twirl it slightly so that it does not stick to the sides.
      NOTE: A spinning float will not stick to the sides of the urinometer jar or cylinder.
   d. Make sure the float is away from the sides of the jar and that it is *not* touching the bottom of the jar or cylinder. The urinometer must be free floating.

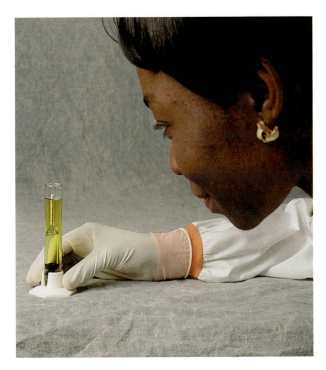

FIGURE 18-40 Read the specific gravity of urine at eye level at the lower line of the meniscus.

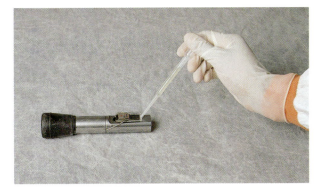

FIGURE 18-41A Place one drop of well-mixed urine on the glass plate of the refractometer.

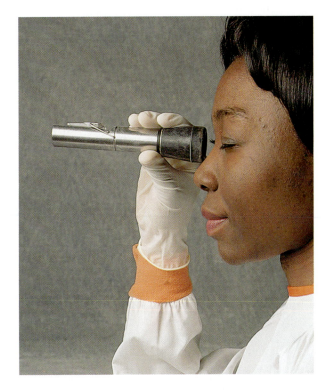

FIGURE 18-41B Look through the eyepiece to read the specific gravity on the refractometer scale.

e. When the urinometer float stops spinning, take the reading at eye level at the lower line of the meniscus (see figure 18-40).

   NOTE: Do *not* read above the meniscus. This is inaccurate. Normal specific gravity is 1.005 to 1.030.

   ✔ **CHECKPOINT:** Your instructor will check the accuracy of your reading.

7. To check specific gravity using a refractometer, proceed as follows:

   a. Use a transfer pipette or eye dropper to place one drop of well-mixed urine on the glass plate of the refractometer (see figure 18-41A).

   b. Close the lid gently.

   c. Look through the eyepiece and read the specific gravity on the scale (see figure 18-41B).

   ✔ **CHECKPOINT:** Your instructor will check the accuracy of your reading.

8. Record the reading.

9. Recheck the reading, if necessary.

10. Clean and replace all equipment. To clean the urinometer and jar or cylinder, pour the urine into a toilet or sink. If a sink is used, flush the sink with water and wipe with a disinfectant. Wash the urinometer and jar or cylinder thoroughly, rinse or soak with a disinfectant, and dry both pieces completely.

To clean the refractometer, follow manufacturer's instructions. Most manufacturers recommend using lens paper on the glass to prevent scratches. A disinfectant can be put on the lens paper to clean the glass, and another sheet of lens paper can be used to dry the glass. Put all contaminated disposable supplies in the infectious-waste bag. Use a disinfectant to wipe the counter and any contaminated areas.

11. Remove gloves. Wash hands thoroughly.

12. **C** Record all required information on the patient's chart or the agency form,

for example, date; time; SpGr: 1.011; and your signature and title. Report any abnormal readings to your supervisor immediately.

Practice *Go to the workbook and use the evaluation sheet for 18:13, Measuring Specific Gravity, to practice this procedure. When you feel you have mastered this skill, sign the sheet and give it to your instructor for further action.*

18:14 INFORMATION Preparing Urine for Microscopic Examination

Microscopic testing of urine is done to examine all the solid materials suspended in the urine. These materials are called **urinary sediment.** Presence of certain substances, such as blood cells, casts, and bacteria, can indicate disease conditions.

A fresh, early-morning first-voided specimen is preferred. This type of specimen is usually the most concentrated; thus, it is more likely to contain abnormal substances. The specimen should be examined immediately, if at all possible. Certain elements, such as red cells and casts, disintegrate rapidly in warm specimens. If the urine cannot be examined immediately, it should be kept cold to preserve these substances.

Only a portion of the urine specimen is actually examined under a microscope. The entire specimen is first mixed well. A small amount, usually 10 to 15 cubic centimeters, is then placed in a centrifuge tube. This tube is then put into a centrifuge. The centrifuge spins the urine, causing any solid materials to settle to the bottom of the tube. These solid materials

are called *sediment*. The clear urine on the top of the tube is poured off, leaving approximately 1 cubic centimeter of sediment in the bottom of the tube. This procedure results in concentrated urine, which is then examined under a microscope.

The size of the drop of concentrated urine examined is important. The drop of sediment placed on a slide for viewing will be covered with a coverslip. The drop should be large enough so that there is no empty space under the coverslip but not so large as to cause the coverslip to float.

The urinary sediment should be examined immediately after it is placed on the slide. Drying of the specimen occurs quickly, and this can result in distortions in the shapes and sizes of any substances present.

Learning to identify various substances detected during a microscopic examination of the urine requires training and experience. Some of the substances that may be seen in urinary sediment are shown in figure 18-42. Elements such as epithelial cells and certain casts can be seen with the low-power objective. Other elements, such as blood cells, bacteria, and crystals, can be seen only with the high-power objective. When recording the elements seen, it is important to note the objective used. This is usually recorded as *per low-power field* (lpf) or *per high-power field*

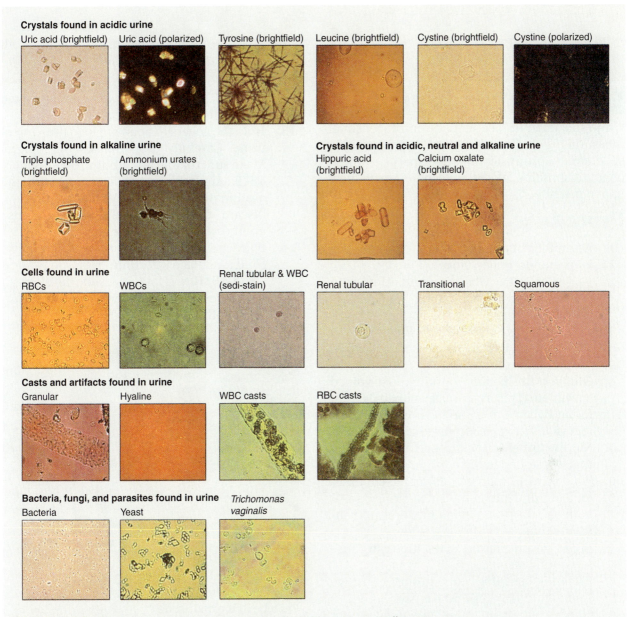

Crystals found in acidic urine
Uric acid (brightfield) Uric acid (polarized) Tyrosine (brightfield) Leucine (brightfield) Cystine (brightfield) Cystine (polarized)

Crystals found in alkaline urine
Triple phosphate (brightfield) Ammonium urates (brightfield)

Crystals found in acidic, neutral and alkaline urine
Hippuric acid (brightfield) Calcium oxalate (brightfield)

Cells found in urine
RBCs WBCs Renal tubular & WBC (sedi-stain) Renal tubular Transitional Squamous

Casts and artifacts found in urine
Granular Hyaline WBC casts RBC casts

Bacteria, fungi, and parasites found in urine
Bacteria Yeast *Trichomonas vaginalis*

FIGURE 18-42 Some elements that may be found in urinary sediment.

(hpf). For example, a recording might state, *epithelial cells: mod/lpf.* In many settings, the laboratory assistant prepares the urine for microscopic examination and a specially trained individual examines the sediment and identifies the elements present. Follow your agency's policy regarding this procedure. If you are responsible for examining the sediment, never hesitate to ask questions or obtain assistance if you are unable to identify the elements present.

STUDENT: *Go to the workbook and complete the assignment sheet for 18:14, Preparing Urine for Microscopic Examination of Urinary Sediment. Then return and continue with the procedure.*

PROCEDURE 18:14

Preparing Urine for Microscopic Examination

Equipment and Supplies

Urine specimen in a container, centrifuge, small measuring cup, centrifuge tube, microscopic slide, coverslip, transfer pipette, urinary-sediment chart, disposable gloves, infectious-waste bag, paper, pen or pencil

Procedure

1. Assemble equipment.
2. Wash hands. Put on gloves.

    CAUTION: Observe standard precautions while obtaining and testing urine.

3. **C** Introduce yourself. Identify the patient. Explain the procedure. Obtain the patient's consent.

4. Obtain a fresh, early-morning, first-voided specimen. This type of specimen is preferred because it is the most concentrated and yields the most accurate results.

5. Mix the urine well to suspend any sediment that has settled to the bottom.

6. Pour 10 to 15 milliliters (or cubic centimeters) of urine into a small measuring cup.

7. Pour the measured urine into a clean centrifuge tube.

    NOTE: Residue or dirt in the tube can cause inaccurate results.

8. Place the centrifuge tube in the centrifuge (see figure 18-43A). Make sure there is another tube containing an equal amount of urine or water opposite this centrifuge tube; the second tube acts to counterbalance the weight of the first.

9. Centrifuge the urine for 4 to 5 minutes.

10. Carefully pour off 9 to 14 milliliters (or cubic centimeters) of the clear urine. Leave 1 milliliter of urine and the sediment in the bottom of the tube.

11. Gently shake the tube to resuspend the sediment in the bottom of the remaining 1 milliliter of urine.

12. Using care, transfer one drop of the well-mixed sediment to a clean glass slide (see figure 18-43B).

    NOTE: The size of the drop is important. If it is too large, it will cause the coverslip to float. If it is too small, it will not fill the area under the coverslip.

13. Hold the coverslip at an angle to the drop of urine. Carefully drop the slip into place. Make sure that *no* air bubbles are present.

    NOTE: Air bubbles will interfere with the examination. If any air bubbles are present, discard the drop on the slide and use another drop of the urine.

14. Place the slide on the microscope stage. Hold it in place with slide clips.

    CAUTION: Hold the slide level at all times to prevent the urine from running off the slide.

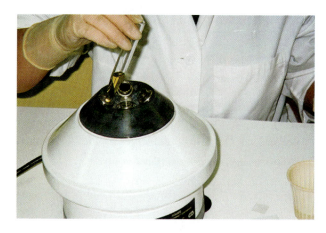

FIGURE 18-43A After pouring 10 to 15 millimeters of urine into the centrifuge tube, place the tube in the centrifuge.

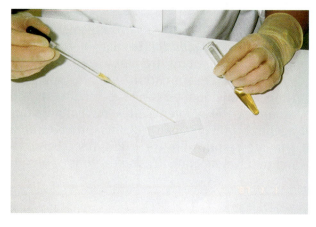

FIGURE 18-43B Transfer one drop of well-mixed sediment to a clean glass slide.

15. Use the low-power (10X) objective and the coarse adjustment to bring the slide into focus.

    ⚠️ **CAUTION:** Watch the stage while using the coarse adjustment to move the objective down toward the slide.

16. Adjust the lighting to allow the best viewing of the slide. A dimmer light usually provides a clearer view under low power.

17. Use a chart on urinary sediment or refer to figure 18-42 to identify some of the substances present in the urinary sediment.

    NOTE: The examination should be completed within 3 minutes. Drying occurs after this time, and can lead to inaccurate identification.

18. Switch to the high-power objective and examine the specimen again. Note which substances are best viewed under high power according to the chart.

19. Clean and replace all equipment. Pour the urine into a toilet or down a sink. If a sink is used, flush the sink with water and wipe with a disinfectant. Place all contaminated disposable supplies in the infectious-waste bag. Use a disinfectant to wipe the counter and any contaminated areas. Cover the microscope.

20. Remove gloves. Wash hands thoroughly.

21. **C** Record all required information on the patient's chart or the agency form, for example, date; time; Microscopic Exam: epithelial: few/lpf, WBCs: 4–6/hpf, RBCs: few/hpf, casts: neg, crystals: few/hpf; and your signature and title. Report any abnormal observations to your supervisor immediately.

Practice *Go to the workbook and use the evaluation sheet for 18:14, Preparing Urine for Microscopic Examination of Urinary Sediment, to practice this procedure. When you feel you have mastered this skill, sign the sheet and give it to your instructor for further action.*

✔ **Final Checkpoint** Using the criteria listed on the evaluation sheet, your instructor will grade your performance.

UNIT 18 SUMMARY

Laboratory assistant skills are utilized not only in medical laboratories, but also in medical offices and nursing care facilities. A basic knowledge of the major types of tests performed is beneficial for many different health care workers.

Because the microscope is used in many laboratory tests, the health care worker should be familiar with how to operate it.

Obtaining culture specimens and preparing them for examination helps the health care professional determine the cause of a disease and, often, the proper way to treat the disease. Many of the specimens contain communicable pathogens (germs capable of spreading disease), so care must be taken while performing these procedures.

Blood tests are performed for a variety of reasons. Some of the more common tests include typing, hemoglobin, hematocrit, blood cell counts for erythrocytes and leukocytes, erythrocyte sedimentation rate, blood smear or film, and blood glucose. Following proper techniques and striving for accuracy is essential because these tests are used to determine the presence or absence of disease.

Urine tests are performed to check the function of various body organs. The presence of abnormal substances in the urine is frequently the first indication of disease. A urinalysis, or examination of the urine, usually involves three areas of testing: physical, chemical, and microscopic. The health care worker should be familiar with each of these areas and be able to perform the tests with precision and accuracy.

Standard precautions must be followed at all times while performing laboratory tests. Many diseases are transmitted by blood and body fluids, so extreme care must be taken while handling these substances.

INTERNET SEARCHES

Use the suggested search engines in Unit 11:4 of this textbook to search the Internet for additional information on the following topics:

1. *Organizations:* locate web sites for the American Medical Technologists Association, International Society for Clinical Laboratory Testing, American Red Cross (blood donations), and the American Diabetic Association (blood glucose testing) to research basic laboratory tests.

2. *Science:* research microbiology, bacteria, viruses, microorganisms.

3. *Blood tests:* research erythrocyte, leukocyte, hemoglobin, hematocrit, blood typing, erythrocyte sedimentation rate, and blood glucose tests.

4. *Urine tests:* research urinary reagent strips, urinary sediments, urinalysis, and specific gravity of urine.

5. *Medical supplies:* search for suppliers of medical laboratory equipment such as hemacytometers, hematocrit centrifuges, hemoglobinometers, photometers, glucose meters, refractometers, automated reagent strip readers, and urinometers to compare and contrast the various products available on the market.

6. *Laws:* research the Clinical Laboratory Improvement Amendment (CLIA) to determine legal responsibilities and quality control standards for a medical laboratory.

REVIEW QUESTIONS

1. What is the purpose of a culture and sensitivity study? Differentiate between *sensitive* and *resistant* organisms.

2. List six (6) points that must be checked prior to performing a skin puncture to obtain blood.

3. Differentiate between an erythrocyte count, hematocrit, and hemoglobin.

4. State the normal values or ranges for each of the following tests:
   a. microhematocrit
   b. hemoglobin
   c. erythrocyte count
   d. leukocyte count
   e. erythrocyte sedimentation rate
   f. specific gravity of urine

5. Why is it important to evaluate the Rh status of a pregnant woman?

6. List five (5) precautions that must be observed while storing and/or using urinary reagent strips.

7. Briefly list the components or tests performed during a physical, chemical, and microscopic examination of the urine.

8. List all of the standard precautions that must be observed while performing culture studies, blood tests, or urine tests.

UNIT 18

SUGGESTED REFERENCES

Bonewit-West, Kathy. *Clinical Procedures for Medical Assistants.* 5th ed. Philadelphia, PA: W.B. Saunders, 2000.

Daniels, Rick. *Delmar's Guide to Laboratory and Diagnostic Tests.* Clifton Park, NY: Delmar Learning, 2002.

Davis, Bonnie Karen. *Phlebotomy: A Customer Service Approach.* 2nd ed. Clifton Park, NY: Delmar Learning, 2002.

Dean, Theresa, and Sheryl Whitlock. *Clinical Laboratory Manual Series: Clinical Chemistry.* Clifton Park, NY: Delmar Learning, 1997.

Flynn, John C., and Sheryl Whitlock. *Clinical Laboratory Manual Series: Urinalysis.* Clifton Park, NY: Delmar Learning, 1998.

Grover-Lakomia, Lynn, and Elizabeth Fong. *Microbiology for Health Careers.* 6th ed. Clifton Park, NY: Delmar Learning, 1999.

Hoeltke, Lynn. *Complete Textbook of Phlebotomy.* 2nd ed. Clifton Park, NY: Delmar Learning, 2000.

Kalanick, Kathryn. *Phlebotomy Technical Specialist.* Clifton Park, NY: Delmar Learning, 2003.

Keir, Lucille, Connie Krebs, and Barbara A. Wise. *Medical Assisting: Clinical and Administrative Competencies.* 5th ed. Clifton Park, NY: Delmar Learning, 2003.

Kovanda, Beverly. *Multiskilling: Waived Laboratory Testing for the Health Care Provider.* Clifton Park, NY: Delmar Learning, 1999.

Linne, Jean Jorgenson, and Karen Munson Ringsrud. *Clinical Laboratory Science: The Basics and Routine Tests.* 4th ed. St. Louis, MO: Mosby 1999.

Mahon, Connie, Linda Smith, and Cheryl Burns. *An Introduction to Clinical Laboratory Sciences.* Philadelphia, PA: W. B. Saunders, 1999.

Moisio, Marie, and Elmer Mosio. *Understanding Laboratory and Diagnostic Tests.* Clifton Park, NY: Delmar Learning, 1998.

Pagana, Kathleen, and Timothy Pagana. *Mosby's Diagnostic and Laboratory Test Reference.* 5th ed. St. Louis, MO: Mosby, 2000.

Russell, Allan, P. *Clinical Laboratory Manual Series: Hematology.* Clifton Park, NY: Delmar Learning, 1997.

Shimeld, Lisa. *Essentials of Diagnostic Microbiology.* Clifton Park, NY: Delmar Learning, 1999.

Stepp, Craig, and Mary Ann Woods. *Laboratory Procedures for Medical Office Personnel.* Philadelphia, PA: W. B. Saunders, 1997.

Walters, Norma J., Barbara H. Estridge, and Anna P. Reynolds. *Basic Medical Laboratory Techniques.* 4th ed. Clifton Park, NY: Delmar Learning, 2000.

Zakus, Sharron. *Clinical Skills for Medical Assistants.* 4th ed. St. Louis, MO: C.V. Mosby, 2001.

For additional information about laboratory careers, contact the following associations:

◆ American Medical Technologists' Association
710 Higgins Road
Park Ridge, Illinois 60068
Internet Address: *www.amt1.com*

◆ State Society for Medical Technology

◆ State Society for Medical Technologists

UNIT 19

Medical Assistant Skills

Unit Objectives

After completing this unit of study, you should be able to:

- Measure and record height and weight of infants and adults
- Position and properly drape a patient in the following positions: horizontal recumbent, prone, Sims', knee-chest, Fowler's, lithotomy, dorsal recumbent, Trendelenburg, and jackknife
- Use a Snellen chart to screen for vision problems
- Prepare for and assist with an eye, ear, nose, and throat examination
- Prepare for and assist with a gynecological examination
- Prepare for and assist with a general physical examination
- Set up a minor surgery tray without contaminating equipment or supplies
- Set up a suture removal tray without contaminating equipment or supplies
- Record and mount an electrocardiogram
- Use the *Physicians' Desk Reference* (PDR) to find basic information about various drugs
- Identify methods of administering medications and safety rules that must be observed
- Interpret Roman numerals
- Convert metric measurements
- Convert household (English) measurements
- Define, pronounce, and spell all the key terms

 Observe Standard Precautions

 Safety—Proceed with Caution

 Math Skill

 Science Skill

C Communications Skill

 Instructors Check—Call Instructor at This Point

 **OBRA** OBRA Requirement— Based on Federal Law

 Legal Responsibility

 Career Information

 Technology

616

KEY TERMS

auscultation
(oss″-kull-tay′-shun)

Ayer blade
(a′-ur) A as in "say"

bandage scissors

dorsal recumbent

electrocardiogram
(ee-leck″-trow-car′-dee-oh-
gram)

Fowler's

hemostats
(hee′-mow″-stats)

horizontal recumbent

hyperopia
(high″-puh-row′-pee-ah)

jackknife

knee–chest

laryngeal mirror
(lar″-ren-gee′-ul)

leads

left lateral

lithotomy
(lith″-ought′-eh-me)

medication

myopia
(my″-oh′-pee-ah)

needle holder

observation

ophthalmoscope
(op-thayl′-mow-skope″)

otoscope
(oh′-toe-skope″)

palpation

Papanicolaou
(pah″-pan-ee′-cow-low)

percussion

percussion hammer

Physicians' Desk Reference
(PDR)

prone

retractors

scalpels
(skal′-pelz)

sigmoidoscope
(sig-moy′-doh-skope″)

Sims'

Snellen charts

speculum
(speck′-you-lum)

supine
(sue-pine′)

surgical scissors

sutures

suture removal sets

tissue forceps

tonometer
(tow″-nom′-et-er)

Trendelenburg
(Tren′-dell-en″-burg)

tuning fork

CAREER HIGHLIGHTS

Medical assistants work under the supervision of physicians and they are important members of the health care team. Educational requirements vary from state to state, but can include on-the-job training (less frequent), one- or two-year health occupations education programs, and/or an associate's degree. Certification can be obtained from the American Association of Medical Assistants, and registered credentials can be obtained from the American Medical Technologists Association, each of which has specific requirements. The duties of medical assistants vary depending on the size and type of practice, and on the legal requirements of the state in which they work. Duties are often classified as administrative or clinical. Administrative, or "front office," duties may include tasks such as answering telephones, greeting patients, scheduling appointments, maintaining records, handling correspondence, and bookkeeping. Clinical, or "back office," duties may include taking medical histories, recording vital signs, preparing patients for and assisting with examinations and treatments, and performing basic laboratory tests. Some medical assistants perform both administrative and clinical duties; others specialize in either administrative or clinical work. The procedures discussed in this unit represent clinical duties. In addition to the knowledge and skills presented in this unit, medical assistants must also learn and master skills such as:

◆ Presenting a professional appearance and attitude

◆ Obtaining knowledge regarding health care delivery systems, organizational structure, and teamwork

◆ Meeting all legal responsibilities

- ◆ Communicating effectively
- ◆ Being sensitive to and respecting cultural diversity
- ◆ Comprehending human anatomy, physiology, and pathophysiology
- ◆ Learning medical terminology
- ◆ Observing all safety precautions
- ◆ Practicing all principles of infection control
- ◆ Taking and recording vital signs
- ◆ Performing waived laboratory tests
- ◆ Administering first aid and cardiopulmonary resuscitation
- ◆ Promoting good nutrition and a healthy lifestyle to maintain health
- ◆ Utilizing computer skills
- ◆ Performing administrative duties such as answering the telephone, scheduling appointments, preparing correspondence, completing insurance forms, maintaining accounts, recording medical histories, and maintaining patient records
- ◆ Ordering and maintaining supplies and materials

19:1 INFORMATION Measuring/Recording Height and Weight

OBRA Height and weight measurements are taken in many health care fields. Height and weight measurements are used to determine whether a patient is overweight or underweight. Either of these conditions can indicate disease. Height–weight charts are used as averages. A 10 percent deviation is usually considered normal. Height–weight measurements must be accurate. Always recheck your calculations.

Height–weight measurements are usually routinely done when a patient is admitted to a hospital, long-term care facility, or other health care agency. They are also a part of the general physical examination in a physician's office. In addition, the measurements provide necessary information in performing and evaluating certain laboratory tests and in calculating dosages of certain medications.

The height, weight, and head circumference measurements of infants and toddlers is monitored frequently because growth is rapid. Usually infants are checked every two months to detect any changes that may indicate problems with growth and development. The measurements are usually recorded on a National Center for Health Statistics (NCHS) growth graph (see figure 19-1). The graphed information allows the physician to check the child's growth and compare it to the average percentiles of other children the same age. Abnormal growth patterns may indicate nutritional deficiencies or genetic diseases.

Patients with cancer or patients on chemotherapy are weighed frequently to monitor weight loss. Daily weights are often ordered for patients with edema (swelling) due to heart, kidney, or other diseases. When taking daily weights, note the following points:

- ◆ Use the same scale each day.
- ◆ Make sure the scale is balanced before weighing the patient.
- ◆ Weigh the patient at the same time each day.
- ◆ Make sure the patient is wearing the same amount of clothing each day.

! Careful consideration must be given to the safety of the patient while weight and

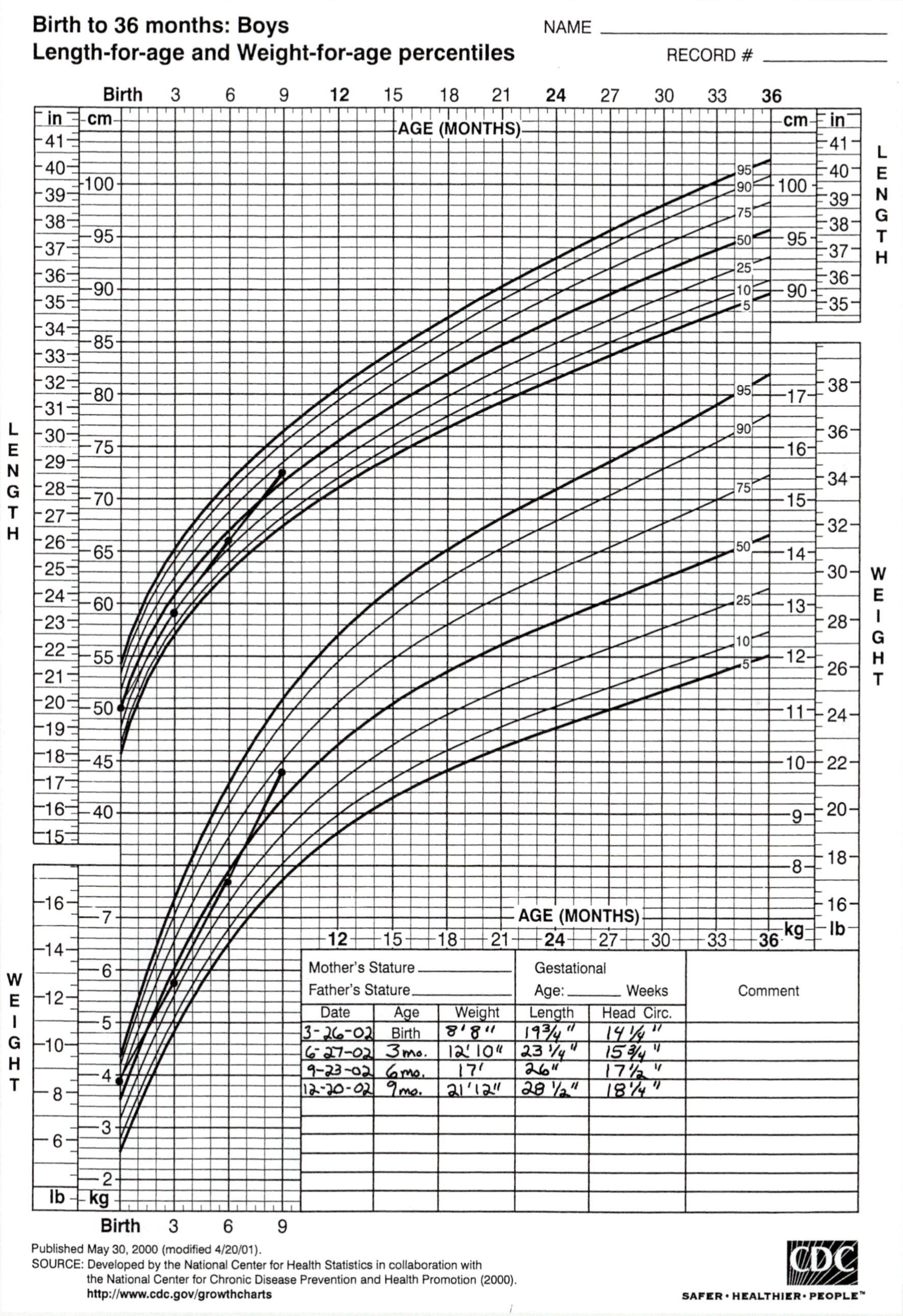
Birth to 36 months: Boys
Length-for-age and Weight-for-age percentiles
NAME
RECORD #
AGE (MONTHS)
LENGTH
WEIGHT
Mother's Stature
Father's Stature
Gestational Age: Weeks
Comment
Date
Age
Weight
Length
Head Circ.
3-26-02 Birth 8'8" 19 3/4" 14 1/4"
6-27-02 3mo. 12'10" 23 1/4" 15 3/4"
9-23-02 6mo. 17' 26" 17 1/2"
12-20-02 9mo. 21'12" 28 1/2" 18 1/4"
Published May 30, 2000 (modified 4/20/01).
SOURCE: Developed by the National Center for Health Statistics in collaboration with the National Center for Chronic Disease Prevention and Health Promotion (2000).
http://www.cdc.gov/growthcharts
CDC
SAFER • HEALTHIER • PEOPLE™

FIGURE 19-1 The National Center for Health Statistics (NCHS) growth graph is used to monitor the growth and development of infants and toddlers.

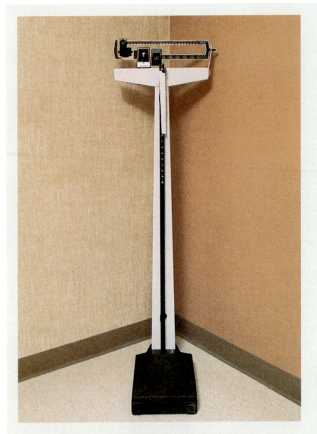

FIGURE 19-2A A sample beam-balance scale.

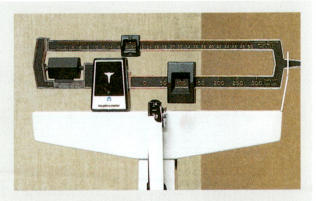

FIGURE 19-2B The weight bars. The bottom weights are in 50-pound increments and the top weights are in ¼-pound increments.

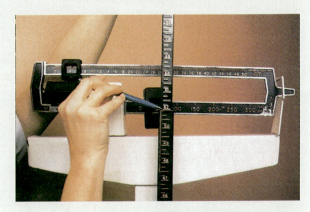

FIGURE 19-2C The height bar. The height is read at the break-point on the movable bar.

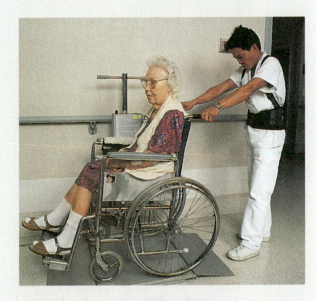

FIGURE 19-3 A wheelchair scale is a convenient scale for weighing a patient who may have difficulty standing on a beam-balance scale.

height are being measured. Observe the patient closely at all times. Prevent falls from the scale and possible injury from the protruding height lever.

C Most patients are very weight conscious. Parents may worry about the weight of their children. Therefore, it is very important for the health care worker to make only positive statements while weighing a patient. In addition, privacy must be provided while weighing a patient.

A wide variety of scales are used to obtain height and weight measurements. Most clinical scales contain a balance beam for measuring weight and a measuring rod for determining height (see figure 19-2A–C). Infant scales provide an area for placing the infant in a lying-down, or flat, position. Institutions, such as hospitals or long-term care facilities, may have special scales for patients who are unable to stand. Such scales include the bed scale with mechanical lift and the wheelchair scale (see figure 19-3). It is important to follow the manufacturer's instructions while using any special scale in order to obtain accurate weight measurements.

Weight is recorded as pounds and ounces or as kilograms (1.0 kilogram = 2.2 pounds). Most scales measure pounds in ¼-pound increments. Metric scales measure in kilograms and have 0.1-kilogram increments.

Height is recorded as feet and inches or as centimeters. The measuring bar measures inches and fractions or ¼-inch increments. A metric measuring bar has 1-centimeter increments. One inch equals 2.5 centimeters.

STUDENT: *Go to the workbook and complete the assignment sheet for 19:1, Measuring/Recording Height and Weight. Then return and continue with the procedures.*

PROCEDURE 19:1A   OBRA

Measuring/Recording Height and Weight

Equipment and Supplies

Balance scale, paper towel, paper, pencil or pen

Procedure

1. Assemble equipment.
2. Wash hands.
3. Prepare the scale. Place a paper towel on the foot stand of the scale. Move both weights to the *zero* position. If the end of the balance bar swings freely, the scale is balanced. If the scale is *not* balanced, follow manufacturer's instructions to balance the scale.

   NOTE: Most scales have a small screw by the end of the balance bar. By adjusting the screw, the scale can be balanced.

   NOTE: The paper towel prevents spread of disease.
4. **C** Introduce yourself. Identify the patient. Explain the procedure. Remember to make only positive statements.
5. Ask the patient to remove shoes, jackets, heavy outer clothing, purses, and heavy objects that may be in the pockets of clothing.

   NOTE: In a hospital or long-term care facility, the patient is usually weighed in a gown or in pajamas.
6. Assist the patient onto the scale. The patient should stand unassisted, with his or her feet centered on the platform and slightly apart (see figure 19-4).

   ⚠ CAUTION: Watch closely at all times to prevent falls.

7. Move the large 50-pound weight to the right until the balance bar drops down on the lower guide. Then move this weight back one notch. Move the smaller

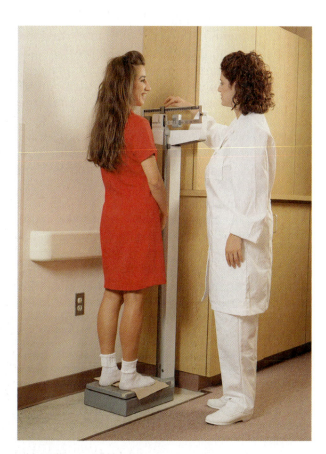

FIGURE 19-4 The patient should stand unassisted on the scale, with her feet centered on the platform and slightly apart.

¼-pound weight until the balance bar swings freely halfway between the upper and lower guides. Add the two weights together to determine the patient's correct weight. Recheck your reading. Record the weight correctly.

✔ **CHECKPOINT:** Your instructor will check your reading for accuracy.

8. Help the patient get off the scale. Raise the height bar higher than the height of the patient. Help the patient get back on the scale with his or her back to the scale.

⚠ **CAUTION:** Watch closely at all times to prevent falls.

9. Instruct the patient to stand as erect as possible (see figure 19-5).

10. Move the bar of the measuring scale down until it just touches the top of the patient's head.

⚠ **CAUTION:** Move slowly. Do *not* hit the patient with the bar.

11. Read the measurement in inches or centimeters. Recheck your reading. Record the height correctly.

NOTE: If the height is difficult to read, assist the patient off the scale without moving the height bar. Then read the correct height measurement.

NOTE: If the reading is in inches, it can be converted to feet and inches after the patient is off the scale.

NOTE: If the height bar is extended above the break point of the movable bar, remember to read the height at the point of the break by reading in a downward direction on the upper bar.

✔ **CHECKPOINT:** Your instructor will check your reading for accuracy.

12. Elevate the height bar.

13. Help the patient get off the scale.

⚠ **CAUTION:** Watch the patient closely to prevent falls.

14. Replace all equipment. Throw the paper towel in a waste can.

15. Return both weight beams to the zero positions. Lower the measurement bar.

16. Convert the inches to feet and inches by dividing by 12. For example 64½ inches divided by 12 equals 5 feet 4½ inches.

17. Wash hands.

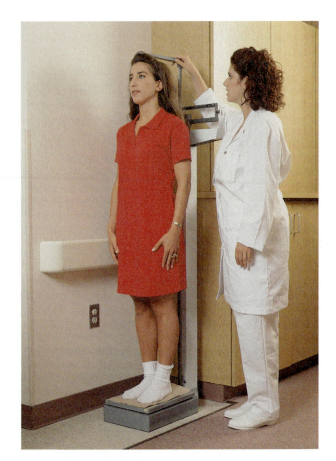

FIGURE 19-5 The patient should stand as erect as possible while height is being measured.

18. **C** Record all required information on the patient's chart, for example, date, time, Wt: 132½ lb, Ht: 5 ft 4½ in., and your signature and title.

Practice *Go to the workbook and use the evaluation sheet for 19:1A, Measuring/ Recording Height and Weight, to practice this procedure. When you feel you have mastered this skill, sign the sheet and give it to your instructor for further action.*

✔ **Final Checkpoint**   Using the criteria listed on the evaluation sheet, your instructor will grade your performance.

PROCEDURE 19:1B

Measuring/Recording Height and Weight of an Infant

Equipment and Supplies

Infant scale, towel or scale paper, tape measure, growth graph, patient's chart or paper, pencil or pen

Procedure

1. Assemble equipment.
2. Wash hands.
3. Prepare the scale. Place a towel or scale paper on the scale to protect the infant from the shock of the cold metal and pathogens (germs). Then balance the scale. Move both weights to the *zero* position. If the end of the balance bar swings freely, the scale is balanced. If the scale is *not* balanced, follow manufacturer's instructions to balance the scale.

   NOTE: Most scales have a small screw by the end of the balance bar. By adjusting the screw, the scale can be balanced.

4. **C** Introduce yourself. Explain the procedure to the parent. Identify the infant by asking the parent for the infant's name. Ask the parent to undress the infant.

   NOTE: An undershirt or pajama is sometimes left on the infant.

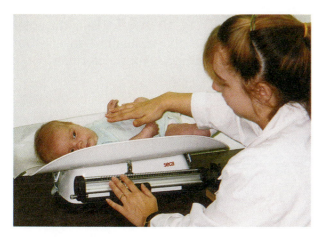

FIGURE 19-6 While keeping one hand slightly above the infant, adjust the scale weights with the other hand.

5. Pick up the infant. Use one arm to support the neck and shoulders and the other arm to support the back and hips.
6. Place the infant on the scale.

   ! CAUTION: Watch closely at all times. To prevent falls, keep one hand over the infant while adjusting the scales (see figure 19-6).

7. Move the large weight to the right until the balance bar drops down on the lower guide. Then move this weight back one notch. Move the smaller weight until the balance bar swings freely halfway between the upper and lower guides. Add the two weights together to determine the infant's correct weight.

   NOTE: If the infant scale contains only one bar and one weight, move the weight to the right until the balance bar swings freely halfway between the upper and lower guide. Read the weight on the bar.

   ✔ CHECKPOINT: Your instructor will check your reading for accuracy.

8. Record the weight in pounds and ounces or in kilograms. Recheck your reading.
9. Pick up and place the infant on a flat surface.

   ! CAUTION: Watch closely at all times. Do not leave the infant unattended. If it is necessary to reach for anything nearby, use one hand to hold the infant and the other hand to reach.

10. Place the zero mark of the measuring tape or rod at the infant's head (see figure 19-7).

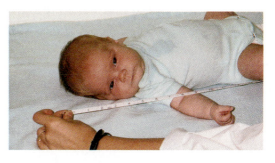

FIGURE 19-7 Hold the tape measure in a straight line to measure an infant's height.

If the measuring bar is a part of the exam table, position the infant so that the infant's head is at the zero mark. Ask the parent or an assistant to hold the head at this mark. Gently straighten the infant's legs. If a measuring tape is used, measure to the infant's heel. If a bar is used, position the heel on the bar while holding the leg straight.

NOTE: If the infant is lying on examining table paper, mark the paper at the infant's head and heel. Then measure the marked area.

✔ **CHECKPOINT:** Your instructor will check your reading for accuracy.

11. Record the height correctly in inches or centimeters. Recheck your reading.

12. The head circumference is frequently measured on an infant. To measure head circumference:

   a. Position the infant on the examination table or ask the parent to hold the infant.

   b. Use a thumb or finger to hold the zero mark of the tape measure against the infant's forehead just above the eyebrows.

   c. Use your other hand to bring the tape around the infant's head, just above the ears, over the occipital bone at the back of the head, and back to the forehead to meet the zero mark on the tape, (see figure 19-8).

   d. Pull the tape snug to compress the hair, but not too tight.

   e. Read the tape measure to the nearest ½ inch or 0.1 centimeter.

   f. Record the reading.

13. Return the infant to the parent.

14. Clean and replace all equipment. Use a disinfectant to wipe the scale. Set the weights at zero. Fold up the tape measure.

15. Wash hands.

16. Record all required information on the infant's chart, for example, date, time, Wt: 9 lb 8 oz, Ht: 23½ in., Head circumference: 16¾ in., and your signature and title. The measurements should also be recorded on the infant's growth graph.

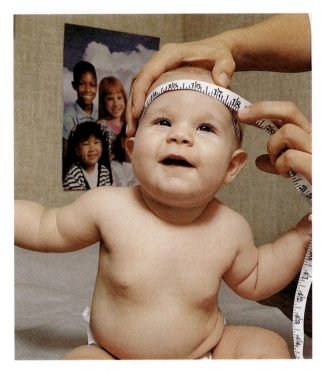

FIGURE 19-8 To measure head circumference, bring the tape around the infant's head, just above the ears, and back to the forehead.

Practice *Go to the workbook and use the evaluation sheet for 19:1B, Measuring/Recording Height and Weight of an Infant, to practice this procedure. When you feel you have mastered this skill, sign the sheet and give it to your instructor for further action.*

✔ **Final Checkpoint** Using the criteria listed on the evaluation sheet, your instructor will grade your performance.

19:2 INFORMATION Positioning a Patient

A wide variety of positions are used for different procedures and examinations. The patient may need to be positioned on a medical examination table or a surgical table. It is important to know how to operate the table before attempting to position a patient. Obtain instruction or read manufacturer's directions carefully. After use, medical examination tables and surgical tables are usually cleaned with disinfectant solution. In addition, table paper is frequently used to cover an examination table prior to the examination and is removed and replaced after the examination.

C **!** During any procedure or examination, reassure the patient. Make sure the patient understands what is being done and grants permission for the procedure. At all times, watch the patient closely for signs of distress. Observe all safety factors to prevent falls and injuries. Use correct body mechanics at all times to prevent injury to yourself.

It is also essential to make sure that the patient is not exposed during any examination or procedure. The door to the room should be closed, and the curtains, if present, should be drawn. Care must be taken to properly drape or cover the patient to avoid unnecessary exposure. At the same time, the drape must be applied so that the doctor or technician has ready access to the area to be examined or treated.

Some of the most common examination positions are listed and described.

Horizontal Recumbent (Supine) Position

◆ Used for examination or treatment of the front, or anterior, part of the body (see figure 19-9).

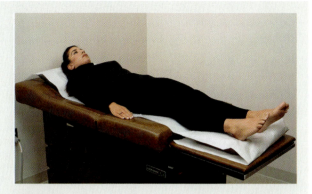

FIGURE 19-9 Horizontal recumbent (supine) position. Draping has been omitted for clarity.

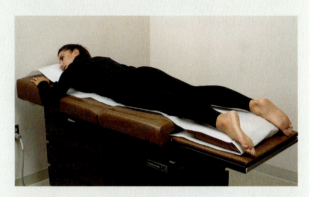

FIGURE 19-10 Prone position.

◆ The patient lies flat on the back with the legs slightly apart.

◆ One small pillow is allowed under the head.

◆ The arms are flat at the side of the body.

◆ The drape is placed over the patient but left loose on all sides to facilitate examination or treatment.

Prone Position

◆ Used for examination or treatment of the back or spine (see figure 19-10).

◆ The patient lies on the abdomen and turns the head to either side. A small pillow may be placed under the head.

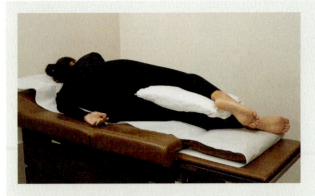

FIGURE 19-11 Sims' (left lateral) position.

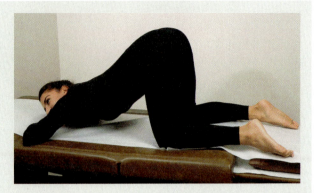

FIGURE 19-12 Knee–chest position.

◆ The arms may be flexed at the elbows and positioned on either side of the head.

◆ One sheet or drape is placed over the patient but left loose on all sides to facilitate examination or treatment.

Sims' (Left Lateral) Position

◆ Used for simple rectal and sigmoidoscopic examinations, enemas, rectal temperatures, and rectal treatments (see figure 19-11).

◆ The patient lies on the left side.

◆ The left arm is extended behind the back.

◆ The head is turned to the side. A small pillow may be used.

◆ The right arm is in front of the patient, and the elbow is bent.

◆ The left leg is bent, or flexed, slightly.

◆ The right leg is bent sharply at the knee and brought up to the abdomen.

◆ Draping can be done with one large sheet or two small sheets that meet at the rectal area. All sheets hang free at the sides.

Knee–chest Position

◆ Used for rectal examinations, usually a sigmoidoscopic examination (see figure 19-12).

◆ The patient rests the body weight on the knees and chest.

◆ The arms are flexed slightly at the elbows and are extended above the head.

◆ The knees are slightly separated, and the thighs are at right angles to the table.

◆ Draping can be done with one large sheet or two small sheets that meet at the rectal area.

A large sheet with a hole at the rectal area can also be used. Sheets hang loose with no tucks.

⚠ **CAUTION:** Never leave a patient alone in this position. This is a very difficult position for the patient to maintain and should be used only as long as absolutely necessary.

Fowler's Positions

◆ Used to facilitate breathing, relieve distress, encourage drainage, and examine the head, neck, and chest.

◆ The patient lies on the back.

◆ The head is elevated to one of three main positions:

   (1) Low Fowler's: the head is elevated to a 25° angle.

   (2) Semi-Fowler's: the head is elevated to a 45° angle (the most frequently used position) (see figure 19-13A).

   (3) High Fowler's: the head is elevated to a 90° angle (see figure 19-13B).

◆ The knees are slightly bent and are sometimes supported on a pillow.

◆ One sheet is used to drape the patient. The sheet is left hanging loose.

Lithotomy Position

◆ Used for vaginal examinations, pap tests, urinary catherization, cystoscopic examinations, and surgery of the pelvic area (see figure 19-14).

◆ The patient is positioned on the back.

◆ The knees are separated and flexed, and the feet are placed in stirrups.

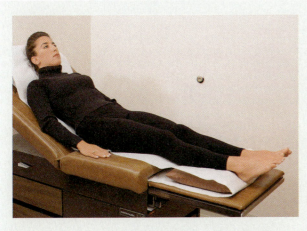

FIGURE 19-13A Semi-Fowler's (mid-Fowler's) position.

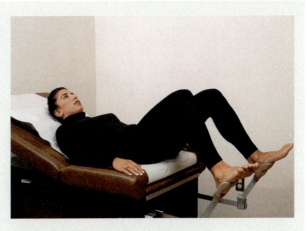

FIGURE 19-14 Lithotomy position.

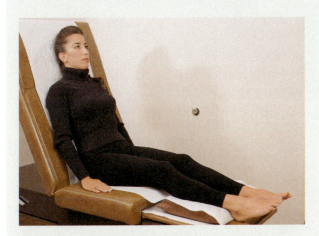

FIGURE 19-13B High Fowler's position.

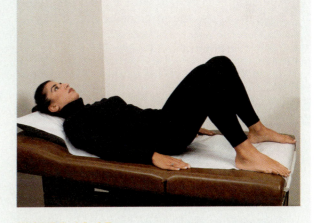

FIGURE 19-15 Dorsal recumbent position.

- The arms rest at the sides.
- The buttocks are at the lower end of the table.
- Draping is done with one large sheet placed over the body in a diamond shape. One corner is at the upper chest, and one corner hangs loose between legs. Each of the other two corners is wrapped around a foot.

Dorsal Recumbent Position

- Similar to the lithotomy position, but the patient is in bed or on a table without stirrups (see figure 19-15).
- The feet are separated but flat on the bed.
- The knees are bent.
- Draping and other points are the same as for the lithotomy position.

Trendelenburg Position

- Increases circulation of blood to the head and brain and can be used for circulatory shock. The entire bed or table is elevated at the feet. The patient lies in the horizontal recumbent position, with the head lower than the feet.
- The surgical Trendelenburg position (see figure 19-16) can be used for surgery on pelvic organs and for pelvic treatments. The patient is flat on the back. The table is lowered at a 45° angle to lower the head, and the feet and lower legs are inclined downward.
- Straps are frequently used to hold the patient in position.

NOTE: Draping for the Trendelenburg position depends on the treatment being performed; usually, one large sheet is used and

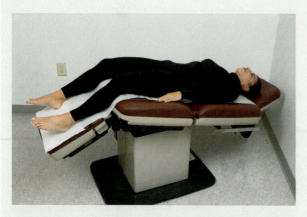

FIGURE 19-16 Surgical Trendelenburg position.

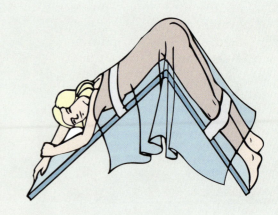

FIGURE 19-17 Jackknife (proctology) position.

left hanging loose. For surgical procedures, the patient is draped with a sheet that has a hole to expose the surgical area.

Jackknife (Proctology) Position

◆ Used mainly for rectal surgery or examinations, and for back surgery or treatments (see figure 19-17).

◆ The patient is in the prone position.

◆ The table is elevated at the center so that the rectal area is at a higher elevation. A special surgical table is required for this position.

◆ The head and chest point downward. The feet and legs hang down at the opposite end of the table.

◆ The patient must be supported to prevent injury. Straps are used to hold the patient in position.

◆ Draping is done with a surgical sheet that has a hole to expose the surgical or treatment area. Two small sheets that meet at the surgical or treatment area can also be used.

⚠ **CAUTION:** It is important to use good body mechanics while positioning the patient to protect both yourself and the patient.

STUDENT: *Go to the workbook and complete the assignment sheet for 19:2, Positioning a Patient. Then return and continue with the procedure.*

PROCEDURE 19:2

Positioning a Patient

Equipment and Supplies

Two to three sheets, bath blankets or drapes, bed or examining table, two small pillows

Procedure

1. Assemble equipment.
2. Wash hands.
3. Ⓒ Introduce yourself. Identify the patient. Explain the procedure. Obtain the patient's consent.

4. Instruct the patient to remove all clothing and to put on an examining gown. Ask the patient to void to prevent bladder discomfort during the examination or treatment.
5. Help the patient get on table.
   NOTE: Positioning of the patient will depend on the examination, treatment, or procedure to be performed.
6. Position the patient in the horizontal recumbent (supine) position as follows:
   a. Lie the patient flat on the back.

b. Place a small pillow under the head.

c. Rest the arms at the sides of the body.

d. Position the legs flat and slightly separated.

e. Use a large sheet or drape to drape the patient. Do *not* tuck the sheet in at the sides or bottom. It should hang loose.

7. Position the patient in the prone position as follows:

a. Ask the supine patient to turn the body in your direction until lying on the abdomen. Hold the drape up while the patient is turning.

b. Turn the head to either side to rest on a small pillow.

c. Flex the arms at the elbows and place at the sides of the head.

d. Use one large sheet or drape to drape the patient. Do *not* tuck in at the sides or bottom.

8. Position the patient in the Sims' (left lateral) position as follows:

a. Ask the prone patient to turn on the left side.

b. Extend the left arm behind the back.

c. Rest the head on a small pillow.

d. Bend the left leg slightly.

e. Bend the right leg sharply to abdomen.

f. Place the right arm bent at the elbow in a comfortable position in front of the body.

g. Drape with one large sheet or drape. Do *not* tuck in at the sides or bottom. Draping can also be done with two small sheets. One sheet covers the upper part of the body and meets the second sheet, which covers the thighs and legs.

9. Position the patient in the knee–chest position as follows:

a. Ask the patient to lie on the abdomen (that is, in the prone position).

b. Raise the buttocks and abdomen until the body weight is resting on the upper chest and knees.

NOTE: Do *not* place the patient in this position until the physician is ready to begin the examination. It is a difficult position for the patient to maintain.

c. Make sure the knees are slightly separated and the thighs are at right angles to the table.

d. Rest the head on a small pillow.

e. Flex the arms slightly and position on the sides of the head.

f. Drape with one large, untucked sheet or drape or two small sheets or drapes that meet at the rectal area. A drape with a hole at the rectal area can also be used.

! CAUTION: *Never* leave the patient alone in the knee–chest position.

g. When the examination is complete, help the patient get into the prone position. Watch closely for signs of dizziness or discomfort and report any such signs immediately after being sure that the patient is in a comfortable, safe position.

10. Position the patient in the Fowler's positions as follows:

a. Place the patient in the horizontal recumbent position.

b. Place a small pillow under the patient's head.

c. Low Fowler's: elevate the head of the bed (or table) to a 25° angle.

d. Mid-, or semi-, Fowler's: elevate the head to a 45° angle.

e. High Fowler's: elevate the head to a 90° angle.

f. Place a second small pillow under the patient's knees after flexing them slightly.

g. Use a large sheet or drape to drape the patient. Do *not* tuck in the sides or end of the sheet or drape.

11. Position the patient in the lithotomy position as follows:

a. Position the patient on the back with the arms at the sides. The feet should be resting on the extension at the lower end of the table.

b. Ask the patient to slide the buttocks down on the table to where the lower end of the table folds down or pulls out.

c. Position a small pillow under the patient's head.

d. Place a sheet or drape over the patient in a diamond position. One corner should be at the chest, the opposite corner at the perineal area, or between the legs. Wrap each side corner around a foot.

e. Flex and separate the knees.

f. Place the feet in the stirrups.

g. Drop the lower end of the table, or push in the extension.

h. To get the patient out of this position, first raise the end of the table or pull out the extension so that it is level. Lift the feet out of the stirrups and place them on the table. Ask the patient to move back up on the table.

12. Position the patient in the Trendelenburg positions as follows:

    NOTE: These positions require a special bed or table and assistance. Care should be taken to prevent the patient from sliding off the table.

    a. Put the patient in the horizontal recumbent position.

    b. Operate the power table or electric bed to raise the foot of the bed so that the patient's head is lower than the rest of the body. The lower frame of the bed is sometimes supported up on blocks.

    c. For the surgical Trendelenburg position, lower the bottom end of the table so that the lower legs are inclined at a downward angle.

    d. Use one large or two small sheets or drapes to drape the patient, or use a drape with a hole at the surgical site.

    e. Use straps to secure the patient in position.

    f. Remain with the patient at all times.

13. Position the patient in the jackknife position as follows:

    NOTE: This position requires a special table and assistance. Care must be taken to prevent the patient from sliding off the table or being injured in any way.

    a. Position the patient in the prone position.

    b. Secure the safety straps on the table.

    c. Lower the top of the table so that the head and upper body are inclined at a downward angle.

    d. Lower the bottom of the table so that the feet and legs are inclined at a downward angle.

    e. Use a large sheet or special drape that has an opening in it to cover the patient. Place the opening over the rectal area. You may also use two small sheets that meet at the rectal area.

    f. Remain with the patient at all times. Observe for any negative reactions to the position, such as dizziness, pain, or discomfort. Immediately report any such signs to your supervisor.

14. When the examination, treatment, or procedure is complete, allow the patient to sit up. Observe for signs of dizzinesss or weakness.

15. Help the patient get off the table. Ask the patient to get dressed or assist if necessary. Inform the patient of how and when he or she will be notified of test results (if tests were conducted during the examination).

    ⚠ CAUTION: Watch the patient closely and prevent falls.

16. Clean and replace all equipment.

17. Wash hands.

18. **C** Record all required information on the patient's chart, for example, date, time, positioned in semi-Fowler's for comfort, appears to be resting well, and your signature and title.

> **Practice** *Go to the workbook and use the evaluation sheet for 19:2, Positioning a Patient, to practice this procedure. When you feel you have mastered this skill, sign the sheet and give it to your instructor for further action.*

✔ **Final Checkpoint** Using the criteria listed on the evaluation sheet, your instructor will grade your performance.

19:3 INFORMATION
Screening for Vision Problems

Vision screening tests are often given as part of a physical examination or to detect eye disease. One method involves the use of Snellen charts. **Snellen charts** are used to test distant vision (see figure 19-18). They come in a variety of types. Some contain pictures for use with small children. Some contain the letter *E* in a variety of positions. The patient points in the direction that the *E* points. This type of chart is used for non-English-speaking people or nonreaders. Some contain letters of the alphabet. It is important to make sure the patient knows all the letters of the alphabet when using this type of chart.

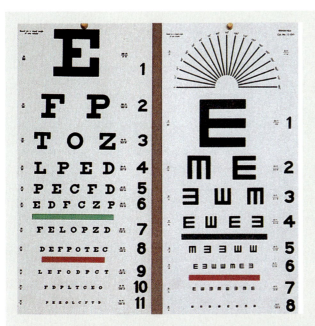

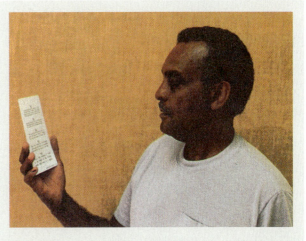

FIGURE 19-19 The patient holds the card 14 to 16 inches from the eyes when testing for defects in close vision.

FIGURE 19-18 Snellen charts are used for vision screening.

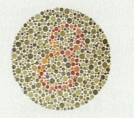 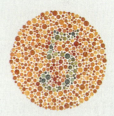

FIGURE 19-20 People with color blindness are not able to see the numbers in these Ishihara color plates.

Characters (that is, letters or pictures) on the Snellen chart have specific heights, ranging from small, on the bottom of the chart, to large, on the top of the chart. When standing 20 feet from the chart, a person with so-called normal vision should be able to see characters that are 20 millimeters high. Such a person is said to have 20/20 vision. When referring to 20/20 vision, the top number represents the distance the patient is from the chart. For this screening test, then, the patient is placed 20 feet from the chart. The bottom number represents the height of the characters that the patient can read at that distance.

◆ *Example 1:* If a patient has 20/30 vision, this means that when standing 20 feet from the chart, the patient can see characters 30 millimeters high. It can also be stated that this patient, who is standing 20 feet from the chart, can see what a patient with normal vision can see standing 30 feet from the chart.

◆ *Example 2:* If a patient has 20/100 vision, this means that when standing 20 feet from the chart, the patient can only see characters that are 100 mm high. This finding represents a defect in distant vision. A person with normal vision would be able to see the same figures while standing 100 feet from the chart.

It is important to note that Snellen charts test only for defects in distant vision, or for nearsightedness (myopia). Defects in close vision (problems with reading small print and seeing up close), known as farsightedness (hyperopia), are tested by using a printed book or cards in which the characters are certain heights. The patient holds the book or cards approximately 14 to 16 inches away from the eyes (see figure 19-19). The patient then reads printed text or identifies pictures that gradually become smaller. The smallest print or character that the patient can read or identify without error is recorded.

Defects in color vision, or color blindness, are usually tested by the Ishihara method. The Ishihara book contains a series of numbers printed in colored dots against a background of dots in contrasting color (see figure 19-20). Patients with normal color vision are able to readily identify the numbers. Patients with color blindness either are unable to see the numbers or identify incorrect numbers. This test is most accurate when it is conducted in a room illuminated by natural daylight but not by bright sunlight.

C When screening for vision problems, there are some special terms or abbreviations to remember:

◆ **OD:** abbreviation for *oculus dexter,* or right eye.

◆ **OS:** abbreviation for *oculus sinister,* or left eye.

◆ **OU:** abbreviation for *oculus uterque,* or each eye; both eyes.

◆ **myopia:** nearsightedness, defect in distant vision.

◆ **hyperopia:** farsightedness, defect in close vision.

◆ **ophthalmoscope:** instrument for checking the eye.

◆ **tonometer:** instrument to measure intraocular tension or pressure; increased pressure often indicates glaucoma.

STUDENT: *Go to the workbook and complete the assignment sheet for 19:3, Screening for Vision Problems. Then return and continue with the procedure.*

PROCEDURE 19:3

Screening for Vision Problems

Equipment and Supplies

Snellen eye chart, pointer, tape, card or eye shield, paper, pen or pencil

Procedure

1. Assemble equipment.
2. Attach the Snellen chart to the wall or place it in a lighted stand. Measure a distance of 20 feet directly away from the front of the chart. Place a piece of tape on the floor at the 20-foot mark.

   NOTE: Most medical offices will have a mark on the floor to indicate the 20-foot distance.
3. Wash hands.
4. **C** Introduce yourself. Identify the patient. Explain the procedure.

   NOTE: If using a chart with letters, make sure the patient knows the letters of the alphabet. If using a picture chart, make sure small children know what each picture represents.
5. Instruct the patient to stand facing the chart. Make sure the patient's toes are on the taped line; the patient's eyes will be 20 feet from the chart.
6. Point to various letters or pictures on the chart. Ask the patient to identify the letters or pictures. If the patient wears corrective lenses (glasses or contact lenses), check the vision with the corrective lenses first. Then ask the patient to remove the corrective lenses. Check the vision again. Record both readings. Observe the following points:

   a. Start with the larger letters or pictures and proceed to the smaller ones.

   b. Make sure the pointer you are using does not block the letters or pictures.

   c. Select letters or pictures at random in each row. Do *not* start at one end of the row and go straight across the line. Patients may memorize order; random sampling makes the patient focus on individual letters or pictures.

   NOTE: If you are sure the patient has not memorized the letters, you may ask the patient to read a row of letters. If the patient is able to read all letters correctly, proceed to a smaller row.

   d. Watch to be sure the patient is not leaning forward or squinting to see the letters or pictures (see figure 19-21A).

   NOTE: Some examiners do the left or right eye first, the opposite eye second, and both eyes last. Follow your agency's policy.
7. Ask the patient to correctly identify all the letters or pictures in the 20/20 line. If the patient

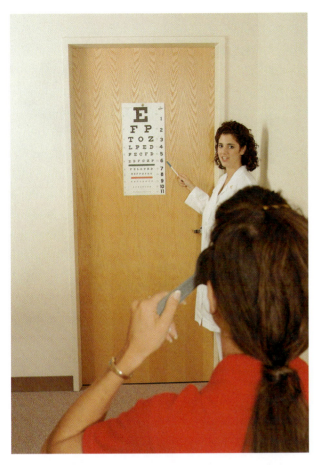

FIGURE 19-21A Watch to make sure the patient is not leaning forward or squinting to see the letters.

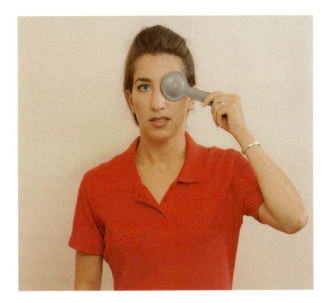

FIGURE 19-21B The patient should keep the eye open while covering it with an eye shield or card.

is unable to do so, note the line that the patient *can* read with 100-percent accuracy.

8. Give the patient an eye shield or card with which to cover the left eye (see figure 19-21B). Warn the patient not to close the left eye while it is covered, because doing so can cause blurred vision. Repeat steps 6 and 7 to test the vision in the right eye (OD).

   ! CAUTION: Warn the patient against pressing on the covered eye to avoid injuring the eye with the card or shield. Do *not* use the card or shield on another patient. Discard it after use.

9. Ask the patient to cover the right eye. Repeat steps 6 and 7 to test the vision in the left eye (OS).

   NOTE: Remind the patient to keep the right eye open while it is covered.

10. Record the test results for both eyes, the right eye, and the left eye. Use abbreviations of *OU, OD,* and *OS* and readings of *20/20, 20/30,* or the correct reading.

11. Thank the patient for being cooperative.

    NOTE: This is a screening test only. Unfavorable results indicate the need for additional testing or referral to an eye specialist.

12. Clean and replace all equipment. If the eye shield is not disposable, wash it thoroughly and clean it with a disinfectant solution.

13. Wash hands.

14. **C** Record all required information on the patient's chart or the agency form, for example, date, time, vision screening with Snellen chart: OU 20/30, OD 20/40, OS 20/30; and your signature and title.

Practice *Go to the workbook and use the evaluation sheet for 19:3, Screening for Vision Problems, to practice this procedure. When you feel you have mastered this skill, sign the sheet and give it to your instructor for further action.*

✔ Final Checkpoint Using the criteria listed on the evaluation sheet, your instructor will grade your performance.

19:4 INFORMATION Assisting with Physical Examinations

A large variety of physical examinations are performed. The methods used and the equipment available vary from physician to physician. However, there are some basic principles that apply to all examinations.

Three major kinds of examinations are:

◆ *EENT:* An eye, ear, nose, and throat examination. Special equipment should be available to examine these areas of the body.

◆ *GYN:* An examination of the female reproductive organs; a gynecological examination. The physician usually examines the vagina, cervix, and other pelvic organs as well as the breasts. A Pap, or **Papanicolaou,** test frequently is done to detect cancer of the cervix or reproductive organs.

◆ *General,* or *complete, physical:* All areas of the body are examined. Blood and urine tests frequently are done. X rays and an electrocardiogram (ECG) may also be part of the examination. An EENT and/or GYN exam may be performed. Necessary equipment and tests are determined by the physician doing the examination.

Four main techniques used during the examination are observation, palpation, percussion, and auscultation.

◆ **Observation** (inspection): The physician looks at the patient carefully to observe things such as skin color, rash, growths, swelling, scars, deformities, body movements, and general appearance (see figure 19-22).

◆ **Palpation:** The physician uses the hands and fingers to feel various parts of the body (see figure 19-23). The physician can determine whether a part of the body is enlarged, hard, out of place, or painful to the touch.

◆ **Percussion:** The physician taps and listens for sounds coming from various body organs (see figure 19-24). The physician may place one or several fingers of one hand on a part

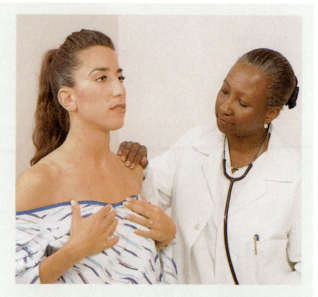

FIGURE 19-22 The physician uses observation to inspect the body for signs of disease.

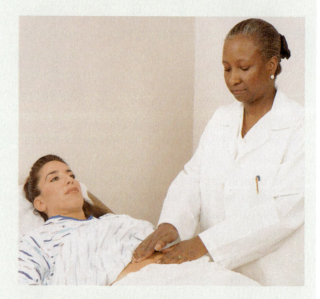

FIGURE 19-23 For palpation, the physician uses the hands and fingers to feel various parts of the body.

of the body, then use the fingers of the other hand to tap the body part. The sounds emitted allow a trained individual to determine the size, density, and position of underlying organs.

◆ **Auscultation:** The physician listens to sounds coming from within the patient's body (see figure 19-25). A stethoscope is used in most cases. The physician listens to

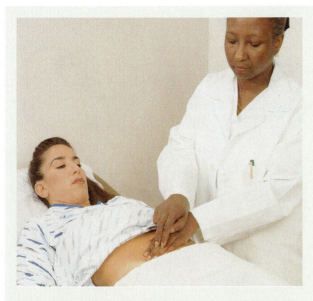

FIGURE 19-24 Percussion involves tapping on body parts and listening to sounds coming from body organs.

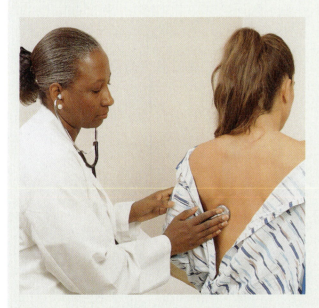

FIGURE 19-25 The physician is using a stethoscope and auscultation to listen to posterior lung and heart sounds.

sounds produced by the heart, lungs, intestines, and other body organs.

All necessary equipment should be assembled prior to the examination. The equipment needed will vary depending on the body areas to be examined. Try to anticipate what the physician will need, and assemble the items for convenient use. Some of the instruments used

for different examinations (see figure 19-26) include:

◆ **Ayer blade:** a wooden or plastic blade used to scrape cells from the cervix, or lower part of the uterus; it is usually a part of a pap kit that also contains slides, swabs, and a cytology brush; used to perform a Pap test to check for cancer of the cervix.

◆ **Laryngeal mirror:** an instrument with a mirror at one end; used to examine the larynx, or voice box, in the throat.

◆ **Ophthalmoscope:** a lighted instrument used to examine the eyes.

◆ **Otoscope:** a lighted instrument used to examine the ears.

◆ **Percussion hammer:** an instrument used to test tendon reflexes.

◆ **Sigmoidoscope:** a lighted instrument used to examine the sigmoid colon, or inside of the lower part of the large intestine; used during sigmoidoscopic examinations.

◆ **Speculum:** an instrument used to examine internal canals of the body; a nasal speculum is used to examine the nose; a vaginal speculum is used to examine the vagina; a rectal speculum is used to examine the rectum.

◆ **Sphygmomanometer:** an instrument used to measure blood pressure.

◆ **Stethoscope:** an instrument used for listening to internal body sounds.

◆ **Tongue blade/depressor:** a wood or plastic stick used to depress, or hold down, the tongue so that the throat can be examined.

◆ **Tonometer:** an instrument used to measure intraocular pressure (pressure inside the eye).

◆ **Tuning Fork:** an instrument with two prongs that is used to test hearing acuity.

C Preparation of the patient must include carefully explaining all procedures. Thorough explanations can help alleviate some fear. Patients often are apprehensive and need reassurance. The patient usually must remove all clothing and put on an examining gown. It is important to tell the patient to void before the examination so that the bladder will be empty and internal organs in the area of the

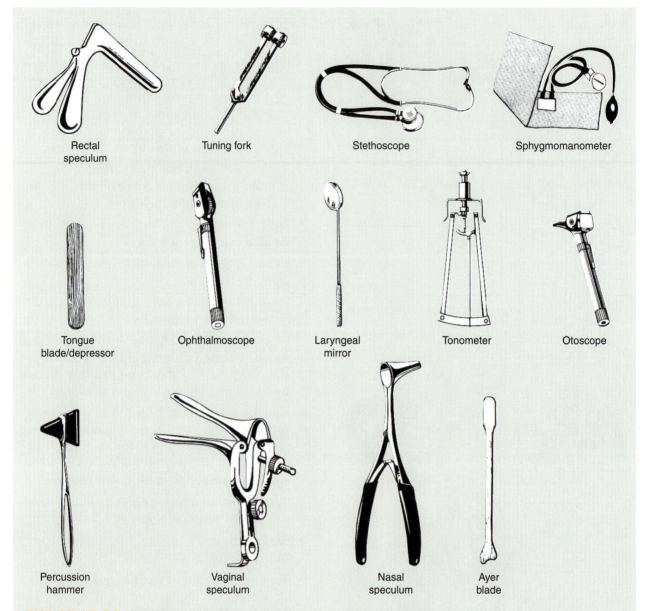

Rectal speculum

Tuning fork

Stethoscope

Sphygmomanometer

Tongue blade/depressor

Ophthalmoscope

Laryngeal mirror

Tonometer

Otoscope

Percussion hammer

Vaginal speculum

Nasal speculum

Ayer blade

FIGURE 19-26 Instruments used for a variety of physical examinations.

bladder can be palpated. If a urinalysis is ordered, the urine specimen can be obtained at this time. Correct positioning and draping is also essential.

Some tests frequently done prior to the physical examination might include the following:

◆ *Height and weight:* record all information accurately.

◆ *Vital signs:* including TPR and BP; record all information accurately.

◆ *Vision screening:* test as previously instructed.

◆ *Audiometric screening:* a special hearing test requiring additional training to administer.

◆ *Blood tests:* various tests may be ordered by the physician

◆ *Electrocardiogram:* a test to check the electrical conduction pattern in the heart; performed if ordered by the physician

During the examination, be prepared to assist as necessary. Hand equipment to the physician as needed. Position the patient correctly for each part of the examination. Pay attention so that you are ready to help with each procedure.

 Standard precautions (discussed in Unit 13:3) must be followed at all times while

assisting with physical examinations. Hands must be washed frequently, and gloves must be worn if contact by blood or body fluids is likely. If splashing or spraying of blood or body fluids is possible, other personal protective equipment (PPE) such as a mask, eye protection, and/or a gown must be worn. Any instruments or equipment contaminated by blood or body fluids must be correctly cleaned and disinfected or sterilized after use. The medical assistant must always be aware of and take steps to prevent the spread of infection.

STUDENT: *Go to the workbook and complete the assignment sheet for 19:4, Assisting with Physical Examinations. Then return and continue with the procedures.*

PROCEDURE 19:4A

Eye, Ear, Nose, and Throat Examination

NOTE: This is a basic guideline. Methods and equipment will vary from physician to physician.

Equipment and Supplies

Tray covered with a towel, basin lined with a paper towel, cotton-tipped applicators, ophthalmoscope, otoscope, tonometer, tuning fork, nasal speculum, laryngeal mirror, glass of warm water, tongue blades or depressors, flashlight or penlight, Snellen chart, culture tubes and slides (as needed), disposable gloves, infectious-waste bag, patient's chart, lab requisition forms, pen or pencil

Procedure

1. Assemble equipment.
2. Wash hands. Put on gloves for any procedure that involves contact with blood or body fluids.

   CAUTION: Observe standard precautions at all times.
3. Introduce yourself. Identify the patient. Explain the procedure. Remember that this procedure has multiple steps.
4. Screen for vision problems with a Snellen chart, as required. Record all results accurately.
5. Place the patient in a sitting position.

   NOTE: If an eye, ear, nose, and throat exam is the only examination being done, the patient can remain dressed.
6. Ask the patient to remove glasses and/or hearing aid(s). Tell the patient to place these items in a safe place.

NOTE: Hearing aids are sometimes *not* removed until the actual ear examination. This is particularly true if the patient cannot hear questions without a hearing aid.

7. Notify the physician that the patient is ready. Have disposable gloves available for the physician to use. The physician may put the gloves on at the start of the examination or at the point during the examination when contact with body fluids may occur.
8. Eyes are usually examined first. Turn the ophthalmoscope light on and hand the ophthalmoscope to the physician. When the physician hands the ophthalmoscope back, turn the light off.

   NOTE: Some physicians want the room light turned off during the eye examination.
9. If the intraocular pressure of the eye is to be checked, hand the physician the tonometer. If the physician is not doing the recording, record the pressure reading stated by the physician.
10. The nose is usually examined next. Have the nasal speculum and flashlight ready for use. Also have cotton-tipped applicators ready. If a culture is taken, handle the culture stick correctly.

    NOTE: Refer to Procedure 18:2A, Obtaining a Culture Specimen, if necessary.
11. The ears are usually examined next. Pass the otoscope with its light on to the physician. Have a cotton-tipped applicator ready for use. When the examination is done, turn off the otoscope light. Place the otoscope tip in the towel-lined basin. If the physician wants

to test hearing acuity, hand the physician the tuning fork. Hold the tuning fork in the middle so the physician can grasp it at the stem end.

12. The mouth and throat are usually examined last. Pass the tongue blade or depressor by holding it in the center. Turn on the flashlight or penlight and hand it to the physician, as needed.

13. Have culture sticks and tubes available. Hand these to the physician correctly.

    ⚠ **CAUTION:** Avoid contaminating the tip of the culture stick.

14. If a laryngeal mirror is used, warm the mirror end by placing it in a glass of warm water. Dry the mirror and hand it to the physician.

    NOTE: This prevents fogging during use.

15. Place the used mirror in the towel-lined basin.

16. Take hold of the used tongue blade in the center. Without touching either end, place it in the infectious-waste bag.

17. When the examination is complete, help the patient replace glasses, hearing aid(s), and so forth. Help the patient get off the examining table. Inform the patient of how and when he or she will be notified of test results.

18. Label all specimens correctly with the patient's name, identification number, and doctor's name. Print all information on the lab requisition form. This might include date, time, patient's name, address, identifi-

cation number, doctor's name and identification number, type or site of specimen, and test ordered. Send to the laboratory as soon as possible.

19. ☣ Clean and replace all equipment. Put on gloves while disinfecting and sterilizing contaminated instruments or equipment. Put all contaminated disposable supplies in the infectious-waste bag. Use a disinfectant to wipe any contaminated areas.

20. Remove gloves. Wash hands.

21. Ⓒ Record all required information on the patient's chart, for example, date, time, EENT exam, throat culture sent to lab, and your signature and title. Place a copy of any lab requisitions in the patient's chart. The physician sometimes records the required information.

Practice *Go to the workbook and use the evaluation sheet for 19:4A, Assisting with an Eye, Ear, Nose, and Throat Examination, to practice this procedure. When you feel you have mastered this skill, sign the sheet and give it to your instructor for further action.*

✔ **Final Checkpoint** Using the criteria listed on the evaluation sheet, your instructor will grade your performance.

PROCEDURE 19:4B

Assisting with a Gynecological Examination

NOTE: The equipment and steps of this procedure can vary from physician to physician.

Equipment and Supplies

Tray covered with a towel, sheet or drape, patient gown, cotton-tipped applicators; sterile cotton-tipped applicators, gloves, lubricant, vaginal speculum, Ayer blades, cytology brush, culture tubes, slides and fixative, examining light, cotton balls, basin lined with a paper towel, tissues, infectious-waste bag, patient's chart, lab requisition forms, pen or pencil

Procedure

1. Assemble equipment and arrange on a tray (see figure 19-27).

2. Wash hands. Put on gloves.

     CAUTION: Gloves should be worn when any contact with vaginal secretions is possible.

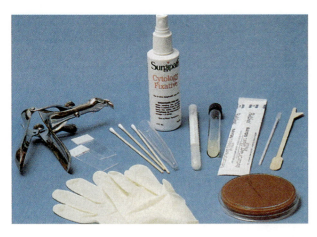

FIGURE 19-27 Basic equipment for a gynecological examination.

3. **C** Introduce yourself. Identify the patient. Explain the procedure. Remember that this procedure has multiple steps.

4. Ask the patient to void. If a urinalysis is ordered, obtain the urine specimen at this time.

5. Ask the patient to remove all clothing and put on an examination gown. The gown is usually open in the front.

6. Make sure the extension of the examining table is pushed in or dropped down. Then assist the patient into a sitting position on the table. Use the drape to cover the patient's lap and legs.

7. Notify the physician that the patient is ready for examination.

8. The breasts are usually examined first. After the physician has examined the breasts, place the patient in the horizontal recumbent position. Drape correctly. The physician will usually complete the breast examination at this point.

   NOTE: The patient should be taught how to do a breast self-examination or BSE (refer to figure 6-66). This can be done before or after the examination. Pamphlets describing the procedure, available from the American Cancer Society, can be given to the patient.

9. Place the patient in the lithotomy position. Drape correctly. Position the examining light for proper lighting.

10. Warm the vaginal speculum by placing it in warm water or rubbing it with a clean towel. Hand the speculum in the closed position to the physician. Be ready to apply lubricant to the speculum. Have cotton-tipped applicators ready for use.

NOTE: If a culture is to be taken, the lubricant may interfere with the organism. Lubricant is not placed on the speculum in such a case.

11. If a culture is to be taken, hand the sterile applicator to the physician. Take care to avoid contaminating the tip. Have the culture tube or slide available to receive the culture.

12. If a Pap test is to be done, hand the physician the Ayer blade. Grasp the blade in the center and place the blunt end in the physician's hand. The V-shaped end is inserted in the patient by the physician.

   NOTE: A cytology brush may be used in place of or in addition to the Ayer blade. Again, grasp the brush in the center, with the brush end directed toward the patient, to hand the brush to the physician.

   NOTE: A Pap test is done to detect cancer of the cervix.

13. Have a slide ready for use. The physician will place the smear on the slide or hand the Ayer blade or cytology brush to you. If the latter, spread the smear evenly and moderately thin on the slide. Put the Ayer blade or cytology brush in the infectious-waste bag.

   NOTE: If the smear is too thick, the cells cannot be seen.

   NOTE: Frequently, two or three slides are prepared: a cervical smear, a vaginal smear, and/or an endocervical smear. Label each slide with the patient's name and place a *c* on the cervical slide, a *v* on the vaginal smear, and an *e* on the endocervical smear.

14. Apply fixative to the slide(s). The fixative is usually a spray that is applied to the entire slide. Sometimes the entire slide is placed in a specimen jar containing fixative solution.

   NOTE: Fixative makes the cells adhere (stick) to the slide until the slide is examined.

15. When the physician hands you the vaginal speculum, place it in the towel-lined basin. If it is disposable, place it in the infectious-waste bag.

16. The digital (finger) examination is usually done next. Place lubricant on the physician's gloved fingers without touching the gloves. The physician usually does a digital examination of both the vagina and rectum.

17. When the examination is complete, assist the patient out of the lithotomy position. Offer tissue to the patient to remove excess

lubrication. Place the tissue in the infectious-waste bag. If no signs of weakness or dizziness are noted, help the patient get off the table.

⚠ **CAUTION:** Watch the patient closely to prevent falls.

18. Inform the patient how and when she will be notified of test results. Ask the patient to get dressed or assist with dressing if necessary.

19. Ⓒ Completely label all cultures and slides with the patient's name, identification number, and doctor's name. Print all information on the lab requisition form. This might include date, time, patient's name, address, identification number, doctor's name and identification number, type or site of specimen, test ordered, date of last menstrual period, and information on any hormone therapy. Be sure you have all required information before the patient leaves the office.

20. Send all specimens to the laboratory as soon as possible.

21. ☣ Wear gloves while cleaning and sterilizing the speculum and any contaminated instruments or equipment. Put all contaminated disposable supplies in the infectious-waste bag. Use a disinfectant to wipe any contaminated areas.

22. Remove gloves. Wash hands.

23. Ⓒ Record all required information on the patient's chart, for example: date, time, GYN exam, Pap smear sent to lab, and your signature and title. Place a copy of any lab requisitions in the patient's chart. The physician sometimes records the required information.

Practice *Go to the workbook and use the evaluation sheet for 19:4B, Assisting with a Gynecological Examination, to practice this procedure. When you feel you have mastered this skill, sign the sheet and give it to your instructor for further action.*

✓ **Final Checkpoint** Using the criteria listed on the evaluation sheet, your instructor will grade your performance.

PROCEDURE 19:4C
Assisting with a General Physical Examination

NOTE: The equipment and steps of this procedure can vary from physician to physician.

Equipment and Supplies

Tray or stand and cover, patient gown, drape or sheet, basin lined with paper towels, tissues, scale, Snellen chart, thermometer, stethoscope, sphygmomanometer, ophthalmoscope, otoscope, nasal speculum, tuning fork, tongue depressors, laryngeal mirror, glass with warm water, percussion hammer, new safety pin or sensory wheel, rectal speculum or proctoscope, Pap test kit and vaginal speculum (female), culture tubes, slides, fixative solution, sterile applicators, lubricant, alcohol swabs, gloves, penlight or examining light, infectious-waste bag, patient's chart, lab requisition forms, pen or pencil

Procedure

1. Assemble equipment. Arrange equipment conveniently on the stand or tray (see figure 19-28).

2. Wash hands. Put on gloves or have gloves available for later use.

   ☣ **CAUTION:** Gloves should be worn anytime contact with blood or body fluids is possible. Observe standard precautions at all times.

3. Ⓒ Introduce yourself. Identify the patient. Explain the procedure. Remember that this procedure has multiple steps.

4. Ask the patient to remove all clothing and put on an examining gown. Ask the patient to void. If a urinalysis is ordered, collect the urine specimen at this time.

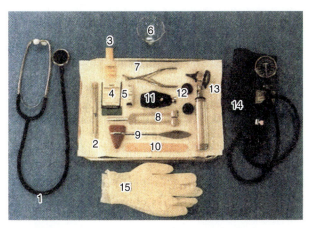

1. stethoscope
2. penlight
3. guaiac/occult blood test developer
4. guaiac/blood test
5. flexible tape measure
6. urine specimen container
7. metal nasal speculum
8. tuning fork
9. percussion hammer
10. tongue depressor
11. opthalmascope (head)
12. okastic ear/nose speculum
13. otoscope head attached to base handle
14. sphygmomanometer
15. gloves

FIGURE 19-28 Equipment and supplies for a physical examination should be arranged in a convenient order.

5. Do any of the required following procedures:
   a. Record height and weight
   b. Take and record TPR and/or BP
   c. Use a Snellen chart to test vision; record results
   d. Perform an audiometric screening if ordered
   e. Run an electrocardiogram if ordered
   f. Obtain all required blood samples for tests ordered
6. Seat the patient on the examining table. Drape the patient correctly.
7. Notify the physician that the patient is ready.
8. Assist with eye, ear, nose, and throat exam as previously instructed.
9. Give the physician the stethoscope and/or sphygmomanometer. Remain quiet while the patient's heart and lungs are examined.
   NOTE: The physician may check the blood pressure.
   NOTE: The physician may also do an initial examination of the breasts, legs, and feet.
10. Place the patient in the horizontal recumbent or supine position. Drape correctly.
11. The physician will examine the chest and abdomen. Draw the drape down to the pubic area. Replace the drape after the abdomen has been examined.

12. The legs and feet are examined next. Have the percussion hammer ready. In addition, have an open new safety pin or sensory wheel ready in case the doctor wants to use it to check sensation in the feet.
13. The back and spine are usually examined next. Turn the patient to the prone position and let the drape hang loose. Assist as needed.
    NOTE: The back and spine can also be examined with the patient in a sitting position.
14. On a female patient, a vaginal examination is usually done next. Put the patient in the lithotomy position. Drape correctly. Assist as taught for a gynecological examination. The male patient can be placed in the horizontal recumbent position for a genital organ examination.
    NOTE: Male patients should be taught how to do a testicular self-examination. This can be done at this point or at the end of the examination.
15. The rectal area is examined last in most cases. A female can be examined while still in the lithotomy position or in the Sims' position. A male is usually placed in the Sims' position. Hand gloves and lubricant to the physician, as needed. Have the rectal speculum or anoscope in a closed position ready for use.
16. When the examination is complete, assist the patient into a sitting position on the examination table. Allow the patient to rest for a few minutes. If no signs of weakness or dizziness are noted, help the patient get off the table. Inform the patient how and when he or she will be notified of test results. Ask the patient to get dressed or assist with dressing if necessary.
    ⚠ **CAUTION:** Watch closely to prevent falls.
17. Label all specimens and cultures with the patient's name, identification number, and doctor's name. Print all information on the lab requisition form(s). This might include date, time, patient's name, address, identification number, doctor's name and identification number, type or site of specimen, and test ordered. Send specimens to the laboratory as soon as possible.
18. ☣ Wear gloves while cleaning and sterilizing any contaminated instruments or equipment. Put all contaminated disposable supplies in the infectious-waste bag.

Use a disinfectant to wipe any contaminated areas.

19. Remove gloves. Wash hands.

20. Record all required information on the patient's chart, for example, date, time, Physical exam, Pap smear sent to lab, and your signature and title. Place a copy of any lab requisition forms in the patient's chart. The physician sometimes records the required information.

Final Checkpoint Using the criteria listed on the evaluation sheet, your instructor will grade your performance.

19:5 INFORMATION
Assisting with Minor Surgery and Suture Removal

As a health care worker, you may be required to prepare for and assist with minor surgery or suture removal in a medical, dental, or health care facility. Minor surgery includes removing warts, cysts, tumors, growths, or foreign objects; suturing wounds; incising and draining body areas; and other similar procedures.

Instruments and equipment used depend on the type of surgery or procedure being done. Some basic instruments and supplies that may be used (see figure 19-29) include the following:

◆ **Scalpels:** instruments with a handle attached to knife blades; used to incise (cut) skin and tissue. Disposable scalpels with a protective retractable blade to prevent sharps injuries, are also available for use (see figure 19-30).

◆ **Surgical scissors:** special scissors with blunt ends or sharp points or a combination; used to cut tissue.

◆ **Hemostats:** special group of curved or straight instruments, usually striated at the ends; used to compress (clamp) blood vessels to stop bleeding or grasp tissue.

◆ **Tissue forceps:** instruments with one or more fine points (or teeth) at the tip of the blades; used to grasp tissue.

◆ **Retractors:** instruments used to hold or draw back the lips, or sides, of a wound or incision.

◆ Suture materials: special materials used for stitches **(sutures)**; applied to hold a wound or incision closed; absorbable suture material such as surgical gut or vicryl is digested by tissue enzymes and absorbed by the body; nonabsorbable suture materials such as silk, nylon, Dacron, stainless steel, and metal skin clips or staples, are removed after the tissue or skin has healed.

◆ **Needle holder:** special instrument used to hold or support the needle while sutures are being inserted.

◆ Needle: pointed, slender instrument with an eye at one end; used to hold suture material while sutures are being inserted into an incision or wound; usually curved for easier insertion into the skin; *swaged* needles have the suture material attached to the needle as one unit.

◆ **Bandage scissors:** special scissors with blunt lower ends; used to remove dressings and bandages; the blunt ends prevent injury to the skin directly next to the dressing material.

Preparation of the surgery tray requires the use of strict sterile technique to prevent infection. Instruments and supplies must be sterilized. Care must be taken to avoid contaminating the instruments and supplies when they are placed on the tray. Complete sterile setups are also available in commercially prepared, disposable packages. Examples include

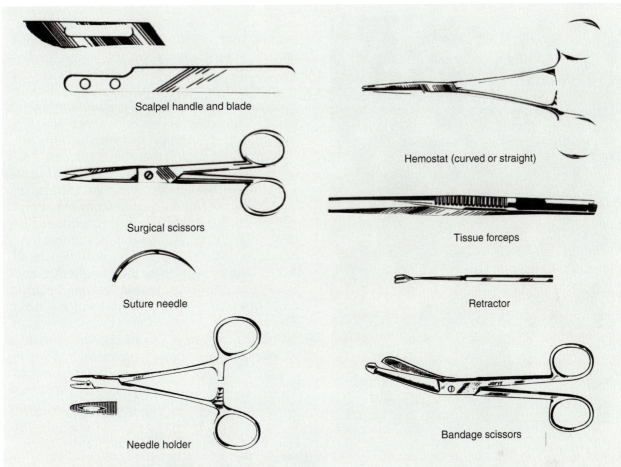

Scalpel handle and blade

Surgical scissors

Suture needle

Needle holder

Hemostat (curved or straight)

Tissue forceps

Retractor

Bandage scissors

FIGURE 19-29 Some sample surgical instruments.

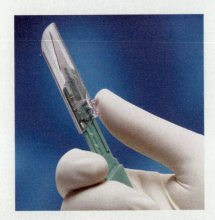

FIGURE 19-30 Disposable scalpels with a protective retractable blade help prevent sharps injuries. *(Photo reprinted courtesy of BD [Becton, Dickinson and Company])*

setups for insertion of sutures and for removal of sutures. It is important to follow sterile technique (see Unit 13:7) while opening the packages in order to maintain sterility of all materials in the package.

During surgery, the medical assistant will be expected to assist as needed. The procedure will depend on the physician doing the surgery. Be alert to all points of the procedure and be ready to help as needed.

Sterile dressings must be available for use. These are usually placed directly on the surgical tray so that they are readily accessible. Some physicians prefer that sterile dressings be left in the original sterile wrappers and placed in the immediate area.

Suture removal (removal of stitches) also requires that sterile technique be followed. Infection is an ever present threat and must be prevented. Again, instruments and supplies will vary. The main instruments used for this procedure are suture scissors and thumb forceps (see figure 19-31). The two instruments are frequently packaged in sterilized, disposable kits called **suture removal sets.** The thumb forceps is used to grasp and hold the suture. It is compressed with the thumb and forefinger. The suture scissors have a curved blade that is

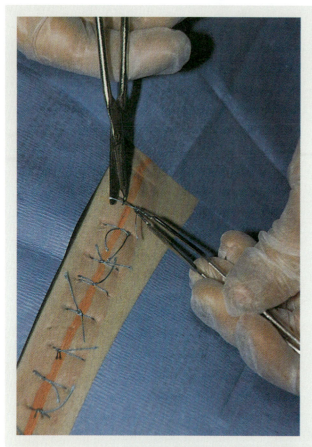

FIGURE 19-31 A suture removal set consists of suture scissors and thumb forceps.

inserted under the suture material so that the stitch can be cut and removed. Basic guidelines are provided in Procedure 19:5B.

C Patients who are undergoing minor surgery or suture removal are often fearful and apprehensive. Reassure the patient to the best of your ability. Refer specific questions regarding the surgery or procedure to the physician.

Body tissues, abnormal growths, and other specimens removed during surgery are usually sent to a laboratory for examination. Place each specimen in an appropriate container immediately to avoid loss. Label the containers correctly and complete the lab requisition form. Send them to the laboratory as soon as possible.

Because contamination from blood and body fluids is possible during minor surgical procedures, standard precautions (discussed in Unit 13:3) must be observed at all times. Hands must be washed frequently, and gloves must be worn. Instruments and equipment must be properly cleaned and sterilized after use. Contaminated areas must be wiped with a disinfectant. Contaminated disposable supplies must be placed in an infectious-waste bag prior to being disposed of according to legal requirements. Sharp objects such as scalpel blades (or disposable scalpels) and needles must be placed in a leakproof puncture-resistant sharps container immediately after use. The medical assistant must always be aware of and take steps to prevent the spread of infection.

STUDENT: *Go to the workbook and complete the assignment sheet for 19:5, Assisting with Minor Surgery and Suture Removal. Then return and continue with the procedures.*

PROCEDURE 19:5A

Assisting with Minor Surgery

NOTE: Instruments and procedures vary depending on the type of surgery and the physician.

Equipment and Supplies

Tray with cover or Mayo stand, infectious-waste bag, sharps container, disposable gloves, tape, patient's chart, lab requisition forms, pen or pencil
NOTE: All the following equipment should be sterile: towels, drapes and drape clamps, two to three pairs of sterile gloves, needle and syringe, anesthetic medication, basin, antiseptic solution, gauze pads, scalpel, surgical scissors, hemostat forceps (straight and curved), tissue forceps, retractors, needle holder, needle, suture material, dressings (gauze and pads).

Procedure

1. Assemble equipment required.
2. Wash hands.

3. Check dates and sterilization indicators on all sterile supplies to make sure the supplies are still sterile.
   NOTE: Many sterile supplies are good for 1 month only.
4. Place the tray or stand in an area where there is freedom of movement and limited chance of contamination.
5. Open a sterile towel and place it on the tray so that the entire tray is covered.
   NOTE: Follow the correct procedure to avoid contamination (see Unit 13:8).
6. Open the other sterile towels or drapes and place them on the tray.
7. Open a sterile basin. Place it on the tray. Put the sterile gauze in the basin. Obtain the correct antiseptic solution and pour a small amount of the solution in a sink or separate container to rinse the lip of the bottle. Then hold the solution bottle approximately 6 inches above the sterile basin and carefully pour the required amount of solution into the sterile basin.
   NOTE: Read the label three times to be sure you have the correct solution.
   CAUTION: Avoid handling the inside of the solution bottle cap. If the cap is placed on a counter, make sure the open end, or inside, is facing up. This prevents contamination of the inside of the cap.
   CAUTION: Do *not* splash the solution onto the tray.
8. Open all wrapped instruments and place them on the tray in a convenient order, usually the order of use (see figure 19-32).
   NOTE: Number and type of instruments will depend on the type of surgery and the physician.
9. Open the needle and syringe and place it on the tray. Unless the physician has specified a certain size, have a variety of needles of different gauges available.
10. Open the suture packages. Place them on the tray. If specific sizes and types have not been requested by the physician, a variety of materials should be made available.
11. Place the sterile dressings on the tray. The outer dressings should be placed on the bottom of the pile. This way, the dressings are in the order of use.
12. Check the tray to be sure everything is present. Use a sterile towel to cover the tray.
   CAUTION: Do *not* leave the tray unattended because contamination of the materials may occur.

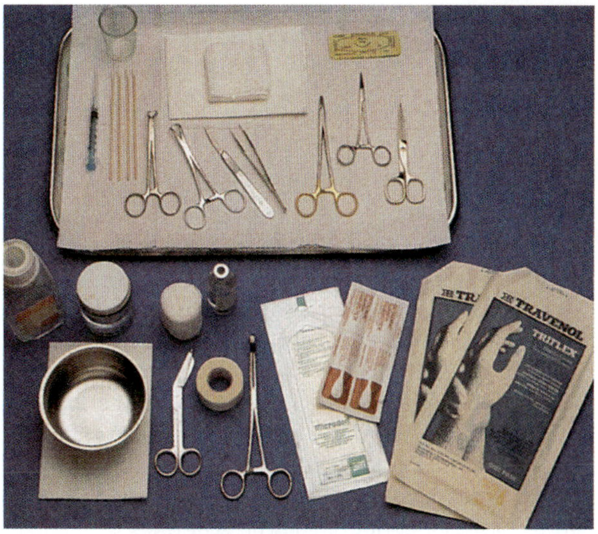

FIGURE 19-32 Instruments and supplies for minor surgery should be arranged in a convenient order.

13. Place the anesthetic solution, sterile gloves, tape, and infectious-waste bag close to the tray.
   NOTE: Several pairs of gloves should be available in case one pair becomes contaminated.
14. **C** Introduce yourself. Identify the patient. Confirm that the patient observed all preoperative instructions. Explain the procedure and preview postoperative orders. Obtain the patient's written consent.
15. Position and drape the patient according to the surgery to be performed.
16. During the surgery, assist as needed:
   a. Uncover the tray when ready for use.
   b. Give the sterile gloves to the physician.
   c. Use a gauze pad saturated with alcohol to clean the top of the anesthetic solution vial. Hold the vial in a convenient position so the physician can fill the syringe (see figure 19-33).
   d. If required, put on sterile gloves and assist as needed. Hold retractors, hand instruments, and assist with the procedure.
   e. Get additional supplies or equipment as needed.
17. After the surgery, assist as needed with placement of dressings and bandages. Observe for any signs of distress. If no signs of weakness or dizziness are noted, help the patient get off the table. Review postoperative orders with the patient. Provide the patient with a written copy of postoperative orders if this is office policy. Inform the

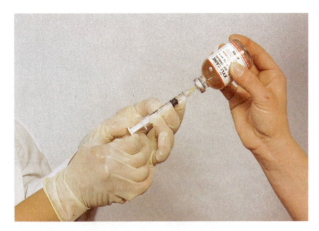

FIGURE 19-33 Hold the anesthetic solution in a convenient position so the physician can fill the syringe without contaminating the needle.

patient how and when he or she will be notified of test results.

18. Label all specimens correctly with the patient's name, identification number, and doctor's name. Print all information on the lab requisition form. This might include date, time, patient's name, address, identification number, doctor's name and identification number, type or site of specimen, and test ordered. Make sure each specimen is in the correct specimen container or bottle. Send specimens to the laboratory as soon as possible.
    NOTE: Pathologists will provide special containers in some agencies.

19. Wear gloves to clean and sterilize all instruments and equipment. Put sharp objects such as the needle and syringe and scalpel blade (or disposable scalpel) in the sharps container immediately after use. Put contaminated disposable supplies in the infectious-waste container. Use a disinfectant to wipe any contaminated areas. Put all equipment in its correct place.

20. Remove gloves. Wash hands.

21. Record all required information on the patient's chart, for example, date, time, Surgical removal of tumor on right forearm, Specimen sent to pathology lab, verbal and written postoperative instructions given to patient, and your signature and title. Place a copy of any lab requisitions in the patient's chart. The physician sometimes records the required information.

Practice Go to the workbook and use the evaluation sheet for 19:5A, Assisting with Minor Surgery, to practice this procedure. When you feel you have mastered this skill, sign the sheet and give it to your instructor for further action.

✔ **Final Checkpoint** Using the criteria listed on the evaluation sheet, your instructor will grade your performance.

PROCEDURE 19:5B
Assisting with Suture Removal

NOTE: The procedure for suture removal varies according to the physician. The following serves as a basic guideline only.

Equipment and Supplies

Tray or stand, suture removal set, sterile towel, sterile gloves, drapes (as needed), dressings (as indicated), sterile basin, sterile gauze, antiseptic solution, tape, infectious-waste bag, patient's chart, pen or pencil

Procedure

1. Assemble required equipment.
2. Wash hands.
3. Check the dates and sterilization indicators on all sterile supplies to make sure the supplies are still sterile.
4. Place a sterile towel on the tray.
    NOTE: Follow the correct procedure for unwrapping and placing all supplies.
5. Place a sterile basin on the tray. Put gauze and antiseptic solution in the basin.

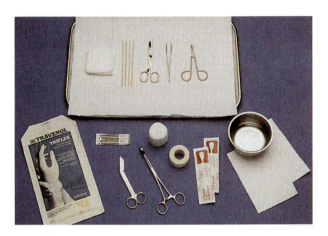

FIGURE 19-34 A sample suture removal tray setup.

6. Place dressings on the tray. Outer dressings should be on the bottom. This way, dressings are in order of use.
7. Place the sterile suture removal set on the tray.
8. Place a sterile towel or needed drapes on the tray.
9. Check the tray to be sure all equipment is present (see figure 19-34).

   (!) CAUTION: Do *not* leave the tray unattended.

10. Put the infectious-waste bag, tape, and sterile gloves near the tray.
11. **(C)** Introduce yourself. Identify the patient. Explain the procedure. Obtain the patient's consent.
12. Position and drape according to location of sutures. Reassure the patient as needed.
13. Assist the physician as necessary during the procedure.

NOTE: Frequently, medical assistants are trained and authorized to remove sutures.

14. When the sutures have been removed, place a clean dressing and bandages on the wound.
15. Instruct the patient on wound care and provide written instructions if this is office policy. Watch closely for signs of distress. If no signs of weakness or dizziness are noted, help the patient get off the table.
16. Wear gloves to clean and sterilize all instruments. If the suture set is disposable, place it in a sharps container. Put all contaminated disposable supplies in the infectious-waste bag. Use a disinfectant to wipe any contaminated areas.
17. Remove gloves. Wash hands.
18. **(C)** Record all required information on the patient's chart or the agency form, for example, date, time, Sutures removed from right forearm, Sterile dressing applied, and your signature and title. The physician sometimes records the required information.

Practice *Go to the workbook and use the evaluation sheet for 19:5B, Assisting with Suture Removal, to practice this procedure. When you feel you have mastered this skill, sign the sheet and give it to your instructor for further action.*

✔ Final Checkpoint Using the criteria listed on the evaluation sheet, your instructor will grade your performance.

19:6 INFORMATION *Recording and Mounting an Electrocardiogram*

In order to understand an **electrocardiogram (ECG),** it is essential to understand the electrical conduction pattern in the muscles of the heart (see figure 19-35). The contraction of the heart muscles is controlled by electrical impulses within the heart. The electrical impulse originates in the sinoatrial (SA) node of the heart, located near the top of the right atrium. The impulse moves through the atria, causing the muscles of the atria to contract. The impulse next travels to the atrioventricular (AV) node, through a band of fibers called the bundle of His, and then through the right and left bundle branches to the final branches, called the Purkinje fibers. The Purkinje fibers distribute the impulse to the muscles of the right and left ventricles, which then contract. The movement of

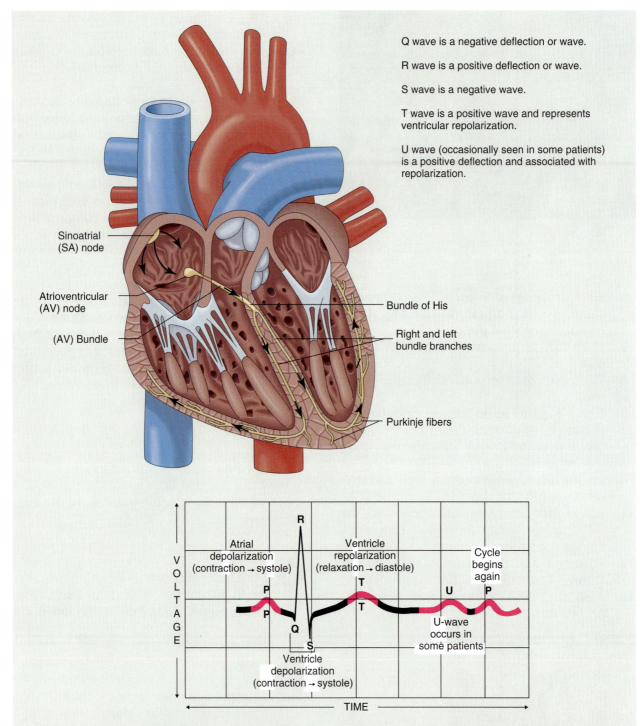

Q wave is a negative deflection or wave.

R wave is a positive deflection or wave.

S wave is a negative wave.

T wave is a positive wave and represents ventricular repolarization.

U wave (occasionally seen in some patients) is a positive deflection and associated with repolarization.

Sinoatrial (SA) node

Atrioventricular (AV) node

(AV) Bundle

Bundle of His

Right and left bundle branches

Purkinje fibers

FIGURE 19-35 As the electrical impulse passes through the conduction pathway in the heart, it creates a pattern recorded as an electrocardiogram.

the electrical impulse is recorded by an electrocardiograph machine as a series of waves known as a *PQRST complex*. The P wave occurs as the impulse originates in the SA node and travels through the atria. The QRS wave represents the movement of the impulse through the AV node, bundle of His, bundle branches, and Purkinje fibers. The T wave represents the repolarization of the ventricles, or the period of recovery in the ventricles before another contraction occurs.

The pattern of electrical current in the heart is recorded by an electrocardiograph machine

Lead Arrangement and Coding

Standard limb leads

Standard or bipolar limb leads	Sensors connected	Marking code
Lead 1	LA & RA	.
Lead 2	LL & RA	..
Lead 3	LL & LA	...

Augmented limb leads

Augmented unipolar limb leads		
aVR	RA & (LA-LL)	-
aVL	LA & (RA-LL)	--
aVF	LL (RA-LA)	---

Chest leads

Chest or precordial leads		
V	C & (LA-RA-LL)	V1 – .
		V2 – ..
		V3 – ...
		V4 – .... .
		V5 – .... ..
		V6 – ....

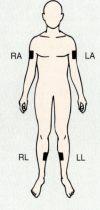

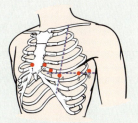

V₁ Fourth intercostal space at right margin of sternum

V₂ Fourth intercostal space at left margin of sternum

V₃ Midway between position V₂ and position V₄

V₄ Fifth intercostal space at junction of left midclavicular line

V₅ At horizontal level of position V₄ at left anterior axillary line

V₆ At horizontal level of position V₄ at left midaxillary line

FIGURE 19-36 The lead arrangement and coding for a standard electrocardiogram.

as an ECG. Each PQRST pattern represents the electrical activity that occurs during each contraction of the heart muscle; thus, each PQRST complex represents one heartbeat. Because an abnormal pattern of the electrical impulses will be evident on an ECG, the ECG can be used to diagnose disease and/or damage to the muscles of the heart.

Using special electrodes, the electrical activity is recorded from different angles, called **leads.** The different leads give the physician a more complete picture of the heart. By noting an electrical disturbance in any of the leads, the physician can determine which parts of the heart are diseased or malfunctioning.

A complete ECG normally consists of twelve leads. Electrodes are placed at specific locations on the body to pick up the voltage present. Connections between the various electrodes create the various leads. The leads are labeled as 1 (I), 2 (II), 3 (III), aVR, aVL, aVF, V_1, V_2, V_3, V_4, V_5, and V_6. There are three classifications: standard, augmented, and chest leads (see figure 19-36).

◆ Standard, or limb, leads: Include leads 1 (I), 2 (II), and 3 (III) (see figure 19-37). Each records the voltage between two extremities.

Lead 1 (I) connects the right arm and the left arm.

Lead 2 (II) connects the right arm and the left leg.

Lead 3 (III) connects the left arm and the left leg.

◆ Augmented voltage leads: Include aVR, aVL, and aVF (see figure 19-38). They are different angles of the standard leads 1 (I), 2 (II), and 3 (III). The aVR stands for augmented voltage

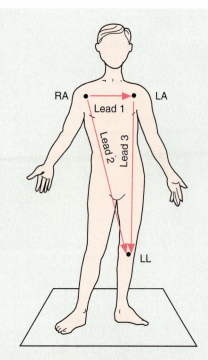

FIGURE 19-37 Standard limb leads.

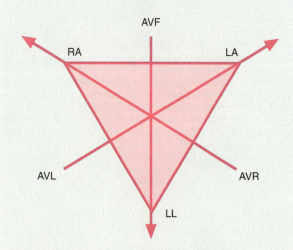

FIGURE 19-38 Augmented voltage (AV) leads.

right arm, aVL stands for augmented voltage left arm, and aVF stands for augmented voltage left foot.

♦ Chest leads: The six chest, or precordial, leads record angles of the electrical impulse from a central point within the heart to specific sites on the front of the chest (see figure 19-39). To obtain these angles, chest electrodes are placed at six specific locations on the chest (refer back to figure 19-36).

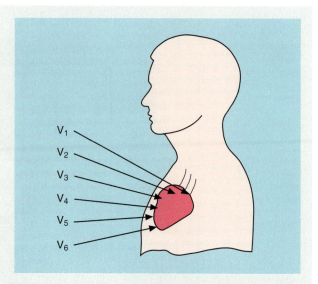

FIGURE 19-39 Heart angles recorded by chest leads.

V_1: Fourth intercostal (between ribs) space on the right side of the sternum (breastbone).

V_2: Fourth intercostal space on the left side of the sternum.

V_3: Midway between the V_2 and V_4 positions.

V_4: Fifth intercostal space at the junction of the mid-clavicular line (line drawn from the middle of the clavicle).

V_5: Same level as 4 but at left anterior axillary line.

V_6: Same level as 4 but at left midaxillary line.

In order to record these twelve leads, electrodes are placed on various parts of the body. The electrodes are coded so that each is put in the proper place. Codes are as follows:

♦ *RA* for right arm: Placed on the fleshy outer area of the upper part of the right arm.

♦ *LA* for left arm: Placed on the fleshy outer area of the upper part of the left arm.

♦ *RL* for right leg: Placed on the fleshy part of the lower right leg. This does not record a lead, but serves as a ground for electrical interference.

♦ *LL* for left leg: Placed on the fleshy part of the lower left leg.

♦ *C* or *V* for chest: Placed at six different locations on the chest (see figure 19-36).

The ECG paper is marked with a code so that the physician knows which lead is being recorded. Some machines record this code automatically, but others must be coded manually. The code for each lead is as follows:

. Lead 1 (I)	—. V1
. . Lead 2 (II)	—.. V2
. . . Lead 3 (III)	—... V3
– aVR	—.... V4
– – aVL	—..... V5
– – – aVF	—...... V6

Some newer ECG machines print the name of the lead (I, II, AVR, etc.) on the paper instead of using the codes.

Electrocardiograph machines vary slightly, but most have the same basic parts. It is important to read the specific manufacturer's instructions with each machine. There are two main classes of electrocardiographs: single-channel and multiple-channel. The single-channel electrocardiograph produces a narrow strip of paper showing one lead at a time. The multiple-channel electrocardiograph produces a full sheet of paper showing all twelve leads (see figure 19-40). All electrocardiograph machines have most of the following basic parts:

- ♦ **Main switch:** Turns the machine on and off.
- ♦ 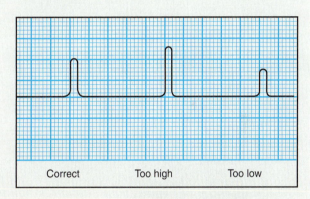 **Pilot light:** A red light that indicates that the machine is on. On newer, computerized machines, this may be indicated by a *ready* signal on the computer readout.
- ♦ **ST'D (standard control):** Used to perform a quality control check and to ensure that the machine is calibrated correctly to record electrical impulses. One millivolt electrical input should cause the stylus (recording needle) to move 10 millimeters on the graph (10 small squares or 2 large squares on the paper) (see figure 19-41). If the standard is not the correct height during the standard check, the ST'D must be adjusted. Follow the manufacturer's instructions to adjust the standard to the proper height.
- ♦ **Stylus heat control:** Used to adjust stylus temperature (see figure 19-42). The heat

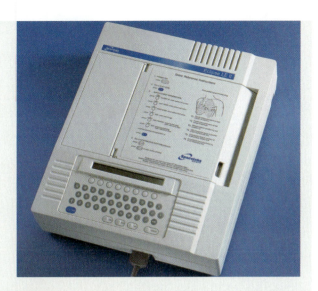

FIGURE 19-40 A multiple-channel electrocardiograph produces a full sheet of paper showing all twelve leads. *(Courtesy of Spacelabs Medical, Inc.)*

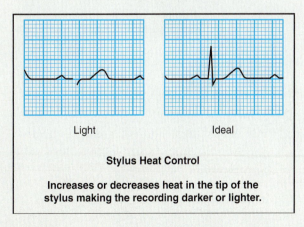

Correct	Too high	Too low

FIGURE 19-41 Standardization: correct, too high, too low.

Light	Ideal

Stylus Heat Control

Increases or decreases heat in the tip of the stylus making the recording darker or lighter.

FIGURE 19-42 Stylus heat control: light and ideal.

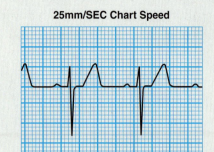

25mm/SEC Chart Speed

SPEED 25 enganges the paper drive to run at an internationally-accepted standard of 25 mm per second. This is the "normal" speed for recording.

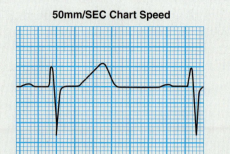

50mm/SEC Chart Speed

SPEED 50 doubles the speed of the paper to 50 mm per second. Useful when heart rate is rapid or when certain segments of a complex are close together, since it extends the recording to twice its normal width.

FIGURE 19-43 Speed settings for an ECG.

from the stylus melts the plastic coating on the ECG paper, forming the black line. At the same time, the coating lubricates the stylus. If the tracing is too light, the heat must be increased. If the tracing is too dark, the heat must be decreased. Follow manufacturer's instructions to adjust the heat.

◆ **Stylus position control:** Used to move the recording up and down on the paper. In most cases, this control should be adjusted to center the ECG on the paper.

◆ **Record, or speed, control:** Has three or four separate functions to control the amplifier and paper drive, or the speed.

(1) Amp off: The unit remains inactive; used when changing chest lead positions.

(2) Amp on: The amplifier is activated, causing the stylus to move, but the paper remains stationary. This position is useful for chest leads. After the chest electrode is in position, turn the machine to amp on, allow the stylus to stabilize or settle, and turn to Run 25.

(3) Run 25: The position normally used when recording an ECG. The paper moves at a rate of 25 millimeters per second (see figure 19-43).

(4) Run 50: The position used when the complexes of the ECG are so close together that they are difficult to examine. It increases the speed of the paper to 50 millimeters per second, stretching the ECG out on the paper. Often used for extremely fast tachycardias (pulse rate above 100). To make the physician aware of the increased speed, "Run 50" must be written on the paper with a pen or pencil (if not recorded automatically by the machine).

◆ **Lead coding marker:** Places a mark or code on the paper to identify the lead being recorded. On most electrocardiograph machines, this is done automatically. On some machines, the lead mark is recorded manually at the start of each lead recording. Many of the multiple-channel ECG machines print the name of the lead on the paper instead of the code.

◆ **Lead selector switch:** Allows selection of the lead to be run. It has a position for checking the standard and other positions for running each of the twelve leads of a standard ECG.

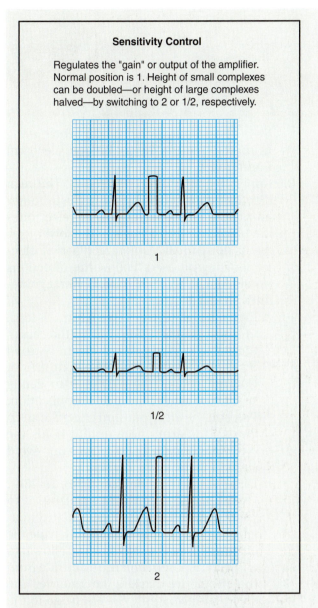

Sensitivity Control

Regulates the "gain" or output of the amplifier. Normal position is 1. Height of small complexes can be doubled—or height of large complexes halved—by switching to 2 or 1/2, respectively.

1

1/2

2

FIGURE 19-44 Sensitivity control on an ECG.

♦ *Sensitivity switch:* Controls amplification (see figure 19-44). It is usually set at position *1*. In position 1, the standard is ten small blocks or two large blocks high. Other positions are as follows:

(1) Position 2: Increases the size of the complex, making it twice as large. The standard will then be twenty small blocks or four large blocks high. Used when the PQRST pattern is too small to be easily seen.

(2) Position 1/2: Decreases the size of the complex to one-half its normal size. The standard will then be five small blocks or one large block high. Used when the PQRST pattern is too large.

C Many patients are frightened or apprehensive about having an ECG taken. It is important to explain this procedure to the patient. Stress that it is not a painful or uncomfortable test. Position the patient comfortably with all body parts supported. Encourage the patient to relax and to avoid moving while the ECG is being taken. Muscle movement can cause electrical interference and will be displayed on the ECG recording. Nervous tension can also interfere with the recording.

After all the ECG leads have been recorded, a section of each recorded lead is mounted. Most newer multiple-channel machines produce complete mounts. These mounts are sometimes attached to firmer backings using self-stick tape. For ECGs from single-channel machines, many different types of mounts are used. Some contain slots for inserting the individual leads. Some contain tape or self-stick areas for placement of each of the leads. Others utilize clamps. The final mount should be neat, with each lead in the correct area on the mount. The mount should be labeled with the patient's name and address, doctor's name, date, and any other pertinent information.

STUDENT: *Go to the workbook and complete the assignment sheet for 19:6, Recording and Mounting an Electrocardiogram. Then return and continue with the procedure.*

PROCEDURE 19:6

Recording and Mounting an Electrocardiogram

NOTE: This procedure provides basic information about recording and mounting an ECG. It is important to read the specific operating instructions provided with each electrocardiograph machine.

Equipment and Supplies

Electrocardiograph machine, electrodes and straps, chest electrode and chest strap (if used), electrocardiograph cables and cords, examination gown, drape, gel or electro pads, gauze pads and/or tongue depressors, pen or pencil

Procedure

1. Assemble required equipment.
2. Wash hands.
3. **C** Introduce yourself. Identify the patient. Explain the procedure. Reassure the patient. Tell the patient that you will be recording the activity of the heart. Stress that the patient will not feel any discomfort from the procedure. Explain that the patient must lie perfectly still because muscle movement will interfere with the recording.
4. Ask the patient to remove clothing and put on an examination gown.
   NOTE: In some offices, the patient is asked to remove clothing from the waist up and to uncover the lower legs.
5. Position the patient. Patient should be lying on a firm bed or examination table. A small pillow can be placed under the head. Use the drape to cover the patient.
6. Position the machine in a convenient location. It may be easier to work from the left side because this is where most of the chest leads are positioned.
7. Connect the power cord to the machine. Do *not* let the power cord pass under the bed or examination table. Plug it in so that it is pointing away from the patient.
   ⚠ CAUTION: Check the three prongs and the cord before using the power cord. Never use a defective cord for any procedure.

NOTE: Positioning the power cord away from the patient helps reduce electrical interference.

8. Apply the four limb electrodes. The arm electrodes are placed on the fleshy outer areas of the upper arms. The leg electrodes are placed on fleshy parts of the lower legs. Avoid bony areas. Different types of electrodes may be used. Follow the directions provided with the electrode. General guidelines are as follows:
   a. Electrodes and straps (see figure 19-45A): Connect the electrode strap to the ears of the electrode. Put gel or an electrolyte pad on the electrode to increase conduction. Use the end of the electrode to gently scrape the skin at the area of application. Position the electrode and bring the strap around the arm or leg until it holds the electrode snugly against the skin. Avoid stretching the strap too tightly.
   b. Disposable electrodes (see figure 19-45B): Use a tongue depressor or gauze pad to vigorously rub the site to stimulate circulation. If the patient's skin is oily, wipe the electrode area with alcohol and allow it to air dry. Then, separate the electrode from the protective backing to uncover the sticky surface. Apply the electrode to the correct site using a smooth, even motion to make sure all parts of the electrode adhere to the skin. The disposable electrodes can only be used with ECG machines that have an alligator clip attached to the ends of the cable wires.
   NOTE: If the skin surface is hairy, it may be necessary to shave small areas at the application sites to allow for better attachment and conduction of the electrodes.
9. Apply the chest electrodes. Refer to figure 19-36 for the exact location for each electrode. Different types of electrodes may be used. Follow the directions provided with the electrode. General guidelines include:
   a. Single chest electrode with strap: Position the anchor plate of the chest strap under

the patient's left side. Adjust the strap so the curved-weight end lies against the right side of the chest. Use an electrolyte pad or gel to cover the chest electrode. Locate the correct site for placement for the V_1 position. Twist the electrode slightly while applying it to the correct site. Hold the electrode in place with the chest strap.

b. Suction bulb electrodes: These are small rubber bulbs each with a suction cup (see figure 19-45C). Electrolyte gel is squeezed into the suction cup. The rubber bulb is depressed to create a suction effect when the cup is placed on the proper position on the chest. If one electrode is used, it is moved from position to position as the ECG chest leads are run. If six electrodes are used, each is placed in position before the chest leads are run. The chest strap is not used with this type of electrode.

c. Disposable electrodes: Use a tongue depressor or gauze pad to vigorously rub the site to stimulate circulation. If the patient's skin is oily, wipe the electrode area with alcohol and allow it to air dry. Then, separate the electrode from its protective backing to uncover the sticky surface. Apply the electrode to the site using a smooth, even motion to make sure all parts of the electrode adhere to the skin. Position all six chest electrodes in the correct locations.

NOTE: If the skin surface is very hairy, it may be necessary to shave small areas at the application sites to allow for better attachment and conduction of the electrodes.

10. Connect the cable wires to the electrodes. The lead wires should follow body contour (see figure 19-46). If there is excess wire, coil it in a loop and fasten with tape or a band. Pay particular attention to the labels and color codes to connect the cable ends to the correct electrodes. Make sure all connections are tight and in the same direction.

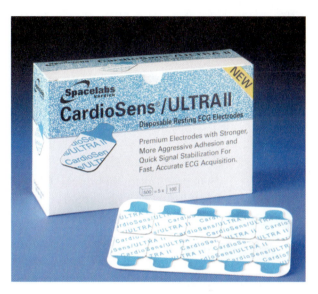

FIGURE 19-45B A disposable electrode has a sticky surface that allows the electrode to adhere to the skin. *(Courtesy of Spacelabs Medical, Inc.)*

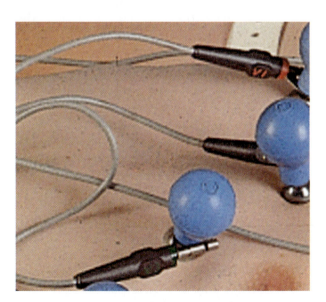

FIGURE 19-45C A suction bulb electrode is squeezed as it is applied, creating suction to hold the electrode in place.

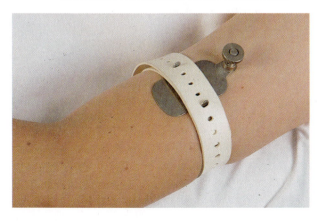

FIGURE 19-45A A limb electrode is positioned on the fleshy outer part of the arm or leg and held in place with a limb strap.

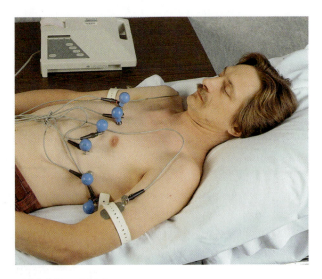

FIGURE 19-46 The lead cables should follow body contour when they are connected to the electrodes.

NOTE: Labels are: RA, for right arm; LA, for left arm; RL, for right leg; LL, for left leg; and C or V, for chest.

NOTE: Color codes are: white for RA, black for LA, green for RL, red for LL, and brown or multicolored for chest or V depending on the model of the ECG machine.

11. Turn on the main switch.

12. Check standardization of the machine. Put the lead selector in the ST'D position. Set the record switch to Run 25. Make sure sensitivity is set at 1. Center the stylus. Momentarily press the ST'D button. Check the standard. It should be ten small blocks or two large blocks high.

NOTE: If the standard is not correct, adjust it to the correct height by following manufacturer's instructions.

13. Check the color of the line. It should be clearly visible but not too dark. Adjust the stylus heat control, if necessary.

NOTE: Remember, the stylus heat melts the coating on the paper to form the line.

14. Record the leads. Set sensitivity at 1. Put the record switch at Run 25. Record several complexes. Insert a standard mark between the complexes, if required. In some agencies, a standard mark is placed at the beginning of the ECG. In other agencies, a standard mark is centered in each lead of the ECG. Follow agency policy.

NOTE: The standard mark should not be on any part of the complex. It should be on the base line between complexes, or after the T wave of one ECG cycle and before the P wave of the next ECG cycle. Repeat the process until a correct standard is present.

15. On a computerized electrocardiograph, set the control to Auto and run the twelve-lead ECG. When all twelve leads are complete, proceed to step 19 of this procedure. On a manual electrocardiograph, set the lead selector switch to each lead and allow the machine to record an adequate amount for each lead. While running the leads, make sure the following points are noted:

a. The recording should be centered on the paper.

b. Record a sufficient amount for each lead. Leads 1, 2, and 3 each usually require 8 to 10 inches. Each of the remaining leads usually require 5 to 6 inches.

c. An ST'D mark is in the center of each lead. Some agencies and physicians prefer an ST'D mark at the start of each lead. Others prefer ST'D marks on the first limb lead and the first chest lead. Follow agency or physician preference.

d. Make sure that the amplitude of the complexes is correct. If complexes are too small, set sensitivity to 2. If complexes are too large, set sensitivity to ½. If the sensitivity is changed, be sure to insert a standard in the lead. A standard that is five small blocks or one large block high indicates a sensitivity setting of ½. A standard that is twenty small blocks or four large blocks high indicates a sensitivity setting of 2.

e. Make sure complexes are not too close together. For severe tachycardias, it is often necessary to increase the speed to Run 50. Alert the physician by marking "Run 50" on the paper with pen or pencil.

f. Make sure that no electrical interference or artifact is present. Watch patient movement. Use a ground wire, as needed.

16. Run leads 1, 2, 3, aVR, aVL, aVF, and V$_1$ as instructed in steps 14 and 15. There is no need to turn off the machine between leads. Simply move the lead selector switch to the next position.

    NOTE: Some machines code each lead automatically; others require manual coding when leads are run; and newer machines record the name of the lead instead of the code.

17. Turn the record switch to Amp off. Place a chest electrode at the V$_2$ position. Twist the electrode slightly while applying. Set the selector switch at V$_2$. Turn the machine to Amp on. Allow the stylus to settle. Center the stylus. Switch to Run 25. Run lead V$_2$.

    NOTE: If six suction bulb or disposable electrodes are in place for the chest leads, the leads can be run without stopping the machine. Simply move the lead selector switch to the next chest lead position.

18. Repeat step 17 for the remaining 4 chest leads (V$_3$, V$_4$, V$_5$, and V$_6$).

19. When all twelve leads have been run, turn the lead selector to the standard position. Allow all of the recording to run out of the machine. Then turn the record switch to Off.

    NOTE: Make sure that all of the recording is out of the machine's window before stopping the movement of the machine.

20. Turn the power button off. Remove the electrodes from the patient. Use warm water to wash the patient's skin, and dry the skin thoroughly. Help the patient get off the examination table or bed.

21. Discard all disposable electrodes. Wash suction bulb electrodes thoroughly and disinfect, if necessary. Use cleanser to clean metal electrodes thoroughly. Rinse each electrode well. Dry and replace in the proper container.

    NOTE: The metal electrodes should be cleaned until they are bright and shiny, because dirty or corroded electrodes are poor electricity conductors.

22. Clean straps as needed. Coil all wires and replace in the proper box. Coil power cord and replace in the proper box.

    NOTE: If wires are bent, they will break.

23. Write the patient's name, the date, and the doctor's name on the ECG. If the ECG has been recorded with all twelve leads on one sheet of paper, it may be necessary to attach it to a self-stick mount. Follow manufacturer's instructions. This type of ECG is sometimes simply placed in the patient's chart without mounting. If the ECG is one long roll, cut into leads and attach to a mount. It is important to follow instructions provided with the mounts, and to make sure that the length for each lead is cut correctly. Look for the lead marking code to determine the lead represented. Use scissors or an ECG cutter to cut a section of the lead to the correct length. Attach the lead to the correct area of the mount. Make sure you match the lead markings on the ECG strip with those on the mount to place each section in its correct location (see figure 19-47). Most mounts have adhesive backs for easy attachment. When all twelve leads are mounted in their correct areas, recheck the ECG. Make sure it is neat and labeled correctly.

    NOTE: Some physicians prefer to read the strip before it is mounted in order to mark specific areas or arrhythmias to mount.

24. Wash hands.

25. Record all required information on the patient's chart or the agency form, for example, date, time, ECG recorded, and your signature and title.

Practice *Go to the workbook and use the evaluation sheet for 19:6, Recording and Mounting an Electrocardiogram, to practice this procedure. When you feel you have mastered this skill, sign the sheet and give it to your instructor for further action.*

✔ **Final Checkpoint** Using the criteria listed on the evaluation sheet, your instructor will grade your performance.

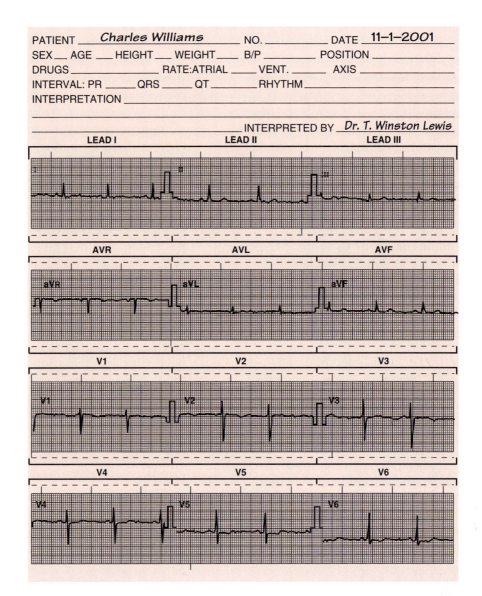

FIGURE 19-47 A mounted single-channel ECG. Check the lead markings on the ECG mount to be sure each strip is in its correct location.

19:7 INFORMATION Using the Physicians' Desk Reference (PDR)

The **Physicians' Desk Reference,** or PDR, is a book that provides essential information about drugs and medications currently in use. It is published yearly and has periodic supplements that provide up-to-date information on new products available. The *Physician's Desk Reference for Nonprescription Drugs* is another resource that can be used to obtain information about over-the-counter (OTC) medications that can be purchased without a prescription.

The PDR contains six main sections. Each section has a specific purpose and provides certain types of information. The main sections are as follows:

◆ *Manufacturers' index:* The initial white section. Major drug manufacturers in the United States are listed in alphabetical order.

Company names, addresses, telephone numbers, and departments to contact are listed. A partial list of each manufacturer's products is also included.

◆ **Brand and generic names:** The second main section, usually pink in color. It provides an alphabetical listing of products by *brand* name or *generic (chemical)* name. All drugs listed by generic name are followed by a list of brand names. The manufacturer's name is given in parentheses after each product. In addition, if drug information is found in a later section, the page number for the information is provided.

◆ **Product classification, or category, index:** The third main section, blue in color. It is a quick-reference section for drugs available for various conditions. For example, if a patient has an infection, a physician can readily find a long list of drugs that can be used to treat the condition by looking under the heading *antibiotics.* Drugs in each group are listed by brand names, with the manufacturers in parentheses. If additional information on the drug is provided in a later section, the page number is listed.

◆ **Product identification guide:** The next main section, it provides color, actual-size pictures of a variety of drugs. Drugs shown are listed alphabetically by manufacturers. Identification numbers may be given for some drugs, but these numbers may be changed by the manufacturer.

◆ **Product information:** The largest section in the book, white in color. It contains a detailed list of drugs and information on the chemical nature, indications for use, contraindications, warnings, and dosage and administration routes for each drug. Drugs are listed by manufacturers. All page number references in preceding sections refer to this section.

◆ **Diagnostic product information section:** Green in color, this section lists all diagnostic products, such as X-ray dyes, by manufacturers.

Several smaller information sections can be found in the back of the PDR. These include:

◆ *Poison control centers:* A list of certified poison control centers arranged alphabetically by state.

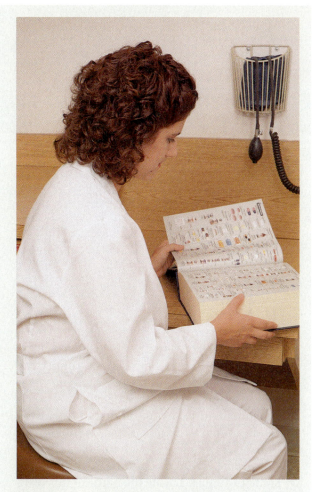

FIGURE 19-48 Check the PDR for information regarding actions, dosages, side effects, and other vital facts for any medication.

◆ *Discontinued products:* An alphabetical listing of products withdrawn from the market during the past year.

◆ *U.S. Food and Drug Administration telephone directory:* The numbers for key reporting programs and information services.

It is important to check the PDR for information regarding actions, dosages, side effects, and other vital facts for any medication (see figure 19-48). You must be familiar with this reference and be able to use it readily.

STUDENT: *Read Procedure 19:7, Using the* Physicians' Desk Reference *(PDR). Then go to the workbook and complete the three assignment sheets for 19:7, Using the* Physicians' Desk Reference *(PDR).*

PROCEDURE 19:7

Using the Physicians' Desk Reference (PDR)

Equipment and Supplies

Physicians' Desk Reference, pen or pencil

Procedure

1. Read Information section 19:7 on the PDR. Locate the various sections in the PDR while you are reading this section. Become familiar with each section and what it contains.

2. Think of the name of a major drug manufacturer. Turn to the manufacturers' index and find this name. Note the address of the company, the telephone number, and the department to contact.

3. Think of the common brand name of a drug with which you are familiar. Turn to the brand and generic name index (pink section) and locate this drug. If it refers to a page number, turn to that page in the product information section and read the information provided on the drug.

4. Think of the generic, or chemical, name of a drug. You may want to look in journals for some examples. Locate the name of this drug in the brand and generic name index. If a list of brand names appears, choose one or two of the names. Refer to the noted page number in the product information section to read about the properties of these drugs. Note how they are alike and how they might differ.

5. Think of any type of illness or disease. Find this disease in the blue product classification, or category, index. Note the list of drugs available to treat the condition. Look up product information on several of the drugs listed.

6. Glance through the product identification guide. Note the pictures of the many drugs listed. Pay particular attention to size, manufacturers' marks such as numbers or letters, and coloring. These signs might help you identify a drug for which you do not know the name. After finding a drug that looks interesting, look up the name in the brand and generic name index, where an alphabetical list is provided. This list provides a page number in the product information section, where more information about the drug can be obtained. Turn to the correct page and read the product information provided.

7. Go to the workbook and complete the first assignment sheet for 19:7, Using the *Physicians' Desk Reference* (PDR). Use Information Section 19:7 and the steps in this procedure to complete the assignment sheet. When you are done, give the assignment sheet to your instructor.

8. Your instructor will grade assignment sheet 1. Note any changes or corrections. Then complete assignment sheet 2. Give this sheet to your instructor for grading. Note any changes or corrections on assignment sheet 2 before completing assignment sheet 3.

 Final Checkpoint After reviewing your completed assignment sheets for 19:7, Using the *Physicians' Desk Reference* (PDR), your instructor will grade your performance.

19:8 INFORMATION Working with Math and Medications

A **medication** is a drug used to treat or prevent a disease or condition. The following discussion provides only basic information about the preparation and administration of medications. Even so, it should make you aware of the need for extreme care in handling all medications. *Only authorized persons can administer medications.*

Medications are available in various forms, usually liquids, solids, or semi-solids.

◆ *Liquids:*

(1) Aqueous suspension: dissolved in water

(2) Suspension: solid mixed with solution; usually must be shaken well

(3) Syrup: concentrated solution of sugar, water, and medication

(4) Tincture: medication dissolved in alcohol

◆ *Solids:*

(1) Capsule: gelatinlike shell with medication inside

(2) Pill: powdered medication mixed with a cohesive substance and molded into shape

(3) Tablet: compressed or molded preparation

(4) Troche or lozenge: large, flat disc that is dissolved in the mouth

(5) Enteric coated: medication with a special coating that does not dissolve until the substance reaches the small intestine

◆ *Semi-solids:*

(1) Ointment: medication in a fatty base

(2) Paste: ointment with an adhesive substance

(3) Cream: medication with water-soluble base

(4) Suppository: medication mixed with substances that melt at body temperature; cocoa butter is often the base material; usually inserted into the rectum, vagina, or urethra

Medications may be given in a variety of ways. Some of the routes of administration are:

◆ *Oral:* given by mouth; for liquid and solid forms.

◆ *Rectal:* given in the rectum; liquids and suppositories.

◆ *Injections:* given with a needle and syringe; often called "parenteral," which means any route other than the alimentary canal (digestive tract) (see figure 19-49).

(1) Subcutaneous (SC or SQ): injected into the layer of tissue just under the skin

(2) Intramuscular (IM): injected into a muscle

(3) Intravenous (IV): injected into a vein

(4) Intradermal: injected just under the top layer of skin; the skin tests for allergies and tuberculosis (TB) are examples

◆ *Topical or local:* applied directly to the top of the skin; ointments, sprays, liquids, and adhesive patches; transdermal adhesive patches applied to the skin can be used to provide a continuous dosage of medication for motion sickness, heart disease, hormonal imbalance, and nicotine withdrawal

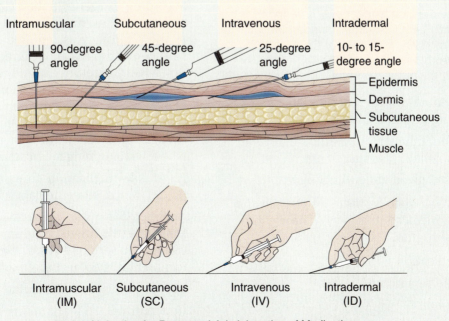

Angle of Injection for Parenteral Administration of Medications

FIGURE 19-49 Types of injections and the correct angles for administration of parenteral medications.

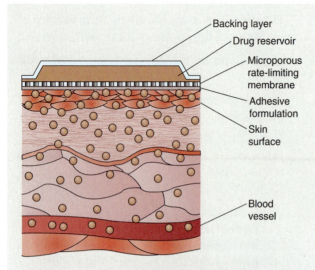

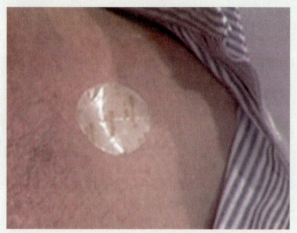

FIGURE 19-50A & B (A) The layers of a transdermal patch allow the medication to be absorbed into the bloodstream over a period of time, frequently 24 hours. (B) A transdermal patch is applied to the skin. *(Courtesy of CIBA Pharmaceutical Company)*

(for individuals who are trying to stop smoking), see figure 19-50A and B.

◆ ***Inhalation:*** inhaled, or breathed in, by way of sprays, inhalers, or special machines.

◆ ***Sublingual:*** given under the tongue.

There are six main points to watch each and every time a medication is given. These can be called the "six rights."

◆ Right medication

◆ Right dose, or amount

◆ Right patient

◆ Right time

◆ Right method or mode of administration

◆ Right documentation

Certain safety rules must be observed when giving medication.

◆ Read the order carefully. Note all six *rights*.

◆ Check for patient allergies before administering any medication.

◆ Check the label three times to be sure it is the correct medication. The label must be read: when the bottle is taken from the shelf, as the medication is poured, and when the bottle is replaced on the shelf.

◆ Prepare or administer medication only on the order of a physician.

◆ Never administer a medication you did not personally prepare.

◆ Know the action of the drug, the usual dosage, the route of administration, and the side effects.

◆ Store medications in a safe, cool, dry area. Make sure they are out of the reach of children.

◆ Check expiration dates on all medications. Medications must *never* be used beyond the expiration date and must be destroyed. It is best to flush them down the toilet to destroy them. Record all required information regarding the destruction of the medication according to agency policy. Controlled substances, such as narcotics, *must* be returned to the pharmacy as required by law. Make sure you complete all required documentation when you return expired controlled substances to the pharmacy. If a partial amount of a unit dose (single dose package) of a controlled substance is used because of the dosage ordered, witnesses must co-sign when the remaining medication is destroyed.

◆ *Never* use medication from an unmarked bottle. Make sure the label is clear. If in doubt, throw it out.

◆ Do *not* return medication to a bottle. This can lead to serious errors. Discard any medication that is *not* used.

◆ Report all mistakes immediately.

◆ Concentrate while handling any medication. Avoid distractions.

◆ Use paper and pencil to calculate dosages. Avoid "mental" math because it can cause errors.

Use the PDR or the literature that comes with each medication to learn the basic information about the medication. *Question dosages or uses that do not seem correct.*

STUDENT: *Go to the workbook and complete the assignment sheet for 19:8, Working with Math and Medications.*

19:8A INFORMATION Using Roman Numerals

Roman numerals are used for some drugs and solutions. In addition, they are sometimes used when ordering supplies. The following chart shows Arabic numerals and their Roman numeral equivalents.

Arabic	Roman	Arabic	Roman
1	I	10	X
2	II	20	XX
3	III	30	XXX
4	IV	40	XL
5	V	50	L
6	VI	100	C
7	VII	500	D
8	VIII	1,000	M
9	IX		

The key numerals are I, V, X, L, C, D, and M. By using these numerals, any number can be formed.

Usually, no more than three of any one Roman numeral is used to represent a number. For example, III represents the number 3. To represent the number 4, an I is placed before the V to form the Roman numeral IV. Thus, IV is used in place of IIII for the number 4.

If the numeral for a smaller number is used after the numeral for a larger number, all of the numbers are added together. See the following examples:

◆ VII = 5 + 1 + 1 = 7
◆ LXX = 50 + 10 + 10 = 70

If the numeral for a smaller number is used in front of the numeral for a larger number, the smaller number is subtracted from the larger number. See the following examples:

◆ IX = 1 before 10 = 10 − 1 = 9
◆ XC = 10 before 100 = 100 − 10 = 90
◆ CD = 100 before 500 = 500 − 100 = 400

STUDENT: *Go to the workbook and complete the assignment sheet for 19:8A, Using Roman Numerals.*

19:8B INFORMATION Converting Metric Measurements

The metric system is used in many health care fields. There are three basic units of measurement in the metric system:

◆ *gram:* measures mass or weight

◆ *liter:* measures volume or liquid
◆ *meter:* measures length or distance

The metric system is based on the power of ten. Units other than the basic units are created by either multiplying or dividing the basic units of measurement by the correct power of ten. The other units and the powers of ten that they represent are as follows:

◆ *kilo (k):* thousands, or 10^3, or 1,000 (multiply the base unit by 1,000)

- *hecto (h):* hundreds, or 10^2, or 100 (multiply the base unit by 100)

- *deka (dk):* tens, or 10^1, or 10 (multiply the base unit by 10)

- *base unit of measurement* (gram, liter, meter): ones, or 10^0

- *deci (d):* tenths, or 10^{-1}, or 0.1 (divide the base unit by 10)

- *centi (c):* hundredths, or 10^{-2}, or 0.01 (divide the base unit by 100)

- *milli (m):* thousandths, or 10^{-3}, or 0.001 (divide the base unit by 1,000)

As an example, if the gram (g) is used as the base unit of measurement, other units are formed as follows:

- *kilogram (kg):* 1 kg = 1,000 g

- *hectogram (hg):* 1 hg = 100 g

- *dekagram (dkg):* 1 dkg = 10 g

- *grams (g):* base unit of measurement, so 1 g = 1 g

- *decigram (dg):* 1 dg = 0.1 g

- *centigram (cg):* 1 cg = 0.01 g

- *milligram (mg):* 1 mg = 0.001 g

NOTE: The same order is used for meters and liters. The word *meter* or *liter* is simply used in place of the word *gram* in the previous example.

Metric measurements are easy to convert from unit to unit because the units represent multiples of ten. Placement of a number in relation to the decimal point represents the powers of ten, so metric measurements can be converted by moving the decimal point according to the power of ten required. Note the following examples:

- How many grams (g) are in 40 kilograms (kg)? First, list the measurements in order from largest to smallest:

kg   hg   dkg   g   dg   cg   mg

To go from kilograms (kg) to grams (g), movement is three places to the right. The decimal point should therefore be moved three places to the right.

Write 40 as 40.000 and then move the decimal point:

4 0.0 0 0 = 40000.0

The answer is that 40 kilograms (kg) equal 40,000 grams (g).

- How many dekaliters (dkL) are in 14,500 milliliters (mL)?

First, list the measurements in order from largest to smallest:

kL   bL   dkL   L   dL   cL   mL

To go from milliliters (mL) to dekaliters (dkL), movement is four places to the left. The decimal point should therefore be moved four places to the left.

Write 14,500 as 14,500.0 and then move the decimal point:

1 4 5 0 0.0 = 1.45000

The answer is that 14,500 milliliters (mL) equal 1.45 dekaliters (dkL).

As can be seen from the previous examples, the first step in converting metric measurements is to list the units in order from largest to smallest, using the prefixes along with the base unit of measurement. If movement is from left to right, the decimal point is moved the same number of places to the right. If movement is from right to left, the decimal point is moved the same number of places to the left. This principle can also be expressed as follows:

- To move from a larger unit of measurement in the metric system to a smaller unit of measurement, the decimal point is moved the correct number of places to the right. **NOTE:** Each unit change moves the decimal point one place to the right.

- To move from a smaller unit of measurement in the metric system to a larger unit of measurement, the decimal point is moved the correct number of places to the left. **NOTE:** Each unit change moves the decimal point one place to the left.

There is also interrelationship between units in the metric system. One important example is that a cube that measures 1 centimeter on all sides will hold 1 milliliter of water. So, 1 cubic centimeter holds 1 milliliter. Therefore, cubic centimeters and milliliters are sometimes interchanged. It is important to remember that 1 cubic centimeter (cc) is the same as 1 milliliter (mL), or that 1 cc is equal to 1 mL.

STUDENT: *Go to the workbook and complete the assignment sheet for 19:8B, Converting Metric Measurements.*

19:8C INFORMATION Converting Household (English) Measurements

The household, or English, system of measurement is the common system used in the United States, but the metric system is used in many health care fields. Therefore, it is sometimes necessary to convert from the household system to the metric system.

The household system of measurement uses many different units of measurement. The metric conversions for the most common household units of measurement are:

◆ *Units for measuring mass or weight:*
  1 ounce (oz) = 0.028 kilograms (kg), or
    28 grams (g)
  1 pound (lb) = 0.454 kilograms (kg), or
    454 grams (g)

◆ *Units for measuring length or distance:*
  1 inch (in) = 0.025 meters (m)
  1 foot (ft) = 0.31 meters (m)
  1 yard (yd) = 0.91 meters (m)
  1 mile = 1601.6 meters (m)

◆ *Units for measuring volume or liquid:*
  1 drop (gtt) = 0.0667 milliliters (mL) or
    cubic centimeters (cc)
  15 drops (gtts) = 1 milliliter (mL) or cubic
    centimeter (cc)
  1 teaspoon (tsp) = 5 milliliters (mL) or
    cubic centimeters (cc)
  1 tablespoon (tbsp) = 15 milliliters (mL) or
    cubic centimeters (cc)
  1 ounce (oz) = 30 milliliters (mL) or cubic
    centimeters (cc)

  1 pint (pt) = 500 milliliters (mL) or cubic
    centimeters (cc)
  1 quart (qt) = 1,000 milliliters (mL) or cubic
    centimeters (cc), or 1 liter (L)

NOTE: Remember, 1 milliliter (mL) equals 1 cubic centimeter (cc).

To convert household measurements to metric measurements, multiply the amount of the household measurement by the number of metric units equal to one of the household units.

Rule to remember: When converting from household (English) to metric, multiply.

Examples:

◆ How many cubic centimeters are in 3 ounces?
  There are 30 cc in 1 oz.
  Multiply $3 \times 30 = 90$
  There are 90 cubic centimeters in 3 ounces.

◆ How many cubic centimeters are in 5 teaspoons?
  There are 5 cc in 1 tsp.
  Multiply $5 \times 5 = 25$
  There are 25 cc in 5 tsp.

◆ How many cubic centimeters are in 3 pints?
  There are 500 cc in 1 pt.
  Multiply $500 \times 3 = 1,500$ cc
  There are 1,500 cc in 3 pt.

◆ How many kilograms are in 120 pounds?
  There are 0.454 kg in 1 lb.
  Multiply $0.454 \times 120 = 54.48$ kg
  There are 54.48 kg in 120 lb.

◆ How many meters are in 12 feet?
  There are 0.31 m in 1 ft.
  Multiply $0.31 \times 12 = 3.72$ m
  There are 3.72 m in 12 ft.

To convert metric measurements to household measurements, divide the amount of the metric measurement by the number of metric units equal to one of the household units.

Rule to remember: When converting from metric to household, divide.

Examples:

◆ How many ounces are in 300 cubic centimeters?
There are 30 cc in 1 oz.
$300 \div 30 = 10$
There are 10 oz in 300 cc.

◆ How many teaspoons are in 20 cubic centimeters?
There are 5 cc in 1 tsp.
$20 \div 5 = 4$ teaspoons
There are 4 tsp in 20 cc.

◆ How many pints are in 1,250 cubic centimeters?
There are 500 cc in 1 pt.

$1,250 \div 500 = 2.5$
There are 2.5 pt in 1,250 cc.

◆ How many ounces are there in 1.232 kilograms?
There are 0.028 kg in 1 oz.
$1.232 \div 0.028 = 44$
There are 44 oz in 1.232 kg.

◆ How many feet are in 62 meters?
There are 0.31 m in 1 ft.
$62 \div 0.31 = 200$
There are 200 ft in 62 m.

STUDENT: *Go to the workbook and complete the assignment sheet for 19:8C, Converting Household (English) Measurements.*

UNIT 19 SUMMARY

A basic knowledge of the main skills used by medical assistants is beneficial for many health care workers, because many of these skills are used in other health care areas.

Height and weight measurements are important in evaluating basic health status of patients. Thus, knowing how to correctly measure height and weight is important for every health care worker.

Proper positioning of patients for examinations and other procedures is another skill needed by the medical assistant. By following correct techniques, the medical assistant can properly prepare patients, as well as provide patients with comfort and privacy.

A knowledge of the basic instruments used and procedures performed during physical examinations, minor surgery, and suture removal is essential. This knowledge allows the medical assistant to work with the physician to provide quality health care to the patient in an efficient manner. Understanding the basic principles of electrocardiography allows the medical assistant to efficiently perform an electrocardiogram.

A knowledge of how to find information on medications and of correct mathematical calculation techniques is also an important responsibility of the medical assistant. By mastering these basic skills, the medical assistant can become an important part of the medical office team.

INTERNET SEARCHES

Use the suggested search engines in Unit 11:4 of this textbook to search the Internet for additional information on the following topics:

1. *Organizations:* find web sites for the American Medical Association, American Association of Medical Assistants, American Society of Podiatric Assistants, Registered Medical Assistants of the American Medical Technologists, and the American Optometric Association to research medical assisting careers and duties.

2. *Vision:* search for information on Snellen charts, Ishihara color plates, myopia, hyperopia, and ophthalmic and optometric treatments and care.

3. *Electrocardiogram:* research electrocardiographs, myocardial infarctions, and cardiac arrhythmias.

4. *Medications:* research the *Physician's Desk Reference,* other medication references, prescription medications, and sites of drug manufacturers.

5. *Suppliers:* research medical and pharmaceutical suppliers to evaluate the types of supplies and equipment available for medical offices. Compare and contrast different types of ECG machines. Locate on-line pharmacies to determine services available.

REVIEW QUESTIONS

1. Why are height and weight measurements important?

2. Identify at least six (6) different positions that can be used for examinations and/or treatments. For each position, list at least two (2) types of treatments or examinations that are performed when a patient is in the position.

3. Differentiate between a Snellen chart and an Ishihara plate by stating the type of eye defects evaluated with each method.

4. Interpret or define each of the following:
   a. OU
   b. OS
   c. OD
   d. myopia
   e. hyperopia

5. Name the areas of the body examined and the type of tests performed during each of the following examinations:
   a. ear, eye, nose, and throat:
   b. gynecological:
   c. general physical:

6. Explain at least five (5) standard precautions that must be observed while assisting with minor surgery and/or suture removal.

7. Name the twelve (12) leads for an electrocardiogram and the code that is used for each lead.

8. List the six (6) rights that must be observed while administering any medication.

9. Interpret or convert each of the following measurements:
   a. XXIV
   b. MMCMXCIII
   c. 300 cc =   oz
   d. 5 lb =   kg
   e. 1750 cc =   pt
   f. 6 tsp =   mL
   g. 5 ft. =   m

10. Use a *Physician's Desk Reference* to find the medication *Celebrex.* List the main action of this drug, suggested dosage, route of administration, and warnings/side effects.

UNIT 19

SUGGESTED REFERENCES

American Medical Association. *Physician's Office Letters.* Chicago, IL: American Medical Association, 2001.

Association of Surgical Technologists. *Surgical Care for the Surgical Technician: A Positive Care Approach.* Clifton Park, NY: Delmar Learning, 2001.

Bonewit-West, Kathy. *Clinical Procedures for Medical Assistants.* 5th ed. Philadelphia, PA: W.B. Saunders, 2000.

Brisendine, Karen. *Multiskilling: Electrocardiographs for the Health Care Provider.* Clifton Park, NY: Delmar Learning, 1998.

Brunner, Lillian Sholtis, and Dorris Smith Suddarth. *The Lippincott Manual of Nursing Practice.* 6th ed. Philadelphia, PA: J.B. Lippincott, 1996.

Durgin, June, and Zachary Hanan. *Pharmacy Practice for Technicians.* 2nd ed. Clifton Park, NY: Delmar Learning, 1999.

Flight, Myrtle R. *Law, Liability, and Ethics for Medical Office Personnel.* 3rd ed. Clifton Park, NY: Delmar Learning, 1998.

Fordney, Marilyn, and Joan Follis. *Administrative Medical Assisting.* 4th ed. Clifton Park, NY: Delmar Learning, 1998.

Keir, Lucille, Connie Krebs, and Barbara A. Wise. *Medical Assisting: Clinical and Administrative Competencies.* 5th ed. Clifton Park, NY: Delmar Learning, 2003.

Lewis, Kathryn, and Kathleen Handal. *Pocket Reference to Sensible Analyses of the ECG.* Clifton Park, NY: Delmar Learning, 2001.

Lewis, Kathryn, and Kathleen Handal. *Sensible ECG Analyses.* Clifton Park, NY: Delmar Learning, 2000.

Lewis, Kathryn, and Kathleen Handal. *Sensible 12-Lead Interpretation.* Clifton Park, NY: Delmar Learning, 2000.

Lindh, Wilburta, Marilyn Pooler, Carol Tamparo, and Joanne Cerrato. *Delmar's Comprehensive Medical Assisting.* 2nd ed. Clifton Park, NY: Delmar Learning, 2002.

Nobles, Sylvia. *Delmar's Drug Reference for Health Care Professionals.* Clifton Park, NY: Delmar Learning, 2002.

Physicians' Desk Reference. Oradell, NJ: Medical Economics Co., updated annually.

Rice, Jane. *Principles of Pharmacology for Medical Assisting.* 3rd ed. Clifton Park, NY: Delmar Learning, 1999.

Shea, Donna, and Adrienne Carter-Ward. *Telephone Triage Card Deck.* Clifton Park, NY: Delmar Learning, 1996.

Simmers, Louise. *Practical Problems in Mathematics for Health Occupations.* Clifton Park, NY: Delmar Learning, 1996.

Spratto, George, and Adrienne Woods. *PDR: Nurse's Drug Handbook.* Clifton Park, NY: Delmar Learning, Updated annually.

Woodrow, Ruth. *Essentials of Pharmacology for Health Occupations.* Clifton Park, NY: Delmar Learning, 2002.

Zakus, Sharron. *Clinical Skills for Medical Assistants.* 4th ed. St. Louis, MO: C.V. Mosby, 2001.

For additional information on medical assisting careers, contact the following association:

◆ American Association of Medical Assistants
20 North Wacker Drive, Suite 1575
Chicago, Illinois 60606
Internet address: *www.aama-ntl.org*

UNIT 20

Nurse Assistant Skills

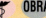

Unit Objectives

After completing this unit of study, you should be able to:

- Admit, transfer, or discharge a patient, demonstrating proper care of patient's belongings
- Position a patient in correct alignment and with no bony prominences exposed
- Move and turn a patient in bed, using correct body mechanics
- Perform the following transfer techniques (using correct body mechanics): dangling, wheelchair, chair, and stretcher
- Transfer a patient by way of a mechanical lift and observe all safety points
- Make closed, open, and occupied beds, using correct body mechanics
- Administer routine, denture, and special oral hygiene
- Administer hair care and nail care
- Administer a backrub, using the five major movements
- Shave a patient, using a safety or an electric razor, and observe all safety precautions
- Change a patient's bedclothes
- Administer a partial bed bath and a complete bed bath with perineal care
- Help a patient take a tub bath or shower, observing all safety points
- Measure and record intake and output
- Assist a patient with eating; feed a patient
- Administer a bedpan or urinal
- Provide catheter care
- Empty a urinary-drainage unit without contaminating the catheter or unit
- Provide ostomy care

 Observe Standard Precautions

 Safety—Proceed with Caution

 Math Skill

 Science Skill

 C Communications Skill

 Instructors Check—Call Instructor at This Point

 OBRA OBRA Requirement— Based on Federal Law

 Legal Responsibility

 Career Information

 Technology

◆ Collect urine and stool specimens
◆ Administer tap-water, soap-solution, disposable, and oil retention enemas
◆ Insert a rectal tube
◆ Apply restraints, observing all safety precautions
◆ Administer preoperative care as directed
◆ Shave an operative site, observing all safety precautions
◆ Prepare a postoperative unit with all equipment in correct position
◆ Apply surgical (elastic) hose
◆ Apply binders
◆ Safely administer oxygen with an oxygen mask, nasal cannula, or tent
◆ Give postmortem care
◆ Define, pronounce, and spell all the key terms

KEY TERMS

alignment
  (ah-line'-ment)
anesthesia
  (an-es-thee'-sha)
bed cradle
binders
catheter
closed bed
colostomy
complete bed bath (CBB)
contracture
  (kon-track'-tyour")
dangling
defecate
  (deaf'-eh-kate")
dehydration
  (dee"-high-dray'-shun)
edema
  (eh-dee'-mah)
enema

fanfolding
ileostomy
impaction
intake and output
mechanical lifts
micturate
  (mick'-chur-rate")
midstream specimen
mitered corners
  (my'-terd corn"-urz)
Montgomery straps
occult blood
  (ah-kult')
occupied bed
open bed
operative care
oral hygiene
ostomy
partial bed bath
personal hygiene

postmortem care
postoperative care
preoperative care
pressure (decubitus) ulcer
  (deh-ku'-beh-tuss uhl"-sir)
rectal tube
restraints
stoma
stool specimen
suppository
  (sup-poz'-ih-tor-ee)
surgical (elastic) hose
surgical shave
24-hour urine specimen
ureterostomy
urinary-drainage unit
urinate
urine specimen
void

CAREER HIGHLIGHT

Nurse assistants, also called nurse aides, nurse technicians, patient care technicians (PCT), and orderlies, work under the supervision of registered nurses or licensed practical nurses. They are important members of the health care team. Educational requirements vary with states, but many assistants obtain training through health occupations education programs.

Assistants who work in long-term care facilities or home health must complete a minimum of 75 hours in a mandatory, state-approved program and pass a written and/or competency examination to obtain certification or registration. Additional educational requirements include continuing education, periodic evaluation of performance, and retraining if the assistant is not employed for two or more years.

Geriatric aides or assistants provide care for patients in environments such as extended care facilities, nursing homes, retirement or assisted-living centers, and adult day care agencies.

Home health assistants or aides perform many of the duties of nurse assistants, but they provide care in the patient's home, usually for an extended period of time. Examples of patients requiring home care include patients who have just been discharged from a hospital or long-term care facility, patients with a disability, elderly patients who require assistance, and patients receiving hospice care. In addition to performing many of the personal care duties of the nurse assistant, home health assistants may also shop for food and prepare meals, maintain and clean the home environment, wash laundry, and accompany patients shopping or to medical appointments. Throughout this unit, special notes are provided to help a home health assistant adapt the procedure to home care.

The duties of nurse assistants vary depending on the facility in which they work and on the nursing practice laws of the state in which they work. *Every nurse assistant must know and follow the legal requirements of the state in which he or she is employed.* In addition to the knowledge and skills presented in this unit, nurse assistants must also learn and master skills such as:

- Presenting a professional appearance and attitude
- Obtaining knowledge regarding health care delivery systems, organizational structure, and teamwork
- Meeting all legal responsibilities
- Communicating effectively
- Being sensitive to and respecting cultural diversity
- Comprehending anatomy, physiology, and pathophysiology
- Learning medical terminology
- Observing all safety precautions
- Practicing all principles of infection control
- Taking and recording vital signs
- Administering first aid and cardiopulmonary resuscitation
- Promoting good nutrition and a healthy lifestyle to maintain health
- Measuring and recording height and weight
- Positioning patients for and assisting with examinations and treatments
- Administering basic physical therapy including range-of-motion exercises, ambulation with assistive devices, and warm or cold applications
- Performing basic laboratory tests such as monitoring glucose or testing urine with reagent strips
- Utilizing computer skills
- Recording information on patient records

20:1 INFORMATION
Admitting, Transferring, and Discharging Patients

OBRA As a health care worker in a hospital or long-term care facility, one of your responsibilities may be to admit, transfer, and discharge patients or residents. Although these procedures vary slightly in different facilities, basic principles apply in all facilities.

C Admission to a health care facility can cause anxiety and fear in many patients and their families. Even a transfer from one room or unit in a facility to another room or unit can cause anxiety, because the individual has to adjust to another new environment. It is essential for the health care worker to create a positive first impression. By being courteous, supportive, and kind, the health care worker can do much to alleviate fear and anxiety. Giving clear instructions on how to operate equipment and on the type of routine to expect, such as mealtimes, helps the patient or resident become familiar with the environment. It is also important not to rush while admitting, transferring, or discharging a patient. Allow the individual to ask questions and to express concerns. If you do not know the answers to specific questions, refer these questions to your immediate supervisor.

Most facilities have specific forms that are used during an admission, transfer, or discharge. A sample admission form is shown in figure 20-1. The forms list the procedures that must be performed and will vary slightly from facility to facility. It is important for the health care worker to become familiar with the information required on such forms. Much of the information on an admission form is used as a basis for the nursing care plan. Therefore, this information must be complete and accurate. If the patient is unable to answer the questions, a relative or the person responsible for the patient is usually able to provide the information. In some facilities, questions regarding medications and allergies are the responsibility of the nurse. Follow agency policy regarding these sections on the form.

When a patient is admitted to a facility, certain procedures are performed. These usually include vital signs, height and weight measurements, and collection of a routine urine specimen. Follow correct techniques while performing these procedures.

In order to protect a patient's possessions, a personal inventory list is made of clothing, valuables, and personal items. In a hospital, a family member frequently will take clothing home. Any clothing or personal items (such as radios) kept in the room should be noted on the list. The list should be checked and signed by both the health care worker and the patient (or the person responsible for the patient). At the time of transfer or discharge, the personal inventory list of clothing and personal items should be checked to make sure that the patient has all belongings.

If the family does not take valuables home, these should be put in a safe place. Most facilities require that they be kept in a safe. A description of the valuables is usually written on a valuables envelope, and the items are placed inside. If money is left in the patient's wallet, it should be counted, and the exact amount recorded on the envelope. Both the health care worker and the patient (or the person responsible for the patient) should check the items and sign the valuables envelope. The valuables are then put in the safe, and a receipt is given to the patient or put on the patient's chart. If a patient is transferred or discharged, the valuables are taken from the safe and checked by both the health care worker and the patient. Again, both individuals sign the envelope to indicate that valuables have been returned to the patient.

C Patients and family members should be oriented to the facility. Instructions on how to operate the call signal, bed controls, television remote control (if present), telephone, and other similar equipment should be provided. Visiting hours, location of lounges, smoking regulations, availability of services such as religious services and activities, mealtimes, and other rules or routines in the facility should be explained. Many facilities give patients and family members pamphlets or papers listing such information, but it is still important to explain the main information.

PATIENT PREFERS TO BE ADDRESSED AS:

_____

FROM: ❑ E.R.   ❑ E.C.F.   ❑ Home   ❑ M.D.'s Office

COMMUNICATES IN ENGLISH: ❑ Well   ❑ Minimal   ❑ Not At All   ❑ Other Language (Specify) _____

❑ INTERPRETER (Name Person)   ❑ None

_____

MODE OF TRANSPORTATION:

❑ Ambulatory   ❑ Other   Smoker: Y❑ N❑

❑ Wheelchair   _____

❑ Stretcher   _____

Home Telephone No. ( ) _____

Work Telephone No. ( ) _____

ORIENTATION TO ENVIRONMENT:

❑ Armband Checked   ❑ Call Light
❑ Bed Control   ❑ Phone
❑ TV Control   ❑ Side Rail Policy
❑ Bath Room   ❑ Visitation Policy
❑ Personal Property Policy ❑ Smoking Policy

PERSONAL BELONGINGS: (Check and Describe)

❑ Clothing   _____
❑ Jewelry   _____
❑ Money   _____
❑ Walker   _____
❑ Wheelchair _____
❑ Cane   _____
❑ Other   _____

DENTURES:

❑ Upper   ❑ Partial
❑ Lower   ❑ None

CONTACT LENSES:

❑ Hard   ❑ LT   ❑ RT
❑ Soft

GLASSES: ❑ Y ❑ N   **HEARING AID:** ❑ Y ❑ N

PROSTHESIS: ❑ Y ❑ N

(Describe) _____

DISPOSITION OF VALUABLES:

❑ Patient
❑ Home   Given To: _____

❑ Placed in   Relationship: _____
Safe _____
          (Claim No.)

IN CASE OF EMERGENCY NOTIFY:

Name: _____

Relationship: _____

Home Telephone No. ( ) _____

Work Telephone No. ( ) _____

VITAL SIGNS:

TEMP: _____ ❑ Oral ❑ Rectal ❑ Axillary

PULSE: _____ ❑ Radial ❑ Apical   Respiratory
                                                      Rate _____
          ❑ RT
B/P: _____ ❑ LT ❑ Standing ❑ Sitting ❑ Lying

HEIGHT: _____ WEIGHT: _____ ❑ Bedside
                                                      ❑ Standing

ALLERGIES:

Medications: ❑ None Known   Food: ❑ None Known
❑ Penicillin   ❑ Tape
❑ Sulfa   ❑ Other (List)   (Shellfish, Eggs, Milk, etc.)
❑ Iodine   _____
❑ Aspirin   _____
❑ Morphine   _____
❑ Demerol   _____

MEDICATIONS: (Prescription Non-Prescription)   Dose/Frequency   Last Dose (Date/Time)

1. _____   _____   _____
2. _____   _____   _____
3. _____   _____   _____
4. _____   _____   _____
5. _____   _____   _____
6. _____   _____   _____

DISPOSITION OF MEDICATIONS:

❑ None Brought to Hospital
❑ Sent Home _____
                    With _____
❑ To Pharmacy: (List)
_____
_____

ADMITTING DIAGNOSIS: _____

NURSE'S SIGNATURE: _____   RN/LVN   Date _____   Time _____

FIGURE 20-1 A sample admission form.

Transfers are done for a variety of reasons. A transfer is sometimes related to a change in the patient's condition. For example, a person may be transferred from or to an intensive care unit. Other times, a transfer is made at the patient's request, such as a request to be moved to a private room. Agency policy must be followed during any transfer. The reason for the transfer should be explained to the patient and family. This is usually the responsibility of the doctor or nurse. The new room or unit must be ready to receive the patient. Clothing, personal items, and certain equipment must be transferred with the patient. The health care worker should also find out how to transport the patient. Wheelchairs, stretchers, and even the patient's bed can be used for the transfer. An organized and efficient transfer helps prevent fear and anxiety in the patient.

A physician's order is usually required before a patient or resident can be discharged from a facility. If an individual plans to leave the facility without permission, report this immediately to your supervisor. Facilities have special policies that must be followed when a person leaves against medical advice (AMA). When an order for discharge has been received, the health care worker must check and pack the patient's belongings. A careful check of the unit, including any drawers, closets, and storage areas helps ensure that all items are found. Most facilities require that a staff member accompany the individual to a car. Some facilities allow patients to walk, but many prefer to transport patients by wheelchair. If a patient is to be transferred by ambulance, the ambulance attendants will bring a stretcher to the room. In this case, it is important for the health care worker to have the patient's belongings ready for the transport. Again, most agencies have forms or checklists that are used during discharge to ensure that all procedures are followed.

STUDENT: *Go to the workbook and complete the assignment sheet for 20:1, Admitting, Transferring, and Discharging Patients. Then return and continue with the procedures.*

PROCEDURE 20:1A   OBRA

Admitting the Patient

Equipment and Supplies

Admission form and/or personal inventory list, valuables envelope, admission kit (if used), thermometer, stethoscope, sphygmomanometer, watch with second hand, scale, urine-specimen container, patient gown (if needed), paper, pen or pencil

Procedure

1. Obtain orders from your immediate supervisor or check orders to obtain permission for the procedure.
2. Wash hands.
3. Assemble equipment. Prepare the room for the admission. Fanfold the top bed linen down to open the bed. If an admission kit is used, unpack the kit and place the items in the bedside stand or table. The admission kit usually includes a water pitcher, cup, soap dish, bar of soap, lotion, and mouthwash (see figure 20-2). Place a bedpan and/or urinal, bath basin, and emesis basin in the bedside stand. Check the room to be sure all equipment and supplies are in their proper places.
4. You may be required to go to the admissions office to get the new patient or resident, or the patient may be brought to the room by other personnel.
5. **C** Greet and identify the patient. Ask the patient if he or she prefers to be called by a particular name. Introduce yourself to the patient and to any family members present. If another patient is in the room, introduce the new patient.

   NOTE: Be friendly and courteous at all times. Do not rush or hurry the patient.

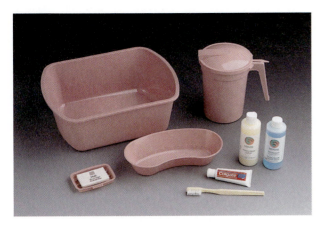

FIGURE 20-2 A sample admission kit. *(Courtesy of Medline Industries, Mundelein, IL)*

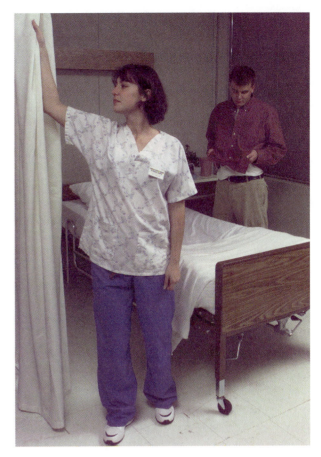

FIGURE 20-3 Close the door and screen the unit to provide privacy while the patient undresses.

6. Ask the family or visitors to wait in the lounge or lobby while you complete the admission process, if this is facility policy.
   NOTE: If a patient is not able to answer questions, a family member or other person responsible for the patient can remain in the room to complete the admission process.

7. Close the door and screen the unit (see figure 20-3). Ask the patient to change into a gown or pajamas. Assist the patient as necessary.
   NOTE: In long-term care facilities, residents usually wear street clothes during the day. In this case, gowns or pajamas are not used.

8. Position the patient comfortably in the bed or in a chair.

9. **C** Complete the admission form. Ask questions slowly and clearly. Provide time for the patient to answer the questions.
   NOTE: Observe the patient carefully during the admission process. Record all observations noted. If the patient expresses certain concerns, be sure to record and report these concerns.

10. Measure and record vital signs. Follow the procedures outlined in Unit 14.

11. Weigh and measure the patient. Follow Procedure 19:1A. Record the information on the admission form.

12. Complete a personal inventory list. Be sure to list all personal items that will be kept in the patient's unit such as clothing, shoes, clocks, radios, religious items, and books. Make sure the patient or a responsible individual checks and signs the list. Assist the patient as necessary in hanging up clothing or putting away personal items.

13. Complete a valuables list. If a family member takes the valuables home, be sure to obtain a signature on the proper form. If the valuables are to be placed in a safe, fill out the form and obtain the patient's and/or a relative's signature. Follow agency policy for placing the valuables in the safe.

14. Obtain a routine urine specimen if ordered. Follow Procedure 20:10A.

15. Orient the patient to the facility by demonstrating or explaining the following:
   a. Call signal or light
   b. Bed controls
   c. Television remote control and/or television rental policy
   d. Telephone
   e. Bathroom facilities and special call signal in bathroom
   f. Visiting hours
   g. Mealtimes and menu selections
   h. Activities or services available

16. Fill the water pitcher, if the patient is allowed to have liquids.

17. Observe all checkpoints before leaving the patient. Make sure the patient is comfortable and in good body alignment; the siderails are up, if indicated; the bed is at its lowest level; the call signal and supplies are in easy reach; and the area is neat and clean.

18. Clean and replace all equipment.

19. Wash hands.

20. When the admission process is complete, allow family members to return to the unit. Answer any questions they may have regarding facility policies. If you do not know answers to their questions, obtain the correct answers from your immediate supervisor.

21. **C** Record all required information on the patient's chart or the agency form, for example, date; time; admission form complete, valuables placed in safe, patient tolerated procedure well; and your signature and title. Report any abnormal observations to your immediate supervisor.

Practice *Go to the workbook and use the evaluation sheet for 20:1A, Admitting the Patient, to practice this procedure. When you feel you have mastered this skill, sign the sheet and give it to your instructor for further action.*

✔ Final Checkpoint Using the criteria listed on the evaluation sheet, your instructor will grade your performance.

PROCEDURE 20:1B `OBRA`

Transferring the Patient

Equipment and Supplies

Transfer checklist (if used), personal inventory list, valuables list, cart (if needed), wheelchair or stretcher, paper, pen or pencil

Procedure

1. Obtain permission from your immediate supervisor or check orders to obtain permission for the procedure. Find out the new unit or room number. Check to be sure that the unit is ready or ask your immediate supervisor to check. Check the method of transport to be used and obtain a wheelchair or stretcher, or use the patient's bed.

2. Assemble equipment.

3. Knock on the door and pause before entering. Introduce yourself. Identify the patient. Explain the procedure to the patient.
   NOTE: Reassure the patient as necessary. Patients are often apprehensive.

4. Wash hands.

5. Collect the patient's clothing and personal items. Check all items against the admission personal inventory list to be sure all items are present. Put the items in a bag or place them on a cart for transport. If the patient wears dentures and/or a hearing aid, make sure he or she has these items.

6. Put any bedside equipment to be transferred on a cart. This may include items such as the water pitcher, cup, soap dish, soap, emesis basin, bedpan, and bath basin. Check whether special equipment is to be transferred. Follow agency policy regarding transfer of equipment.

7. If valuables are to be transferred, they must be checked and signed for by both the patient and the health care worker. The valuables are usually kept in the facility safe, and the room or unit number of the patient is changed on the valuables bag.

8. Assist the patient into a wheelchair or stretcher. Follow the appropriate procedure as outlined in Information Section 20:2.

9. Transport the patient and the cart of supplies to the new unit or room (see figure 20-4). If help is not available, the patient may be taken to the new room first and the belongings taken afterward.
   ⚠ CAUTION: Observe all safety precautions while transporting the patient.

10. Introduce the patient to the new staff members. Assist the staff members in getting the

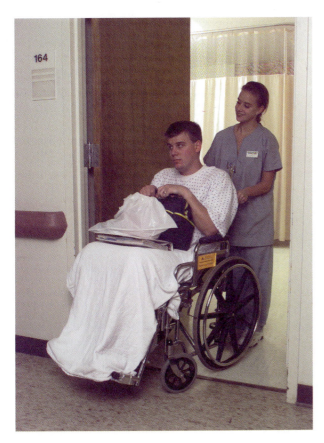

FIGURE 20-4 The patient is usually transferred in a wheelchair to the new unit.

patient positioned comfortably in bed or in a chair. If another patient is in the room, introduce the patient. Orient the patient to the new room or unit by explaining or demonstrating the use of the equipment and supplies.

NOTE: The staff members of the new unit may orient the patient.

11. Check the patient's belongings with the new staff member. Use the personal inventory and/or valuables checklist as needed. Be sure to obtain correct signatures according to agency policy.

12. Help put away the patient's clothing and personal items.

13. Observe all checkpoints before leaving the patient. Make sure the patient is comfortable and in good body alignment, the siderails are up (if indicated), the bed is at its lowest level, the call signal and supplies are in easy reach, and the area is neat and clean.

14. Replace all equipment.

15. Wash hands.

16. **C** Complete the transfer checklist. Record all required information on the patient's chart or the agency form, for example, date; time; Transferred to room 239-A by wheelchair, patient tolerated procedure well, transfer checklist complete; and your signature and title.

17. Return to the patient's previous room. Strip the bed and remove any equipment that was not transferred. Follow agency policy for cleaning the room.

    NOTE: This may be the responsibility of the housekeeping department. If so, notify housekeeping that the patient has been transferred.

18. Wash hands.

19. **C** Report to your immediate supervisor that the transfer has been completed.

Practice *Go to the workbook and use the evaluation sheet for 20:1B, Transferring the Patient, to practice this procedure. When you feel you have mastered this skill, sign the sheet and give it to your instructor for further action.*

 Final Checkpoint Using the criteria listed on the evaluation sheet, your instructor will grade your performance.

PROCEDURE 20:1C   OBRA

Discharging the Patient

Equipment and Supplies

Discharge checklist (if used), personal inventory list, valuables list, wheelchair (if needed), cart (if needed), paper, pen or pencil

Procedure

1. Obtain orders from your immediate supervisor or check orders to obtain permission for the procedure. Check with the patient to

determine when relatives or other individuals will be there to discharge patient.

NOTE: If the patient is to be discharged to another facility by ambulance, determine the time the ambulance will arrive.

2. Assemble equipment.

3. **C** Knock on the door and pause before entering. Introduce yourself. Identify the patient. Explain the procedure.

4. Wash hands.

5. Close the door and screen the unit. Help the patient dress, if assistance is needed.

6. Assemble all of the patient's personal belongings. If the patient wears dentures and/or a hearing aid, make sure he or she has these items. Check drawers, closets, the bedside stand or table, and storage areas. Check all items against the personal inventory list to be sure everything is present. Obtain the patient's signature according to agency policy.

7. Assemble any equipment that is to be given to the patient. Examples include the supplies in the admission kit, such as the pitcher and cup.

8. **C** Check to make sure that the patient has received final instructions from the nurse and/or physician. These may include discharge instructions and prescriptions.

9. Obtain the patient's valuables, if they are in a safe. Check the valuables with the patient. Obtain the correct signature to indicate that the valuables were returned to the patient.

NOTE: In some agencies, the patient or a responsible person obtains the valuables directly from the safe. In such a case, tell the patient how to obtain the valuables.

10. Complete a discharge checklist, if one is used, to be sure all procedures are complete.

11. Place all of the patient's belongings on a cart, if needed. Packed items sometimes are taken to the car by a relative.

12. Assist the patient into a wheelchair. Follow Procedure 20:2F.

NOTE: Most facilities require the use of wheelchairs to transport patients. Some facilities allow patients to walk, but health care workers must accompany patients. Follow agency policy.

13. In some facilities, the patient must go to the business office if financial arrangements are not complete. Check with your immediate supervisor or check the discharge slip to determine whether the patient must stop at the business office. If this is necessary, transport the patient to the business office.

14. Transport the patient to the exit area. Help the patient into the car.

NOTE: If a cart is used to transfer the patient's belongings, another staff member should take the cart to the car.

! CAUTION: Observe all safety factors while transporting the patient.

15. Help put the patient's belongings in the car.

16. Say good-bye to the patient.

17. Return to the unit. Strip the bed and remove any equipment in the unit. Follow agency policy for cleaning the unit. Replace equipment.

NOTE: In some facilities, this is the responsibility of the housekeeping department. If so, notify housekeeping that the patient has been discharged.

18. Wash hands.

19. **C** Record all required information on the patient's chart or the agency form, for example, date; time; patient discharged, taken to husband's car by wheelchair, tolerated procedure well; and your signature and title. Report to your immediate supervisor that the discharge has been completed.

Practice *Go to the workbook and use the evaluation sheet for 20:1C, Discharging the Patient, to practice this procedure. When you feel you have mastered this skill, sign the sheet and give it to your instructor for further action.*

 Final Checkpoint Using the criteria listed on the evaluation sheet, your instructor will grade your performance.

20:2

INFORMATION
Positioning, Turning, Moving, and Transferring Patients

OBRA As a health care worker, you may be responsible for positioning, turning, moving, and transferring many patients. If these procedures are done correctly, you will provide the patient with optimum comfort and care. In addition, you will prevent injury to yourself and the patient.

It is essential to remember that improper moving, turning, or transferring of a patient can result in serious injuries to the patient. Some patients cannot be moved safely without special assistance or mechanical devices. If a patient has restrictions for moving or transferring, the restrictions should be posted outside the door. If you are not sure if a patient can be moved or transferred safely, *always* ask your supervisor before attempting any procedure. Remember, you are *legally* responsible for the safety and well being of the patient.

Correct body mechanics are required for all procedures discussed here. Review and practice all of the rules of correct body mechanics as outlined in Information Section 12:1. If you are unable to move or turn a patient by yourself, always get help.

Alignment

Patient care must be directed toward maintaining normal body alignment. **Alignment** is defined as "positioning body parts in relation to each other in order to maintain correct body posture." Benefits of proper alignment include:

◆ *Prevent fatigue:* Correct alignment helps the patient feel more comfortable and prevents fatigue,

◆ *Prevent pressure ulcers:* A **pressure ulcer,** also called a **decubitus ulcer,** *pressure sore,* or *bedsore,* is caused by prolonged pressure on an area of the body that interferes with circulation. Pressure ulcers are common in areas where bones are close to the skin, such as the tailbone, or coccygeal area; hips; knees; ankles; heels; and elbows. The tissue breakdown of a pressure ulcer occurs in four stages. In stage I (see figure 20-5A), a red or blue-gray discoloration appears on the intact skin. The discoloration does not disappear after pressure has been relieved. In stage II (see figure 20-5B), abrasions, bruises, and/or open sores develop as a result of tissue damage to the top layers of the skin (epidermis and dermis). In stage III (see figure 20-5C), a deep open crater forms when all layers of the skin are destroyed. Fat and muscle tissues are exposed. In stage IV (see figure 20-5D), damage extends into muscle, tendon, and bone tissue. It is easier to prevent pressure ulcers than it is to treat them. In addition, if pressure ulcers are detected in early stages, immediate treatment can help prevent further damage. Effective ways to prevent pressure ulcers include providing good skin care; prompt cleaning of urine and feces from the skin; massaging in a circular motion around a reddened area; frequent turning; positioning to avoid pressure on irritated areas; keeping linen clean, dry, and free from wrinkles; applying protectors (of sheepskin, lamb's wool, or foam) to bony prominences such as heels and elbows; and using egg crate, alternating-pressure mattresses (see figure 20-6A), or water- or gel-filled mattresses (see figure 20-6B). Careful observation of the skin during bathing or turning is essential. If a pale, reddened, or blue-gray area is noted, this should be reported immediately.

◆ *Prevent contractures:* A **contracture** (see figure 20-7) is a tightening or shortening of a muscle usually caused by lack of movement or usage of the muscle. Foot drop is a common contracture. It can be prevented in part by keeping the foot at a right angle to the leg

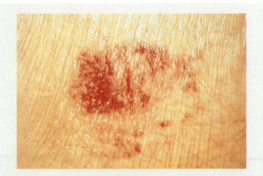

FIGURE 20-5A A Stage I pressure ulcer has a red or blue-gray discoloration that does not disappear after pressure has been relieved. *(Permission to reproduce this copyrighted material has been granted by the owner, Hollister Incorporated)*

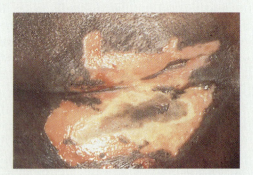

FIGURE 20-5B A Stage II pressure ulcer is characterized by abrasions, bruises, and/or open sores as a result of tissue damage to the top layers of skin. *(Permission to reproduce this copyrighted material has been granted by the owner, Hollister Incorporated)*

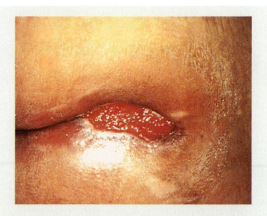

FIGURE 20-5C In a Stage III pressure ulcer, a deep open crater forms when all layers of the skin are destroyed. *(Permission to reproduce this copyrighted material has been granted by the owner, Hollister Incorporated)*

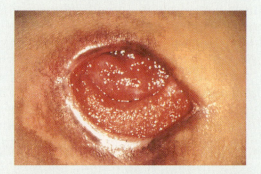

FIGURE 20-5D In a Stage IV pressure ulcer, damage extends into muscle, tendon, and bone tissue. *(Permission to reproduce this copyrighted material has been granted by the owner, Hollister Incorporated)*

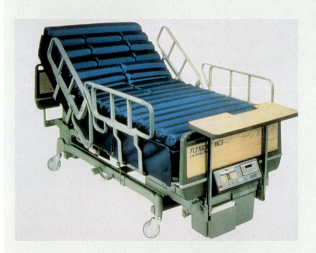

FIGURE 20-6A An alternating air pressure mattress constantly changes the pressure points against a patient's skin. *(Courtesy of Hill-Rom, Charleston, SC)*

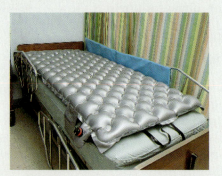

FIGURE 20-6B A water-filled mattress helps relieve pressure on the patient's skin.

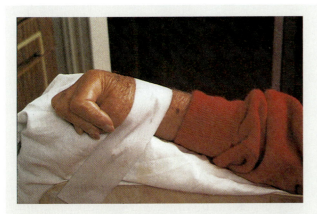

FIGURE 20-7 A contracture is a tightening of a muscle caused by lack of movement or usage of the muscle.

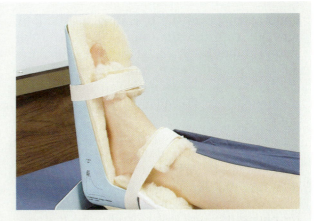

FIGURE 20-8 Foot supports can be used to hold the feet at right angles and prevent foot drop, a common contracture. *(Courtesy of J.T. Posey Company)*

(see figure 20-8). Footboards, foot supports, and high-top tennis shoes can be used to keep the foot in this position. Range of motion (ROM) exercises, discussed in Information section 21:1, also help prevent contractures from developing.

Turning

The patient confined to bed must be turned frequently. The patient's position should be changed at least every 2 hours, if permitted by the physician. Some agencies post a turning position schedule by the patient's bed. For example: 6AM: Right side, 8AM: Back, 10AM: Left side, and 12NOON: Abdomen. Frequent turning provides exercise for the muscles. It also stimulates circulation, helps prevent pressure ulcers and contractures, and provides comfort to the patient. Correct turning procedures must be followed to prevent injury to both the patient and the health care worker.

Dangling

If a patient has been confined to bed for a period of time, the patient is frequently placed in a dangling position prior to being transferred from the bed. **Dangling** means sitting with the legs hanging down over the side of the bed. This allows the patient some time to adjust to the sitting position. The pulse rate is checked at least three times during this procedure: before, during, and after the dangling period. It is taken just before the patient is moved to the dangling position; this pulse rate serves as a control, or resting, rate. The pulse rate is checked again immediately after positioning the patient in the dangling position. The third check occurs after the patient is returned to a lying-down (supine) position in the bed. By noting changes in the pulse rate, the health care worker can determine how well the patient tolerates the procedure. In addition to taking the pulse, observe the patient's respiratory rate, balance (the patient may complain of vertigo or dizziness), amount of perspiration, color, and other similar characteristics. If the pulse rate shows an abnormal increase, respirations become labored, color becomes pale, increased perspiration is noted, or the patient gets dizzy or very weak, the patient should be returned immediately to the supine, resting position.

Transfers

Patients are frequently transferred to wheelchairs, chairs, or stretchers. Again, correct procedures must be followed to prevent injury to both the patient and the worker. Many different models of wheelchairs and stretchers are available. It is important to read the manufacturer's instructions regarding the operation of any given piece of equipment. If no instructions are available, ask your immediate supervisor to demonstrate the correct operation of a particular wheelchair or stretcher.

Mechanical lifts are frequently used to transfer weak or paralyzed patients. Again, it is important to read the operating instructions provided with the lift. Straps, clasps, and the sling should be checked carefully for any defects. Smooth, even movements must be used while operating the lift. Patients are often frightened of the lift and must be reassured that it is safe.

In home care situations, it is important to move unnecessary furniture out of the way during transfers. If the bed does not raise or lower, it is essential for the health care worker to observe correct body mechanics and to bend at the hips and knees instead of the waist. It is possible to rent hospital beds, wheelchairs, mechanical lifts, and other similar items for home care.

⚖️ Before a patient is moved or transferred, the health care worker must obtain approval or orders from his or her immediate supervisor. *Never* move or transfer a patient without correct authorization.

❗ During any move or transfer, it is important to watch the patient closely. Note changes in pulse rate, respirations, and color. Observe for signs of weakness, dizziness, increased perspiration, or discomfort. If you note any abnormal changes, return the patient to a safe and comfortable position and check with your immediate supervisor. The supervisor will determine whether the move or transfer should be attempted.

STUDENT: *Go to the workbook and complete the assignment sheet for 20:2, Positioning, Turning, Moving, and Transferring Patients. Then return and continue with the procedures.*

PROCEDURE 20:2A   OBRA

Aligning the Patient

Equipment and Supplies

Three pillows, two to three bath blankets, two to three large towels, two to three washcloths or small towels, protectors for bony prominences, footboard, pen or pencil

Procedure

1. Obtain orders from your immediate supervisor or check orders to obtain permission for the procedure.
2. Assemble equipment.
3. Ⓒ Knock on the door and pause before entering. Introduce yourself. Identify the patient. Explain the procedure to the patient.
4. Provide privacy. Close the door and screen the unit.
5. Wash hands.
6. Lock the wheels on the bed. Elevate the bed to a comfortable height. Lower the bedrail or siderail on the side of the bed where you are working.

   ❗ **CAUTION:** If the bed does not raise to a working height, use correct body mechanics and bend from the hips and knees, not the waist, to get close to the patient.

7. Align the patient who is lying on the back (in a supine position) as follows (see figure 20-9):
   a. Position the head in a straight line with the spine.
   b. Place a pillow under the head and neck to provide support.
   c. A pillow or rolled blanket may be placed under the lower legs, from the knees to 2 inches above the heels to provide support and keep the heels off the bed.
   d. Protector pads may be placed on the heels or elbows (see figure 20-10).
   e. Toes should point upward. You may place a footboard, pillow, or rolled blanket against the soles of the feet to achieve this. High-top tennis shoes can also be placed on the feet to keep them at this angle.
   NOTE: Check the patient for comfort, safety, and support before leaving. Make sure no bony prominences are exposed and all body parts are supported.

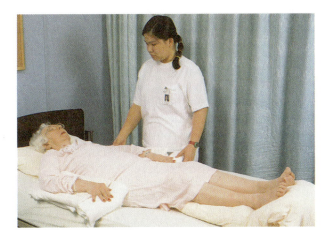

FIGURE 20-9 Correct alignment for a patient positioned on the back in the horizontal recumbent or supine position.

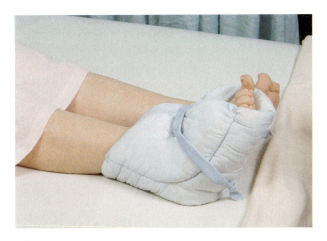

FIGURE 20-10 Foot protectors can help prevent pressure ulcers on the heels.

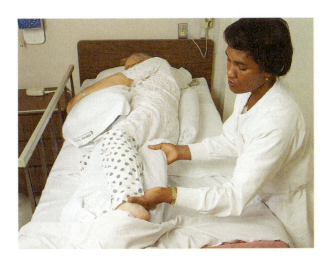

FIGURE 20-11 Correct alignment for a patient positioned on the side.

8. Align the patient who is lying on the side (see figure 20-11) as follows:
   a. Place a small pillow under the head and neck for support.
   b. Flex the lower arm at the elbow. It can be placed in line with the face.
   c. Support the upper arm, flexed at the elbow, on a pillow or rolled blanket.
   d. Flex both knees slightly. Place a firm pillow or rolled blanket between the legs. The pillow should extend from the upper leg to the ankle.
   e. Use a footboard, pillow, rolled blanket, or high-top tennis shoes to keep the feet at right angles (90°) to the legs.
   f. Rolled washcloths or foam rubber balls may be placed in paralyzed hands to prevent contractures.
   g. Use pillows to support the back and/or abdomen.
   h. Protector pads may be placed on the ankles, heels, and elbows.

   ❗ CAUTION: Make sure that the patient's body is not twisted and that any one body part is not applying direct pressure on any other body part.

   NOTE: Check all aspects of the patient's position prior to leaving.

9. Align the patient who is lying on the abdomen (in the prone position) as follows:
   a. Place the head in direct line with the spine.
   b. Turn the head to one side. It may be supported with a small pillow. Placing the pillow at an angle will keep it away from the patient's face.
   c. A small pillow may be placed under the waist for support.
   d. Place a firm pillow under the lower legs. This will slightly flex the knees.
   e. The feet can be extended over the end of the mattress so that they will remain at right angles to the legs. They can also be supported in this position by pillows or rolled blankets (see figure 20-12).
   f. Place the arms in line on either side of the head. Use pads to protect the elbows. Flex the elbows slightly for comfort.

   NOTE: Check all aspects of position, comfort, and safety before leaving the patient.

10. Observe all checkpoints prior to leaving the patient. Make sure the siderails are elevated (if indicated), the bed is at its lowest level,

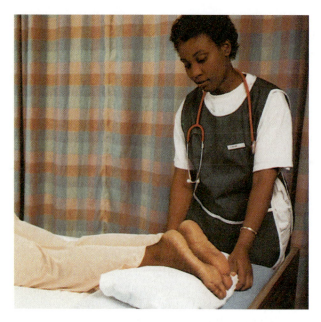

FIGURE 20-12 A large pillow can be used to support the feet when the patient is lying in the prone position.

the call signal and supplies are in easy reach, the patient is comfortable and in good body alignment, and the area is neat and clean.

11. Properly replace all equipment not being used.
12. Wash hands.
13. **C** Report that the procedure is complete and/or record all required information on the patient's chart or the agency form, for example, date; time; positioned on left side in correct alignment, patient appears to be resting comfortably; and your signature and title. Note any unusual observations.

Practice *Go to the workbook and use the evaluation sheet for 20:2A, Aligning the Patient, to practice this procedure. When you feel you have mastered this skill, sign the sheet and give it to your instructor for further action.*

✔ **Final Checkpoint** Using the criteria listed on the evaluation sheet, your instructor will grade your performance.

PROCEDURE 20:2B OBRA
Moving the Patient Up in Bed

Equipment and Supplies

Pen or pencil

Procedure

1. Obtain permission from your immediate supervisor or check orders to make sure that the patient can be moved.
2. **C** Knock on the door and pause before entering. Introduce yourself. Identify the patient. Explain the procedure to the patient.
3. Provide privacy. Close the door and screen the unit.
4. Wash hands.
5. Lock the bed (usually by way of wheel locks) to prevent movement of the bed. Elevate the bed to a comfortable height. Lower the siderail nearest to you.

NOTE: Locks and siderails on beds vary. If you do not know how to lock a bed or operate siderails, check with your immediate supervisor.

6. Lower the head of the bed. Remove all pillows. One pillow can be placed against the headboard of the bed to prevent injury to the patient's head while moving the patient up in bed.

NOTE: Observe the patient for respiratory distress.

⚠ **CAUTION:** If any breathing difficulty is noted, immediately raise the head of the bed. Check with your supervisor before proceeding.

7. Ask the patient to flex the knees and brace both feet firmly on the bed.

NOTE: If necessary, help by flexing the patient's knees and bracing the patient's feet on the bed.

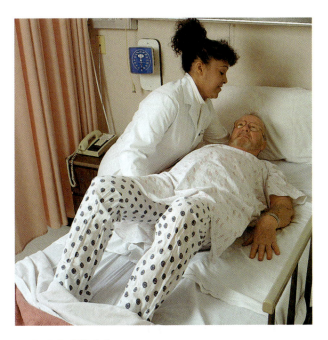

FIGURE 20-13 Get close to the patient and bed while moving a patient up in bed.

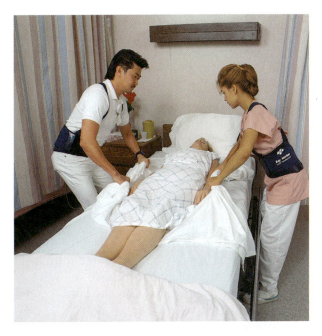

FIGURE 20-14 A turning sheet or lift sheet can also be used to move the patient up in bed.

8. Face the head of the bed. Get a broad base of support by putting one foot ahead of the other. Get close to the patient and bed (see figure 20-13).

   NOTE: Use proper body mechanics throughout the procedure.

9. Place your arm that is closest to the head of the bed under the patient's head and shoulders. Place your other arm under the patient's hips.

   ! CAUTION: If the patient is unable to help, get someone else to assist you. Do not risk injury to yourself or to the patient.

   NOTE: Sometimes, two people, one on each side of the patient, can move the patient to the head of the bed. Other times, two people can use a turning sheet or a lift sheet rolled close to both sides of the patient's body to lift the patient up in bed (see figure 20-14).

10. If the patient can assist, arrange a signal. For example, say, "On the count of three, push with your feet."

11. Use the signal. Slide the patient toward the head of the bed. Shift your weight from the rear leg to the forward leg at the same time that you slide the patient.

    NOTE: Use the weight of your body to move the patient. Avoid back strain.

    ! CAUTION: If you are *not* able to move the patient, get help.

12. Leave the patient in good body alignment. Make sure the patient is comfortable.

13. Elevate the siderails (if indicated). Place the call signal and any needed supplies within easy reach of the patient. Lower the bed to its lowest level.

14. Replace all equipment. Make sure the area is neat and clean.

15. Wash hands.

16. **C** Report that the patient has been moved up in bed and/or record all required information on the patient's chart or the agency form, for example, date; time; moved to head of bed, tolerated procedure well; and your signature and title. Note any unusual observations.

Practice *Go to the workbook and use the evaluation sheet for 20:2B, Moving the Patient Up in Bed, to practice this procedure. When you feel you have mastered this skill, sign the sheet and give it to your instructor for further action.*

 Final Checkpoint Using the criteria listed on the evaluation sheet, your instructor will grade your performance.

PROCEDURE 20:2C   OBRA

Turning the Patient Away to Change Position

Equipment and Supplies

Pen or pencil

Procedure

1. Obtain permission from your immediate supervisor or check orders to make sure that the patient can be turned.

2. **C** Knock on the door and pause before entering. Introduce yourself. Identify the patient. Explain the procedure.

3. Provide privacy. Close the door and screen the unit.

4. Wash hands.

5. Lock wheels to prevent movement of the bed. Elevate the bed to a comfortable height.

6. Lower the siderail nearest to you. Make sure the opposite siderail is raised and locked securely.

7. The patient should be lying on the side of the bed close to you. If so, proceed to step 8. If the patient is at the center or close to the far side of the bed, move the patient as follows:

   a. Place one hand under the patient's head and neck. Place your other hand under the patient's upper back. Slide the upper part of the patient's body toward you.

   b. Place both hands under the patient's hips. Slide the hips toward you.

   c. Place both hands under the patient's upper and lower legs. Slide the legs toward you.

   ⚠ **CAUTION:** If you are not able to move the patient, get help.

   ⚠ **CAUTION:** Check the opposite siderail. Make sure it is up before proceeding.

8. Ask the patient to place his or her arms across the chest and move the proximal leg (the one closest to you) over the other leg (see figure 20-15A).

   NOTE: This will make it easier to turn the patient and helps prevent injury.

   ⚠ **CAUTION:** Do *not* cross the legs if the patient had hip replacement surgery.

9. Get close to the patient by bending your knees and keeping your back straight. Position your feet to provide a broad base of

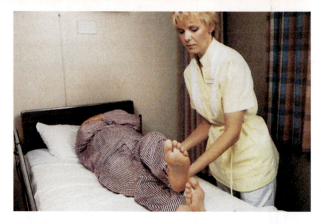

FIGURE 20-15A Cross the patient's near leg over the far leg before turning, unless the patient had hip replacement surgery.

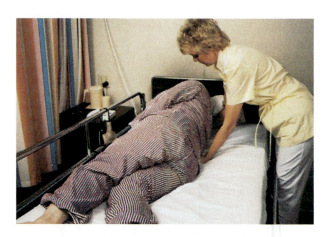

FIGURE 20-15B After rolling the patient away from you, pull the patient's hips back to the center of the bed.

support. Place one arm under the patient's shoulders. Place your opposite hand under the patient's hips.

10. Use a smooth, even motion to roll the patient away from you and onto his or her side.

    C **NOTE:** Explain what you are doing to the patient.

11. Place your hands under the patient's head and shoulders. Draw the head and shoulders back toward the center of the bed.

12. Place your hands under the patient's hips and gently pull them back toward the center of the bed (see figure 20-15B).

13. Place your hands under the patient's legs and pull them back toward the center of the bed.
14. Place a pillow behind the patient's back, between the legs to align the hips, and under the upper arm. Make sure the patient is comfortable and in good alignment.
15. Elevate the siderails (if indicated) before leaving the patient. Make sure that the call signal and other needed supplies are within easy reach of the patient. Lower the bed to its lowest level.
16. Replace all equipment. Leave the area neat and clean.
17. Wash hands.
18. **C** Report that patient has been turned and/or record all required information on the patient's chart or the agency form, for example, date, time, turned on right side and positioned in correct alignment, and your signature and title. Note any unusual observations.

> **Practice** *Go to the workbook and use the evaluation sheet for 20:2C, Turning the Patient Away to Change Position, to practice this procedure. When you feel you have mastered this skill, sign the sheet and give it to your instructor for further action.*

✔ **Final Checkpoint** Using the criteria listed on the evaluation sheet, your instructor will grade your performance.

PROCEDURE 20:2D **OBRA**

Turning the Patient Inward to Change Position

Equipment and Supplies

Pen or pencil

Procedure

1. Obtain permission from your immediate supervisor or check orders to make sure that the patient can be turned.
2. Knock on the door and pause before entering. Introduce yourself. Identify the patient. Explain the procedure.
3. Provide privacy. Close the door and screen the unit.
4. Wash hands.
5. Lock the wheels of the bed to prevent movement. Elevate the bed to a comfortable height.
6. Lower the siderail nearest to you.
7. If the patient is too close to the near side of the bed, move him or her to the opposite side as follows:
   a. Place one hand under the patient's head and shoulders and the other hand under the patient's back. Slide the upper part of the body toward the opposite side of the bed.
   b. Place both hands under the patient's hips. Slide the hips toward the opposite side of the bed.
   c. Place both hands under the patient's legs. Slide the legs toward the opposite side of the bed.
8. Instruct the patient to cross his or her arms on the chest. Place the patient's leg that is farthest from you on top of the leg that is nearest to you.
   NOTE: This prevents injury to the patient's arms and legs.
   ⚠ **CAUTION:** Do *not* cross the legs if the patient had hip replacement surgery.
9. Get close to the patient by bending your knees and keeping your back straight. Position your feet to provide a broad base of support. Place your hand that is closest to the head of the bed on the patient's far shoulder. Place your other hand behind the patient's hip. Use your knee to brace your body against the side of the bed.
10. Use a gentle, smooth motion to roll the patient toward you (see figure 20-16A).
    ⚠ **CAUTION:** Observe proper body mechanics at all times.

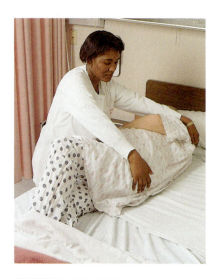

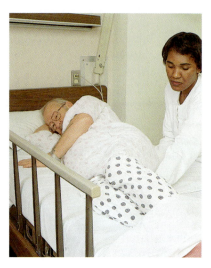

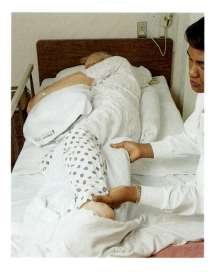

FIGURE 20-16A With your hands on the patient's far shoulder and hip, use a gentle, smooth motion to roll the patient toward you.

FIGURE 20-16B Place your hands under the patient's hips and draw them toward the center of the bed.

FIGURE 20-16C Place a pillow behind the patient's back, between the legs to align the hips, and under the upper arm.

11. Raise and secure the siderail. Go to the opposite side of the bed and lower the siderail.
12. Place your hands under the patient's head and shoulders and draw the head and shoulders back toward the center of the bed.
13. Place your hands under the patient's hips and draw them toward the center of the bed (see figure 20-16B).
14. Place your hands under the patient's legs and draw them toward the center of the bed.
15. Place pillows behind the patient's back, between the legs, and under the upper arm to position the patient in good body alignment (see figure 20-16C). Make sure that the patient is comfortable.
16. Elevate the siderail, if indicated. Place the call signal and other necessary supplies within easy reach of the patient. Lower the bed to its lowest level.
17. Replace all equipment. Leave the area neat and clean.
18. Wash hands.

19. Report that patient has been turned and/or record all required information on the patient's chart or the agency form, for example, date, time, turned on left side and positioned in correct alignment, and your signature and title. Note any unusual observations.

Practice *Go to the workbook and use the evaluation sheet for 20:2D, Turning the Patient Inward to Change Position, to practice this procedure. When you feel you have mastered this skill, sign the sheet and give it to your instructor for further action.*

✔ **Final Checkpoint** Using the criteria listed on the evaluation sheet, your instructor will grade your performance.

PROCEDURE 20:2E

OBRA

Sitting Up to Dangle

Equipment and Supplies

Footstool (if needed), bath blanket, robe and/or slippers, pen or pencil

Procedure

1. Check orders or obtain authorization from your immediate supervisor. Orders usually state the length of time the patient should dangle.
2. Assemble equipment.
3. **C** Knock on the door and pause before entering. Introduce yourself. Identify the patient. Explain the procedure.
4. Provide privacy. Close the door and screen the unit.
5. Wash hands.
6. Lock bed wheels to prevent movement of the bed.
7. Lower the bed to its lowest level. Lower the siderail on side where the patient is to dangle.
8. Check the patient's radial pulse. This reading will serve as a guideline on how the patient tolerates the procedure.

9. Slowly elevate the head of the bed to a sitting position. Provide time for the patient to adjust to this position.
10. Put a bedjacket or robe on the patient. Prevent unnecessary exposure.
11. Get close to the patient by bending your knees and keeping your back straight. Position your feet to provide a broad base of support. Place your arm that is nearest to the head of the bed around the patient's shoulders. Place your other arm under the patient's knees (see figure 20-17A). Slowly and smoothly rotate the patient toward the side of the bed (see figure 20-17B).

    (!) CAUTION: Use proper body mechanics at all times.

    (!) CAUTION: Stand in front of the patient to prevent falls.
12. Use the bath blanket to cover the patient's lap and legs. Put slippers on the patient. Rest the patient's feet on a footstool (if necessary).
13. Check the patient's radial pulse. Note any signs of distress, such as pale color, increased perspiration, labored respirations, weakness, dizziness, or nausea.

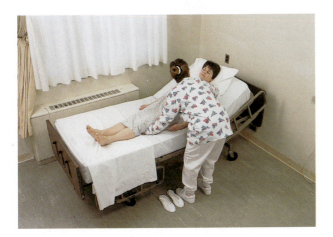

FIGURE 20-17A Place one arm around the patient's shoulders and the other arm under the patient's knees.

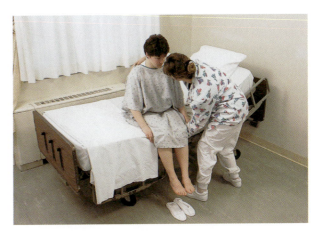

FIGURE 20-17B Slowly rotate the patient toward the side of the bed.

⚠ **CAUTION:** If any of these signs are noted, go immediately to step 17 and return the patient to the original position in bed.

14. Instruct the patient to flex and extend the legs and feet. This increases circulation to the area and stimulates the muscles.

15. Have the patient dangle for the time ordered or as the patient's condition permits.

16. When the time is up, remove the patient's slippers and the bath blanket.

17. Place one arm around the patient's shoulders and your other arm under the patient's knees. Gently and slowly return the patient's body to the bed.

⚠ **CAUTION:** Use correct body mechanics.

18. Remove the patient's robe.

19. Slowly lower the head of the bed.

20. Position the patient in good alignment.

21. Check the patient's radial pulse. Note any major changes. Report any changes *immediately*.

22. Observe all checkpoints before leaving the patient. Make sure the siderails are elevated (if indicated), the bed is at its lowest level, the call signal and other supplies are within easy reach, and the area is neat and clean.

23. Wash hands.

24. Ⓒ Report that the patient has dangled and/or record all required information on the patient's chart or the agency form, for example, date; time; sat on side of bed for 15 minutes, P 72 strong and regular at start of procedure, P 78 strong and regular at end, knees and legs flexed and extended, tolerated procedure well; and your signature and title. Note any unusual observations.

> **Practice** *Go to the workbook and use the evaluation sheet for 20:2E, Sitting Up to Dangle, to practice this procedure. When you feel you have mastered this skill, sign the sheet and give it to your instructor for further action.*

✔ **Final Checkpoint** Using the criteria listed on the evaluation sheet, your instructor will grade your performance.

PROCEDURE 20:2F   OBRA
Transferring a Patient to a Chair or Wheelchair

NOTE: Wheelchairs vary slightly. Read the manufacturer's instructions or ask your immediate supervisor to demonstrate correct operation of the footrests, wheel locks, and other parts.

Equipment and Supplies

Wheelchair or chair, bathrobe, transfer belt, one to two bath blankets, slippers, pen or pencil

Procedure

1. Obtain orders from your immediate supervisor or check physician's orders to obtain authorization.

2. Assemble equipment.

3. Knock on the door and pause before entering. Introduce yourself. Identify the patient. Explain the procedure to the patient.

4. Close the door and screen the unit to provide privacy for the patient.

5. Wash hands.

6. Position the wheelchair or chair. It can be placed at the head of the bed facing the foot or at the foot of the bed facing the head. Positioning often depends on other equipment in the room.

   NOTE: Whenever possible, the chair should be positioned so that it is secure against a wall or solid furniture and will *not* slide backward.

7. Securely lock the wheels of the wheelchair. Raise the footrests so that they are out of the way.

   ⚠ **CAUTION:** Double-check the locks on the wheelchair.

   NOTE: For additional comfort and warmth, a bath blanket can be folded lengthwise and placed in the chair or wheelchair.

8. Lock the bed to prevent movement. Lower the bed to its lowest level.

9. Slowly elevate the head of the bed.

10. Lower the siderail on the side that the patient is to exit from the bed.

11. Put the robe on the patient. Fanfold the bed linen to the foot of the bed.

    NOTE: Avoid exposing the patient during this procedure.

12. Assist the patient to a sitting position on the side of the bed with his or her feet flat on the floor. Observe for any signs of distress. Note color, pulse rate, breathing, and other similar signs. Put socks and shoes or slippers with nonslip soles on the patient. Put a transfer (gait) belt on the patient following procedure 21:2A.

    NOTE: Refer to Procedure 20:2E on dangling.

    ! **CAUTION:** If the patient is weak or too heavy, get help.

    ! **CAUTION:** If distress is noted, return the patient to bed immediately.

    ! **CAUTION:** Use proper body mechanics.

13. Keep your back straight. Place one hand on each side of the belt using an underhand grasp. Face the patient and stand close to the patient. Position your feet to provide a broad base of support. If the patient has a weak leg, support the leg by positioning your knee against the patient's knee or by blocking the patient's foot with your foot.

    NOTE: If the use of a transfer belt is contraindicated, place your hands under the patient's arms and around to the back of the shoulders to provide support.

14. **C** Arrange a signal with the patient, such as counting to three. Instruct the patient to push against the bed with his or her hands to rise to a standing position.

15. At the given signal, assist the patient to a standing position. Lift up on the belt while the patient pushes up from the bed (see figure 20-18A). Place your knees and feet firmly against the patient's knees and feet to provide support.

16. Keeping your hands in the same position, help the patient turn by using several pivot steps until the back of his or her legs are touching the seat of the chair (see figure 20-18B).

17. Ask the patient to place his or her hands on the armrests and to bend at the knees as you

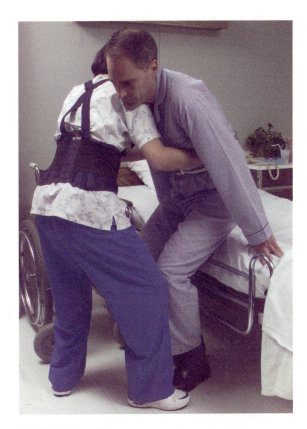

FIGURE 20-18A Lift up on the belt while the patient pushes up from the bed.

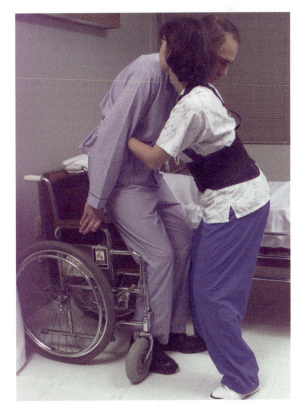

FIGURE 20-18B Help the patient turn until the back of his legs are touching the seat of the chair.

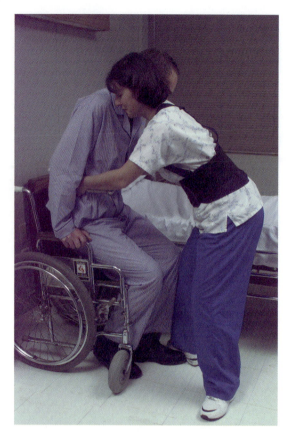

FIGURE 20-18C Gradually and slowly lower the patient to a sitting position in the chair.

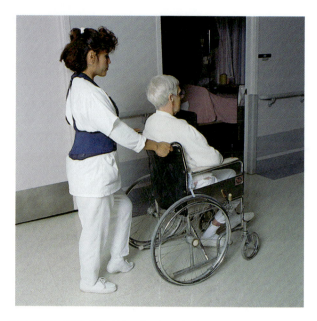

FIGURE 20-19 Watch closely for other traffic at doorways and intersections.

gradually and slowly lower the patient to a sitting position in the chair (see figure 20-18C).

> **⚠ CAUTION:** Bend at the hips and knees and keep your back straight.

18. Position the patient comfortably. Remove the transfer belt. Use a bath blanket to cover the patient's lap and legs. Lower the footrests on the wheelchair, taking care not to hit the patient's feet.

    NOTE: Observe for any signs of distress.

19. Remain with the patient until you are sure there are no problems. If you leave the patient seated in a wheelchair or chair, make sure that the call signal and other supplies are within easy reach. Leave the area neat and clean. Check on the patient at frequent intervals.

20. If you are transporting the patient in the wheelchair, observe the following rules:
    a. Walk on the right side of the hall or corridor.
    b. Slow down and look for other traffic at doorways and intersections (see figure 20-19).
    c. To enter an elevator, turn the chair around and back into the elevator.
    d. To go down a steep ramp, turn the chair around and back down the ramp.
    e. Use the weight of your body to push the chair. Stand close to the chair.
    f. Watch the patient closely for signs of distress while transporting.

21. To return the patient to bed, reverse the procedure, beginning by putting a transfer belt on the patient and raising the footrests (step 18).

    > **⚠ CAUTION:** Be sure the wheels are locked before helping the patient out of the wheelchair. Lock the bed to prevent movement.

22. Position the patient in good body alignment after returning him or her to bed.

23. Observe all checkpoints before leaving the patient: elevate the siderails (if indicated), lower the bed to its lowest level, place the call signal and other supplies within easy reach of the patient.

24. Replace all equipment used. Wipe the wheelchair with a disinfectant and return it to its proper place. Leave the area neat and clean.

25. Wash hands.

26. **C** Report that the patient was transferred to a wheelchair and/or record all required information on the patient's chart or the agency form, for example, date;

time; transferred to chair, sat in chair for 30 minutes, tolerated well; and your signature and title. Note any unusual observations.

✔ **Final Checkpoint** Using the criteria listed on the evaluation sheet, your instructor will grade your performance.

Practice Go to the workbook and use the evaluation sheet for 20:2F, Transferring a Patient to a Chair or Wheelchair, to practice this procedure. When you feel you have mastered this skill, sign the sheet and give it to your instructor for further action.

PROCEDURE 20:2G
OBRA

Transferring a Patient to a Stretcher

Equipment and Supplies

Stretcher with siderails and safety belt(s), bath blanket, pen or pencil
NOTE: Because this procedure requires more than one person, it is best to determine what tasks each of the assistants will perform before beginning the procedure.

Procedure

1. Check physician's orders or obtain authorization from your immediate supervisor for the transfer.
2. Assemble equipment. Cover the stretcher with a clean sheet.
3. **C** Knock on the door and pause before entering. Introduce yourself. Identify the patient. Explain the procedure to the patient.
4. Provide privacy. Close the door and screen the unit.
5. Wash hands.
6. Elevate the bed to the level of the stretcher. Lock the bed wheels to prevent movement of the bed. Lower the siderail on the side of the transfer.
7. Place a bath blanket over the patient. Fold bed linen to the foot of the bed.
   NOTE: Avoid exposing the patient.
8. Place the stretcher next to the bed. The bed and the stretcher should be parallel.
9. Lock the wheels of the stretcher.

(!) **CAUTION:** In addition to the locks, use the weight of your body to hold the stretcher against the bed during this procedure.

(!) **CAUTION:** Use correct body mechanics at all times.

10. If the patient is conscious and capable of moving unassisted, proceed as follows:
    a. Reach across the stretcher and hold up the bath blanket.
    b. Ask the patient to slide from the bed to the stretcher. Hold the stretcher against the bed (see figure 20-20).

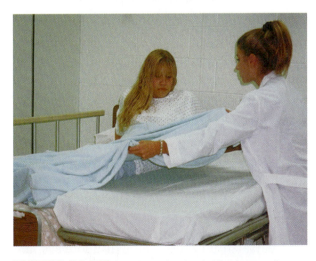

FIGURE 20-20 Hold up the bath blanket and use the weight of your body to hold the stretcher against the bed while the patient is moving to the stretcher.

c. If the patient needs assistance, help by moving first the patient's head and shoulders, then the patient's hips, and finally the patient's legs and feet.

> **CAUTION:** Make sure that the bed and stretcher wheels are locked and stabilized while the patient is being moved toward you.

> **CAUTION:** If the patient is too heavy or unable to assist with the move, obtain help.

11. If the patient is very weak, paralyzed, semiconscious or unconscious, proceed as follows:

   a. Obtain the assistance of three or four other people.

   b. Position a lifting sheet or blanket under the patient extending from the patient's head and neck to the feet.

   c. Position two or three people by the stretcher and one or two people on the open side of the bed.

   d. Roll the sides of the lifting sheet or blanket close to the patient's body.

   e. Using overhand grasps, one assistant should grasp the sheet by the patient's head and shoulders. The second assistant should grasp the sheet by the waist and lower hip. The third assistant should grasp the sheet by the patient's thighs and legs. The assistant(s) on the open side of the bed should grasp the sheet at the patient's head and hips (see figure 20-21).

   f. At a given signal, all assistants should lift the sheet slightly to gently slide the patient from the bed to the stretcher.

   NOTE: Some facilities use slider boards instead of a lifting sheet or blanket.

12. Position the patient comfortably on the stretcher.

13. Lock the safety belt(s). Raise both siderails of the stretcher.

14. To transport the patient, two persons should direct the stretcher (one at the head and one at the foot).

   a. Unlock the wheels of the stretcher. Move slowly.

   b. The stretcher patient always travels feet first.

   c. Walk on the right side of the hall.

   d. Watch for cross traffic at doorways and intersections.

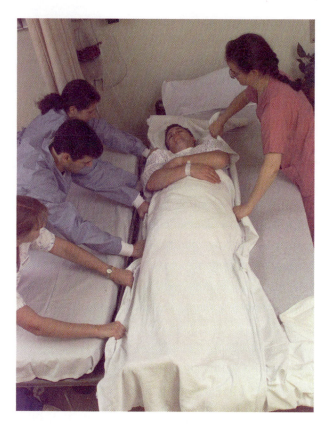

FIGURE 20-21 Three to five people can use a lift sheet or blanket to move a patient from the bed to the stretcher.

   e. When going down an incline, the person at the foot of the stretcher should go backward and use body weight to control the stretcher.

   f. To enter an elevator, push the correct button to keep the elevator door open. Back the stretcher into the elevator so that the head end enters first. To leave the elevator, push the button to keep the door open, and push the stretcher out feet-end first.

15. To return the patient to bed, reverse the procedure, beginning with locking the wheels of the stretcher and bed and unlocking the safety belt(s), step 13.

> **CAUTION:** Always check the wheel locks before transferring patients.

16. Observe all checkpoints before leaving the patient: position the patient in correct alignment, elevate the siderails (if indicated), lower the bed to its lowest level, place the call signal and other supplies within easy reach of the patient, and leave the area neat and clean.

17. Remove the sheet from the stretcher and place the sheet in a linen hamper. Use a disinfectant to wipe the stretcher. Replace all equipment used. Leave the area neat and clean.
18. Wash hands.
19. **C** Report that the patient was transferred to a stretcher and/or record all required information on the patient's chart or the agency form, for example, date; time; transferred to stretcher and transported to X-ray department, tolerated procedure well; and your signature and title. Note any unusual observations.

Practice *Go to the workbook and use the evaluation sheet for 20:2G, Transferring a Patient to a Stretcher, to practice this procedure. When you feel you have mastered this skill, sign the sheet and give it to your instructor for further action.*

✔ **Final Checkpoint** Using the criteria listed on the evaluation sheet, your instructor will grade your performance.

PROCEDURE 20:2H

OBRA

Using a Mechanical Lift to Transfer a Patient

NOTE: Mechanical lifts vary slightly. Read the manufacturer's instructions or ask your immediate supervisor to demonstrate the correct operation of the lift.

⚠ **CAUTION:** The manufacturer will indicate the weight limits for the mechanical lift. Do *not* use the mechanical lift if the patient weighs more than the weight limit.

Equipment and Supplies

Mechanical lift with straps and sling, bath blanket, chair or wheelchair, pen or pencil

NOTE: If the lift is being used to transfer a patient to a bathtub or shower area, a chair or wheelchair is not required.

⚠ **CAUTION:** Some facilities require that two health care providers perform this procedure. One person operates the lift while the second person guides the movements of the patient. Follow agency policy for this procedure.

Procedure

1. Obtain orders from your immediate supervisor or check physician's orders to obtain authorization.
2. Assemble equipment. Read the operating instructions provided with the mechanical lift or ask your immediate supervisor to demonstrate operation of the lift. Check the straps, sling, and any clasps to make sure there are no defects. Check the hydraulic unit and look for evidence of oil leaks.

⚠ **CAUTION:** Do not use the lift if straps or sling are torn or defective, if clasps are not secure, or if oil is leaking from the hydraulic unit. Serious injury may result. Label the defective mechanical lift with a warning or lock-out and notify your supervisor immediately.

3. **C** Knock on the door and pause before entering. Introduce yourself. Identify the patient. Explain the procedure. Reassure the patient, as needed.
   NOTE: Patients are often apprehensive about being transferred by lift. It is important that they be as relaxed as possible for the transfer. Constant reassurance and encouragement are necessary.
4. Close the door and screen the unit for privacy during the transfer.
5. Wash hands.
6. Position the chair or wheelchair next to the foot of the bed, with the open seat facing the head of the bed. Lock the wheels of the wheelchair or ask another health team member to hold the chair in position.

7. Lock the wheels of the bed. Lower the siderail on the side of the transfer.

8. Turn or move the patient to position the sling under the patient. The sling should be positioned under the shoulders, buttocks, and thighs. Make sure that the sling is smooth and that the center is near the center of the patient's back (see figure 20-22A).

9. Attach the suspension straps to the sling. Insert the hooks from the inside of the sling to the outside to keep the open end of the hooks away from the patient's body (see figure 20-22B). Make sure that the straps are not tangled or twisted. If clasps are present on the hooks, make sure they are secure.

10. Position the mechanical lift over the bed so that the straps can be attached to the frame of the lift (see figure 20-22C). Check to make sure that the suspension straps are locked to the frame or attached securely. Make sure that the straps are not tangled or twisted. Position the patient's arms inside the straps. Encourage the patient to keep his or her arms folded across the chest to keep the arms inside the straps.

11. **C** Tell the patient that he or she will be lifted from the bed. Constantly reassure the patient.

12. Turn the crank or use the hydraulic control to slowly raise the patient slightly above the bed. Check the straps, sling, and position of the patient to be sure that the patient is suspended securely by the lift. Then, continue to raise the patient as needed until you can slowly turn the lift to move the patient away from the bed and into position over the chair or wheelchair. Keep all movements as smooth and even as possible (see figure 20-22D).

    (!) CAUTION: Move slowly to prevent jerking motions that may frighten the patient.

13. Slowly lower the lift to position the patient in the chair or wheelchair. Guide the patient's legs into position on the chair (see figure 20-22E).

14. Unhook the suspension straps from the sling. The sling is usually left in position under the patient. Carefully move the lift away from the patient.

    (!) CAUTION: Be careful not to injure the patient with the straps or lift while moving the lift away from the chair.

15. Use the blanket to cover the patient. Lower the footrests of the wheelchair and position the patient's feet in a comfortable position. If the patient is in a chair, slippers can be put on the patient's feet.

16. To return the patient to bed, reverse the procedure. Begin by making sure the wheels of

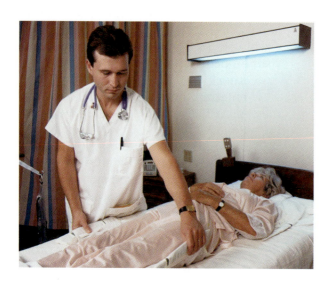

FIGURE 20-22A Position the sling under the patient's shoulders, buttocks, and thighs.

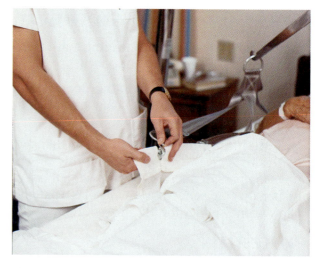

FIGURE 20-22B Insert the hooks from the inside of the sling to the outside.

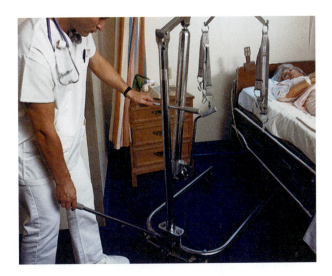

FIGURE 20-22C Position the mechanical lift over the bed.

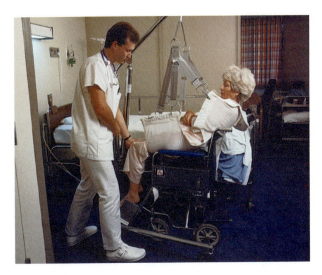

FIGURE 20-22E Lower the lift slowly to position the patient in the wheelchair.

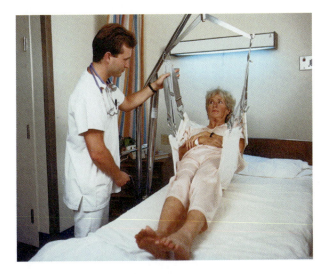

FIGURE 20-22D Use a smooth motion to lift the patient out of the bed.

the chair and bed are locked. Attach the suspension straps securely to the sling.

17. Observe all checkpoints before leaving the patient: position the patient in correct alignment, elevate the siderails (if indicated), lower the bed to its lowest level, place the call signal and other supplies within easy reach of the patient, and leave the area neat and clean.

18. Use a disinfectant to wipe the mechanical lift. Properly replace all equipment used. Leave the area neat and clean.

19. Wash hands.

20. **C** Report that the patient was transferred to a chair or wheelchair using a mechanical lift and/or record all required information on the patient's chart or the agency form, for example, date; time; transferred to chair with mechanical lift, patient seemed slightly apprehensive at start of procedure but relaxed while in chair; and your signature and title. Note any unusual observations.

Practice *Go to the workbook and use the evaluation sheet for 20:2H, Using a Mechanical Lift to Transfer a Patient, to practice this procedure. When you feel you have mastered this skill, sign the sheet and give it to your instructor for further action.*

 Final Checkpoint Using the criteria listed on the evaluation sheet, your instructor will grade your performance.

20:3 INFORMATION Bedmaking

OBRA Making beds correctly is a task performed by many health care workers. A correctly made bed provides comfort and protection for the patient confined to bed for long periods of time. Therefore, care must be taken when beds are made. The bed linen must be free of all wrinkles. Wrinkles cause discomfort and can lead to the formation of pressure ulcers.

Mitered corners are used to hold the linen firmly in place. Mitering corners is a special folding technique that secures the linen under the mattress. Mitered corners are also used for linen placed on stretchers and examination tables. Some agencies and homes use fitted contour sheets for bottom sheets. Mitered corners would not be used with these sheets, but would be used with top sheets.

Following are examples of the types of beds that you may be required to make:

◆ **Closed bed:** A bed made following the discharge of a patient and after terminal cleaning of the unit. Its purpose is to keep the bed clean until a new patient is admitted.

◆ **Open bed:** A closed bed is converted to an open bed by **fanfolding** (folding like accordion pleats) the top sheets. This is done to "welcome" a new patient. It is also done for patients who are ambulatory or out of bed for short periods of time.

◆ **Occupied bed:** A bed made while the patient is in the bed. This is usually done after the morning bath.

◆ **Bed cradle:** A cradle is placed on a bed under the top sheets to prevent bed linen from touching parts of the patient's body. A cradle frequently is used for patients with burns, skin ulcers, lesions, blood clots, circulatory disease, fractures, surgery on legs or feet, and other similar conditions.

Draw sheets are half sheets that are frequently used on beds. A draw sheet extends from the patient's shoulders to the patient's knees. The draw sheet is used to protect the mattress. If soiled, the draw sheet can be changed readily without changing the bottom sheet of the bed. In some settings, disposable bed protectors, frequently called *underpads*, are placed under the patient to protect the sheets instead of using draw sheets. Draw sheets are sometimes used as lift sheets.

To prevent injury to yourself, it is essential that you observe correct body mechanics while making beds. It is also important to conserve time and energy. Keeping linen arranged in the order of use is one way to conserve time and energy. In addition, most beds are made completely first on one side and then on the other side. This limits unnecessary movement from one side of the bed to the opposite side.

It is also important to limit the movement of organisms and, therefore, the spread of infection while making beds. Roll dirty or soiled linen while removing it from the bed. Hold dirty linen away from your body and place it in a linen hamper, cart, or bag immediately. Never place dirty linen on the floor. Some facilities do not allow linen hampers or carts in a patient's room. The hamper or cart is left in the hall. Soiled linen is placed in a pillowcase or plastic bag, carried to the hall, and placed in the hamper or cart. Wash your hands after handling dirty linen and before handling clean linen. Clean linen should be stored in a closed closet or on a covered linen cart. Never allow clean linen to contact your uniform. Never bring extra linen to the patient's room because it is then considered contaminated and cannot be used for another patient. Avoid shaking clean sheets. Unfold them gently. Place the open end of the pillowcase away from the door. This looks neater and also helps prevent the entrance of organisms from the hall.

If linen is contaminated by blood, body fluids, secretions, excretions, urine, or feces, observe standard precautions (discussed in Unit 13:3). Wash your hands frequently and wear gloves while handling contaminated linen. Follow agency policy for proper disposal of linen. Many agencies have special self-dissolving plastic laundry bags that dissolve during the washing process. The contaminated linen is placed in the bag, and sealed. The bag is then placed inside another plastic bag and labeled before being sent to the laundry department.

The second bag is necessary because wet linen may dissolve the water-soluble bag before it reaches the laundry department. The health care worker must be alert at all times to prevent the spread of infection by contaminated linen.

STUDENT: *Go to the workbook and complete the assignment sheet for 20:3, Bedmaking. Then return and continue with the procedures.*

PROCEDURE 20:3A   OBRA
Making a Closed Bed

Equipment and Supplies

Two large sheets (or one large sheet and one fitted sheet), draw sheet (if used), spread, pillow, pillowcase, blanket (as necessary), linen hamper, cart, or bag

Procedure

1. Assemble equipment.
2. Wash hands.
3. Arrange the linen on a chair in the order in which the linen is to be used.

   NOTE: This simplifies the procedure and prevents excessive handling of linen.
4. Elevate the bed to a comfortable height. Lock the wheels to prevent movement.
5. If dirty linen is on the bed, remove the linen. Roll it into a compact bundle. Hold the linen away from your body. Place it in the linen hamper, bag, or cart.

   CAUTION: Prevent spread of organisms and infection. Wear gloves and observe standard precautions if linen is contaminated with blood, body fluids, secretions, or excretions. If the mattress is soiled, wipe it with a disinfectant. After removing contaminated linen, remove the gloves and wash your hands before handling clean linen.

   NOTE: Some facilities do not allow linen hampers or carts in a patient's room. The hamper or cart is left in the hall. Soiled linen is placed in a pillowcase or plastic bag, carried to the hall, and placed in the hamper or cart.
6. Unfold the bottom sheet right side up. Place the small hem even with the foot of the mattress (see figure 20-23A). The center fold should be at the center of the bed. The wide hem should be at the head of the bed.

   CAUTION: Avoid shaking the sheet because doing so spreads germs.

   NOTE: If a fitted sheet is used, it is positioned on the bed, with the contour corners positioned at the head and foot of the mattress. Fit one contour corner smoothly around the foot of the mattress. Then fit the contour corner around the head of the mattress.

   NOTE: Complete one side of the bed entirely before going to the opposite side. This saves time and energy.
7. Tuck 12 to 18 inches of the sheet under the mattress at the head of the bed.
8. Make a mitered corner as follows:
   a. Pick up the sheet approximately 12 inches from the head of the bed.
   b. Form a triangle with a 45° angle on top of the mattress (see figure 20-23B).
   c. Tuck the lower portion under the mattress (see figure 20-23C).
   d. Hold the fold with one hand and bring the triangle down with the other.
   e. Tuck the folded part under the mattress (see figure 20-23D).
9. Tuck in the side of the sheet by working from the head to the foot of the bed (see figure 20-23E).

   CAUTION: Avoid injury. Use correct body mechanics. Work close to the bed and with a broad base of support.
10. Place a draw sheet, if used, in the center of the bed, approximately 14 to 16 inches from the head of the bed. Tuck the draw sheet in at the side of the bed.

    NOTE: Make sure the tucks are secure and as far under the mattress as possible. This helps hold the sheets in place.

    NOTE: Not all agencies use draw sheets. Underpads may be placed on the bed to prevent soiling of the linen.

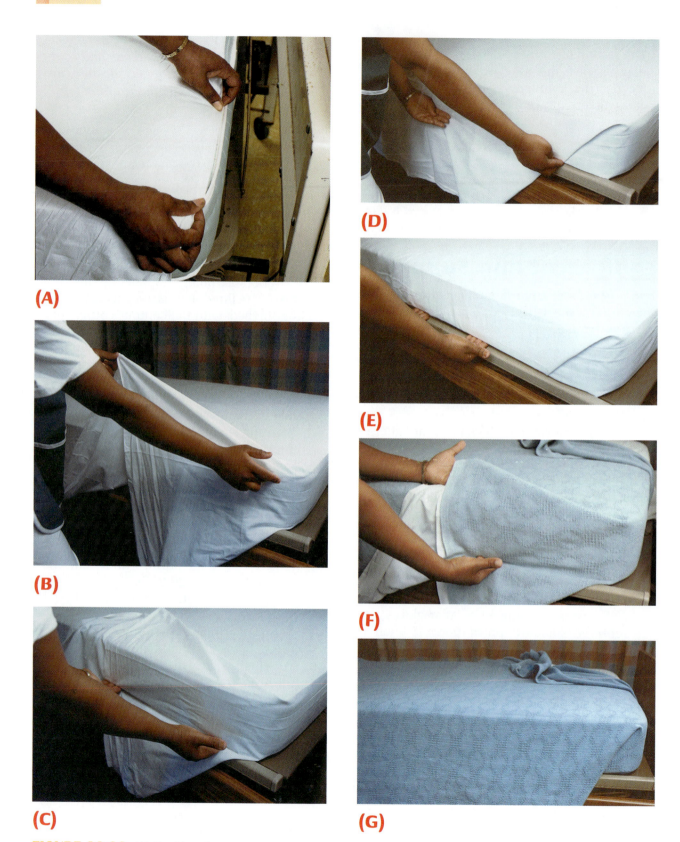

(A)

(B)

(C)

(D)

(E)

(F)

(G)

FIGURE 20-23 (A) Position the small hem of the bottom sheet even with the foot of the mattress. (B) To make a mitered corner, pick up the sheet approximately 12 inches from the head of the bed and form a triangle with a 45° angle. (C) Tuck the bottom part of the triangle under the mattress. (D) Bring the triangle down and tuck it firmly under the mattress to finish the mitered corner. (E) Tuck the side of the sheet under the mattress. (F) The top sheet, blanket, and spread can be tucked under the mattress as one unit and secured with a single mitered corner. (G) After making a mitered corner, allow the top sheet, blanket, and spread to hang free on the side of the mattress.

11. Place the top sheet on the bed, wrong side up. Use the center fold to center the sheet. The wide hem should be even with the top edge of the mattress.

12. Tuck the top sheet over the foot of the mattress.

13. Make a mitered corner as previously instructed.

14. Tuck the side of the sheet under the mattress to the center of the bed only.

15. If a blanket is used, it can be placed on the bed in the same manner as the top sheet. The top sheet and blanket can be tucked in at the same time.

16. Place the spread on the bed right side up. The top edge should be even with the top edge of the mattress. Use center fold to center the spread.

17. Tuck the spread under the mattress at the foot of the bed.
    NOTE: The top sheet, blanket, and spread can all be placed on the bed at the same time. They are then tucked in as one unit at the bottom of the bed, and a mitered corner is made with all of the linen (see figure 20-23F).

18. Make a mitered corner but do *not* tuck the final end under the side of the mattress. Let the triangle hang loose (see figure 20-23G).

19. Go to the opposite side of the bed. From the side, fanfold the top covers to the center of the bed so you can work with the bottom sheet.

20. Tuck the bottom sheet under the head of the mattress. Make a mitered corner.

21. Work from the head of the bed to the foot to tuck in the side of the sheet. Pull the sheet gently to remove all wrinkles before tucking in the side.

22. Grasp the draw sheet in the center. Pull gently to remove wrinkles. Tuck in firmly at the side.

23. Tuck in the top sheet (and blanket) at the foot of the bed. Make a mitered corner. Remove all wrinkles and tuck in at the side up to the center of the bed only.

24. Tuck in the spread at the foot of the bed. Make a mitered corner but do not tuck in the final fold. Let it hang.

25. Line up all sheets so they are smooth and free of wrinkles. If a blanket is used, the top sheet can be folded back over the blanket, making a cuff. This protects the patient from the edge of the blanket.

26. Insert the pillow into the pillowcase as follows:
    a. Place hands in the clean pillowcase and loosen the corners.
    b. Use one hand to grasp the center of the end seam on the outside. Turn the case back over the hand and lower arm (see figure 20-24A).
    c. Using the hand that is covered by the case, grab the end of the pillow at the center of the pillow (see figure 20-24B).
    d. Using your free hand, unfold the case over the pillow (see figure 20-24C).
    e. Adjust the end corners of the pillow into the corners of the case.
    f. Adjust the pillowcase on the pillow. It may be necessary to make a lengthwise pleat for a better fit.
    ! CAUTION: Do not hold the pillow under your chin or against your body. Rather, place it on the bed for support.

27. Place the pillow on the bed, with the open end pointed away from the door.

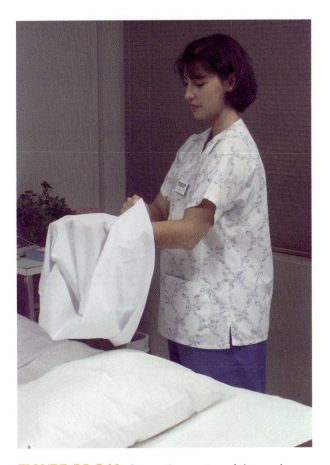

FIGURE 20-24A Grasp the center of the end seam on the pillowcase and turn the case back over the hand and lower arm.

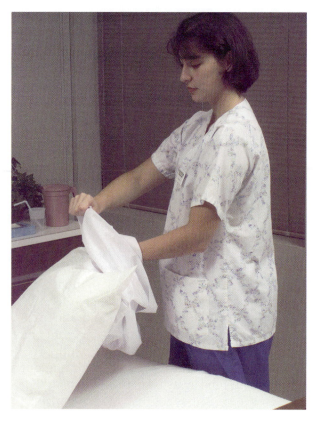

FIGURE 20-24B Using the pillowcase-covered hand, grab the end of the pillow.

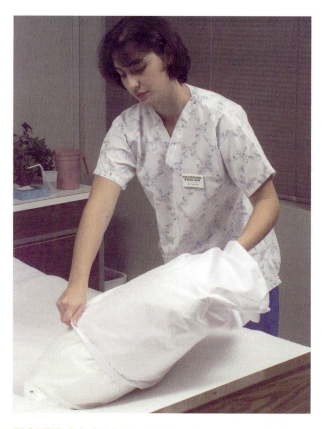

FIGURE 20-24C Unfold the pillowcase over the pillow.

NOTE: This position looks neater and allows fewer organisms from the hall to enter the pillow.

28. Lower the bed to its lowest position. Replace all other equipment (bedside table, call signal, chair, etc.).
29. Before leaving the area check to make sure it is neat and clean.
30. Wash hands.
31. **C** Record or report that a closed bed was made.

Practice *Go to the workbook and use the evaluation sheet for 20:3A, Making a Closed Bed, to practice this procedure. When you feel you have mastered this skill, sign the sheet and give it to your instructor for further action.*

✔ **Final Checkpoint** Using the criteria listed on the evaluation sheet, your instructor will grade your performance.

PROCEDURE 20:3B — OBRA

Making an Occupied Bed

Equipment and Supplies

Laundry hamper, cart, or bag; two large sheets (or one large sheet and one fitted sheet); draw sheet (if used); spread; pillow; pillowcase; blanket (if needed); bath blanket; disposable protective pads; pen or pencil

Procedure

1. Assemble equipment.
2. **C** Knock on the door and pause before entering. Introduce yourself. Identify the patient. Explain the procedure.
3. Close the door and screen the unit for privacy.

4. Wash hands.

   ☣ **CAUTION:** Put on gloves and observe standard precautions if linen on bed is contaminated with blood, body fluids, secretions, or excretions.

5. Arrange the linen on a chair in the order in which the linen will be used.

6. Lock the wheels of the bed. Elevate the bed to a comfortable working position.

7. Lower the headrest and footrest so that the bed is flat, if permissible.

   NOTE: Make sure the patient can tolerate this position before going on with the procedure.

8. Lower the siderail on the side where you are working.

   ⚠ **CAUTION:** Make sure the siderail on the opposite side is elevated.

9. Loosen the top bedclothes at the bottom of the mattress. Remove the spread and blanket. If they are to be reused, fold and place them over the chair.

10. Replace the top sheet with a bath blanket. Have the patient hold the top edge of the bath blanket, if able, while you slide the soiled top sheet out from top to bottom. Place the soiled sheet in the linen hamper, cart, or bag.

    ⚠ **CAUTION:** Avoid shaking the linen because doing so spreads germs. Hold the linen away from your body.

11. Remove the pillow. If this makes the patient uncomfortable, leave the pillow under the patient's head.

12. Assist the patient in turning to the opposite side of the bed.

13. Fanfold the cotton draw sheet up to the patient's body.

14. Fanfold the bottom sheet up to and under the draw sheet (see figure 20-25A). Make sure all of the sheets are as close to the patient as possible.

15. Place the clean bottom sheet on the bed right side up. Place the narrow hem even with the foot of the bed. Center using the center fold. Fanfold the opposite side close to patient.

    ⚠ **CAUTION:** Avoid injury. Use correct body mechanics, including a broad base of support.

16. Tuck in the clean bottom sheet at the head of the bed. Make a mitered corner. Working from the head to the foot of the bed, tuck in the entire side.

    NOTE: If a fitted sheet is used, it is positioned on the bed, with the contour corners positioned at the head and foot of the mattress.

17. Place the clean draw sheet on the bed. Center using the draw sheet's center fold. Fanfold the opposite half close to the patient. Tuck the draw sheet firmly under the mattress at the side (see figure 20-25B).

18. Turn the patient toward you. Caution the patient that he or she will be turning over the top of the fanfolded linen. Elevate the siderail.

19. Go to the opposite side of the bed. Lower the siderail.

20. Remove the soiled bottom sheet and draw sheet. Place in the linen hamper, cart, or bag.

21. Pull the clean bottom sheet into place. Tuck it under the mattress at the head of the bed. Make a mitered corner.

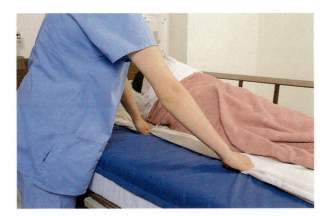

FIGURE 20-25A Fanfold the bottom sheet up to and under the draw sheet in the center of the bed.

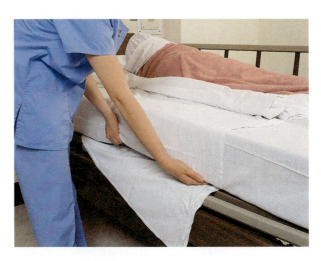

FIGURE 20-25B Tuck the clean bottom sheet and draw sheet firmly under the mattress.

22. Pull gently to remove all wrinkles. Tuck the side of the sheet under the mattress, working from top to bottom.

23. Pull the clean draw sheet into place. Remove all wrinkles and tuck it firmly under the side of the mattress.

24. Assist the patient to turn on his or her back in the center of the bed.

25. Place the top sheet, wrong side up, over the bath blanket. Center using the sheet's center fold. Ask the patient to hold the top edge of the clean sheet. Remove the bath blanket by pulling it from the top to the bottom of the bed.

   🛑 **CAUTION:** Avoid exposing the patient during this procedure.

26. If a blanket is to be used, place it over the top sheet.

27. Place the spread on top, right side up. Center it on the bed.

28. Tuck the top sheet, blanket, and spread into the bottom of the mattress. Make a mitered corner. Before tucking in the final fold, form a toe pleat by making a 3-inch fold in the top of the linen (see figure 20-26). The fold should be made toward the foot of the bed. Complete the mitered corner.

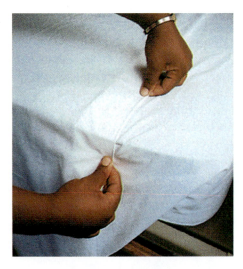

FIGURE 20-26 Make a toe pleat in the top linen to provide more room for the patient's feet and toes.

NOTE: The toe pleat provides more room for the patient's feet and toes and prevents pressure on the toes from the sheets.

29. Raise the siderail and go to the opposite side of the bed. Lower the siderail and complete the top sheets on the opposite side of the bed.

30. Fold the top edge of the spread over and under the top of the blanket. Bring the top sheet over the top of the spread and blanket and make a 6- to 8-inch cuff.

31. Insert the pillow into a clean pillowcase as instructed in Procedure 20:3A.

32. Place the pillow on the bed, with the open end away from the door.

33. Position the patient comfortably in good body alignment.

34. Observe all checkpoints before leaving the patient: place the call signal and other supplies within easy reach of the patient, lower the bed to its lowest level, elevate the siderails (if necessary), and leave the area neat and clean.

35. Dispose of dirty linen in the appropriate location. Properly replace all equipment.

36. Wash hands.

37. Report that an occupied bed was made and/or record all required information on the patient's chart or the agency form, for example, date, time, occupied bed made, and your signature and title. Note any unusual observations.

> **Practice** *Go to the workbook and use the evaluation sheet for 20:3B, Making an Occupied Bed, to practice this procedure. When you feel you have mastered this skill, sign the sheet and give it to your instructor for further action.*

✔ **Final Checkpoint** Using the criteria listed on the evaluation sheet, your instructor will grade your performance.

PROCEDURE 20:3C

Opening a Closed Bed

OBRA

Equipment and Supplies

Closed bed with linen in place, pen or pencil

Procedure

1. Wash hands.
2. Check the closed bed to be sure it was made correctly. Lock the wheels and elevate the height of the bed to a comfortable working position.
   NOTE: For an ambulatory patient, the bed is made as a closed bed and then converted to an open bed.
3. Place the pillow on a chair or overbed table.
4. Go to the head of the bed and work from its side. Fold the top edge of the spread over and under the blanket. Fold the top sheet down over the blanket and spread to form a cuff.
5. Face the foot of the bed. Hold the upper edge of the top layers of linen (spread, blanket, and sheet) with both hands.
6. Fanfold the linen into three even layers down to the foot of the bed (see figure 20-27).
   NOTE: The top of the fold should be facing the head of the bed. In this manner, the patient will be able to pull the top covers up more readily after getting into the bed.
7. Place the pillow back at the head of the bed. Make sure the open end is away from the door.
8. Observe all checkpoints before leaving the area: place the call signal within easy reach of the bed, lower the bed to its lowest level, lock the bed wheels, correctly position all equipment, leave the area neat and clean.
9. Wash hands.
10. Report that an open bed was made and/or record all required information

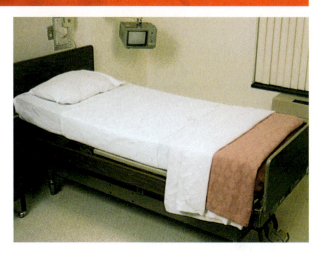

FIGURE 20-27 In an open bed, the top sheets are fanfolded to the foot of the bed.

on the patient's chart or the agency form, for example, date, time, open bed made, and your signature and title.

Practice *Go to the workbook and use the evaluation sheet for 20:3C, Opening a Closed Bed, to practice this procedure. When you feel you have mastered this skill, sign the sheet and give it to your instructor for further action.*

✔ **Final Checkpoint** Using the criteria listed on the evaluation sheet, your instructor will grade your performance.

PROCEDURE 20:3D

Placing a Bed Cradle

OBRA

Equipment and Supplies

Laundry hamper, cart, or bag; bed cradle; two large sheets (or one large sheet and one fitted sheet), draw sheet (if used); spread; pillow; pillowcase; blanket (if needed); bath blanket; pen or pencil

Procedure

1. Assemble equipment.
2. **C** Knock on the door and pause before entering. Introduce yourself. Identify the patient. Explain the procedure.
3. Close the door and screen the unit to provide privacy.
4. Wash hands.

   CAUTION: Wear gloves and observe standard precautions if bed linen is contaminated with blood, body fluids, secretions, or excretions.

5. Lock the bed wheels. Elevate the bed to a comfortable working height. Lower the siderail on the side of the bed where you are working.

   CAUTION: Check the opposite siderail to make sure it is raised and secured.

6. Use a bath blanket to cover the patient. Remove soiled top linen and place it in the linen hamper, cart, or bag.
7. Turn the patient toward the opposite side of the bed.
8. Loosen the bottom sheet and draw sheet and fanfold them to the center of the bed.
9. Place the clean bottom sheet and draw sheets on the bed as described in Procedure 20:3B, Making an Occupied Bed. Finish changing bottom linen on both sides of the bed.
10. Position the patient in the center of the bed and on his or her back.
11. Place the bed cradle into position (see figure 20-28).

    CAUTION: To prevent injury, make sure the cradle is not touching any part of the patient's skin.

12. Tie or anchor the cradle to the bed as necessary. Many bed cradles have metal clamps

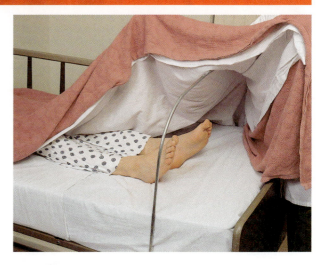

FIGURE 20-28 A bed cradle supports the top linen and prevents the linen from coming into contact with the patient's legs and feet.

that attach to the mattress and/or bed frame. If no clamps are present, roller gauze or straps can be attached to the cradle and then fastened to the bedframe under the mattress.

NOTE: A restless or confused patient may knock the cradle off of the bed. To prevent this, the cradle should be clamped or tied in place.

13. Place the top sheet, blanket, and spread over the top of the cradle and patient. Remove the bath blanket. Tuck in the top sheets at the foot of the bed.
14. Miter the corners and tuck them into place. A larger fold can be made near the lower edge of the cradle in order to form a neater mitered corner.
15. Make a cuff by folding the top sheet over the blanket and spread.
16. Insert the pillow into a clean pillowcase. Position the pillow on the bed, with the open end away from the door.
17. Observe all checkpoints before leaving the patient: the patient is safe, comfortable, and in good body alignment; the call signal and other supplies are within easy reach of the patient; the siderails are elevated (if indicated); the bed is at its lowest level; the area is neat and clean.

18. Check placement of the bed cradle at the end of the procedure and at intervals afterward. Make sure it keeps the bed linen away from the patient. Make sure it is securely in place.
19. Replace all equipment.
20. Wash hands.
21. **C** Report that a bed with cradle was made and/or record all required information on the patient's chart or the agency form, for example, date, time, bed with cradle made, and your signature and title. Note any unusual observations.

Practice *Go to the workbook and use the evaluation sheet for 20:3D, Placing a Bed Cradle, to practice this procedure. When you feel you have mastered this skill, sign the sheet and give it to your instructor for further action.*

Final Checkpoint Using the criteria listed on the evaluation sheet, your instructor will grade your performance.

20:4 INFORMATION Administering Personal Hygiene

OBRA Administering personal care and hygiene may be one of your responsibilities as a health care worker. Ill patients often depend on health care workers for all aspects of personal care. The health care worker must be sensitive to the patient's needs and respect the patient's right to privacy while personal care is administered.

Personal hygiene usually includes bathing, back care, perineal care, oral hygiene, hair care, nail care, and shaving, when necessary. Such care promotes good habits of personal hygiene, provides comfort, and stimulates circulation. Providing such care also gives the health worker an excellent opportunity to develop a good and caring relationship with the patient.

Different types of baths are given to patients. The type of bath depends on the patient's condition and ability to help.

◆ **Complete bed bath (CBB):** The health care worker bathes all parts of the patient's body and also provides oral hygiene, back care, hair care, nail care, and perineal care. A complete bath is usually given to the patient who is confined to bed and is too weak or ill to bathe.

◆ **Partial bed bath:** The health care worker bathes some parts of the patient's body. The term *partial bath (PB)* has two meanings, both related to the patient's ability to help. If the patient is too weak to help, a partial bath means that only the face, arms, hands, back, and perineal area are bathed by the health care worker. If the patient is able to wash most of his or her body, a partial bath means that the health care worker completes the bath, usually bathing the patient's legs and back. In both types of partial baths, the health care worker prepares the supplies needed by the patient (see figure 20-29).

◆ *Tub bath or shower:* Some patients are allowed to take tub baths or showers. The health care worker helps as needed by providing towels and supplies, preparing the tub or shower area, and assisting the patient as much as the situation demands.

◆ *Waterless bath:* Some facilities are using prepackaged disposable cleansing cloths instead of basins of water for baths (see figure 20-30). The cleansing cloths contain a rinse-free cleanser and moisturizer and are warmed in a microwave (follow package instructions) or in a special warmer. Most packages contain from 8 to 10 cloths. Usually one cloth is used for the face, neck and ears; one for each arm and each leg; one for the chest and abdomen; one for the perineum; and one for the back and buttocks. The solution dries quickly on the skin, but a towel can be used to gently remove excess moisture.

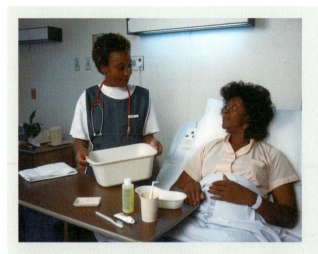

FIGURE 20-29 Position supplies conveniently when assisting a patient with a partial bath.

Extreme care must be taken to avoid overheating the cloths. Read and follow manufacturer's instructions.

Oral hygiene means care of the mouth and teeth. Oral hygiene should be administered at least three times a day. If the patient's condition requires frequent oral care, it should be administered more often, usually at least every two hours. Proper oral hygiene prevents disease and dental caries, stimulates the appetite, and provides comfort. In addition, it aids in the prevention of halitosis (bad breath).

◆ *Routine oral hygiene* refers to regular, every-day toothbrushing and flossing. Many times, patients are able to provide their own care. In such cases, the health care worker provides all of the necessary equipment and supplies. In other cases, the worker helps the patient brush and care for the teeth and mouth.

◆ *Denture care* is necessary when a patient has dentures or artificial teeth. In such cases, the health care worker must help clean the dentures. Patients may be sensitive about dentures. Therefore, it is important that the health care worker provide privacy and reassure the patient. Extreme care must also be taken to prevent damage to the dentures.

◆ *Special oral hygiene* is usually provided for the unconscious or semiconscious patient. Because many of these patients breathe through their mouths, extra care must be taken to clean all parts of the mouth. Special supplies are used for this procedure.

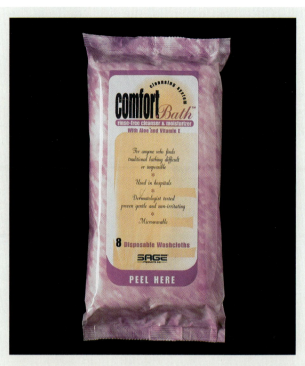

FIGURE 20-30 Packages of cleansing cloths containing a rinse-free cleaner and moisturizer can be used to give a waterless bath. *(Courtesy of Sage Products, Inc.)*

Hair care is an important aspect of personal care that is, unfortunately, frequently neglected. Patients confined to bed often have tangles and knots in their hair. Brushing stimulates circulation to the scalp and helps prevent scalp disease. It is also important to observe the condition of the hair and scalp. Signs of disease, redness, scaling, scalp irritation, or any other conditions should be reported. Shampooing must be approved by the physician. Various types of dry or fluid shampoos are available for patients confined to bed. Read all instructions carefully before using any of these products. Special devices are also available for use while giving a shampoo to a patient confined to bed (see figure 20-31).

Nail care is another often-neglected area in the personal care of the patient. Nails harbor dirt, which can lead to infection and disease. In addition, rough or sharp nails can cause injury. It is important that nail care be included as a part of the daily personal care provided to the patient. However, nails should never be cut unless you receive specific orders to do so from the physician or your immediate supervisor. Cutting of the nails may cause injury. In some

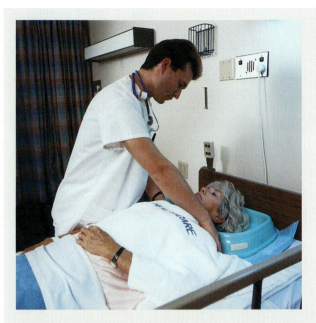

FIGURE 20-31 Special devices are available for use when shampooing the hair of a patient confined to bed.

facilities, only licensed or advanced practice personnel are allowed to cut fingernails. If you are permitted to cut fingernails, use nail clippers, not scissors, and clip the nails straight across. Clip slowly and carefully to avoid accidentally damaging the skin around the nail. Then file the nails straight across to remove rough edges. *Never* cut toenails because injuries to the feet are prone to infection and slow healing. File toenails straight across. Learn and follow your agency policy on nail care.

Shaving is a normal daily routine for most men. It is important to provide this care when the patient is unable to shave himself. Either regular or electric razors may be used. The type used usually depends on the patient's personal preference. Correct technique must be used to prevent injury to the patient. Females usually appreciate shaving of the legs and underarms. Be sure you have specific orders from the physician or your immediate supervisor before shaving any patient. Shaving may be prohibited or special precautions may be required for patients on anticoagulants, or medications that prevent the blood from clotting.

Unless contraindicated by the patient's condition, a *back rub* is given as part of the daily bath. It can also be given at other times during the day and should be done at least once every 8 hours for a patient confined to bed. A good back rub takes at least 4 to 7 minutes and stimulates circulation, prevents pressure ulcers, and leads to relaxation and comfort. It is important that the health care worker's nails be short to prevent injury.

Changing a patient's gown or pajamas is also important. Most patients prefer to wear their own gowns or pajamas. However, hospital gowns are frequently used on very ill patients or on patients with limited movement. These gowns usually open down the back and are easier to position and remove. If the patient has a weak or injured arm, or if an intravenous solution is being infused in one arm, the gown or pajama top must be positioned with care. Usually, the sleeve of the soiled gown or pajama top is removed from the uninjured or untreated arm first. This allows more freedom of movement while removing the sleeve from the injured or treated arm. Likewise, the sleeve of the clean gown or pajama top is placed on the affected arm first, and then is placed on the unaffected arm. It is sometimes necessary to leave one arm out of the gown, and place the sleeve on the unaffected arm only. Some agencies have gowns with openings at the shoulders. Such a gown can be placed over a treated arm and then closed with snaps, ties, or Velcro strips at the shoulder area. In home care, gowns or pajama tops can be opened at the arm seam for easy application. Velcro strips or ties can then be applied so that the gown or pajama top can be closed after being put on the patient. In long-term care facilities, most residents wear regular clothing during the day. It is important to help the resident as needed in choosing and dressing in appropriate clothing. If a resident has difficulty moving one side or is paralyzed, always put the clothing on the affected side first and remove it from the affected side last.

When administering personal hygiene, it is important that the health care worker be alert for any signs that might be unusual. When performing any personal hygiene procedure, watch for and report any unusual observations, including the following:

◆ *Sores, cuts, injuries:* Any noted on the skin, mouth, or scalp must be reported.

◆ *Rashes:* Any type of rash should be reported. Many times, a rash is the first sign of an allergic reaction to a medication.

◆ *Color:* Any unusual color should be noted. Redness (erythema) of the skin is often the first sign of a pressure sore, or decubitus ulcer. A blue color (cyanosis) is a sign of poor circulation. A yellow color (jaundice) is a sign of liver disease, bile obstruction, or destruction of red blood cells.

◆ *Swelling, or edema:* Can indicate poor circulation or disease and should be reported immediately. Pay particular attention to the hands, feet, ankles, and toes.

◆ *Other signs of distress:* Difficult breathing (dyspnea), dizziness (vertigo), unusual weakness, excessive perspiration (diaphoresis), extreme pallor, or abnormal drowsiness or sluggishness (lethargy) should be reported immediately.

When administering personal hygiene, standard precautions (described in Unit 13:3) must be observed at all times. Hands must be washed frequently, and gloves must be worn when contact with blood, body fluids, secretions, or excretions is likely. A gown must be worn if contamination of a uniform or clothing is likely. A mask and protective eyewear, or a face shield, must be worn if droplets of blood or body fluids are present, such as when a patient is coughing excessively. Health care workers with cuts, sores, or dermatitis on their hands must wear gloves for all patient contact. Preventing the spread of infection is a major responsibility of the health care provider.

Always be sensitive to the patient's feelings and respect the patient's rights. Knock on the door and pause before entering a patient's or resident's room. Provide privacy during procedures by closing the door and screening the unit. Avoid exposing the patient when administering personal hygiene. Explain all procedures and reassure the patient as needed. Observe professional ethics at all times.

STUDENT: *Go to the workbook and complete the assignment sheet for 20:4, Administering Personal Hygiene. Then return and continue with the procedures.*

PROCEDURE 20:4A

OBRA

Providing Routine Oral Hygiene

Equipment and Supplies

Toothbrush, toothpaste or powder, mouthwash solution (if used) in cup, cup of water, straw, emesis basin, bath towel, tissues, dental floss, plastic bag or plastic-lined waste can, disposable gloves, pen or pencil

Procedure

1. Obtain proper authorization and assemble equipment.
2. **C** Knock on the door and pause before entering. Introduce yourself. Identify the patient. Explain the procedure.
3. Wash hands. Put on gloves. If spraying or splashing of oral fluids is possible, wear a face mask and eye protection.

CAUTION: Observe standard precautions when contamination by body fluids is possible.

4. Position the patient comfortably. Close the door and screen the unit to provide privacy. Raise the head of the bed, if permitted. Elevate the bed to a comfortable working height. Lower the siderail on the side where you are working. Position the overbed table containing all equipment in a convenient location (see figure 20-32A).

    NOTE: If the patient can brush his or her own teeth, the overbed table is usually positioned over the patient's lap.

5. Place the bath towel on the bedclothes and over the patient's shoulders.

    NOTE: A disposable bed protector can also be used to drape the patient.

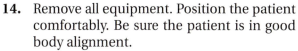
6. Put water on the toothbrush. Add toothpaste. Give the brush to the patient.
   NOTE: Before adding the toothpaste, ask how much the patient uses.

7. If the patient cannot brush, brush the patient's teeth. Carefully insert the brush into the patient's mouth. Start at the rear of the upper teeth. Place the brush at a slight angle to the gum, rotate gently, and then use a slight vibrating motion to thoroughly clean all of the upper teeth. Repeat this process on the lower teeth.

8. Give the patient water from the cup to rinse the mouth. Provide a straw, if needed.

9. Hold the emesis basin under the patient's chin. Instruct the patient to expel the mouth secretions into the basin (see figure 20-32B).

10. Repeat steps 8 and 9, as necessary.

11. Offer tissues to allow the patient to wipe the mouth and chin. Discard tissues in the plastic bag.

12. Provide dental floss. Allow the patient to floss the teeth. Assist as needed. If the patient is not able to floss, obtain a piece of floss about 12 to 18 inches long. Gently insert the floss between the teeth. Curve the floss into a C-shape. Use a gentle up-and-down motion to clean the sides of the teeth. Repeat for both sides of every tooth.

13. Provide mouthwash, if desired by the patient. Mouthwash is sometimes diluted to a proportion of one-half mouthwash to one-half water. Use the emesis basin and tissues, as necessary.

14. Remove all equipment. Position the patient comfortably. Be sure the patient is in good body alignment.

15. Rinse the toothbrush thoroughly. Use cool water and towels to clean the emesis basin. Properly replace all equipment.

16. Observe all checkpoints before leaving the patient: elevate the siderails (if indicated), place the call signal and other supplies within easy reach of the patient, lower the bed to its lowest level, and leave the area neat and clean.

17. Remove gloves. Remove mask and eye protection, if worn. Wash hands.

18. **C** Report that routine oral hygiene was given to the patient and/or record all required information on the patient's chart or the agency form, for example, date, time, oral hygiene given, and your signature and title. Note any unusual observations.

Practice *Go to the workbook and use the evaluation sheet for 20:4A, Providing Routine Oral Hygiene, to practice this procedure. When you feel you have mastered this skill, sign the sheet and give it to your instructor for further action.*

✔ **Final Checkpoint** Using the criteria listed on the evaluation sheet, your instructor will grade your performance.

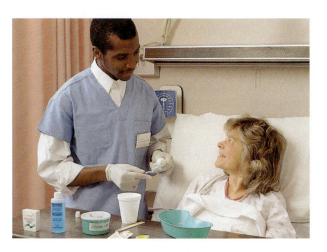

FIGURE 20-32A Position all supplies in a convenient location when assisting a patient with routine oral hygiene.

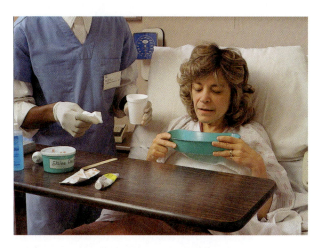

FIGURE 20-32B Instruct the patient to expectorate (spit) into the emesis basin.

PROCEDURE 20:4B

OBRA

Cleaning Dentures

Equipment and Supplies

Toothbrush and toothpaste or denture brush and denture cleaner, denture cup, tissues, cup with mouthwash (if used), straw, applicators, bath towel, paper towels, emesis basin, plastic bag or plastic-lined waste can, disposable gloves, pen or pencil

Procedure

1. Obtain proper authorization and assemble equipment.
2. **C** Knock on the door and pause before entering. Introduce yourself. Identify the patient. Explain the procedure.
   NOTE: The patient may be sensitive about dentures. Provide privacy and reassurance.
3. Close the door and screen the unit for privacy.
4. Wash hands. Put on gloves.
   CAUTION: Observe standard precautions when contamination by body fluids is possible.
5. Elevate the bed to a comfortable working height. Raise the head of the bed, if permitted. Lower the siderail on the side where you are working.
6. Offer tissues to the patient. Ask the patient to remove the dentures. If the patient is unable to do so, use tissues or a gauze sponge to grasp the dentures between your thumb and index finger (see figure 20-33A). Gently apply downward and forward pressure to loosen and remove the top denture. Remove the lower denture by grasping it with your thumb and forefinger and turning it slightly to lift it out of the mouth.
   CAUTION: Never force dentures loose. They can break.
7. Carefully place the dentures in a denture cup. Raise the siderails for patient safety. Carry the dentures to the sink.
8. Line the sink with paper towels.
   NOTE: This provides a protective cushion for the dentures should they be dropped.
9. Put toothpaste or powder on the toothbrush. Place the dentures in the palm of one hand. Holding them under a gentle stream

of cool or lukewarm water, brush all surfaces thoroughly (see figure 20-33B).
   CAUTION: Do *not* use hot water. This can cause breakage.
NOTE: Clean all parts of the dentures, not just the teeth.
NOTE: Dentures can be soaked in a solution containing a cleansing tablet prior to brushing.

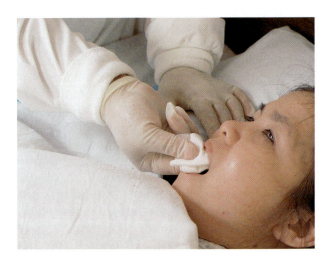

FIGURE 20-33A Use tissues or a gauze sponge to grasp the dentures and ease them down and forward to remove them from the mouth.

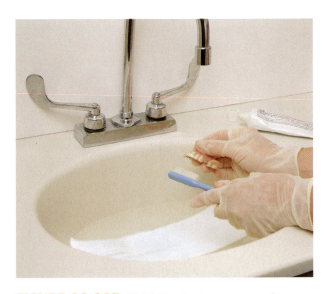

FIGURE 20-33B Hold the dentures securely while brushing all surfaces.

10. Rinse dentures thoroughly in cool water.

    ⚠ CAUTION: Do *not* use very cold water. This can also cause breakage.

11. Put clean, cool water in the denture cup. Place the cleaned dentures in the cup.

12. Return to the patient's bedside. Lower the siderail on the side where you will be working.

13. Help the patient to rinse the mouth with cool water and/or mouthwash. Use the emesis basin and tissues. Place used tissues in the plastic bag.

    NOTE: Some patients want to brush their gums with a soft toothbrush or applicator moistened with mouthwash before inserting clean dentures. Assist the patient, as necessary.

14. Hand the dentures to the patient. Help the patient insert the dentures, as needed. The upper denture is inserted first.

    NOTE: If the patient desires adhesive, line the palates of the dentures with denture adhesive.

    NOTE: If dentures are not immediately returned to the patient, they should be stored inside the denture cup and in a safe area (such as a drawer), and labeled with the patient's name and room number. At times, a denture cleansing or soaking tablet is placed in the water when dentures are stored.

15. Observe all checkpoints before leaving the patient: position the patient in correct body alignment; elevate the siderails (if necessary); lower the bed to its lowest level; place the call signal, tissues, water, and supplies within easy reach of the patient; clean and replace all equipment; leave the area neat and clean.

16. Remove gloves. Wash hands thoroughly.

17. **C** Report that denture care was given and/or record all required information on patient's chart or the agency form, for example, date, time, dentures cleaned, and your signature and title. Note any unusual observations.

> **Practice** *Go to the workbook and use the evaluation sheet for 20:4B, Cleaning Dentures, to practice this procedure. When you feel you have mastered this skill, sign the sheet and give it to your instructor for further action.*

✓ Final Checkpoint Using the criteria listed on the evaluation sheet, your instructor will grade your performance.

PROCEDURE 20:4C OBRA

Giving Special Mouth Care

Equipment and Supplies

Glycerine and lemon juice prepared swabs, tissues, emesis basin, bath towel or underpad (protective pad), cotton-tipped applicator sticks, water-soluble lubricant for lips, mouth solution as ordered (optional), plastic bag or plastic-lined waste can, disposable gloves, pen or pencil

Procedure

1. Check physician's orders or obtain authorization from your immediate supervisor.

2. Assemble equipment.

3. **C** Knock on the door and pause before entering. Introduce yourself. Identify the patient by checking the wristband and addressing the patient by name. Explain the procedure.

   NOTE: Semiconscious or unconscious patients can sometimes hear.

4. Close the door and screen the unit for privacy.

5. Wash hands. Put on gloves.

   ⚠ CAUTION: Observe standard precautions when contamination by body fluids is possible.

6. Elevate the bed to a comfortable working height. Raise the head of the bed if permissible. Lower the siderail on the side where you are working.

7. Turn the patient's head to the side toward you. Place the bath towel or underpad under the patient's head and chin.

8. Open the package of mouth swabs containing lemon and glycerine.

   NOTE: Toothettes are a common brand name of mouth swabs.

   NOTE: Some prepared swabs contain hydrogen peroxide in place of the lemon and glycerine.

9. Use the prepared swab to cleanse all parts of the patient's mouth (see figure 20-34). Do the teeth, gums, tongue, and roof of the mouth thoroughly. Work from the gums to the cutting edges of the teeth. Use a gentle motion.

10. Discard used swabs in the plastic bag. Use fresh swabs until the entire mouth is clean.

11. If the patient is able to help, have him or her rinse the mouth with mouthwash, if allowed. Then follow with a fresh-water rinse. If the patient is unconscious, use clean applicators moistened with clear water to rinse the patient's mouth. Use a soft towel to dry the area around the mouth.

    ⬠**CAUTION:** Never give an unconscious or semiconscious patient mouthwash or any other liquids.

12. Use the cotton-tipped applicator sticks to apply water-soluble lubricant lightly to the tongue and lips.

    NOTE: This keeps the tissues soft and moist.

13. Reposition the patient in correct body alignment.

14. Replace all equipment used. A tray with supplies for special mouth care is sometimes kept at the bedside. If so, restock supplies on the tray so it is always ready for use.

15. Observe all checkpoints before leaving the patient: elevate the siderails (if indicated), place the call signal within easy reach of the patient, lower the bed to its lowest level, leave the area neat and clean.

16. Remove gloves. Wash hands.

17. Report that special mouth care was given and/or record all required

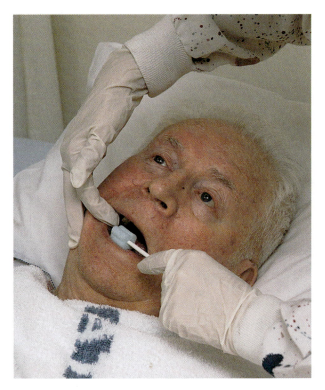

FIGURE 20-34 Use the prepared swab to cleanse all parts of the patient's mouth while providing special oral hygiene.

information on the patient's chart or the agency form, for example, date; time; special mouth care given, lips appear dry and chapped; and your signature and title. Immediately report any problems noted, including sores, irritated areas in the mouth, bleeding gums, and/or cuts.

Practice *Go to the workbook and use the evaluation sheet for 20:4C, Giving Special Mouth Care, to practice this procedure. When you feel you have mastered this skill, sign the sheet and give it to your instructor for further action.*

✔ **Final Checkpoint**   Using the criteria listed on the evaluation sheet, your instructor will grade your performance.

PROCEDURE 20:4D

OBRA

Administering Daily Hair Care

Equipment and Supplies

Comb and/or brush, towel, alcohol or petroleum jelly, pen or pencil

Procedure

1. Obtain proper authorization and assemble equipment.
2. **C** Knock on the door and pause before entering. Introduce yourself. Identify the patient. Explain the procedure.
3. Close the door and screen the unit to provide privacy.
4. Wash hands.
5. Elevate the bed to a comfortable working height. Raise the head of the bed, if permissible. Lower the siderail on the side where you are working.
6. Cover the pillow with the towel.
7. Ask the patient to move to the side of the bed nearest you. Assist as necessary.

   ⬡ CAUTION: Use proper body mechanics, including a broad base of support. Bend from hips.
8. Part or section the hair. Start at one side and work around to the other side.
9. Comb or brush the hair thoroughly. Keep the fingers of your hand between the scalp and comb whenever possible.

   NOTE: This prevents pulling and decreases discomfort.
10. Do each section completely. To do the back of the head, turn the patient or lift the head slightly.
11. If the hair is tangled or knotted, do the following:

    a. For dry hair, put a very small amount of petroleum jelly on your hands and rub it into the hair. Then, comb or brush gently. Start close to the scalp and work to the ends of the hair.

    b. For oily hair, put a small amount of alcohol or water on your hands and apply it to the hair. Comb or brush.

    ⬡ CAUTION: Be careful not to get alcohol near the patient's eyes.
12. When all areas of the hair have been brushed or combed, arrange the hair attractively

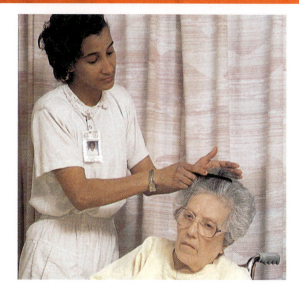

FIGURE 20-35 Arrange the hair attractively after brushing or combing it.

(see figure 20-35). After obtaining the patient's permission, braid long hair to prevent tangling.

   NOTE: Bands or hairpins can be used to hold the hair in place. Take care that they will *not* injure the scalp.
13. Throughout the entire procedure, closely observe the condition of the scalp and hair. Report any abnormal conditions immediately.
14. Observe all checkpoints before leaving the patient: position the patient in correct body alignment, elevate the siderails (if indicated), lower the bed to its lowest level, place the call signal and supplies within easy reach of the patient.
15. Clean and replace all equipment used. It is sometimes necessary to remove hair from the brush and comb. Wash the comb and brush in a mild, soapy solution. Rinse thoroughly. Leave the area neat and clean.
16. Wash hands.
17. **C** Report that hair care was given and/or record all required information on the patient's chart or the agency form, for example, date, time, hair combed and braided, and your signature and title. Note any unusual observations.

Practice *Go to the workbook and use the evaluation sheet for 20:4D, Administering Daily Hair Care, to practice this procedure. When you feel you have mastered this skill, sign the sheet and give it to your instructor for further action.*

 Final Checkpoint Using the criteria listed on the evaluation sheet, your instructor will grade your performance.

PROCEDURE 20:4E   OBRA

Providing Nail Care

Equipment and Supplies

Orange stick, emeryboard, nail clippers (if permitted), water and mild detergent in basin, towel, plastic bag, pen or pencil

⚖️ **CAUTION:** In some facilities, only licensed or advance practice personnel are permitted to cut fingernails. In addition, cutting nails may be prohibited for some patients, such as diabetics. It is important to learn and follow agency policy regarding nail care.

Procedure

1. Check physician's orders or obtain authorization from your immediate supervisor.
2. Assemble equipment.
3. **C** Knock on the door and pause before entering. Introduce yourself. Identify the patient. Explain the procedure.
4. Close the door and screen the unit to provide privacy.
5. Wash hands.
6. Elevate the bed to a comfortable working height. Lower the siderail on the side where you are working.
7. Clean the nails by soaking them in a solution of mild detergent and water at a temperature of 105° to 110°F (40.6° to 43.3°C). This loosens the dirt in the nailbeds.
   NOTE: Oil is sometimes used in place of detergent.
8. Use the slanted or blunt edge of the orange stick to clean dirt out of the nailbeds under the nails (see figure 20-36).

🛑 **CAUTION:** Using the pointed edge can result in a puncture wound. Using a metal instrument such as a nail file can roughen the nail, causing it to harbor dirt.

9. Use the emeryboard to file the nails and shorten them. Use short strokes. Work from the side of the nail to the top of the nail. Repeat for the opposite side.
   NOTE: Do *not* use a back-and-forth motion. Such a motion can split the nails.
10. If the fingernails are very long, and you are allowed to cut them, use nail clippers to cut the nails straight across. Be careful not to injure the skin around the nail. *Never* cut toenails. File them straight across.

🛑 **CAUTION:** Do *not* use scissors. They can cut the patient.

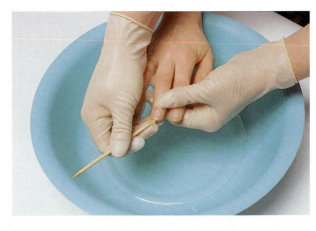

FIGURE 20-36 After soaking the nails, use the blunt edge of an orange stick to remove any dirt from under the nails.

11. When the nails are the correct length, use the smooth side of the emeryboard to eliminate rough edges. Make sure that the nails are filed straight across.

    ⚠ **CAUTION:** Pointed nails may cause injuries.

12. When the nails have been cleaned and filed short, apply lotion or another emollient, such as cold cream. This helps keep the nails and cuticles in good condition.

    NOTE: Nail care can be carried out for fingernails and toenails.

13. Apply lotion to the hands and/or feet.

14. Position the patient in correct body alignment.

15. Observe all checkpoints before leaving the patient: elevate the siderails (if indicated); place the call signal, water, and tissues within easy reach of the patient; lower the bed to its lowest level; leave the area neat and clean.

16. Clean and properly replace all equipment used.

17. Wash hands.

18. **C** Report that nail care has been given and/or record all required information on patient's chart or the agency form, for example, date, time, nail care given to fingers and toes, and your signature and title. Report any observations that may signify problems.

> **Practice** *Go to the workbook and use the evaluation sheet for 20:4E, Providing Nail Care, to practice this procedure. When you feel you have mastered this skill, sign the sheet and give it to your instructor for further action.*

✔ **Final Checkpoint** Using the criteria listed on the evaluation sheet, your instructor will grade your performance.

PROCEDURE 20:4F **OBRA**

Giving a Backrub

Equipment and Supplies

Lotion, bath towel, washcloth, soap and water, disposable gloves (if needed), basin, pen or pencil

Procedure

1. Obtain authorization from your immediate supervisor or check physician's orders.

   NOTE: Some patients *cannot* receive a backrub because of heart disease. A backrub would be too stimulating and affect the circulation. Other patients with burns, back injuries, back surgeries, and similar conditions may not be able to tolerate a backrub.

2. Assemble equipment.

3. Knock on the door and pause before entering. Introduce yourself. Identify the patient. Explain the procedure.

4. Close the door and screen the unit to provide privacy.

5. Wash hands. Put on gloves if contact with nonintact skin is possible.

6. Elevate the bed to a comfortable working height. Lower the siderail on the side where you are working.

7. Position the patient. The patient can lie on the abdomen (prone), or, if this is not comfortable, on his or her side, facing away from you.

8. Place a bath towel lengthwise next to the patient's body.

9. Fill the basin with water at a temperature of 105° to 110°F (40.6° to 43.3°C). Wash the patient's back thoroughly. Rinse and dry the back.

   NOTE: If the patient has had a bed bath, this step is not necessary, because the back has already been washed.

   NOTE: Be alert for any abnormal condition of the skin. Note any red areas, rash, sores, or cuts. Pay particular attention to bony parts.

10. Rub a small amount of lotion into your hands.

NOTE: This warms the solution slightly. The container of lotion can also be placed in a basin of warm water prior to use.

11. Begin at the base of the spine. Rub *up* the center of the back to the neck, around the shoulders, and down the sides of the back. Rub *down* over the buttocks, around, and circle back to starting point. Use long, soothing strokes (see figure 20-37). Use firm pressure on the upward strokes and gentle pressure on the downward strokes. Repeat this step four times.

    NOTE: See figure 20-38A.

    ⚠ **CAUTION:** Long nails may scratch the patient. File your nails short before giving a backrub.

    ⚠ **CAUTION:** Use proper body mechanics. Get close to the patient by bending at your hips and knees, and keep your back straight. Position your feet to provide a broad base of support.

12. Repeat the long, upward strokes but on the downward strokes, use a circular motion. Pay particular attention to bony prominences. Repeat this motion four times.

    NOTE: See figure 20-38B.

    ⚠ **CAUTION:** Take care not to rub skin tags as this might cause them to bleed. Also avoid massaging directly over reddened areas. Massage around these areas.

13. Repeat the long, upward strokes but on the downward strokes, use very small circular motions. Use the palm of your hand to apply firm pressure. Pay particular attention to the bony prominences. Do this motion one time.

    NOTE: See figure 20-38C.

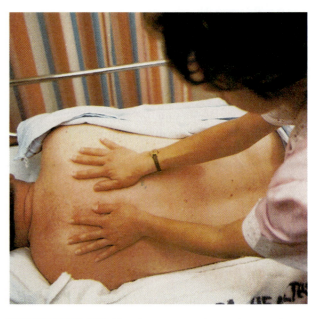

FIGURE 20-37 Use long, smooth strokes and firm pressure when giving a backrub.

14. Repeat the long, soothing strokes used initially. Do this for 3 to 5 minutes.

    NOTE: See figure 20-38D.

15. End the backrub with up-and-down motions over the entire back. Do this for 1 to 2 minutes. This provides relaxation after stimulation.

    NOTE: See figure 20-38E.

16. Dry the back thoroughly with the towel.

17. Straighten the bed linen. Change the patient's gown, if necessary.

18. Position the patient in good body alignment.

19. Observe all checkpoints before leaving the patient: elevate the siderails (if indicated), lower the bed to its lowest level, and place

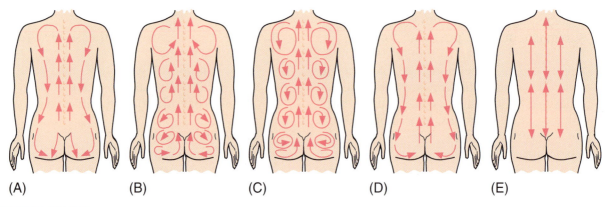

(A)   (B)   (C)   (D)   (E)

FIGURE 20-38 Motions for a backrub.

the call signal, water, and tissues within easy reach of patient.

20. Clean and replace all equipment. Leave the area neat and clean.
21. Remove gloves if worn. Wash hands.
22. **C** Report that a backrub was given and/or record all required information on patient's chart or the agency form, for example, date, time, back massage given, patient states he feels very relaxed; and your signature and title. Report any abnormal observations immediately.

Practice *Go to the workbook and complete the evaluation sheet for 20:4F, Giving a Backrub, to practice this procedure. When you feel you have mastered this skill, sign the sheet and give it to your instructor for further action.*

Final Checkpoint Using the criteria listed on the evaluation sheet, your instructor will grade your performance.

PROCEDURE 20:4G   OBRA

Shaving a Patient

Equipment and Supplies

Razor with blade, shaving lather, gauze pad, basin with water, towel, washcloth, mirror, electric razor (for some patients), aftershave lotion (optional), disposable gloves, sharps container, pen or pencil

Procedure

1. Obtain proper authorization.

   ! CAUTION: If the patient is taking anticoagulants to prevent blood clots, shaving may be prohibited or restricted to the use of an electric razor. Always check with your immediate supervisor to see if a patient is on anticoagulants before shaving a patient.

2. Assemble equipment. Examine the razor blade closely. Make sure there are no nicks or damaged edges. Carefully rub the razor blade over a folded gauze pad to check for damage.

3. **C** Knock on the door and pause before entering. Introduce yourself. Identify the patient. Explain the procedure.

4. Close the door and screen the unit to provide privacy.

5. Wash hands. Put on gloves if you are using a safety razor.

 CAUTION: Observe standard precautions. A safety razor can nick the skin and cause bleeding.

6. Elevate the bed to a comfortable working height. Raise the head of the bed. Lower the siderail on the side where you are working. Put the patient in a comfortable position. Arrange all needed equipment on the overbed table.

   NOTE: Allow the patient to help as much as possible.

7. Place a towel over the patient's chest and near the patient's shoulders.

8. Fill the basin with water at a temperature of 105° to 110°F (40.6° to 43.3°C). Use the washcloth to moisten the face.

9. Apply lather. Put it on your fingers first and then apply it to the patient's cheek.

   NOTE: It is usually best to do one area of the face at a time.

10. Start in front of the ear. Hold the skin taut (stretched tightly) to prevent cuts (see figure 20-39). Bring the razor down over the cheek and toward the chin.

    ! CAUTION: Always shave in the direction of hair growth.

11. Rinse the razor after each stroke. Repeat until the lather is removed and the area is shaved.

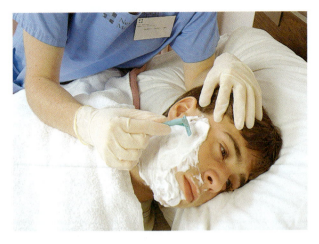

FIGURE 20-39 Hold the skin taut and shave in the direction of hair growth while shaving the patient.

12. Repeat steps 9 to 11 for the opposite cheek, the chin and neck area, and under the nose. When shaving the chin and under the nose, instruct the patient to hold the skin taut. Use firm, short strokes. Rinse the razor frequently.

> ⬣ **CAUTION:** If the skin is accidentally nicked, use a gauze pad to apply pressure directly over the area. Then, apply an antiseptic or follow the policy of your agency. Be sure to report the incident to your immediate supervisor.

> ☣ **CAUTION:** Observe standard precautions when controlling bleeding.

13. Wash and thoroughly dry the face and neck.
14. Apply aftershave lotion, if the patient desires.
15. To use an electric razor, read the instructions that come with the razor.
    a. Some patients prefer dry skin when using an electric razor. Others prefer to use a preshave lotion.
    b. Hold the skin taut before using the razor.
    c. Some razors require short circular strokes. Others require short strokes in the direction of hair growth.
    d. Shave all areas of the face.
    e. Wash and dry the face thoroughly when done.

f. Apply aftershave lotion, if desired.
g. Clean the razor thoroughly after use. Use a small brush (which usually comes with the razor) to clean out all the hair.

16. Observe all checkpoints before leaving the patient: position the patient in correct body alignment, elevate the siderails (if indicated), lower the bed to its lowest level, and place the call signal and supplies within easy reach of the patient.

17. Clean and replace all equipment used. Wash the safety razor thoroughly. Discard the blade in a puncture-resistant sharps container. If a disposable razor was used, discard the entire razor in the sharps container.

18. Remove gloves. Wash hands.

19. Report that the patient was shaved and/or record all required information on the patient's chart or the agency form, for example, date, time, shaved with electric razor, and your signature and title. Report any observations that may signify problems.

NOTE: Female patients sometimes want facial, underarm, and/or leg hair shaved. Obtain proper authorization before doing any of these procedures. Follow the same steps: check the razor, moisten the area, apply lather or a soapy solution, hold the skin taut, shave in the direction of hair growth, rinse the area, do small sections at a time, and finish by thoroughly washing and drying the areas shaved.

Practice *Go to the workbook and use the evaluation sheet for 20:4G, Shaving a Patient, to practice this procedure. When you feel you have mastered this skill, sign the sheet and give it to your instructor for further action.*

✔ **Final Checkpoint** Using the criteria listed on the evaluation sheet, your instructor will grade your performance.

PROCEDURE 20:4H

OBRA

Changing a Patient's Gown or Pajamas

Equipment and Supplies

Gown or pajamas, towel or bath blanket, linen hamper, cart, or bag; disposable gloves (if needed), pen or pencil

Procedure

1. Obtain proper authorization and assemble equipment.
2. **C** Knock on the door and pause before entering. Introduce yourself. Identify the patient. Explain the procedure to the patient.
3. Close the door and screen the unit to provide privacy.
4. Wash hands. If necessary, put on gloves.

    CAUTION: Wear gloves and observe standard precautions if the gown is contaminated by blood, body fluids, secretions, or excretions, such as drainage from an incision.
5. Elevate the bed to a comfortable working height. Lower the siderail on the side where you are working.

    NOTE: It is easier to change the patient's clothing if you first fold the bed covers to the foot of the bed and cover the patient with a bath blanket.
6. Loosen the patient's bedclothes:
    a. If the patient is wearing a hospital gown, untie the tapes by having the patient turn on his or her side or by reaching under the neck. Then, gently pull out any part of the gown that is under the patient.
    b. If the patient is wearing a gown of her own, loosen any buttons or ties. Gently ease the gown upward from the hemline to the neck. Prevent unnecessary exposure by using the towel or bath blanket, as necessary.
    c. If the patient is wearing pajamas, first untie or unbutton the pants at the waist. Gently ease the pants down over the legs

and feet. Use the towel or bath blanket to drape the patient. Avoid exposing the patient. Unbutton the pajama top.

7. Take off the soiled clothing, one sleeve at a time. Gently grasp the edge of the sleeve near the shoulder. Ease the arm out. Do the far arm first. If the patient has an affected arm (injured, paralyzed, weak, etc.) or is receiving an intravenous (IV) infusion, remove the sleeve from the unaffected arm first and from the affected arm or arm with the IV second. Place the soiled clothing on a chair.

    NOTE: If an IV is in place, ease the sleeve off of the upper arm, taking care not to disturb the infusion site, where the needle is inserted. Then, gently ease the sleeve over the tubing by keeping your hand and arm in the sleeve; holding the solution bottle above the infusion site; and passing the container through the sleeve (see figure 20-40A to C).

    NOTE: Many facilities use gowns that open at the shoulder when a patient has an IV. The gown is positioned over the shoulder and closed with snaps, ties, or Velcro strips.
8. Unfold the clean gown or pajama top and place it over the patient.
9. Put the patient's arms into the sleeves one at a time. Gather the sleeve of the gown or pajama top into your hands. Then put your arm through the sleeve, take the patient's hand in yours, and slip the sleeve up the patient's wrist and arm and to the shoulder.

    NOTE: If one arm is affected or has an IV, do this arm first. This places less strain on the arm. For an IV, pass the solution container and tubing through the sleeve first. Keep the solution container above the level of the infusion site at all times.

    CAUTION: Sometimes, a sleeve cannot be placed because of an IV infusion machine, bulky dressing, or other similar problem. If this is the case, leave the sleeve

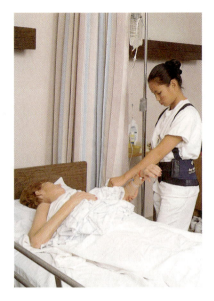

FIGURE 20-40A After removing the gown from the unaffected arm, gather the gown together on the arm with the IV infusion site.

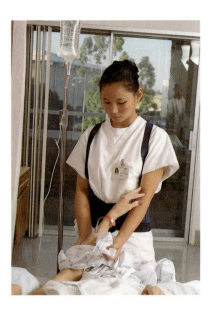

FIGURE 20-40B Ease the gown over the IV tubing, taking care to prevent displacement of the tubing.

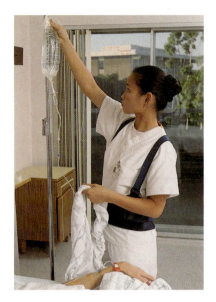

FIGURE 20-40C Keeping the IV container above the level of the infusion site, pass the IV container through the arm of the gown.

off of the one arm, or use a gown that opens at the shoulders.

10. Pull the body of the gown down over the patient or position the pajama top correctly. Make sure that the gown or top is smooth and free from wrinkles or folds.

11. Tie the tapes or ties on the gown, or button the buttons on the pajama top. Make sure that the tied knot is *not* on a bony prominence.

> ⚠ **CAUTION:** Knots or wrinkles can lead to pressure ulcers.
>
> **NOTE:** Avoid exposing the patient during the procedure. Continue to use the towel or bath blanket to drape the patient.

12. If the patient is wearing pajamas, put on the pants after the pajama top. Gently ease the pants over the feet and up the legs. Adjust them into position at the waist. Use the towel or bath blanket to cover the patient during this procedure. Tie or button the pants. Make sure the pants are smooth and free from wrinkles or folds.

13. Observe all checkpoints before leaving the patient: position the patient comfortably and in good body alignment; elevate the siderails (if indicated); place the call signal, water, and supplies within easy reach of the patient; lower the bed to its lowest level; leave the area neat and clean.

14. Place a soiled hospital gown in the laundry hamper or bag. Place a soiled personal gown or pajamas in a drawer, the closet, or other location specified by patient.

> ☣ **CAUTION:** If the gown is contaminated with blood or body fluids, follow agency policy for handling contaminated linen.

15. Remove gloves, if worn. Wash hands thoroughly.

16. Report that the patient's gown has been changed and/or record all required information on the patient's chart or the agency form, for example, date, time, pajamas changed, and your signature and title. Report any observations that may signify problems.

Practice *Go to the workbook and use the evaluation sheet for 20:4H, Changing a Patient's Gown or Pajamas, to practice this procedure. When you feel you have mastered this skill, sign the sheet and give it to your instructor for further action.*

✔ **Final Checkpoint** Using the criteria listed on the evaluation sheet, your instructor will grade your performance.

PROCEDURE 20:41
Giving a Complete Bed Bath

OBRA

Equipment and Supplies

Bed linen (complete set); laundry hamper, bag, or cart; bath blanket; two to three washcloths; face towel; one to two bath towels; soap and soap dish; basin; bath thermometer; clean gown or pajamas; supplies for hair care; supplies for nail care; shaving supplies; oral hygiene supplies; lotion; disposable gloves; pen or pencil

Procedure

1. Obtain authorization from your immediate supervisor or check physician's orders to obtain authorization for the procedure.
2. Assemble equipment.
3. **C** Knock on the door and pause before entering. Introduce yourself. Identify the patient. Explain the procedure.
4. Screen the unit. Close all doors and windows. Eliminate drafts. Adjust the thermostat to a comfortable room temperature, if possible.
5. Wash hands.
   NOTE: Gloves can be put on either at this point or during parts of the procedure when contact with blood and body fluids is likely, such as when administering oral hygiene and perineal care. If the patient has a draining wound or the patient's skin is soiled with urine and feces, gloves must be worn. Observe standard precautions.
6. Arrange all equipment conveniently. Put linen on the chair in the order of use. Position the laundry bag, hamper, or cart conveniently.
   NOTE: Proper preparation saves time and energy.
7. Elevate the bed to a comfortable working height. Lower the siderail on the side where you are working.
8. Replace the top linen with a bath blanket (see figure 20-41). If the same linen is to be reused, fanfold it to the bottom of the bed. If the linen is to be replaced, remove it and place in the hamper.
9. Provide oral hygiene as previously instructed.
10. Shave the male patient, if necessary.

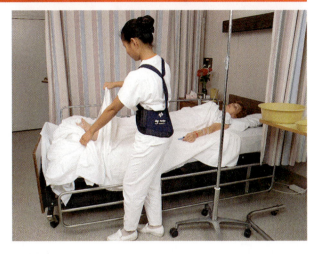

FIGURE 20-41 Replace the top linen with a bath blanket.

NOTE: Some patients prefer to be shaved after the face is washed.

11. Fill the basin approximately two-thirds full with warm water at a temperature of 105° to 110°F (40.6° to 43.3°C). Check the temperature with a bath thermometer.
12. Help the patient move to the side of the bed nearest to you. Remove the patient's bedclothes as previously instructed.
13. Place a towel over the upper edge of the bath blanket.
14. With the washcloth, form a mitten around your hand. Tuck in the loose edges (see figure 20-42).
    NOTE: This prevents the loose edges of the cloth from striking the patient as you work. It also keeps water from dripping on the patient and the bed.
15. Wet the washcloth and squeeze out excess water. Wash the patient's eyes first. Start at the inner area and wash to the outside of the eye. Use a different section of the cloth when you wash the second eye.
16. Rinse the washcloth. Ask whether the patient uses soap on the face and use soap if desired. Wash the face, neck, and ears. Rinse. Dry well.
17. Place a bath towel lengthwise under the patient's arm that is farthest from you. Place the basin of water on the bed and on the towel, at the lower end. Put the patient's

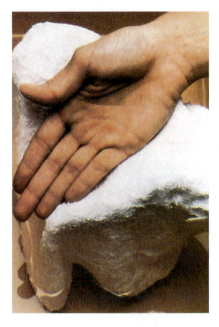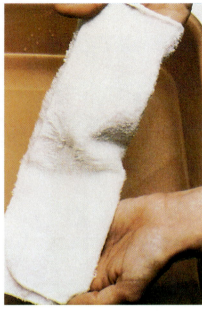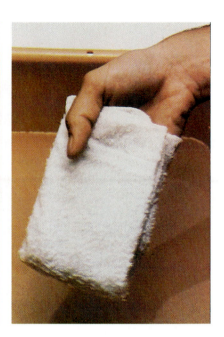

FIGURE 20-42 Fold the washcloth to form a bath mitten around your hand.

hand and nails into the water. Wash, rinse, and dry the arm, from the axilla to the hand. Repeat for the other arm.

NOTE: If the patient desires deodorant, it can be applied after the axillae are clean and dry.

18. Provide nail care as previously instructed.
19. Put a bath towel over the patient's chest. Fold the bath blanket down to the patient's waist.
20. Wash, rinse, and dry the chest and breasts (see figure 20-43). Pay particular attention to the areas under a female's breasts. Dry these areas thoroughly.

NOTE: A small amount of lotion may be placed under the breasts. Put the lotion in your hand first and then apply it smoothly to the skin.

21. Turn the bath towel lengthwise to cover the patient's chest and abdomen. Fold the bath blanket down to the pubic area. Wash, rinse, and dry the abdomen. Replace the bath blanket. Remove the towel.
22. Fold the bath blanket up to expose the patient's leg that is farthest from you. Place a towel lengthwise under the leg and foot. Place the basin on the bed and on top of the towel. Place the patient's foot in the basin by flexing the leg at the knee. Wash and rinse the leg and foot, remove the basin, and dry the leg and foot. Repeat for the other leg.

NOTE: Support the patient's leg and foot with your hand and lower arm when moving

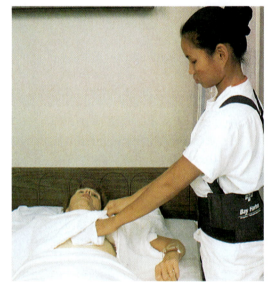

FIGURE 20-43 Avoid exposing the patient when washing the breasts.

the foot in and out of the basin (see figure 20-44).

23. Provide nail care to the toes, as needed. *Never* cut the toenails. File them straight across. Apply lotion to the feet, if the skin is dry.

CAUTION: Observe for any color changes or irritated areas that may signify problems.

24. Elevate the siderail. Change the water in the basin.

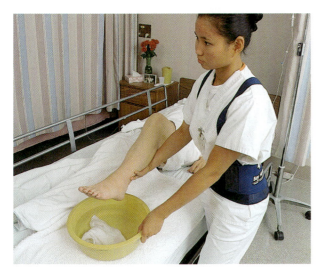

FIGURE 20-44 Support the leg when placing the patient's foot in the basin.

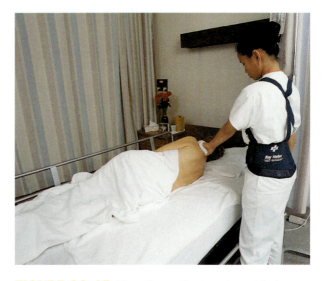

FIGURE 20-45 Turn the patient on her side to wash, rinse, and dry the back.

NOTE: Water should always be changed at this point in the bath. However, it can be changed anytime it becomes too cool, dirty, or soapy.

25. Lower the siderail.
26. Turn the patient on his or her side or into the prone position. Place the towel lengthwise on the bed and along the patient's back. Wash, rinse, and dry the entire back (see figure 20-45).

    CAUTION: Observe the back closely for any changes that may signify problems. Pay particular attention to bony areas.
27. Give a backrub as previously instructed.
28. Help the patient turn onto his or her back. Keep the patient draped with the bath blanket.
29. If the patient is able to wash the perineal area, place the basin with water, the soap, the washcloth, the towel, and the call signal within easy reach. Raise the siderail and wait outside the unit while the patient completes this procedure.
30. If the patient is not able to wash the perineal area, put on gloves. Drape and position the patient in the dorsal recumbent position. Put a towel or disposable underpad under the patient's buttocks and upper legs. For a female patient, always wash from the front to the back, or rectal, area. Separate the labia, or lips, and cleanse the area thoroughly with a front-to-back motion (see figure 20-46). Use a clean area of the washcloth or rinse the cloth between each wipe. For a

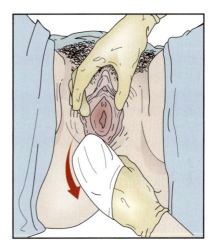

FIGURE 20-46 To provide perineal care to a female, separate the labia and cleanse the area with a front-to-back motion.

male patient, cleanse the tip of the penis using a circular motion and starting at the urinary meatus and working outward. Cleanse the penis from top to bottom (see figure 20-47A). If the male is not circumcised, gently draw the foreskin back to wash the area (see figure 20-47B). After rinsing and drying the area, gently return the foreskin to its normal position. Wash the scrotal area, taking care to clean under the scrotum. To wash the rectal area, turn the male patient on his side. Rinse and dry all areas thoroughly on both the male and female. When the perineal area is clean, reposition the patient on his or her back and remove

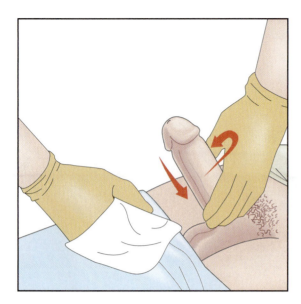

FIGURE 20-47A Use a circular motion to cleanse the penis from the top to the base.

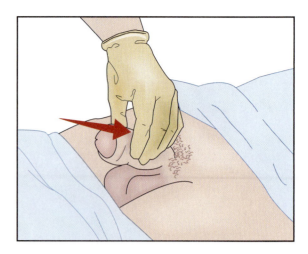

FIGURE 20-47B If the male is not circumcised, gently draw the foreskin back to wash the area. After rinsing and drying the area, gently return the foreskin to its normal position.

the towel or underpad from under the buttocks. Remove gloves and wash hands.

NOTE: In some facilities, disposable washcloths or large gauze pads are used to clean the perineal area. These are discarded in an infectious-waste bag and a fresh washcloth or pad is used for each area. Follow agency policy.

31. Place clean bedclothes on the patient as previously instructed.
32. Provide hair care as previously taught.
33. Make the bed according to Procedure 20:3B, Making an Occupied Bed.
34. Observe all checkpoints before leaving the patient: position the patient in correct body alignment; elevate the siderails (if indicated); lower the bed to its lowest level; place the call signal, water, tissues, and supplies within easy reach of the patient.
35. Clean and replace all equipment. Wash the emesis basin and bath basin thoroughly.
36. Put the bag or hamper of dirty linen in the proper area or send it to the laundry according to agency policy. Replace all remaining equipment.

37. Remove gloves, if worn. Wash hands.
38. Report that a complete bed bath was given and/or record all required information on the patient's chart or the agency form, for example, date; time; complete bed bath given, occupied bed made, patient stated he was tired at end of procedure; and your signature and title. Report any observations that may signify problems.

Practice *Go to the workbook and use the evaluation sheet for 20:4I, Giving a Complete Bed Bath, to practice this procedure. When you feel you have mastered this skill, sign the sheet and give it to your instructor for further action.*

✓ **Final Checkpoint** Using the criteria listed on the evaluation sheet, your instructor will grade your performance.

PROCEDURE 20:4J   **OBRA**

Helping a Patient Take a Tub Bath or Shower

Equipment and Supplies

Washcloth, two to three towels, soap and soap dish, bathmat, rubber mat, bath thermometer, chair or stool (placed in bath area), bedclothes, robe, slippers, disposable gloves, pen or pencil

Procedure

1. Check physician's orders or obtain authorization from your immediate supervisor. A physician's order is generally required before a tub bath or shower is allowed, unless the patient is considered able to take care of this need (for example, in the case of a totally ambulatory patient).

2. Assemble equipment.

3. **C** Knock on the door and pause before entering. Introduce yourself. Identify the patient. Also, check to make sure the time is appropriate for taking a shower or bath.

   NOTE: If the patient has visitors or is receiving another treatment, time and energy would be wasted in preparing the tub or shower.

4. Wash hands. Put on gloves if necessary.

   CAUTION: Wear gloves and observe standard precautions if contact with blood, body fluids, secretions, or excretions is possible.

5. Take the supplies to the bath or shower area. Make sure the tub or shower is clean. If it is dirty, put on gloves to clean the tub or shower. Wipe it with a disinfectant (see figure 20-48). When the tub or shower is clean, remove gloves and wash your hands. If nonskid strips are not present, put a rubber mat in the tub or shower to prevent the patient from slipping. Place the bathmat on the floor. Fill the tub half full with water at 105°F, or 40.6°C.

6. Help the patient put on a robe and slippers. Take the patient to the bath or shower area.

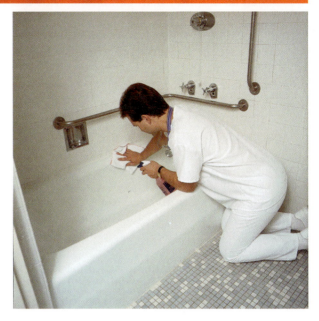

FIGURE 20-48 The tub should be cleaned and wiped with a disinfectant before and after each use.

   CAUTION: Use a wheelchair, if necessary.

7. If necessary, help the patient undress. Help the patient into the tub or shower.

   CAUTION: Before the patient enters the shower, adjust the temperature of the shower water.

8. If necessary, remain with the patient and assist with the bath or shower. If the patient can manage without assistance, explain how to use the emergency call signal, leave the room, and check on the patient at frequent intervals.

   CAUTION: If the patient shows any signs of weakness or dizziness, use the call button to get help. If the patient is in a tub, remove the plug and let the water drain. If the patient is in a shower, turn off the shower and seat the patient in the chair. Keep the patient covered with a towel or bath blanket to prevent chilling.

! **CAUTION:** Most long-term care facilities require that you always stay with the patient.

NOTE: In a home care situation, a small bell (such as a dinner bell) can be left with the patient.

9. When the patient is finished bathing, help as needed. Dry all areas of the patient's body thoroughly. Put clean bedclothes or clothing on the patient.

10. Assist the patient back to the bedside. Administer a backrub. Help with hair or nail care, if necessary.

NOTE: Observe all checkpoints before leaving the patient: position the patient in correct body alignment, elevate the siderails (if indicated), lower the bed to its lowest level, place the call signal and supplies within easy reach of the patient, and leave the area neat and clean.

11. Return to the bath or shower area. Replace all supplies and equipment used. Put on gloves. Clean the tub or shower thoroughly and wipe with a disinfectant.

12. Remove gloves. Wash hands.

13. **C** Report that a tub bath or shower was given and/or record all required information on the patient's chart or the agency form, for example, date; time; assisted with tub bath, patient tolerated procedure well; and your signature and title. Report any observations that may signify problems.

Practice *Go to the workbook and use the evaluation sheet for 20:4J, Helping a Patient Take a Tub Bath or Shower, to practice this procedure. When you feel you have mastered this skill, sign the sheet and give it to your instructor for further action.*

✔ **Final Checkpoint** Using the criteria listed on the evaluation sheet, your instructor will grade your performance.

20:5 INFORMATION
Measuring and Recording Intake and Output

OBRA A record of how much fluid is taken in and eliminated by a patient often helps a physician provide care to the patient. A large part of the body is fluid, so there must be a balance between the amount of fluid taken into the body and the amount lost from the body. In a healthy individual, the fluid balance is usually maintained by the body structures. However, if an individual has heart or kidney disease, or loses large amounts of fluids through vomiting, diarrhea, excessive perspiration, or bleeding, the fluid balance may be abnormal. If excessive fluid is retained by the body, swelling, or **edema,** results. If excessive fluid is lost from the body, **dehydration**

occurs. Either condition can lead to death if not treated. In such cases, physicians may order that a record be kept of all fluids taken in and discharged from the body. This record is usually called an *intake and output (I & O) record.*

An **intake and output** record is a means of recording all fluids a person takes in and eliminates during a certain period of time. Each agency has its own form, but most contain the following information:

Intake refers to all fluids taken in by the patient. The following routes and liquids must be considered:

◆ *Oral* is intake by way of the mouth. Liquids taken in orally include water, coffee, tea, milk, juices, and other beverages. In addition, soups, gelatin, ice cream, and other similar foods that are liquid at room temperature also qualify for measurement. The nurse assistant often measures and records or reports these amounts.

◆ *Tube feedings,* or *enteral feedings,* are recorded as oral intake or in a special column. They are used for patients who are unable to swallow, for unconscious or comatose patients, or when certain digestive diseases occur. The solution given contains all of the nutrients required by the body and is more nourishing than an intravenous feeding. Enteral feedings may be administered through a nasogastric tube or a gastrostomy tube. A *nasogastric tube* is a tube inserted through the nose, down the esophagus, and into the stomach (see figure 20-49A). A *gastrostomy tube* is surgically inserted through the abdominal skin and into the stomach (see figure 20-49B). A feeding pump is usually used to administer the solution (see figure 20-49C). A nurse or another legally authorized team member will administer the enteral feeding. The nurse assistant must keep the patient's head elevated 30° to 45° during the feeding and for approximately 30 to 60 minutes after the feeding; make sure there are no kinks in the tubing; use extreme caution when turning or positioning the patient to avoid dislodging the tubing; provide frequent oral hygiene; and notify the nurse immediately if the alarm sounds on the feeding pump, if the solution is not flowing through the tubing, or if the solution container is low or empty.

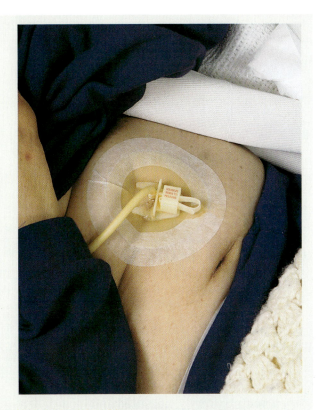

FIGURE 20-49B A gastrostomy tube is surgically inserted through the abdominal skin and into the stomach.

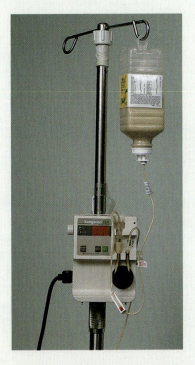

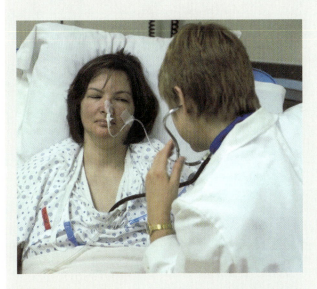

FIGURE 20-49A A nasogastric tube is inserted through the nose, down the esophagus, and into the stomach.

FIGURE 20-49C A feeding pump is usually used to administer tube or enteral feedings.

◆ *Intravenous (IV)* refers to fluids given into a vein. Blood units, plasma, and other intravenous solutions are measured. This measurement is the responsibility of the nurse or another legally authorized team member.

◆ *Irrigation* refers to fluid placed into tubes that have been inserted in the body. Any fluid removed is not considered to be intake and is not recorded. For example, if a nasogastric tube is irrigated with 80 milliliters of solution and the same exact amount is immediately drawn back out of the tube, this is not recorded as intake. However, if 60 milliliters is withdrawn, the intake is recorded as 20 milliliters (80 minus 60 is 20). This measurement is also the responsibility of the nurse or another legally authorized team member.

Output refers to all fluids eliminated by the patient. The following routes and liquids must be considered:

◆ *Bowel movement (BM):* Liquid bowel movements are usually measured and recorded. A solid or formed BM is usually noted in the *remarks* column or described under *feces*. The nurse assistant may measure and record or report this elimination.

◆ *Emesis:* Anything that is vomited is measured and recorded. Color, type, and other facts are usually noted in the *remarks* column. The nurse assistant often measures and records or reports emesis.

◆ *Urine:* All urine voided or drained via a catheter is measured and recorded. This measurement may be the responsibility of the nurse assistant.

◆ *Irrigation:* Any irrigation or suction drainage, including drainage from nasogastric tubes, hemo-vacs, chest tubes, and other drainage tubes, is measured (see figure 20-50). The type, amount, color, and other facts are noted in the *remarks* column. If an irrigating solution is injected into a tube and more solution returns, the excess amount is considered output. This measurement is the responsibility of the nurse or another legally authorized team member.

Records must be accurate. All amounts must be measured in graduates. A *graduate* is a container that is made of plastic or stainless steel and has calibrations for milliliters/cubic centimeters and/or ounces on the side. It is similar to a measuring cup and is used to obtain accurate measurements. The graduate should be held at eye level to accurately record amounts (see figure 20-51). In addition, care must be taken when adding or totaling the columns on the I&O record. Most records contain totals for 8-hour and 24-hour periods. See figure 20-52 on the next page and study it carefully.

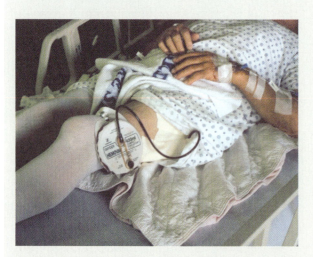

FIGURE 20-50 Suction drainage from a hemovac, one type of wound drainage system, is recorded as irrigation output on an I&O record.

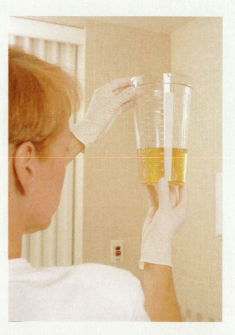

FIGURE 20-51 Hold the graduate at eye level to obtain an accurate measurement.

INTAKE AND OUTPUT RECORD

Family Name	First Name	Attending Physician	Room No.	Hosp. No.
JOHNSON, ROBERT		DR. MIKE SMITH	238	54-3201

Date 9/30 TIME	INTAKE Oral	I.V.	Blood		OUTPUT Urine	Tube	Emesis	Feces		OTHER				REMARKS
7 - 8 a.m.	100													
8 - 9 a.m.	320						200							EMESIS– GREEN LIQUID
9 - 10 a.m.					420									
10 - 11 a.m.	100													
11 - 12 noon			10											NG IRRIGATION NS
12 - 1 p.m.	240				310									
1 - 2 p.m.		850				200								NASOGASTRIC GOLD–BROWN
2 - 3 p.m.	60													
8 HOUR TOTAL	820	850		10	730	200	200							
3 - 4 p.m.														
4 - 5 p.m.	320	150						120						BROWN LIQUID
5 - 6 p.m.					280									
6 - 7 p.m.	180													
7 - 8 p.m.														
8 - 9 p.m.	100													
9 - 10 p.m.		500				240								NASOGASTRIC BROWNISH
10 - 11 p.m.					310									
8 HOUR TOTAL	600	650			590	240		120						
11 - 12 p.m.														
12 - 1 a.m.			10											NG IRRIGATION NS
1 - 2 a.m.	180				420									
2 - 3 a.m.														
3 - 4 a.m.							650							EMESIS– GREEN LIQUID
4 - 5 a.m.														
5 - 6 a.m.		600				180								NASOGASTRIC GOLD–BROWN
6 - 7 a.m.	100				380									
8 HOUR TOTAL	280	600		10	800	180	650							
24 HOUR TOTAL	1700	2100		20	2120	620	850	120						
	TOTAL INTAKE 3820				TOTAL OUTPUT 3170									

FIGURE 20-52 A sample intake and output (I&O) record.

For I&O records, fluids are usually measured in metric units. Approximate equivalents for units of the metric system are as follows:

Metric		Household
1 cc or 1 mL	=	15 gtts (drops)
5 mL or cc	=	1 tsp (teaspoon)
15 mL or cc	=	1 tbsp (tablespoon)
30 mL or cc	=	1 oz (ounce)
240 mL or cc	=	1 cup (8 oz)
500 mL or cc	=	1 pt (pint) (16 ounces)
1,000 mL or cc	=	1 qt (quart) (32 oz)

NOTE: Remember, 1 cubic centimeter and 1 milliliter are the same amount. Therefore, 30 cubic centimeters equals 30 milliliters.

Various agencies have different policies for recording I&O. In some agencies, the I&O record is kept at the bedside. Team members note the I&O of the patient and record the measurements on the record. At times, the patient is even taught to measure and write down the amounts. In other agencies, the I&O record is kept on the patient's chart. Measurements are noted on a slip of paper and reported. The nurse, unit secretary or clerk, or an authorized team member then records the information on the chart's I&O form. Ascertain and follow the policy of your agency.

C Patients should be given careful instructions when an I&O record is being kept. The patient must inform health care providers when he or she drinks fluids not provided by the health care team. Sometimes, the patient records how many glasses of water or other liquids are consumed. Other times, the health care worker fills a water pitcher and then checks the quantity remaining before refilling the pitcher. The worker then subtracts this quantity from the total amount originally in the pitcher and records the difference as water intake. To avoid missing any amounts of oral intake, the health care worker must also think about fluid intake every time a glass, cup, or water pitcher is removed from the unit. If visitors bring milkshakes or other liquids, the amounts of these must also be recorded. Females should be asked to urinate in a bedpan or to use a special urine collector that can be placed under the seat on the toilet (see figure 20-53). The female must be

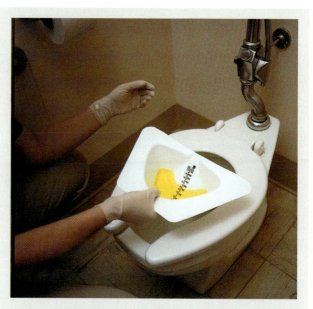

FIGURE 20-53 A specimen collector to collect urine can be placed under the seat on the toilet.

told not to place toilet tissue or expel a bowel movement into the bedpan or urine collector. Males can be told to use a urinal. If patients are given correct instructions, they can cooperate, and accurate records can be maintained.

Standard precautions (discussed in Unit 13:3) must be followed at all times when body fluids are measured for I&O records. Body fluids include urine, emesis, liquid bowel movements, and drainage. Gloves must be worn while the fluids are being measured and discarded. Hands must be washed frequently and must always be washed immediately after gloves are removed. If splashing or spraying of fluids is possible, a mask, eye protection, and gown must be worn. The graduate or measuring device for monitoring a patient's output must be used for that patient only. It should be discarded or sterilized according to agency policy when output is no longer measured. Any areas contaminated by body fluids when measurements are being obtained must be wiped with a disinfectant. The health care provider must constantly take steps to prevent the spread of infection.

STUDENT: *Go to the workbook and complete the assignment sheet for 20:5A, Measuring Intake and Output. Then return and continue with the procedure.*

PROCEDURE 20:5

OBRA

Recording Intake and Output

NOTE: Competency will be evaluated by way of successful completion of several assignment sheets rather than by way of the usual evaluation sheet. (Follow the procedure steps to complete the assignment sheets.)

Equipment and Supplies

Assignment sheets for this topic (assignment sheets 1 to 5 for 20:5B), scrap paper, pen

Procedure

1. Review the preceding Information section, figure 20-52, and your completed assignment sheet for 20:5A, Measuring Intake and Output.
2. Assemble equipment.
3. Go to the workbook and carefully read assignment sheet 1 for 20:5B, Recording Intake and Output. *It will be part of this procedure.* After reading it through once, do the assignment based on the following guidelines and instructions.
4. Use a pen to record all information.
   a. Find the correct time line on the I&O record.
   b. Find the correct column: for example, *oral intake* or *urine output.*
   c. Record the amounts stated on the assignment sheet in the correct block. Number of cubic centimeters (cc) for a coffee cup and other containers are at the top of the I&O sheet.
5. When the information on the assignment sheet has been recorded in the appropriate places on the I&O record, recheck all areas of the record.
6. Make sure you have entered observations about color, type, and other facts in the *remarks* columns. Make sure the observations are on the right time lines (by checking the times against the assignment sheet).

7. Under *intake,* add each column for 8-hour totals. For example, add all of the amounts for oral intake between 7 AM and 3 PM. Do the same for each of the other columns for all three 8-hour periods.

   ⚠ CAUTION: Recheck your addition. The totals must be accurate.

8. Now add the three 8-hour totals together for each column (7 AM to 6 AM) to get the 24-hour total at the bottom of the page. Do this for each column in *intake* and each column in *output.*

   NOTE: You should have a 24-hour total for oral intake and another total for IV intake.

9. Recheck all work.

   NOTE: If you make an error, draw one red line through the error. Place your initials in red by the error line. Then use a blue or black pen to write the correct information on the record.

10. Give the paper to your instructor for grading. Replace all equipment used.

    NOTE: The record must be neat and legible. All figures must be recorded in metric units.

Practice *Your instructor will grade assignment sheet 1 for 20:5B, Recording Intake and Output. When it is returned to you, note all comments or corrections. Then complete assignment sheet 2 for 20:5B, Recording Intake and Output. Give it to your instructor to grade. Again note comments or corrections. Repeat the process for assignment sheets 3, 4, and 5.*

✔ **Final Checkpoint** Based on the grades earned on the completed assignment sheets, your instructor will grade your performance.

20:6 INFORMATION
Feeding a Patient

OBRA Good nutrition is an important part of a patient's treatment. It may be one of your responsibilities to make mealtimes as pleasant as possible for the patient. Mealtimes are often regarded as a time for social interaction. Most people prefer to eat with others. People who eat alone often have poor appetites and poor nutrition. In long-term care facilities, patients are encouraged to eat in the dining room. This provides an opportunity for social interaction with others. If a patient is confined to bed, it is important to talk with the patient while serving the food tray or feeding the patient.

Proper mealtime preparation is important. If the patient is ready to eat when the tray arrives, mealtime is likely to be more pleasant. Preparation before the tray is delivered includes:

◆ Offering the bedpan or urinal or assisting the patient to the bathroom. Clear the room of any offensive odors by using a deodorizer or opening a window.

◆ Allowing the patient to wash his or her hands and face, if desired.

◆ Providing oral hygiene, if desired. Many individuals want to brush their teeth before meals, especially before breakfast.

◆ Positioning the patient comfortably and in a sitting position, if possible.

◆ Clearing the overbed table and positioning it for the tray.

◆ Removing objects such as an emesis basin or bedpan from the patient's view. Place such objects in the bedside stand, if they will not be needed.

If a meal will be delayed because of X-rays or other treatments, be sure to explain this to the patient.

Check the tray carefully against the patient's name and room number and the type of diet ordered (see figure 20-54A). If anything seems out of place (for example, a salt shaker provided with a salt-free diet, or sugar with a diabetic diet), check with your immediate supervisor or the dietitian. Never add any food to the tray without checking the diet order first.

Allow patients to feed themselves whenever possible. If necessary, assist by cutting meat, opening beverage cartons, and buttering bread (see figure 20-54B). If a patient is blind or visually impaired, tell the patient what food is on the plate by comparing the plate to a clock. For example, say, "Swiss steak is at 12 o'clock, peas and carrots are at 4 o'clock, and mashed potatoes are at 9 o'clock." Make sure all food and utensils are conveniently placed.

Before feeding any patient, test the temperature of all hot foods. A small amount can be placed on your wrist to check temperature. Never blow on hot food to cool it.

Points to observe when feeding a patient include:

◆ Alternate the foods by giving sips of liquids between solid foods.

◆ Use straws for liquids unless the patient has *dysphagia* (difficulty in swallowing). Straws can force liquids down the throat faster and cause choking. A product called "Thick-It" can be added to liquids to solidify them slightly and make them easier to swallow. A physician or dietitian must approve the use of this product.

◆ Hold the spoon or fork at right angles to the patient's mouth so you are feeding the patient from the tip of the utensil.

◆ Encourage the patient to eat as much as possible.

◆ Provide a relaxed, unhurried atmosphere.

◆ Give the patient sufficient time to chew the food.

C Observe how much the patient eats so that a record of nutritional intake can be kept (see figure 20-55). If the patient does not like certain foods on the tray, ask your immediate supervisor or the dietitian whether a substitute can be provided. Record intake if an intake and output (I&O) record is being kept for the patient.

⚠ CAUTION: Always be alert to signs of choking while feeding a patient. Take every effort to prevent choking by feeding small

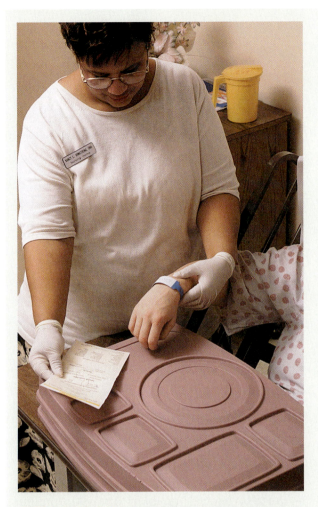

FIGURE 20-54A Check the food tray carefully against the patient's name, room number, and type of diet ordered.

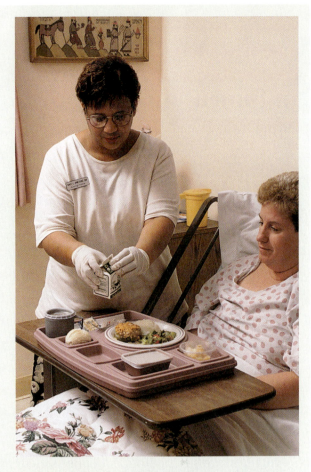

FIGURE 20-54B Assist the patient by cutting meat, opening beverage cartons, and positioning the food conveniently.

quantities, allowing the patient time to chew and swallow, and providing liquids to keep the mouth moist and make chewing and swallowing easier. If a patient had a stroke, one side of the mouth may be affected. As you feed the patient, direct food to the unaffected side. Watch the patient's throat to check swallowing. Watch for food that may be lodged in the affected side of the mouth. If a patient chokes on food, be prepared to provide abdominal thrusts (Heimlich maneuver) as described in Procedures 15:2E and 15:2F, CPR for Conscious and Unconscious Choking Victims.

STUDENT: *Go to the workbook and complete the assignment sheet for 20:6, Feeding a Patient. Then return and continue with the procedure.*

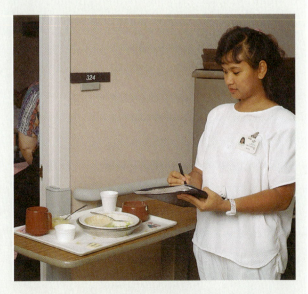

FIGURE 20-55 It is important to observe how much a patient eats so that a record of nutritional intake can be maintained.

PROCEDURE 20:6

OBRA

Feeding a Patient

Equipment and Supplies

Food tray with diet card, flex straws, towel, pen or pencil

Procedure

1. Obtain proper authorization and assemble equipment.
2. **C** Knock on the door and pause before entering. Introduce yourself. Identify the patient. Explain that it is almost time to eat. Close the door and screen the unit to provide privacy.
3. Wash hands. Put on gloves if contact with oral fluids is possible.
4. Prepare the patient for mealtime. Provide oral hygiene, if desired. Help the patient use the bedpan, as needed. Position the patient in a sitting position, if permitted. Allow the patient to wash his or her hands and face. Position the overbed table.

   NOTE: Make sure the patient is not scheduled for X-ray or any other treatment requiring the tray to be withheld.
5. Check the tray. Make sure the diet card, patient's name, and food are correct. Do not add anything to the tray without first checking with your supervisor.

   NOTE: If any foods seem to be incorrect for the diet ordered, check immediately with your supervisor.
6. Place the tray on the overbed table. Place a towel or napkin under the patient's chin.
7. If the patient can feed him- or herself, arrange all food and silverware conveniently. Cut meat, butter bread, and open beverage cartons.
8. To feed a patient, proceed as follows:
   a. Follow the patient's preference for the order of foods eaten.
   b. Test hot liquids on your wrist before giving them to the patient (see figure 20-56A). Wipe away any food placed on your wrist.
   c. Use drinking straws for liquids unless the patient has dysphagia. Use a separate straw for each liquid offered. Give the patient a drink of water to wet the palate and make swallowing easier.
   d. Hold utensils at a right angle (90°) to the patient's mouth (see figure 20-56B). Feed the patient from the tip of the utensil.
   e. Place a small amount of food on the utensil. Fill the spoon or fork about 1/3 to 1/2 full.
   f. Tell the patient what he or she is eating.
   g. If the patient had a stroke, place food in the unaffected side of the mouth. Watch the throat to make sure the patient is swallowing.
   h. Allow time for the patient to chew. Do not hurry the patient.
   i. Alternate foods, but don't mix foods together. Provide liquids at intervals to keep the mouth moist and make chewing and swallowing easier.
   j. Allow the patient to hold bread and to help to the extent that he or she is able.
   k. Use a towel or napkin to wipe the patient's mouth, as necessary.

   ! **CAUTION:** Be alert at all times to signs of dysphagia and/or choking.
9. Encourage the patient to eat as much as possible.

   NOTE: If the patient does not like a particular food, check with your immediate supervisor or the dietitian about substitute foods.
10. When the meal is complete, allow the patient to wash his or her hands. Provide oral hygiene. Position the patient comfortably and in correct body alignment.
11. Observe all checkpoints before leaving the patient: elevate the siderails, if indicated; lower the bed to its lowest level; place the call signal and supplies within easy reach of the patient; leave the area neat and clean.
12. Note how much food was eaten. Record amounts on the I&O record, if one is being kept.

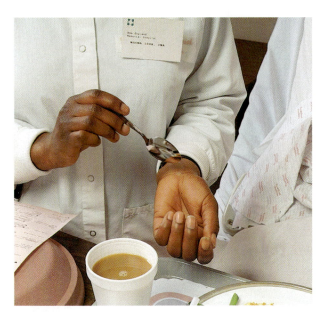

FIGURE 20-56A Test hot liquids before feeding them to a patient.

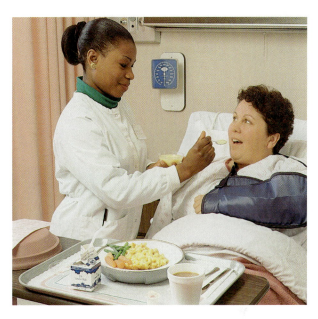

FIGURE 20-56B Hold utensils at a right angle to the mouth to feed the patient from the tip of the utensil.

13. Clean and replace all equipment. Place the tray in the correct area.
14. Wash hands.
15. Report that the patient has been fed and/or record all required information on the patient's chart or the agency form, for example, date; time; fed breakfast, ate everything except one-half slice toast; and your signature and title.

Practice *Go to the workbook and use the evaluation sheet for 20:6, Feeding a Patient, to practice this procedure. When you feel you have mastered this skill, sign the sheet and give it to your instructor for further action.*

✔ **Final Checkpoint** Using the criteria listed on the evaluation sheet, your instructor will grade your performance.

20:7 INFORMATION Assisting with a Bedpan/Urinal

OBRA Regular elimination of body wastes contributes to good health. Patients confined to bed must rely on the health care worker's help in meeting this important physical need.

Elimination of body wastes is essential. Death will occur if wastes are not eliminated. The following terms are used in reference to elimination:

◆ **Urinate, micturate,** or **void:** Emptying of the bladder, which stores the liquid waste, or urine, produced by the kidney. A urinal is used by male patients when they need to urinate, micturate, or void; a bedpan is used by females. Two main types of bedpans are the

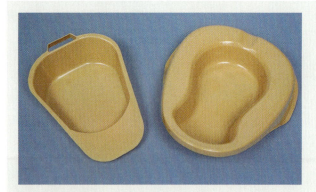

FIGURE 20-57 Two types of bedpans: the fracture, or orthopedic, bedpan (at left) and the standard bedpan (at right).

fracture, or orthopedic, bedpan and the standard bedpan (see figure 20-57).

◆ **Defecate:** Having a bowel movement, or BM; the discharge of the waste through the rectum. The material is called *feces* or *stool*.

Many patients are sensitive about using bedpans or urinals. It is important that the health care worker provide privacy by closing the door, privacy curtain, and window curtain. Make the patient as comfortable as possible during this procedure. It is also important to provide the bedpan or urinal immediately when the patient requests it. In addition, a bedpan or urinal should be offered frequently to any patient confined to bed.

Accurate observations of the frequency, amount, and appearance of urine and stool are important. Abnormalities in any of these factors may indicate disease or complications. Any abnormality must be reported immediately, and a specimen must be saved for examination.

Prior to emptying a bedpan or urinal, it is the health care worker's responsibility to check whether specimens are needed. In addition, amounts must be measured and recorded if an intake and output (I&O) record is being kept for the patient. Check with your immediate supervisor or note physician's orders for this information.

Standard precautions must be observed when handling urine or feces. Hands must be washed frequently, and gloves must be worn. Eye protection must be worn if splashing or spraying is possible while emptying the bedpan.

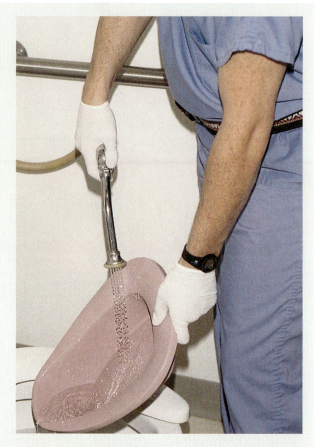

FIGURE 20-58 Some agencies have special spray units in the bathrooms to rinse and clean bedpans and urinals.

Some agencies have special spray units in the bathrooms to rinse and clean bedpans and urinals (see figure 20-58). After rinsing, the bedpan or urinal must be disinfected. It must be used for only one patient. After the patient is discharged, it must be sterilized according to agency policy before being used for another patient. Some bedpans are disposable and are discarded in an infectious-waste container when the patient is discharged. Any areas contaminated by urine or feces must be wiped with a disinfectant. In addition, patients should have the opportunity to wash their hands and receive perineal care after using bedpans or urinals.

STUDENT: *Go to the workbook and complete the assignment sheet for 20:7, Assisting with a Bedpan/Urinal. Then return and continue with the procedures.*

PROCEDURE 20:7A

OBRA

Assisting with a Bedpan

Equipment and Supplies

Bedpan with cover, toilet tissue, basin, soap, washcloth, towel, disposable gloves, pen or pencil

Procedure

1. Obtain proper authorization and assemble equipment.
2. **C** Knock on the door and pause before entering. Introduce yourself. Identify the patient. Explain the procedure.
3. Wash hands. Put on gloves.

    CAUTION: Observe standard precautions when handling urine or feces.
4. Close the door and screen the unit. Place the bedpan on a chair. Place the tissue within easy reach of the patient. Raise the bed to a comfortable working height. Lower the head of the bed, if tolerated by the patient.

    CAUTION: Use correct body mechanics during this procedure. Bend from the hips, not the waist. Maintain a broad base of support.
5. If the bedpan is metal, warm it by running hot water into it and then emptying it. If no water is available, rub the bedpan briskly with a cloth.
6. Lower the siderails on the side where you are working.
7. Fold the top bedcovers back at a right angle. Raise the patient's gown.

    NOTE: Avoid exposing the patient. If the patient is wearing pajama pants, help lower the pants.
8. **C** Ask the patient to flex the knees and rest his or her weight on the heels, if able. Discuss a signal such as, "On the count of three, raise up."
9. At the signal, assist the patient to raise his or her hips by putting one of your hands under the small of the patient's back (see figure 20-59A).

    CAUTION: If the patient is too heavy, get help.
10. With your other hand, slide the bedpan under the patient's hips. The narrow end should face the foot of bed. Adjust to the correct placement.

NOTE: The patient's buttocks should rest on the rounded portion of the pan.

11. The patient who is too weak to get on the pan may be rolled away from the health care worker and onto his or her side. The bedpan

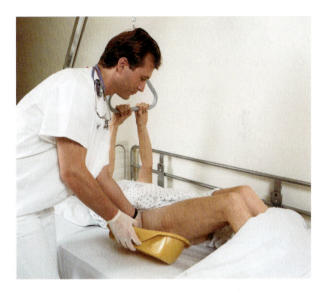

FIGURE 20-59A Ask the patient to raise his or her hips so that the bedpan can be put in position.

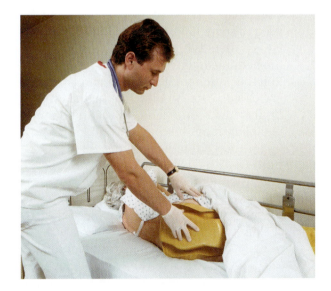

FIGURE 20-59B The patient can also turn onto his or her side so that the bedpan can be positioned. The patient then rolls back onto the bedpan.

can then be placed against the patient's buttocks (see figure 20-59B). The patient is then rolled back onto the bedpan. The bedpan must be held in place during this procedure. **NOTE:** Lower bedpans, called fracture (or orthopedic) bedpans, can also be used by patients who are unable to help (refer again to figure 20-57).

12. Replace the top bedcovers. Position the patient in a comfortable position. Raise the head of the bed, as needed.

13. Place the call signal and tissue within easy reach of the patient.
    NOTE: If a urine specimen is needed or the patient is on Intake and Output, instruct the patient not to put toilet tissue in the pan. Provide a small plastic bag for discarding the soiled tissue.

14. Raise the siderail before leaving the patient.
    NOTE: If you leave to do another task while the patient is on the bedpan, remove gloves and wash hands. Wash hands again and put on gloves when you return.

15. Answer the patient's call signal immediately. Lower the siderail.

16. Ask the patient to flex the knees and put his or her weight on the heels. Place one hand under the small of the patient's back. Assist in raising the patient's buttocks off the pan. With your other hand, remove the bedpan carefully.

17. Cover the bedpan and place it on the chair.
    NOTE: If a bedpan cover is not available, cloth, paper bags, or tissue paper can be used to cover the bedpan.

18. If the patient is unable to assist in getting off the bedpan, it may be necessary to get help. Roll the patient off the bedpan and onto his or her side while holding the bedpan firmly in place with one hand. Cover the bedpan and place it on the chair.

19. Clean the genital area, as necessary. Wipe from front to back. Drop the soiled tissue into the bedpan, unless a specimen is needed or output is being measured. In these situations, temporarily place the tissue in a plastic bag until you can discard it in the toilet or trash can in the utility room.

20. Fill a basin with warm water. Allow the patient to wash his or her hands. Wash the patient's perineal area, if necessary, or assist the patient, as needed.

21. Replace all bedcovers. Observe all checkpoints before leaving the patient: position the patient in correct body alignment; elevate the siderails (if indicated); lower the bed to its lowest level; and place the call signal, water, and tissues within easy reach of the patient.

22. Take the bedpan to the bathroom. Note the contents. Check amount, color, type. If an I&O record is being kept for the patient, measure and record the amount.
    NOTE: Check to see whether a specimen is needed before emptying the bedpan.
    (!) CAUTION: Save a sample of the contents if there are any abnormalities.

23. Empty the bedpan. Use a paper towel to cover your gloved hand while turning on the faucet or flushing the toilet. Put on eye protection if spraying or splashing is possible. Rinse the bedpan with cold water and a disinfectant. Rinse and dry.
    NOTE: Follow your agency's policy for cleaning bedpans.

24. Return the covered pan to the patient's unit. Replace all equipment used.

25. Remove gloves. Wash hands thoroughly.

26. **C** Report and/or record all required information on the patient's chart or the agency form, for example, date; time; used bedpan, voided 250 cc of straw yellow urine; and your signature and title. Always report unusual observations immediately.

Practice *Go to the workbook and use the evaluation sheet for 20:7A, Assisting with a Bedpan, to practice this procedure. When you feel you have mastered this skill, sign the sheet and give it to your instructor for further action.*

✔ Final Checkpoint Using the criteria listed on the evaluation sheet, your instructor will grade your performance.

PROCEDURE 20:7B

OBRA

Assisting with a Urinal

Equipment and Supplies

Urinal with cover, basin, soap, washcloth, towel, toilet tissue, disposable gloves, pen or pencil

Procedure

1. Obtain proper authorization and assemble equipment. Make sure the urinal has a lid or cover of some type (see figure 20-60).
2. **C** Knock on the door and pause before entering. Introduce yourself. Identify the patient. Explain the procedure.
3. Wash hands. Put on gloves.
   CAUTION: Observe standard precautions when handling urine or feces.
4. Close the door and screen the unit. Elevate the bed to a comfortable working height. Lower the siderail on the side where you are working.
5. If the patient is weak or helpless, lift the top bedcovers and help the patient grasp the handle and position the urinal.
6. Make sure the call signal and toilet tissue are within easy reach of the patient. Leave the patient alone, if possible, to ensure privacy. Elevate the siderail before leaving.
   NOTE: If you leave to do another task while the patient is using the urinal, remove gloves and wash hands. Wash hands again and put on gloves when you return.
7. Answer the patient's call signal immediately.
8. Ask the patient to hand you the urinal. If the patient needs assistance, reach under the covers and take hold of the urinal handle. Close the lid or cover the top of the urinal and place it on a chair.
   NOTE: Avoid exposing the patient.
9. Fill the basin with warm water. Assist the patient to wash his hands, as needed. Wash the patient's perineal area, if necessary, or assist the patient, as needed.
10. Observe all checkpoints before leaving the patient: position the patient in correct body alignment, elevate the siderails, if indicated; lower the bed to its lowest level; and place the call signal and supplies within easy reach of the patient.
11. Take the urinal to the bathroom. Observe the contents. Measure and record the amount if an I&O record is being kept for the patient.
    NOTE: Check to see whether a specimen is needed before emptying the urinal.
    CAUTION: Save a specimen if there are any abnormalities. Report unusual observations immediately to your supervisor.
12. Empty the urinal. Use a paper towel to cover your gloved hand while turning on the faucet or flushing the toilet. Put on eye protection if spraying or splashing is possible. Rinse the urinal with cold water and a disinfectant. Rinse and dry.
    NOTE: Follow agency policy for cleaning the urinal.
13. Return the urinal to the patient's unit. Place it in the bedside stand or in the urinal holder on the bed.
14. Remove gloves. Wash hands.
15. **C** Report and/or record all required information on the patient's chart or the agency form, for example, date; time; used urinal, voided 250 cc of straw yellow urine; and your signature and title. Always report unusual observations immediately.

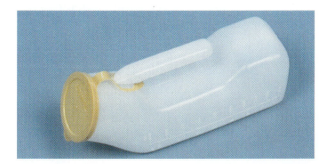

FIGURE 20-60 A urinal should have a lid or cover.

Practice *Go to the workbook and use the evaluation sheet for 20:7B, Assisting with a Urinal, to practice this procedure. When you feel you have mastered this skill, sign the sheet and give it to your instructor for further action.*

 Final Checkpoint Using the criteria listed on the evaluation sheet, your instructor will grade your performance.

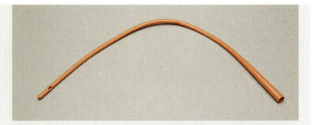

FIGURE 20-61A A straight catheter is inserted into the bladder to drain urine but is not left in the bladder.

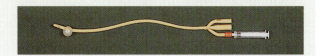

FIGURE 20-61B A Foley catheter has a small balloon on the end that is inserted in the bladder. The balloon is inflated with sterile water to hold the catheter in place.

20:8 INFORMATION
Providing Catheter and Urinary-Drainage-Unit Care

OBRA Some patients are unable to urinate, or void. In these cases, a catheter may be inserted into the bladder to drain the urine. The catheter is usually connected to a drainage unit to collect the urine.

A **catheter** is a hollow tube, usually made of soft rubber or plastic. There are different kinds of catheters. A French, or straight, catheter is inserted into the bladder to drain urine but is not left in the bladder (see figure 20-61A). It is usually used to collect a sterile urine specimen. A Foley catheter (also called an indwelling, or retention, catheter) is usually used to drain the bladder over an extended period of time. It has a small balloon on the end that is inserted in the bladder (see figure 20-61B). Once the catheter is inserted, the balloon is inflated with sterile water to keep the catheter in place. The catheter must be kept sterile at all times. Insertion of a catheter is a sterile technique performed by a nurse, physician, or other authorized person. If a male patient requires urinary drainage, external condom catheters may be used (see figure 20-61C). The condom catheters eliminate the need for an internal catheter and decrease the chance of urinary infection. The condom catheter is placed on the penis and attached to the urinary-drainage tubing and collection bag. The condom must be removed at least every 24 hours and the skin must be checked for any signs of irritation.

A **urinary-drainage unit** or bag is attached to the catheter to collect drained urine. This is usually a closed unit to keep microorganisms from entering the catheter and, therefore, prevent infection. The unit consists of plastic or rubber tubing attached to the catheter and extending to a bag in which the urine is collected.

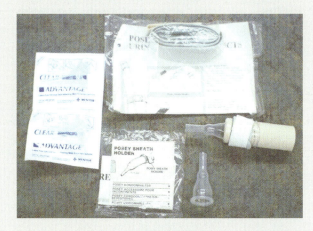

FIGURE 20-61C Condom catheters are used to provide an external urinary drainage system for males.

Careful observation of the catheter and drainage unit is required. The following should be checked frequently:

◆ The connection between the catheter and drainage unit is secure.

◆ The tubing is free from kinks or bends that stop the urine flow.

◆ The drainage bag is always below the level of the bladder. If it is raised above the level of the bladder, a backflow of urine into the bladder can occur. This can, in turn, lead to infection.

◆ The urine is flowing freely into the drainage bag. The system usually relies on gravity for drainage. Therefore, the drainage bottle or bag should be kept low enough to make use of the force of gravity.

◆ The catheter is taped, strapped, or tied to the patient's leg. This prevents pull on the catheter, which might dislodge it or cause irritation.

◆ The drainage unit is emptied frequently. Stagnant urine encourages the growth of microorganisms. The units are usually emptied every 8 hours, but they may be emptied more frequently, if required.

◆ The drainage bag is *not* lying on the floor. It should be attached to the bed frame.

◆ No loops of the drainage tube are hanging below the drainage bag. Such loops interfere with the gravitational flow of urine into the bag.

◆ The drainage tubing leading to the drainage bag is always above the level of urine in the unit. This prevents infection and microorganisms in the urine from traveling back up the tubing and into the patient's bladder.

◆ The patient complains of burning, pain, irritation, or tenderness in the urethral area. Any such complaints should be reported immediately to your supervisor.

When a catheter and urinary-drainage unit is in place, it is preferable to never disconnect the drainage unit. However, it may sometimes be necessary to disconnect the catheter from the unit. For example, when a urine-collection area is not present on the drainage unit, and a sterile or fresh urine specimen is required (because the urine in the bag is not fresh and is contaminated). Careful sterile technique must be followed to prevent infection. Both the catheter and top connection of the drainage unit must be kept sterile. Special clamps, plugs, and other equipment are available for disconnecting the catheter (see figures 20-62A and B). Most drainage units have special

urine-collection areas on the tubing. The catheter does not have to be disconnected when a specimen is obtained from this type of unit. Follow the specific instructions provided with the unit or follow agency policy to maintain sterility during this procedure. A clamp is usually placed on the tubing below the collection unit to allow urine to collect in the tubing and/or bladder. The collection unit is wiped with a disinfectant, and a sterile needle and syringe is inserted into the unit to obtain the

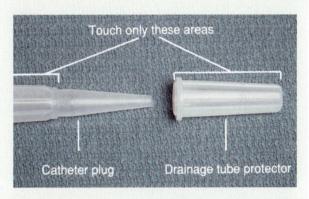

FIGURE 20-62A A sterile catheter plug and protective cap.

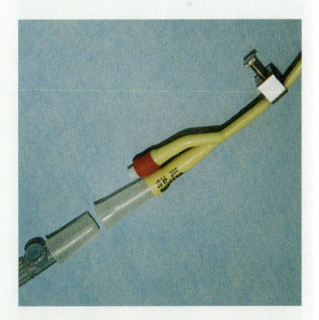

FIGURE 20-62B A catheter disconnected from the drainage tube and protected with the catheter plug. Note the protective cap on the drainage tube.

urine specimen (see figures 20-63A and B). The urine is then placed in a specimen container. Gloves must be worn during this procedure, and the contaminated needle and syringe must be placed in a sharps container immediately after use.

When a Foley, or indwelling, catheter is in place, the urinary meatus must be kept clean and free of secretions to help prevent bladder and kidney infections. Catheter care is provided for this purpose and it should be administered at least once every 8 hours, and more frequently, if ordered. This care is usually provided during the bath and as part of perineal care. Disposable catheter-care kits containing applicators and antiseptic solution are used in many agencies. Other agencies use soap and water. Some kits also contain disposable bed protectors or underpads and gloves. Follow the instructions provided with the kit or the procedure recommended by your agency. Procedure 20:8A describes one method of catheter care.

C Careful observations of the urine drained should be made. The amount, color, type, presence of other substances, and other observations should be noted. Unusual observations should be reported immediately.

Correct procedure must be followed when emptying the drainage unit to prevent contamination and infection. Procedure 20:8B describes one way of emptying a drainage unit.

If a patient has had an indwelling catheter in place over a period of time, a bladder-training program may be instituted before the catheter is removed. The purpose of a bladder-training program is to develop voluntary control of urination and prevent incontinence, or the inability to control urination. At first, the catheter is clamped for 1 to 2 hours at a time to allow urine to accumulate in the bladder. The clamp is then released, and urine is allowed to drain into the urinary-drainage-unit bag. The time is gradually increased until the catheter is clamped for 3 to 4 hours at a time. After the catheter is removed, the patient is encouraged to void every 3 to 4 hours or whenever necessary to regain bladder control. Bladder-training programs can also be used for incontinent patients who do not have indwelling catheters in place. This type of program encourages the patient to attempt to void at regularly scheduled intervals. A record is kept of times of incontinence to establish when the patient should be encouraged to void. Staff members then assist the patient to the bathroom or offer the bedpan or urinal before the expected time of incontinence. The support, understanding, and cooperation of all staff members is important when a bladder-training program is used for a patient.

Standard precautions (discussed in Unit 13:3) must be observed at all times when handling urine. Gloves must be worn when providing catheter care, obtaining urine specimens from a urine-collection unit, and emptying a urinary-drainage unit. Hands must be washed frequently, and immediately after

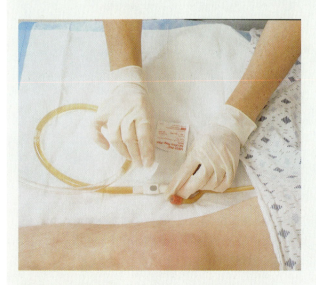

FIGURE 20-63A The urine collection area is first wiped with a disinfectant.

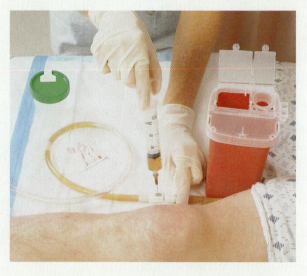

FIGURE 20-63B A sterile needle and syringe are then used to obtain the urine specimen.

removing gloves. If splashing or spraying of body fluids is possible, eye protection must be worn. Any areas contaminated by urine must be wiped with a disinfectant.

STUDENT: *Go to the workbook and complete the assignment sheet for 20:8, Providing Catheter and Urinary-Drainage-Unit Care. Then return and continue with the procedures.*

PROCEDURE 20:8A   OBRA

Providing Catheter Care

Equipment and Supplies

Catheter-care kit (or sterile applicators, bowl, and antiseptic solution or soap and water), bath blanket, disposable underpad or bed protector, catheter strap or tape (if needed), disposable gloves, plastic waste bag, pen or pencil

NOTE: Catheter care is usually administered after the perineal area has been washed and cleaned during the bath. If administered at a different time, equipment must be obtained to wash and clean the perineal area before providing catheter care.

Procedure

1. Obtain proper authorization and assemble equipment.
2. **C** Knock on the door and pause before entering. Introduce yourself. Identify the patient. Explain the procedure.
3. Close the door and screen the unit for privacy.
4. Wash hands.
   CAUTION: Wear gloves and observe standard precautions when providing catheter care.
5. Elevate the bed to a comfortable working height. Lower the siderail on the side where you are working.
6. Cover the patient with a bath blanket. Without exposing the patient, fanfold the top bed linen to the foot of the bed.
7. Position the patient in the dorsal recumbent position, if possible, with the legs separated and knees bent. Drape the patient so that only the perineal area is exposed.
8. Open the catheter-care kit and place it on the overbed table. Position the plastic waste bag conveniently.

9. Place the disposable underpad or bed protector under the patient's buttocks and upper legs.
10. Put on gloves.
    NOTE: Sterile gloves are required by some agencies. Follow agency policy.
11. Obtain a sterile applicator (usually a cotton ball or gauze pad) moistened with antiseptic solution or soap and water.
    NOTE: Some kits contain premoistened sterile applicators. Other kits contain containers of antiseptic solution that must be poured into small bowls provided with the kits. The sterile applicator is then placed in the antiseptic.
12. For a female patient:
    a. Use the thumb and forefinger of one hand to gently separate the labia, or lips, and expose the urinary meatus (opening).
    b. Wipe from front to back with the sterile applicator.
    c. Place the used applicator in the plastic waste bag.
    d. Using a clean sterile applicator each time, continue to wipe from front to back until the area is clean.
13. For a male patient:
    a. Gently grasp the penis and draw the foreskin back.
    b. Use the sterile applicator to wipe from the meatus down the shaft.
    c. Place the used applicator in the plastic waste bag.
    d. Using a clean sterile applicator each time, continue to wipe from the meatus down the shaft until the area is clean.
    e. After the area is clean, gently return the foreskin to its normal position.
14. Without pulling on the catheter, use a sterile applicator to clean the catheter from the

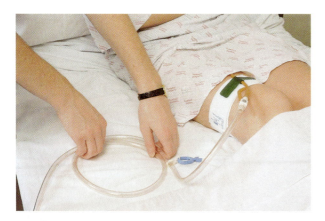

FIGURE 20-64A Check the catheter to be sure it is strapped to the leg.

meatus down approximately 4 inches. Place the used applicator in the plastic waste bag. Repeat as necessary, using a fresh applicator for each stroke.

15. Observe the area carefully for any signs of irritation, abnormal discharge, or crusting.

16. Remove the bed protector or underpad and place it in the plastic waste bag.

17. Remove gloves and discard in the plastic waste bag. Wash hands.

18. Check the catheter to be sure it is strapped or taped to the leg (see figures 20-64A and B). Reposition the strap or replace the tape, if necessary.

   ⚠ **CAUTION:** Make sure there is no strain or pull on the catheter.

19. Position the patient comfortably and in correct body alignment.

20. Replace the top bed linen and remove the bath blanket.

21. Observe all checkpoints before leaving the patient: elevate the siderails (if indicated); place the call signal, water, and supplies within easy reach of the patient; lower the bed to its lowest level; leave the area neat and clean.

22. Perform a final check of the catheter and drainage unit to ensure the following:
   a. The tubing is free of kinks and bends.
   b. The tubing is positioned to allow for proper flow of urine.
   c. The drainage bag is attached to the bed-frame.
   d. The drainage bag is below the level of the bladder.

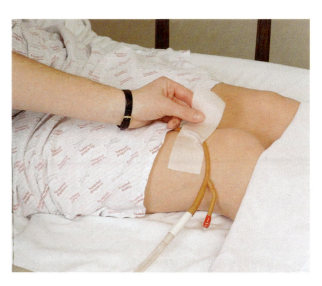

FIGURE 20-64B The catheter may also be taped to the leg. If possible, use hypoallergenic tape.

   e. The drainage tubing is above the level of the urine in the bag.
   f. Urine is flowing into the drainage bag.

23. Place all disposable supplies in the plastic waste bag. Seal properly and dispose of in the correct area. Clean and properly replace any other equipment used.

24. Wash hands thoroughly.

25. ⓒ Report and/or record all required information on the patient's chart or the agency form, for example, date; time; catheter care given, urine flowing into drainage bag; and your signature and title. Report any unusual observations immediately.

Practice *Go to the workbook and use the evaluation sheet for 20:8A, Providing Catheter Care, to practice this procedure. When you feel you have mastered this skill, sign the sheet and give it to your instructor for further action.*

 Final Checkpoint Using the criteria listed on the evaluation sheet, your instructor will grade your performance.

PROCEDURE 20:8B

OBRA

Emptying a Urinary-Drainage Unit

Equipment and Supplies

Paper towels, graduated cylinder or pitcher, antiseptic or disinfectant swab, disposable gloves, paper, pen or pencil

Procedure

1. Obtain proper authorization and assemble equipment.
2. **C** Knock on the door and pause before entering. Introduce yourself. Identify the patient. Explain the procedure.
3. Wash hands. Put on gloves. Wear eye protection if spraying or splashing of body fluids is possible.

   CAUTION: Observe standard precautions when measuring urine.
4. Place paper towels on the floor. Place the measuring graduated cylinder on top of the towels.
5. Remove the drainage outlet from the drainage bag. Place the end of the outlet in the measuring pitcher.

   CAUTION: Do not allow the end of the outlet to touch the graduated cylinder.
6. Release the clamp to allow the urine to drain. Empty all the urine (see figure 20-65A).

NOTE: If necessary, tilt the bag to remove all the urine.

7. Clamp the drainage tube. Wipe the drainage outlet with an antiseptic or disinfectant swab (see figure 20-65B). Replace the tube in the unit (see figure 20-65C).
8. Observe all checkpoints before leaving the patient: position the patient comfortably and in correct body alignment, elevate the siderails (if indicated), lower the bed to its lowest level, place the call signal and supplies within easy reach of the patient, and leave the area neat and clean.
9. Perform a final check of the catheter and unit to ensure the following:
   a. The catheter is strapped or taped to the patient's leg.
   b. The tubing is free of kinks and bends.
   c. The tubing does not loop down below the drainage bag.
   d. The drainage bag is attached to the bedframe.
   e. The drainage bag is below the level of the bladder.
   f. The drainage tubing is above the level of the urine in the bag.
   g. Urine is flowing into the bag.

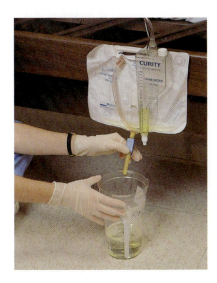

FIGURE 20-65A Drain the urine from the urinary-drainage unit.

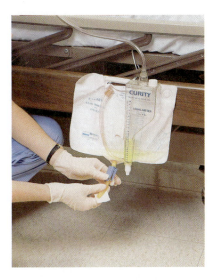

FIGURE 20-65B Wipe the drainage outlet with a disinfectant.

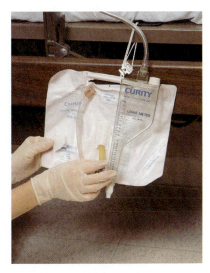

FIGURE 20-65C Replace the drainage tube in the drainage unit.

10. Take the graduate to the patient's bathroom. Record the amount and color of urine in the graduate. Record any unusual observations and report such observations immediately.
    NOTE: Save a specimen if needed, or if anything unusual is noted about the urine.

11. Empty the graduate into the toilet. Rinse it with cold water. Wash with soap and warm water. Clean with a disinfectant. Rinse and dry. Return to its proper place.
    NOTE: The graduate is usually kept in the patient unit. It should be used for one patient only. Most agencies use disposable graduates. If the graduate is not disposable, it should be sterilized according to agency policy before being used for another patient.

12. Remove gloves. Wash hands.

13. **C** Report and/or record all required information on the patient's chart or the agency form, for example, date; time; emptied urinary-drainage unit, 580 cc of light yellow urine; and your signature and title. Report any unusual observations immediately.

> **Practice** *Go to the workbook and use the evaluation sheet for 20:8B, Emptying a Urinary-Drainage Unit, to practice this procedure. When you feel you have mastered this skill, sign the sheet and give it to your instructor for further action.*

✔ **Final Checkpoint** Using the criteria listed on the evaluation sheet, your instructor will grade your performance.

20:9 INFORMATION Providing Ostomy Care

An **ostomy** is a surgical procedure in which an opening, called a **stoma,** is created in the abdominal wall. This allows wastes such as urine or stool (feces) to be expelled through the opening. In most cases, an ostomy is performed because of tumors and/or cancer in the urinary bladder or intestine. An ostomy may also be done as a treatment for birth defects, ulcerative colitis, bowel obstruction, or injury. At times, an ostomy is permanent. At other times, an ostomy is temporary and is repaired when the injury heals or the condition necessitating the ostomy improves.

 There are different types of ostomies. A **ureterostomy** is an opening into one of the two ureters that drain urine from the kidney to the bladder. The ureter is brought to the surface of the abdomen, and urine drains from the stoma, or opening. An **ileostomy** is an opening into the ileum, a section of the small intestine. A loop of the ileum is brought to the surface of the abdomen. Because the entire large intestine is bypassed, the stools expelled are frequent and liquid and contain digestive enzymes that irritate the skin. A **colostomy** is an opening into the large intestine, or colon. There are different kinds of colostomies, depending on the area of large intestine involved (see figure 20-66). Stool expelled through an ascending colostomy tends to be liquid, while stool expelled through a transverse or descending colostomy is more solid and formed. Stool expelled through a sigmoid colostomy is similar to normal stool, because the digestive products have moved through most of the intestine, and water and other substances have been reabsorbed.

Most patients with ostomies wear a bag or pouch over the stoma to collect the drainage (see figure 20-67). The pouch is held in place with a belt or an adhesive seal. Problems that can occur include leakage, odor, and irritation of the skin surrounding the stoma. The pouch must be emptied frequently. Many pouches have areas that can be opened to allow urine or stool to drain. The drainage end of the bag is placed in a bedpan (see figure 20-68). If the patient is up, the patient can sit on the toilet and position the drainage end of the bag over the toilet. The clamp at the drainage end of the

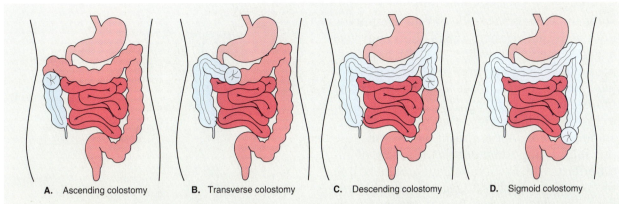

A. Ascending colostomy   **B.** Transverse colostomy   **C.** Descending colostomy   **D.** Sigmoid colostomy

FIGURE 20-66 The type of colostomy depends on which part of the intestine is removed. Areas of intestine that remain after each type of colostomy are shown in blue.

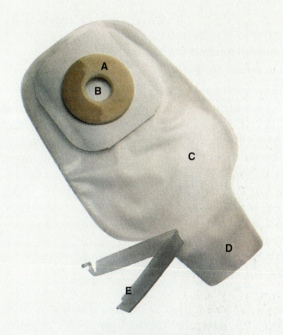

A. Adhesive ring seals around stoma to prevent leakage
B. Opening placed over stoma
C. Collection bag
D. Drainage end of bag
E. Secures drainage end of bag to prevent leakage

FIGURE 20-67 Most patients with ostomies wear a bag or pouch over the stoma, or opening, to collect the drainage.

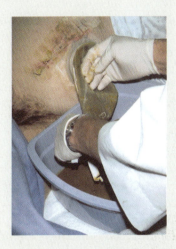

FIGURE 20-68 To empty the ostomy pouch, place the drainage end in a bedpan.

bag is opened to allow the stool or urine to drain. The drainage end is then cleaned to prevent odors and the clamp is resealed. Some pouches are disposable and are removed and replaced. Good stoma and skin care is essential because of irritation caused by urine or stool drainage. Skin barriers such as wafers, pastes, powders, and liquid films frequently are applied to the skin around the stoma to prevent irritation from the removal of the pouch.

When an ostomy is first performed, care is provided by a registered nurse. For "older" ostomies, other trained and qualified health care workers may provide routine stoma care. It is essential to check the policy of your facility and to know your legal responsibilities before providing ostomy care. Eventually, most patients are taught to care for their own ostomies, if they are capable.

Patients with ostomies may experience psychological reactions. They may feel loss of personal worth and dignity because they are unable to eliminate body wastes in a routine manner. Even though clothing conceals the ostomy and pouch, the patient feels different.

Some individuals have difficulty in maintaining normal sexual relationships. Others may feel anger, anxiety, depression, fear, or hopelessness. If the ostomy is done because of a malignant tumor (cancer), fear and anxiety can be more severe. It is essential to allow the patient to express feelings and verbalize fears. Understanding and support from all health care providers is important during the period of initial adjustment. Eventually, patients realize that thousands of people with ostomies live normal lives. Through ostomy support groups, made up of people with ostomies, and help from health care providers, most individuals learn to cope and live with their ostomies.

Careful observation is essential when providing care to the patient with an ostomy. The stoma is mucous membrane with no nerve endings. It is bright- to dark-red in color and looks wet because of the exposed mucosa (see figure 20-69). Rubbing or pressure can cause the stoma to bleed. Any abnormalities in appearance should be reported immediately. A blue to black color indicates interference with the blood supply. A pale or pink color can indicate a low hemoglobin level. A dry or dull appearance signifies dehydration. Profuse bleeding, ulcerations or cuts, or the formation of crystals on the stoma also indicate problems. The discharge in the ostomy bag or pouch should also be observed. It is important to note the amount, color, and type (liquid, semiformed, formed) of discharge. Any unusual observations should be reported to your immediate supervisor and/or recorded on the patient's chart or the agency form.

 Standard precautions (discussed in Unit 13:3) must be observed at all times when

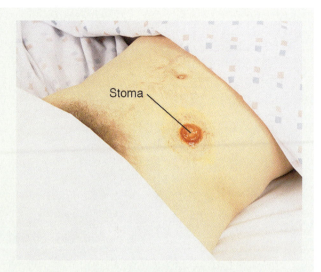

FIGURE 20-69 A stoma should be bright- to dark-red in color and look wet because of the exposed mucous membrane.

handling urine or stool. Gloves must be worn when emptying the pouch or providing stoma care. Hands must be washed frequently, and immediately after removing gloves. Eye protection must be worn if splashing or spraying of body fluids is possible. The pouch must be discarded in an infectious-waste or plastic waste bag. If a bedpan is used, it must be cleaned and disinfected. Any areas contaminated with urine or stool must be wiped with a disinfectant. Taking proper precautions can help prevent the spread of infection.

STUDENT: *Go to the workbook and complete the assignment sheet for 20:9, Providing Ostomy Care. Then return and continue with the procedure.*

PROCEDURE 20:9

Providing Ostomy Care

Equipment and Supplies

Washcloth, towel, soap, basin, bed protector or underpad, bath blanket, ostomy pouch or bag, ostomy belt, adhesive (if needed), skin barrier or wafer (as ordered), toilet tissue, bedpan, disposable gloves, infectious-waste bag, pen or pencil

Procedure

1. Check physician's orders or obtain authorization from your immediate supervisor.

   CAUTION: Know your legal responsibilities before providing ostomy care.

2. Assemble equipment.

3. **C** Knock on the door and pause before entering. Introduce yourself. Identify the patient. Explain the procedure.

4. Close the door and screen the unit for privacy.

5. Wash hands.

6. Lock the wheels of the bed. Elevate the bed to a comfortable working height. Lower the siderail on the side where you are working.

7. Cover the patient with a bath blanket. Without exposing the patient, fanfold the top bed linen to the foot of the bed.

8. Place a bed protector or underpad under the patient's hips on the side of the stoma.

9. Fill the basin with water at a temperature of 105° to 110°F (40.6° to 43.3°C). Place the bedpan and plastic waste bag within easy reach.

10. Put on disposable gloves.

    CAUTION: Observe standard precautions at all times when handling urine or feces.

11. Open the belt and carefully remove the ostomy bag. Be gentle when peeling the bag away from the stoma. Note the amount, color, and type of drainage in the bag. Place the bag in the bedpan or infectious-waste bag. Follow agency policy.

    NOTE: Most ostomy bags are disposable, but some are reusable. To reuse a bag, drain the fecal material (or urine from a ureterostomy) by placing the clamp end of the bag over a bedpan. Then release the clamp and allow the fecal material to empty into the bedpan. Wash the inside of the bag with soap and water and allow it to dry before reapplying the bag. Most people use a second bag while the first bag is drying.

12. Use toilet tissue to gently wipe around the stoma to remove feces or drainage. Put the tissue in the bedpan or infectious-waste bag.

    NOTE: If the patient has a ureterostomy, wipe urine from the stoma area to prevent the urine from contacting the skin.

13. Carefully examine the stoma and surrounding skin. Check for irritated areas, bleeding, edema (or swelling), or discharge. Make sure you report any unusual observations to your immediate supervisor at the end of the procedure.

14. Wash the ostomy area gently with soap and water. Use a circular motion, working from the stoma outward.

15. Rinse the entire area well to remove any soapy residue. Dry the area gently with a towel.

NOTE: Make sure soap is removed. It has a drying effect and may irritate the skin.

16. Use a measuring chart to check the size of the stoma and determine the correct size barrier or wafer (see figure 20-70A). If the wafer is not self-adhesive, apply adhesive stoma paste to the skin around the stoma. Some pastes must dry a few minutes; follow manufacturer's instructions. Peel the paper backing from the wafer. Position the wafer, adhesive side down, over the adhesive paste (see figure 20-70B).

NOTE: The wafer serves as a barrier between the ostomy pouch or bag and the skin. It is not changed every time the pouch is changed.

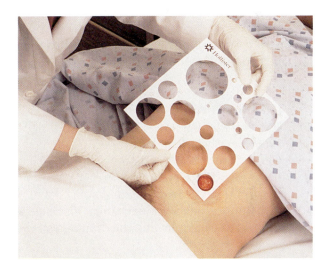

FIGURE 20-70A Check the size of the stoma to determine the correct size for the barrier or wafer.

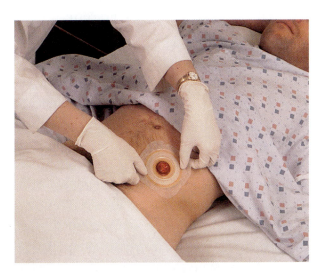

FIGURE 20-70B Position the wafer, adhesive side down, around the stoma.

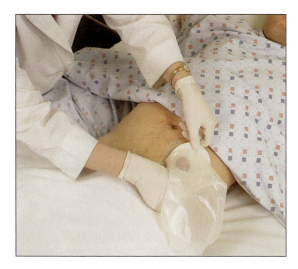

FIGURE 20-70C Gently press the ostomy bag in place over the wafer.

NOTE: Some types of ostomy pouches and bags do not use wafers. Instead, barriers in the forms of pastes, liquids, or powders are applied to the skin to protect it. Follow manufacturer's instructions.

17. Position the belt around the patient. If necessary, apply a clean belt.
18. Gently press a clean ostomy bag in place over the wafer (see figure 20-70C). Seal the bag tightly to the wafer to prevent leakage.
19. If the pouch has a drainage area, make sure the clip or clamp sealing the drainage site is secure.
20. Remove the underpad or bed protector. If any linen on the bed is soiled, change the linen.
21. Replace the top bed linen and remove the bath blanket. Make sure the patient is comfortable and positioned in correct body alignment.
22. Observe all checkpoints before leaving the patient: elevate the siderails (if indicated); lower the bed to its lowest level; and place the call signal, water, tissues, and other supplies within easy reach of the patient.
23. Take the bedpan and waste bag to the bathroom. Follow agency policy for disposal of the ostomy pouch or bag. In some agencies, the bag is emptied into the bedpan. The contents of the bedpan are then flushed down the toilet. The ostomy pouch or bag is then placed in an infectious-waste bag. In other agencies, the full bag is put in an infectious-waste bag. Rinse the bedpan with cool water and a disinfectant. Then rinse and dry it. Discard any other contaminated supplies in an infectious-waste bag.
24. Return the covered bedpan to the patient's unit. Replace all equipment used. Leave the area neat and clean.
25. Remove gloves. Wash hands thoroughly.
26. **C** Report and/or record all required information on the patient's chart or the agency form, for example, date; time; provided ostomy care, pouch 3/4 full of semi-formed light brown stool; and your signature and title. Always report unusual observations immediately.

Practice *Go to the workbook and use the evaluation sheet for 20:9, Providing Ostomy Care, to practice this procedure. When you feel you have mastered this skill, sign the sheet and give it to your instructor for further action.*

✔ **Final Checkpoint** Using the criteria listed on the evaluation sheet, your instructor will grade your performance.

20:10 INFORMATION
Collecting Stool/ Urine Specimens

As a health care worker, you may be responsible for collecting stool and urine specimens. Laboratory tests are performed on the specimens to aid in diagnosis of disease. In order for the tests to be accurate, the specimens must be collected correctly. Types of specimens include:

Routine Urine Specimen

◆ A routine **urine specimen** is one of the most common specimens. It is used for a variety of laboratory tests such as urinalysis (described in Information Section 18:11).

The specimen is usually collected from the first urine voided in the morning because this urine is more concentrated and may reveal more abnormalities. In addition, a first-voided specimen usually has an acidic pH, which helps preserve any cells present. However, for tests such as glucose and acetone, the specimen is usually collected just before mealtime or bedtime and is a fresh specimen. Check with the physician, team leader, laboratory technologist, or other person in charge to find out when the specimen should be collected.

◆ The specimen can be collected in a bedpan, urinal, or special urine collector (refer back to figure 20-53) and then poured into the specimen container. It may also be collected by instructing the patient to void directly into the specimen container.

◆ Usually, 120 cubic centimeters of urine is sufficient for this test. If the patient is unable to void this amount, obtain what is available and send this amount to the laboratory.

◆ The specimen should be sent to the laboratory immediately. If this is not possible, refrigerate the specimen until it can be sent to the laboratory.

◆ If a specimen container is not available, any clean container can be used. Wash the container thoroughly with soap and water, then rinse and dry it. Patients should be cautioned against using containers that previously held medications, however, because using such containers can alter the results of the test.

Clean-Catch, or Midstream-Voided, Specimen

◆ A **midstream specimen** is a urine specimen that is free from contamination. Because microorganisms are present on the genital area and on the specimen containers, special precautions are used to obtain a specimen.

◆ A sterile urine-specimen container, free from all microorganisms, is used to collect a midstream specimen.

◆ The genital area is cleansed thoroughly. This can be done by the health care worker, or the patient can be given careful instructions on how to do this procedure. Clean cotton sponges or gauze squares and a mild antiseptic solution are used.

◆ On a female patient, the genital area includes the perineum and the vulva. The vulva consists of two prominent folds, called the labia majora, and the structures within them: the labia minora, the urinary opening, the clitoris, and the vagina. Moist cotton or gauze wipes are used to clean the external lips of the vulva. They are wiped from front to back. After each wipe, the cotton or gauze square is discarded. The internal lips are then cleaned. Finally, the center area is cleaned from front to back. The center area contains the urinary opening (meatus).

◆ On a male patient, a circular motion is used. Starting at the urinary meatus (opening) at the tip of the penis, the end is cleaned thoroughly in a circular downward motion. Each cotton or gauze square is discarded after each wipe.
NOTE: On uncircumcised males, the foreskin should be pushed back before cleaning. After the end of the penis is clean, gently push the foreskin back into its normal position.

◆ After the area has been cleaned, the patient is told to urinate, or void. Allow a few drops of urine to flow into the bedpan or toilet bowl; then, use the sterile container to catch the urine that follows. Avoid collecting the last few drops of urine. In this way, you discard the first and last part and collect only the middle, or midstream, urine.

◆ The sterile lid of the container should be placed on this specimen immediately to prevent contamination. The specimen should be sent to the laboratory immediately or be refrigerated.

Catheterization for Sterile Urine Specimen

◆ It is sometimes necessary to obtain a sterile urine specimen from a patient. In order to do this, the patient is catheterized. A narrow, hollow, sterile tube is inserted directly into the bladder. Urine from the tube is then placed in a sterile urine-specimen container.

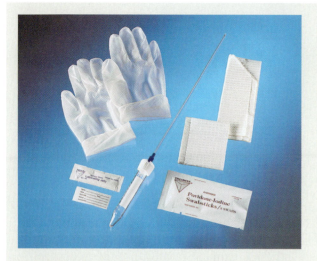

FIGURE 20-71 This Speci-Cath kit is designed to obtain a sterile urine specimen from a male. *(Courtesy of Medline Industries, Inc., Mundelein, IL. [800-MEDLINE.])*

◆ Specimen collection catheters are also available for obtaining a sterile urine specimen (see figure 20-71). These units contain a very small catheter attached to a collection test tube. The catheter is inserted into the bladder and urine drains directly into the tube. When the tube is full, the catheter is withdrawn. The catheter is then separated from the tube and discarded in a sharps container. The tube is sealed by pressing on the spout.

◆ ⚖ Only a trained person should insert the catheter. However, if a catheter is already in place, you may collect a urine specimen for the sterile container (refer back to figures 20-63A and B). It is important that you work under supervision and use sterile technique to prevent contamination of the catheter when obtaining the specimen.

24-Hour Urine Specimens

◆ Special tests require a **24-hour urine specimen.** This means that all of the urine produced by the patient during a 24-hour period must be saved. This urine is used to check kidney function and components

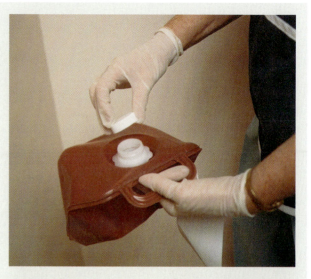

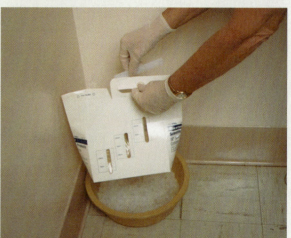

FIGURE 20-72 Different types of specimen collectors for collecting 24-hour urine specimens.

such as protein, creatinine, urobilinogen, hormones, and calcium.

◆ The urine is preserved by way of chemicals and/or cold storage. The laboratory sends the correct container and instructions for preserving the specimen (see figure 20-72).

◆ To start, the patient voids to empty the bladder. This urine is discarded because it was produced before the start of the 24-hour period. The time of voiding is noted as the start of the 24-hour period. All urine voided in the next 24 hours is saved in the special container. At the end of the 24-hour period, the patient voids again for the final collection of urine.

Routine Stool Specimen

◆ A **stool** (feces) **specimen** is examined by the lab, usually to check for ova and parasites (eggs and worms). Stool can also be examined for the presence of fats, microorganisms, and other abnormal substances. A new experimental stool test, currently being researched by Johns Hopkins Cancer Center in Baltimore, checks for a gene that is usually faulty in the earliest stages of colon cancer. If this test is approved, it will help physicians detect colon cancer at its earliest stages when it can be treated much more effectively.

◆ The stool is placed in a special stool-specimen container.

◆ The container should be kept at body temperature, and the specimen sent to the laboratory immediately. For the most accurate results, it should be examined within 30 minutes.

Stool for Occult Blood

◆ Sometimes **occult blood** (blood from areas of the intestinal tract) can be found in the stool. Testing for occult blood requires only a small amount of stool.

◆ A special card is usually used for this test. The small specimen of stool is placed on a certain part of the card (see figure 20-73).

◆ The card is sent to the laboratory. A few drops of a special developing solution, such as Hemoccult, is added to the area. A color change indicates a positive result.

◆ A positive test means that blood is present in the stool.

◆ The test for occult blood does not require that the stool be kept warm or that it be examined immediately. However, it should be sent to the laboratory as soon as possible so that the specimen is not misplaced.

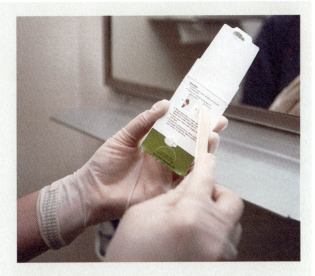

FIGURE 20-73 A small specimen of stool is placed on the Hemoccult card to test for occult blood.

C All specimens must be labeled correctly, including the kind of specimen (urine or stool), the test ordered, the patient's name and address, the date and time, and the physician's name. Print required information on the correct lab requisition or obtain the requisition from your immediate supervisor. A lab requisition must be sent with the labeled specimen.

Standard precautions (discussed in Unit 13:3) must be observed when obtaining and handling urine or stool specimens. Gloves must be worn. Hands must be washed frequently and are always washed immediately after removing gloves. Eye protection must be worn if splashing or spraying of body fluids is possible. Any areas contaminated by urine or stool must be wiped with a disinfectant. To avoid contamination from spills, all urine or stool specimens are placed in special biohazard bags before being transported to the laboratory for testing. Taking proper precautions can help prevent the spread of infection.

STUDENT: *Go to the workbook and complete the assignment sheet for 20:10, Collecting Stool/Urine Specimens. Then return and continue with the procedures.*

PROCEDURE 20:10A
Collecting a Routine Urine Specimen

Equipment and Supplies

Bedpan with cover/urinal, urine-specimen container and label, toilet tissue, graduated or measuring pitcher, disposable gloves, plastic waste bag, biohazard bag, pen or pencil

Procedure

1. Check physician's orders or obtain authorization from your immediate supervisor to be sure you are collecting the right type of specimen.
2. Assemble equipment.
3. **C** Knock on the door and pause before entering. Introduce yourself. Identify the patient. Explain the procedure to the patient. Advise the patient not to put toilet tissue in the bedpan or urinal. Provide a plastic waste bag for disposal of soiled toilet tissue.
4. Wash hands. Put on gloves.

   CAUTION: Observe standard precautions when obtaining and handling urine specimens.
5. Offer the bedpan or urinal as previously instructed.

   NOTE: The patient may urinate directly into the urine-specimen container. Be sure all instructions are understood by the patient.

   NOTE: A special specimen collector is also available for use. This device fits directly under the seat on the toilet bowl (refer back to figure 20-53). The patient must be instructed to throw toilet tissue into the toilet and not into the specimen collector.

   NOTE: In most cases, the first-voided specimen of the day is collected.
6. When the specimen has been obtained, allow the patient to wash his or her hands.
7. Observe all checkpoints before leaving the patient: position the patient comfortably and in correct body alignment, elevate the siderails (if indicated), place the call signal and supplies within easy reach of the patient, lower the bed to its lowest level, and leave the area neat and clean.
8. Take the bedpan or urinal to the patient's bathroom. Pour the urine into a measuring pitcher.

   NOTE: Record the amount if an intake and output (I&O) record is being kept for the patient.
9. Pour approximately 120 cubic centimeters into the urine-specimen container.
10. Wash the outside of the container to remove any spilled urine. Remove gloves. Wash hands.

    CAUTION: Do not allow water to enter the container. Water will dilute the urine specimen and affect the accuracy of the test results.
11. Place the cover on the container.
12. **C** Label the container. Include the date, time, patient's name and room or hospital number or address, specimen type, test required, and physician's name. Print required information on the correct lab requisition or obtain the requisition from your immediate supervisor. A lab requisition must be sent with the labeled specimen.
13. Clean and replace all equipment.

    CAUTION: Remember to wear gloves and observe standard precautions when cleaning any equipment or area contaminated by urine.
14. Put the specimen in a protective biohazard bag for transport (see figure 20-74). Take or

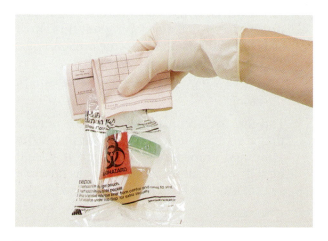

FIGURE 20-74 All specimens must be placed in protective biohazard bags before being transported to the laboratory.

send the specimen to the laboratory immediately. Report the arrival of the specimen to laboratory personnel. If this is not possible, refrigerate the specimen until it can be sent to the laboratory.

15. Wash hands thoroughly.
16. **C** Report and/or record all required information on patient's chart or the agency form, for example, date, time, routine urine specimen collected and sent to lab, and your signature and title.

Practice *Go to the workbook and use the evaluation sheet for 20:10A, Collecting a Routine Urine Specimen, to practice this procedure. When you feel you have mastered this skill, sign the sheet and give it to your instructor for further action.*

✔ **Final Checkpoint** Using the criteria listed on the evaluation sheet, your instructor will grade your performance.

PROCEDURE 20:10B

Collecting a Midstream Urine Specimen

Equipment and Supplies

Sterile urine-specimen bottle and label, gauze or cotton squares, antiseptic solution, small basin, plastic waste bag, biohazard bag, disposable gloves, underpad or bed protector (if needed), pen or pencil

Procedure

1. Check physician's orders or obtain authorization from your immediate supervisor to be sure you are collecting the correct type of specimen.
2. Assemble equipment.
3. **C** Knock on the door and pause before entering. Introduce yourself. Identify the patient. Explain the procedure to the patient.
4. Wash hands.
5. Close the door and screen the unit to provide privacy for the patient. Elevate the bed to a comfortable working height. Lower the siderail on the side where you are working. If the patient is able, the specimen can be collected in the bathroom.
6. Place the gauze or cotton squares in the basin. Pour the required amount of antiseptic solution into the basin. In many agencies, a special kit is available for collecting midstream specimens. Follow the instructions that come with the kit, if one is used.

NOTE: In some agencies premoistened antiseptic pads are used. Under these circumstances, the basin and antiseptic solution would not be necessary.

7. Put on disposable gloves.
    CAUTION: Wear gloves and observe standard precautions when obtaining urine specimens.
8. Wash the genital area correctly or instruct the patient on how to do so.
   a. For a female patient, use antiseptic and gauze squares. Clean the outer folds from front to back. Use a clean gauze for each wipe. Discard each gauze in the plastic waste bag after one use. Clean the inner folds (lips) from front to back, using a clean gauze for each wipe. Discard each gauze after use. Finally, clean the innermost (middle) area from front to back. Discard soiled gauze.
   b. For a male patient, use a circular motion to clean from the urinary meatus outward and downward. Discard each gauze after one wipe in the plastic waste bag. Repeat at least two times or until the area is clean.
      NOTE: On uncircumcised males, the foreskin should be pushed back before cleaning. After cleaning, gently push the foreskin back to its normal position.
9. Instruct the patient to void. Allow the first part of the stream to escape. Catch the middle

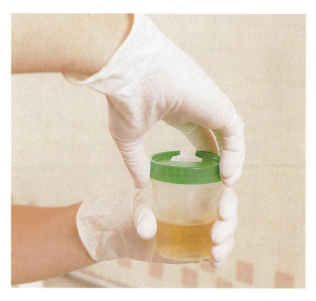

FIGURE 20-75 Place the sterile cap on the container immediately after collecting the urine specimen.

of the stream in the sterile specimen container. Allow the last part of the stream to escape.

NOTE: If the amount must be measured because an I&O record is being kept for the patient, catch the first and last urine in a bedpan or urinal.

10. Place the sterile cap on the container immediately to prevent contamination of the specimen (see figure 20-75).

    CAUTION: Do not touch the inside of the specimen container or the inside of the lid because this will contaminate the specimen.

    NOTE: Some midstream-specimen containers have a funnel that aids in the collection of the specimen. This is removed and discarded in the plastic waste bag before the sterile cap is placed on the container.

11. Allow the patient to wash his or her hands.

12. Observe all checkpoints before leaving the patient: position the patient in correct body alignment, elevate the siderails (if indicated), lower the bed to its lowest level, place the call signal and supplies within easy reach of the patient, and leave the area neat and clean.

13. Wash the outside of the container. Remove gloves and wash hands.

14. **C** Label the container as a "Midstream" or "Clean-Catch" specimen. Print the name of the ordered test, the patient's name and room number or address, the date and time, and physician's name on the label. Print required information on the correct lab requisition or obtain the requisition from your immediate supervisor. A lab requisition must be sent with the labeled specimen.

15. Clean and replace all equipment.

    CAUTION: Remember to wear gloves and observe standard precautions when cleaning any equipment or area contaminated by urine.

16. Put the specimen in a protective biohazard bag for transport. Take or send the specimen to the laboratory immediately. Report the arrival of the specimen to laboratory personnel. If this is not possible, refrigerate the specimen until it can be sent to the laboratory.

    NOTE: For most accurate results, the specimen should be examined as soon as possible.

17. Wash hands thoroughly.

18. **C** Report and/or record all required information on the patient's chart or the agency form, for example, date, time, midstream urine specimen collected and sent to lab, and your signature and title.

Practice *Go to the workbook and use the evaluation sheet for 20:10B, Collecting a Midstream Urine Specimen, to practice this procedure. When you feel you have mastered this skill, sign the sheet and give it to your instructor for further action.*

 Final Checkpoint Using the criteria listed on the evaluation sheet, your instructor will grade your performance.

PROCEDURE 20:10C

Collecting a 24-Hour Urine Specimen

Equipment and Supplies

24-hour specimen container and label, sign for patient's bed, graduate (if urine is to be measured), disposable gloves, plastic waste bag, biohazard bag, pen or pencil

Procedure

1. Check physician's orders or obtain authorization from your immediate supervisor to be sure you are collecting the correct specimen.

2. Check on the type of container and preservative required.

   NOTE: Some containers for certain tests contain chemical preservatives. Others must be kept on ice or refrigerated during the 24 hours. The laboratory will supply information on the correct method for preserving the specimen.

3. Assemble equipment.

4. Label the container with the patient's name and room number or address, the test ordered, the specimen type, the date, and the physician's name.

5. **C** Knock on the door and pause before entering. Introduce yourself. Identify the patient. Explain the procedure. Tell the patient not to discard toilet tissue in the urine specimen. Provide a plastic waste bag for disposal of toilet tissue.

   NOTE: Make sure the patient understands the entire procedure. Stress the importance of saving all urine.

6. Wash hands. Put on disposable gloves.

   CAUTION: Remember to wear gloves and observe standard precautions when obtaining urine and placing it in a 24-hour specimen container.

7. Allow the patient to void. Assist with the bedpan or urinal, if necessary. Measure the amount, if an I&O record is being kept for the patient. Discard this specimen. Note the time of voiding as the start of the 24-hour period.

   NOTE: Urine voided at this time has been produced before the 24-hour time period. The patient must begin the 24-hour period with an empty bladder.

   NOTE: For female patients allowed to use the bathroom, a special urine-specimen collector can be placed under the seat in the toilet (refer back to figure 20-53). The patient must be told not to discard toilet tissue or defecate in the specimen collector.

8. Remove gloves. Wash hands thoroughly.

9. Place a sign on the patient's bed to alert others that a 24-hour specimen is being collected. The sign usually states, "Save all urine—24-hour specimen."

10. During the 24-hour period, use the specimen container to collect all urine voided (see figure 20-76).

    NOTE: If any urine is discarded, the procedure must be stopped and started again.

11. At the end of the 24-hour period, ask the patient to void. Add this urine to the specimen container. It is the final voiding of the procedure.

12. Remove the sign from the patient's bed.

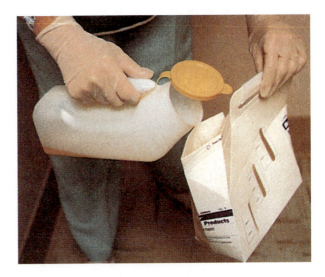

FIGURE 20-76 All urine voided during the 24-hour period must be placed in the specimen container.

13. **C** Check the specimen label to make sure it is accurate and contains all required information. Print required information on the correct lab requisition or obtain the requisition from your immediate supervisor. A lab requisition must be sent with the labeled specimen.

14. Put the specimen in a protective biohazard bag for transport. Take or send the specimen to the laboratory immediately. Notify laboratory personnel of the specimen's arrival.
    NOTE: For the most accurate results, urine should go to the laboratory as soon as possible.

15. Replace all equipment used.

16. Remove gloves. Wash hands thoroughly.

17. **C** Report and/or record all required information on the patient's chart or the agency form, for example, date, time, 24-hour urine specimen completed and sent to lab, and your signature and title.

Practice *Go to the workbook and use the evaluation sheet for 20:10C, Collecting a 24-Hour Urine Specimen, to practice this procedure. When you feel you have mastered this skill, sign the sheet and give it to your instructor for further action.*

✔ **Final Checkpoint** Using the criteria listed on the evaluation sheet, your instructor will grade your performance.

PROCEDURE 20:10D
Collecting a Stool Specimen

Equipment and Supplies

Bedpan with cover, stool-specimen container, tongue blades, label, disposable gloves, plastic waste bag, biohazard bag, pen or pencil

Procedure

1. Check physician's orders or obtain authorization from your immediate supervisor; verify the type of specimen needed.

2. Assemble equipment.

3. **C** Knock on the door and pause before entering. Introduce yourself. Identify the patient. Explain the procedure to the patient. Ask the patient to use the bedpan for his or her next bowel movement because a specimen is needed. Ask the patient not to void or place toilet tissue in the bedpan. Provide a plastic waste bag for soiled toilet tissue.
   NOTE: In some agencies, special collection containers that fit directly under the toilet seat are used (refer back to figure 20-53).

4. Wash hands. Put on disposable gloves.
    CAUTION: Wear gloves and observe standard precautions when obtaining stool specimens.

5. Obtain the specimen in the bedpan. Allow the patient to wash his or her hands.
   NOTE: Assist with the bedpan, as necessary.

6. Take the bedpan to the bathroom.

7. Use two tongue blades to remove the stool from the bedpan. Place the stool in the specimen container. Discard the tongue blades in the plastic waste bag.

8. Remove gloves and wash hands thoroughly.
   ⬡ **CAUTION:** Avoid contaminating the outside of the container.

9. Place the lid on the container. Make sure it is tightly in place.

10. **C** Label the container correctly, including specimen type, test ordered, patient's name and room number or address, date and time, and physician's name. Print required information on the correct lab requisition or obtain the requisition from your immediate supervisor. A lab requisition must be sent with the labeled specimen.

11. Put on gloves to clean the bedpan. Rinse the bedpan with cool water. Clean with a disinfectant, and rinse and dry. Replace all equipment used. Leave the area neat and clean.

12. Remove gloves and wash hands.
13. Keep the specimen warm. Put the specimen in a protective biohazard bag for transport. Take or send it to the laboratory immediately. Report the arrival of the specimen to laboratory personnel.

    NOTE: The specimen should be examined within 30 minutes for most accurate results.
14. Wash hands.
15. **C** Report and/or record all required information on the patient's chart or the agency form, for example, date, time, stool specimen collected and sent to lab, and your signature and title.

> **Practice** *Go to the workbook and use the evaluation sheet for 20:10D, Collecting a Stool Specimen, to practice this procedure. When you feel you have mastered this skill, sign the sheet and give it to your instructor for further action.*

 Final Checkpoint Using the criteria listed on the evaluation sheet, your instructor will grade your performance.

PROCEDURE 20:10E
Preparing and Testing a Hemoccult Slide

NOTE: Legal requirements regarding who can perform this procedure vary from state to state. Check your legal responsibilities before performing this procedure.

Equipment and Supplies

Bedpan with cover/specimen collector, Hemoccult slide packet, Hemoccult developer, tongue blade, paper towel, disposable gloves, plastic waste bag, biohazard bag, pen or pencil

Procedure

1. Obtain proper authorization to be sure of the type of specimen needed.
2. Assemble equipment. Read the manufacturer's instructions for the use of the Hemoccult slide packet and developer.
3. **C** Knock on the door and pause before entering. Introduce yourself. Identify the patient. Explain the procedure to the patient. Ask the patient to use the bedpan for his or her next bowel movement because a specimen is needed. Tell the patient not to void or place toilet tissue in the specimen in the bedpan. If necessary, provide a plastic waste bag for disposal of soiled toilet tissue.

    NOTE: In some agencies, special collection containers that fit directly under the toilet seat are used (refer back to figure 20-53).
4. Wash hands. Put on gloves.

CAUTION: Wear gloves and observe standard precautions when obtaining stool specimens.

5. Obtain the specimen in the bedpan. Assist the patient, as necessary. Allow the patient to wash his or her hands.
6. Take the bedpan and specimen to the bathroom.
7. Place a paper towel on the counter. Put the Hemoccult slide packet on top of the towel.
8. Open the front cover or flap of the Hemoccult packet.
9. Use the tongue blade to smear a small amount of the stool specimen on the correct areas of the slide (refer back to figure 20-73). Use different parts of the stool specimen to obtain sample smears for each of the two areas.

    NOTE: Read the instructions. One or two small areas of exposed guaiac paper are present under the cover. Stool is placed on these areas.
10. Discard the tongue blade in a plastic waste bag.
11. Remove gloves and wash hands.
12. Close the cover or flap of the Hemoccult packet.
13. **C** Label the outside of the Hemoccult packet with all required information, usually the date and time, patient's name and address or room number, and physician's name. Print required information on

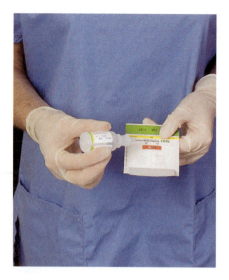

FIGURE 20-77A Place the required number of drops of Hemoccult developing solution on the exposed guaiac paper.

READING AND INTERPRETING THE HEMOCCULT® TEST

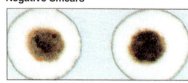

Negative Smears

Sample report: negative
No detectable blue on or at the edge of the smears indicates the test is negative for occult blood.

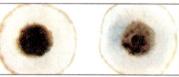

Negative and Positive Smears

Positive Smears

Sample report: positive
Any trace of blue on or at the edge of one or more of the smears indicates the test is positive for occult blood.

FIGURE 20-77B A change in color indicates that blood is present in the stool.

the correct lab requisition or obtain the requisition from your immediate supervisor. A lab requisition must be sent with the labeled specimen.

14. Send the Hemoccult packet to the laboratory for developing. Put the specimen in a protective biohazard bag for transport. In some agencies, you may be required to complete the test. To develop the test, proceed as follows:

a. Open the back tab of the Hemoccult packet to expose the back of the guaiac paper.

b. Place the required number of drops (usually one to two) of Hemoccult developer on the exposed guaiac paper (see figure 20-77A). Some packets also have test areas to which developer is applied.
NOTE: Read and follow manufacturer's instructions.

c. Wait the correct amount of time, usually 30 to 60 seconds.

d. Check the areas for color change. A positive test usually causes a blue or purple discoloration of the smear (see figure 20-77B).
NOTE: A positive test indicates the presence of blood in the stool.

15. Put on gloves to clean the bedpan. Discard any remaining stool in the toilet. Rinse the bedpan with cool water. Clean with a disinfectant, then rinse and dry. Replace all equipment used. Leave the area neat and clean.

16. Remove gloves and wash hands.

17. Report and/or record all required information on the patient's chart or the agency form, for example, date, time, Hemoccult stool specimen obtained and sent to lab, and your signature and title.

Practice *Go to the workbook and use the evaluation sheet for 20:10E, Preparing and Testing a Hemoccult Slide, to practice this procedure. When you feel you have mastered this skill, sign the sheet and give it to your instructor for further action.*

✔ **Final Checkpoint** Using the criteria listed on the evaluation sheet, your instructor will grade your performance.

20:11 INFORMATION Enemas and Rectal Treatments

⚖️ **NOTE:** Responsibility for performing these procedures varies from agency to agency. Check your agency's policy.

As a health care worker, you may be required to perform a number of rectal treatments. Equipment and solutions will vary from agency to agency, but the same basic principles are followed.

An **enema** is an injection of fluid into the large intestine and through the rectum. The main purpose of an enema is to remove feces and flatus (gas) from the colon and rectum. In addition, enemas can be used to relieve intestinal congestion and give medication. Before some surgeries, X-ray procedures, and childbirth, enemas may be ordered to clear the bowel of fecal material. The order may state, "enemas until clear." This means that enemas are given until the return solution is the same as that injected, and no fecal material is present. Check with your immediate supervisor to determine how many enemas can be given.

⚖️ A physician's order is required. The order usually states the type of enema and the amount of solution; it may also give other information such as time, purpose, or special instructions.

Enemas are frequently classified as retention or nonretention enemas:

- *Retention enemas* are small amounts of solution that are retained, or kept, in the intestine for a specified period of time after they are given. They are used to instill medications, soften stool, aid in elimination of intestinal parasites, lubricate the rectum, or expel flatus.

- *Nonretention enemas* are usually expelled in 5 to 10 minutes. Larger quantities of solution are usually given, and the enemas are generally used to clean the bowel of feces and flatus (gas).

Types of enemas in frequent use are cleansing enemas, disposable enemas, and oil retention enemas.

- *Cleansing enema:* Usually a soap-solution, tap-water enema, or saline solution. Soap-solution enemas irritate the intestine, so they are no longer used as frequently as tap-water enemas. A large amount of the solution, from 750 to 1,000 cubic centimeters, is usually given. The main purpose is to remove stool and flatus.

- *Disposable enema:* Also a cleansing enema, in most cases. However, these enemas come in prepared, disposable containers, each usually containing 4 to 6 ounces (120 to 180 cubic centimeters). The solution tends to be hypertonic, meaning that it draws fluid from the body to stimulate peristalsis and elimination of stool and flatus.

- *Oil retention enema:* Mineral or olive oil may be used. Commercially prepared enemas containing oil are also available. Four to six ounces is the usual amount. These enemas are retained for at least 30 to 60 minutes. The main purpose is to soften fecal material so that it can be expelled. An oil retention enema is sometimes followed with a cleansing enema.

The patient receiving an enema is usually placed in the Sims' (left lateral) position. This encourages the solution to flow from the rectum to the sigmoid portion of the colon. The patient should be encouraged to breathe deeply during enema administration. Deep breathing encourages relaxation and increases retention of the solution for more effective results.

C Results must be observed after an enema is given. Amount, type, and color of stool, and/or the amount of flatus expelled should be recorded.

An **impaction** is a large, hard mass of fecal material lodged in the intestine or rectum. Oil-retention enemas are frequently ordered to soften the impaction so it can be expelled. If it cannot be removed by an enema, it is sometimes necessary to insert a lubricated, gloved finger into the rectum to break up the fecal material. The licensed supervisor or advanced care provider usually performs this procedure.

Gas (flatus) accumulation in the intestine is a frequent problem for surgical patients. A **rectal tube** may be inserted to aid in the expulsion of flatus. The tube is usually left in place for 20 to 30 minutes. Because fecal material may drain out of the tube, it is wise to place the open end of the tube in a basin or container. This procedure also is ordered by the physician.

A **suppository** is a cone-shaped object that usually has a base material of cocoa butter or glycerine. It is inserted into the rectum and melts as a result of body heat. Suppositories are used to stimulate peristalsis and aid in expelling feces. Medicated suppositories have medication added to the base material. They can be used to relieve pain, decrease body temperature (aspirin suppositories), stop vomiting (anti-emetics), and treat other conditions, depending on the medication given. A health care worker is *not* permitted to administer medications, so insertion of the medicated suppositories would *not* be your responsibility.

Feces is contaminated with many microorganisms, so standard precautions (discussed in Unit 13:3) must be observed when giving enemas and rectal treatments. Gloves must be worn. Hands must be washed frequently, and are always washed immediately when gloves are removed. Eye protection must be worn if spraying or splashing of body fluids is possible. Any areas or equipment contaminated by fecal material must be cleaned with a disinfectant or sterilized. Most agencies use disposable enema kits and rectal tubes. These are discarded in an infectious-waste bag after use. Precautions must be taken at all times to prevent the spread of infection.

STUDENT: *Go to the workbook and complete the assignment sheet for 20:11, Enemas and Rectal Treatments. Then return and continue with the procedures.*

PROCEDURE 20:11A
Giving a Tap-Water or Soap-Solution Enema

Equipment and Supplies

Disposable enema kit (or irrigation container or bag with tubing, rectal tube, and liquid soap for a soap-solution enema), graduated pitcher, bath thermometer, paper towels, lubricating jelly, tray, two towels, toilet tissue, bedpan with cover, bath blanket, underpad or bed protector, disposable gloves, basin, washcloth, soap, infectious-waste bag, pen or pencil

Procedure

1. Check physician's orders or obtain authorization from your immediate supervisor.
   NOTE: The physician's order usually states the type of enema and amount to be given.
2. Assemble equipment.
3. Wash hands.
   CAUTION: Wear gloves and observe standard precautions when giving an enema.

4. Prepare the tray in the utility room or bathroom.
5. If necessary, attach the tubing to the irrigation container or bag (see figure 20-78A). Adjust the clamp to the proper position on the tubing (see figure 20-78B). Snap the clamp shut.
   NOTE: If the tubing does *not* have a rectal tube tip, attach a rectal tube.
6. Fill the irrigation container with water to the 1,000-cubic-centimeter line (or to the level ordered by physician), see figure 20-78C. Use a bath thermometer to check the temperature of the water; it should measure 105°F or 41°C (see figure 20-78D).
   CAUTION: Be sure the temperature is accurate. If the solution is too hot, it will burn the mucous membrane of the patient. If it is too cold, it could cause cramps and discomfort.
   NOTE: If the irrigation container does not have measurement markings, use a graduated

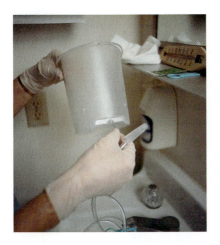

FIGURE 20-78A Attach the tubing to the enema container.

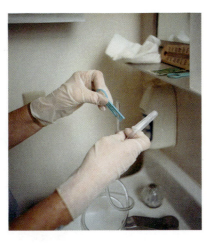

FIGURE 20-78B Slip the clamp into position on the tubing.

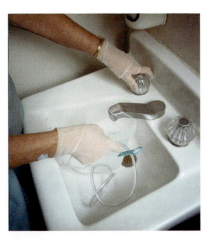

FIGURE 20-78C Fill the container with water to the 1,000-cubic-centimeter line (or the level ordered by the physician).

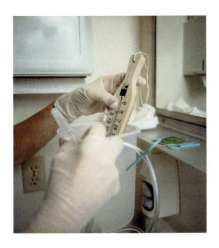

FIGURE 20-78D Use a bath thermometer to check the temperature of the water; it must measure 105°F.

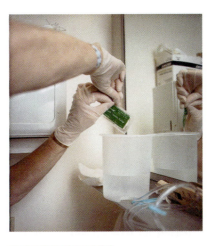

FIGURE 20-78E Add the packet of soap to the container, if a soap-solution enema is ordered.

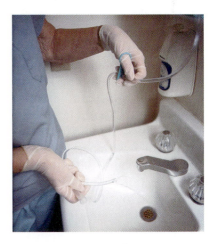

FIGURE 20-78F Run the solution through the tubing to remove air from the tubing.

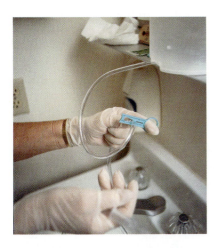

FIGURE 20-78G Clamp the tubing.

pitcher to measure the amount needed. Then, pour the solution into the irrigation container or bag.

7. Put the liquid soap (usually 20 to 30 cubic centimeters) into the water if a soap-solution enema is ordered (see figure 20-78E). Stir gently to prevent sud formation.
   NOTE: If a saline solution is given, 2 teaspoons of salt are usually added to the 1,000 cubic centimeters of water. For a tap-water enema, nothing is added.

8. Run the solution through the tubing to remove air from the tubing (see figure 20-78F). Clamp the tubing closed (see figure 20-78G).
   NOTE: This step can also be done immediately before insertion of the enema.

9. Place a small amount of lubricant on a paper towel. Place the tip of the tubing into the towel.

   NOTE: Even prelubricated tips usually require additional lubrication.

10. Place all equipment on the tray. Check to be sure all equipment is there. Cover the tray with a towel.

11. Take the tray to the patient's unit.

12. **C** Knock on the door and pause before entering. Introduce yourself. Identify the patient. Explain the procedure to the patient. Close the door and screen the unit.

13. Wash hands. Put on gloves.

   CAUTION: Observe standard precautions when giving an enema.

14. Place the bedpan on a chair by the bed. Position all equipment conveniently.

15. Elevate the bed to a comfortable working height. Lower the siderail on the side where you are working.

16. Cover the patient with a bath blanket. Fanfold the top bed linens to the foot of the bed.

17. Place the underpad or bed protector under the patient's buttocks.

   CAUTION: Use correct body mechanics. Bend at the hips and maintain a wide base of support.

18. Position the patient in the Sims' (left lateral) position. Fold the bath blanket back at an angle to expose the buttocks.

   NOTE: For patients who have difficulty retaining the enema, it is permissible to position them on the bedpan and in the dorsal recumbent position. Check with your immediate supervisor if you do not know which position to use.

19. Check to be sure the tip is lubricated. Loosen the clamp and let some solution flow through the tubing and into the bedpan. Clamp off but make sure the solution is at the end of the tubing.

20. **C** Use one hand to raise the upper buttock and expose the anus (the opening to the rectum). With your other hand, gently insert the tip 2 to 4 inches into the rectum. Tell the patient you are inserting the tube. Encourage deep breathing and relaxation.

   NOTE: If unable to insert the tube, pull back slightly and attempt to reinsert. If still unable to insert, discontinue the procedure and check with your immediate supervisor. A fecal impaction may be present.

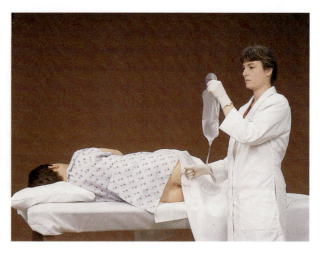

FIGURE 20-79 Raise the irrigation bag 12 inches above the level of the anus to allow the solution to slowly flow into the rectum.

21. Open the clamp. Raise the irrigation container or bag 12 inches above the level of the anus (see figure 20-79). Make sure the solution flows in slowly. Encourage the patient to breathe deeply.

   NOTE: If the patient complains of cramping or discomfort, clamp the tube to stop the flow and wait until the cramping stops.

   NOTE: Regulate the rate of flow by raising (for a faster flow) or lowering (for a slower flow) the container or bag. The container may also be placed on an adjustable IV pole or stand.

22. When all of the solution has been drained, clamp the tubing before air enters the rectum.

23. Remove the tubing gently. Tell the patient what you are doing. Wrap the tubing in tissue and place it in the empty irrigation container.

24. Position the patient on the bedpan as previously instructed or escort the patient to the bathroom or onto a bedside commode, if the patient is ambulatory. Encourage the patient to retain the enema as long as possible. If the patient is ambulatory and will use the toilet, caution the patient *not* to flush the toilet until results are noted.

   NOTE: Retention yields more effective results.

25. Raise the patient's head to a comfortable position. Leave the call signal and toilet tissue within easy reach of the patient.

26. If the patient can be left alone, take the equipment to the bathroom for cleaning; if not, remain with the patient. Observe for

signs of distress, weakness, excessive perspiration, paleness, or discomfort.

27. Answer the call signal immediately. Remove the bedpan. Assist with cleaning the rectal area, if necessary.

28. Provide a towel and washcloth so that the patient can wash his or her hands. Assist with perineal care as needed.

29. Reposition bed linens. Remove the bath blanket and underpad or bed protector.

30. Observe all checkpoints before leaving the patient: position the patient comfortably and in correct body alignment, elevate the siderails (if indicated), lower the bed to its lowest level, place the call signal and supplies within easy reach of the patient, and leave the area neat and clean.

31. Take the bedpan to the bathroom. Observe contents before emptying the bedpan. Note the amount, type, and color of stool expelled, and the effectiveness of the enema.

    C **NOTE:** Words such as *good, poor, small,* or *no results* are used to describe the effectiveness of an enema.

32. Empty the bedpan. Rinse it with cold water. Clean it with a disinfectant. Rinse, dry, and return the bedpan to the patient's unit.

33. Clean and replace all other equipment used. If the irrigation container is disposable, place it in an infectious-waste bag.

34. Remove gloves and wash hands thoroughly.

35. **C** Report and/or record all required information on the patient's chart or the agency form, for example, date; time; 1000 cc tap-water enema given with good results, retained 10 minutes, expelled 4 large dark-brown formed stools, tolerated procedure well; and your signature and title. Report any unusual observations immediately.

> **Practice** *Go to the workbook and use the evaluation sheet for 20:11A, Giving a Tap-Water or Soap-Solution Enema, to practice this procedure. When you feel you have mastered this skill, sign the sheet and give it to your instructor for further action.*

✔ **Final Checkpoint** Using the criteria listed on the evaluation sheet, your instructor will grade your performance.

PROCEDURE 20:11B

Giving a Disposable Enema

NOTE: Approximately 4 ounces (120 milliliters) of hypertonic solution is usually contained in a plastic bottle with a prelubricated tip (for example, a Fleet's enema).

Equipment and Supplies

Disposable enema unit, lubricating jelly, paper towels, tray with cover, bath blanket, underpad or bed protector, bedpan with cover, toilet tissue, disposable gloves, basin, towel, washcloth, soap, infectious-waste bag, pen or pencil

Procedure

1. Check physician's orders or obtain authorization from your immediate supervisor; verify the type of enema.

2. Assemble equipment.

3. Remove the enema from its package. Remove the cover from the tip. Add additional lubrication as needed by placing the tip in a paper towel with lubricating jelly.

   NOTE: Even prelubricated tips often need additional lubrication.

   NOTE: If the enema is to be warmed, place it in a basin of water at a temperature of 105°F (41°C). Disposable enemas are usually given at room temperature.

4. Place all equipment on the tray and cover with a towel. Go to the patient's unit.

5. **C** Knock on the door and pause before entering. Introduce yourself. Identify the patient. Explain the procedure.

6. Close the door and screen the unit.

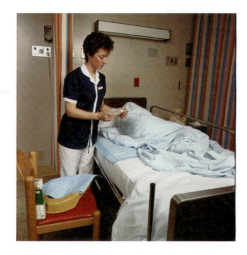

FIGURE 20-80 Squeeze the container slightly to get the solution to the top of the tip of a disposable enema.

7. Wash hands. Put on gloves.

   CAUTION: Wear gloves and observe standard precautions when giving an enema.

8. Place the bedpan on a chair near the bed. Position all equipment conveniently.

9. Elevate the bed to a comfortable working height. Lower the siderail on the side of the bed where you are working.

10. Cover the patient with a bath blanket. Fanfold the top bed linens to the foot of the bed. Place an underpad or bed protector under the patient's buttocks.

11. Position the patient in the Sims' position. Fold the bath blanket at an angle to expose the buttocks.

12. Squeeze the container slightly to get the solution to the top of the tip and eliminate air in the container (see figure 20-80).

13. **C** Use one hand to raise the upper buttock and expose the anus (the opening to the rectum). With your other hand, gently insert the tip approximately 2 inches. Explain each step to the patient to reduce anxiety and apprehension.

    NOTE: If unable to insert the tip, pull it back slightly and try again. Sometimes, releasing a small amount of solution eases insertion. If still unable to insert, discontinue the procedure and check with your immediate supervisor.

14. To expel the solution, gently squeeze the container, starting from the bottom and progressing toward the tip in a spiral manner. Hold the container at a slight upward angle to prevent air bubbles. Encourage the patient to breathe deeply and to retain the enema solution.

15. When the solution has been injected and the container is empty, gently remove the tip from the rectum. Inform the patient as you do this. Place the container in an infectious-waste bag.

16. Place the bedpan under the patient or assist the patient to the bathroom or onto a bedside commode. Encourage 5 to 10 minutes of retention.

17. Position the patient comfortably. Leave the call signal and toilet tissue within easy reach of the patient. Wash hands and remove gloves before leaving the room.

    NOTE: Remain with the patient, if necessary.

18. Answer the call signal immediately. Wash hands and put on gloves. Remove the bedpan. Assist the patient in cleaning the anal area, as needed.

19. Provide a washcloth and towel. Allow the patient to wash his or her hands with soap and water. Assist with perineal care as needed.

20. Replace the top bed linens. Remove the bed protector and bath blanket. Position the patient comfortably and in correct body alignment.

21. Observe all checkpoints before leaving the patient: elevate the siderails (if indicated), lower the bed to its lowest level, place the call signal and supplies within easy reach of the patient, and leave the area neat and clean.

22. Take the bedpan to the bathroom. Observe the contents of the bedpan before emptying. Note amount, color, type, and any abnormalities. Record the results or effectiveness of the enema.

23. Empty the bedpan and rinse it with cold water. Clean it with a disinfectant. Rinse, dry, and return the bedpan to the patient's unit.

24. Clean and replace other equipment used.

25. Remove gloves. Wash hands.

26. **C** Report and/or record all required information on the patient's chart or the agency form, for example, date; time; Fleet's enema given with poor results, expelled 1 small formed dark-brown stool, patient complaining of "gas pains"; and your signature and title. Report any unusual observations immediately.

Practice *Go to the workbook and use the evaluation sheet for 20:11B, Giving a Disposable Enema, to practice this procedure. When you feel you have mastered this skill, sign the sheet and give it to your instructor for further action.*

 Final Checkpoint Using the criteria listed on the evaluation sheet, your instructor will grade your performance.

PROCEDURE 20:11C

Giving an Oil Retention Enema

Equipment and Supplies

Commercially prepared oil retention enema (or 4 to 6 ounces mineral oil, olive oil, or other oil specified by physician; irrigation container with tubing, rectal tube, and clamp), lubricating jelly, paper towels, disposable gloves, tray with cover, bath blanket, underpad(s) or bed protector(s), toilet tissue, bedpan with cover, basin, towel, washcloth, infectious-waste bag, pen or pencil

Procedure

1. Check physician's orders or obtain authorization from your immediate supervisor; verify the type and amount of enema.
2. Assemble equipment.
3. If a commercial enema unit is used, remove the enema from the outer package. Remove the protective cap from the tip and add lubrication as needed by rolling the tip in a paper towel with lubricating jelly.

   NOTE: If a commercial unit is not used, use 4 to 6 ounces of mineral oil, olive oil, or other oil specified in the order. Warm the oil by placing the container in a pan of warm water. Measure the correct amount of oil and place it in the irrigation container. Make sure the tubing is free of air and the clamp is shut. Lubricate the tip of the rectal tube.
4. Place all equipment on a tray. Cover and take to the patient's unit.
5. **C** Knock on the door and pause before entering. Introduce yourself. Identify the patient. Explain the procedure.
6. Close the door and screen the unit.
7. Wash hands. Put on gloves.

CAUTION: Wear gloves and observe standard precautions when giving an enema.

8. Place the bedpan on a chair near the bed. Position all equipment conveniently.
9. Elevate the bed to a comfortable working height. Lower the siderail on the side where you are working.
10. Cover the patient with a bath blanket. Fanfold the top bed linens to the foot of the bed. Place an underpad or bed protector under the patient's buttocks.
11. Position the patient in the Sims' position. Fold the bath blanket at an angle to expose the buttocks.
12. Squeeze the container slightly to bring the oil to the tip and remove air.

    NOTE: If an irrigation container and tubing are used, open the clamp to allow oil to fill the tubing.
13. **C** Use one hand to raise the upper buttock and expose the anus (the opening to the rectum). With your other hand, gently insert the tip 2 to 4 inches into the rectum. Tell the patient what you are doing.
14. Squeeze the container in a spiral fashion to expel the solution. Instill the solution slowly and gently. Encourage the patient to breathe deeply and to retain the enema solution.

    NOTE: If a container and tubing are used, raise the container 12 inches to control the flow rate.
15. When the container is empty, gently remove the tip. Tell the patient what you are doing. Place the container in an infectious-waste bag.

16. Encourage the patient to retain the solution for at least 30 to 60 minutes. Leave the call signal within easy reach. Remove gloves and wash hands thoroughly.

    NOTE: If the oil seeps, an additional underpad may be necessary.

17. Answer the call signal immediately. Wash hands and put on gloves. Position the patient on the bedpan or assist him or her to the bathroom or onto a bedside commode. Make sure toilet tissue and the call signal are within easy reach.

    NOTE: Remain with the patient, if necessary.

18. Answer the call signal immediately. Remove the bedpan. Assist the patient in cleaning the anal area, as needed.

    NOTE: A tap-water or soap-solution enema is sometimes ordered to follow an oil retention enema, if the results are poor or the patient cannot expel the oil retention enema.

19. Provide a washcloth and towel for the patient to wash his or her hands. Assist with perineal care as needed.

20. Position the patient comfortably and in correct body alignment. Replace top bed linens. Remove underpad and bath blanket. If necessary, put a clean underpad under the patient's buttocks.

    NOTE: Because some oil may continue to seep from the rectum after cleaning, it is usually wise to place a clean underpad under the patient's buttocks.

21. Observe all checkpoints before leaving the patient: elevate the siderails (if indicated),

lower the bed to its lowest level, place the call signal and supplies within easy reach of the patient, and leave the area neat and clean.

22. Take the bedpan to the bathroom. Note amount, color, and type of stool before emptying.

23. Empty the bedpan and rinse it with cold water. Clean with a disinfectant. Rinse, dry, and return the bedpan to the patient's unit.

24. Clean and replace all other equipment used.

25. Remove gloves. Wash hands.

26. Report and/or record all required information on the patient's chart or the agency form, for example, date; time; oil retention enema given with good results, retained 30 minutes, expelled large amount of light-brown semi-formed stool and flatus, patient stated "I feel much better"; and your signature and title. Report any abnormal observations immediately.

Practice *Go to the workbook and use the evaluation sheet for 20:11C, Giving an Oil Retention Enema, to practice this procedure. When you feel you have mastered this skill, sign the sheet and give it to your instructor for further action.*

✔ **Final Checkpoint** Using the criteria listed on the evaluation sheet, your instructor will grade your performance.

PROCEDURE 20:11D

Inserting a Rectal Tube

Equipment and Supplies

Rectal tube and flatus bag, lubricating jelly, paper towel, tissue, underpad or protective bed cover, basin or specimen bottle (if needed), disposable gloves, tape, infectious-waste bag, pen or pencil

Procedure

1. Check physician's orders or obtain authorization from your immediate supervisor. Note time ordered.

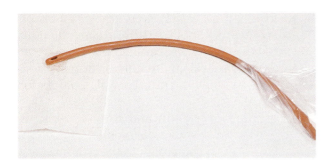

FIGURE 20-81 Place the tip of the rectal tube in lubricating jelly on a paper towel. Connect the opposite end to the flatus bag.

NOTE: This procedure may be ordered for a specific time, for example, 1/2 hour after administration of a medication.

2. Assemble equipment. Place the tip of the rectal tube in lubricating jelly on a paper towel. Connect the opposite (open) end to the flatus bag (see figure 20-81).

   NOTE: Instead of connecting it to a flatus bag, the open end may be placed in a disposable glove and taped or in a basin or specimen bottle. Follow agency policy.

   NOTE: Many agencies now use disposable rectal tubes with flatus bags attached. The tip of the tube must still be lubricated. The tube and bag are discarded in an infectious-waste bag after one use.

3. **C** Knock on the door and pause before entering. Introduce yourself. Identify the patient. Explain the procedure to the patient.

4. Close the door and screen the unit.

5. Wash hands. Put on gloves.

   CAUTION: Wear gloves and observe standard precautions when giving an enema.

6. Elevate the bed to a comfortable working height. Lower the siderail on the side where you are working.

7. Position the patient in the Sims' position. Place an underpad under the patient's buttocks. Fold the bed linen at an angle to expose the buttocks.

8. Use one hand to raise the upper buttock and expose the anus (the opening to the rectum). With your other hand, insert the rectal tube 2 to 4 inches into the rectum. Tell the patient what you are doing.

9. Tape the tube to the patient's buttocks to hold the tube in place.

10. If a flatus bag is *not* in use, place the free end of the tube in a basin, bedpan, or specimen bottle.

    NOTE: Fecal material may seep from tube.

11. Make sure the patient is as comfortable as possible before leaving. Elevate siderails, if indicated. Leave the call signal within easy reach of the patient.

12. Remove gloves and wash hands thoroughly.

13. Return at intervals to check the patient and rectal tube.

    CAUTION: Do *not* leave if the patient is unconscious or not alert to surroundings.

14. Wash hands and put on gloves. Remove the tube promptly at the end of the time period, usually 20 to 30 minutes. Tell the patient what you are doing. Remove the tube gently.

    CAUTION: The tube can irritate sensitive tissue if left in place too long.

15. Place the rectal tube and bag in the infectious-waste bag. Clean the patient, as needed. Remove the underpad and replace the bed linens.

16. **C** Ask the patient how much flatus (gas) was expelled or if the patient feels better.

    NOTE: Licensed personnel may listen to bowel sounds immediately after the rectal tube is removed. Inform the correct person that you have removed the rectal tube.

17. Observe all checkpoints before leaving the patient: position the patient in correct body alignment, elevate the siderails (if indicated), lower the bed to its lowest level, place the call signal and supplies within easy reach of the patient, and leave the area neat and clean.

18. Note any result including collection of air (flatus) in the bag, drainage, and patient's comments following the procedure.

19. Clean and replace all equipment.

20. Remove gloves. Wash hands.

21. **C** Report and/or record all required information on the patient's chart or the agency form, for example, date; time; rectal tube inserted for 20 minutes, expelled large amount of flatus, no drainage noted, Patient stated "I feel much better"; and your signature and title. Report any unusual observations immediately.

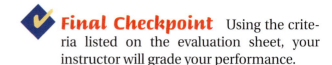

20:12 INFORMATION Applying Restraints

OBRA Although sick people are usually quiet and need encouragement to move, there are times when it is necessary to limit the movement of overactive patients. **Restraints** are used to limit movement. There are two kinds of restraints: chemical and physical. Chemical restraints are medications that affect the patient's behavior. Examples include tranquilizers, sedatives, and mood-altering medications. Licensed personnel are responsible for administering any chemical restraints.

Physical restraints are protective devices that limit a patient's movements. They should be used *only* to protect patients from harming themselves or others and when all other measures to correct the situation have failed. OBRA legislation clearly defines the limitations of using restraints. All resident behavior that may necessitate the use of restraints must be documented. Alternatives must be tried and carefully documented. If alternate solutions are not successful, the resident and/or resident's family or legal guardian must give approval and written consent for the use of a restraint or safety device. A physician must write the order for the restraint, and the order must state the type of restraint, the reason for its use, the length of time it can be used, and where or when it can be used. The least restrictive device must always be used first. A restraint applied unnecessarily can be considered false imprisonment. A health care worker should *never* apply a restraint without proper authorization.

Circumstances and conditions that may necessitate the use of restraints include:

◆ *Irrational or confused patients:* Patients can become irrational or confused because of medications, senility, and other factors. They may attempt to climb out of bed or over siderails, or may wander about. Because they could fall and injure themselves, restraints must sometimes be applied to limit their movements.

◆ *Skin conditions:* Patients, especially small children, with itching skin conditions must sometimes have their hands restrained or encased in protective mittens to prevent scratching.

◆ *Paralysis or limited muscular coordination:* Patients under anesthesia or who are paralyzed by strokes are often unable to coordinate or control their muscular movements. They may require restraints.

There are different kinds of physical restraints. It is important to follow the manufacturer's recommendations when applying any kind of restraint. Some common kinds include:

◆ *Straps or safety belts:* Usually found on wheelchairs, some are designed to be utilized interchangeably on wheelchairs, beds, and stretchers (see figure 20-82). A strap or safety belt is used to prevent a patient from falling out of the device. The strap or belt should not be applied too tightly because it can restrict breathing and/or interfere with circulation.

◆ *Limb restraints:* Usually, soft, padded restraints that are wrapped around the arm or leg to limit movement of the limb. The restraint straps are then attached to the frame

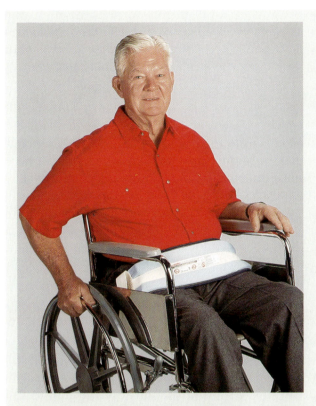

FIGURE 20-82 A belt restraint can be used to support a patient sitting in a wheelchair. *(Courtesy of J.T. Posey Company)*

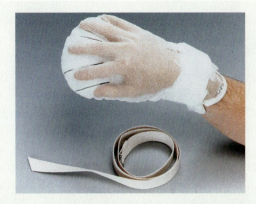

FIGURE 20-83 Hand mitts can be applied to prevent the patient from scratching or injuring the skin.

of the bed or stretcher to secure the limb into position. At least two fingers should be slipped between the restraint and skin to make sure the restraint is not too tight.

◆ *Restraint jackets:* Used to prevent a patient from sitting up, rolling, getting out of bed, or falling out of a wheelchair. Jacket restraints are available in different sizes. It is important to follow manufacturer's directions and measure the patient carefully to make sure the correct size jacket restraint is used. Jacket restraints must also be applied so that they do not interfere with breathing or circulation.

◆ *Hand mitts:* devices similar to mittens that are applied to the hands to prevent the patient from scratching or injuring the skin (see figure 20-83).

There are some important points to remember when using restraints:

◆ Use only when all other means of obtaining the patient's cooperation have failed.

◆ Restraints should be as unnoticeable to the patient as possible.

◆ Patients should be allowed to move as much as possible without danger of self-injury.

◆ The patient should always be told why his or her movements are being restricted, even when the patient is irrational or confused.

◆ The restrained patient feels both physical and mental frustration. Therefore, it is important to reassure the patient frequently.

◆ Restraints should be checked frequently after they have been applied. Circulation below a limb restraint should be checked every 15 to 30 minutes. Signs of poor circulation include paleness, cyanosis (blue discoloration), cold skin, edema (or swelling), weak or absent pulse, poor return of pink color after the nail beds are pressed lightly (or blanched), and the patient complaining of pain, numbness, or tingling. If any signs of poor circulation are noted, the restraint must be removed immediately and your supervisor notified. All restraints *must* be removed every 2 hours for at least 10 minutes. The patient should be repositioned, and range of motion (ROM) exercises and skin care to the skin under the restraint should be provided.

◆ Remove restraints as soon as there is adequate supervision or as soon as the danger of the patient injuring him- or herself has passed.

Some complications that can occur when restraints are applied include:

◆ *Physical and mental frustration* on the part of the patient. The loss of freedom imposed by restraints can cause disorientation, depression, hostility, agitation, and/or withdrawal. Provide reassurance and supportive care to the patient.

◆ *Impaired circulation.* Check skin color and skin temperature frequently.

◆ *Pressure ulcers* from the pressure applied by restraints.

◆ *Loss of muscle tone; joint stiffness;* and *discomfort from immobility.* The inability to go to the bathroom at will can lead to incontinence and constipation. Provide frequent ROM exercises, and offer to take the patient to the bathroom at regular intervals.

◆ *Respiratory or breathing problems,* especially when jacket restraints are applied.

Most health care facilities have specific rules and policies regarding the use of restraints. All patients have the right to maintain their dignity and independence as much as possible. It is important for the staff to evaluate whether the risk of potential injury to the patient and/or others is greater than the risk of complications from the use of restraints. It is essential that the health care worker knows and follows all rules and policies, and is aware of legal responsibilities regarding the use of restraints.

STUDENT: *Go to the workbook and complete the assignment sheet for 20:12, Applying Restraints. Then return and continue with the procedures.*

PROCEDURE 20:12A   OBRA

Applying Limb Restraints

Equipment and Supplies

Adjustable limb restraint(s), pen or pencil

Procedure

1. Check physician's orders or obtain authorization from your immediate supervisor.

   CAUTION: A restraint *cannot* be applied without a physician's order.

2. Assemble equipment.

3. **C** Knock on the door and pause before entering. Introduce yourself. Identify the patient. Explain the procedure even if the patient is irrational or confused.

4. Wash hands.

5. Close the door and screen the unit to provide privacy. If the patient is in a bed, elevate the bed to a comfortable working height, and lower the siderail on the side where you are working. If the patient is in a wheelchair, lock the wheels of the chair. Position the patient in a comfortable position and in good body alignment.

6. Place the soft edge of the restraint against the patient's skin (see figure 20-84). Wrap the restraint smoothly around the limb. Make sure there are no wrinkles.

7. Pull the ends of the straps through the tabs or rings on the restraint. Then, pull the restraint secure, but not too tight, against the patient's skin.

   CAUTION: If applied too tightly, the restraint could stop circulation or cause a pressure sore.

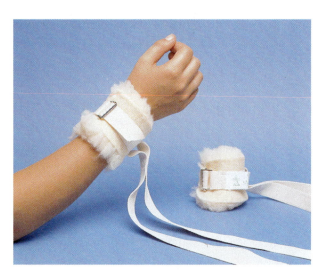

FIGURE 20-84 Place the soft edge of the limb restraint against the patient's skin. *(Courtesy of J.T. Posey Company)*

8. Test for fit and comfort by inserting two fingers between the restraint and the patient's skin.

9. Position the arm or leg in a comfortable position. Limit movement only as much as is necessary.

10. Use a quick-release tie to secure the straps to the movable part of the bedframe, stretcher frame, or other frame. To make the quick-release tie, bring the end of the strap around the frame. Then, bring the loose end up behind and around the back of the strap to create a hole. Fold the loose end of the strap into a loop and tuck the loop into the hole formed. Pull up on the descending part of the strap to tighten the loop in the hole. To release the tie, simply pull on the loose, exposed end of the strap.

11. Recheck the patient before leaving.

    ! CAUTION: Make sure the restraint is secure but not too tight.

12. Observe all checkpoints before leaving the patient: position the patient in correct body alignment, place the call signal and supplies within easy reach of the patient, elevate the siderails (if indicated), lower the bed to its lowest level, and leave the area neat and clean.

13. Check the circulation below the limb restraint every 15 to 30 minutes. Note color and temperature of skin, return of color after pressing lightly on nail beds, edema (or swelling), and patient complaints of pain, numbness, or tingling.

    ! CAUTION: If any signs of impaired circulation are noted, remove the restraint immediately and notify your supervisor.

14. Remove the restraint every 2 hours for at least 10 minutes. Reposition the patient. Provide ROM exercises to the restrained limb. Administer skin care to the skin under the restraint.

15. Remove the restraint when authorized to do so by your supervisor or the physician.
    NOTE: Restraints are removed when the physician or supervisor feels that the danger of self-injury to the patient has passed. Restraints must always be removed as soon as is possible.

16. Replace all equipment.

17. Wash hands.

18. **C** Report and/or record all required information on the patient's chart or the agency form, for example, date; time; limb restraints applied to both arms while patient positioned in wheelchair, P 82 strong and regular at both wrists, patient appears to be resting quietly; and your signature and title. Report any unusual observations immediately.

> **Practice** *Go to the workbook and use the evaluation sheet for 20:12A, Applying Limb Restraints, to practice this procedure. When you feel you have mastered this skill, sign the sheet and give it to your instructor for further action.*

✔ **Final Checkpoint** Using the criteria listed on the evaluation sheet, your instructor will grade your performance.

PROCEDURE 20:12B   OBRA

Applying a Jacket Restraint

Equipment and Supplies

Sleeveless jacket restraint, pen or pencil

Procedure

1. Check physician's orders or obtain authorization from your immediate supervisor.

   ⚖ CAUTION: A restraint *cannot* be applied without a physician's order.

2. Assemble equipment. Obtain the correct size restraint for the patient.

   ! CAUTION: Follow manufacturer's instructions and carefully measure the patient to make sure the correct size jacket/vest restraint is used. If an incorrect size is used, the restraint will *not* provide proper support and could injure the patient.

3. Knock on the door and pause before entering. Introduce yourself. Identify

the patient. Explain the procedure even if the patient is irrational or confused.

4. Wash hands.

5. Close the door and screen the unit to provide privacy. If the patient is in a bed, elevate the bed to a comfortable working height, and lower the siderail on the side where you are working. If the patient is in a wheelchair, lock the wheels of the chair. Position the patient in a comfortable position and in good body alignment.

6. Slip the sleeves of the jacket restraint onto the patient's arms. The solid part of the jacket restraint goes on the back, and the open or V-neck part of the restraint goes on the front (see figure 20-85A). It is essential to follow manufacturer's instructions.

   ⊘ CAUTION: A restraint applied incorrectly may cause suffocation or injury.

7. Crisscross the straps in the back. Check all of the material to make sure it is free from wrinkles.

8. Bring the loose ends of the straps through the hole in the jacket. The jacket should now completely encircle the patient.

9. Check the restraint to be sure it is not too tight against the patient.

   ⊘ CAUTION: Excessive tightness could interfere with breathing.

10. Position the patient in a comfortable position. Allow as much movement as possible without risk of injury.

11. On each side of a bed or stretcher, use a quick-release tie to bring the straps down and secure them to the movable part of the frame.

12. Straps should be brought down between the wheelchair and side plate. In a wheelchair, the straps can be attached to the kick bars at the rear of the wheelchair. Note, the kick bars must have their plastic end-caps in place to ensure that the ties won't slip off (see figure 20-85B).

    ⊘ CAUTION: Never attach the straps to any parts of the wheels.

13. Recheck the restraint before leaving the patient. Check the patient's respirations.

14. Observe all checkpoints before leaving the patient: position the patient comfortably and in correct body alignment, place the call signal and supplies within easy reach of the patient, elevate the siderails (if indicated), lower the bed to its lowest level, and leave the area neat and clean.

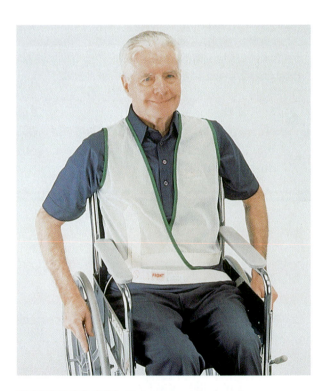

FIGURE 20-85A Follow manufacturer's instructions to measure a patient to make sure the jacket or vest is the correct size. Position the jacket restraint with the open or V-neck part of the restraint on the front. *(Courtesy of J.T. Posey Company)*

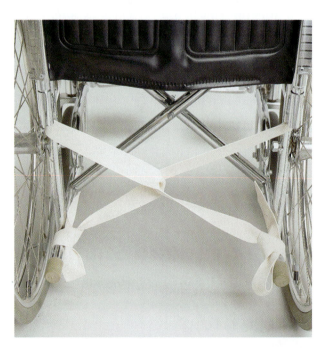

FIGURE 20-85B Use a quick-release tie to secure the straps to the back frame of a wheelchair. *(Courtesy of J.T. Posey Company)*

15. Return every 15 to 30 minutes to check the patient. Check count and character of respirations, and the color and temperature of the skin.

   ⬡! **CAUTION:** If any signs of impaired circulation or respiration are noted, remove the restraint immediately and notify your supervisor.

16. Remove the restraint every 2 hours for at least 10 minutes. Reposition the patient. Provide ROM exercises. Administer skin care to the skin under the restraint.

17. Remove the restraint when authorized to do so by your supervisor or the physician.

   NOTE: A restraint is removed when the danger of self-injury has passed. Restraints must always be removed as soon as is possible.

18. Replace all equipment.

19. Wash hands.

20. ⒸReport and/or record all required information on the patient's chart or the agency form, for example, date; time; jacket restraint applied, patient seated in wheelchair; and your signature and title.

> ***Practice*** *Go to the workbook and use the evaluation sheet for 20:12B, Applying a Jacket Restraint, to practice this procedure. When you feel you have mastered this skill, sign the sheet and give it to your instructor for further action.*

✔ **Final Checkpoint** Using the criteria listed on the evaluation sheet, your instructor will grade your performance.

20:13 INFORMATION
Administering Pre- and Post-Operative Care

Providing care to patients scheduled for surgery may be one of your responsibilities as a health care worker. Surgical care is divided into three phases:

◆ **Preoperative care** (pre-op): care provided before the surgery

◆ **Operative care:** care provided during the surgery

◆ **Postoperative care** (post-op): care provided following surgery

NOTE: Unless you work in an operating room, your major responsibilities will likely involve the pre-op and post-op phases.

Ⓒ Every patient scheduled for surgery, no matter how minor, has some fears. Fears regarding disfigurement, pain, loss of control, the unknown, length of recovery time, costs and financial problems, a poor diagnosis after surgery, and even death create concerns for many patients. It is important to provide emotional support in addition to physical care. Answer all questions you can to the best of your ability. However, specific questions about the surgery, outcome, or anesthesia should be referred to the physician or your supervisor. Be sure to report these questions and the patient's fears to your immediate supervisor.

Preoperative care involves many aspects of care. Most of the preparation is ordered by the physician, depending on the type of operation. Possible aspects of preparation are:

◆ *Operative permit:* A form signed by the patient to give permission for the anesthesia and surgery. It must be witnessed by a legally authorized individual.

◆ *Laboratory tests:* May include blood tests, urine tests, chest or other X-rays, ECG, and special tests ordered by the physician.

◆ *Enemas or vaginal irrigations:* Ordered by the physician in preparation for certain types of surgery.

◆ *Baths:* May be given both the night before surgery and the morning of surgery. The purpose is to remove as many microorganisms as possible in an effort to prevent infections. It also gives the patient a chance to talk and relieve some anxiety.

◆ *Vital signs:* These are taken and recorded. They are used as a standard to check vital signs during and after the surgery.

◆ *NPO:* The patient is allowed nothing by mouth for 8 to 12 hours before the surgery. The order is usually started at 12:00 AM (midnight). A sign is usually placed on the patient's bed. Water is removed from the area at the appointed time.

◆ *Valuables:* All the patient's valuables, including money and jewelry, should be placed in a hospital safe to prevent loss. A patient is sometimes allowed to wear a wedding ring. However, it must be taped or tied to the finger to prevent loss.

◆ *Remove prosthetics:* All artificial parts are removed. This includes dentures, contact lenses or glasses, artificial arms or legs, and hearing aids.

◆ *Remove cosmetics:* Nail polish, make-up, hair pins, and wigs are all removed prior to surgery.

Presence of cosmetics can mask skin or nail bed color changes.

◆ **Surgical shave** *or skin preparation:* Includes shaving and cleaning of the operative site. This may or may not be done. Some physicians feel that shaving the skin can cause superficial cuts that lead to infection, a concern supported by the Centers for Disease Control and Prevention (CDC). If a surgical shave is done, it can be done by a special skin-prep team or by the surgical staff immediately before the surgery or, sometimes, by the nurse assistant before the patient is transferred to the operating room. Skin preparation sites for some specific surgeries are shown in figure 20-86. Each agency has its own policy regarding what area is to be prepared. Sometimes, the physician specifies the area. The skin is shaved in order to prevent infection in and around the surgical site, and to remove longer hair that would interfere with surgery.

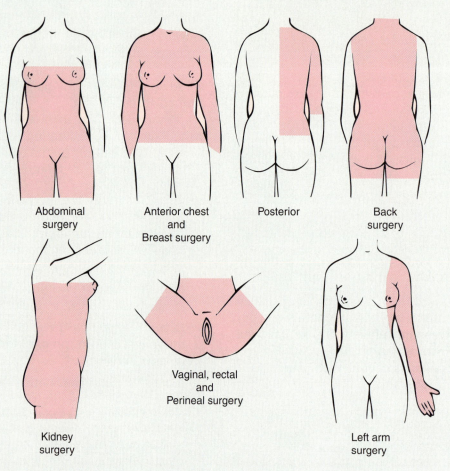

Abdominal surgery

Anterior chest and Breast surgery

Posterior

Back surgery

Kidney surgery

Vaginal, rectal and Perineal surgery

Left arm surgery

FIGURE 20-86 Shaded areas represent skin-preparation sites for some specific surgeries.

◆ *Clothing:* Usually, the patient must remove all clothing, including undergarments. A hospital gown is placed on the patient. Most agencies also place a surgical cap on the patient to cover the hair.

◆ **C** *Name band:* Prior to surgery, the patient's name band or identification band should be checked for accurate information. Because the patient frequently is unconscious during surgery, the name band is the only method of identifying the patient.

◆ *Voiding:* To make sure the bladder is empty during surgery, the patient should void immediately before being brought to the operating room. For some surgeries, a catheter is inserted in the bladder to constantly drain all urine. Only a qualified person should insert the catheter.

◆ *Surgical checklist:* Most agencies use surgical checklists to track most of the previously noted preparation items. As these items are completed, they are checked off the checklist. This provides a method for determining that the patient has been properly prepared for surgery. The checklist is usually attached to the patient's chart.

Frequently patients are not admitted to the hospital or surgical clinic until the morning of the surgery. In this case, many of the tests such as blood work, X-rays, and ECG, are performed on an outpatient basis.

Anesthesia is prevention of pain by way of loss of sensation. Medication is administered by an anesthesiologist, anesthetist, or physician. The type of anesthetic used and the method of administration depends on the type of surgery, the length of time needed, and the physical condition of the patient. Three main kinds are as follows:

◆ *General anesthesia:* Medication is given intravenously or is inhaled through a mask. This causes unconsciousness, which continues throughout surgery. A common postoperative problem is nausea or vomiting.

◆ *Local anesthesia:* Medication is injected into the area around the operative site to stop the sensation of pain. The patient is awake when local anesthesia is used.

◆ *Spinal anesthesia:* Medication is injected into the spinal canal and causes loss of sensation

(feeling) in all areas below the injection. This is often used for abdominal surgery because it produces good muscle relaxation. Patients must be told that they will not have any feeling or movement in the legs for a period of time. Patients sometimes complain of headaches after this type of anesthesia. This symptom should be reported.

While the patient is in surgery, the postoperative room or bed unit is prepared in such a way that all necessary equipment will be available when the patient returns from surgery. A recovery bed is made, an IV pole or stand and equipment for taking vital signs is put in place, and an emesis basin and tissues are placed at the bedside. Necessary special equipment, such as a suction machine for drainage tubes or equipment for administering oxygen, is also placed in the unit. All unnecessary supplies or equipment are removed from the area. For example, the water pitcher and cup are removed until postoperative orders state that the patient can have fluids.

Postoperative care is an important aspect of surgical care. Some of the factors to be considered in immediate postoperative care are:

◆ *Vital signs:* These must be checked frequently and as ordered. They are sometimes taken every 15 minutes until the patient is stable. A sudden drop in blood pressure or change in pulse rate or character are often the first signs of hemorrhage and/or shock, so any changes or abnormal readings must be reported immediately.

◆ *Dressings:* These must be checked frequently (see figure 20-87). Color, amount, and type of drainage must be noted. Any unusual observations should be reported immediately.

◆ *IV:* Flow rate and injection site must be checked only by an authorized individual.

◆ *Level of pain:* An assessment must be made on the amount of pain a patient is experiencing. Frequently patients are asked to describe pain on a scale of 1 to 10, with 1 being mild pain and 10 being extreme pain. *Patient controlled analgesics (PCAs)* are often used to control pain. An analgesic pump is attached to an intravenous (IV) line. The patient is taught to push a button when pain is felt. The

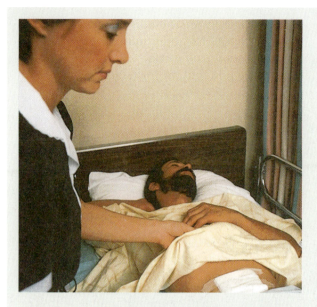

FIGURE 20-87 Dressings must be checked frequently after surgery.

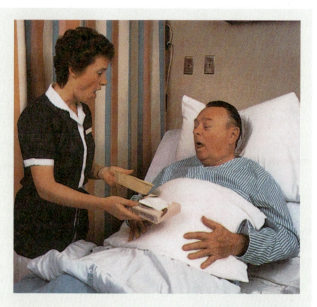

FIGURE 20-88 A pillow across the abdomen provides support when the patient is coughing and deep breathing.

pump delivers a specific dose of pain medication directly into the bloodstream to provide immediate relief. The patient cannot overdose on the medication because the pump locks out delivery of medication for a set period of time. A change in position, if allowed, can also help alleviate pain. If patients do not seem to be able to get pain relief, this should be reported immediately.

- ◆ *Observations:* Restlessness, color and temperature of skin, nausea and/or vomiting, and similar observations should be noted and reported.

- ◆ *Position:* The patient's position must be changed when possible. Be sure you are aware of all movement restrictions. Some operations limit movement and positioning. Turn or move patients only after obtaining correct authorization.

- ◆ *Cough and deep breathe:* Most patients need to be encouraged to cough and deep breathe after general anesthesia (see figure 20-88). This exercise helps remove mucus from the lungs and respiratory tract and helps prevent pneumonia and other lung disorders.

- ◆ **C** *Tubes:* Surgical patients frequently have drainage tubes in place. The tubes are connected to drainage bottles or special drainage collectors. If the tubes are not draining, if they are clamped, if the drainage solution changes or seems unusual, if a tube is not connected to a drainage source, or if any unusual observations are noted, they should be reported immediately. Care must also be taken when turning or moving the patient to make sure that the tubes are not disconnected, twisted, or pulled out.

Binders are special devices that are ordered to hold dressings in place or provide support. (See Information Section 20:14 for information about binders.)

Surgical (elastic) hose may be ordered to support the veins of the legs and increase circulation. These hose help prevent formation of blood clots in the legs. The hose must be applied correctly. If they are applied too tightly, they can interfere with circulation.

Montgomery straps are special adhesive strips that are applied when dressings must be changed frequently at the surgical site (see figure 20-89). The skin around the surgical site is cleaned thoroughly. A skin barrier, such as a liquid or paste, is applied to the skin to protect it from irritation from the tape. The Montgomery straps are then applied on either side

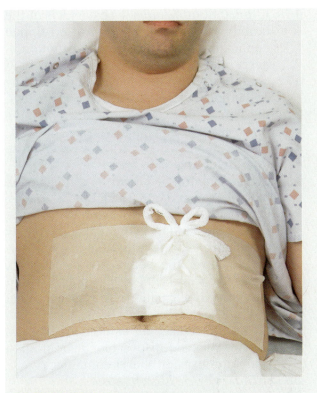

FIGURE 20-89 Montgomery straps are special adhesive strips that are applied when dressings must be changed frequently at the surgical site.

of the surgical site. The centers of the straps are nonadhesive and tied together. To change dressings, the straps are untied, the dressings are changed, and the straps are then tied in place on top of the dressings. This eliminates the need to remove and reapply adhesive tape during each dressing change.

It is essential that the nurse assistant follow all standard precautions whenever contact with blood or body fluids is possible. This helps prevent the spread of infection, including infection in the surgical patient after surgery.

In order to properly care for the surgical patient, it is essential for the nurse assistant to know and understand all aspects of care that have been ordered. Good operative care can mean a faster recovery with fewer complications for the patient.

STUDENT: *Go to the workbook and complete the assignment sheet for 20:13, Administering Pre- and Postoperative Care. Then return and continue with the procedures.*

PROCEDURE 20:13A
Shaving the Operative Area

NOTE: Disposable kits contain a bowl, razor, and most of the other supplies.

Equipment and Supplies

Skin-preparation kit, two bowls (if a kit is *not* used), razor and blades, ordered cleansing soap, gauze sponges, paper towels, applicator sticks, bath blanket, underpads or bed protectors, washcloth, towel, tray with cover, disposable gloves, gooseneck light or good light source, puncture-resistant sharps container, plastic waste bag, pen or pencil

Procedure

1. Check physician's orders or obtain authorization from your immediate supervisor. Clarify any questions about the area to be shaved.

   NOTE: Sometimes, the physician orders what area is to be shaved; other times agency policy is followed.

2. Assemble equipment.

3. Prepare equipment in the utility room or bathroom. Fill both bowls (or sections of the skin-preparation kit) with water at 105°F, or 41°C. Add liquid cleansing soap to one bowl. Place the bowls on the tray.

   NOTE: Some kits contain sponges saturated with soap. Soap does not have to be added when using these kits.

4. Check razor and blades carefully. Carefully rub the blades over a folded gauze pad to

check for damaged edges. Make sure there are no rough edges on the blades.

⚠️ **CAUTION:** Rough or damaged blades can nick or cut the patient's skin. Discard any defective blades.

5. Check the tray for all equipment and take it to the patient's unit.

6. **C** Knock on the door and pause before entering. Introduce yourself. Identify the patient. Explain the procedure.

7. Close the door and screen the unit.

8. Wash hands.

NOTE: Gloves may be put on at this point or immediately before shaving the patient.

9. Elevate the bed to a comfortable working height. Lower the siderail on the side where you are working. Cover the patient with a bath blanket. Fanfold the top bed linens to the foot of the bed. Place an underpad near the area to be shaved.

10. Position the gooseneck light or other light source so that the skin area is clearly illuminated. Make sure there are no glares or shadows.

11. Put on disposable gloves.

☣️ **CAUTION:** If you nick the skin, observe standard precautions while controlling bleeding.

12. Start at the top of the area to be shaved. Apply soapy lather to a small area of skin.

13. Hold the skin taut. Shave in the direction of hair growth. If the hair is long, as may be the case with pubic, axillary, or chest hair, it may be clipped with scissors first. Take care to avoid cutting the patient's skin with the scissors.

NOTE: When scalp hair must be cut before brain or skull surgery, it is usually done in the operating room because it can be very traumatic for the patient.

⚠️ **CAUTION:** Watch out for areas with moles or warts. Shave carefully around these areas.

14. Rinse the razor in the bowl of clean water. Remove excess hairs by rubbing the razor edge against a gauze square.

15. Repeat steps 12 to 14 on small areas until the entire operative site has been shaved. Work from top to bottom, side to side.

16. If the abdominal area is shaved, clean the umbilicus (navel) with cotton-tipped applicators. Shave with circular motion, if necessary.

17. Carefully check the shaved area for any remaining hairs. Hold a light at an angle to the skin to see reflections of any remaining hairs. Remove all remaining hairs.

18. Wash the area with warm soapy water. Rinse thoroughly and dry.

19. Replace the top bed linens and remove the bath blanket and underpad.

20. Observe all checkpoints before leaving the patient: position the patient in correct body alignment, elevate the siderails (if indicated), lower the bed to its lowest level, place the call signal and supplies within easy reach of the patient, and leave the area neat and clean.

21. Clean and replace all equipment. Put the used blades or disposable razor(s) in a puncture-resistant sharps container.

22. Remove gloves. Wash hands.

23. **C** Report and/or record all required information on the patient's chart or the agency form, for example, date; time; abdominal skin prep completed, patient resting quietly; and your signature and title. Report any cuts, nicks, or unusual observations immediately.

Practice *Go to the workbook and use the evaluation sheet for 20:13A, Shaving the Operative Area, to practice this procedure. When you feel you have mastered this skill, sign the sheet and give it to your instructor for further action.*

 Final Checkpoint Using the criteria listed on the evaluation sheet, your instructor will grade your performance.

PROCEDURE 20:13B
Administering Preoperative Care

Equipment and Supplies

Thermometer, stethoscope and sphygmomanometer, surgical gown and cap, nail polish remover, valuables envelope, tape or gauze (if needed), paper, pencil or pen

Procedure

1. Check physician's orders or obtain authorization from your immediate supervisor. Check the time of surgery.

    NOTE: Care should be completed 1 hour prior to surgery.

2. Assemble equipment.

3. **C** Knock on the door and pause before entering. Introduce yourself. Identify the patient. Explain the procedure.

    NOTE: The patient may be frightened; reassure as needed.

4. Close the door and screen the unit.

5. Wash hands.

6. Elevate the bed to a comfortable working height. Lower the siderail on the side where you are working.

7. Check the patient's identification band. Make sure it is secure. Verify name, room number, and other facts.

8. Assist with or instruct the patient to complete oral hygiene and bath.

    NOTE: The bed is *not* made prior to surgery.

    ⬡ CAUTION: Because the patient is NPO (nothing by mouth), do *not* allow the patient to swallow any water when performing oral hygiene.

9. Put a surgical gown on the patient. No other clothing is permitted. Make sure the patient's underwear is removed.

10. Remove all hairpins, wigs, and other hair ornaments. Put a cap on the patient. Make sure all hair is inside the cap.

11. Remove nail polish. Check to be sure the patient is not wearing any make-up.

12. Remove all of the patient's jewelry and place it in a valuables envelope. Also place money and other valuables in the envelope. Follow hospital procedure for placing the valuables in a safe.

    NOTE: Wedding rings may be tied or taped in place. Follow hospital procedure.

    ⚖ CAUTION: In some agencies, only certain health care workers are permitted to handle valuables. Follow agency policy.

13. Remove full or partial dentures. Place these in a denture cup labeled with the patient's name and room number. Place the cup in a drawer or safe area to prevent breakage.

14. Have the patient remove contact lenses, glasses, hearing aids, and all other prostheses (artificial parts). Place in a safe area.

15. Offer a bedpan and encourage the patient to void. If a catheter and urinary-drainage unit is in place, empty the urinary-drainage unit and record the measurement.

16. Take vital signs and record correctly (see figure 20-90).

    ⬡ CAUTION: These must be accurate and correct. If in doubt about the results, ask your supervisor to check them.

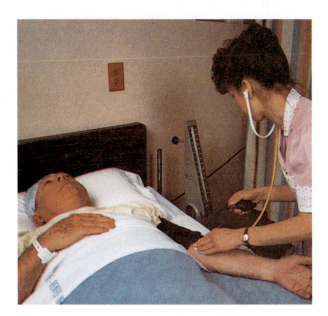

FIGURE 20-90 Vital signs must be taken and recorded as part of preoperative care.

17. Elevate the siderail immediately after preoperative medication has been given by an authorized person.

    NOTE: Preoperative medication is usually given 1 hour before surgery. It helps the patient relax, and often contains medication to dry up nose and mouth secretions. Because the patient could become drowsy and fall out of bed, the siderails must be elevated immediately.

18. Place the patient in a comfortable position. Encourage the patient to rest.

19. Observe all checkpoints before leaving the patient: make sure the water pitcher has been removed from the unit, lower the bed to its lowest level, place the call signal within easy reach of the patient, and leave the area neat and clean.

    NOTE: Many hospitals use pre-op checklists, which are placed on patients' charts. If this is hospital policy, complete the checklist.

20. Clean and replace all equipment.

21. Wash hands.

22. **C** Report and/or record all required information on the patient's chart or the agency form, for example, date; time; pre-op care complete and noted on checklist, siderails elevated, patient resting quietly; and your signature and title. Report any unusual observations immediately.

Practice *Go to the workbook and use the evaluation sheet for 20:13B, Administering Preoperative Care, to practice this procedure. When you feel you have mastered this skill, sign the sheet and give it to your instructor for further action.*

✔ **Final Checkpoint** Using the criteria listed on the evaluation sheet, your instructor will grade your performance.

PROCEDURE 20:13C

Preparing a Postoperative Unit

Equipment and Supplies

Bed linen for an unoccupied bed; extra draw sheet; underpads or protective covers; emesis basin; tissues; plastic bag and tape; gauze bandage; intravenous (IV) pole or stand; vital signs equipment (thermometer, blood pressure apparatus, watch with second hand); linen bag, hamper, or cart; pen or pencil

Procedure

1. Assemble equipment.

    NOTE: The post-op unit is prepared immediately after the patient leaves the area for the operating room.

2. Wash hands. Put on gloves if needed.

     CAUTION: Wear gloves if the linen is contaminated with blood, body fluids, secretions, or excretions. Remove the gloves and wash hands thoroughly after removing the dirty linen and before applying the clean linen.

3. Remove any used linen from the bed and place in the linen bag, hamper, or cart.

4. Make the foundation (bottom sheet and draw sheet) of the bed as previously instructed for an unoccupied bed.

5. Place a cotton draw sheet over the head of the bed. Tuck in at the head of the bed as was done for bottom sheet. Make mitered corners and tuck in at the sides.

    NOTE: This protects the bed should the patient vomit.

    NOTE: Some agencies use underpads instead of draw sheets.

6. Place a top sheet and a spread on the bed. Let them fall loose.

7. Go to the foot of the bed and fold the top linen back. Make a cuff so that the top linen is even with the end of the mattress.

    NOTE: The top linen is *not* tucked in.

8. Go to the head of the bed. Make a cuff with the top linen.

9. Fanfold the top linen to the side of the bed opposite from where the patient will be brought in on the stretcher.

   NOTE: In some agencies, the sheets are folded to the foot of the bed. Follow agency policy.

10. Elevate the siderail on the far side of the bed.

11. Cover the pillow with a pillowcase. Position the pillow in an upright position at the head of the bed. Use gauze bandage to tie it to the head of the bed.

    NOTE: This protects the patient's head against injury during the transfer to the bed.

12. Estimate the height of the stretcher and elevate the bed to this height.

13. Put a cuff on the plastic bag. Tape it to the side of the bed or bedside table.

14. Place underpads on the bed near where the operated body part will be resting.

15. Remove all unnecessary articles from the bedside stand. Place the emesis basin, tissues, and equipment for taking vital signs on the stand.

    NOTE: Make sure the water pitcher and cup are *not* on the bedside stand. Patients may be NPO (nothing by mouth) postoperatively.

16. Position the overbed table, chair, and other furniture so it will not be in the way of the stretcher.

17. Place the intravenous (IV) stand and/or pump in the most convenient location. It should be ready for the intravenous when the patient is transferred to the bed.

18. Check the area before leaving. Make sure that all equipment and supplies are ready for the patient's return from surgery (see figure 20-91).

19. Replace all equipment used.

20. Wash hands.

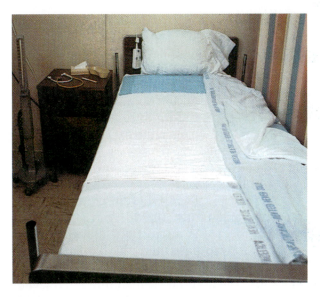

FIGURE 20-91 Before leaving the post-op unit, check to make sure that all equipment and supplies are ready for the patient's return from surgery.

21. Report and/or record all required information on the patient's chart or the agency form, for example, date, time, post-op unit prepared, and your signature and title.

Practice *Go to the workbook and use the evaluation sheet for 20:13C, Preparing a Postoperative Unit, to practice this procedure. When you feel you have mastered this skill, sign the sheet and give it to your instructor for further action.*

✔ **Final Checkpoint** Using the criteria listed on the evaluation sheet, your instructor will grade your performance.

PROCEDURE 20:13D OBRA

Applying Surgical Hose

NOTE: Surgical hose come in various sizes and lengths. This procedure deals with the application of knee-length surgical stockings.

Equipment and Supplies

Correct size surgical hose, measuring tape, pen or pencil

Procedure

1. Check physician's orders or obtain authorization from your immediate supervisor.
2. Assemble equipment.
3. **C** Knock on the door and pause before entering. Introduce yourself. Identify the patient. Explain the procedure.
4. Wash hands.
5. Check the hose to be sure they are clean and the correct size.

   NOTE: Hose from different companies are sized differently. Use the measuring tape and follow the instructions that came with the hose to determine the correct size for the patient.
6. Close the door and screen the unit. Elevate the bed to a comfortable working height. Lower the siderail on the side where you are working. Expose the patient's legs.
7. Insert your hand into the top of the hose. Turn the hose so that the smooth side is on the outside.

   NOTE: This makes application easier and leaves the rough edge on the outside of the foot.
8. Grasp the heel area of the hose. Smoothly tuck the foot portion back into the stocking.
9. Stretch the hose open at the heel. Support the patient's leg and slide the foot and pocket of the heel into position on the patient's foot (see figure 20-92A).

   ⚠ CAUTION: Use correct body mechanics when applying hose. Stand with your feet apart and one leg ahead of the other, bending at the hips rather than the waist.
10. Make sure the heel of the stocking is secure over the patient's heel.
11. Grasp the top of the stocking. Pull it over the foot. Gather the material at the ankle. Use two hands and gentle pressure.
12. Begin gently pulling the hose up the leg to the area below the knee (see figure 20-92B). Work slowly to prevent wrinkles. Use both hands to smooth the hose into place.

    ⚠ CAUTION: Do not pull and stretch the hose. This will make it too tight and interfere with circulation.
13. Check the position of the hose. The top should be just below the knee. Smooth any excess material with your hands.
14. Pull the toe forward slightly to provide "toe room."
15. Repeat steps 7 to 14 for the opposite leg.

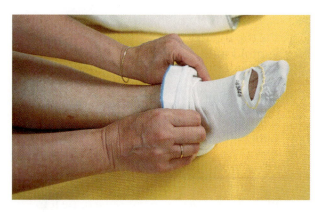

FIGURE 20-92A Slide the foot of the hose into position.

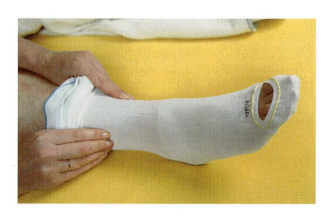

FIGURE 20-92B Draw the hose gently up the leg to the area below the knee.

16. Observe all checkpoints before leaving the patient: position the patient in correct body alignment, elevate the siderails (if indicated), lower the bed to its lowest level, place the call signal and supplies within easy reach of the patient, and leave the area neat and clean.
17. Check the hose at intervals. Look for signs of impaired circulation, including abnormal skin color or temperature, swelling, and other abnormalities. Report any abnormalities to your supervisor immediately. Remove the hose at intervals, at least once every 8 hours. Administer skin care to the skin under the hose. If the hose become soiled, they can be washed.
18. Wash hands.
19. **C** Report and/or record all required information on the patient's chart or the agency form, for example, date, time, surgical hose applied to both legs, and your signature and title. Report any unusual observations immediately.

Practice *Go to the workbook and use the evaluation sheet for 20:13D, Applying Surgical Hose, to practice this procedure. When you feel you have mastered this skill, sign the sheet and give it to your instructor for further action.*

 Final Checkpoint Using the criteria listed on the evaluation sheet, your instructor will grade your performance.

20:14 INFORMATION Applying Binders

Binders are usually made of heavy cotton or flannelette with elastic sides or supports. They are applied to various parts of the body, but mainly to the abdomen and breasts. Functions of binders include the following:

◆ Provide support and relief from pain following surgery.

◆ Hold dressings in place.

◆ Provide support for engorged breasts.

◆ Limit motion.

◆ Apply pressure to specific body parts.

Binders must be applied smoothly to prevent pressure areas, which can lead to the formation of pressure ulcers. Binders should fit snugly for support but not be so tight as to cause discomfort. No wrinkles or creases should be present.

Different types of binders are available for use (see figure 20-93). The type used most frequently is a straight binder. It can be applied to the abdomen, back, or rib cage. Some straight binders have Velcro tabs; others are pinned in place. If pins are used, they should be placed no more than 2 inches apart for optimal support. If the waist on a straight binder is too large, darts can be made to ease the excess material. Breast binders are used to support the breasts of a female patient. They can be used to support engorged breasts (breasts full of milk) after childbirth. Single T-binders are used for female patients, and double T-binders are used for

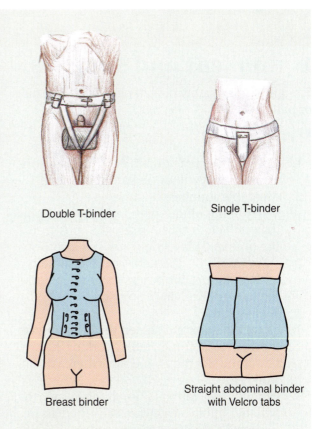

Double T-binder

Single T-binder

Breast binder

Straight abdominal binder with Velcro tabs

FIGURE 20-93 Different types of binders.

male patients. The binder is placed around the patient's waist, and the tail(s) is passed between the patient's legs. The tail(s) is then pinned at the waist. This type of binder is used to hold perineal dressings in place or provide support. In most instances, T-binders have been replaced by scrotal supports for men and self-adhesive sanitary napkins for women.

Binders are applied from bottom to top for optimal support. In this way, organs can be supported correctly. Circulation and breathing should always be checked after binders are applied. A binder that is too tight can cause severe complications. In addition, binders should be removed at intervals and skin care should be provided to the skin under the binder.

STUDENT: *Go to the workbook and complete the assignment sheet for 20:14, Applying Binders. Then return and continue with the procedure.*

PROCEDURE 20:14

Applying a Straight Binder

Equipment and Supplies

Straight binder, safety pins (if needed), soap, pen or pencil

Procedure

1. Check physician's orders or obtain authorization from your immediate supervisor.
2. Assemble supplies.
   NOTE: If the binder requires the use of pins (has no Velcro tabs), insert the pins in the bar of soap. This allows for easier insertion.
3. **C** Knock on the door and pause before entering. Introduce yourself. Identify the patient. Explain the procedure.
4. Wash hands.
5. Close the door and screen the unit. Elevate the bed to a comfortable working height. Lower the siderail on the side where you are working.
6. Fanfold the top bed linen down to the patient's pubic area. Arrange the bedclothes so that the abdomen is exposed.
7. Assist the patient to move to the near side of the bed.
   ⚠ CAUTION: Use correct body mechanics when applying binders.
8. With the inside facing out, fold the binder in half to determine where the center is.
9. Ask the patient to flex the knees, place his or her weight on the heels, and raise the hips.
   NOTE: The patient can also turn on his or her side, if this is easier.
10. Unfold the binder and slide it under the patient (see figure 20-94A). Keep your thumbs at the edge of the center fold. Position the binder by putting the center fold at the center of the patient's spine. The bottom

edge should be at the base of the spine but not so low as to interfere with the use of a bedpan.
11. Open the binder completely. Check placement. Make sure the binder is smooth and even, with no wrinkles.
12. Fasten the binder from the bottom to the top.
    a. For Velcro tabs, pull the sides together firmly. Start at the bottom edge and seal in an upward direction (see figure 20-94B).
    b. For pins, start at the lower edge. Overlap the edges. Place pins no more than 2 inches apart.
       ⚠ CAUTION: To avoid sticking the patient with pins, place your hands between the binder and the patient's skin before inserting the pins.

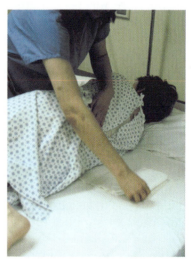

FIGURE 20-94A Position the binder under the patient with the center fold at the patient's spine and the bottom edge at the base of the spine.

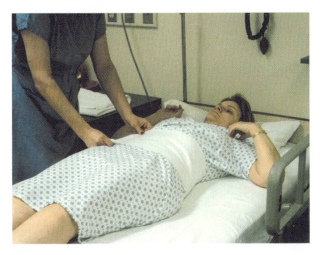

FIGURE 20-94B Secure the Velcro tabs of the binder by starting at the bottom edge and working in an upward direction.

13. Check the waist of the binder. If it is too large, make darts for a better fit. Insert pins vertically to hold the darts in place.

   ⚠️ **CAUTION:** Avoid placing pins over bony prominences.

14. Check the entire binder. Make sure it is snug but not too tight. Make sure it is smooth and positioned correctly. Check to be sure that it is not restricting breathing and/or circulation.

15. Replace all bed linens.

16. Observe all checkpoints before leaving the patient: position the patient in correct body alignment, elevate the siderails (if indicated), lower the bed to its lowest level, place the call signal and supplies within easy reach of the patient, leave the area neat and clean.

17. Replace equipment.

18. Wash hands.

19. Report and/or record all required information on the patient's chart or the agency form, for example, date, time, straight binder applied to abdomen, and your signature and title. Report any unusual observations immediately.

> **Practice** *Go to the workbook and use the evaluation sheet for 20:14, Applying a Straight Binder, to practice this procedure. When you feel you have mastered this skill, sign the sheet and give it to your instructor for further action.*

✔️ **Final Checkpoint** Using the criteria listed on the evaluation sheet, your instructor will grade your performance.

20:15 INFORMATION Administering Oxygen

⚖️ This section provides facts about administering oxygen. *Check your legal responsibilities with regard to this procedure.* Some states prohibit administration of oxygen by a health care assistant.

The blood must have oxygen. The blood's supply of oxygen is normally obtained from the air. Air is approximately 20 percent oxygen. As a result of accident, injury, or respiratory disease, however, the body may be unable to take in enough oxygen or to use oxygen effectively. In such cases, oxygen can be given to the patient by various means.

The signs of an oxygen shortage are rapid and shallow respirations, rapid pulse, restlessness, and cyanosis. A deficiency of oxygen is called *hypoxia*. Lack of oxygen can cause brain damage in 4 to 6 minutes.

⚖️ A physician's order is usually required for the administration of oxygen. The order will include the method of administration and the concentration to be given. In cases of extreme emergency, oxygen can be started with standard concentrations, and the physician notified as soon as possible. Most rescue teams, ambulance personnel, and others involved in emergency work follow specific orders regarding oxygen administration.

Oxygen is usually administered by one of the following methods:

◆ *Mask* (see figure 20-95A): The mask should cover the mouth and the nose. It should fit snugly to prevent loss of oxygen, but it should not be so tight as to cause discomfort to the patient. Oxygen by mask is the method of administration used most frequently by rescue personnel. It provides the highest concentration of oxygen. However, some patients are frightened by the mask. A careful explanation of its purpose along with constant reassurance are necessary. The rate of flow by mask is usually 6 to 10 liters per minute.

◆ *Cannula* (see figure 20-95B): The cannula consists of two small, curved, plastic tubes, which are placed one in each nostril. The other end of the cannula is attached to an oxygen tank or unit. The patient must be instructed to breathe through the nose. If the patient opens the mouth to breathe, the concentration of oxygen is reduced. The rate of flow by cannula is usually 2 to 6 liters per minute.

◆ *Catheter* (see figure 20-95C): The catheter is a long, narrow, plastic or rubber tube that is passed through a nostril and to the pharynx. It is inserted by a physician, registered nurse, respiratory therapist, or other specially trained individual. The rate of flow is usually 2 to 6 liters per minute.

◆ *Tent:* The tent surrounds the patient with a high concentration of oxygen. It is often used for small children or restless patients who are not able to cooperate well with other methods. Oxygen and humidity are provided. A common example is a croupette used with infants and small children. The flow rate is usually 10 to 12 liters per minute.

Pure oxygen is very drying and can damage or irritate mucous membranes. Therefore, oxygen must be moisturized by passing it through water before it is administered to the patient. A humidifier is used to moisturize oxygen (see figure 20-96). The humidifier must be filled with distilled water to the proper level, usually one-half to two-thirds of the container. Most humidifiers are marked for the proper level. Distilled water is usually used to prevent mineral deposits on the equipment. In emergency

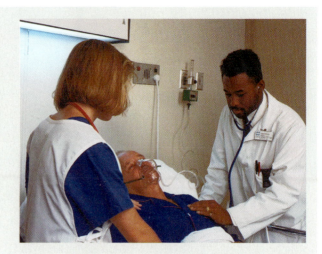

FIGURE 20-95A The oxygen mask covers the nose and mouth and provides a high concentration of oxygen.

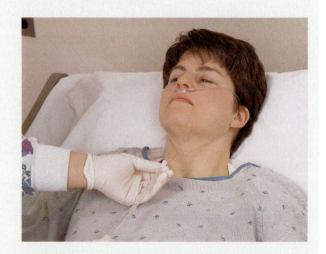

FIGURE 20-95B When a nasal cannula is used to provide oxygen, the patient must breathe through the nose.

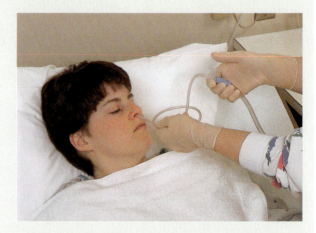

FIGURE 20-95C A nasal catheter is passed through a nostril and to the pharynx, or throat, to administer oxygen.

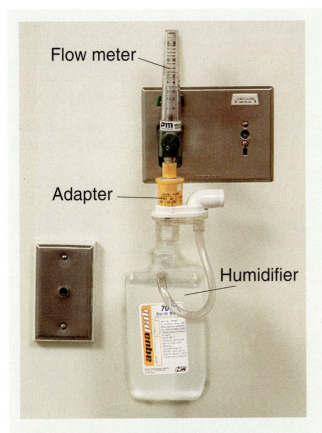

FIGURE 20-96 A humidifier is used to moisturize oxygen.

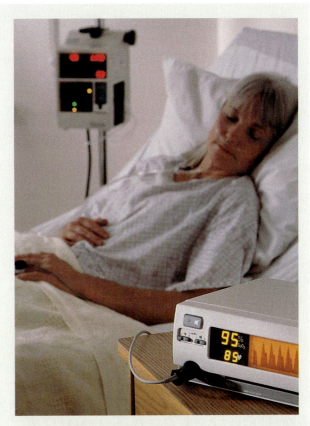

FIGURE 20-97 Pulse oximeters may be used to monitor the patient who is receiving oxygen. The oximeter measures the level of oxygen in arterial blood.

situations when oxygen is given for short periods of time during transportation to a medical facility, the oxygen may not be humidified.

Safety precautions must be observed when oxygen is in use. Although oxygen does not explode, burning is more rapid and intense in the presence of oxygen. Flammable materials (those that burn) will burn much more rapidly in the presence of oxygen. The following precautions should be taken whenever oxygen is in use:

◆ Smoking, lighting cigarettes or matches, burning candles, and the use of open flames are prohibited when oxygen is in use. In patient-care areas, a warning sign reading, for example, "No Smoking—Oxygen" is placed on the door to the patient's room, on the bed, or on the wall nearby. Warning labels are also sometimes placed on tanks used by emergency rescue personnel.

◆ The sign is not enough. The patient must be cautioned against smoking. Observers at the scene of an accident or emergency situation, and visitors in a patient-care area must also be told to avoid smoking.

◆ The use of electrically operated equipment, which could cause sparks, should be avoided.

◆ Never use flammable liquids such as nail polish remover or adhesive tape remover.

◆ Cotton blankets should be used in place of wool or nylon. In addition, all bed linen, bedspreads, and gowns or pajamas should be cotton instead of synthetic materials. Cotton is static-free, and its use decreases the danger of static electricity.

◆ Frequent inspections must be made of any area where oxygen is in use. Sources of sparks or static electricity should be removed.

Pulse oximeters may be used to monitor the patient who is receiving oxygen (see figure 20-97). An oximeter measures the level of oxygen in arterial blood. A photo-detector probe is clipped on the patient's finger or ear lobe. The percentage of oxygen in the arterial blood is displayed on the monitor screen of the oximeter. If the oxygen level falls below the minimum percentage programmed into the oximeter, an alarm will sound. Licensed personnel are responsible for programming and monitoring the oximeter. The health care assistant should make sure the probe is not disturbed and notify a supervisor if the alarm sounds.

A patient who is receiving oxygen must be checked frequently. Quality of respirations should be noted. Mouth and nose care must be provided if a mask, catheter, or cannula is used. The rate of flow of oxygen should be checked. Watch to make sure that the patient and/or visitors do *not* change the liter flow. If a humidifier is used, water (preferably distilled) must be added to the humidifier as needed. Safety precautions should be checked. In many facilities, oxygen administration is the responsibility of the respiratory therapy department. However, the health care worker, who is with the patient more frequently, should always be aware of safety precautions and check patients carefully. Any abnormal observations should be reported immediately.

STUDENT: *Go to the workbook and complete the assignment sheet for 20:15, Administering Oxygen. Then return and continue with the procedure.*

PROCEDURE 20:15

Administering Oxygen

Equipment and Supplies

Oxygen mask, cannula, or tent; tubing and gauge; oxygen tank or supply; distilled water (if humidifier is used); pen or pencil

CAUTION: Some states prohibit the administration of oxygen by a health care assistant. Check your legal responsibilities in regard to this procedure.

Procedure

1. Read the physician's orders or obtain orders from your immediate supervisor. In emergency rescue situations, standard orders are usually provided for victims requiring oxygen. The orders should state the method of administration and liter flow per minute.
2. Assemble equipment.
3. **C** Knock on the door and pause before entering. Introduce yourself. Identify the patient. Explain the procedure to the patient. Patients are often apprehensive. Reassure as needed.
4. Wash hands. In emergency situations, this may not be possible.
5. Connect the tubing from the oxygen supply (tank or wall unit) to the tubing on the mask or cannula. If a humidifier is used, check the water level to make sure the water supply is adequate.
   NOTE: Fill the container with distilled water, if needed. Distilled water prevents mineral deposits from forming.
6. Turn on the oxygen supply.
   CAUTION: Do not insert the nasal cannula or apply the mask at this time. Regulate the gauge to the correct liter flow rate per minute. See figure 20-98.
   CAUTION: Make sure to follow specific manufacturer's instructions or agency policy for connecting and turning on the oxygen supply. Do *not* operate any oxygen equipment until you have been specifically instructed on how to use it.
7. Check to be sure that oxygen is passing through the tubing. Place your hand by the outlet on the mask or cannula.
8. Put on disposable gloves.

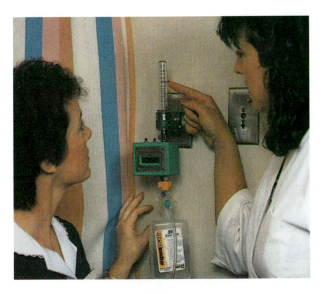

FIGURE 20-98 Regulate the gauge to provide the correct liter flow rate for oxygen.

CAUTION: Observe all standard pre-cautions if contact with the patient's oral or nasal secretions is possible.

9. With the oxygen still flowing, apply the mask or cannula to the patient. If a mask is used, position it over the patient's nose and mouth. Adjust the strap so that it fits snugly but does not apply pressure to the face. If a cannula is used, place the two tips in the patient's nostrils and loop the tubing around each ear. Adjust the straps at the neck so that the tips remain in position. Instruct the patient to breathe through the nose.

10. If a tent is used, it is first filled with oxygen; then, the prescribed liter flow is set. The humidifier is filled to the marked level with distilled water. The tent is placed over the bed or crib, and the edges are tucked in on all sides to prevent oxygen loss. A cotton blanket, bath blanket, or sheet can be used to provide a cuff around the loose end covering the patient.

11. Check the surrounding area to make sure all safety precautions are being observed. Eliminate any sources of sparks or flames. Caution any visitors and the patient against smoking while the oxygen is in use. In a patient-care area, make sure a sign is posted on the door or in the immediate area.

12. Check the patient at frequent intervals. Note respirations, color, restlessness, or discomfort. Provide skin care to the face and/or nose, if a mask or cannula is used. Check the skin behind the ears and provide skin care if a nasal cannula is used. At times, it may be necessary to use a towel or cloth to dry the inside of the mask, because moisture will accumulate in the mask. If a nasal cannula is used, check the tips to make sure they are open and not plugged by mucus. Provide oral hygiene frequently. Check the water level, if a humidifier is used. Check the gauge and make sure the liter flow rate is correct. Report any abnormal conditions immediately.

13. When the oxygen is discontinued, make sure that the oxygen supply is turned off. Follow specific manufacturer's instructions or agency policy. Clean and replace all equipment. Most masks and cannulas are disposable and are discarded after use. If the items are not disposable, they should be cleaned and disinfected according to established agency policy.

14. Wash hands.

15. **C** Report and/or record all required information on the patient's chart or the agency form, for example, date; time; oxygen per mask at 6 L/min, R 16 deep and even; and your signature and title. Report any unusual observations immediately.

Practice *Go to the workbook and use the evaluation sheet for 20:15, Administering Oxygen, to practice this procedure. When you feel you have mastered this skill, sign the sheet and give it to your instructor for further action.*

 Final Checkpoint Using the criteria listed on the evaluation sheet, your instructor will grade your performance.

20:16 INFORMATION Giving Postmortem Care

OBRA Providing care after death is a difficult but essential part of patient care. As a health care worker, you may perform or assist with this care.

Postmortem care is care given to the body immediately after death. It begins when a physician has pronounced the patient dead.

Dealing with death and dying is a difficult part of providing care. If a health care worker has cared for a patient over a period of time, it is natural for the worker to feel grief and a sense of loss upon the patient's death. Crying is a natural expression of grief, and you should not feel embarrassed if you cry. However, it is also important for health care workers to try to control emotions because family members and other patients will need their support.

The patient's rights continue to apply after death. The body should be treated with dignity and respect. Privacy should be provided at all times.

If family members are not present when death occurs and want to view the body before it is taken to the morgue or funeral home, the body should be prepared for viewing. The patient should be positioned naturally, with the limbs straight. If dentures were removed, they should be returned to the mouth. The bed linen should be neat and clean, and extra equipment should be removed from the unit. Provide privacy while the family views the body, unless they request that you remain with them.

After the family has viewed the body, postmortem care is completed. The procedure for this care varies in different facilities. In some facilities, morgue personnel prepare the body and remove it to the morgue. In other facilities, the body is prepared and remains in the unit until the funeral home personnel arrive. In yet other facilities, funeral home personnel remove the body and provide postmortem care. Know and follow the procedure established by your facility.

Morgue kits often are used for postmortem care (see figure 20-99). Each kit usually contains a shroud or body bag, a gown, chin strap, pads,

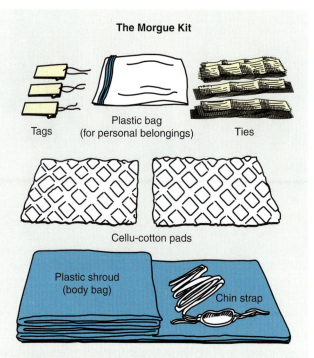

The Morgue Kit

Tags

Plastic bag (for personal belongings)

Ties

Cellu-cotton pads

Plastic shroud (body bag)

Chin strap

FIGURE 20-99 Supplies needed for postmortem care.

gauze squares, ties, two or three tags to identify the body, and safety pins. Procedure 20:16 describes one method of using these supplies to provide postmortem care.

Care of the patient's valuables and belongings are an important part of postmortem care. Each facility has a policy that should be followed. The personal inventory and valuables lists prepared on admission are often used to make sure that all items are present. These items are checked according to facility policy. Valuables in the safe usually remain there until a family member signs for them. Jewelry is usually removed from the body, listed, and placed in the safe until received by a family member. A wedding ring is frequently left on the body, but it should be taped in place and noted on the chart.

Frequently, two people work together to complete postmortem care. Some aspects of care, such as removal of tubes or IVs, may be the responsibility of the nurse or another authorized person. Follow your agency's policy and know your legal responsibilities with regard to giving or assisting with postmortem care.

STUDENT: *Go to the workbook and complete the assignment sheet for 20:16, Giving Postmortem Care. Then return and continue with the procedure.*

PROCEDURE 20:16 OBRA

Giving Postmortem Care

Equipment and Supplies

Postmortem kit (shroud or clean sheet, gown, tags, gauze squares, cotton balls, safety pins), underpads or bed protectors, basin, towels, washcloth, personal inventory and valuables lists, disposable gloves, plastic waste bag, pen or pencil

Procedure

1. Obtain proper authorization and assemble equipment.
2. Identify the patient by checking the armband.
3. Close the door and screen the unit to provide privacy.
4. Wash hands. Put on gloves, if needed.

    CAUTION: If the body is contaminated with blood or body fluids, observe standard precautions.
5. Elevate the bed to a comfortable working height. Lower the siderail on the side where you are working.
6. Position the body lying flat on the back, with the arms and legs straight. Place a pillow under the head and shoulders.

    NOTE: Handle the body gently and with respect.
7. If the eyes are open, close them by gently pulling the eyelids over the eyes (see figure 20-100). Put a moist cotton ball on each eye if the eyes do not remain shut.
8. Replace dentures in the mouth, if they have been removed. Use a chin strap to hold the jaw shut. A rolled towel or padding can also be used under the chin to keep the mouth closed.
9. Remove soiled dressings and replace with clean ones, as necessary. If tubes, IVs, catheters, or drainage bags are in place, follow agency policy for removal. This is often the responsibility of the nurse. If an autopsy is to be performed, some tubes may have to be left in place.
10. Use warm water to bathe any soiled body areas. Dry all areas thoroughly. Comb the hair, if needed.
11. Place an underpad or padding under the buttocks at the anal area.

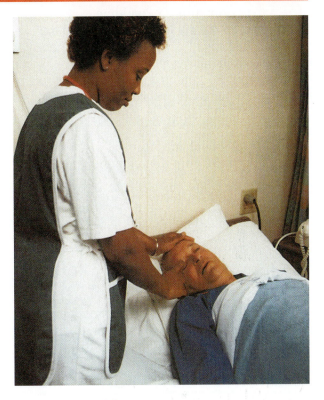

FIGURE 20-100 If the eyes are open after death, close them by gently pulling the eyelids over the eyes.

NOTE: The bowels and bladder may empty after death.

12. If gloves are worn, remove gloves and wash hands.
13. Put a clean gown on the body.
14. If jewelry is present, follow agency policy. Jewelry is usually removed, listed on a valuables list, and stored in a safe until signed for by a family member. A wedding ring frequently is left on the body, but it should be taped in place and noted on the chart or postmortem form.
15. Fill out the identification card or tag. One tag is usually placed on the patient's right ankle or right big toe.
16. If the family is to view the body, use a sheet to cover the body to the shoulders. Make sure the room is neat and clean. Provide privacy for the family unless they request that you remain with them.
17. After the family's visit, place the body in the shroud or body bag. Use safety pins or tape

to hold the shroud in place. If a shroud is not available, use a sheet to cover the body.

! CAUTION: Handle the body carefully. Pressure from your hands can leave marks on the body.

NOTE: Sometimes, padding is placed between the ankles and knees, and the legs are tied together lightly before the body is placed in the shroud.

18. If required, attach a second identification card or tag to the outside of the shroud.

19. Collect all belongings and make a list. This list frequently is checked against the admission personal inventory and/or valuables list to make sure that all items are present. Put the items in a bag or container and attach an identification card or tag. Follow agency policy for care of belongings until they are signed for by a family member.

20. Obtain assistance and transfer the body to a stretcher. Make sure doors to other patient's rooms are closed and the corridor is empty before transporting the body to the morgue.

NOTE: In some facilities, morgue personnel transport the body to the morgue. In other facilities, the body remains in the unit until funeral home personnel arrive.

21. Return to the unit. Strip the linen from the bed. Follow agency policy for cleaning the unit and equipment. Leave the area neat and clean.

22. Wash hands.

23. **C** Report and/or record all required information on the patient's chart or the agency form, for example, date; time; postmortem care given, body transported to morgue, belongings placed in locked closet by nurses' station; and your signature and title.

> **Practice** *Go to the workbook and use the evaluation sheet for 20:16, Giving Postmortem Care, to practice this procedure. When you feel you have mastered this skill, sign the sheet and give it to your instructor for further action.*

✓ **Final Checkpoint**   Using the criteria listed on the evaluation sheet, your instructor will grade your performance.

UNIT 20 SUMMARY

Many nurse assistant skills are directed toward providing quality personal care for the patient. Examples include bathing, caring for hair and nails, gowning or dressing the patient, giving backrubs, providing oral hygiene, shaving, feeding, assisting with bedpans or urinals, and bedmaking. It is essential that the nurse assistant learn and follow correct procedures to provide for the safety, comfort, and privacy of the patient.

Other nurse assistant skills include positioning, turning, moving, and transferring patients. During any move or transfer, the use of correct body mechanics is essential.

 Nurse assistant skills are also used in other special procedures. Examples of these procedures include measuring intake and output, collecting stool and urine specimens, giving enemas, assisting the surgical patient, administering oxygen, applying restraints, providing catheter care, applying binders or surgical hose, and giving postmortem care. It is important to determine legal responsibility before performing some of the special procedures, because some states or agencies do not allow all nurse assistants to perform the procedures.

☣ While performing any nurse assistant skill, it is essential to use approved procedures and make every effort to provide quality care to the patient. In addition, if any contact with blood, body fluids, secretions, or excretions is possible, standard precautions should be observed. Finally, it is important to make careful observations of the patient while providing care, and to record or report these observations correctly. In this way, you will use nurse assistant skills to become an important member of the health care team.

INTERNET SEARCHES

Use the suggested search engines in Unit 11:4 of this textbook to search the Internet for additional information on the following topics:

1. *Organizations*: research nurse assisting careers, educational requirements, and duties at organizational sites such as the American Health Care Association, American Hospital Association, American Nurse's Association, Association of Surgical Technologists, Foundation for Hospice and Homecare, National Association for Practical Nurse Education and Service, National League for Nursing, and the National Federation of Licensed Practical Nurses.

2. *Patient care*: research patient's rights, hospice care, home health care, oncology care, surgical care, and postmortem care.

3. *Suppliers*: find suppliers of hospital and medical equipment to compare the different products available.

REVIEW QUESTIONS

1. List six (6) specific tasks that must be performed while admitting a patient to a hospital or long-term-care facility.

2. Describe four (4) ways to prevent pressure sores and/or contractures from developing.

3. Name three (3) main ways to make beds and explain when each type is made.

4. Identify all the areas of care that may be included to provide personal hygiene to a patient.

5. Why is it important to constantly observe a patient while providing personal care? Identify six (6) observations that might be indicative of a medical problem.

6. What is a urinary catheter? Why is it used?

7. Differentiate between a routine, midstream or clean catch, sterile, and 24-hour urine specimen.

8. Why is stool tested for occult blood?

9. Define each of the following words:
   a. ostomy
   b. suppository
   c. fecal impaction
   d. enema
   e. flatus

10. Differentiate between a retention and a nonretention enema. Give an example for each type.

11. List four (4) specific rules that OBRA legislation has placed on the use of restraints.

12. Identify five (5) specific aspects of care for both pre-op and post-op patients.

13. Name the three (3) main methods for administering oxygen. List the average flow rate for each method.

14. Explain five (5) standard precautions that must be observed while performing any nurse assisting procedure.

UNIT 20

SUGGESTED REFERENCES

Acello, Barbara. *Advanced Patient Care Skills.* Clifton Park, NY: Delmar Learning, 2000.

Acello, Barbara. *Nursing Assisting: Essentials of Long-Term Care.* Clifton Park, NY: Delmar Learning, 1999.

Acello, Barbara. *Patient Care: Basic Skills for the Health Care Provider.* Clifton Park, NY: Delmar Learning, 1998.

Acello, Barbara. *Restorative Care: Fundamentals for Certified Nursing Assistants.* Clifton Park, NY: Delmar Learning, 2000.

Acello, Barbara, and Barbara Kast. *Competency Exam Preparation and Review for Nursing Assistants.* 3rd ed. Clifton Park, NY: Delmar Learning, 2001.

Altman, Gaylene, Patricia Buchsel, and Valerie Coxon. *Delmar's Fundamental and Advanced Nursing Skills.* Clifton Park, NY: Delmar Learning, 2000.

DeLaune, Sue, and Patricia Ladner. *Fundamentals of Nursing: Standards and Practices.* 2nd ed. Clifton Park, NY: Delmar Learning, 2002.

Hegner, Barbara, and Joan Needham. *Assisting in Long-Term Care.* 4th ed. Clifton Park, NY: Delmar Learning, 2002.

Hegner, Barbara, Esther Caldwell, and Joan Needham. *Nursing Assistant: A Nursing Process Approach.* 8th ed. Clifton Park, NY: Delmar Learning, 1999.

Hogstel, Mildred. *Nursing Care of the Older Adult.* Clifton Park, NY: Delmar Learning, 2001.

Huber, Helen, and Audree Spatz. *Homemaker–Home Health Aide.* 5th ed. Clifton Park, NY: Delmar Learning, 1998.

Netting, Sandra. *The Lippincott Manual of Nursing Practice.* 7th ed. Philadelphia, PA: Lippincott, Williams, and Wilkins, 2000.

Potts, Nicki, and Barbara Mandleco. *Pediatric Nursing: Caring for Children and Their Families.* Clifton Park, NY: Delmar Learning, 2002.

Simmers, Louise. *Practical Problems in Mathematics for Health Occupations.* Clifton Park, NY: Delmar Learning, 1996.

Smeltzer, Suzanne, and Brenda Bare. *Brunner and Suddarth's Textbook of Medical Surgical Nursing.* 9th ed. Philadelphia, PA: Lippincott, Williams, & Wilkins, 1999.

Townsend, Carolyn E., and Ruth A. Roth. *Nutrition and Diet Therapy.* 7th ed. Clifton Park, NY: Delmar Learning, 2000.

White, Lois. *Basic Nursing: Foundations of Concepts and Skills.* Clifton Park, NY: Delmar Learning, 2002.

White, Lois. *Foundations of Nursing: Caring for the Whole Person.* Clifton Park, NY: Delmar Learning, 2000.

White, Lois, and Gena Duncan. *Medical–Surgical Nursing: An Integrated Approach.* Clifton Park, NY: Delmar Learning, 1998.

For additional information on nursing careers, contact the following associations:

◆ American Health Care Association
1201 L Street NW
Washington, DC 20005
Internet address: *www.ahca.org*

◆ American Nurses' Association
600 Maryland Avenue SW
Washington, DC 20024
Internet address: *www.ana.org*

◆ National Association for Practical Nurse Education and Service
1400 Spring Street, Suite 330
Silver Spring, MD 20910
Internet address: *www.napnes.org*

◆ National Federation of Licensed Practical Nursing
893 U.S. Highway 70, Suite 202
Garner, NC 27529
Internet address: *www.nflpn.org*

◆ State nurses' associations

Physical Therapy Skills

Unit Objectives

After completing this unit of study, you should be able to:

- ◆ Perform range-of-motion (ROM) exercises on all body joints, observing all safety precautions
- ◆ Ambulate a patient using a transfer (gait) belt
- ◆ Check the correct measurements of patients for canes, crutches, and walkers
- ◆ Ambulate a patient using the following crutch gaits: four point, three point, two point, swing to, swing through
- ◆ Ambulate a patient using a cane
- ◆ Ambulate a patient using a walker
- ◆ Apply an ice bag or ice collar, observing all safety precautions
- ◆ Apply a warm-water bag, observing all safety precautions
- ◆ Apply an aquamatic pad, observing all safety precautions
- ◆ Apply a moist compress, observing all safety precautions
- ◆ Administer a sitz bath
- ◆ Define, pronounce, and spell all the key terms

 Observe Standard Precautions

 Instructors Check—Call Instructor at This Point

 Safety—Proceed with Caution

 OBRA Requirement— Based on Federal Law

 Math Skill

 Legal Responsibility

 Science Skill

 Career Information

 C Communications Skill

 Technology

KEY TERMS

aquamatic pads
   (ak″-wah-mat′-ik)

cane

compresses
   (cahm′-press-ez)

contracture
   (kun-track′-shure)

crutches

dry cold

dry heat

hydrocollator packs

hypothermia blankets
   (high″-poh-thur′-me-ah)

ice bags

ice collars

moist cold

moist heat

paraffin wax treatment

range of motion (ROM)

sitz bath

transfer (gait) belt

vasoconstriction
   (vay″-zow″-kon-strik′-shun)

vasodilation
   (vay″-zow″-di-lay′-shun)

walker

warm-water bags

CAREER HIGHLIGHT

Physical therapist assistants provide treatment to improve mobility and prevent or limit permanent disability of patients with disabling injuries or disease. They are important members of the health care team. They work under the supervision of a physical therapist who has a bachelor's or master's degree (master's required as of 2001) from an accredited program, and is licensed (required in all states). Most physical therapist assistants have an associate's degree from an accredited program. Licensure is required in most states.

The duties of physical therapist assistants vary but usually include performing exercises, providing ultrasound or electrical stimulation treatments, administering heat, cold, or moist applications, ambulating patients with assistive devices, and informing the physical therapist of patient's response and progress. In addition to the knowledge and skills presented in this unit, physical therapist assistants must also learn and master skills such as:

- ◆ Presenting a professional appearance and attitude
- ◆ Obtaining knowledge regarding health care delivery systems, organizational structure, and teamwork
- ◆ Meeting all legal responsibilities
- ◆ Communicating effectively
- ◆ Being sensitive to and respecting cultural diversity
- ◆ Comprehending anatomy, physiology, and pathophysiology with an emphasis on the skeletal, muscular, nervous, and circulatory systems
- ◆ Learning medical terminology
- ◆ Observing all safety precautions
- ◆ Practicing all principles of infection control
- ◆ Administering first aid and cardiopulmonary resuscitation
- ◆ Promoting good nutrition and a healthy lifestyle to maintain health
- ◆ Utilizing computer skills
- ◆ Cleaning and maintaining equipment
- ◆ Ordering and maintaining supplies and materials
- ◆ Performing duties such as answering the telephone, scheduling appointments, completing insurance forms, and maintaining patient records

21:1 INFORMATION *Performing Range-of-Motion (ROM) Exercises*

OBRA Activity and exercise are important for all individuals. When patients have limited ability to move, range-of-motion exercises help keep muscles and joints functioning.

Range-of-motion (ROM) exercises are done to maintain the health of the musculoskeletal system. Each joint and muscle in the body is moved through its full range of motion. Range-of-motion exercises are frequently ordered by physicians for patients with limited ability to move. These exercises are administered by a physical therapist, nurse, health care assistant, or other authorized person. Range-of-motion exercises can be done during the daily bath or at other times during the day.

Range-of-motion exercises are done to prevent the problems caused by lack of movement and by inactivity (see figure 21-1). Some of these problems include:

♦ **Contracture:** A tightening and shortening of a muscle, resulting in a permanent flexing of a joint. Foot drop is a common contracture, but contractures can also affect the knees, hips, elbows, and hands.

♦ *Muscle and joint function:* Muscles atrophy (shrink) and become weak. Joints become stiff and difficult to move.

♦ *Circulatory impairment:* The circulation of blood is affected, and blood clots and pressure ulcers (pressure sores) can develop.

♦ *Mineral loss:* Inactivity causes mineral loss, especially of calcium from the bones. The bones become brittle, and fractures occur. As the blood calcium level increases, renal calculi (kidney stones) are more likely to form.

♦ *Other problems:* Lack of exercise can also cause poor appetite, constipation, urinary infections, respiratory problems, and hypostatic pneumonia.

There are four main types of ROM exercises:

♦ *Active ROM exercises:* performed by patients who are able to move each joint without assistance (see figure 21-2). This type of ROM

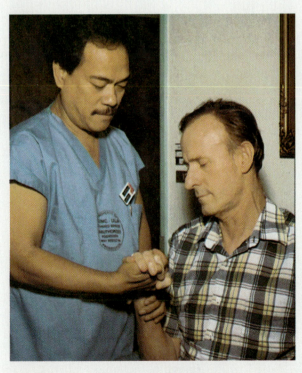

FIGURE 21-1 Range-of-motion (ROM) exercises are done to prevent problems caused by lack of movement and by inactivity.

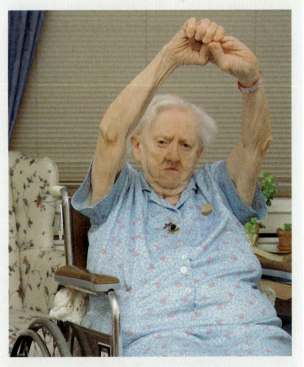

FIGURE 21-2 Patients who are able to move each joint without assistance perform active ROM exercises.

strengthens muscles, maintains joint function and movement, and helps prevent deformities.

◆ *Active assistive ROM exercises:* the patient actively moves the joints but receives assistance to complete the entire ROM. This type of ROM strengthens muscles, maintains joint function and movement, and helps prevent deformities. At times, equipment, such as a pulley, is used to complete the ROM.

◆ *Passive ROM exercises:* another person moves each joint for a patient who is not able to exercise. This type of ROM maintains joint function and movement, and helps to prevent deformities. However, it does not strengthen muscles.

◆ *Resistive ROM exercises:* administered by a therapist, and the exercises are performed against resistance provided by the therapist. This type of ROM helps the patient develop increased strength and endurance.

The health care worker should find out what type of ROM exercises are to be performed and determine whether any limitations to the exercises exist before administering or assisting the patient with the exercises. In some states and health care facilities, only physical therapists or registered nurses may perform range of motion exercises to the head and neck, especially if stretching is involved. After hip or knee replacement surgeries, some ROM exercises may be restricted or limited. Patients with osteoporosis, a condition in which the bones become porous and are prone to fracture, may have limitations on ROMs. It is your responsibility to check legal requirements regarding ROM exercises.

Various movements are used when performing ROM exercises. The health care worker must be aware of the terms used for movements of each joint. The main movements are shown in figure 21-3 and include:

◆ *Abduction:* moving a part away from the midline of the body

◆ *Adduction:* moving a part toward the midline of the body

◆ *Flexion:* bending a body part

◆ *Extension:* straightening a body part

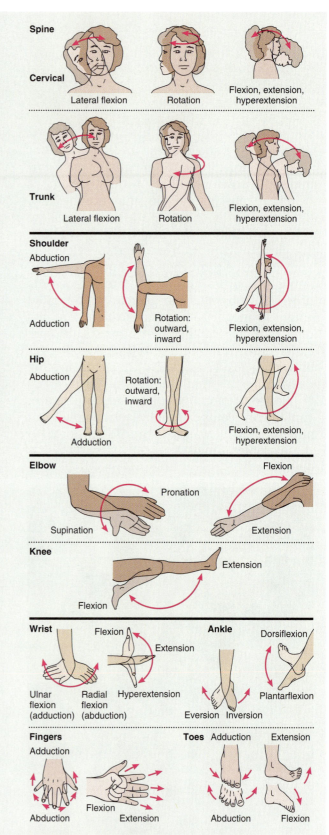

FIGURE 21-3 Range-of-motion (ROM) exercises for specific joints.

◆ *Hyperextension:* excessive straightening of a body part

◆ *Rotation:* moving a body part around its own axis, for example, turning the head from side to side

◆ *Circumduction:* moving in a circle at a joint, or moving one end of a body part in a circle while the other end remains stationary, such as swinging arm in a circle; involves all the movements of flexion, extension, abduction, adduction, and rotation

◆ *Pronation:* turning a body part downward (turning palm down)

◆ *Supination:* turning a body part upward (turning palm up)

◆ *Opposition:* touching each of the fingers with the tip of the thumb

◆ *Inversion:* turning a body part inward

◆ *Eversion:* turning a body part outward

◆ *Dorsiflexion:* bending backward (bending the foot toward the knee)

◆ *Plantar flexion:* bending forward (straightening the foot away from the knee)

◆ *Radial deviation:* moving toward the thumb side of the hand

◆ *Ulnar deviation:* moving toward the little finger side of the hand

Certain principles must be observed at all times when performing ROM exercises:

◆ Movements should be slow, smooth, and gentle to prevent injury.

◆ Support should be provided to the parts above and below the joint being exercised.

◆ A joint should never be forced beyond its ROM or exercised to the point of pain, resistance, or extreme fatigue.

◆ If a patient complains of pain, stop the exercise and report this fact to your immediate supervisor.

◆ Each movement should be performed three to five times or as ordered.

◆ The patient should be encouraged to assist as much as possible.

◆ Prevent unnecessary exposure of the patient. Only the body part being exercised should be exposed.

◆ The door should be closed and the unit screened to provide privacy.

◆ Use correct body mechanics at all times to prevent injury.

STUDENT: *Go to the workbook and complete the assignment sheet for 21:1, Performing Range-of-Motion (ROM) Exercises. Then return and continue with the procedure.*

PROCEDURE 21:1 — OBRA

Performing Range-of-Motion (ROM) Exercises

Equipment and Supplies

Bath blanket, pen or pencil

Procedure

1. Obtain proper authorization. Determine the type of ROM exercises and any limitations to movement.

    ⚖ **CAUTION:** Remember it is your responsibility to check legal requirements regarding ROMs.

2. Assemble supplies.

3. **C** Knock on the door and pause before entering. Introduce yourself. Identify the patient. Explain the procedure.

4. Close the door and screen the unit. Lock the wheels of the bed to prevent movement.

5. Wash hands.

6. Elevate the bed to a comfortable working height. Lower the siderail on the side where you are working.

7. Position the patient in the supine position (on the back) and in good body alignment.

NOTE: Some ROM exercises can be done while patient is sitting in a chair.

8. Use the bath blanket to drape the patient. Fanfold the top bed linens to the foot of the bed.

9. Administer the exercises in an organized manner. Start at the head and move to the feet. Complete one side of the body first and then work on the opposite side of the body. Perform each movement three to five times or as ordered. Provide support for the body parts above and below the joint being exercised. *Never* force any joint beyond its ROM or cause pain while exercising a joint.

   ⚠ **CAUTION:** Use proper body mechanics when administering ROM exercises. Get close to get the patient by bending at your hips and knees and keeping your back straight. Stand with your feet apart and one foot slightly forward to provide a good base of support.

   ⚠ **CAUTION:** If the patient complains of pain or discomfort during any exercise, stop the exercise and report the fact to your immediate supervisor.

10. Exercise the neck, if you have specific orders to do so:

    ⚖ **CAUTION:** In some states and health care facilities, only physical therapists or registered nurses may perform ROMs to the head and neck. Check your legal responsibilities.

    a. Support the patient's head by placing one hand under the chin and the other hand on the top-back part of the head.
       NOTE: Hands can also be placed on either side of the patient's head.
    b. Rotate the neck by turning the head gently from side to side.
    c. Flex the neck by moving the chin toward the chest (see figure 21-4).
    d. Extend the neck by returning the head to the upright position.
    e. Hyperextend the neck by tilting the head backward.
    f. Laterally flex or rotate the neck by moving the head first toward the right shoulder and then toward the left shoulder.

11. Exercise the shoulder joint nearest you:
    a. Support the patient's arm by placing one hand at the elbow and the other at the wrist.
    b. Abduct the shoulder by bringing the arm straight out at a right angle to the body (see figure 21-5A).

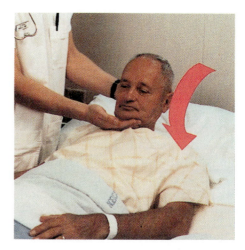

FIGURE 21-4 Flex the neck by moving the chin toward the chest.

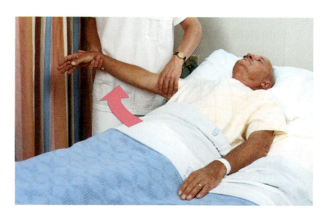

FIGURE 21-5A Abduct the shoulder by bringing the arm straight out at a right angle to the body.

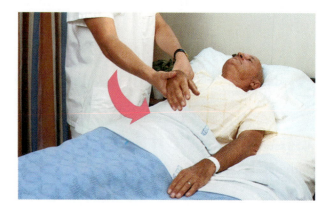

FIGURE 21-5B Adduct the shoulder by moving the arm straight in to the body.

    c. Adduct the shoulder by moving the arm straight in to the side (see figure 21-5B).
    d. Flex the shoulder by raising the arm in front of the body and then above the head (see figure 21-6).

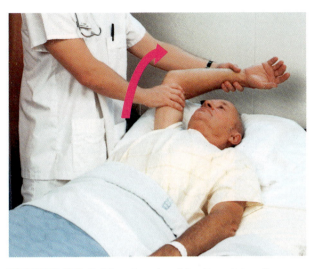

FIGURE 21-6 Flex the shoulder by raising the arm in front of the body and then above the head.

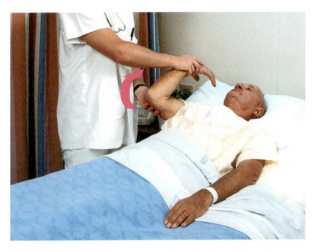

FIGURE 21-7A Flex the elbow by bending the forearm and hand up to the shoulder.

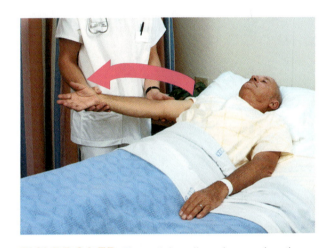

FIGURE 21-7B Extend the elbow by moving the forearm and hand down to the side. *(Courtesy of Sunrise Medical)*

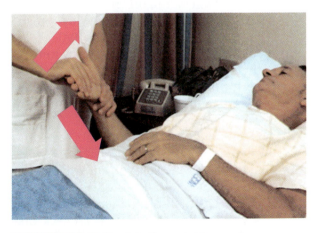

FIGURE 21-8 Deviate the wrist in an ulnar direction by moving the hand toward the little finger side and in a radial direction by moving it toward the thumb side.

   e. Extend the shoulder by bringing the arm back down to the side from above the head.
12. Exercise the elbow joint nearest you:
   a. Support the patient's arm by placing one hand on the elbow and the other hand on the wrist.
   b. Flex the elbow by bending the forearm and hand up to the shoulder (see figure 21-7A).
   c. Extend the elbow by moving the forearm and hand down to the side, or straightening the arm (see figure 21-7B).
   d. Pronate by turning the forearm and hand so that the palm of the hand is down.
   e. Supinate by turning the forearm and hand so that the palm of the hand is up.
13. Exercise the wrist nearest you:
   a. Support the patient's wrist by placing one hand above it and the other hand below it.
   b. Flex the wrist by bending the hand down toward the forearm.
   c. Extend the wrist by straightening the hand.
   d. Hyperextend the wrist by bending the top of the hand back toward the forearm.
   e. Deviate the wrist in an ulnar direction by moving the hand toward the little finger side (see figure 21-8).
   f. Deviate the wrist in a radial direction by moving the hand toward the thumb side.
14. Exercise the fingers and thumb on the hand nearest you:
   a. Support the patient's hand by placing one hand at the wrist.

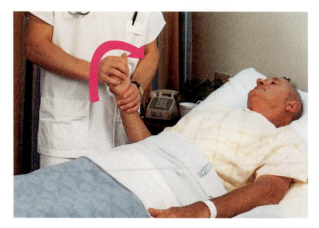

FIGURE 21-9A Flex the thumb and fingers by bending them toward the palm.

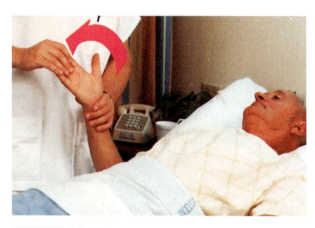

FIGURE 21-9B Extend the thumb and fingers by straightening them.

b. Flex the thumb and fingers by bending them toward the palm (see figure 21-9A).
c. Extend the thumb and fingers by straightening them (see figure 21-9B).
d. Abduct the thumb and fingers by spreading them apart (see figure 21-10A).
e. Adduct the thumb and fingers by moving them together (see figure 21-10B).
f. Perform opposition by touching the thumb to the tip of each finger (see figure 21-10C).
g. Circumduct the thumb by moving it in a circular motion.

15. Uncover the leg nearest you and exercise the hip:

⚠ **CAUTION:** If the patient had hip or knee replacement surgery, check first for any limitations or restrictions to ROMs.

a. Support the patient's leg by placing one hand under the knee and the other hand under the ankle.

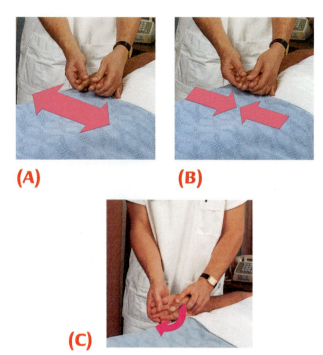

(A) **(B)**

(C)

FIGURE 21-10 (A) Abduct the thumb and fingers by spreading them apart. (B) Adduct the thumb and fingers by moving them together. (C) Perform opposition by touching the thumb to the tip of each finger.

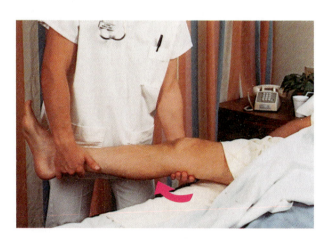

FIGURE 21-11A Abduct the hip by moving the entire leg out to the side.

b. Abduct the hip by moving the entire leg out to the side (see figure 21-11A).
c. Adduct the hip by moving the entire leg back toward the body (see figure 21-11B).
d. Flex the hip by bending the knee and moving the thigh up toward the abdomen (see figure 21-12A).
e. Extend the hip by straightening the knee and moving the leg away from the abdomen (see figure 21-12B).

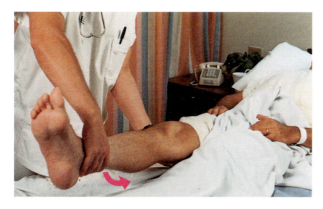

FIGURE 21-11B Adduct the hip by moving the entire leg back toward the body.

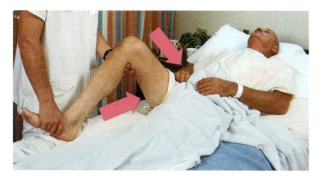

FIGURE 21-12A Flex the hip by bending the knee and moving the thigh up toward the abdomen.

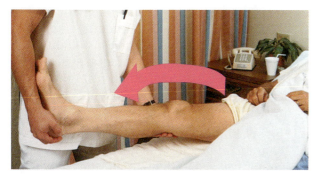

FIGURE 21-12B Extend the hip by straightening the knee and moving the leg away from the abdomen.

f. Medially rotate the hip by bending the knee and turning the leg in toward the midline.

g. Laterally rotate the hip by bending the knee and turning the leg out away from the midline.

16. Exercise the knee nearest you:
   a. Support the patient's leg by placing one hand under the knee and the other hand under the ankle.

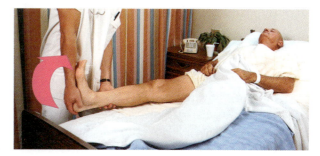

FIGURE 21-13A Dorsiflex the ankle by moving the toes and foot up toward the knee.

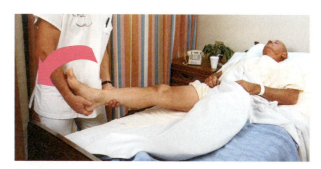

FIGURE 21-13B Plantar flex the ankle by moving the toes and foot down away from the knee.

   b. Flex the knee by bending the lower leg back toward the thigh.
   c. Extend the knee by straightening the leg.
17. Exercise the ankle nearest you:
   a. Support the patient's foot by placing one hand under the foot and the other hand behind the ankle.
   b. Dorsiflex the ankle by moving the toes and foot up toward the knee (see figure 21-13A).
   c. Plantar flex the ankle by moving the toes and foot down away from the knee (see figure 21-13B).
   d. Invert the foot by gently turning it inward.
   e. Evert the foot by gently turning it outward.
18. Exercise the toes on the foot nearest you:
   a. Rest the patient's leg and foot on the bed for support.
   b. Abduct the toes by separating them, or moving them away from each other.
   c. Adduct the toes by moving them together.
   d. Flex the toes by bending them down toward the bottom of the foot.
   e. Extend the toes by straightening them.
19. Use the bath blanket to cover the patient. Raise the siderail and move to the opposite side of the bed. Lower the siderail.
20. Repeat steps 11 to 18.

21. When ROM exercises are complete, comfortably position the patient in good body alignment. Replace the top bed linens and remove the bath blanket.

22. Observe all checkpoints before leaving the patient: elevate the siderails (if indicated), lower the bed to its lowest level, place the call signal and supplies within easy reach of the patient, and leave the area neat and clean.

23. Wash hands.

24. **C** Report and/or record all required information on the patient's chart or the agency form, for example, date; time; ROM exercises performed on all joints, patient assisted with movements of arms and hands; and your signature and title. Report any unusual observations immediately.

Practice *Go to the workbook and use the evaluation sheet for 21:1, Performing Range-of-Motion (ROM) Exercises to practice this procedure. When you feel you have mastered this skill, sign the sheet and give it to your instructor for further action.*

✔ **Final Checkpoint** Using the criteria listed on the evaluation sheet, your instructor will grade your performance.

21:2

INFORMATION
Ambulating Patients Who Use Transfer (Gait) Belts, Crutches, Canes, or Walkers

 OBRA Many patients require aids, or assistive devices, when ambulating. The type used depends on the injury and the patient's condition. However, certain points must be observed when a patient uses crutches, canes, or a walker.

Transfer (Gait) Belt

A **transfer (gait) belt** is a band of fabric or leather that is positioned around the patient's waist. During transfers or ambulation, the health care worker can grasp the transfer belt to provide additional support for the patient. The transfer belt helps provide the patient with a sense of security and helps to stabilize the patient's center of balance. Some important facts to remember when ambulating a patient with a transfer belt include the following:

- The transfer belt must be the proper size. It should fit securely around the waist for support but must not be too tight for comfort.

- Some transfer belts contain loops that are grasped when ambulating the patient. If loops are not present, an underhand grasp should be used to hold on to the belt during ambulation. The underhand grasp is more secure than grasping the belt from the top, because the hands are less likely to slip off the belt.

- The belt should be grasped at the back during ambulation, and the health care worker should walk slightly behind the patient. When assisting a patient to stand, or during transfers such as transferring a patient to a wheelchair, grasp the belt on both sides while facing the patient.

- The transfer belt is applied over the patient's clothing. It should not be applied over bare skin because it can irritate the skin.

The use of a transfer belt is contraindicated in patients who have an ostomy, gastrostomy tube, abdominal pacemaker, severe cardiac or respiratory disease, fractured ribs, or recent surgery on the lower chest or abdominal area. It is also contraindicated for pregnant women.

Crutches

Crutches are artificial supports that assist a patient who needs help walking. Crutches are usually prescribed by a physician. A therapist or other authorized individual fits the crutches to the patient and teaches the appropriate gait. In addition, exercises to strengthen the muscles of the shoulders, arms, and hands are frequently prescribed by the physician or therapist. Health care workers should be aware of the criteria for fitting and of the gaits so that they can properly ambulate patients.

There are three main types of crutches:

◆ *Axillary crutches* (see figure 21-14A): made of wood or aluminum and used for patients who need crutches for a short period of time. The patient must be taught to bear weight on the hand bars instead of the axillary supports. If pressure is applied on the axillary bar, it can injure axillary blood vessels and nerves. They are *not* recommended for weak or elderly patients since axillary crutches require good upper body and arm strength, and a good sense of balance and coordination.

◆ *Forearm or Lofstrand crutches* (see figure 21-14B): attach to forearms; used for patients with weakness or paralysis in both legs; recommended for patients who need crutches permanently or for a long period of time; require upper arm strength and good coordination.

◆ *Platform crutches* (see figure 21-14C): used for patients who cannot grip handles of

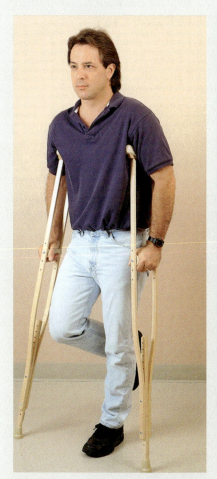

FIGURE 21-14A A patient using an axillary crutch must be taught to bear weight on the hand bars instead of on the axillary supports.

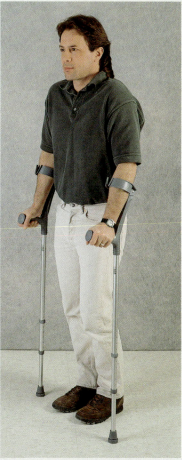

FIGURE 21-14B Forearm or Lofstrand crutches are recommended for patients who need crutches permanently or for a long period of time.

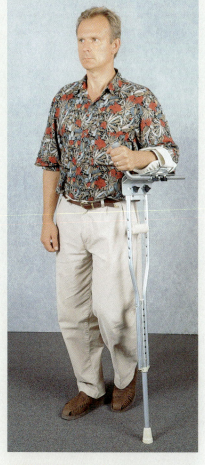

FIGURE 21-14C Platform crutches are used by patients who cannot grip the handles of other crutches or bear weight on the wrist and hands.

other crutches or bear weight on wrist and hands; do not require as much upper body strength, but do require a good sense of balance and coordination; require that elbows be flexed at 90° or right angle so patient can bear weight on forearm.

The following points should be observed when fitting crutches to a patient.

◆ The patient should wear walking shoes that fit well and provide good support. The shoes should have low, broad heels approximately 1 to 1½ inches high and nonskid soles.

◆ The crutches should be positioned 4 to 6 inches in front of and 4 to 6 inches to the side of the patient's foot (see figure 21-15).

◆ The length of axillary crutches should be adjusted so that there are 2 inches between the armpit and the axillary bar of the crutch (see figure 21-16).

◆ The handpieces of axillary or forearm crutches should be adjusted so that each elbow is flexed at a 25° to 30° angle.

Some of the more common crutch-walking gaits are described. The gait taught by the therapist or authorized person depends on the injury and the patient's condition.

◆ *Four-point gait:* Used when both legs can bear some weight. It is a slow gait. Patients often are taught the four-point gait as the first gait and are then taught faster gaits when this one is mastered.

◆ *Two-point gait:* Often taught after the four-point gait is mastered. It is a faster gait and is usually used when both legs can bear some weight. The two-point gait is closest to the natural rhythm of walking.

◆ *Three-point gait:* Used when only one leg can bear weight. It too is a gait taught initially.

◆ *Swing-to gait:* This is a more rapid gait. It is taught after other gaits are mastered, in most cases. It requires that the patient have more shoulder and arm strength.

◆ *Swing-through gait:* This is the most rapid gait. However, it requires the most strength and skill. It is usually taught as a more advanced method of crutch walking.

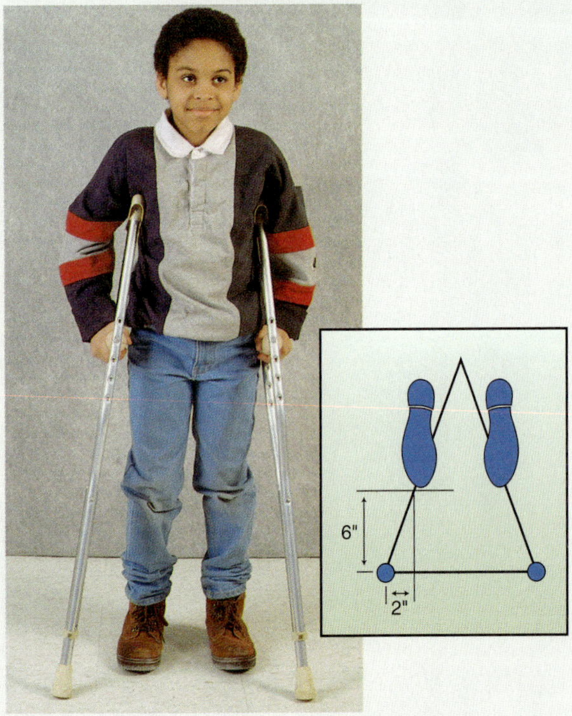

Cane

A **cane** is an assistive device that provides balance and support. There are several different types of canes (see figure 21-17A). *Standard* canes are single-tipped canes. They can have

FIGURE 21-15 Crutches should be positioned 4 to 6 inches in front of and 4 to 6 inches to the side of the patient's foot.

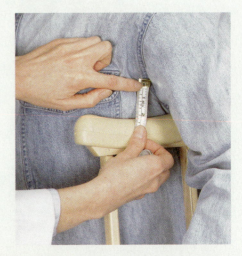

FIGURE 21-16 The length of axillary crutches should be adjusted so that there are 2 inches between the axillary area and the top of the crutches.

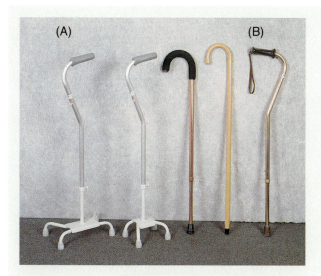

FIGURE 21-17A Different types of canes: (A) Quad canes; (B) Single-tipped canes.

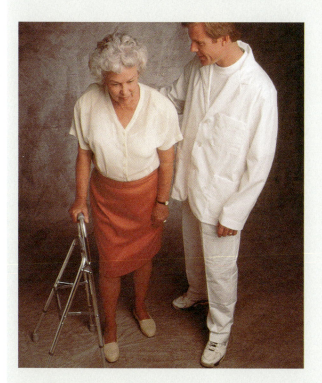

FIGURE 21-17B A walkcane has four legs and a handlebar that the patient can grip. *(Courtesy of Sunrise Medical)*

curved handles, T-handles, or J-handles with a handgrip. *Tripod* canes with three tips and *quad* canes with four tips provide a wider base of support and more stability for the patient. A *walkcane,* also called a Hemiwalker, has four legs and a handlebar that the patient can grip (see figure 21-17B). It is used with patients who

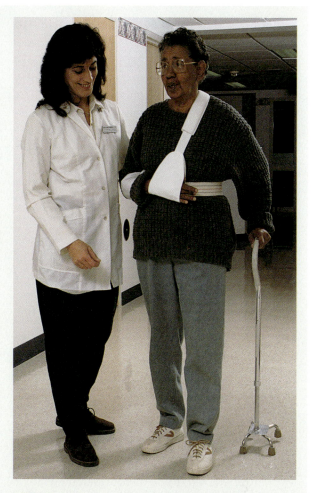

FIGURE 21-17C A cane is used on the unaffected (good) side to provide a wider base of support.

have *hemiplegia,* or paralysis on one side of the body. The bottom tip(s) of all canes should be fitted with a 1½-inch rubber-suction tip to provide traction and prevent slipping. Basic principles for using canes include:

◆ A cane is used on the unaffected (good) side (see figure 21-17C). In this way, a wider base of support is provided to increase stability. This prevents the patient from leaning toward the cane and falling because of the weak or injured leg. In addition, in normal walking, the leg and opposite arm move together, so the cane and leg will follow the same pattern.

◆ Canes must be correctly fitted. The bottom tip of the cane should be positioned approximately 6 to 10 inches from the side of the unaffected foot. The cane handle should be level with the top of the femur at the hip joint. The patient's elbow should be flexed at a 25° to 30° angle.

◆ Several gaits for cane walking can be taught. In one gait, the patient is taught to move the cane and affected leg together, and then move the unaffected leg. In another gait, the patient is taught to move the cane, then the affected or involved leg, and finally the unaffected leg. The therapist or other authorized person determines the correct gait.

Walker

A **walker** is a four-legged device that provides support. Walkers are available in several styles, including standard, folding, rolling, and platform. Walkers often are used for weak patients who have a poor sense of balance even though no leg injuries may be present. Basic principles for using a walker include:

◆ The walker should be fitted to the patient. The handles should be level with the top of the femurs at the hip joints. Each elbow should be flexed at a 25° to 30° angle.

◆ The patient must be taught to lift the walker and place it in front of the body. It should be positioned so that the back legs of the walker are even with the toes of the patient. The patient then walks "into" the walker.

◆ All legs of the walker should be fitted with rubber tips to prevent slipping.

◆ The patient should be cautioned against sliding the walker. A sliding technique may be dangerous because it can very easily tip over the walker. Most walkers are made of lightweight aluminum, so most patients are capable of lifting them.

Ambulation Precautions

⚠ CAUTION: It is essential that the health care worker remain alert at all times when ambulating a patient. Always walk on the patient's weak side and slightly behind the

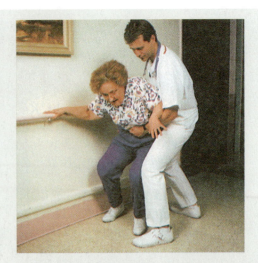

FIGURE 21-18 Ease a falling patient to the floor as slowly as possible. Try to protect the patient's head and neck.

patient, and be alert for signs that the patient may fall. If the patient starts to fall, do *not* try to hold the patient in an upright position. Use your body to brace the patient, if at all possible: keep your back straight, bend from the hips and knees, maintain a broad base of support, and try to grasp the patient under the axillary (armpit) areas. If the patient is wearing a transfer belt, keep a firm hold on the belt. The patient should be eased to the floor as slowly as possible (see figure 21-18). The patient's head and neck should be protected, and the head should be prevented from striking the floor. Stay with the patient and call for help. Patients should not be moved until they have been examined for injuries. After a fall has occurred, most agencies require a written incident report. Follow agency policy for correct documentation of the incident.

STUDENT: *Go to the workbook and complete the assignment sheet for 21:2, Ambulating Patients Who Use Transfer (Gait) Belts, Crutches, Canes, or Walkers. Then return and continue with the procedures.*

PROCEDURE 21:2A

Ambulating a Patient with a Transfer (Gait) Belt

Equipment and Supplies

Transfer or gait belt, pen or pencil

Procedure

1. Check orders or obtain authorization from your immediate supervisor for ambulating the patient.
2. Assemble supplies.
3. **C** Knock on the door and pause before entering. Introduce yourself. Identify the patient and explain the procedure.
4. Close the door and screen the unit to provide privacy.
5. Wash hands.
6. Lock the wheels on the bed to prevent movement. Lower the siderail on the side where you are working.
7. Assist the patient into a sitting position. If the patient is wearing bedclothes, put a robe on the patient.
8. Check to be sure the transfer belt is the correct size. Position the belt around the patient's waist and on top of the clothing (see figure 21-19A). Position the buckle or clasp so that it is slightly off center in the front. Make sure the belt is smooth and free of wrinkles.

   NOTE: Unless loops are present on the back side, the clasp or buckle can also be positioned slightly off center in the back.
9. Tighten the belt so that it fits snugly; secure the clasp or buckle. Place fingers under the belt to make sure it is not too tight (see figure 21-19B). Make sure the belt is comfortable and does not interfere with breathing. On a female patient, make sure the breasts are not under the belt.

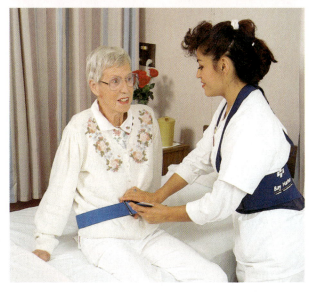

FIGURE 21-19A Position the transfer belt around the patient's waist and on top of the clothing.

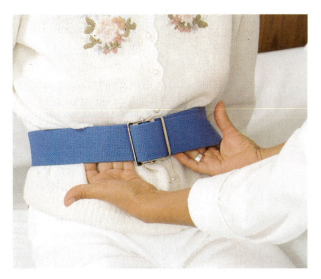

FIGURE 21-19B Check the transfer belt to make sure it is not too tight.

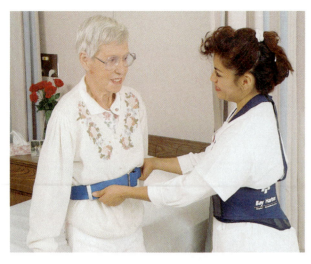

FIGURE 21-19C Place your hands under the sides of the belt and use proper body mechanics as you help the patient to a standing position.

10. Put shoes or slippers on the patient. For the most security, shoes should be worn. The shoes should have low, broad heels approximately 1 to 1½ inches high and nonskid soles.

11. Assist the patient to a standing position. Face the patient and get a broad base of support. Grasp the loops on the side of the belt or place your hands under the sides of the belt. Ask the patient to assist by pushing against the bed with his/her hands at a given signal, such as "one, two, three, stand." Bend at your knees and give the signal for the patient to stand. Keep your back straight and straighten your knees as the patient stands (see figure 21-19C).

12. To ambulate the patient, support the patient in a standing position. Keep one hand on one side of the belt while moving the other hand to the loops or the back of the belt. Then, move the second hand from the side to the loops or the back of the belt while you move behind the patient.

    ⚠ **CAUTION:** Keep one hand firmly on the belt at all times when changing position.

13. Ambulate the patient. Encourage the patient to walk slowly and use handrails, if available. Walk slightly behind the patient at all times and keep a firm, underhand grip on the belt or keep your hands firmly in the loops.

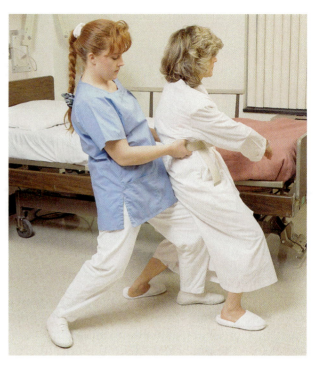

FIGURE 21-20 Keep your back straight and use your body to brace the patient if the patient starts to fall.

14. If the patient starts to fall, keep a firm grip on the belt. Use your body to brace the patient; keep your back straight (see figure 21-20). Gently ease the patient to the floor, taking care to protect his or her head. Stay with the patient and call for help. Do not try to stand the patient up until help arrives and the patient has been examined for injuries.

15. When ambulation is complete, assist the patient in returning to bed. Remove the transfer belt.

16. Observe all checkpoints before leaving the patient. Make sure the patient is comfortable and in good body alignment. Elevate the siderails (if indicated), lower the bed to its lowest level, place the call signal and supplies within easy reach of the patient, and leave the area neat and clean.

17. Replace all equipment.

18. Wash hands.

19. **C** Report and/or record all required information on the patient's chart or the agency form, for example, date; time; ambulated with a transfer belt, walked down to lounge and back; and your signature and title. Report any problems immediately.

Practice *Go to the workbook and use the evaluation sheet for 21:2A, Ambulating a Patient with a Transfer (Gait) Belt, to practice this procedure. When you feel you have mastered this skill, sign the sheet and give it to your instructor for further action.*

 Final Checkpoint Using the criteria listed on the evaluation sheet, your instructor will grade your performance.

PROCEDURE 21:2B
Ambulating a Patient Who Uses Crutches

Equipment and Supplies

Adjustable crutches, pen or pencil

Procedure

1. Check orders or obtain authorization from your immediate supervisor. Ascertain which gait the therapist taught the patient.
2. Assemble equipment.
3. Check the crutches. Make sure there are rubber-suction tips on the bottom ends and that the tips are not worn down or torn. Check to be sure the axillary bars and hand rests are covered with padding.
   NOTE: Foam-rubber pads are usually placed on crutches.
4. **C** Knock on the door and pause before entering. Introduce yourself. Identify the patient. Explain the procedure.
5. Wash hands.
6. Help the patient put on good walking shoes. The shoes should have low, broad heels approximately 1 to 1½ inches high and non-skid soles.
7. Place a transfer (gait) belt on the patient. Use an underhand grasp on the belt and assist the patient to a standing position. Advise the patient to bear his or her weight on the unaffected leg. Position the crutches correctly.
8. Check the fit of the crutches.
   a. Position the crutches 4 to 6 inches in front of the patient's feet.
   b. Move the crutches 4 to 6 inches to the sides of the feet.
   c. Make sure there is a 2-inch gap between the axilla (armpit) and the axillary bar or rest. If the length must be adjusted, check with your immediate supervisor.
   d. Each elbow must be flexed at a 25° to 30° angle. If the hand rests must be adjusted to achieve this angle, check with your immediate supervisor.
   NOTE: In some agencies, the trained health care worker is permitted to adjust the crutches as necessary. The adjustments are then checked by the therapist or other authorized person. Follow your agency's policy.
9. Assist the patient with the required gait. The gait used depends on the patient's injury and condition and is determined by the therapist or other authorized person.
   CAUTION: Remain alert at all times. Be ready to catch the patient if there are any signs of falling.
10. Four-point gait (see figure 21-21):
    a. The patient can bear weight on both legs. Start the patient in a standing position, with crutches at the sides.
    b. Move the right crutch forward.
    c. Move the left foot forward.
    d. Move the left crutch forward.
    e. Move the right foot forward.
    NOTE: This is a slow gait taught initially when both legs can bear weight.
11. Three-point gait (see figure 21-22):
    a. The patient can bear weight on one leg only. Start the patient in a standing position, with crutches at the sides.

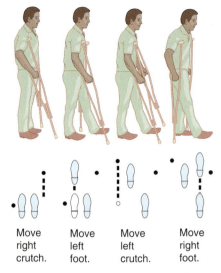

FIGURE 21-21 Four-point gait for crutches.

Move right crutch. Move left foot. Move left crutch. Move right foot.

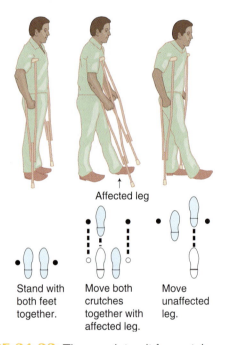

Affected leg

Stand with both feet together. Move both crutches together with affected leg. Move unaffected leg.

FIGURE 21-22 Three-point gait for crutches.

b. Advance both crutches and the weak or affected foot.
c. Transfer the patient's body weight forward to the crutches.
d. Advance the unaffected, or good, foot forward.

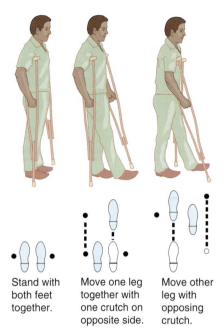

Stand with both feet together. Move one leg together with one crutch on opposite side. Move other leg with opposing crutch.

FIGURE 21-23 Two-point gait for crutches.

NOTE: This is a slow gait taught initially when only one leg can bear weight.

12. Two-point gait (see figure 21-23):
   a. The patient can bear weight on both legs. Start with the crutches at the sides.
   b. Move the right foot and left crutch forward at the same time.
   c. Move the left foot and right crutch forward at the same time.
   NOTE: This is a more advanced and a more rapid gait used when the four-point gait has been mastered.

13. Swing-to gait:
   a. One or both of the patient's legs can bear weight. Start with the crutches at the sides.
   b. Balance weight on foot or feet. Move both crutches forward.
   c. Transfer weight forward.
   d. Use shoulder and arm strength to swing feet up to crutches.
   NOTE: This is a more rapid gait and requires more shoulder and arm strength and a good sense of balance and coordination.

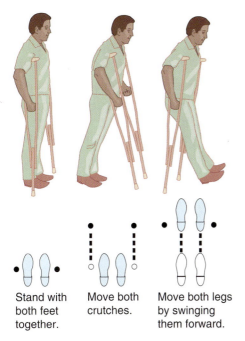

| Stand with both feet together. | Move both crutches. | Move both legs by swinging them forward. |

FIGURE 21-24 Swing-through gait for crutches.

14. Swing-through gait (see figure 21-24):
    a. One or both of the patient's legs can bear weight. Start with the crutches at the sides. Balance weight on foot or feet.
    b. Advance both crutches forward at the same time.
    c. Transfer weight forward.
    d. Use shoulder and arm strength to swing up to and through the crutches, stopping slightly in front of the crutches.
       NOTE: This is the most rapid and advanced gait. It requires a great deal of shoulder and arm strength. It also requires an excellent sense of balance because at one point only the crutches are in contact with the ground.

15. When using crutches, the patient must *not* rest his or her body weight on the axillary rests. Shoulder and arm strength should provide movement on the crutches.
    CAUTION: Warn the patient that nerve damage can occur if weight is supported constantly on the axillary rest.

16. Check to make sure that the patient is not moving too far forward at one time. Distances should be limited. If the patient attempts to move the crutches too far forward, he or she can very easily lose balance and fall forward.

17. Check the patient's progress. Report the progress to the therapist or your immediate supervisor. The therapist will determine when to teach the patient more advanced gaits.

18. When the patient is finished using the crutches, replace all equipment.

19. Assist the patient back to bed or position the patient in a chair. Remove the transfer belt. Observe all checkpoints before leaving the patient. Make sure the patient is comfortable and in good body alignment. If the patient is in bed, elevate the siderails (if indicated), lower the bed to its lowest level, place the call signal and other supplies within easy reach of the patient, and leave the area neat and clean.

20. Wash hands.

21. Report and/or record all required information on the patient's chart or the agency form, for example, date; time; ambulated with crutches, walked down the hall two times using two-point gait, no problems noted; and your signature and title. Report any problems immediately.

Practice *Go to the workbook and use the evaluation sheet for 21:2B, Ambulating a Patient Who Uses Crutches, to practice this procedure. When you feel you have mastered this skill, sign the sheet and give it to your instructor for further action.*

Final Checkpoint Using the criteria listed on the evaluation sheet, your instructor will grade your performance.

PROCEDURE 21:2C   OBRA

Ambulating a Patient Who Uses a Cane

Equipment and Supplies

Adjustable cane, pen or pencil

Procedure

1. Check orders or obtain authorization from your immediate supervisor. Ascertain which gait the therapist taught the patient.
2. Assemble equipment.
3. Check the cane. Make sure the bottom has a rubber-suction tip. If the patient needs extra stability, use a tripod (three-legged) or quad (four-legged) cane.
4. **C** Knock on the door and pause before entering. Introduce yourself. Identify the patient. Explain the procedure.
5. Wash hands.
6. Help the patient put on good walking shoes. The shoes should have low, broad heels approximately 1 to 1½ inches high and non-skid soles.
7. Place a transfer (gait) belt on the patient. Use an underhand grasp on the belt and assist the patient to a standing position. Advise the patient to bear his or her weight on the unaffected leg.
8. Check the height of the cane:
   a. Position the cane on the unaffected (good) side and approximately 6 to 10 inches from the side of the foot.
   b. The top of the cane should be level with the top of the femur at the hip joint.
   c. The patient's elbow should be flexed at a 25° to 30° angle.
      NOTE: If the height of the cane needs adjustment, follow agency policy. In some agencies, only the therapist adjusts canes. In other agencies, the trained health care worker can adjust canes.
9. Instruct the patient to use the cane on the good, or unaffected, side.
   NOTE: This prevents leaning toward the weak or affected side and provides a broader base of support.
10. Assist the patient with the gait ordered. For a three-point gait (see figure 21-25A):
    a. Balance the body weight on the strong or unaffected foot. Move the cane forward approximately 12 to 18 inches.

b. Move the weak or affected foot forward.
c. Transfer the weight to the affected foot and cane. Bring the unaffected foot forward.

For a two-point gait (see figure 21-25B):
a. Balance the weight on the strong or unaffected foot.
b. Move the cane and the weak or affected foot forward. Keep the cane fairly close to the body to prevent leaning.
c. Transfer body weight forward to the cane.
d. Move the good, or unaffected, foot forward.

   ⚠ CAUTION: Remain alert at all times. Be ready to catch the patient if there are any signs of falling.

11. A common sequence to follow when assisting the patient up and down stairs is that of always starting with the good (unaffected) leg:
    a. Step up with the unaffected leg.
    b. Bring the cane and weak or affected leg up.

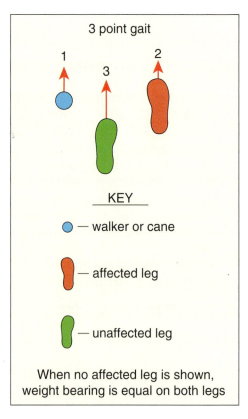

FIGURE 21-25A Three-point gait for canes.

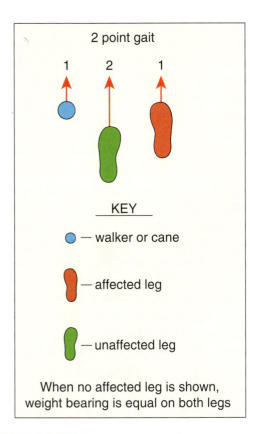

FIGURE 21-25B Two-point gait for canes.

c. To go down steps, reverse this procedure. Step down on the good leg and follow with the cane and affected or weak foot. **NOTE:** Remember this sequence by saying, "Good Guys Go First."

12. When walking with a cane, the patient should not try to take large steps. Smaller steps are recommended to prevent leaning and/or loss of balance.

13. Note the patient's progress. Pay particular attention to any problems the patient experiences during ambulation. Report this information to your immediate supervisor or the therapist.

14. Assist the patient back to bed or position the patient in a chair. Remove the transfer belt. Observe all checkpoints before leaving the patient. Make sure the patient is comfortable and in good body alignment. If the patient is in bed, elevate the siderails (if indicated), lower the bed to its lowest level, place the call signal and other supplies within easy reach of the patient, and leave the area neat and clean.

15. Replace all equipment.

16. Wash hands.

17. Report and/or record all required information on the patient's chart or the agency form, for example, date; time; ambulated with tripod cane, walked to visitor's lounge and back to room, no problems noted; and your signature and title. Report any problems immediately.

Practice *Go to the workbook and use the evaluation sheet for 21:2C, Ambulating a Patient Who Uses a Cane, to practice this procedure. When you feel you have mastered this skill, sign the sheet and give it to your instructor for further action.*

Final Checkpoint Using the criteria listed on the evaluation sheet, your instructor will grade your performance.

PROCEDURE 21:2D   OBRA

Ambulating a Patient Who Uses a Walker

Equipment and Supplies

Adjustable walker, pen or pencil

Procedure

1. Check orders or obtain authorization from your immediate supervisor for ambulating the patient.

2. Assemble equipment.

3. Check the walker. Make sure rubber-suction tips are secure on all of the legs. Check for rough or damaged edges on the hand rests.

4. Knock on the door and pause before entering. Introduce yourself. Identify the patient. Explain the procedure.

5. Wash hands.

6. Help the patient put on good walking shoes. The shoes should have low, broad heels approximately 1 to 1½ inches high and non-skid soles.

7. Place a transfer (gait) belt on the patient. Use an underhand grasp on the belt and assist the patient to a standing position. Position the walker correctly and ask the patient to grasp the hand rests securely.

8. Check the height of the walker to see whether the following requirements are met:
   a. The hand rests are level with the tops of the femurs at the hip joints.
   b. The elbows are flexed at 25° to 30° angles.
   NOTE: If the height of the walker needs adjustment, follow agency policy. In some agencies, only the therapist makes such adjustments. In other agencies, a trained health care worker may adjust walkers.

9. Start with the walker in position. The patient should be standing "inside" the walker.

10. Tell the patient to lift the walker and place it forward so that the back legs of the walker are even with the patient's toes.
    ⚠ **CAUTION:** Tell the patient to avoid sliding the walker. The walker could fall forward and cause the patient to fall.

11. Instruct the patient to transfer his or her weight forward slightly to the walker.

12. Instruct the patient to use the walker for support and to walk "into" the walker. Do *not* allow the patient to "shuffle" his or her feet (see figure 21-26).

13. Repeat steps 10 to 12. While the patient is using the walker, walk to the side and slightly behind the patient. Be alert at all times. Be ready to catch the patient if there are any signs of falling.

14. Check constantly to make sure the patient is lifting the walker to move it forward. Also make sure the patient is placing the walker forward just to his or her toes and not attempting too large a step.

15. Note the patient's progress. Pay particular attention to any problems the patient experiences during ambulation. Report this information to your immediate supervisor or the therapist.

16. Assist the patient back to bed or position the patient in a chair. Remove the transfer belt. Observe all checkpoints before leaving the patient. Make sure the patient is comfortable and in good body alignment. If the patient is in bed, elevate the siderails (if indicated),

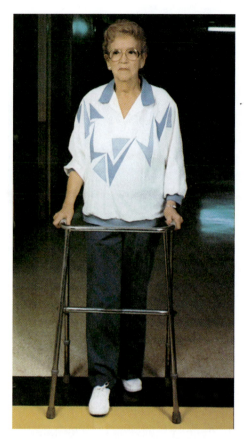

FIGURE 21-26 Instruct the patient to use the walker for support while walking "into" the walker.

lower the bed to its lowest level, place the call signal and other supplies within easy reach of the patient, and leave the area neat and clean.

17. Replace all equipment.

18. Wash hands.

19. Ⓒ Report and/or record all required information on the patient's chart or the agency form, for example, date; time; ambulated with walker, walked down the hall and back two times, needs encouragement to pick up walker and not slide it; and your signature and title. Report any problems immediately.

Practice *Go to the workbook and use the evaluation sheet for 21:2D, Ambulating a Patient Who Uses a Walker, to practice this procedure. When you feel you have mastered this skill, sign the sheet and give it to your instructor for further action.*

 Final Checkpoint Using the criteria listed on the evaluation sheet, your instructor will grade your performance.

21:3 INFORMATION Administering Heat/Cold Applications

As a health care worker, you may be responsible for administering a variety of heat and cold applications. Some of the main principles involved are described in this section.

Cold applications (cryotherapy) are administered to relieve pain, reduce swelling, reduce body temperature, and control bleeding.

◆ **Moist cold** applications are cold and moist or wet against the skin. Examples are cold **compresses,** packs, and soaks. These applications are more penetrating than are dry cold applications.

◆ **Dry cold** applications are cold and dry against the skin. Examples are **ice bags, ice collars, hypothermia blankets,** and similar devices. Hypothermia blankets are used to reduce high body temperatures.

Heat applications (thermotherapy) are administered to relieve pain, increase drainage from an infected area, stimulate healing, increase circulation to an area, combat infection, and relieve muscle spasms or increase muscle mobility before exercise.

◆ **Moist heat** applications are warm and wet against the skin. These applications are more penetrating and more effective in relieving pain in deeper tissues than are dry heat applications. Examples are the **sitz bath,** hot soaks, compresses, **hydrocollator packs,** and **paraffin wax treatments.** The sitz bath is used to provide warm moist heat to the perineal and rectal area. It is used postpartum (after birth) and after rectal surgery to provide comfort and promote healing. Hydrocollator packs are gel-filled packs which are warmed in a water bath at a temperature of 150° to 170°F. The gel maintains the warmth for approximately 30 to 40 minutes and the pack can be contoured to fit smoothly over any area of the body (see figure 21-27). The pack must be covered with a thick terry cloth or flannel cover before being applied to the skin. Hydrocollator packs are frequently used prior to ROM exer-

cises. Paraffin wax treatments are often used for chronic joint disease, such as arthritis, or prior to ROM exercises. A mixture of paraffin and a small amount of mineral oil are heated to the melting point. The physical therapist dips the patient's hand(s) or other body part into the warm paraffin three or four times to create a "glove" of wax (see figure 21-28A). The wax is left in place for 20 to 30 minutes before being peeled off (see figure 21-28B).

◆ **Dry heat** applications are warm and dry against the skin. Examples are **warm-water bags,** heating pads, **aquamatic pads** or aquathermia pads, and heat lamps.

Heat and cold applications are effective because of the reactions they cause in the blood vessels.

◆ Heat applications cause **vasodilation.** The blood vessels in the area become larger (dilated). More blood comes to the area. Therefore, more oxygen and nutrients are

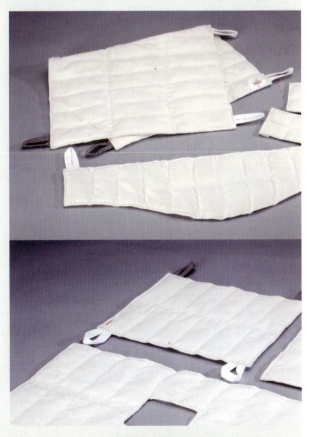

FIGURE 21-27 Hydrocollator packs are gel-filled packs that are warmed in a water bath. *(Courtesy of Briggs Corporation, Des Moines, IA)*

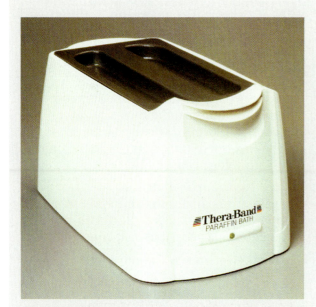

FIGURE 21-28A A body part is dipped into the paraffin bath three or four times to create a layer of warm wax on the skin. *(Courtesy of Briggs Corporation, Des Moines, IA)*

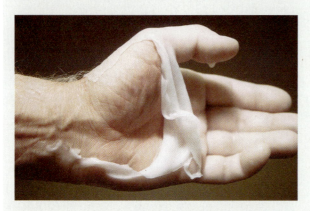

FIGURE 21-28B After the wax has been in place for 20 to 30 minutes, it is peeled off and discarded.

available to stimulate healing. Heat applications ease pain by allowing the blood to carry away fluids that cause inflammation and pain.

◆ Cold applications cause **vasoconstriction.** The blood vessels become smaller (constricted). Less blood comes to the area. Swelling decreases because fewer fluids are present. The cold also has a numbing effect, which decreases local pain.

A physician's order is required for a heat or cold application. The order should state the type of application, duration of treatment, temperature (if not standard), and area of application. In some states and agencies, health care assistants are not allowed to administer heat or cold applications. It is important to check your agency's policy and be aware of your legal responsibilities.

CAUTION: The patient must be checked frequently when an application is in place. Color and temperature of the skin, amount of pain and bleeding, effect on circulation, and other signs and symptoms must be noted. Special attention must be given to infants, young children, and elderly patients, because the skin of these patients is less resistant and burns or injuries can occur rapidly. Metal objects, such as rings, bracelets, necklaces, watches, and zippers, readily conduct heat or cold. Patients should be asked to remove all metal objects in the treated area before a heat or cold application. When administering heat or cold applications, the rubber or plastic should never come in contact with the skin. All rubber or plastic applications should be covered with a towel or special cloth cover. If any abnormal symptoms are noted, the application should be discontinued and the immediate supervisor notified. The health care worker must be alert at all times and observe all safety precautions when administering heat and cold applications.

Standard precautions (discussed in Unit 13:3) must be observed if any contact with blood, body fluids, secretions, or excretions is possible. An example is a moist heat application placed on a draining wound. Gloves must be worn. Hands must be washed frequently and are always washed immediately after removing gloves. A mask and eye protection must be worn if splashing or spraying of body fluids is possible. A health care worker must always use proper precautions to prevent the spread of infection.

STUDENT: *Go to the workbook and complete the assignment sheet for 21:3, Administering Heat/Cold Applications. Then return and continue with the procedures.*

PROCEDURE 21:3A
Applying an Ice Bag or Ice Collar

Equipment and Supplies

Ice collar or ice bag and cap, cover or towel, tape, ice in basin, scoop or paper cup, pen or pencil

Procedure

1. Check physician's orders or obtain authorization from your immediate supervisor for the application.
2. Assemble equipment.
3. Wash hands.
4. Fill the ice bag or collar with water. Check for leaks. Empty if no leaks are present.

   NOTE: Ice bags come in various sizes for different parts of the body. An ice collar is narrow and is used on the throat.
5. Use the scoop to fill the ice bag or collar half full (see figure 21-29A). To assist in filling, a paper cup with the bottom cut out can be placed in the neck of the bag and used as a funnel. Ice can then be scooped into the bag.

   NOTE: If ice cubes are used, rinse them with water to remove sharp edges.

   NOTE: In some agencies, disposable cold packs are used. To activate the chemicals in the cold pack, squeeze the pack or strike it against a solid surface. It does not need to be filled with ice. A cover must still be placed on the disposable cold pack because the plastic and cold can injure the skin.

   (!) CAUTION: Chemical ice packs are *not* recommended for use on the face or head because of the danger of leaking chemicals.
6. Place the bag on a table or flat surface. Push gently on the bag to expel all air (see figure 21-29B). Tighten the cap.

   NOTE: If a rubber ring is present on the cap, make sure the ring is secure; it prevents leakage.
7. Wipe the outside of the bag dry.
8. Place a cover on the bag. If an ice bag or ice collar cover is not available, use a towel. Tape the towel in place.

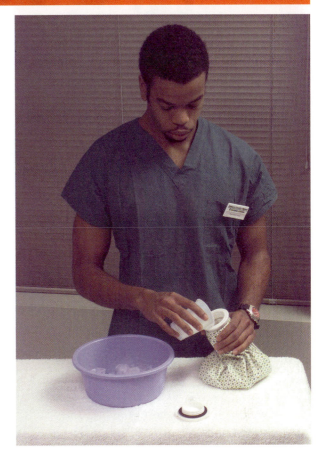

FIGURE 21-29A Fill the ice bag half full.

(!) CAUTION: The bag *must* be covered. The rubber or plastic and the extreme cold can injure the skin.

9. **(C)** Knock on the door and pause before entering. Introduce yourself. Identify the patient. Explain the procedure.
10. Wash hands. Put on gloves if necessary.

    (☣) CAUTION: Wear gloves and observe standard precautions if the area to be treated has any drainage of blood, body fluids, secretions, or excretions.
11. Place the ice bag gently on the affected area as ordered. Make sure the metal cap is not on the patient's skin.
12. Make sure the patient is comfortable and the ice application is positioned correctly before leaving. Place the call signal within

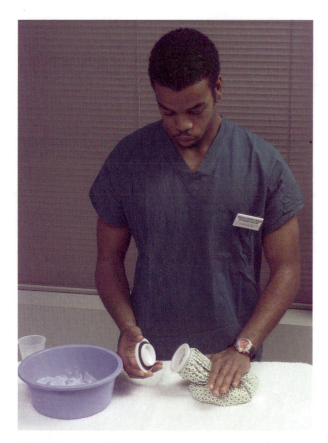

FIGURE 21-29B Push gently on the bag to expel all air before tightening the cap.

easy reach of the patient. Remove gloves, if worn, and wash hands before leaving the room.

13. Recheck the patient at frequent intervals. Make sure the bag is cold and refill it as needed. Check the condition of the skin. Check for pale or white skin, cyanosis (bluish color), or a mottled appearance. Ask the patient about numbness and pain.

> ⬣ **CAUTION:** If the skin is mottled or very discolored, or the patient complains of pain, remove the bag immediately and inform your immediate supervisor.

14. Leave the ice application in place for the length of time ordered. In some cases, continuous application is ordered; in others, a specific time period, such as 20 minutes, is ordered. Remove the bag when the designated time has elapsed.

15. Carefully check the condition of the patient's skin. Note any comments the patient makes about the treatment. Report these to your supervisor.

16. Observe all checkpoints before leaving the patient: position the patient in correct body alignment, elevate the siderails (if indicated), lower the bed to its lowest level, place the call signal and supplies within easy reach of the patient, and leave the area neat and clean.

17. Empty the ice bag and clean it thoroughly. Wipe it with a disinfectant, rinse, and dry. Inflate it with air before storing. This prevents the sides from sticking. Replace all equipment. Discard a disposable pack.

18. Remove gloves if worn. Wash hands.

19. Report and/or record all required information on the patient's chart or the agency form, for example, date; time; ice bag applied to right forearm for 20 minutes, patient states arm feels better; and your signature and title. Report any unusual observations immediately.

> **Practice** *Go to the workbook and use the evaluation sheet for 21:3A, Applying an Ice Bag or Ice Collar, to practice this procedure. When you feel you have mastered this skill, sign the sheet and give it to your instructor for further action.*

✔ **Final Checkpoint** Using the criteria listed on the evaluation sheet, your instructor will grade your performance.

PROCEDURE 21:3B

Applying a Warm-Water Bag

Equipment and Supplies

Warm-water bag, cover or towel for bag, tape, measuring graduate or pitcher, bath thermometer, pen or pencil

Procedure

1. Check physician's orders or obtain authorization from your immediate supervisor for the application.
2. Assemble equipment.
3. Wash hands.
4. Check for leaks by filling the warm-water bag with tap water or air. Expel the water or air if no leaks are present.
5. Fill the pitcher with water at a temperature of 110° to 120°F, or 43° to 49°C. Use the bath thermometer to check the temperature (see figure 21-30A).

   ⚠ CAUTION: The temperature should *not* exceed 120°F, or 49°C.

NOTE: Temperatures may vary. Follow agency policy.

NOTE: In some agencies, disposable heat packs are used. To activate the chemicals in the heat pack, squeeze the pack or strike it against a solid surface. It does not need to be filled with hot water. A cover must still be placed on the disposable heat pack because the plastic and heat can injure the skin.

   ⚠ CAUTION: Chemical heat packs are *not* recommended for use on the face or head because of the danger of leaking chemicals.

6. Pour the measured hot water into the warm-water bag. Fill the bag one-third to one-half full (see figure 21-30B).
7. Expel remaining air by placing the warm-water bag on a flat surface, lifting and holding the neck portion of the bag upright, and pushing gently on the bag until the water reaches the neck (see figure 21-30C). Apply the screw cap or fold over the end.

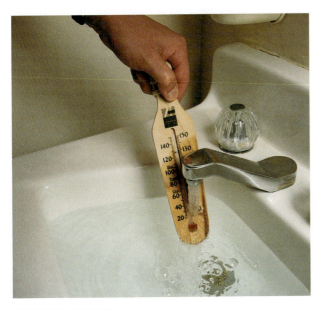

FIGURE 21-30A Use a bath thermometer to verify that the temperature of the water is 110° to 120°F.

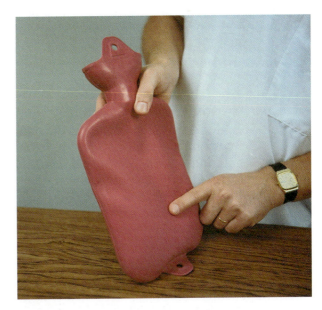

FIGURE 21-30B Fill the warm-water bag one-third to one-half full.

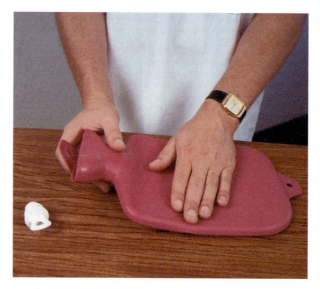

FIGURE 21-30C Expel air from the warm-water bag by placing it on a flat surface and gently pressing it until the water reaches the neck of the bag.

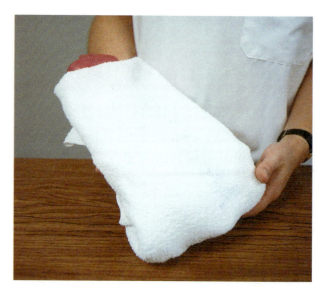

FIGURE 21-30D Cover the warm-water bag with a towel or standard cover.

NOTE: If the bag has a fold end, note the letters *A, B,* and *C.* Fold *A* to *B, B* to *C,* and *C* to seal.

8. Wipe the outside of the bag dry. Check again for any signs of leaks.

   ! CAUTION: Never use a warm-water bag or cap that leaks. The patient can be scalded.

9. Place a cover on the warm-water bag (see figure 21-30D). Use a standard cover, if available. If not, use a towel and tape the towel in place. The towel should be smooth and should completely cover the warm-water bag.

   ! CAUTION: The warm-water bag *must* be covered to prevent injury to the skin.

10. **C** Knock on the door and pause before entering. Introduce yourself. Identify the patient. Explain the procedure.

11. Wash hands. Put on gloves if necessary.

    ☣ CAUTION: Wear gloves and observe standard precautions if the area to be treated has any drainage of blood, body fluids, secretions, or excretions.

12. Apply the bag gently to the affected area as ordered. Make sure it is placed on top of the area. Never place heat under the body.

    ! CAUTION: Do *not* allow any part of the patient's body to lie on top of the warm-water bag. Weight of the body part could intensify the heat.

13. Before leaving, check to be sure the patient is comfortable and the bag is properly positioned. Place the call signal within easy reach of the patient. Remove gloves, if worn, and wash hands before leaving the room.

14. Recheck the patient at frequent intervals. Refill the bag as needed to maintain warm temperature. Note any pain, extreme redness, or other conditions.

    ! CAUTION: If signs of a burn are noted, remove the application immediately and report to your immediate supervisor.

15. Remove the heat application when the time ordered has elapsed. Closely check the patient's skin.

16. Observe all checkpoints before leaving the patient: position the patient in correct body alignment, elevate the siderails (if indicated), lower the bed to its lowest level, place the call signal and supplies within easy reach of the patient, and leave the area neat and clean.

17. Empty the warm-water bag and clean thoroughly. Wipe it with a disinfectant, rinse, and dry. Fill it with air before storing. This keeps the sides from sticking together. Replace all equipment. Discard a disposable heat pack.

18. Remove gloves if worn. Wash hands.

19. **C** Report and/or record all required information on the patient's chart or the agency form, for example, date; time; warm-water bag applied to right knee for 20 minutes, patient stated pain relieved in knee; and your signature and title. Report any unusual observations immediately.

Final Checkpoint Using the criteria listed on the evaluation sheet, your instructor will grade your performance.

PROCEDURE 21:3C

Applying an Aquamatic Pad

NOTE: Aquamatic or aquathermia pads can vary. Read the manufacturer's instructions before using.

Equipment and Supplies

Aquamatic unit and pad, cover, distilled water, pen or pencil

Procedure

1. Check physician's orders or obtain authorization from your immediate supervisor for the application.
2. Assemble equipment.
3. **C** Knock on the door and pause before entering. Introduce yourself. Identify the patient. Explain the procedure to the patient.
4. Wash hands. Put on gloves if necessary.
   CAUTION: Wear gloves and observe standard precautions if the area to be treated has any drainage of blood, body fluids, secretions, or excretions.
5. Place the aquamatic control unit on a solid table or stand. Check the cord. Attach the tubing to the main unit and aquamatic pad, if necessary.
   NOTE: Follow specific manufacturer's instructions. Some agencies use disposable pads. Tubing must be attached to these pads.
6. Unscrew the reservoir cap on the top of the unit. Use distilled water to fill the unit to the *fill* line.
   NOTE: Distilled water prevents formation of mineral deposits.
7. Screw the cap in place and then loosen it one-quarter turn. This allows for overflow of water and escape of steam.

8. Plug in the cord. Set the desired temperature by inserting the special key into the center of the dial or follow manufacturer's instructions. Temperature is usually set at 95° to 105°F, or 35° to 41°C. Turn the unit on.
   NOTE: Set the temperature according to physician's orders or agency policy.
9. Check the pad for leaks (see figure 21-31). Also check that the unit is getting warm. Make sure the tubing is not bent or kinked.

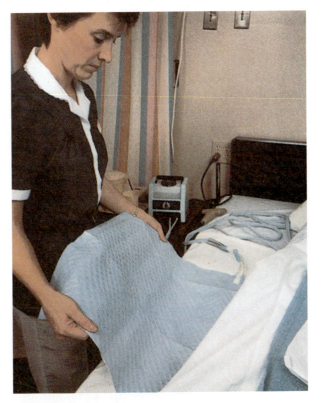

FIGURE 21-31 Check the aquamatic pad for leaks before applying it to the patient.

Recheck the level of water in the reservoir. A large amount of water is used when the pad is filled with water.

10. Cover the pad. If a custom cover is not available, a pillowcase or towel can be used. Use tape to hold the cover in place. (Pins could puncture the pad.)

   ! **CAUTION:** The pad must *never* be placed directly on the patient's skin. It can cause burns.

11. Place the pad on the correct area as ordered. Coil the tubing on the bed to facilitate the flow of water through the tubing. Do not allow the tubing to hang below the level of the bed. Check that the patient is comfortable. Place the call signal within easy reach of the patient. Remove gloves, if worn, and wash hands before leaving the room.

12. Recheck the patient at intervals. Note the condition of the skin. If the skin is red or shows evidence of burns, or the patient complains of pain, remove the pad and inform your immediate supervisor.

13. Refill the water unit with distilled water as necessary.

14. When the ordered time has elapsed, remove the pad from the patient. Note the condition of the skin. Note the patient's comments to determine whether the application was effective.

   NOTE: The physician's orders may prescribe continuous application of the pad. If so, check the patient periodically.

15. Observe all checkpoints before leaving the patient: position the patient in correct body alignment, elevate the siderails (if indicated), lower the bed to its lowest level, place the call signal and supplies within easy reach of the patient, and leave the area neat and clean.

16. Empty the pad. Empty the control unit. Clean all equipment thoroughly. Disinfect the pad and unit according to agency policy or discard if disposable. Replace all equipment.

   ! **CAUTION:** Do *not* put the electric control unit in water.

17. Remove gloves, if worn. Wash hands.

18. **C** Report and/or record all required information on the patient's chart or the agency form, for example, date; time; aquamatic pad applied to left elbow and forearm for 20 minutes, patient stated pain relieved; and your signature and title. Report any unusual observations immediately.

Practice *Go to the workbook and use the evaluation sheet for 21:3C, Applying an Aquamatic Pad, to practice this procedure. When you feel you have mastered this skill, sign the sheet and give it to your instructor for further action.*

 Final Checkpoint Using the criteria listed on the evaluation sheet, your instructor will grade your performance.

PROCEDURE 21:3D

Applying a Moist Compress

Equipment and Supplies

Basin; bath thermometer; underpads or bed protectors; washcloth, towel, or gauze pads (for compress); bath towel; plastic sheet; pen or pencil

Procedure

1. Check physician's orders or obtain authorization from your immediate supervisor for the application.

2. Assemble equipment.

3. **C** Knock on the door and pause before entering. Introduce yourself. Identify the patient. Explain the procedure to the patient.

4. Wash hands. Put on gloves.

   ☣ **CAUTION:** Observe standard precautions if any contact with blood or body fluids is likely, such as when a compress is applied to a draining wound.

5. Screen the unit. Elevate the bed to a comfortable working height. Fold the sheets back to expose the area to be treated.
   NOTE: A bath blanket can be used to drape the patient during the procedure.

6. Position an underpad or bed protector near the area to be treated. This will keep the patient's bedclothes and bed linens dry.

7. Fill the basin with water at the correct temperature. Use the bath thermometer to check the temperature.
   a. If a cold compress is to be applied, fill the basin with cold water. Ice cubes are sometimes added to the water. Do not add ice cubes unless you are told to do so.
   b. If a hot compress is to be applied, fill the basin with water at a temperature of 100° to 105°F, or 37.8° to 41°C.
   NOTE: Temperatures may vary. Follow physician's orders or agency policy.

8. Put the compress (washcloth, towel, or gauze pad) in the water. Wring out the compress to remove excess liquid (see figure 21-32A).

9. Apply the compress to the correct area (see figure 21-32B). Use a plastic sheet to cover the area. Then wrap a bath towel around the treated area.
   NOTE: The plastic sheet helps keep the compress moist and hot or cold.
   NOTE: An underpad or bed protector is sometimes used instead of a plastic sheet.

10. An ice bag or aquamatic pad is sometimes placed over the compress to help maintain the temperature. Follow agency policy or physician's orders.

11. Check the compress at frequent intervals. Change the compress and remoisten it as necessary. Check the condition of the skin under the compress. If the skin is discolored or the patient complains of pain, remove the compress immediately and inform your immediate supervisor.

12. Continue the treatment for the required period of time as ordered by the physician or per agency policy. Most compresses are left in place for 15 to 20 minutes.

13. When the ordered time has elapsed, remove the compress from the patient. Note the condition of the skin. Note the patient's comments to determine whether the application was effective.

14. Observe all checkpoints before leaving the patient: position the patient in correct body

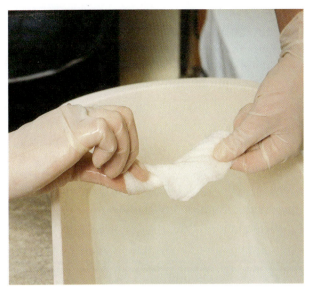

FIGURE 21-32A After putting the compress in the water, wring it out to remove excess liquid.

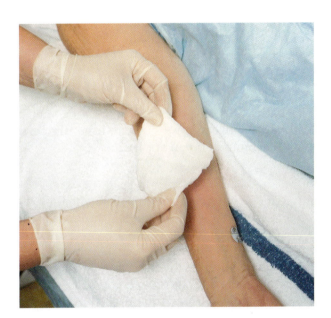

FIGURE 21-32B Apply the compress to the correct area.

alignment, elevate the siderails (if indicated), lower the bed to its lowest level, place the call signal and supplies within easy reach of the patient, and leave the area neat and clean.

15. Clean and replace all equipment used. Discard gauze pads used as compresses. Place linen in a hamper or the laundry area.

16. Remove gloves. Wash hands.

17. **C** Report and/or record all required information on the patient's chart or the agency form, for example, date; time;

cold moist compresses applied to right knee for 20 minutes, no change in skin color noted, patient states knee still hurts; and your signature and title. Report any unusual observations immediately.

✔ **Final Checkpoint** Using the criteria listed on the evaluation sheet, your instructor will grade your performance.

PROCEDURE 21:3E

Administering a Sitz Bath

Equipment and Supplies

Sitz-bath chair, disposable unit, or tub; one to two bath blankets; towels; gown; robe; slippers; bath thermometer; pen or pencil

Procedure

1. Check physician's orders or obtain authorization from your immediate supervisor for the treatment.
2. Assemble equipment.
3. **C** Knock on the door and pause before entering. Introduce yourself. Identify the patient. Explain the procedure. Ask the patient to put on a hospital gown. Assist as necessary.
4. Wash hands.
5. Prepare the sitz-bath unit:
   a. A *sitz chair* has an automatic temperature control, set at 105°F, or 41°C (see figure 21-33A). Fill the chair with water. Plug in the cord. Drape the bottom with a towel or bath blanket.
   b. Fill a *tub* or *sitz tub* to the correct level with water at 105°F, or 41°C (see figure 21-33B). Place a towel or bath blanket in the bottom of the tub.
   c. Fill the container on a *portable unit* with water at 105°F, or 41°C. Place the container on a commode chair or toilet (lift the seat before positioning), see figure 21-33C. Connect the tubing to the container. Make sure the holes on the tubing are facing the sides of the container. Clamp the tubing with its clamp. Fill the bag with water at 110° to 115°F, or 43° to 46°C.
   NOTE: Temperatures may vary. Follow physician's orders or agency policy.

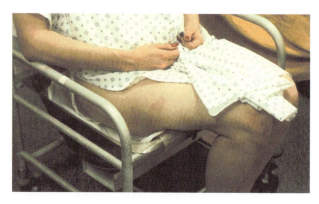

FIGURE 21-33A The sitz chair has an automatic control to maintain the correct temperature while the patient is seated in the chair.

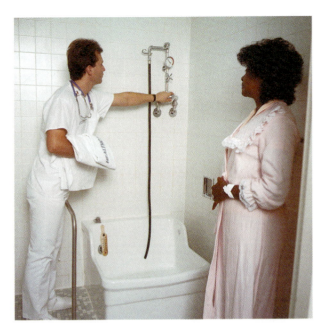

FIGURE 21-33B Stationary sitz-bath tubs are available in many health care facilities.

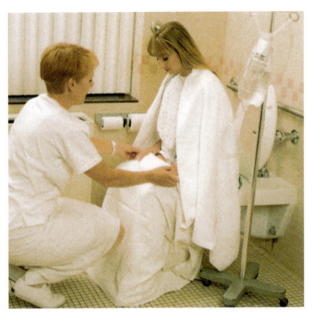

FIGURE 21-33D After the patient is seated in the sitz bath, cover the patient's legs and shoulders with a bath blanket.

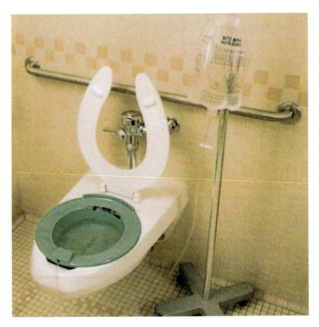

FIGURE 21-33C A portable sitz-bath unit is positioned on the base of the toilet after the seat is elevated.

6. Position the patient in the sitz bath. Raise the patient's gown above the water level. Make sure the perineal area is in the water. Use bath blankets to cover the patient's legs and/or shoulders (see figure 21-33D).

NOTE: The gown can be removed if the patient is in a tub. Drape the patient with a bath blanket to prevent exposure.

7. Observe the patient closely for signs of weakness or dizziness.

CAUTION: If excessive weakness or dizziness is noted, discontinue the treatment and inform your immediate supervisor.

8. If a portable unit is used, add water from the bag when the water in the container gets cool. In a tub, drain some water and then add additional water as necessary to maintain the temperature at 105°F, or 41°C.

9. If the patient tolerates the procedure, leave the patient in the sitz bath for 20 minutes or the length of time ordered by the physician.

10. When the treatment is complete, assist the patient out of the chair, tub, or unit. Dry the patient with a towel. Put clean, dry clothing on the patient.

11. Assist the patient in returning to bed.

12. Observe all checkpoints before leaving the patient: position the patient in correct body alignment, elevate the siderails (if indicated), lower the bed to its lowest level, position the call signal and supplies within easy reach of the patient, and leave the area neat and clean.

13. Clean and replace all equipment used. Wear gloves to disinfect the tub, sitz tub, or sitz chair according to agency policy. Portable units are usually charged to the patient and kept in the patient's unit.

14. Remove gloves. Wash hands.

15. **C** Report and/or record all required information on the patient's chart or the agency form, for example, date; time; sitz bath taken in sitz tub for 20 minutes, patient states she feels much better; and your signature and title. Report any unusual observations immediately.

Practice *Go to the workbook and use the evaluation sheet for 21:3E, Administering a Sitz Bath, to practice this procedure. When you feel you have mastered this skill, sign the sheet and give it to your instructor for further action.*

Final Checkpoint Using the criteria listed on the evaluation sheet, your instructor will grade your performance.

UNIT 21 SUMMARY

Physical therapy techniques are utilized by a wide variety of health care workers. Physical therapy involves using physical means to treat the patient.

Range-of-motion (ROM) exercises are done to maintain the health of the muscles and skeletal system. They are frequently ordered for patients with limited ability to move. Each joint and muscle in the body is moved through its full ROM. By following the correct procedures and using proper body mechanics, the health care worker can help the patient maintain as much mobility as possible.

Proper techniques must also be used when ambulating patients using transfer (gait) belts, crutches, canes, or walkers. By understanding the different gaits, proper ways of fitting the devices to patients, and safety precautions, the health care worker can provide support and guidance for patients relying on these aids.

Heat and cold applications are administered for a wide variety of conditions. In order to prevent injury to the patient, careful observation of temperature and condition of the skin is essential. Again, correct techniques must be used at all times when these applications are administered.

Physical therapy is frequently an important part of the patient's treatment. By learning and understanding basic principles, the health care worker can help provide this part of the patient's care.

INTERNET SEARCHES

Use the suggested search engines in Unit 11:4 of this textbook to search the Internet for additional information on the following topics:

1. *Organizations:* research physical therapy careers, educational requirements, and duties at sites such as the American Athletic Trainer's Association, American Physical Therapy Association, and the American Massage Therapy Association.

2. *Physical therapy:* research range-of-motion exercises, massage therapy, ultrasound therapy, cryotherapy, thermotherapy, and physical therapy.

3. *Suppliers:* find suppliers of physical therapy equipment to compare the different types of equipment available.

REVIEW QUESTIONS

1. What are the four (4) main types of ROM exercises? How is each type performed?

2. List eight (8) different types of joint movements and briefly describe each movement.

3. What are the basic rules that must be followed while measuring a patient for crutches?

4. You are ambulating a patient with a transfer belt. The patient starts to fall. What do you do?

5. Differentiate between a three-point and a two-point gait for canes.

6. What is the different between moist heat and dry heat? Give two (2) examples for each type of application.

7. Define each of the following:
   a. vasodilation
   b. vasoconstriction

8. Identify five (5) safety measures or checkpoints that must be observed whenever a heat or cold application is applied to a patient.

UNIT 21

SUGGESTED REFERENCES

Acello, Barbara. *Restorative Care: Fundamentals for Nursing Assistants.* Clifton Park, NY: Delmar Learning, 2000.

Connor, LeAnne, Daniel Snyder, and Gregory Lorenz. *Kinesiology for the Health Care Professional.* Clifton Park, NY: Delmar Learning, 2002.

Hegner, Barbara R., and Joan Needham. *Assisting in Long-term Care.* 4th ed. Clifton Park, NY: Delmar Learning, 2002.

Hegner, Barbara, Esther Caldwell, and Joan Needham. *Nursing Assistant: A Nursing Process Approach.* 8th ed. Clifton Park, NY: Delmar Learning, 1999.

Weiss, Roberta. *The Physical Therapy Aide.* 2nd ed. Clifton Park, NY: Delmar Learning, 1999.

Wyatt, Kathy. *Multiskilling: Rehabilitation Services for the Health Care Provider.* Clifton Park, NY: Delmar Learning, 1999.

For additional information on physical therapy careers, contact the following:

◆ American Physical Therapy Association
1111 North Fairfax Street
Alexandria, VA 22314
Internet address: *www.apta.org*

UNIT 22

Business and Accounting Skills

Unit Objectives

After completing this unit of study, you should be able to:

- ◆ File records using both the alphabetical and numerical systems
- ◆ Utilize correct telephone techniques when using a business telephone
- ◆ Schedule appointments using a standard appointment ledger or a computer program
- ◆ Complete registration and history records
- ◆ Compose and print letters of consultation, collection, appointment, recall, and inquiry
- ◆ Complete basic insurance forms accurately, neatly, and thoroughly
- ◆ Maintain a bookkeeping system
- ◆ Write checks, deposit slips, and receipts
- ◆ Define, pronounce, and spell all the key terms

	Observe Standard Precautions		Instructors Check—Call Instructor at This Point
	Safety—Proceed with Caution	OBRA	OBRA Requirement—Based on Federal Law
	Math Skill		Legal Responsibility
	Science Skill		Career Information
C	Communications Skill		Technology

KEY TERMS

answering service

appointments

automated routing unit (ARU)

block style

body

buffer period

cellular telephone

charge slip

check

collection

complimentary close

confidential

consultation
(con-sul-tay'-shun)

cross indexes/references

day sheet (daily journal)

deposit slips

electronic mail

enclosure notation

endorsement
(en-dors'-ment)

fax (facsimile) machine

filing

heading

indexed

inquiry
(in-kwy'-ree or in'-kwih-ree")

inside address

insurance forms

ledger card

letterhead

medical history

memorandums
(meh-mow-ran'-dumbz)

modified-block style

originator (maker)

paging system

payee

pegboard system

recall

receipt

reference initials

salutation

screen

signature

statement–receipt

statistical data

subject line

triage

voice mail

22:1 INFORMATION Filing Records

Filing is the systematic or orderly arrangement of papers, cards, or other materials so that they are readily available for future reference. Correct filing methods for health care records and other information are necessary for two main reasons. First, it must be possible to quickly locate the material when it is needed. Second, the material must be stored safely and protected as legal records. Various filing systems are in use. It is important that you become thoroughly familiar with your agency's method and that you follow all instructions carefully.

Types of Filing Systems

Four main filing systems are:

◆ *Alphabetical:* The most common method in use. Items are filed in alphabetical order according to the same rules followed in the telephone directory.

◆ *Numerical:* The second most common system. Materials to be filed, such as names, are each assigned a number. The numbers are then placed in order and filed according to numerical order. This system requires a cross-index or cross-reference list. An index card file is usually used for this purpose. The patient's name is placed on the index card along with the assigned number. The index cards are filed alphabetically according to last name. When a patient comes to the health care agency, his or her index card is pulled. The patient's file is then located in the numerical file by using the number on the card. If patients have the same name, the numerical system can eliminate errors because each patient has his or her own number.

◆ *Geographic:* In this system, items are filed according to location. Cities, states, or countries are used as the key filing units. For example, in a rural agency that cares for patients from several areas, charts might be filed by area or location. Within each specific area, the charts might be filed alphabetically. A cross-reference system is usually required to prevent loss of charts. The use of geographic filing is usually reserved for large companies or corporations.

◆ *Subject:* In this system, material is filed by subject or topic. For example, all material concerning diabetes might be filed under the topic *Diabetes.* A cross-reference system is sometimes required. For example, if several pieces of correspondence are received on an aspect of diabetes, all the material obtained might be filed in the diabetes folder. However, another (alphabetical) file with the correspondent's name and a cross reference saying "see diabetes" might be kept in case the employer wants to refer to a specific piece of correspondence.

Cross Indexes or References

Cross indexes or **references** are essential in a filing system to avoid misplacing or losing records. Some uses of cross references were discussed in the descriptions of filing systems. Cross references might be kept on index cards in a separate file, or colored sheets of paper might be placed in file folders. For example, if a letter contains information about three or four patients, the letter might be filed under the topic or under the name of the patient about whom the letter contains the most information. A cross reference should be placed in each of the other patients' files. Usually a colored sheet of paper so that it will stand out in the file, the cross reference would state, "See . . ." If a reference paper contains information about two topics, such as diabetes and glaucoma, the paper might be filed under *Diabetes.* In this case, a cross reference that says, "See diabetes" should be filed in the folder labeled *Glaucoma.* Many agencies have special cross-reference sheets that are used for this purpose.

Color-Coded Filing Systems

Color-coded indexing is an innovative method of filing that helps prevent errors (see figure 22-1A). Each folder is marked with a series of colors representing the letters in the patient's name. For example, all *A*s might be red, and all *B*s might be dark blue (see figure 22-1B). A

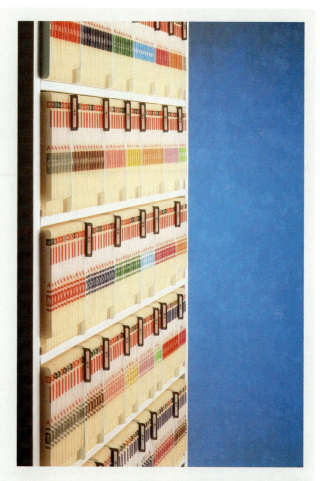

FIGURE 22-1A A color-coded filing system helps prevent errors because a chart with different color-coding will stand out if placed in an incorrect position. *(Courtesy of Smead Manufacturing Company)*

series of two to eight colors is used to represent the letters in the patient's last name. The colors provide a second means of verifying placement of folders in the file. Because a chart with different color coding will stand out, a quick glance at the folders allows the person filing to immediately locate a file that is out of place.

Color-coded folder systems are frequently used in larger agencies. This system utilizes different colored file folders. For example, in an office with several doctors, each doctor's patients would have a different color file folder. One doctor's patients would have yellow file folders, a second doctor's patients would have green file folders, and a third doctor's patients would have red file folders. This system can also be used to identify types of insurance, with each type of medical insurance having its own

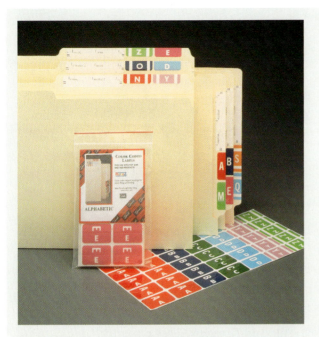

FIGURE 22-1B Color letter labels are available for both top- and side-cut files. *(Courtesy of Smead Manufacturing Company)*

unique color of file folder. For example, patients on Medicare would have blue file folders, patients in HMOs would have yellow file folders, and patients with private insurance would have green folders. Some agencies use a different color folder to represent the first letter of a patient's last name. For example, last names starting with *S* are assigned a pink folder, and last names starting with *T* are assigned a green folder. This system requires 26 colors of folders, one for each letter of the alphabet.

Storage of Files

In a manual filing system, records are stored in file folders and the folders are stored in filing cabinets or shelves. File folders must be durable and of good quality. Filing cabinets or shelves must be conveniently located, fireproof, and equipped with locks. Sufficient file space must be available so that records are not packed tightly in the drawers or shelves of the filing cabinets. Because thousands of records can accumulate in a busy agency, most facilities have a policy to classify records as active, inactive, or closed. An *active* record is one that is currently being used because the patient is seen by the agency. An *inactive* record is a

record for a patient who has not been seen for a number of years, usually 2 to 3 years. A *closed* record is usually a record for a patient who has died or a file that is no longer required. States have different time requirements for retention of records. For this reason, most health care agencies keep all records in case they are needed for legal or research purposes. To facilitate storage of these records, inactive or closed records are frequently put on optical disks or microfiche. The computer has simplified the storage of this type of record. The record can be copied with a laser beam and placed on an optical disk or scanned into a computer and saved on magnetic tape or disk. The record can then be retrieved from the optical disk or magnetic tape, displayed on the computer, and printed in hard copy form if it is needed. It is important to note that the original record must be destroyed by shredding or burning to protect the confidentiality of the patient.

In an electronic filing system, agencies use computers and "paperless" files. A database is created with the name, address, and case number of the patient. The database will automatically file all patient names in correct alphabetical order. When the patient arrives at the agency, the patient's name is entered into the computer and the database information with the case number appears. Some computer programs will retrieve the patient's file by name; others require the case number. Once the file is retrieved, a printout can be obtained with pertinent information. When the health care provider sees the patient, current information is entered into the computerized patient file. This information can be stored in the hard drive, or on magnetic tape reels, disks, or CD-ROMs so it can be retrieved when needed. A back-up tape must be made frequently when an electronic system is used because if the computer fails, or the hard drive crashes, all information would be lost. Most offices using an electronic system have automatic back-ups scheduled on an hourly or daily basis to prevent losing information. Maintaining the confidentiality of patient's records is also essential when an electronic system is used. Passwords, limited access, and locked storage of disks and tapes are methods used to prevent access to the records by unauthorized individuals.

An efficient filing system is an important part of any health care agency. Follow all instructions carefully as you learn the system your agency uses. Ask questions when you do not understand a particular procedure.

STUDENT: *Go to the workbook and complete the assignment sheet for 22:1, Filing Records. Then return and continue with the section Filing Records Using the Alphabetical or Numerical System.*

FILING RECORDS USING THE ALPHABETICAL OR NUMERICAL SYSTEM

Alphabetical Filing

Alphabetical filing is one of the main methods used to file names and materials. It is the system used in the telephone book. If you question a particular order, check similar examples in a telephone book. The main rules for this system are as follows:

◆ Before names can be filed alphabetically, they must be put into units and indexed. Dividing a name into units simply involves separating each name. For example, the name *John Robert Davis* has three units: *John, Robert,* and *Davis.* The name *Mary K. Kasper* also has three units: *Mary, K.,* and *Kasper.* In the second example, the middle initial is considered to be one unit. After dividing the name into units, the units are **indexed,** or placed in order for filing. The most general method of indexing is to place the surname (last name) first, followed by the first name, and then the middle name or initial. Note the following examples:

   (1) John Robert Davis would be indexed and filed as *Davis, John Robert.*

   (2) Mary K. Kasper would be indexed and filed as *Kasper, Mary K.*

◆ Names of organizations and businesses are usually filed in the same order as they are written. For example, *American Medical Association* is filed with *American* as the first

indexing unit, *Medical* as the second indexing unit, and *Association* as the third indexing unit.

NOTE: An exception is when the owner's initials or first name form part of the name. For example, *E. J. Thomas Company* would be filed as *Thomas, E. J., Company.*

◆ Words such as *of, and, at, the, on, a,* and *an* are not counted as indexing units. Each such word is placed next to the word to which it belongs, and in parentheses. For example, the company *The National Company of Medical Supplies* is indexed as *National (the), Company (of), Medical, Supplies.* This would be filed under *N* for *National* instead of *T* for *The.*

◆ After a name or company is indexed, strict alphabetical order is followed. Use as many letters as needed. Use the telephone book, if needed, to check order. Examples are as follows:

   (1) *Brooks* comes before *Corey,* because *B* comes before *C.*

   (2) *Tournovsky* comes before *Tournowsky. Tourno* is the same in both names. The first letter that is different is used. Because *v* comes before *w, Tournovsky* is filed first.

   (3) *Jones, Betty* comes before *Jones, Mary.* Surnames (last names) are the same, so the first letter of the first name determines the order for filing. The *B* in *Betty* comes before the *M* in *Mary.*

   (4) *Jones, Betty C.* comes before *Jones, Betty F.* Here, the middle initial is used to determine filing position. *C* comes before *F.*

◆ Nothing comes before something. For example, *Brook* comes before *Brooks* (with the additional letter *s*). Also, *Brown, W.* would come before *Brown, William.*

◆ Prefixes, such as *De, Del, La, Le, Mac, Mc, O, San, St, Van,* and *Von,* are treated as parts of names. They are *not* used as separate indexing units. For example, in *Van Dyke* and *O'Leary, VanDyke* is one unit, not *Van* and *Dyke;* and *O'Leary* is one unit, not *O* and *Leary. O'Leary* would be filed before *Oliver.*

◆ Hyphenated names are each considered one unit, for example, *Lans-Worth, Miller-Jones,* and *Smith-Ville.* Therefore, *Smith-Ville* would be filed before *Smithworth.*

◆ Familiar abbreviations are treated as though the word is spelled out in full. Therefore, *St.* is filed under *Saint,* and *Mt.* is filed under *Mount.* A correct filing order is: *Saccerin, St. James, Samson.* Other abbreviations include *Co.* for *Company, Inc.* for *Incorporated, Ltd.* for *Limited,* and *U.S.* for *United States.*

◆ If two or more individuals have the exact same name, the geographic location is used for filing purposes. In geographic order, items are filed alphabetically first by state, then by city, and finally by street address. For example, three individuals are named *John William Smith.* One lives on Ash Street in Charleston, West Virginia; another lives on Elm Street in Charleston, West Virginia; and the third lives on Brook Street in Charleston, South Carolina. Correct indexing and filing order is: *Smith, John William (Charleston, South Carolina); Smith, John William (Ash Street, Charleston, West Virginia);* and *Smith, John William (Elm Street, Charleston, West Virginia).*

◆ Titles or degrees are usually not considered in filing, but are written in parentheses at the end of indexed names for identification purposes. Some common titles or degrees include *MD, BS, RN, DDS,* and *Professor. James Robert Jones, DDS* would be indexed as *Jones, James Robert (DDS).* If two individuals have the same name, geographic location is used for filing. For example, *Jones, James Robert (MD) (Cleveland, Ohio)* is filed before *Jones, James Robert (DDS) (Columbus, Ohio).* An exception to this rule occurs with religious or special titles followed by one name. These are filed as they are written. For example, *Father John, Sister Ann,* and *Prince Phillip* are filed as *Father, John; Prince, Phillip;* and *Sister, Ann.* Titles in a firm name are also filed as written, for example, *Dr. John's Medical Supply Company.*

◆ Terms of seniority such as *Jr, Sr,* or *II* are usually used as the last indexing unit. *Hayden Kobelak, Jr* is indexed as *Kobelak, Hayden, Jr.* If names are identical, the seniority terms are filed in alphabetical or numerical order. For example, *Kobelak, Hayden, Jr,* is filed before *Kobelak, Hayden, Sr,* and *Kobelak, Hayden, II* is filed before *Kobelak, Hayden, III.* In addition, numerical seniority terms are filed before alphabetical terms. For example, *Kobelak, Hayden, II* is filed before *Kobelak, Hayden, Jr.*

◆ If a woman is married and uses her husband's name, her name is indexed with her husband's surname as the first unit, her first name, and then her middle or maiden name. A *Mrs.* is often placed in parentheses at the end. The husband's first name is often also placed in parentheses. So, *Mrs. Kaleigh Simmers Nartker* is indexed as *Nartker, Kaleigh, Simmers (Mrs. Brian).*

◆ Numbers in a name are indexed as though the number were spelled in letters. For example, *3rd Street Supply House* is indexed as *Third, Street, Supply, House.*

Numerical Filing

Numerical filing is also a common method of filing. Basic principles for this system are as follows:

◆ If a numerical system is used, cross indexing or referencing is required. Patient's names are usually indexed as for alphabetical filing. Each name is then placed on a card or in a computer database, and a number is assigned. Numbers in an agency usually run in order, and a record is kept of which numbers have been assigned. If cards are used, the card with the name and number is kept in an alphabetical file. When the patient comes to the agency, the alphabetical card is located or the patient's name is entered into the computer database to determine the patient's number. The numbered file is then located.

◆ Numbers always go in order from small to large. Number *23* is filed before number *230.*

By simply numbering from 1 on, a large number of patients can be accommodated.

◆ Many offices use digit-numbering systems in which a series of numbers similar to Social Security numbers is used. Numbers such as *32-444-5609* allow for a great variety of charts. Each office establishes a preferred method that should be followed.

◆ If a zero falls *before* other numbers, the zero is usually disregarded when filing. For example, the number *00230* would be filed as if it were *230* and before the number *231*. Most offices use the same number of digits for each number assigned. That is why initial zeros are left in; they are used in place of other numbers.

◆ All of the numbers listed must be checked carefully. It is essential that numbers be written clearly if this type of system is used. Most offices prefer that numbers be typed to eliminate errors; otherwise, a written *1* can look like a *7*.

◆ Many systems use the same terminal, or last, digit for certain shelves or drawers. For example, a series of charts might contain *58* as the last digit. Another series might contain *62* as the last digit. Charts labeled *08-92-58, 18-99-58, 19-34-58,* and *02-41-58,* are placed in one group separate from charts labeled *04-45-62, 05-98-62,* and *03-78-62.* Then, all charts with the terminal digit *58* are filed in correct numerical order. The order for the numbers listed previously is *02-41-58, 08-92-58, 18-99-58,* and *19-34-58.* These are placed on the shelf or drawer labeled *58* in the terminal system. Charts ending with *62* are then placed in numerical order. The correct order for the numbers listed previously is *03-78-62, 04-45-62,* and *05-98-62.* Therefore, in a terminal-number system, first check the last digit and then put all same last digits together. Then place this series in numerical order.

STUDENT: *Go to the workbook and complete assignment sheet number 1 for Filing Records Using the Alphabetical or Numerical System. Give the sheet to your instructor. Note any corrections or changes to the assignment sheet. Then complete assignment sheet number 2 to be sure you understand the principles outlined in this section. Then return and continue with the procedure.*

PROCEDURE 22:1

Filing Records Using the Alphabetical or Numerical System

Equipment and Supplies

Labeled file cards or folders, file drawer or index rack.

Procedure

1. Assemble equipment.
2. Review the Information section on filing and refer to it as necessary throughout the procedure.

   NOTE: If labeled file cards or folders are not available for practice, make your own. Use 3-by-5-inch index cards (which are less expensive than file folders). Create three sets with forty to fifty cards in each set. Make one set for alphabetical filing. Make sure you include examples of all of the rules given in the preceding Information section. Use the telephone book to find sample names, or make up your own names. Make a second set of cards for numerical filing. List a variety of numbers on the cards. Be sure you include examples of the principles stated in the preceding Information section. Make a third set of cards using a terminal-digit numerical filing system. Divide the cards into three or more groups. Label each group with a different terminal digit (last number). Then place a variety of numbers before the terminal digits.

3. Assemble all of the folders or cards with names in place for alphabetical filing. Check all names to be sure they are indexed correctly. Then file according to the following steps.
   a. Separate all folders or cards into letters of the alphabet. Place all *A*s together, *B*s together, and so forth through the end of the alphabet.
   b. Next, file just the *A*s. Start with the second letters of all of the *A*s and place them in alphabetical order. Proceed to the third letter, fourth letter, and additional letters as needed.
   c. When the *A*s are complete and in order, follow the same procedure for all remaining letters.
   d. Recheck the files. Note common errors. Make sure you filed abbreviations such as *St.* or *Mt.* as though they are spelled out. Make sure that you considered prefixes such as *Mc* or *Van* each as a part of the name and not as a separate unit. Make sure that you treated numbers as though they were spelled out in letters.

      ✔ **CHECKPOINT:** Your instructor will check the filed folders or cards for accuracy.

4. Work with the numerical folders or cards. Note only actual numbers on each card. For example, *0023* would be regarded as a two-digit number, or *23;* but *0300* would be regarded as a three-digit number, or *300.* Ignore any zeros that come before the first number. Proceed as follows to file the numerical folders or cards:
   a. Divide the cards or folders into sets according to digits. Put all two-digit numbers (for example, *23, 68, 0023, 078,* and *010*) in one pile.

      NOTE: Remember to ignore any zeros *before* the number.
   b. Place all three-digit numbers in a second pile. These would include numbers such as *893, 0938, 00567, 0800,* and *901.*
   c. Continue to separate the folders or cards in this manner. Create a four-digit stack, a five-digit stack, and so forth, as needed.
   d. Next, place all two-digit numbers in order. Start with the smallest number and proceed to the largest.

   e. Repeat step d with all remaining digit groups. Working with smaller groups of cards makes the process easier.
   f. Recheck the entire series of filed cards or folders. Make sure they are in correct order by number.

      ✔ **CHECKPOINT:** Your instructor will check the filed folders or cards for accuracy.

5. Work with the terminal-number system folders or cards according to the following steps:
   a. Separate the cards or folders into groups by noting the terminal digit (last number). All cards ending with the same last number will be in one group, for example, *19-52, 09-98-52, 54-19-52,* and *00-01-52.* Another group might be *05-77, 09-09-77, 00-66-77,* and *77-77.*
   b. Working with each terminal-number group, arrange each group in numerical order. Ignore any zeros that come before the first number. Order numbers from smallest to largest. For example, the series of cards ending in *52* would be filed in a group before the series of cards ending in *77.*
   c. Recheck all cards or folders filed.

      ✔ **CHECKPOINT:** Your instructor will check the filed folders or cards for accuracy.

6. Repeat steps 3, 4, and 5 until you master the systems. Read the preceding Information section and additional references as needed. For additional practice, make up other folders or cards with names from the telephone book or with number systems, and file these in correct order.

7. Clean and replace all equipment used.

Practice *Go to the workbook and use the evaluation sheet for 22:1, Filing Records Using the Alphabetical or Numerical System, to practice this procedure. When you feel you have mastered this skill, sign the sheet and give it to your instructor for further action.*

 Final Checkpoint Using the criteria listed on the evaluation sheet, your instructor will grade your performance.

Basic Telephone Techniques

C The telephone is an important tool of public relations in any health agency. Because you create an impression every time you talk on the telephone, it is important that you use correct techniques.

Correct use of the telephone requires many different skills. The impression you create on the telephone will influence a patient or other caller. It is essential to be tactful, diplomatic, firm yet flexible, friendly yet professional, and courteous. You must be capable of making decisions and be willing to accept responsibility. Developing the correct tone of voice is essential. Your voice must be pleasant, low pitched, clear, and distinct. Avoid a monotone or indifferent tone. Correct grammar should be used at all times. Practice courtesy and good manners during the entire conversation. Don't forget to use the words *please* and *thank you.*

Always answer the telephone promptly. In addition, answer with a smile (see figure 22-2); doing so helps create a pleasant voice. Even though callers will not see the smile, they will be able to detect it in your voice. While talking on the phone, keep the receiver firmly against your ear. Put the mouthpiece approximately 2 to 3 inches away from the center of your lips. This allows the best transmission of your voice.

Identify the office or agency—and in most cases yourself—when you answer the phone. For example, do not say "Hello," "Yes," or even just "Good Morning," when answering. Use greetings such as "Good Morning, Dr. Smith's office," "Hello, Health Care Hospital, Miss Jones speaking," or "Respiratory Clinic, Miss Jones speaking, may I help you?" In this way, callers know that they have reached the correct party.

In many agencies, it will be your responsibility to **screen** calls. This means that you must determine which calls should be referred to the doctor or other appropriate person and which calls can be handled by you or another worker in the agency. Each agency usually has some policy regarding calls. For example, in some offices, calls from the doctor's immediate family (that is,

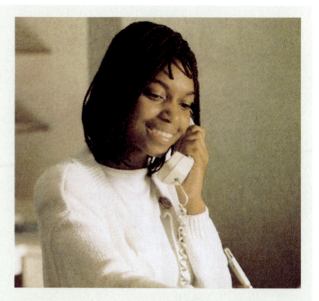

FIGURE 22-2 Answer the telephone with a smile while holding the mouthpiece 2 to 3 inches away from your lips.

wife or husband and children) and calls from other professionals are put through to the doctor. Other calls are screened to determine whether they are emergencies or whether the caller really must speak with the doctor. Experience in screening calls will help you make appropriate decisions.

In order to screen calls, you must find out certain information. First, find out the name of the caller. Avoid statements such as "Who is this?" or "Who are you?" It is better to say, "May I have your name, please?" or "May I ask who is calling, please?" If the caller states "Mrs. Jones," find out which Mrs. Jones she is. Ask for her first name and/or her husband's name. If you are unsure of the name, ask, "Would you please spell that?" It is also important for you to determine the purpose of the call. Many patients simply ask to talk with a particular person. By asking, "May I help you?" or "May I tell Dr. Jones why you are calling?" you can usually determine the nature of the call. At times you may have to say, "Dr. Smith is with a patient at this time, may I take a message?" or "The therapist is not available at present, would you explain your problem to me so I can determine if someone else can assist you?"

Emergency calls must be evaluated. In some cases, a patient is upset and there is really no emergency. Most health care agencies establish a telephone triage procedure to deal with emergency calls. **Triage** is the process of evaluating the situation and prioritizing treatment. A list of questions is often kept by the telephone and used to assist in evaluating the situation. For example, the following questions may be used depending on the situation:

◆ Who is the patient?

◆ What happened? When did it happen?

◆ Is the patient breathing? conscious? bleeding?

◆ Is it possible the patient took or contacted a poison? If so, what, when, and how much?

◆ Have you called emergency medical services?

By asking pertinent questions and remaining calm, you may be able to recognize real emergencies. Most emergencies are referred to the appropriate person if he or she is available. If the appropriate person is not available, obtain important information so that you can help the caller obtain help from the correct source. It may be necessary to refer the patient to an emergency medical service, emergency room, or hospital. A list of emergency numbers should be readily available so the correct number can be provided to the caller. Most agencies have procedures to follow when appropriate people are not available during emergencies.

Telephone triage can also be used to determine how quickly a patient should be scheduled for an appointment. Specific questions will help provide information on the seriousness of the patient's condition. Questions that might be asked include:

◆ What symptoms are you experiencing?

◆ How long have you had the symptoms?

◆ Do you have a fever or elevated temperature?

◆ Are you having any difficulty in breathing?

◆ Are you in pain? Where? How severe?

Evaluating a patient's responses will allow you to determine if the patient should be seen immediately or if the patient can be scheduled at the next convenient appointment time. Never hesitate to ask others for advice if you are not certain about the seriousness of the patient's condition.

Use discretion at all times when using the telephone. You should not say, "Doctor is having coffee down the hall," "He isn't in yet, and I don't know where he is," "The therapist is playing golf," or similar comments. Statements such as, "He is not available at present" or "I expect her to return at four o'clock; may I take a message?" are more appropriate.

At the end of a conversation, always close with, "Thank you for calling. Good-bye," and replace the receiver gently. If possible, allow the caller to hang up first. If you hang up first, you might miss something the patient wanted to say. In most agencies, **memorandums,** or written messages, are made of all calls that require action. In other agencies, telephone logs are kept, and all calls are recorded. The log must be accurate because it can be subpoenaed as a legal record. Telephone messages should always contain the following information (see figure 22-3):

◆ *Name of the caller:* Note the full name. Make sure it is spelled correctly.

◆ *Telephone number of the caller:* Be sure to note the area code and extension number, if needed. If there is a specific time when the caller can be reached, include this information.

◆ *Message:* Briefly summarize the reason for the call, but include all important information.

◆ *Date and time of the call.*

◆ *Action taken:* If any action was taken, record what was done.

◆ *Initials of the person taking the message:* If the message receiver has any questions, he or she will know whom to ask.

It is essential to keep a pencil or pen and paper by the telephone. Most agencies use telephone message pads. If a copy of the message is needed for the patient's record, message pads that provide a duplicate copy of each memorandum recorded can be purchased. When recording any memorandum, always print clearly. Include all important facts and spell words correctly.

Problem calls can occur in any agency. Some individuals may refuse to give their names or state the purposes of their calls. At times, they may try to intimidate or threaten the person answering the phone. Try to remain calm and to control your temper. Do not hesitate to say, "Dr. Smith cannot be disturbed unless I can tell her who is calling." Be polite but

TELEPHONE MESSAGE LOG

Date _____ Time Of Call _____

Caller _____ Patient _____

Address _____ Age ____

Complaint _____

_____

Medication Taken _____ How Long Sick _____

Cough _____ Productive _____ Temp _____

Vomiting _____ Diarrhea _____

Pain _____ Location _____

Bleeding ____ How Long _____ From _____ How Much _____

Nurse Return Call ____ Doctor Return Call ____ Phone No. ____

Appointment Made _____
and
Response or/Prescription given _____

_____

_____

PHONE MESSAGE

FOR _____

M _____

OF _____

TELEPHONE NO _____

☐ Telephoned   ☐ Please Return Call
☐ Will Call Again   ☐ Came In
☐ Returned Your Call   ☐ Important
☐ See Me   ☐ Wants To See You

MESSAGE _____

_____

_____

_____

_____

_____

_____

DATE _____ TIME_____ BY _____

FIGURE 22-3 A sample telephone message log and sample telephone message form.

firm in dealing with this type of caller. If a caller gives his or her name but refuses to state the general purpose of the call, this situation also requires tact. When in doubt, you can put the call on *hold* and check with the person whom the caller wants. That person can then determine whether or not to take the call.

If a call must be put on *hold* or you know there will be a slight delay before the appropriate person answers the call, be sure to inform the caller of this fact. Never leave a caller on *hold* for long periods. If there is a delay, offer to take the caller's number and have the individual return the call. Be considerate of all callers.

Correct telephone techniques require practice and experience. Think about the kind of impression you want to create; practice correct responses. At all times, think before you speak. Avoid comments that might offend a caller. Treat callers as you would want to be treated if you were the caller.

Automatic Routing Telephone Systems

Larger health care facilities frequently have telephone systems with an **automated routing unit (ARU).** This type of system allows a large number of telephone calls to be answered at the same time. The automated routing unit answers the telephone and a recorded voice provides directions to the caller. Most ARU systems provide a menu with a series of numbers. The caller presses the correct number to connect with a specific department or individual. The ARU system can be programmed so a caller with an emergency can be transferred immediately to an individual who can handle the emergency.

Voice mail is a common feature of most ARU systems. Voice mail is similar to the recording on an answering machine. If the individual is not available, the caller is instructed to leave a message and/or directed to contact another person. It is essential that individuals with voice mail check messages frequently. Most telephones will provide a signal, such as a beep, to alert the individual that messages are on the voice mail system. An individual who does not respond to voice mail messages creates poor public relations.

Answering Services and Machines

An **answering service** is used by many health care agencies to respond to telephone calls when the agency is closed. This allows the patient to talk with an operator at the answering service who can transfer the call to the appropriate individual, contact the individual and ask them to call the patient, or record a message. The health care agency provides the operator with procedures to follow in case of emergency, telephone numbers of individuals who may have to be contacted, and guidelines for a variety of calls. The health care agency usually pays a monthly fee for this service.

An *answering machine* is used in some health care agencies, but it is not as efficient as an answering service. The recording on the answering machine usually identifies the agency and asks the caller to leave a message. Some health care agencies also include the hours they are open on the recording. If an answering machine is used, the message on the machine should tell patients what to do in case of an emergency. Most agencies provide an alternative number a patient can call for an emergency. The answering machine must be checked frequently for messages. A designated individual should check for messages immediately after the agency opens and at frequent intervals if the machine is used during the time the agency is open.

Paging Systems

A **paging system** allows an individual to be contacted through the use of a *pager* or "beeper." The pager can provide a voice message, a signal such as a beep that alerts the individual to call a designated number to receive the message, or a digital message on a display screen with the telephone number of the caller or a message. The type of message received depends on the paging system used. Pagers are used to contact an individual. They do not allow for two-way communication, but they do allow access to the individual 24 hours a day. The individual receiving the pager message must use a telephone in order to contact the caller. The health care agency usually pays a monthly fee for each pager in use.

Cellular Telephones

A **cellular telephone** allows two-way communication between people in almost any location. Car phones or portable phones operate through cellular communications and do not require a telephone line. This provides much more flexibility for an individual to receive calls. It is more efficient than a pager, because the individual does not have to use another telephone to respond. A major drawback to cellular communication is that other people can hear the cellular signal by using scanners. For this reason, confidential patient information should *never* be discussed on a cellular phone. A cellular telephone is more expensive than a pager. In addition to a monthly charge, many cellular telephone service providers charge for each minute of phone use.

Electronic Mail

Electronic mail, or e-mail, allows an individual to use a computer and telephone modem to send, receive, and forward messages in digital form. The e-mail message can be sent to another individual in place of a telephone call or letter. Insurance companies, billing services, and health care agencies use e-mail messages to communicate with each other. In large health care agencies where computers are networked (electronically connected to each other), an e-mail message can be forwarded to many staff members at the same time and take the place of a written interoffice message. If an e-mail message is transmitted though the Internet on a modem that is not secure, it can be intercepted and read by others. For this reason, confidential patient information should *not* be sent. There is no expense for e-mail on networked computers in a health care agency. There is a monthly charge for Internet service that allows e-mail communication with others.

Fax (Facsimile) Machines

A **fax (facsimile) machine** is an essential piece of equipment in many health care facilities. This machine transmits data or information electronically over the telephone lines. For the system to work, the sending and receiving facilities must each have a fax machine and a telephone line designated for the fax machine. To fax information to another facility, use the telephone connected to the fax machine to dial the fax number of the other facility. Place the paper containing the information to be transmitted in the fax machine. When the fax number is answered at the other facility, the sending fax machine works similarly to a photocopy machine but transmits the information electronically. When information is being sent to a fax machine, a signal such as a beep or light is usually given by the receiving fax machine. The receiving fax machine then answers the fax phone, and prints a copy of the information being sent. Rapid transmission of information is possible with a fax machine.

Legal and confidentiality issues must be considered when faxing a patient's medical records. Some newer facsimile machines are password protected. If both the sender and receiver have this type of machine, a password can be used. Material will not be transmitted until the receiver enters the password. Other ways to meet legal and confidentiality requirements include:

◆ Always have written authorization from the patient before records are faxed.

◆ Never fax financial information.

◆ Fax only to machines located in secure locations. Never fax to machines in public areas where others might gain access to the records.

◆ Use a cover sheet that contains a confidentiality statement such as "This information is confidential. Be advised that you can be prosecuted under federal and state law for sharing this information with unauthorized individuals."

◆ Contact the receiver before faxing the material so he or she will be ready to receive it.

◆ Check with the receiver after the material has been faxed to make sure that it was transmitted correctly.

◆ When in doubt, mail the records or send them by a messenger.

STUDENT: *Go to the workbook and complete the assignment sheet for 22:2, Using the Telephone. Then return and continue with the procedure.*

PROCEDURE 22:2   C

Using the Telephone

Equipment and Supplies

Telephone message pad, pen or pencil, telephone set-up

Procedure

1. Assemble equipment. Review the Information section on telephone techniques. Prepare a list of sample triage questions to use while answering the telephone. Refer to these questions as you practice obtaining information from the caller.
2. Answer the telephone promptly and with a smile.
3. Identify yourself and the agency to the caller.
4. Determine the caller's name and the purpose of the call. Be sure you have all the facts.
5. Watch your tone of voice, manners, grammar, and responses during the conversation.
6. Deal with the call or refer the call to the appropriate person, if this is indicated.

7. At the end of the conversation, thank the caller and say, "Good-bye." Allow the caller to hang up the phone first. Replace the receiver gently.
8. Immediately record a memorandum of the call. Be sure to print clearly. Record all important facts.
   NOTE: In some agencies, the message is recorded during the conversation.
9. Practice the following situations with a partner. Assume the roles of both the caller and the receptionist receiving the call.
   a. A patient calls to make an appointment.
   b. Another doctor calls to discuss his findings on a referred patient.
   c. A mother calls. Her child is ill.
   d. A salesperson calls. She has some new equipment she wants to demonstrate and discuss.
   e. A man calls. He states that his wife just fell to the floor unconscious.

f. A mother calls and states that her two-year-old child took an entire bottle of baby aspirin.

10. Think about other situations and role-play those situations. Use correct telephone techniques. Evaluate your partner's responses and let your partner evaluate you. Discuss different ways of dealing with the preceding and other situations.

11. Replace all equipment used.

Practice *Go to the workbook and use the evaluation sheet for 22:2, Using the Telephone, to practice this procedure. When you feel you have mastered this skill, sign the sheet and give it to your instructor for further action.*

 Final Checkpoint Using the criteria listed on the evaluation sheet, your instructor will grade your performance.

22:3 INFORMATION Scheduling Appointments

One of the most frequent complaints that patients voice regarding doctor's offices, clinics, and other health agencies is having to spend a lot of time sitting in waiting rooms before getting to see doctors or other appropriate health personnel. To prevent this as much as possible, a carefully planned appointment book is used. Correct scheduling of **appointments** is essential for good public relations.

Appointment books or logs vary from office to office (see figure 22-4). However, most contain one or one-half page for each day. Time is usually blocked off in units of 10 to 15 minutes in order that all time can be used wisely. Become familiar with the type of appointment book you will use and know what block of time each line represents.

An organized approach is needed to avoid scheduling patients at times when the appropriate person is not available. Before scheduling any appointments, block out periods of time when individuals are not available. These include time periods for lunches, meetings, or afternoons off. A large *X* is usually drawn through each of these time periods so that no scheduling errors can occur.

In most agencies a pencil is used to record appointments. In this way, if an appointment is canceled, names can be erased, and the time can be assigned for another patient. Follow your agency's procedure.

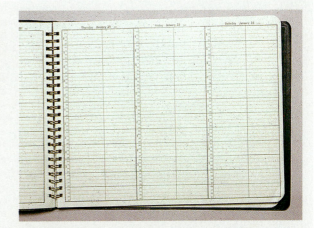

FIGURE 22-4 A sample appointment book. *(Courtesy of Control-o-fax Office Systems, Waterloo, IA)*

Learn how long various procedures in your agency take. If an examination takes 1 hour and you schedule a 15-minute appointment, you will be 45 minutes behind for later appointments. Many agencies keep lists of standard procedures and average time required for each near the appointment book.

Appointments should be scheduled as close together as possible, but not so close that patients will feel rushed in the office or be required to wait for long periods. Long periods of unscheduled time are wasteful and cost money. Some agencies schedule a 15- to 30-minute **buffer period** in the middle of each morning and afternoon. This allows time to catch up if some appointments run over. If the appointments run as scheduled, this time can be used for other business such as returning telephone calls or seeing patients with emergencies.

C When a patient calls for an appointment, find out the reason for the appointment. Then try to accommodate the patient by scheduling an appointment convenient for him or her. Questions such as, "Do you prefer morning or afternoon?" "Which day is most convenient?" and "Would two o'clock or four o'clock be more convenient?" give the patient a choice and help you select the correct time and day. Sometimes, choices are limited because the appointment book is full. However, by giving patients as much choice as possible, you let them know that you are trying to accommodate them.

C Make sure you have the required information before closing your conversation with the patient. Obtain the full name of the patient. Do not hesitate to ask the patient to spell the name if you are not sure of the correct spelling. Determine the reason for the appointment. It is also wise to get the patient's telephone number in case an emergency requires cancellation of the appointment. Writing the telephone number in the appointment ledger eliminates having to find the number in the patient's record and, saves time. Repeat the date, day, and exact time of the appointment to the patient. By giving both date and day, you provide a double check and prevent errors. Make sure the patient understands all information. Before hanging up the phone, you can again repeat the information by saying, "We will expect you Friday, March 1st at two o'clock. Thank you for calling, Mrs. Clark. Good-bye."

After scheduling an appointment, make sure you mark the full amount of time in the book. In many agencies, arrows that extend down from the patient's name to fill in the entire time block the patient will require are used. This also prevents scheduling errors.

If a patient calls to cancel an appointment, be polite. Ask the patient if he or she would like to reschedule the appointment. Erase the appointment or remove it from the book by drawing a single line through the entry. Then record all new information in the correct time block. It is not necessary to pry and ask patients why they must cancel. Many patients will offer explanations; if they do not, however, do not question them.

Chronic scheduling problems occur in every agency. Some patients schedule appointments and then do not show up for them. If a patient becomes a chronic offender, there are several methods of dealing with the problem. One method is to schedule the patient at the end of the day. This way, if the patient does not keep the appointment, other patients and the schedule will be minimally affected. In some agencies, bills for time scheduled are sent to patients who do not keep appointments. In these agencies, patients must be told that if they cannot keep appointments, they must notify the office 24 hours in advance or they will be charged for the time scheduled. In many agencies, broken appointments or "no-shows" are noted on patients' charts. The final decision on how to deal with these situations rests with the individual in charge. Be sure you know and follow his or her policy.

Emergencies occur in every agency. In the case of an emergency, appointments may run later than scheduled. Sometimes, it is necessary to cancel all appointments scheduled. If possible, patients should be notified by telephone before they come to the office or agency. When you call to cancel an appointment, make every effort to reschedule the patient at a time convenient to him or her. If a patient arrives at the office, and appointments are behind schedule, offer the patient a choice between waiting or scheduling another appointment. If told that an emergency has occurred (the full nature of the emergency need not be explained) and they will have to wait, many patients will be willing to do so. However, patients should never be left waiting without an explanation.

In many health care agencies, appointment scheduling is done by computer. The computer automatically locates the next available date and time, provides a record of appointments already scheduled, can be programmed to schedule a set block of time for a particular procedure, and prints out copies of the daily schedule. Although computerized scheduling can be efficient and convenient, an alternate system must exist for downtime, or times when the computer is not functioning.

Correctly scheduling appointments takes practice. If your present system is resulting in long waits for patients, review your system. Determine whether longer time periods are necessary for each patient. Add additional buffer times for overlap or emergency patients, if indicated. Constantly be willing to try to correct problems and create a good impression of the agency.

STUDENT: *Study Procedure for 22:3, Scheduling Appointments, before completing any assignment sheets.*

PROCEDURE 22:3

Scheduling Appointments

Equipment and Supplies

Appointment book ledger or worksheet, pencil, assignment sheets numbers 1 and 2, 22:3, Scheduling Appointments.

NOTE: If you are using a computer program to schedule appointments, follow the instructions provided with the software. The same principles will apply, but the computer will identify available appointment times and allocate the correct amount of time based on the procedure entered.

Procedure

1. Assemble equipment. Check the appointment book ledger or worksheet. Note how much time each line represents. Examine the sample appointment schedule in figure 22-5.
   NOTE: Appointment books vary. Many contain lines that each represent a 15-minute period. In these books, the line labeled *9:00* represents the time from 9:00 to 9:15.
2. Place the day and date on the top of each of the daily columns. This provides a double check.
3. Block off those periods of time when the person for whom appointments are being scheduled will not be in. Put a large *X* through each of these time periods. If the reason is known, write a brief explanation such as *medical meeting* to block out the time period.
4. If your agency requires a buffer time, mark this time period. It can be used for emergency patients or catch-up time.
5. Begin working with assignment sheet 1, 22:3 Scheduling Appointments, in your workbook. Read each case listed. Note the

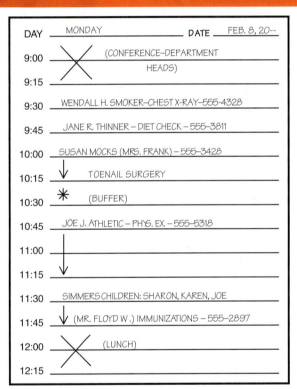

FIGURE 22-5 A sample appointment schedule.

time required and time preferred. Using a worksheet, schedule each of the cases. Check each case and notation to be sure of the following:
a. Full name of the patient is listed and, if a female is married and uses her husband's name, the spouse's name is in parentheses. Spelling must be correct.
b. The patient is in the correct time slot. Draw arrows downward from the name to indicate the time needed. Draw only to the end of the patient's appointment.
c. The reason for the appointment is briefly listed. Abbreviations can be used.

d. The telephone number of the patient is noted. Check to be sure the number is correct.

e. The entry is printed and easy to read.

6. Double-check each entry. Some time periods may have to vary slightly.

7. Turn in assignment sheet number 1 or print a copy of a computer-generated schedule to be graded. Your instructor will correct it and note changes to be made.

   ✔ **CHECKPOINT:** Your instructor will grade assignment sheet number 1 according to the criteria listed on the evaluation sheet.

8. When assignment sheet number 1 has been graded, note all changes and corrections. If you do not understand a change, be sure to ask your instructor for help before doing assignment sheet number 2.

9. Complete assignment sheet number 2 for 22:3, Scheduling Appointments, in your workbook. Follow steps 1 to 6. When you have checked all entries, turn the sheet in or print a computer-generated schedule to be graded.

10. Replace all equipment.

> **Practice** *Go to the workbook and use the evaluation sheet for 22:3, Scheduling Appointments, to practice this procedure and to complete the two assignment sheets for 22:3, Scheduling Appointments.*

✔ **Final Checkpoint**   Your instructor will grade the assignment sheets according to the criteria listed on the evaluation sheet.

22:4 INFORMATION Completing Medical Records and Forms

 Medical records vary but some forms are used for certain purposes. Two common forms are **statistical data** sheets or cards and **medical history** records. All records are considered to be **confidential.** *No* information can be released from the records without the written consent of the patient. These forms belong to the physician or agency. They should be locked up when not in use.

Statistical data sheets are also called *registration forms, patient information forms,* or other similar names (see figure 22-6). This form is usually completed on a patient's first visit to an office or health agency. It contains basic reference information about the patient. The form may be a sheet of paper, an index card, or even the inside of the patient's folder. In many offices, the information is entered into a computer database. A sample entry screen is shown in figure 22-7. No matter what type of form is used, most contain the following information:

- patient's name in full
- patient's address, including city and zip code
- patient's telephone number
- patient's marital status, gender, and birthdate
- patient's place of employment
- name of the person responsible for the account
- insurance company information including address, policy and group numbers, and other pertinent information
- name of referring physician or other person

In most agencies this information is typed on the form or keyed into a computer database. If a computer is used, a printed copy may be placed in the patient's record. Care must be taken to ensure that all information is accurate. Double-check numbers and spelling.

A **medical history** record is another important form used in almost all agencies. Information on this form helps the practitioner provide better care and, at times, even make a diagnosis. These forms also vary but most forms contain the following basic parts (see figure 22-8):

PATIENT INFORMATION   DATE:

PATIENT'S NAME		MARITAL STATUS	DATE OF BIRTH	SOCIAL SECURITY NO.	
		S | M | W | DIV | SEP			

STREET ADDRESS ☐ PERMANENT ☐ TEMPORARY	CITY AND STATE		ZIP CODE	HOME PHONE NO.

PATIENT'S EMPLOYER	OCCUPATION (INDICATE IF STUDENT)	HOW LONG EMPLOYED?	BUSINESS PHONE NO.

EMPLOYER'S STREET ADDRESS	CITY AND STATE	ZIP CODE

IN CASE OF EMERGENCY CONTACT:	DRIVERS LIC. NO.

SPOUSE'S NAME

SPOUSE'S EMPLOYER	OCCUPATION (INDICATE IF STUDENT)	HOW LONG EMPLOYED?	BUSINESS PHONE NO.

EMPLOYER'S STREET ADDRESS	CITY AND STATE	ZIP CODE

WHO REFERRED YOU TO THIS PRACTICE?

IF THE PATIENT IS A MINOR OR STUDENT

MOTHER'S NAME	STREET ADDRESS, CITY, STATE AND ZIP CODE		HOME PHONE NO.
MOTHER'S EMPLOYER	OCCUPATION	HOW LONG EMPLOYED?	BUSINESS PHONE NO.
EMPLOYER'S STREET ADDRESS	CITY AND STATE		ZIP CODE
FATHER'S NAME	STREET ADDRESS, CITY, STATE AND ZIP CODE		HOME PHONE NO.
FATHER'S EMPLOYER	OCCUPATION	HOW LONG EMPLOYED?	BUSINESS PHONE NO.
EMPLOYER'S STREET ADDRESS	CITY AND STATE		ZIP CODE

INSURANCE INFORMATION

PERSON RESPONSIBLE FOR PAYMENT, IF NOT ABOVE	STREET ADDRESS, CITY, STATE AND ZIP CODE		HOME PHONE NO.
☐ COMPANY NAME & ADDRESS	NAME OF POLICYHOLDER	CERTIFICATE NO.	GROUP NO.
☐ COMPANY NAME & ADDRESS	NAME OF POLICYHOLDER	POLICY NO.	
☐ COMPANY NAME & ADDRESS	NAME OF POLICYHOLDER	POLICY NO.	

☐ MEDICARE	MEDICARE NO.	☐ MEDICAID	PROGRAM NO.	COUNTY NO.	ACCOUNT NO.

In order to control our cost of billing, we request that office visits be paid at the time service is rendered. We would rather control our billing costs than be forced to raise our fees.

AUTHORIZATION: I hereby authorize the physician indicated above to furnish information to insurance carriers concerning this illness/accident, and I hereby irrevocably assign to the doctor all payments for medical services rendered. I understand that I am financially responsible for all charges whether or not covered by insurance.

_____
Responsible Party Signature

FIGURE 22-6 A sample statistical data sheet or patient information form.

```
                                    Screen ID # 5-1 _____
ACCOUNT INFORMATION    Account Number _____
Last Name _____  First Name _____ M.I. __
Address _____  Social Security # ___-__-__
City _____  State _____ Zip Code _____
Home Phone _____  Business Phone _____
Account Date __/__/__ Pri. Doctor __ Referring Doctor _____
Type Account ___ Fee Group ___  Number of Plans ___ Number of Dependents ___
Monthly Payment _____.00  Percentage of Discount __%

PERSONS COVERED BY ACCOUNT         FINANCIAL INFORMATION
Name                    S R Birth date
First Name  Last Name   E E MM/DD/YY  Balance        $ _____
                        X L          Date Last Pay   __/__/__
                                     Amount Last Pay $ _____
_____ _____ _ _ __/__/__       Balance Current $ _____
_____ _____ _ _ __/__/__       Balance 30 Day  $ _____
_____ _____ _ _ __/__/__       Balance 60 Day  $ _____
_____ _____ _ _ __/__/__       Balance 90 Day  $ _____
_____ _____ _ _ __/__/__       Balance 120 Day $ _____

E - Edit, S - Save, A - Abandon, F - Finish, M - Account Message _____
F1-New F2-Daily F3-Report F4-Update F5-Post F6-Pull F7-Mail F8-Recall F9-Notes
```

FIGURE 22-7 Statistical data about the patient can be entered into a computer database by using a patient entry screen.

◆ *General statistical data:* name, address, age, and other similar information.

◆ *Family history:* Information on members of the patient's immediate family, including parents, grandparents, sisters, and brothers. Questions are asked regarding heart disease, cancer, mental disorders, diabetes, epilepsy, kidney disease, and allergies. If a family member has died, the cause of death and age at time of death are recorded. Only information regarding blood relatives is obtained. Information regarding relatives by marriage, such as a mother-in-law, is not obtained because the patient cannot inherit diseases from these individuals.

◆ *Patient's past history:* Past illnesses, treatments, operations, accidents, physical defects, allergies, childhood diseases, and other similar items. For each past illness, the year of the illness or the patient's age at the time of the illness is recorded. For each past operation, the date of the operation or the age of the patient at the time of the operation and the type of operation are recorded.

◆ *Personal/social history:* May include questions about the patient's diet, sleep, or exercise routines and personal habits such as smoking or alcohol use. In the case of a female, information regarding pregnancies, number of children, abortions, and menstrual pattern is also recorded.

◆ *Present illness or ailment:* An exact description of the signs and symptoms the patient is currently experiencing. Information about when the illness first occurred, any previous treatment, and other pertinent information offered by the patient should be noted. This section is sometimes designated as *chief complaint.*

◆ *Physical examination or Review of Systems (ROS):* The physician performs an examination of all body systems and records both positive and negative findings. This section may also include results from laboratory tests (although there is sometimes a separate section for laboratory tests).

◆ *Diagnosis, prognosis, treatment rendered:* These sections can be separate or combined on the form. They are completed by the physician after all of the previous information is reviewed. The diagnosis is the physician's judgment regarding what disease or condition the patient has. Sometimes a tentative diagnosis is listed, or the physician may write "R/O" followed by the name of one or more diseases to indicate that tests should be done to rule out the diseases listed. The prognosis is the physician's opinion regarding the course and expected outcome of the disease or condition, such as "terminal in 3 to 6 months" or "full recovery in 1 to 2 weeks." Any specific treatment given is also listed.

In most agencies, the health care worker will complete only the statistical data information and/or family history, past history, and personal history sections. The physician or another authorized person will do all other parts of the medical history.

The patient must have privacy when being questioned. A separate room should be used, and the door to the room should be closed. Specific questions must be asked. It is essential that questions be asked in a professional rather than prying manner. It is also important to make sure the patient understands the meaning of all questions. For example, diabetes may have to be explained as "sugar." Information obtained must be accurate and complete. Facts should be rechecked as necessary. The patient should be given time

MEDICAL HISTORY FORM

Date _____
Patient's name _____

Age	Date of birth	Sex
Address	City	State Zip code

Phone ( ) _____

Insurance company	Policy number
Place of employment	Address
Phone ( )	Job responsibilities

Parent/Guardian if minor _____

Address	City	State Zip code

Phone ( ) _____

Family History:

List family members: (mother, father, brothers, sisters, grandparents, etc.)—ages and health status (if deceased write their age at the time of their death and the cause). List allergies and/or any conditions or diseases they may have or have had, such as asthma, arthritis, tuberculosis, diabetes, cancer, heart disease, hypertension, kidney disease, mental illness, depression, or any other health problems that you know of in your family.

_____
_____
_____

Patient's Past History: Mark the boxes to the right either "yes" or "no" for the following questions:*

Do you ever have or have you ever had any of the following: **(yes) (no)**

SKIN
Rashes, hives, itching or other skin irritations ( ) ( )

EYES, EARS, NOSE, THROAT
Headaches, dizziness, fainting ( ) ( )
Blurred or impaired vision ( ) ( )
Hearing loss or ringing in the ears ( ) ( )
Discharge from eyes or ears ( ) ( )
Sinus trouble/colds/allergies ( ) ( )
Asthma or hay fever ( ) ( )
Sore throats/hoarseness ( ) ( )

CARDIOPULMONARY
Shortness of breath ( ) ( )
Persistent cough or coughing up blood or other secretions ( ) ( )
Chills and/or fever ( ) ( )
Night sweats ( ) ( )
Tuberculosis or exposed to TB ( ) ( )

Scarlet fever or rheumatic fever ( ) ( )
Chest pain ( ) ( )
Heart palpitations or rapid heart-beat or pulse ( ) ( )
High blood pressure ( ) ( )
Swelling of hands and/or feet ( ) ( )

GASTROINTESTINAL
Heartburn or indigestion ( ) ( )
Nausea and/or vomiting ( ) ( )
Loss of appetite ( ) ( )
Belching or gas ( ) ( )
Peptic ulcer, gallbladder or liver disease ( ) ( )
Yellow jaundice or hepatitis ( ) ( )
Diarrhea or constipation ( ) ( )
Dysentery ( ) ( )
Rectal bleeding, hemorrhoids (piles) ( ) ( )
Tarry or clay-colored stools ( ) ( )

GLANDS
Weight gain or loss ( ) ( )

Diabetes ( ) ( )
Thyroid or goiter ( ) ( )
Swollen glands ( ) ( )

GENITOURINARY
Kidney disease or stones, or Bright's disease ( ) ( )
Painful, frequent or urgent urination ( ) ( )
Blood or pus in urine ( ) ( )
Sexually transmitted disease (venereal disease) ( ) ( )
Been sexually active with anyone who has AIDS or HIV or hepatitis ( ) ( )

NEUROMUSCULAR
Problems with becoming tired and/or upset easily ( ) ( )
Nervous breakdown/depression ( ) ( )
Poliomyelitis (infantile paralysis) ( ) ( )
Convulsions ( ) ( )
Joint and/or muscular pain ( ) ( )
Back pain or injury/osteomyelitis/rheumatism ( ) ( )

Are you currently taking any medications? Yes ( ) No ( )
If yes, please list them _____
Have you ever had or been treated for cancer or any tumors? ( ) ( )
Are you anemic or have you ever had to take iron medication? ( ) ( )
Do you use tobacco? ( ) ( )
What type? _____
Do you use IV drugs or alcohol? ( ) ( )

WOMEN ONLY
Painful menstrual periods ( ) ( )
Pregnancy/abortion/miscarriage ( ) ( )
Vaginal infection or discharge/abnormal bleeding ( ) ( )

Last menstrual period _____
Birth control _____
List dates of all operations/surgeries, injuries, and illnesses that required hospitalization:

_____

Did you ever receive benefits from a medical insurance claim due to illness or injury? Yes ( ) No ( )
Were you ever rejected from the military or for employment? ( ) ( )
Were you absent from school/work in the past 10 years because of illness or injury? ( ) ( )
Did you ever file a Workers' Compensation claim? ( ) ( )
Did you ever seek psychological or psychiatric treatment? ( ) ( )

*Please use the back of this form to explain any "yes" answers. Thank you.

FIGURE 22-8 A sample medical history form.

to think about each question. It is important that the patient feels relaxed and at ease during the questioning. Note any additional information that the patient provides if it seems important to the overall history. If no specific areas are provided on the forms for this type information, be sure the physician or other appropriate person is made aware of the information.

Legal requirements must be observed while working with medical records. It is essential to remember that all information on the record is confidential and cannot be given to any other individual, agency, or insurance company without the written permission of the patient. All records must be maintained for the period of time required by law. If an error is made while recording a medical record, the error should be crossed out in red ink, dated, and initialed. Correct information is then recorded.

An awareness of cultural diversity is essential when information is obtained. In some cultures, individuals feel it is disrespectful to speak of the dead. A patient may hesitate to discuss family history and illness if the person is deceased. A similar situation may exist in cases of adoption where biological family history is not known. An interpreter may be needed if a patient has limited English and speaks a foreign language. Patients may refuse to discuss family problems that may be causing stress and/or physical problems if they believe that this is personal information. If an individual has a cultural belief that illness is caused as a punishment for sin, the patient may not want to discuss specific symptoms or problems. In some cultures, individuals do not discuss pain.

These individuals believe pain is something that must be tolerated and accepted; acknowledging pain is a sign of weakness. Many individuals may be hesitant to discuss cultural or religious remedies they have tried, such as herbal remedies, acupuncture, witchcraft, or religious rituals. The health care worker must show respect, tolerance, and acceptance of a patient's cultural and religious beliefs while obtaining information for the medical record.

The final version of the medical history record is usually typed, or keyed into a computer program and printed for the patient's permanent record. Make sure any handwritten copy is legible and clear. Double-check all information to make sure it has been recorded correctly.

Some common abbreviations used on medical records and forms are as follows:

- *S* for single
- *M* for married
- *W* for widowed
- *D* for divorced
- *O* for negative or none
- *l and w* for living and well
- *d* for died (year of death is usually placed after the symbol)
- *NA* or *N/A* for not applicable, or does not apply

STUDENT: *Go to the workbook and complete the assignment sheet for 22:4, Completing Medical Records and Forms. Then return and continue with the procedure.*

PROCEDURE 22:4
Completing Medical Records and Forms

NOTE: A blank statistical data sheet and blank medical history sheet are in the workbook. Use these sheets to practice this procedure. (You may use other varieties of the sheets and adapt the questions to the information required.)

Equipment and Supplies

Statistical data sheet, medical history sheet, pen or typewriter

 NOTE: If a computer program is used to complete medical records, follow the

instructions provided with the software. Basic principles provided in this procedure are still followed when information is entered into the computer.

Procedure

1. **C** Assemble equipment. Use a private area for questioning the patient (lab partner in a practice situation).

   NOTE: A separate room with the door closed is preferred.

   CAUTION: Patient information is confidential. The patient's legal right to privacy must be observed.

2. Complete the statistical data sheet. Ask questions in a polite manner. Speak clearly and distinctly. Observe all of the following points:

   a. Type or print the name clearly. Check spelling.

   b. Fill in the complete address of the patient's permanent residence. Use the space provided.

   c. List the full telephone number of the patient's residence. If the patient does not have a telephone, put "none." Do not leave blank because doing so indicates that you have omitted the question. If the phone number is not local, list the area code.

   d. Fill in the personal information requested, including age, full birthdate (month, day, and year), and sex.

   e. Circle either *S, M, W,* or *D* to indicate the patient's marital status. The letters stand for *single, married, widowed,* or *divorced.*

   f. List the patient's full Social Security number, placing dashes (-) between sections of the number (for example, 218-40-2593).

   CAUTION: Repeat and check numbers for accuracy.

   g. List the spouse's name (the name of the patient's husband or wife), if this is requested. If the patient is single, widowed, or divorced, put "NA" for "not applicable."

   h. List the patient's place of employment. Include address, telephone number, and other information requested. If the patient is not employed, put "none" or current work status such as "student" or "homemaker."

   i. List the full name of the person responsible for the account. If this is the patient, list "self." If it is a husband, wife, or parent, complete all requested information.

   j. List the full name of the insurance company and the company's address and telephone number. Double-check the policy number to be sure it is accurate. This information is essential for billing.

   NOTE: Be sure to include dashes, letters, and other parts of the policy number.

   NOTE: Most agencies make a copy of both the front and back of the patient's insurance card to place in the patient's file.

   k. In the *referred* by section, place the name of the person who suggested your agency to the patient. This could be another physician, another patient, a friend, a relative, or even the telephone directory.

3. Recheck the information on the statistical data sheet as needed. Be sure all information is printed, typed, or keyed into a computer correctly. If an error occurs on a printed paper copy, draw a single red line through any incorrect entry and put your initials and the date near the line. Then insert the correct information. If an incorrect entry is noted on a computer page, delete the information and replace it with correct information.

4. Complete the medical history form. Ask each question clearly. Obtain all pertinent information such as dates of illnesses, treatments for illnesses, and details of complaint. Be professional. Allow the patient time to think about the answers. Be sure the patient understands all questions. Describe the various symptoms as stated. Make sure the patient has privacy when answering the questions. Note the following points:

   a. Complete all parts of the form. If answers are "no" or "none," the symbol *O* is sometimes used. Some questions may not apply to the patient. An example would be menstrual history, which would not apply to a male patient. Use *NA* for "not applicable."

   b. Complete the first part using information from the statistical data sheet previously completed. If no data sheet was completed, fill in as instructed.

   c. Under *family history,* record information on blood relatives only. Do not include information on the patient's in-laws. Symbols can be used, such as *l and w* for "living and well"; *d. in 1960* indicates the family member died in 1960. Under *sisters and brothers,* list number of each. If any have died, list the date and cause of death. Explain the diseases listed and question the patient about any relatives who have or had the disease.

d. Under *past history,* record any illnesses the patient has had. List the date of the illness or the age of the patient at the time of the illness. The symbol *O* can be used if the patient has not had the disease. List types of operations and dates.

e. Under *personal history,* obtain all pertinent information. Be specific. For example, do not just put "yes" for tobacco use; put "two packs per day."

f. List the *present ailment* or chief complaint in detail. For example, enter "continuous sharp pain in upper right arm" instead of "pain in arm." List any previous treatment, including treatments the patient has tried by him- or herself. List the date of onset (when the problem started).

NOTE: In many agencies, the physician or other authorized person completes the medical history. Make sure that the patient and physician or other authorized person have privacy during this time. Have forms, a pen, and a typewriter readily available.

5. Recheck the medical history record to be sure all parts are complete. Note any additional information provided by the patient. Make sure numbers, dates, spelling, and other information are accurate. If an error is present on a paper copy of the medical history, draw a single red line through the incorrect entry and put your initials and the date near the line. Then insert the correct information. If an incorrect entry is noted on a computer page, delete the information and replace it with correct information. A copy of a computer generated medical history is usually printed and placed in the patient's file.

6. Prepare the patient for the physical examination, if indicated. (This procedure was explained in Information Section 19:4.)

7. Replace all equipment.

Practice *Go to the workbook and use the evaluation sheet for 22:4, Completing Medical Records and Forms, to practice this procedure. When you feel you have mastered this skill, sign the sheet and give it to your instructor for further action.*

 Final Checkpoint Using the criteria listed on the evaluation sheet, your instructor will grade your performance.

22:5 INFORMATION
Composing Business Letters

C There are many different types of business letters. Some types of business letters you may be required to prepare include:

◆ **Collection** letter: Encourages a patient to pay an account that is due. Collection letters frequently are sent to patients who do not respond to bill statements.

◆ **Appointment** letter: Informs a patient of a scheduled appointment. All information including the day, date, and time must be included in the letter.

◆ **Recall** letter: Reminds a patient that it is time to return for a periodic examination. A reminder letter for a 6-month dental checkup is one example. In some agencies, recall cards are sent to patients.

◆ **Consultation** letter: Sent to another professional to request an examination of a particular patient. It is sometimes used as a referral to another physician, therapist, or treatment/diagnostic agency.

◆ **Inquiry** letter: Seeks some information. A letter asking a patient for information about medical insurance is one example.

Every letter must include certain parts. The parts and their components are as follows:

◆ **Heading** or **letterhead:** In most cases, printed stationery is used. The agency's name, address, and telephone number are printed on the paper as a letterhead. The date the letter is being written is keyed (typed) under the letterhead. If there is no printed letterhead, a heading is keyed on the paper. The heading includes the address of the individual sending the letter, including the city, state, and zip code, and the date of writing.

◆ **Inside address:** The name, address, city, state, and zip code of the person or firm to whom the letter is being sent.

◆ **Salutation:** The name of the person to whom the letter is directed. The salutation should include the title such as *Dear Mr., Mrs., Ms.,* or *Dr.* followed by the last name of the person. If the letter is addressed to a company, the salutation should read *Gentlemen.* If the letter is addressed to a title (for example, personnel manager), the salutation should read *Dear Sir* or *Madam.*

◆ **Subject line:** Some letters may include a subject line to reference the reason for writing. This is not present in all letters.

◆ **Body:** The message of the letter. Most letters include three paragraphs. The first paragraph states why the letter is being written. The second paragraph lists the main facts. The third paragraph is the sign off or final reminder.

◆ **Complimentary close:** A courtesy, most commonly *Sincerely, Sincerely yours,* or *Yours truly.*

◆ **Signature:** The name and/or title of the person writing the letter. Leave space after the complimentary close for a handwritten signature, and then key the name and title of the person who is sending the letter.

◆ **Reference initials:** The initials of the person dictating the letter and the initials of the person preparing the letter, or the initials of just the preparer.

◆ **Enclosure notation:** If enclosures are included with the letter, this is noted at the end of the letter with a brief description of the material enclosed.

When keying a letter into a computer, it is important to follow specific rules and use correct spacing. Some of the main points to observe are as follows:

◆ All letters must be neat and professional. Spelling and punctuation must be correct. Use the spelling and grammar checks on the computer to correct errors. Use a dictionary to check medical or dental terms that might not be on the computer spell check.

◆ The style for letters varies. Follow the style desired by your agency. Two common styles are block style and modified-block style. In **block style** (see figure 22-9), all parts of the letter are aligned starting at the left margin of the paper. In **modified-block style** (see figure 22-10), certain parts of the letter are aligned at the center line of the paper and the remaining parts are aligned at the left margin of the paper.

◆ If a letterhead is printed on the paper, space down approximately 15 lines from the top of the document or four to six lines below the letterhead. Begin keying at the center line for modified-block style or at the left margin for block style. Key in the month, day, and year. Do *not* abbreviate the month.

◆ If preprinted letterhead is not used, key a heading on the paper. Start 1½ to 2 inches (nine to twelve blank lines) from the top of the paper. Beginning at the center line for modified-block style or at the left margin for block style, key the street number and name. Do not abbreviate words such as *Road, Avenue, Street,* and *Lane.* On the next line (again starting at the center line or left margin, depending on style) key the full name of the city, the state (full name or correct abbreviation), and zip code. Leave one space after the name of the state before keying the zip code. The third line of the heading includes the full name of the month, the day, and the year.

◆ Space down five lines and begin the inside address on the fifth line below the last line of the heading. Start at the left margin line regardless of style. The inside address should

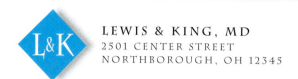

LEWIS & KING, MD
2501 CENTER STREET
NORTHBOROUGH, OH 12345

NORTHBOROUGH
FAMILY MEDICAL GROUP

Date Line

January 12, 20___ (approximately 15th line)

Inside Address

Jeremy Brown, MD (approximately 20th line)
111 S Main
Blossom, UT 10283-1120
(double-space)

Salutation

Dear Dr. Brown:
(double-space)

Subject Line

Blossom Medical Society Meeting
(double-space)

Thank you for inviting me to speak at the Blossom Medical Society
Meeting June 15, 20___. As requested, my topic will describe the
use of the MRI in assisting physicians to make a more accurate
diagnosis without resorting to invasive procedures. The exact
title of my speech will be sent by next Friday.
(double-space)

Please have your office manager send information regarding the
number of participants expected, time of meeting, location, and
any other details that will assist me in preparing my speech.

I will write or call if I have any additional questions.
(double-space)

**Complimentary
Closing**

Yours truly,

Winston Lewis, MD (4-5 line spaces)

Keyed Signature

Winston Lewis, MD
(double-space)

Reference Initials

WL:jg
(double-space)

Enclosure Notation

Enclosure: Handout on MRI

FIGURE 22-9 The form for a block-style letter. All sections are aligned at the left margin.

be at least three lines long. The first line is the name and title (for example, *Mr.* or *Miss*) of the person to whom the letter is being sent. Never use a double title such as *Dr. D.A. Jones, M.D.;* rather, use *D.A. Jones, M.D.* The second line is the street number and address. The third line is the city, state, and zip code. Leave one space but no punctuation after the name of the state before keying the zip code.

◆ Space down two lines (double-space) and begin the salutation on the second line below the inside address. A colon (:) should follow the salutation or subject line. Start on the left margin regardless of style. Capitalize all words in the salutation, for example, *Dear Mr. Brown:, Dear Dr. Jones:,* or *Dear Madam:.*

◆ If a subject line is included in the letter, space down two lines (double-space) below

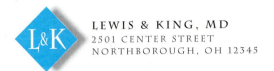

LEWIS & KING, MD
2501 CENTER STREET
NORTHBOROUGH, OH 12345

NORTHBOROUGH
FAMILY MEDICAL GROUP

January 12, 20___ (approximately 15th line)

Jeremy Brown, MD (approximately 20th line)
111 S Main
Blossom, UT 10283-1120

Dear Dr. Brown:

Blossom Medical Society Meeting

Thank you for inviting me to speak at the Blossom Medical Society
Meeting June 15, 20___. As requested, my topic will describe the use of
the MRI in assisting physicians to make a more accurate diagnosis without resorting to invasive procedures. The exact title of my speech will
be sent by next Friday.

Please have your office manager send information regarding the number of
participants expected, time of meeting, location, and any other details
that will assist me in preparing my speech.

I will write or call if I have any additional questions.

Yours truly,

Winston Lewis, MD

Winston Lewis, MD

WL:jg

Enclosure: Handout on MRI

FIGURE 22-10 The form for a modified-block style letter.

the salutation. Begin keying at the left margin to insert the subject of the letter.

♦ Space down two lines and begin keying the body on the second line after the salutation or subject line. Single-space within paragraphs; double-space to separate paragraphs. Start each line of the body on the left margin. In most cases, the first line of any paragraph in either modified-block style or block style is not indented. Some agencies, however, may indent the first line of each paragraph five spaces in a modified-block style letter. Follow agency policy.

♦ Space down two lines after the last sentence in the body and begin keying the close. Start at the center line for modified-block style or at the left margin for block style. Capitalize only the first word of the complimentary close and place a comma at the end of the close, for example, *Sincerely, Sincerely yours,* or *Yours truly.*

◆ Leave four to five blank lines for the written signature and begin the keyed name and title on the fifth or sixth line below the complimentary close. Start at the center line for modified-block style or at the left margin for block style. Key the name and title of the person sending the letter. Long titles may be placed on a second line under the name.

◆ Double-space after the keyed name and title and key the reference initials. Start at the left margin regardless of style. Key either the initials of just the preparer or the initials of the writer and the initials of the preparer. Use either capital or small letters. If two sets of initials are used, use a colon to separate capitalized initials and a slash to separate lower-cased initials, for example, *LMS:WHB* or *lms/whb.* Some agencies use capital initials for the writer, lower-cased initials for the preparer, and a colon to separate the two sets of initials. Follow agency policy.

◆ Leave neat, even margins at both sides of the paper. Margins should be wide enough to be attractive, but not too wide as to distort. An average width for margins is 1 to 1½ inches. Leave a bottom margin of at least 1 inch (six lines).

All letters should be proofread before the sender receives them for signature. Make sure that all words are spelled correctly and that complete sentences and correct punctuation are used. Use the spelling and grammar checks available on most word processing programs. In most agencies, computers and word processing software are used to prepare letters, so it is easy to correct errors on the computer screen prior to printing a hard copy of a letter. In addition, most health care agencies have standard form letters saved in a computer database. When a letter is needed for a specific purpose, such as a letter of appointment, the letter of appointment form letter is retrieved. The patient's name and personal information are keyed into the form letter. If the same letter has to be sent to a large group of people, the mail merge feature (found on

AL	Alabama	NE	Nebraska
AK	Alaska	NV	Nevada
AS	American Samoa	NH	New Hampshire
AZ	Arizona	NJ	New Jersey
AR	Arkansas	NM	New Mexico
CA	California	NY	New York
CO	Colorado	NC	North Carolina
CT	Connecticut	ND	North Dakota
DE	Delaware	MP	No. Mariana Islands
DC	Dist. of Columbia	OH	Ohio
FL	Florida	OK	Oklahoma
GA	Georgia	OR	Oregon
GU	Guam	PA	Pennsylvania
HI	Hawaii	PR	Puerto Rico
ID	Idaho	RI	Rhode Island
IL	Illinois	SC	South Carolina
IN	Indiana	SD	South Dakota
IA	Iowa	TN	Tennessee
KS	Kansas	TX	Texas
KY	Kentucky	TT	Trust Territory
LA	Louisiana	UT	Utah
ME	Maine	VT	Vermont
MD	Maryland	VI	Virgin Islands, U.S.
MA	Massachusetts	VA	Virginia
MI	Michigan	WA	Washington
MN	Minnesota	WV	West Virginia
MS	Mississippi	WI	Wisconsin
MO	Missouri	WY	Wyoming
MT	Montana		

FIGURE 22-11 United States Postal Service abbreviations for states and territories.

most word processing programs) can be used to create a large number of personalized letters. Computer classes can help the health care assistant learn how to utilize the many features present in word processing programs.

At times, using the full name of a state or territory makes a letter seem unbalanced. In such cases, the name of the state or territory is abbreviated. Only the abbreviations shown in figure 22-11 are acceptable. They are recommended by the United States Postal Service. Note that both letters are capitalized and that no periods are used in the abbreviations.

STUDENT: *Go to the workbook and complete the assignment sheet for 22:5, Composing Business Letters. Then return and continue with the procedure.*

PROCEDURE 22:5
Composing Business Letters

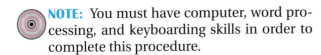 **NOTE:** You must have computer, word processing, and keyboarding skills in order to complete this procedure.

Equipment and Supplies

Computer with word processing software and printer (or typewriter), letterhead or good quality paper, scrap paper, pen or pencil

Procedure

1. Read the preceding Information section, Composing Business Letters.
2. Determine a topic for a business letter or obtain a topic from your instructor. Decide on the style of the letter (that is, modified block or block). Your instructor may specify a style.
   NOTE: In the following steps, *MB* indicates modified-block style, and *B* indicates block style.
3. Use scrap paper to write a rough draft of the letter. Check to be sure all required information is included. Use a dictionary to ensure proper spelling.
   NOTE: Ask your instructor for assistance, as needed.
4. Open a new document. Set the margins for the document. Note the center reading.
   NOTE: Margins should be wide enough to appear attractive, but not so wide as to distort. The average width is 1 to 1½ inches.
5. If a letterhead is preprinted on the paper, space down to the fifteenth line and key in the month, day, and year. Begin at the center line for MB or at the left margin for B.
   NOTE: Most health care agencies use paper with a letterhead. If no letterhead is present, space down approximately fifteen lines from the top of the document. Key the heading (sender's address and date) starting at the center line for MB or at the left margin for B.
6. Space down five lines. On the fifth line, key the inside address, starting at the left margin.
7. Space down two lines (double-space). Key the salutation, starting at the left margin. Insert a colon (:) after the salutation.
8. If a subject line is included in the letter, space down two lines, begin at the left margin, and key in the subject of the letter.
9. Double-space. Start keying the body at the left margin. Single-space within paragraphs; double-space between paragraphs. Do not indent the first lines of paragraphs.
   NOTE: Most letters should contain at least three paragraphs.
10. Double-space after the body. Key the complimentary close starting at the center line for MB or at the left margin for B. If more than one word is used, capitalize only the first word. Insert a comma at the end.
11. Leave four to five blank lines for the written signature.
12. Starting at the center line for MB or at the left margin for B, key the sender's name and title. If it is long, the title can be keyed on a second line.
13. Double-space. Key the reference initials, starting at the left margin. Use either capital or small letters for the initials of either just the preparer or of both the sender and the preparer. If two sets of initials are used, use a colon to separate capitalized initials and a slash to separate lower-cased initials. Some agencies use capital initials for the sender, lower-cased initials for the preparer, and a colon to separate the letters.
14. Read the entire letter. Perform a spelling and grammar check. Use a dictionary as necessary to check spelling of medical and dental terms not included in the computer's dictionary.
15. Print a hard copy of the letter. In most agencies, a second copy of the letter is placed in the patient's file. Save the letter on the computer hard drive or on a disk.
16. Replace all equipment.

Practice *Go to the workbook and use the evaluation sheet for 22:5, Composing Business Letters, to practice this procedure. When you feel you have mastered this skill, sign the sheet and give it to your instructor for further action.*

Final Checkpoint Using the criteria listed on the evaluation sheet, your instructor will grade your performance.

22:6 INFORMATION
Completing Insurance Forms

C Because many patients rely on insurance companies to pay medical and/or dental expenses, completing **insurance forms** may be a part of your duties. In order to obtain prompt payment from the companies, the forms must be completed correctly.

Information regarding a patient's insurance coverage is essential. Such information is usually obtained on the patient's first visit to the agency. The information is usually recorded on the statistical data sheet, on the patient's information card, or in a computer database. In addition, most agencies make a copy of both the front and back of a patient's insurance card and place the copy in the patient's file. It is essential that all names, addresses, and contract numbers be correct. Double-check this information as it is being recorded. It is also wise to periodically check that the patient's coverage has not changed.

If a patient wishes to file an insurance claim, make sure the patient has completed any parts of the form that he or she is required to complete. Also make sure that the patient has signed the form wherever his or her signature is required. If the patient is a dependent, such as a spouse or older child, it is also necessary to obtain the signature of the person to whom the insurance contract has been issued. This person is referred to as the *insured*. Because most agencies now complete insurance forms on a computer and file the claims electronically, the patient and the insured usually sign an "Authorization to Release Information and Assign Benefits" form. This form is kept in the patient's file and the insurance form is marked "patient's signature on file." In some agencies, the form is scanned into the computer and filed electronically with the insurance form.

An all-purpose form is now used in many agencies (see figure 22-12). This form, known as the HCFA-1500, was developed by the Health Care Financing Administration. It must be used for any government sponsored health care claims, such as Medicare or Medicaid. All major insurance companies will also accept this form.

Most insurance forms have two parts that require codes: diagnosis and procedures/services. Numerical codes are used to clearly identify information in a uniform and standard manner. Most insurance companies use computers and optical scanning equipment to process and pay claims, so the numerical codes must be accurate. Use of an incorrect code can lead to rejection and/or delayed payment of a claim. There are two major sources of correct numerical codes:

◆ The United States Department of Health and Human Services publishes the *International Classification of Diseases* (ICD), which is used for diagnosis coding, also referred to as ICD-9-CM coding. The diagnosis is the identification of the disease or condition that the patient has. If a patient is diagnosed as having more than one condition, the most important diagnosis and its corresponding ICD-9-CM code are listed first. Other diagnoses and their ICD-9-CM codes follow in order of importance. The ICD-9-CM codes are three to five digits long. The first three digits represent a single disease or a group of closely related conditions within a given disease classification. A fourth digit further specifies the disease, usually describing the location, cause, or stage of the disease. A fifth digit provides even more information. For example, the code *812* indicates a fracture of the humerus. The code *812.0* indicates a fracture of the humerus, upper end, closed; and the code *812.1* indicates a fracture of the

PLEASE
DO NOT
STAPLE
IN THIS
AREA

☐☐ PICA

HEALTH INSURANCE CLAIM FORM

PICA ☐☐

1. MEDICARE ☐ (Medicare #)   MEDICAID ☐ (Medicaid #)   CHAMPUS ☐ (Sponsor's SSN)   CHAMPVA ☐ (VA File #)   GROUP HEALTH PLAN ☐ (SSN or ID)   FECA BLK LUNG ☐ (SSN)   OTHER ☐ (ID)

1a. INSURED'S I.D. NUMBER   (FOR PROGRAM IN ITEM 1)

2. PATIENT'S NAME (Last Name, First Name, Middle Initial)

3. PATIENT'S BIRTH DATE MM | DD | YY   SEX M ☐ F ☐

4. INSURED'S NAME (Last Name, First Name, Middle Initial)

5. PATIENT'S ADDRESS (No., Street)

6. PATIENT RELATIONSHIP TO INSURED   Self ☐ Spouse ☐ Child ☐ Other ☐

7. INSURED'S ADDRESS (No., Street)

CITY   STATE

8. PATIENT STATUS   Single ☐ Married ☐ Other ☐
Employed ☐ Full-Time Student ☐ Part-Time Student ☐

CITY   STATE

ZIP CODE   TELEPHONE (Include Area Code) (   )

ZIP CODE   TELEPHONE (INCLUDE AREA CODE) (   )

9. OTHER INSURED'S NAME (Last Name, First Name, Middle Initial)

10. IS PATIENT'S CONDITION RELATED TO:

11. INSURED'S POLICY GROUP OR FECA NUMBER

a. OTHER INSURED'S POLICY OR GROUP NUMBER

a. EMPLOYMENT? (CURRENT OR PREVIOUS)   YES ☐ NO ☐

a. INSURED'S DATE OF BIRTH MM | DD | YY   SEX M ☐ F ☐

b. OTHER INSURED'S DATE OF BIRTH MM | DD | YY   SEX M ☐ F ☐

b. AUTO ACCIDENT?   PLACE (State)   YES ☐ NO ☐

b. EMPLOYER'S NAME OR SCHOOL NAME

c. EMPLOYER'S NAME OR SCHOOL NAME

c. OTHER ACCIDENT?   YES ☐ NO ☐

c. INSURANCE PLAN NAME OR PROGRAM NAME

d. INSURANCE PLAN NAME OR PROGRAM NAME

10d. RESERVED FOR LOCAL USE

d. IS THERE ANOTHER HEALTH BENEFIT PLAN?   YES ☐ NO ☐ *If yes*, return to and complete item 9 a-d.

READ BACK OF FORM BEFORE COMPLETING & SIGNING THIS FORM.
12. PATIENT'S OR AUTHORIZED PERSON'S SIGNATURE I authorize the release of any medical or other information necessary to process this claim. I also request payment of government benefits either to myself or to the party who accepts assignment below.

SIGNED _____   DATE _____

13. INSURED'S OR AUTHORIZED PERSON'S SIGNATURE I authorize payment of medical benefits to the undersigned physician or supplier for services described below.

SIGNED _____

14. DATE OF CURRENT: MM | DD | YY   ILLNESS (First symptom) OR INJURY (Accident) OR PREGNANCY(LMP)

15. IF PATIENT HAS HAD SAME OR SIMILAR ILLNESS. GIVE FIRST DATE MM | DD | YY

16. DATES PATIENT UNABLE TO WORK IN CURRENT OCCUPATION MM | DD | YY   FROM   TO MM | DD | YY

17. NAME OF REFERRING PHYSICIAN OR OTHER SOURCE

17a. I.D. NUMBER OF REFERRING PHYSICIAN

18. HOSPITALIZATION DATES RELATED TO CURRENT SERVICES MM | DD | YY   FROM   TO MM | DD | YY

19. RESERVED FOR LOCAL USE

20. OUTSIDE LAB? $ CHARGES   YES ☐ NO ☐

21. DIAGNOSIS OR NATURE OF ILLNESS OR INJURY. (RELATE ITEMS 1,2,3 OR 4 TO ITEM 24E BY LINE)

1. |___|.|___|
2. |___|.|___|
3. |___|.|___|
4. |___|.|___|

22. MEDICAID RESUBMISSION CODE   ORIGINAL REF. NO.

23. PRIOR AUTHORIZATION NUMBER

24. A					B	C	D			E	F		G	H	I	J	K
DATE(S) OF SERVICE From			To		Place of Service	Type of Service	PROCEDURES, SERVICES, OR SUPPLIES (Explain Unusual Circumstances)			DIAGNOSIS CODE	$ CHARGES		DAYS OR UNITS	EPSDT Family Plan	EMG	COB	RESERVED FOR LOCAL USE
MM	DD	YY	MM	DD	YY			CPT/HCPCS	MODIFIER								

25. FEDERAL TAX I.D. NUMBER   SSN ☐ EIN ☐

26. PATIENT'S ACCOUNT NO.

27. ACCEPT ASSIGNMENT? (For govt. claims, see back)   YES ☐ NO ☐

28. TOTAL CHARGE $

29. AMOUNT PAID $

30. BALANCE DUE $

31. SIGNATURE OF PHYSICIAN OR SUPPLIER INCLUDING DEGREES OR CREDENTIALS (I certify that the statements on the reverse apply to this bill and are made a part thereof.)

SIGNED   DATE

32. NAME AND ADDRESS OF FACILITY WHERE SERVICES WERE RENDERED (If other than home or office)

33. PHYSICIAN'S, SUPPLIER'S BILLING NAME, ADDRESS, ZIP CODE & PHONE #

PIN#   GRP#

(APPROVED BY AMA COUNCIL ON MEDICAL SERVICE 8/88)   *PLEASE PRINT OR TYPE*   APPROVED OMB-0938-0008 FORM CMS-1500 (12-90),   FORM RRB-1500, APPROVED OMB-1215-0055 FORM OWCP-1500,   APPROVED OMB-0720-0001 (CHAMPUS)

CARRIER   PATIENT AND INSURED INFORMATION   PHYSICIAN OR SUPPLIER INFORMATION

FIGURE 22-12 Standard medical insurance claim form.

humerus, upper end, open. The code *812.02* indicates a fracture of the humerus, upper end, closed, anatomical neck. Note that if four or five digits are used, a decimal point or period is used to separate the last two digits from the first three digits. Every diagnosis must be coded to the highest level of specificity or the claim will be rejected. Therefore, it is important to use as many digits as possible with each diagnosis. In order to find a diagnosis in the code book, look up the noun or main term in the alphabetical index. For example, look up *hysterectomy* for a diagnosis of *subtotal hysterectomy*. Use the code number in the alphabetical index to find the exact ICD-9-CM number in the tabular list for a *subtotal* hysterectomy. Most computer programs also start with the noun or main term. When the noun is keyed into the computer, a list appears with subheadings and complete codes. By practicing using the code book or computer software, you will find that it is not difficult to use.

◆ The American Medical Association (AMA) annually publishes *The Physician's Current Procedural Terminology* (CPT). This is the major source of numerical codes for procedures and services, called CPT codes. The American Dental Association (ADA) publishes A *Current Dental Terminology* (*ADA-CDT2*) book for use in dental offices. These codes are also available on computer tape for use in agencies where computers are used for billing and insurance purposes (see figure 22-13). It is important to use the latest edition of the book or computer tape to be sure that the codes are accurate and current. Each procedure or service is assigned a five-digit code without decimal points or periods. Modifiers are used to further explain or to change the meaning of a code and are separated from the code by a dash. For example, the code *44950* indicates an appendectomy, or surgical removal of the appendix. Usually, this is the only code required. However, if the appendectomy was very complex and involved much more time or care than is normally required, the modifier *-22* is added to the CPT code for a correct code of *44950-22*. The introduction in the CPT code book provides excellent instructions on the use of the book and on proper coding. By reading the introduction and practicing using the book, you can learn to correctly code procedures and

DOE, JOHN H.		BC		BC / BS OF FLA		BELL	BELLSOUTH	DED.		A
			Select Diagnosis		8,297					
1	271.1						letter and then			
2	794.31	dia			← type		bring up the			
3							al listing of			
4		DIABETES INSIPIDUS			253.5		codes.			
		DIABETES MELLITUS			250					
FROM		DIABETES MELLITUS OF MOTHER, WITH DELIVE			648.0					
11/19/02		DIABETES MELLITUS WITHOUT MENTION OF COM			250.0		INSURANC		PATIENT	
11/26/02		DIABETES WITH HYPEROSMOLAR COMA			250.2		0.00		75.00	
		DIABETES WITH KETOACIDOSIS			250.1		0.00		33.00	
		DIABETES WITH NEUROLOGICAL MANIFESTATION			250.6					
		DIABETES WITH OPHTHALMIC MANIFESTATIONS			250.5					
		DIABETES WITH OTHER COMA			250.3					
		DIABETES WITH OTHER SPECIFIED MANIFESTAT			250.8					
		DIABETES WITH PERIPHERAL CIRCULATORY DIS			250.7					
		DIABETES WITH RENAL MANIFESTATIONS			250.4					
		ENTER TO SELECT	[INS] TO ADD		[F10] TO CHANGE					
HOLD FOR		[DEL] TO DELETE		[F6] VIEW BY NUMBER			0.00		108.00	
							.00			
[INS] Next Proc.	[DEL] Delete	[F10] Done	[F3] Walkout	[F4] HCFA 1500	[F5] Payment	[F6] Transfer	[F7] Hold	[F8]* Recall	[F9] Path/Lab	

FIGURE 22-13 ICD-9-CM and CPT codes are available on computer tapes.

services. In addition, most agencies have lists containing proper CPT codes for the common procedures and services provided. The CPT codes frequently are also printed on the communication form or superbill (discussed in Information Section 22:7), which simplifies the process of completing insurance claims.

Some general rules that apply to completing most insurance forms are as follows:

◆ Make sure you are using the correct form.

◆ Read the form thoroughly or review the software program on a computer to be sure you understand what is required.

◆ Check to be sure that the patient has completed the proper areas. Make sure his or her signature appears in all required spaces. If you are using a computer program to generate the form, make sure the patient and insured have signed an authorization to release information and assign benefits form. This is often kept in the patient's file. *Signature on file* is then keyed in box 12, the area designated for the patient's signature.

◆ Double-check for accuracy all names, addresses, and contract numbers listed on the form.

◆ Policy numbers or contract numbers frequently include a letter or series of letters. Make sure these numbers are accurate and appear on the form in the proper places.

◆ Use correct codes, if codes are required. On some forms, numerical codes are used for *place of services.* For example, *11* indicates provider's office, *12* indicates home, *21* indicates inpatient hospital, *22* indicates outpatient hospital, and *32* indicates nursing home. Numerical codes are also used to describe *type of service.* For example, *1* indicates medical care, *2* indicates surgery, *4* indicates diagnostic X-rays, *5* indicates diagnostic laboratory, and *9* indicates other medical services. The codes required are usually listed on the form or described in the software on a computer program. Refer to these as necessary.

◆ Answer all questions on the form. Do *not* leave blank areas unless specifically instructed to do so. If a question does not apply, put *NA* or a dash in the space.

◆ Answer all questions thoroughly and list specific information. For example, instead of putting *lab tests,* list the tests that have been performed.

◆ Standard abbreviations are allowed on most forms. Ensure the accuracy of all abbreviations used.

◆ Make sure the amounts charged are accurately listed. Double-check all arithmetic.

◆ Make sure the physician or other authorized person has signed the form in the required areas. Many forms require the physician's National Provider Number (NPI) and/or the Physician's Identifying Number (PIN). Medicare requires the use of the NPI number. The NPI is a 10-digit number that is inserted in box 24 K and box 33 of the HCFA-1500 form. Make sure this is entered accurately.

◆ Note the boxed area for *assignment.* If the physician or agency will accept the amount allowed by the insurance company as payment in full, this is marked *yes;* if not, it is marked *no.*

◆ The form is generally copied and a copy placed in the patient's file.

◆ Recheck the entire form before mailing.

In many agencies, computers programmed to complete standard insurance claim forms are used. A sample entry screen for recording information is shown in figure 22-14. Information for the insurance claim is entered into the computer. The computer then prints the information in the proper areas on the insurance form. The form can be printed and mailed, but many agencies now file insurance forms electronically on a secure modem. Electronic filing results in faster processing and payment of the claim. These programs are easy to use and save a great deal of time when processing insurance forms.

STUDENT: *Go to the workbook and complete the assignment sheet for 22:6, Completing Insurance Forms. Then return and continue with the procedure.*

THIS IS A PREVIOUSLY ENTERED FORM 11/19/02   Pt Bal =

Doctor [1]   Assistant [ ]   Assign? [N]   Fee Code [A]
MEDICARE   MEDICAID   CHMPUS   CHMPVA   GROUP   FECA   OTHER   Insured's ID Number
  [X]   [ ]   [ ]   [ ]   [ ]   [ ]   [ ]   123456789A

Patient's Name   Birthdate   Sex (M/F)   Insured's Name
Doe, John H.   05/06/56   M   John H. Doe
Address   Insured's Address
3508 SOUTH ATLANTIC AVE   SelfX   Spouse   Child   Other
NEW SMRYNA BEACH FL 32771
32771   427-0558   (904)   Single   Married   Other
Other Insured's Name   Employd   FullTS   PartTS   Insured's Group

Policy Number   Condition Related to: Ins. DOB   Sex
65913222   Employment   [ ] Yes   [X] No   / /
DOB   Sex   ST   Employer
  / /   Auto Acc.   [ ] Yes   [X] No
Employer   Plan Name
                                       Other Acc.   [ ] Yes   [X] No   BC / BS OF FLA
Plan Name   Date of Disability
BELLSOUTH DED. SERV CENTR   Local
Date of Current   First consulted   Hospitalization
Referring {F5}   Referring ID#

                                                                                  Lab [ ] Yes [X] No
Facility {F5}   Prior Auth
  {F10} = Next Pg   {ESC} = Back Up   {F3} = Pt Info   CTRL + ESC = Abort   11/19/02   1

FIGURE 22-14 A sample computer entry screen for insurance information.

PROCEDURE 22:6   C

Completing Insurance Forms

 NOTE: You must have keyboarding or typing skills in order to complete this procedure.

Equipment and Supplies

Computer with insurance coding software for ICD-9-CM and CPT codes, or typewriter with good ribbon, sample insurance forms, correction tape or fluid, *International Classification of Diseases* (ICD-9-CM) book, *The Physician's Current Procedural Terminology* (CPT) book (or ADA-CDT-2 book for dental claims)

Procedure

1. Assemble equipment. Open the insurance software program on the computer or obtain a sample insurance form from your instructor.

2. Read the insurance form or review the entry areas on the computer program. Make sure you understand all required information.
   NOTE: Ask your instructor to explain areas, as needed.

3. Make sure that the patient has completed his or her portions of the form or has signed an authorization to release information form. Check to be sure that correct signatures are on the form. Signatures should be written in blue or black ink. If the patient is a dependent, make sure the insured person has signed the form, if this is required.
   NOTE: If the form is computer generated, and the patient and/or insured have signed authorization to release information forms, *Signature on file* is keyed in the area designated for the signature.

4. Enter all patient information, usually including the full name and address of the insured (the person to whom the insurance contract is issued); the patient's name, address (including zip code), birthdate (written as six digits, for example, 03/26/67), gender (put an *X* in the correct box), and relationship to insured (put an *X* in the correct box); the group number or name; the contract or identifying number; and other

similar data. Double-check all entries for accuracy.

NOTE: If the contract number has letters, be sure they are included.

5. Most policies require information about other insurance the patient may have. Record this information in the correct spaces. If the patient does not have other insurance, insert *NA,* for "not applicable," or *none* in this space.

6. Most forms contain questions about whether or not the condition is related to employment or an accident. Workers' Compensation may cover an employment-related condition; other insurance may cover a condition caused by an accident. Therefore, it is important to answer these questions correctly. Mark *yes* or *no,* or insert an *X* in the correct box.

7. Enter information regarding dates of care. Correct information is usually obtained from the patient's chart and/or the physician or supervisor. Be sure the sources are accurate.

8. Many forms require dates of total or partial disability. This is determined by the physician or other authorized person (for example, a therapist). The time a patient is disabled and unable to work usually begins with the date of the onset of the condition. Insert this date in the correct area. An authorized person then determines an approximate date when the patient's disability will end and the patient will be able to return to work. Insert this date as the final date. If no disability is determined, type *NA* in all spaces.

9. If the patient was referred by another physician or agency, insert the full name of the referring source. The NPI number of the referring physician is placed in the *ID Number* space. Put *NA* or *none* in the blank if there was no referring source.

10. If services were provided to the patient in a hospital, record the dates of hospitalization in the correct blanks. If a laboratory outside the hospital or health care facility performed tests, note this information along with the charges for the tests.

11. Leave line 19 *Reserved for Local Use* blank.

12. In the *diagnosis* section of the form, list the ICD-9-CM code for the main or primary diagnosis first followed by other diagnoses in order of importance. Use the *International Classification of Diseases* to find the correct ICD-9-CM code for each diagnosis. Make sure each diagnosis is coded to the highest level of specificity. Double-check all entries for accuracy.

NOTE: Payment on a claim can be delayed or rejected if an incorrect or non-specific ICD-9-CM code is used.

13. The CPT codes for any services or procedures provided should be listed in the *services or treatment* section of the form. Each service or procedure should be listed separately with the most important service listed first. Dates should be obtained from the patient's chart or from an authorized person. Numerical codes are frequently used to indicate place of service. Common codes include *11* for office, *21* for inpatient hospital, *22* for outpatient hospital, *12* for patient's home, *31* for skilled-nursing facility, and *32* for nursing home. Numerical codes are also used to describe types of service. Common codes include *1* for medical care, *2* for surgery, *3* for consultation, *4* for diagnostic X-rays, *5* for diagnostic laboratory, and *9* for other medical services. Codes for both type and place of service are listed on the form or defined in the computer software. Use *The Physician's Current Procedural Terminology* to find the correct CPT code for each procedure or service. Double-check the code before inserting it in the correct area. The *diagnosis code* column refers to the diagnoses listed in the *diagnosis* section. The corresponding number of the diagnosis for which the service was given should be inserted in this column.

14. List the charges for services rendered. Make sure the numbers for dollars are lined up in the correct spaces. Place the amounts for cents or *00* in the correct columns. Total all charges. Recheck all math, especially addition. If the patient has paid an amount, note this in the correct place. Subtract any amount paid by the patient from the total charge to obtain the balance due.

15. Insert the physician's social security or tax identification number in the space provided. Mark the appropriate box.

16. Insert the patient's account number in the appropriate space.

17. A boxed area is usually provided for information regarding assignment, or whether

the physician or agency will accept the amount allowed and paid by the insurance company. Check either *yes* or *no,* as determined by the physician or agency.

18. Insert all required information regarding the physician or supplier, including full name and title, address, telephone number (if requested), NIP, PIN, social security and/or ID or license number, and other required information. Be sure the physician or authorized person signs in the correct area.

    ! **CAUTION:** Double-check all numbers for accuracy.

19. Recheck all information on the form. Make sure that all required information is recorded and all answers are provided.

20. Before filing the form electronically or mailing the form to the insurance company,

place a copy in the patient's file for reference, if this is the policy of your agency.

21. Replace all equipment.

Practice Go to the workbook and use the evaluation sheet for 22:6, Completing Insurance Forms, to practice this procedure. When you feel you have mastered this skill, sign the sheet and give it to your instructor for further action.

✔ **Final Checkpoint** Using the criteria listed on the evaluation sheet, your instructor will grade your performance.

22:7 INFORMATION Maintaining a Bookkeeping System

Pegboard System

One common bookkeeping system is the pegboard system. The **pegboard system** is also called a *"write-it-once" system.* Various records are noted simultaneously. The pegboard system usually encompasses the following series of records:

◆ **Day sheet,** or **daily journal:** A daily record of all patients seen, all charges incurred, and all payments received (see figure 22-15). Each day sheet also provides a total column, which can be used for bank deposit slips; a business analysis summary; a section for daily and monthly account totals; a proof of posting section for verifying that account totals are accurate; and a section to record accounts receivable, or total amounts owed by patients. When a month's supply of day sheets is compiled in one folder, a monthly record of all business is available.

◆ **Statement–receipt** record: Information on past balance due, charges for treatment,

payment received, and current balance (see figure 22-16). Many slips also have a space to note the patient's next appointment. When complete, the statement–receipt can be given to the patient to provide a record of payment or of balance due. In some agencies another version of this record is being used. This version is usually a three-layer form that notes all the previous information as well as specific services and corresponding insurance code numbers. Called a communication form, or a superbill (see figure 22-17), this version serves as a statement for the insurance company. One copy can be retained by the agency, the second copy can be sent to the insurance company (or attached to an insurance form) to serve as a claim form, and the third copy can be given to the patient to serve as a payment receipt, a record of treatment or services, a bill for the balance due on the account, and an appointment card, if another appointment is scheduled. Use of this form eliminates the need to type out specific insurance forms.

◆ **Charge slip:** On some pegboard systems, these are a part of the statement–receipt record. When the patient arrives at the agency, his or her name is entered at the top. This section of the record is torn off the statement–receipt and attached to the patient's

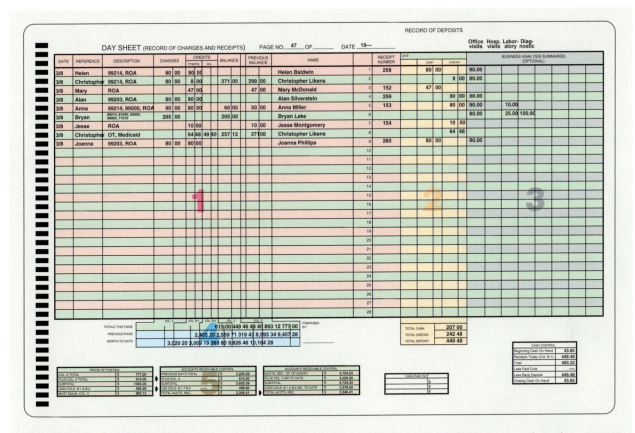
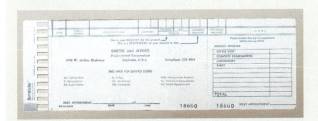
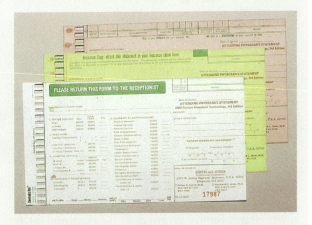

FIGURE 22-15 The day sheet provides a daily record of patients seen, charges incurred, and payments received.

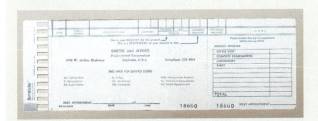

FIGURE 22-16 A statement–receipt provides information on past balance due, charges, payment received, and current balance. *(Courtesy of Control-o-fax Office Systems, Waterloo, IA)*

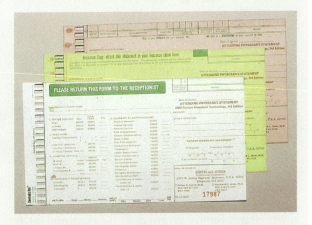

FIGURE 22-17 A three-layer version of the statement–receipt form, the communication form or superbill, also lists treatments and insurance codes. It can be used as the form for insurance claims or attached to insurance forms. *(Courtesy of Control-o-fax Office Systems, Waterloo, IA)*

chart. The physician or other authorized individual then notes the treatments and charges on this slip while treating the patient. The slip is given back to the receptionist, who can then use it to post charges.

◆ **Ledger card:** A total record of care provided to a patient. Also, a financial record of the patient's account. A brief description of services, charges, payments made, and current balance due is noted on the card. In some agencies, copies of the ledger cards are used in place of separate bills. The ledger card is reproduced by photocopy or microfilm and mailed to the patient as a monthly statement (see figure 22-18).

KERRY PEOPLES, M.D.
101 Fitness Lane
Anywhere, U.S.A. 00000

Marsha Leonard
777 Pine Tree Lane
Troy, Ohio 47100

DATE	DESCRIPTION	CHARGE	CREDITS		CURRENT BALANCE
			PAYMENTS	ADJ.	
		BALANCE FORWARD→			
8/31/XX	Marsha Office visit	35.00			35.00
8/31/XX	Marsha SMAC w/CBC & diff	30.00			65.00
9/15/XX	ROA - cash		15.00		50.00

276L   PLEASE PAY LAST AMOUNT IN THIS COLUMN ↑

THIS IS A COPY OF YOUR ACCOUNT AS IT APPEARS ON YOUR LEDGER CARD

FIGURE 22-18 The ledger card serves as a financial record of the patient's account and can be copied and mailed to the patient as a monthly statement.

The procedure for recording patient visits, treatments, charges, and payments on the pegboard system is described in Procedure 22:7 which follows. In addition to recording patients' visits and charges, the pegboard system is also used to record payments received. One example is an insurance company check for payment for services. The same steps are followed, but in place of a treatment, *ROA,* for "received on account," is usually noted under *description.* Balances are then determined, and all information is simultaneously noted on the day sheet and ledger card. A receipt may be mailed to the patient.

At the end of a business day, the day sheet provides a total record of all charges and payments and a method of checking accounts. Daily totals are obtained by adding the amounts of each column on the day sheet. The accuracy of the records can be checked immediately. Small total boxes in the *Proof of Posting* section at the bottom of the sheet provide the correct formulas for determining that all entries are correct. A bank deposit slip is also provided, if payments received are to be deposited.

Because a series of records is recorded at one time, it is important for the recorder to use a ballpoint pen and print neatly while pressing hard enough for all copies to record. If an error is made, it must be lined out neatly. Neither erasers nor correction fluid should be used because these are financial records that may be audited for tax or legal purposes. If a major error is made, it may be best to void the statement–receipt record and start a new record. Neatness and accuracy are essential when using the pegboard system. These are bookkeeping records; therefore, they must be stored for reference. Special folders can be purchased for this purpose.

Computerized Bookkeeping Systems

Most health care facilities use computerized bookkeeping systems. There are many types of software available, but most provide the same basic functions. Most systems used begin with the creation of a patient's account history or a computerized ledger card. Information including the name and address of the patient, the person responsible for the account, family members in the account, and insurance information is entered for each patient. This forms the database for the system. ICD-9-CM and CPT codes used in the agency are also programmed into the computer along with a description of the codes and the fees charged for each. Most software is programmed to indicate a source of payment, such as cash, check, or insurance. When a patient receives a service, the patient's account history is retrieved. Information about the service is entered on a daily transaction screen (see figure 22-19). When the correct CPT codes are entered, the software automatically calculates the current balance by using the past balance in the account history and adding it to the new charges. If payment is made, the software deducts the payment and calculates the new balance. The account history or computerized ledger card is updated automatically as entries are made. Printed copies of the account can be given to the patient to show all charges, payments made, and the current balance due. In addition, the account history can be used for billing patients at regular intervals.

In addition to handling patient accounts, bookkeeping software will also create a daily journal (see figure 22-20). This provides a financial record showing patients seen, services provided, charges, payments made, and outstanding balances. Most software will generate a deposit slip created from the totals entered as payment is made.

Most computerized billing systems are easy to use. The computer guides the user through each step of entering financial information by providing directions or asking the user questions. However, the health care worker must still understand the basic principles of financial management used in the manual bookkeeping method to use the computerized program. In addition, safeguards must be in place when this type of system is used. Most agencies use password protection so only authorized individuals are allowed access to the financial information. In addition, all systems should be programmed to record deleted transactions to prevent someone from deleting a transaction and stealing the money. A final important point is to make sure daily tape, disk, or CD-ROM back-ups are made of all information and stored in a safe area in case of computer failure.

Messages-

Patient and Provider INFORMATION Starting Balance $ ______
Patient Name ______ Account Number ______
Relationship ______ Provider Number ______
Voucher Number ______ Treatment Date ___/___/___
INSURANCE INFORMATION
Covered by Insurance ____ Service Place ____
Plan Covering Treatment____ Last Entered Diagnosis
Description is:

TREATMENT AND PAYMENT INFORMATION

Proc. Code	Description	Charge	Receipt	Primary Diag.	Suffix
	Totals			New Balance	

E - Edit, A - Abandon, S - Save, H - Save/Hold, F - Finished
F1-New F2-Daily F3-Report F4-Update F5-Post F6-Pull F7-Mail F8-Recall F9-Notes

FIGURE 22-19 A daily transactions entry screen allows the health care provider to enter information about a patient's treatments and maintain the patient's account.

STUDENT: *Go to the workbook and complete the assignment sheet for 22:7, Maintaining a Bookkeeping System. Then return and continue with the procedure.*

DAILY CHARGES AND RECEIPTS REPORT - March 8, 2002

Page 1

DATE	ACCNT #	ACCOUNT NAME	PAT NAME PMT. SOURCE	DOCTOR	PROC	DIAG	VOUCHER	CHARGES	RECEIPTS	TODAYS BALANCE	BILLED P	BILLED I	INS
03/08/02	2	Brown	Rachael	1	82996	V22.2	2	$18.00	$0.00	$134.00	N	N	Y
03/08/02	4	Gonzales	Joseph	1	93000	785.1	1	$36.00	$0.00	$36.00	N	N	Y
03/08/02	6	O'Brien	Janet	1	85022	285.9	3	$23.00	$23.00	$75.00	N	N	N
03/08/02	9	Williams	Ryan	1	90071	780.7	7	$44.00	$0.00	$144.00	N	N	Y
03/08/02	1	Takamoto	Credit Adj.	1	MO2		5	−$18.00	$0.00	$78.00	N	N	Y
03/08/02	10	Young	David	2	73090	848.9	6	$54.00	$54.00	$0.00	N	N	N
03/08/02	15	Anderson	Nancy	1	86300	075	4	$18.00	$0.00	$62.00	N	N	Y
03/08/02	12	Lightfoot	James	2	92551	389.9	8	$36.00	$0.00	$36.00	N	N	Y
03/08/02	11	Roberts	Debit Adj.	1	MO1		9	$0.00	−$25.00	$75.00	N	N	N
03/08/02	13	Paulson	Jon	2	95000	477.9	10	$44.00	$0.00	$144.00	N	N	Y
03/08/02	14	Bond	PAYMENT	1	M91		11	$0.00	$75.00	$200.00	N	N	Y
TOTALS								$255.00	$127.00				

Total interest included in Charges $0.00
Total Debit Adjustments - $25.00
Total Credit Adjustments - $18.00
Mode of operation - Daily data only

FIGURE 22-20 Computerized bookkeeping systems will provide a daily transactions report similar to the day sheet.

PROCEDURE 22:7
Maintaining a Bookkeeping System

Equipment and Supplies

Pegboard base, day sheet, ledger cards, statement–receipt forms or communication forms, ballpoint pen, assignment sheet number 1 for 22:7, Maintaining a Bookkeeping System

NOTE: This procedure describes a manual pegboard system of bookkeeping. Computerized bookkeeping systems require the same type of entries. If you are using a computerized program, follow the instructions provided with the software to enter the information and balance the accounts.

Procedure

1. Assemble equipment. Review the various forms and note the areas on each.
2. Place the day sheet on the pegboard. Use the pegs to secure it in position.
3. Place a supply of statement-receipt forms or a communication form on top of the day sheet. Position these so that the top line of each form lines up with the first recording line on the day sheet.
4. Prepare the patient ledger cards. In most agencies, this is done according to the head of the household's name. If this is the case, record the last name and then first name of this individual on each card. Complete the full address. Be sure to include the zip code because it is frequently used for billing purposes. If the agency requires a separate ledger card for each patient, fill out the ledger card for each individual patient.
5. If the patient is new, enter two zeros *(00)* under *Current Balance*. If this is a second card for a patient whose first card is full, place the current balance from the old card in this space.
6. Follow the instructions on assignment sheet number 1 for patients seen and charges incurred. As each patient "enters" the office, do the following:
   a. Pull the correct ledger card for the patient.
   b. Insert the ledger card in position. Make sure the last line of information is above the statement–receipt form.
   c. Fill in the date and the patient's name.
   d. Put the current balance (the amount the patient owes for previously rendered services) noted on the ledger card in the space labeled *Previous Balance* on the charge slip.
   e. Put the receipt number on the statement–receipt form on the day sheet.
   f. Tear off the charge slip or remove the communication form. Attach this to the patient's chart. The person rendering treatment will complete the slip or form when he or she sees the patient.
7. As each patient "leaves" the office, do the following:
   a. Record the treatments and total charges listed on the charge slip or communication form.
   b. Insert the patient's ledger card in the correct position between the day sheet and statement–receipt form (see figure 22-21). Be sure to use the correct statement–receipt form.
   c. Under *Description*, list the services or treatments noted on the charge slip. Services or treatments are already noted on communication forms. Abbreviations are usually used. These often are listed on the statement–receipt form.
   d. Put the charges or amount due in the *Charges* space. Put dollars to the left of the line and cents to the right.
   e. If the patient pays an amount, note this in the *Payment* area.
      NOTE: *Adj,* for "adjustment," is used for discounts or special credits.
   f. If no payment is made, draw lines through these areas.
   g. Record the payment on the day sheet. If a bank deposit slip is to be used, make sure it is folded back under the *Receipts* area of the day sheet or positioned correctly for posting. If the payment is by check, record the amount in the column labeled *Checks*. If the payment is by cash, record the amount in the column labeled *Cash*. Double-check all figures.
      NOTE: Print numbers clearly, so there is no chance of error.

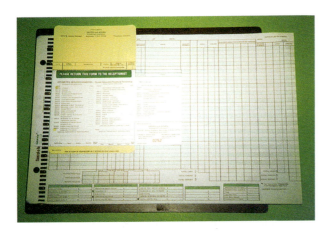

FIGURE 22-21 The ledger card is inserted between the statement–receipt record and the day sheet on the pegboard. *(Courtesy of Control-o-fax Office Systems, Waterloo, IA)*

form can be either given to the patient to use for filing a claim or sent to the insurance company by the agency. The third copy is retained by the agency.

l. Check to make sure all information has been recorded on the day sheet.

8. If money is received on an account, follow the same steps as before. However, record *ROA* (for "received on account") under *Description*. Note the amount as a payment.

9. At the end of the day, total all account columns on the day sheet. Enter the figures in the *Proof of Posting* box and follow the instructions given to catch any possible errors. Total the deposit slips and check these for accuracy.

10. Replace all equipment.

h. Add the previous balance and charges together. Double-check your addition.

i. Subtract any payment made from the total amount due (the amount obtained in step 7h). Record your final figure in *Current Balance*.

j. Remove the ledger card and check to be sure all entries are clear and correct.

k. Tear off the statement–receipt record or remove the communication form and give it to the patient. If the patient needs an appointment, the next appointment can be recorded on this receipt.

NOTE: If a communication form is used, one copy is given to the patient. The insurance copy of the communication

Practice *Use the evaluation sheet for 22:7, Maintaining a Bookkeeping System, to practice this procedure. Complete assignment sheet number 1 in the workbook and give it to your instructor. Note any corrections made to this sheet before completing assignment sheet number 2. Make up additional practice sessions, as needed. When you feel you have mastered this skill, sign the evaluation sheet and give it to your instructor for further action.*

✔ **Final Checkpoint** Using the criteria listed on the evaluation sheet, your instructor will grade your performance.

22:8 INFORMATION Writing Checks, Deposit Slips, and Receipts

Maintaining accurate financial records may be part of your responsibilities as a health care worker. Checks and receipts are important documents, and they must be filled in accurately. Checks and receipts help provide a record of financial transactions.

A **check** is a written order for payment of money through a bank. A check is used in place of cash for payment. Terms associated with checks include the following:

◆ **Payee:** The person receiving payment.

◆ **Originator** or **maker:** The person writing the check, or issuing payment.

◆ **Endorsement:** The signature of the payee. This is usually posted to the back of the check and is required before payment will be made by the bank.

Basic rules for completing checks include the following:

◆ Checks must be written in ink, typed, or printed on a computer printer. Using pencil allows alterations by a dishonest person.

◆ Writing must be legible. All names and numbers must be clear.

◆ Spaces should be avoided in name or amount lines. Begin writing to the far left of the line. This prevents another person from adding another name or increasing the amount of money.

◆ Check stubs or registers should be recorded before the check is written. A check stub or register is a record of information about a check. It states the number of the check, the person to whom the check was written, and the amount of the check.

◆ Use fractions in place of decimals to indicate number of cents. For example, instead of writing $100.00 (easily changed to $1,000.00), write $100 00/100.

◆ The check must include the correct signature of the maker, or originator. This signature is recorded at the bank when a checking account is opened. In an agency, the signature is usually that of the person in authority (for example, the physician, dentist, therapist, or agency head). Only this individual is allowed to sign his or her name. If any other person signs the name, this is forgery.

◆ Before issuing a completed check, all information should be checked again for accuracy and completeness.

When a check is received from a patient, it should be checked closely. Make sure the amount is correct and noted the same way on both parts of the check showing amount. Make sure the patient has listed the correct individual or agency name as the payee. Check the date for accuracy. Make sure the check has been signed by the patient. Patients sometimes want to write checks for more than the amounts due to obtain extra cash. It is usually not wise to accept these types of checks. If the person has insufficient funds in his or her checking account, the agency will lose not only the amount due, but also the additional cash given to the patient. Sometimes a patient will write *Payment in Full* on a check. Do not accept such a check unless it does pay the entire balance due, including previous charges and current charges.

Checks received by an agency are usually stamped *For Deposit Only to the Account of* . . . . This prevents anyone from cashing a check if it is stolen. It also serves as a means of endorsing the check. If the payee wishes to cash the check, it must be endorsed with his or her written signature. If an endorsed check is lost before it can be taken to the bank, however, anyone who finds the check will be able to cash it. If a written signature is used as an endorsement, the check should not be endorsed until the person takes it to the bank. Federal regulations now require that all endorsements be within 1½ inches of the "trailing edge" (on the back and directly behind the left side of the front of the check) of all checks. If an endorsement extends below this area, the financial institution may refuse payment on the check.

A **receipt** is a record of money or goods received. If a patient makes a payment, a receipt can be given to the patient as proof of payment. The receipt stub or a register entry provides the agency with proof that payment has been received. All information must be completed accurately and legibly. Again, ink must be used to prevent any alteration of the receipt. In some agencies, a separate receipt book is used. In other agencies, receipts are part of the daily log record or pegboard system.

Specific instructions for writing checks and receipts are included in Procedures 22:8A and 22:8C. Each step is important. All work should be checked for accuracy.

Deposit slips are also important in maintaining accurate financial records (see figure 22-22). Any cash monies or checks received

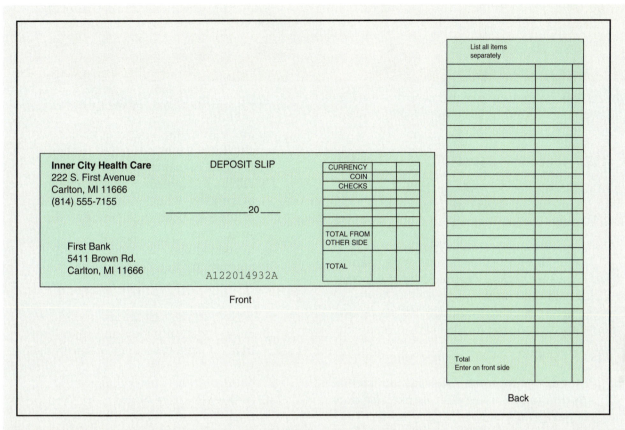

List all items
separately

Inner City Health Care
222 S. First Avenue
Carlton, MI 11666
(814) 555-7155

DEPOSIT SLIP

CURRENCY
COIN
CHECKS

_____ 20 ____

TOTAL FROM
OTHER SIDE

First Bank
5411 Brown Rd.
Carlton, MI 11666

TOTAL

A122014932A

Front

Total
Enter on front side

Back

FIGURE 22-22 Deposit slips usually have an area on the back for recording a large number of checks.

should be deposited in the bank as soon as possible. Most agencies deposit monies on a daily basis. This prevents loss or theft. In addition, most agencies keep a copy of each deposit slip with the financial records. This can be used to verify deposits and/or ascertain that a specific check has been deposited. Deposit slips must be accurate. All addition must be double-checked. Terms used on these slips include the following:

♦ *Currency:* Any money in bill form, such as $1 bills, $10 bills, and other bills. All currency to be deposited is added together and entered as one entry in this section.

♦ *Coins:* All coins to be deposited are added together and entered as one entry in this section.

♦ *Checks:* Usually listed separately and then added together for the total. Most deposit slips have a series of lines on the back for a large number of checks. Here, the checks are again listed separately, and are added together for a subtotal, which is then transferred to the front of the deposit slip in the space indicated. **NOTE:** Specific rules for completing deposit slips are noted in Procedure 22:8B.

STUDENT: *Go to the workbook and complete the assignment sheet for 22:8, Writing Checks, Deposit Slips, and Receipts. Then return and continue with the procedures.*

PROCEDURE 22:8A

Writing Checks

NOTE: This procedure is to be completed using the problems found in assignment sheets numbers 1 and 2 in the workbook.

Equipment and Supplies

Sample blank checks (copies provided in workbook); assignment sheets numbers 1 and 2 for 22:8, Writing Checks, Deposit Slips, and Receipts; pen

NOTE: This procedure describes the manual writing of checks. Computerized check writing systems require the same types of entries. If you are using a computerized program, follow the instructions provided with the software.

Procedure

1. Assemble equipment. Review preceding information about writing checks. Use only ink to write checks.

2. Follow the directions on assignment sheet number 1 for 22:8, Writing Checks, Deposit Slips, and Receipts.

3. First complete the check stub or register entry (see figure 22-23) so that you do not accidentally issue a check without making a written record.

   a. Make sure that the current balance of the checking account is noted in the *Balance Brought Forward* section.

   b. Fill in the number of the check. Most preprinted checks have the number printed on both the check and the check stub.

   c. In the dollar *($)* space, print in the amount of the check. Write the dollar amount close to the dollar sign. Write cents as a fraction, for example, *.50* as *50/100, no cents* as *no/100* or *00/100*.

   d. Fill in the month, day, and year.

   e. In the *To* space, write the name of the person or company to whom the check is being written. This is the payee.

   f. In the *For* space, write a brief reason for the payment, for example, *computer supplies,* or *rent*.

   g. In the *Deposits* space, note the amount of any deposit you make to the account. Add this amount to the balance brought forward to obtain the new total balance. If no

---

No. 444	$ 23 39/100	Happy Doctor, M.D.		No. 444
		1 Healthy Lane		
Date MARCH 8 20__		Fitness, OH 11133		Date MARCH 8 20 --
To ACE SUPPLY CO.				
For ECG PAPER		Pay to the Order of ACE SUPPLY COMPANY		$ 23 39/100

Balance Brought Forward	442	06	TWENTY-THREE AND 39/100 ———————————— dollars
Deposits	–	–	First Money Bank
			1 Rich Lane
Balance	442	06	Wealthy, OH 11133
			0098-5567
Amount this check	23	39	Memo EKG PAPER By *Happy Doctor, M.D.*
Balance Carried Forward	418	67	⑆0119⑈0044⑆ 268 8495⑈ 0101

FIGURE 22-23 A sample check with the check stub or register at the left.

deposit has been made since the last check was written, put dashes in this space. Write the new total balance in the *Balance* space.

h. Fill in the amount of the check you are writing.

i. Subtract the amount of the check you are writing from the new total balance. Record the difference in the *Balance Carried Forward* space.

   NOTE: Double-check all addition and subtraction.

j. Immediately place the final balance amount in the *Balance Brought Forward* space of the next check stub so that the balance will be there when you write the next check.

4. Once the stub has been completed, write the check. Print or write legibly. Use only ink.

   a. If the number is not preprinted on the check, write the number of the check in the *No.* space.

   b. Put the month, day, and year in the *Date* space.

   c. Write the payee's name in the *Pay to the Order of* space. Write the person's name or company name completely. Begin writing to the far left of the line.

   d. In the *$* space, print the amount of the check in numbers. Place the dollar amount numbers close to the dollar sign. Print cents amount as a fraction. Do *not* leave blank spaces where other numbers could be inserted.

   e. In the *dollars* space, write out in words the amount of the check. Start at the far left of the line. Write the number of dollars; express cents as a fraction. Draw a line from the end of your notation to the printed word *dollars* to avoid leaving space for any alterations, for example, *Two hundred thirty-six and 30/100 ——— dollars.*

   f. If there is a *For* or *Memo* space on the check, fill in a brief explanation of why the check is being written, for example, *office supplies, rent,* or *insurance payment.*

g. The check must be signed on the signature line by the person to whom the checking account belongs. Only the authorized person is permitted to sign the check. After you have completed all parts of the check, double-check all entries. If they are accurate, obtain the appropriate signature. The check will *not* be valid without this signature.

    CAUTION: Never sign a check unless you are specifically authorized to do so and your signature is on the account at the bank. Otherwise, signing the check is considered forgery.

h. Recheck all parts of the check and stub for accuracy.

5. If you make an error on any part of the check, do not erase. Write *void* on both the check and the stub. Then start over with a new check and stub.

6. Follow steps 3 to 5 to complete all parts of assignment sheet number 1. Then turn it in to your instructor for grading.

7. Replace all equipment.

Practice *Use the evaluation sheet for 22:8A, Writing Checks, to practice this procedure. Note any changes or corrections to the graded assignment sheet number 1. Then follow the steps in the procedure to complete assignment sheet number 2 for 22:8, Writing Checks, Deposit Slips, and Receipts. When you feel you have mastered this skill, sign the evaluation sheet and give it to your instructor for further action.*

✔ **Final Checkpoint** Using the criteria listed on the evaluation sheet, your instructor will grade your performance.

PROCEDURE 22:8B
Writing Deposit Slips

Equipment and Supplies

Assignment sheets numbers 1 and 2 for 22:8, Writing Checks, Deposit Slips, and Receipts; sample deposit slips (copies provided in workbook); pen

Procedure

1. Assemble equipment. Record all information in ink.
2. Read assignment sheet number 1 to note the amount of the deposit to be made to the checking account.
3. On the deposit slip (see figure 22-24) fill in the correct date. Put the month, day, and year.
4. Write the total amount in bills in the *Currency* space. Because no cents are involved, place two zeros in the far right-hand column.
5. Count the total amount in coins. Write this amount in the *Coin* column.
   NOTE: Write dollar amounts to the left of the line and cent amounts to the right of the line.
6. List each check separately on the *Checks* lines. If additional space is needed, most deposit slips have areas on the back to note checks. The subtotal from the back is then noted on the front of the slip.
7. Add the amounts for currency, coins, and checks together and write the sum in the *Total* space. If none of the total is to be kept as cash (that is, all of the money is to be deposited), enter this total amount two lines down in the *Total Deposit* space.
   NOTE: If some of the total is kept as cash, place this amount in the *Less Cash* space. Subtract this amount from the total to obtain the amount of the total deposit.
   NOTE: If cash is retained, a signature is usually required on the deposit slip. The person to whom the account belongs must sign in the space indicated.
8. Recheck all amounts for accuracy. Recheck all addition and subtraction. Make a copy of the deposit slip to keep with financial records. Take the original deposit slip, cash, and checks to the bank for deposit. Make sure to obtain a deposit receipt from the bank.
9. Note the amount deposited on the check stub of the next check to be written. Add the balance and amount deposited together to get the total current balance. The checkbook and stubs will then be up to date and ready to use.
10. Replace all equipment.

Happy Doctor, M.D. 1 Healthy Lane Fitness, OH 11133		
Currency	21	00
Coin	2	38
Checks	24	50
	182	06
Date ___March 8___ 20 —		
Signature _____		
(If cash received)		
TOTAL	229	94
First Money Bank 1 Rich Lane Wealthy, OH 11133 0098-5567	Less Cash	—	—
	TOTAL DEPOSIT	229	94

FIGURE 22-24 A sample deposit slip.

Final Checkpoint Using the criteria listed on the evaluation sheet, your instructor will grade your performance.

PROCEDURE 22:8C

Writing Receipts

Equipment and Supplies

Assignment sheets numbers 1 and 2 for 22:8, Writing Checks, Deposit Slips, and Receipts; sample receipts; pen

Procedure

1. Assemble equipment. Review preceding information on writing receipts. Use ink to record all transactions.
2. Obtain information to be recorded on the receipts from assignment sheet number 1.
3. First complete the stub or register (see figure 22-25). In this way, you will not forget to record this information and will have a record of the receipt issued.

a. In the *No.* space, write the number of the receipt. On preprinted receipts, this is often already done, and all receipts are numbered consecutively.
b. In the *Date* space, print the month, day, and year.
c. In the *To* space, print the name of the person or company to whom the receipt is being issued.
d. In the *For* space, write a brief explanation of why the receipt is being issued, for example, *POA* (for "payment on account"), *office supplies, ROA* (for "received on account").
e. In the *Amount* space, print the dollar amount for which the receipt is being

No. ____481____	No. ____481____	MARCH 8 _____	20 __ --
Date ____3/8/—____	Received From JOHN W. SMITH		
To ____JOHN W . SMITH____	ONE HUNDRED TWENTY AND $^{10}/_{100}$ ———————		**Dollars**
For ____POA____	For PAYMENT ON ACCOUNT		
Amount ____$120 \frac{10}{100}$ (ck)____	$ ____$120 \frac{10}{100}$ (ck)____	*Louise M. Simmers*	

FIGURE 22-25 A sample receipt with the receipt stub or register at the left.

issued. In most offices, whether the payment was made by check or cash is also noted.

4. Complete the receipt as follows:
   a. Place the correct number of the receipt in the *No.* space. This number may be preprinted.
   b. Fill in the full date, including month, day, and year.
   c. Write the full name of the person or company from whom payment was received in the *Received From* space. Write legibly. Start at the far left of the line.
   d. On the *Dollars* line, write out in words the amount received. Start at the far left of the line. Note any cents as a fraction. Draw a line from the end of your notation to the printed word *dollars.*
   e. In the *For* space, write a brief reason for the payment.
   f. In the *$* space, fill in the amount in numbers. Write close to the dollar sign. Record cents as a fraction. Note whether payment was made by check or cash.

   g. Sign your name to show that you received the money or items.
5. Recheck all parts of the receipt and stub before issuing the receipt. Make sure the amounts are accurate in both places. Be sure all writing is clear, legible, and accurate.
6. Replace all equipment.

Practice *Use the evaluation sheet for 22:8C, Writing Receipts, to practice this procedure. Note any changes or corrections to the graded assignment sheet number 1. Then follow the steps in the procedure to complete assignment sheet number 2. When you feel you have mastered this skill, sign the evaluation sheet and give it to your instructor for further action.*

 Final Checkpoint   Using the criteria listed on the evaluation sheet, your instructor will grade your performance.

UNIT 22 SUMMARY

Business and accounting skills are used in many health care careers. In addition, many of the skills can be used in the personal life of the health care worker.

Proper use of the telephone, composing professional business letters, completing insurance forms, and writing checks, receipts, and deposit slips are skills that can be utilized by any individual. They are also essential skills for those who work in medical or dental offices, private health care facilities, or business offices of major health care providers.

Proper filing techniques result in excellent organization and allow for easy access to records. Proper scheduling of appointments helps a health care facility function efficiently. Maintaining patient records, such as statistical data sheets and medical

histories, is an important aspect of patient care. Accuracy is essential because medical records are considered legal documents. Bookkeeping systems are used to maintain financial records for health care facilities, including records of services rendered, payments made, and balances due on accounts.

By learning business and accounting skills, the health care worker can choose from a variety of health care careers.

INTERNET SEARCHES

Use the suggested search engines in Unit 11:4 of this textbook to search the Internet for additional information on the following topics:

1. *Accounting methods:* research accounting systems, bookkeeping systems, financial records, and fiscal reports.

2. *Insurance:* research specific insurance companies, health maintenance organizations, and preferred provider organizations to determine their requirements for processing claims.

3. *American Medical Association:* find the AMA site to obtain information on insurance forms and other materials available for purchase.

4. *Banks:* research different banks to compare different types of checking and savings accounts.

5. *Suppliers:* research business and accounting supplies to compare the different types of bookkeeping supplies, appointment ledgers, business stationery, and computer software programs for bookkeeping, patient databases, completing insurance forms, scheduling appointments, and writing checks.

REVIEW QUESTIONS

1. List five (5) rules that must be observed while filing records alphabetically. Create one (1) example to describe each of the rules.

2. File the following numbers in correct numerical order: 08532, 008553, 03251, 0325, 0008564, 00038, 081000, and 0566.

3. You work in a medical office for four (4) different doctors. Create a list of triage questions that you can use to determine if a patient needs an immediate appointment.

4. Identify security measures that must be followed when using electronic mail, cellular phones, and fax machines.

5. Lift five (5) sections on a medical history form. Briefly describe the type of information in each section.

6. Differentiate between a modified-block and a block style letter.

7. What is an ICD-9-CM code? a CPT code? a NPI number?

8. Kaleigh Nartker visits the office with a complaint of abdominal pain. Her previous account balance is $234.55. Charges for the office visit are: consultation $45.00, complete blood count $64.00, urinalysis $38.00, and ECG $76.50. She pays $125.00 by check. What is her new account balance?

UNIT 22

SUGGESTED REFERENCES

Alternative Link Systems, Inc. *The CAM Nursing and Coding Manual.* Clifton Park, NY: Delmar Learning, 2002.

American Dental Association. *Dental Letters with Impact.* Chicago, IL: American Dental Association, 2001.

American Medical Association. *ICD-9-CM Code It Fast.* Chicago, IL: American Medical Association, updated annually.

American Medical Association. *Physician's Current Procedural Terminology (CPT) Codebook.* Chicago, IL: American Medical Association, updated annually.

American Medical Association. *Physician's Office Letters.* Chicago, IL: American Medical Association, 2001.

Atkinson, Phillip S. *Medical Office Practice.* 6th ed. Clifton Park, NY: Delmar Learning, 1999.

Baird, Marijo, and Sandi Laferty. *Tele-Nurse: Telephone Triage Protocols.* Clifton Park, NY: Delmar Learning, 2001.

Browning, Doreen, and Lorraine Villemarie. *Writing Skills for Health Care Professionals.* Clifton Park, NY: Delmar Learning, 2001.

Buck, Carol. *Step-by-Step Medical Coding.* 4th ed. Philadelphia, PA: W.B. Saunders, 2002.

Chapman, Shirley. *Medical and Dental Associates P.C.: Insurance Forms Preparation.* 3rd ed. Clifton Park, NY: Delmar Learning, 1998.

Claeys, Terese. *Medical Filing.* 2nd ed. Clifton Park, NY: Delmar Learning, 1997.

Colwell Systems. *Dental Appointment Forms Kit.* Champaign, IL: Colwell Systems, n.d.

Colwell Systems. *Medical Appointment Forms Kit.* Champaign, IL: Colwell Systems, n.d.

Colwell Systems. *Medical Insurance Reference Manual.* Champaign, IL: Colwell Systems, n.d.

Covell, Alice. *Coding Workbook for the Physician's Office.* 4th ed. Clifton Park, NY: Delmar Learning, 2001.

Dietz, Ellen. *Dental Office Management.* Clifton Park, NY: Delmar Learning, 2000.

Flores, Eleanor K. *Medical Office Procedures with Medical Pegboard.* 4th ed. Clifton Park, NY: Delmar Learning, 2000.

Fordney, Marilyn. *Insurance Handbook for The Medical Office.* 7th ed. Philadelphia, PA: W.B. Saunders, 2001.

Fordney, Marilyn, and Joan Follis. *Administrative Medical Assisting.* 4th ed. Clifton Park, NY: Delmar Learning, 1998.

Fosegan, M., and H. Ginn. *Business Records Control.* 8th ed. Cincinnati, OH: South-Western, 2000.

Gartee, Richard. *The Medical Manager, Version 9.20 Windows.* Clifton Park, NY: Delmar Learning, 2001.

Guthrie, Mearl R., and Carolyn V. Norwood. *Alphabetical Indexing.* 6th ed. Cincinnati, OH: South-Western, 1999.

Humphrey, Doris. *Contemporary Medical Office Procedures.* 2nd ed. Clifton Park, NY: Delmar Learning, 1997.

Humphrey, Doris, and Kathie Sigler. *Delmar's Medical Office Reference Manual.* 3rd ed. Clifton Park, NY: Delmar Learning, 1997.

Johnson, Sandra. *Understanding Medical Coding: A Comprehensive Guide.* Clifton Park, NY: Delmar Learning, 2000.

Keir, Lucille, Connie Krebs, and Barbara A. Wise. *Medical Assisting: Clinical and Administrative Competencies.* 5th ed. Clifton Park, NY: Delmar Learning, 2003.

Lindh, Wilburta, Marilyn Pooler, Carol Tamparo, and Joanne Cerrato. *Delmar's Comprehensive Medical Assisting: Administrative and Clinical Competencies.* 2nd ed. Clifton Park, NY: Delmar Learning, 2002.

McWay, Dana. *Legal Aspects of Health Information Management.* 2nd ed. Clifton Park, NY: Delmar Learning, 2003.

Moisio, Marie. *A Guide to Health Insurance Billing.* Clifton Park, NY: Delmar Learning, 2001.

Moss, Edna Jean. *Basic Keyboarding for the Medical Office.* 2nd ed. Clifton Park, NY: Delmar Learning, 1999.

Rizzo, Christina. *Uniform Billing: A Guide to Claims Processing.* Clifton Park, NY: Delmar Learning, 2000.

Rowell, Jo Ann C., and Michael Green. *Understanding Health Insurance: Guide to Professional Billing.* 6th ed. Clifton Park, NY: Delmar Learning, 2002.

St. Anthony's Physician ICD-9-CM Primer. Clifton Park, NY: Delmar Learning, 2002.

Schultheis, K., A. Kalzmarski, and C. Jones. *Applied Business Mathematics.* 15th ed. Cincinnati, OH: South-Western, 2003.

Shea, Donna, and Adrienne Carter-Ward. *Telephone Triage Card Deck.* Clifton Park, NY: Delmar Learning, 1996.

Simmers, Louise. *Practical Problems in Mathematics for Health Occupations.* Clifton Park, NY: Delmar Learning, 1996.

U.S. Department of Health, Education and Welfare. *International Classification of Diseases.* Washington, DC: U.S. Government Printing Office, updated annually.

For additional information on health careers in medical records, contact the following organization:

◆ American Medical Records Association
  875 N. Michigan Avenue, Suite 1850
  Chicago, IL 60611

Appendix A

Career and Technology Student Organizations (CTSO's)

Career and technology student organizations provide both secondary (high school) and postsecondary (after high school) career/technical students with the opportunity to associate with other students enrolled in the same programs or career areas. Some purposes of these organizations are to:

◆ Develop leadership abilities, citizenship skills, social competencies, and a wholesome attitude about life and work

◆ Strengthen creativity, thinking skills, decision-making abilities, and self-confidence

◆ Enhance the quality and relevance of education by developing the knowledge, skills, and attitudes that lead to successful employment and continuing education

◆ Promote quality of work and pride in occupational excellence through competitive activities

◆ Obtain scholarships for post-secondary education from corporations that recognize the importance of these organizations

The United States Department of Education recognizes and supports the following eight vocational student organizations:

◆ Business Professionals of America (BPA)
◆ Distributive Education Clubs of America (DECA)
◆ Future Business Leaders of America (FBLA)
◆ Future Farmers of America (FFA)
◆ Future Homemakers of America/Home Economics Related Occupations (FHA/HERO)
◆ Health Occupations Students of America (HOSA)
◆ Technology Students of America (TSA)
◆ SkillsUSA-VICA

Two organizations that supplement Health Occupations education are discussed: Health Occupations Students of America (HOSA) and SkillsUSA-VICA.

HEALTH OCCUPATIONS STUDENTS OF AMERICA

Health Occupations Students of America (HOSA, pronounced *Ho'sa*) is the national organization for secondary and postsecondary/collegiate students enrolled in Health Occupations programs. HOSA is endorsed by the U.S. Department of Education and the Health Occupations Education Division of the American Vocational Association. Membership begins at the local level, where students who are enrolled in a Health Occupations education program join together under the supervision of their classroom instructor, who serves as the HOSA local chapter advisor. Local chapters associate with the HOSA state association and the HOSA national organization.

Members of HOSA are involved in community-oriented, career-related, team-building, and leadership-development activities. All HOSA activities relate to the classroom instructional program and the health care delivery system. Furthermore, HOSA is an integral part of the Health Occupations education program, meaning that HOSA activities motivate students and enhance what the students learn in the classroom and on the job.

The mission of HOSA is "to enhance the delivery of compassionate, quality health care by providing opportunities for knowledge, skills, and leadership development of all health occupations education students, therefore, helping the student meet the needs of the health care community." The HOSA motto is "The hands of HOSA mold the health of tomorrow." Goals that HOSA believes are vital for each member are:

◆ To promote physical, mental, and social well-being

◆ To develop effective leadership qualities and skills

◆ To develop the ability to communicate more effectively with people

◆ To develop character

◆ To develop responsible citizenship traits

◆ To understand the importance of pleasing oneself as well as being of service to others

◆ To build self-confidence and pride in one's work

◆ To make realistic career choices and seek successful employment in the health care field

◆ To develop an understanding of the importance of interacting and cooperating with other students and organizations

◆ To encourage individual and group achievement

◆ To develop an understanding of current health care issues, environmental concerns, and survival needs of the community, the nation, and the world

◆ To encourage involvement in local, state, and national health care and education projects

◆ To support health occupations education instructional objectives

In addition to providing activities that allow members to develop occupational skills, leadership qualities, and fellowship through social and recreational activities, HOSA also encourages skill development and a healthy competitive spirit through participation in the National Competitive Events Program. Competition is held at the local, district/regional, state, and national levels. Some of the competitive events include contests in prepared and extemporaneous speaking, job-seeking skills, CPR/first aid, dental assisting, dental laboratory technology, emergency medical technician, clinical and administrative medical assisting, medical laboratory assisting, nursing assisting, practical nursing, physical therapy aide, veterinary assisting, dental spelling and terminology, medical spelling and terminology, extemporaneous health poster, community awareness project (of health-

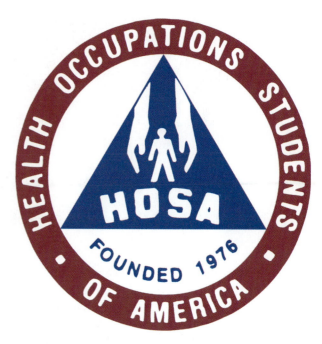

FIGURE A-1 The HOSA emblem. *(With permission of Health Occupations Students of America)*

related issues), creative problem solving, biomedical debate, parliamentary procedure, and the HOSA Bowl.

HOSA has an official emblem, shown in figure A-1. The circle represents the continuity of health care; the triangle represents the three aspects of human well-being: social, physical, and mental; and the hands signify the caring of each HOSA member. The colors of HOSA—maroon, medical white, and navy blue—are represented in the emblem. Navy blue represents loyalty to the health care profession. Medical white represents purity of purpose. Maroon represents the compassion of HOSA members.

The HOSA handbook provides detailed information about the structure, purposes, competitive events, and activities of HOSA. Students interested in further details should refer to this handbook or obtain additional information from the Internet by contacting HOSA at *www.hosa.org*.

SkillsUSA-VICA

Some states do not have HOSA organizations. Students in Health Occupations education programs in these states can participate in SkillsUSA-VICA (pronounced *Vik′a*). It is a national organization for secondary and postsecondary/collegiate students enrolled in training programs in technical, skilled, and service occupations, including health occupations. Examples of these programs include auto mechanics, cosmetology, carpentry, collision repair, computer-aided drafting, electronics, masonry, precision machining, welding, and health occupations. Membership begins with local clubs that affiliate with a state association and then the national organization.

SkillsUSA-VICA's mission is to:

◆ Provide quality education experiences for students in leadership, teamwork, citizenship, and character development

◆ Build and reinforce self-confidence, work attitudes, and communication skills

◆ Emphasize total quality with high ethical standards, superior work skills, life-long education, and pride in the dignity of work

◆ Promote understanding of the free enterprise system and involvement in community service

The SkillsUSA-VICA motto is "Preparing for leadership in the world of work." Some of the purposes include:

◆ To unite in a common bond all students enrolled in technical, skilled, and service occupations, including health occupations

◆ To develop leadership abilities through participation in educational, technical, civic, recreational, and social activities

◆ To foster a deep respect for the dignity of work

◆ To assist students in establishing realistic goals

◆ To help students attain purposeful lives

◆ To create enthusiasm for learning

◆ To promote high standards in trade ethics, workmanship, scholarship, and safety

◆ To develop the ability of students to plan together, organize, and carry out worthy activities and projects through the use of the democratic process

◆ To develop patriotism through a knowledge of our nation's heritage and the practice of democracy

To achieve these purposes, SkillsUSA-VICA offers a *Professional Development Program (PDP), Skills-USA-VICA Total Quality Curriculum,* and SkillsUSA-VICA Championships. The *Professional Development Program (PDP)* is a

self-paced curriculum for students to obtain skills in areas such as effective communication, management, teamwork, networking, workplace ethics, and job interviewing. The *SkillsUSA-VICA Total Quality Curriculum* emphasizes the competencies and essential workplace basic skills identified by employers and the U.S. Secretary of Labor's Commission on Achieving Necessary Skills (SCANS). SkillsUSA-VICA Championships offer skill competition in both leadership and occupational areas. Competition is held at the local, district/ regional, state, and national levels. Examples of leadership contests include prepared and extemporaneous speech, SkillsUSA-VICA ceremonies, club business procedure, job interview, and safety promotion. Examples of career contests for health occupations students include medical assisting, dental assisting, nurse assisting, practical nurse, basic health care skills, first aid and CPR, and a health knowledge bowl.

The official emblem of SkillsUSA-VICA is shown in figure A-2. The shield represents patriotism, or a belief in democracy, liberty, and the American way of life. The torch represents knowledge. The orbital circles represent technology and the training needed to master new technical frontiers along with the need for continuous education. The gear represents the industrial society and the cooperation of the individual working with labor and management for the betterment of humankind. The hands represent the individual

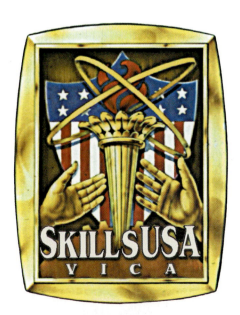

FIGURE A-2 The SkillsUSA-VICA emblem. *(With permission of SkillsUSA-VICA)*

and portray a search for knowledge along with the desire to acquire a skill.

The colors of the SkillsUSA-VICA organization are red, white, blue, and gold. Red and white represent the individual states and chapters. Blue represents the common union of the states and chapters. Gold represents the individual, the most important element of the organization.

The SkillsUSA-VICA Leadership Handbook and other SkillsUSA-VICA publications provide more information on the various activities and programs. Students interested in further details should refer to these sources of information or obtain additional information from the Internet by contacting VICA at *www.skillsusa.org*.

OTHER SOURCES OF INFORMATION

◆ Health Occupations Students of America
6021 Morris Rd., Suite 111
Flower Mound, TX 75028
800-321-HOSA
Internet address: *www.hosa.org*

◆ SkillsUSA-VICA
P.O. Box 3000
Leesburg, Virginia 20177-0300
703-777-8810
Internet address: *www.skillsusa.org*

SUGGESTED REFERENCES

Health Occupations Students of America. *HOSA Handbook: Sections A, B, C.*
SkillsUSA-VICA. *SkillsUSA-VICA Leadership Handbook.*

Appendix B

Metric Conversion Charts

The metric system is gradually replacing other systems of measurement. The following information and charts will assist you in converting measurements.

1. Temperature measurements:
   - To convert Fahrenheit (F) temperatures to Celsius (centigrade) (C) temperatures, subtract 32 from the Fahrenheit temperature and then multiply the result by 5/9, or 0.5556.
   - To convert Celsius (C) temperatures to Fahrenheit (F) temperatures, multiply the Celsius temperature by 9/5, or 1.8, and then add 32 to the total.
   - The chart provides some major temperature equivalents.

2. Linear measurements:
   - To convert inches to centimeters, multiply the number of inches by 2.54 (1 inch = 2.54 centimeters).
   - To convert feet to centimeters, multiply the number of feet by 30.48 centimeters (1 foot = 30.48 centimeters).
   - To convert centimeters to inches, divide the number of centimeters by 2.54.
   - To convert centimeters to feet, divide the number of centimeters by 30.48.

3. Weight measurements:
   - To convert pounds to kilograms, divide the number of pounds by 2.2 (1 kilogram = 2.2 pounds).
   - To convert kilograms to pounds, multiply the number of kilograms by 2.2.

4. Liquid measurements:
   - Note that 1 cubic centimeter (cc) is equal to 1 milliliter (mL).
   - To convert household measurements (e. g., cups, ounces, quarts, or pints) to metric measurements, multiply the household measurement by the equivalent number of cubic centimeters or milliliters. For example, 1 teaspoon equals 5 cubic centimeters. Therefore, 3 teaspoons converted to metric would be 3×5, or 15 cubic centimeters or milliliters.
   - To convert metric measurements to household measurements, divide the metric measurement by the number of metric units in one of the household units. For example, there are 30 cubic centimeters or milliliters in 1 ounce. Therefore, 180 cubic centimeters or milliliters converted to ounces would be $180 \div 30$, or 6 ounces.

FAHRENHEIT–CELSIUS (CENTIGRADE) EQUIVALENTS

F°	C°	F°	C°	F°	C°
32	0	102	38.9	116	46.7
70	21.1	103	39.4	117	47.2
75	23.9	104	40	118	47.8
80	26.7	105	40.6	119	48.3
85	29.4	106	41.1	120	48.9
90	32.2	107	41.7	125	51.7
95	35	108	42.2	130	54.4
96	35.6	109	42.8	135	57.2
97	36.1	110	43.3	140	60
98	36.7	111	43.9	150	65.6
98.6	37	112	44.4	212	100
99	37.2	113	45		
100	37.8	114	45.6		
101	38.3	115	46.1		

LINEAR ENGLISH–METRIC EQUIVALENTS

1 inch (in) = 0.0254 meters (m) = 2.54 centimeters (cm)

12 inches = 1 foot (ft) = 0.3048 meters (m) = 30.48 centimeters (cm)

3 feet = 1 yard (yd) = 0.914 meters (m) = 91.4 centimeters (cm)

5,280 feet = 1 mile = 1601.6 meters (m)

39.372 inches = 3.281 feet = 1 meter (m)

1.094 yards = 1 meter (m)

0.621 miles = 1 kilometer (km)

LIQUID ENGLISH—METRIC EQUIVALENTS

1 drop (gtt) = 0.0667 milliliters (ml)

15 drops (gtts) = 1.0 milliliters (ml)

1 teaspoon (tsp) = 5.0 milliliters (ml)

3 teaspoons = 1 tablespoon (tbsp) = 15.0 milliliters (ml)

1 ounce (oz) = 30.0 milliliters (ml)

8 ounces (oz) = 1 cup (cp) = 240.0 milliliters (ml)

2 cups (cp) = 1 pint (pt) = 500.0 milliliters (ml)

2 pints (pt) = 1 quart (qt) = 1,000.0 milliliters (ml)

Appendix C

24-Hour Clock (Military Time) Conversion Chart

TIME	24-HOUR TIME	TIME	24-HOUR TIME
12:01 AM	0001	12:01 PM	1201
12:05 AM	0005	12:05 PM	1205
12:30 AM	0030	12:30 PM	1230
12:45 AM	0045	12:45 PM	1245
1:00 AM	0100	1:00 PM	1300
2:00 AM	0200	2:00 PM	1400
3:00 AM	0300	3:00 PM	1500
4:00 AM	0400	4:00 PM	1600
5:00 AM	0500	5:00 PM	1700
6:00 AM	0600	6:00 PM	1800
7:00 AM	0700	7:00 PM	1900
8:00 AM	0800	8:00 PM	2000
9:00 AM	0900	9:00 PM	2100
10:00 AM	1000	10:00 PM	2200
11:00 AM	1100	11:00 PM	2300
12:00 NOON	1200	12:00 MIDNIGHT	2400

Glossary

abbreviation—A shortened form of a word, usually just letters.

abdominal—Pertaining to the cavity or area in the front of the body and containing the stomach, the small intestine, part of the large intestine, the liver, the gallbladder, the pancreas, and the spleen.

abduction—Movement away from the midline.

abrasion—Injury caused by rubbing or scraping the skin.

absorption—Act or process of sucking up or in; taking in of nutrients.

abuse—Any care that results in physical harm or pain, or mental anguish.

accelerator—A chemical substance that increases the rate of a chemical reaction.

acceptance—The process of receiving or taking; approval; belief.

acculturation—Process of learning the beliefs and behaviors of a dominant culture and assuming some of the characteristics.

acidosis—A pathological condition resulting from a disturbance in the acid–base balance in the blood and body tissues.

activities of daily living (ADL)—Daily activities necessary to meet basic human needs, for example, feeding, dressing, and elimination.

acute—Lasting a short period of time but relatively severe (e.g., an acute illness).

addiction—State of being controlled by a habit, as can happen with alcohol and drugs.

adduction—Movement toward the midline.

adenitis—Inflammation of a gland or lymph node.

adipose—Fatty tissue; fat.

adolescence—Period of development from 12 to 20 years of age; teenage years.

adrenal—One of two endocrine glands located one above each kidney.

advance directive—A legal document designed to indicate a person's wishes regarding care in case of a terminal illness or during the dying process.

aerobic—Requiring oxygen in order to live and grow.

afebrile—Without a fever.

affection—A warm or tender feeling toward another; fondness.

agar plate—Special laboratory dish containing agar, a gelatinous colloidal extract of a red alga, which is used to provide nourishment for growth of organisms.

agent—Someone who has the power or authority to act as the representative of another.

agglutination—Clumping together, as in the clumping together of red blood cells.

agnostic—Person who believes that the existence of God cannot be proved or disproved.

air compressor—Machine that provides air under pressure; used in dental areas to provide air pressure to operate handpieces and air syringe.

albino—Absence of all color pigments.

alginate—Irreversible, hydrocolloid, dental- impression material.

alignment—Positioning and supporting the body so that all body parts are in correct anatomical position.

alimentary canal—The digestive tract from the esophagus to the rectum.

alopecia—Baldness.

alternative therapy—Method of treatment used in place of biomedical therapies.

alveolar process—Bone tissue of the maxilla and mandible that contains alveoli (sockets) for the roots of the teeth.

alveoli—Microscopic air sacs in the lungs.

Alzheimer's disease—Progressive, irreversible disease involving memory loss, disorientation, deterioration of intellectual function, and speech and gait disturbances.

amalgam—Alloy (mixture) of various metals and mercury; restorative or filling material used primarily on posterior teeth.

ambulate—To walk.

amino acid—The basic component of proteins.

amputation—The cutting off or separation of a body part from the body.

anaerobic—Not requiring oxygen in order to live and grow; able to thrive in the absence of oxygen.

analgesia—The state of inability to feel pain yet still being conscious.

anatomy—The study of the structure of an organism.

anemia—Disease caused by lack of blood or an insufficient number of red blood cells.

anesthesia—The state of inability to feel sensation, especially the sensation of pain.

anger—Feeling of displeasure or hostility; mad.

anorexia—Loss of appetite.

anorexia nervosa—Psychological disorder involving loss of appetite and excessive weight loss not caused by a physical disease.

anoxia—Without oxygen; synonymous with suffocation.

antecubital—The space located on the inner part of the arm and near the elbow.

anterior—Before or in front of.

anterior teeth—Teeth located toward the front of the mouth; includes incisor and cuspids.

antibody—Substance, usually a protein, formed by the body to produce an immunity to an antigen or pathogen.

antibody screen—Test that checks for antibodies in the blood prior to a transfusion.

anticoagulant—Substance that prevents clotting of the blood.

antigen—Substance that causes the body to produce antibodies; may be introduced into the body or formed within the body.

antioxidants—Enzymes or organic molecules; help protect the body from harmful chemicals called free radicals.

antisepsis—Aseptic control that inhibits, retards growth of, or kills pathogenic organisms; not effective against spores and viruses.

anuria—Without urine; producing no urine.

anus—External opening of the anal canal, or rectum.

aorta—Largest artery in the body; carries blood away from the heart.

aortic valve—Flap or cusp located between the left ventricle of the heart and the aorta.

apathy—Indifference; lack of emotion.

apex—The pointed extremity of a conelike structure; the rounded, lower end of the heart, below the ventricles.

aphasia—Language impairment; loss of ability to comprehend or speak normally.

apical foramen—The opening in the apex of a tooth; allows nerves and blood vessels to enter tooth.

apical pulse—Pulse taken with a stethoscope and near the apex of the heart.

apnea—Absence of respirations; temporary cessation of respirations.

apoplexy—A stroke; *see* **cerebrovascular accident.**

appendicular skeleton—The bones that form the limbs or extremities of the body.

application form—A form or record completed when applying for a job.

appointment—A schedule to do something on a particular day and time.

aquamatic pad—Temperature-controlled unit that circulates warm liquid through a pad to provide dry heat.

aqueous humor—Watery liquid that circulates in the anterior chamber of the eye.

arrhythmia—Irregular or abnormal rhythm, usually referring to the heart rhythm.

arterial—Pertaining to an artery.

arteriole—Smallest branch of an artery; vessel that connects arteries to capillaries.

arteriosclerosis—Hardening and/or narrowing of the walls of arteries.

artery—Blood vessel that carries blood away from the heart.

arthritis—Inflammation of a joint.

asepsis—Being free from infection.

aspirate—To remove by suction.

aspirating syringe—Special dental anesthetic syringe designed to hold carpules.

assault—Physical or verbal attack on another person; treatment or care given to a person without obtaining proper consent.

assistant—Level of occupational proficiency where an individual can work in an occupation after a period of education or on-the-job training.

associate's degree—Degree awarded by a vocational–technical school or community college after successful completion of a two-year course of study or its equivalent.

astigmatism—Defect or blurring of vision caused by irregularity of the cornea of the eye.

atheist—Person who does not believe in any deity.

atherosclerosis—Form of arteriosclerosis characterized by accumulation of fats or mineral deposits on the inner walls of the arteries.

atrium—Also called an *auricle;* an upper chamber of the heart.

atrophy—Wasting away of tissue; decrease in size.

audiologist—Individual specializing in diagnosis and treatment of hearing disorders.

audiometer—Instrument used to test hearing and determine hearing defects.

aural temperature—Measurement of body temperature at the tympanic membrane in the ear.

auricle—Also called the *pinna;* external part of the ear.

auscultation—Process of listening for sounds in the body.

autoclave—Piece of equipment used to sterilize articles by way of steam under pressure and/or dry heat.

autonomic nervous system—That division of the nervous system concerned with reflex, or involuntary, activities of the body.

avulsion—A wound that occurs when tissue is separated from the body.

axial skeleton—The bones of the skull, rib cage, and spinal column; the bones that form the trunk of the body.

axilla—Armpit; that area of the body under the arm.

Ayer blade—Wooden or plastic blade used to scrape cells from the cervix of the uterus; used for Pap tests.

B

bachelor's degree—Degree awarded by a college or university after a person has completed a four-year course of study or its equivalent.

bacteria—One-celled microorganisms, some of which are beneficial and some of which cause disease.

bandage—Material used to hold dressings in place, secure splints, and support and protect body parts.

bandage scissors—Special scissors with a blunt lower end used to remove dressings and bandages.

bargaining—Process of negotiating an agreement, sale, or exchange.

Bartholin's glands—Two small mucous glands near the vaginal opening.

basal metabolism—The amount of energy needed to maintain life when the subject is at complete rest.

base—Protective (dental) material placed over the pulpal area of a tooth to reduce irritation and thermal shock.

base of support—Standing with feet 8 to 10 inches apart to provide better balance.

battery—Unlawfully touching another person without that person's consent.

bed cradle—A device placed on a bed to keep the top bed linens from contacting the legs and feet.

benign—Not malignant or cancerous.

bias—A preference that inhibits impartial judgment.

bicuspids—Also called *premolars;* the teeth that pulverize or grind food and are located between cuspids and molars.

bifurcated—Having two roots (as in teeth).

bile—Liver secretion that is concentrated and stored in the gallbladder; aids in the emulsification of fats during digestion.

binders—Devices applied to hold dressings in place, provide support, apply pressure, or limit motion.

biohazardous—Contaminated with blood or body fluid and having the potential to transmit disease.

biopsy—Excision of a small piece of tissue for microscopic examination.

bitewing—Also called a *cavity-detecting X-ray;* a dental X-ray that shows only the crowns of the teeth.

bladder—Membranous sac or storage area for a secretion (gallbladder); also, the vesicle that acts as the reservoir for urine.

bland diet—Diet containing only mild-flavored foods with soft textures.

block style—Letter format in which all parts of the letter start at the left margin.

blood—Fluid that circulates through the vessels in the body to carry substances to all body parts.

blood pressure—Measurement of the force exerted by the heart against the arterial walls when the heart contracts (beats) and relaxes.

blood smear—A drop of blood spread thinly on a slide for microscopic examination.

body—Main content, or message part, of a letter.

body mechanics—The way in which the body moves and maintains balance; proper body mechanics involves the most efficient use of all body parts.

bolus—Food that has been chewed and mixed with saliva.

bowel—The intestines.

Bowman's capsule—Part of the renal corpuscle in the kidney; picks up substances filtered from the blood by the glomerulus.

brachial—Pertaining to the brachial artery in the arm, which is used to measure blood pressure.

bradycardia—Slow heart rate, usually below 60 beats per minute.

bradypnea—Slow respiratory rate, usually below 10 respirations per minute.

brain—Soft mass of nerve tissue inside the cranium.

brand name—Company or product name given to a medication or product.

breast—Mammary, or milk, gland located on the upper part of the front surface of the body.

bronchi—Two main branches of the trachea; air tubes to and from the lungs.

bronchioles—Small branches of the bronchi; carry air in the lungs.

budget—An itemized list of income and expected expenditures for a period of time.

buccal surface—Outside surface of the posterior teeth; surface facing the cheek; facial surface of bicuspids and molars.

buffer period—Period of time kept open on an appointment schedule to allow for emergencies, telephone calls, and other unplanned situations.

bulimarexia—Psychological condition in which person eats excessively and then uses laxatives or vomits to get rid of the food.

bulimia—Psychological condition in which person alternately eats excessively and then fasts or refuses to eat.

burn—Injury to body tissue caused by heat, caustics, radiation, and/or electricity.

burs—Small, rotating instruments of various types; used in dental handpieces to prepare cavities for filling with restorative materials.

C

calcaneous—Large tarsal bone that forms the heel.

calculus—Also called *tartar;* hard, calcium-like deposit that forms on the teeth; a stone that forms in various parts of the body from a variety of different substances.

calorie—Unit of measurement of the fuel value of food.

cane—A rod used as an aid in walking.

capillary—Tiny blood vessel that connects arterioles and venules and allows for exchange of nutrients and gases between the blood and the body cells.

carbohydrate-controlled diet—Diet in which the number and types of carbohydrates are restricted or limited.

carbohydrates—Group of chemical substances including sugars, cellulose, and starches; nutrients that provide the greatest amount of energy in the average diet.

cardiac—Pertaining to the heart.

cardiopulmonary—Pertaining to the heart and lungs.

cardiopulmonary resuscitation (CPR)—Procedure of providing oxygen and chest compressions to a victim whose heart has stopped beating.

cardiovascular—Pertaining to the heart and blood vessels.

caries—Tooth decay, an infectious disease that destroys tooth tissue.

carious lesion—An occurrence of tooth decay.

carpal—Bone of the wrist.

carpule—A glass cartridge that contains a premeasured amount of anesthetic solution; used for dental anesthesia.

cataract—Condition of the eye where the lens becomes cloudy or opaque, leading to blindness.

catheter—A rubber, metal, or other type of tube that is passed into a body cavity and used for injecting or removing fluids.

caudal—Pertaining to any tail or tail-like structure.

cavitation—The cleaning process employed in an ultrasonic unit; bubbles explode to drive cleaning solution onto article being cleaned.

cavity—A hollow space, such as a body cavity (which contains organs) or a hole in a tooth.

cell—Mass of protoplasm; the basic unit of structure of all animals and plants.

cell membrane—Outer, protective, semipermeable covering of a cell.

cellulose—Fibrous form of carbohydrate.

cement—Dental material used to seal inlays, crowns, bridges, and orthodontic appliances in place.

cementum—Hard, bonelike tissue that covers the outside of the root of a tooth.

central nervous system—The division of the nervous system consisting of the brain and spinal cord.

central processing unit (CPU)—Unit that controls all of the work of a computer; frequently called the "brains" of the computer.

centrifuge—A machine that uses centrifugal (driving away from the center) force to separate heavier materials from lighter ones.

centrosome—That area of cell cytoplasm that contains two centrioles; important in reproduction of the cell.

cerebellum—The section of the brain that is dorsal to the pons and medulla oblongata; maintains balance and equilibrium.

cerebrovascular accident—Also called a *stroke* or *apoplexy;* an interrupted supply of blood to the brain, caused by formation of a clot, blockage of an artery, or rupture of a blood vessel.

cerebrospinal fluid—Watery, clear fluid that surrounds the brain and spinal cord.

cerebrum—Largest section of brain; involved in sensory interpretation and voluntary muscle activity.

certification—The issuing of a statement or certificate by a professional organization to a person who has met the requirements of education and/or experience and who meets the standards set by the organization.

cervical—Pertaining to the neck portion of the spinal column or to the lower part of the uterus.

cervix—Anatomical part of a tooth where the crown joins with the root; entrance to or lower part of the uterus.

chain of infection—Factors that lead to the transmission or spread of disease.

character—The quality of respirations (e.g., deep, shallow, or labored).

charge slip—A record on which charges or costs for services are listed.

check—A written order for payment of money through a bank.

chemical—The method of aseptic control in which substances or solutions are used to disinfect articles; does not always kill spores and viruses.

chemical abuse—Use of chemical substances without regard for accepted practice; dependence on alcohol or drugs.

chemotherapy—Treatment of a disease by way of chemical agents.

Cheyne–Stokes respirations—Periods of difficult breathing (dyspnea) followed by periods of no respirations (apnea).

chiropractic—System of treatment based on manipulation of the spinal column and other body structures.

cholelithiasis—Condition of stones in the gallbladder.

cholesterol—Fat-like substance synthesized in the liver and found in body cells and animal fats.

choroid—Middle or vascular layer of the eye, between the sclera and retina.

chromatin network—That structure in the nucleus of a cell that contains chromosomes with genes, which carry inherited characteristics.

chronic—Lasting a long period of time; reoccurring.

cilia—Hairlike projections.

circumduction—Moving in a circle at a joint, or moving one end of a body part in a circle while the other end remains stationary.

citizenship—Status of being a citizen (including associated duties, rights, and privileges).

clavicle—Collarbone.

clean—Free from organisms causing disease.

clear-liquid diet—Diet containing only water-based liquids; nutritionally inadequate.

clinic—Institution that provides care for outpatients; a group of specialists working in cooperation.

closed bed—Bed that is made following the discharge of a patient.

coccyx—The tailbone; lowest bones of the vertebral column.

cochlea—Snail-shaped section of the inner ear; contains the organ of Corti for hearing.

collection—To receive; a letter requesting payment on an account.

colon—The large intestine.

colostomy—An artificial opening into the colon; allows for the evacuation of feces.

communicable disease—Disease that is transmitted from one individual to another.

communication—Process of transmission; exchange of thoughts or information.

compensation—Something given or received as an equivalent for a loss, service, or debt; defense mechanism involving substitution of one goal for another goal to achieve success.

competent—Able, capable.

complementary therapy—Method of treatment used in conjunction with biomedical therapies.

complete bed bath—A bath in which all parts of a patient's body are bathed while the patient is confined to bed.

complimentary close—Courtesy closing of a letter (e.g., *Sincerely*).

composite—The dental restorative or filling material used most frequently on anterior teeth.

compress—A folded wet or dry cloth applied firmly to a body part.

computer-assisted instruction (CAI)—Teaching method in which a computer and computer programs are used to control the learning process and deliver the instructional material to the learner.

computerized tomography (CT)—A scanning and detection system that uses a minicomputer and display screen to visualize an internal portion of the human body; formerly known as *CAT (computerized axial tomography)*.

concave—Curved inward; depressed.

confidential—Not to be shared or told; to be held in confidence, or kept to oneself.

congenital—Present at birth (as in a congenital defect).

conjunctiva—Mucous membrane that lines the eyelids and covers the anterior part of the sclera of the eye.

connective tissue—Body tissue that connects, supports, or binds body organs.

constipation—Difficulty in emptying the bowel; infrequent bowel movements.

constrict—To contract or narrow; to make smaller.

consultation—Process of seeking information or advice from another person.

contamination—Containing infection or infectious organisms or germs.

contra angle—Attachment used on dental handpieces to cut and polish.

contract—To shorten, decrease in size, or draw together; an agreement between two or more persons.

contracture—Tightening or shortening of a muscle.

conventional-speed handpiece—Low-speed handpiece in dental units; used to remove caries and for fine-finishing work.

convex—Curved outward; projected.

convulsion—Also called a *seizure;* a violent, involuntary contraction of muscles.

cornea—The transparent section of the sclera; allows light rays to enter the eye.

cortex—The outer layer of an organ or structure.

cost containment—Procedures used to control costs or expenses.

Cowper's glands—The pair of small mucous glands near the male urethra.

cranial—Pertaining to the skull or cranium.

cranium—Part of the skull; the eight bones of the head that enclose the brain.

criticism—Judgment regarding worth; censure, disapproval; evaluation.

cross index/reference—A paper or card used in filing systems to prevent misplacement or loss of records.

cross-match—A blood test that checks the compatibility of the donor's blood and the recipient's blood before a transfusion.

crown—The anatomical portion of a tooth that is exposed in the oral cavity, above the gingiva, or gums.

crust—A scab; outer covering or coat.

crutches—Artificial supports that assist a patient in walking.

cryotherapy—Use of cold applications for treatment.

cultural assimilation—Absorption of a culturally distinct group into a dominant or prevailing culture.

cultural diversity—Differences among individuals based on cultural, ethnic, and racial factors.

culture—Values, beliefs, ideas, customs, and characteristics passed from one generation to the next.

culture specimen—A sample of microorganisms or tissue cells taken from an area of the body for examination.

cuspid—Also called a *canine* or *eyetooth;* the type of tooth located at angle of lips and used to tear food.

custom tray—Dental impression tray specially made to fit a particular patient's mouth.

cyanosis—Bluish color of the skin, nail beds, and/or lips due to an insufficient amount of oxygen in the blood.

cystitis—Inflammation of the urinary bladder.

cystoscope—Instrument for examining the inside of the urinary bladder.

cytoplasm—The fluid inside a cell; contains water, proteins, lipids, carbohydrates, minerals, and salts.

D

dangling—Positioning the patient in a sitting position with his or her feet and legs over the side of the bed prior to ambulation.

day sheet—A daily record listing all financial transactions and/or patients seen.

daydreaming—Defense mechanism of escape; dreamlike musing while awake.

deciduous teeth—Also called *primary teeth;* the first set of 20 teeth.

decubitus ulcer—*See* **pressure (decubitus) ulcer.**

deduction—Something subtracted or taken out (e.g., monies taken out of a paycheck for various purposes).

defamation—Slander or libel; a false statement that causes ridicule or damage to a reputation.

defecation—Evacuation of fecal material from the bowel; a bowel movement.

defense mechanism—Physical or psychological reaction of an organism used in self-defense or to protect self-image.

dehydration—Insufficient amounts of fluid in the tissues.

dementia—Loss of mental ability characterized by decrease in intellectual ability, loss of memory, impaired judgment, and disorientation.

denial—Declaring untrue; refusing to believe.

dental chair—Special chair designed to position a patient comfortably while providing easy access to the patient's oral cavity.

dental hygienist—A licensed individual who works with a dentist to provide care and treatment for the teeth and gums.

dental light—Light used in dental units to illuminate the oral cavity.

dentin—Tissue that makes up the main bulk of a tooth.

dentist—A doctor who specializes in diagnosis, prevention, and treatment of diseases of the teeth and gums.

dentition—The number, type, and arrangement of teeth in the mouth.

denture—An entire set of teeth; usually refers to artificial teeth designed to replace natural teeth.

dependable—Capable of being relied on; trustworthy.

deposit slip—A bank record listing all cash and checks that are to be placed in an account, either checking or savings.

depression—Psychological condition of sadness, melancholy, gloom, or despair.

dermis—The skin.

diabetes mellitus—Metabolic disease caused by an insufficient secretion or utilization of insulin and leading to an increased amount of glucose (sugar) in the blood and urine.

diabetic coma—An unconscious condition caused by an increased level of glucose (sugar) and ketones in the bloodstream of a person with diabetes mellitus.

diagnosis—Determination of the nature of a person's disease.

dialysis—Removal of urine substances from the blood by way of passing solutes through a membrane.

diaphoresis—Profuse or excessive perspiration, or sweating.

diaphysis—The shaft, or middle section, of a long bone.

diarrhea—Frequent bowel movements with watery stool.

diastole—Period of relaxation of the heart.

diastolic pressure—Measurement of blood pressure taken when the heart is at rest; measurement of the constant pressure in arteries.

diencephalon—The section of the brain between the cerebrum and midbrain; contains the thalamus and hypothalamus.

dietitian—An individual who specializes in the science of diet and nutrition.

differential count—Blood test that determines the percentage of each kind of leukocyte (white blood cell).

digestion—Physical and chemical breakdown of food by the body in preparation for absorption.

digital—Pertaining to fingers or toes; examination with the fingers.

dilate—Enlarge or expand; to make bigger.

direct smear—A culture specimen placed on a slide for microscopic examination.

disability—A physical or mental handicap that interferes with normal function; incapacitated, incapable.

discretion—Ability to use good judgment and self-restraint in speech or behavior.

disease—Any condition that interferes with the normal function of the body.

disinfection—Aseptic-control method that destroys pathogens but does not usually kill spores and viruses.

dislocation—Displacement of a bone at a joint.

disorientation—Confusion with regard to the identity of time, place, or person.

displacement—Defense mechanism in which feelings about one person are transferred to someone else.

distal—Most distant or farthest from the trunk; center or midline.

distal surface—Side surface of teeth that is toward the back of the mouth, or away from the midline of the mouth.

diuretics—Drugs that increase urinary output; "water pills."

doctorate—Degree awarded by a college or university after completion of a prescribed course of study beyond a bachelor's or master's degree.

dorsal—Pertaining to the back; in back of.

dorsal recumbent position—The patient lies on the back with the knees flexed and separated; used for vaginal and pelvic examinations.

douche—*See* **vaginal irrigation.**

dressing—Covering placed over a wound or injured part.

dry cold—Application that provides cold temperature but is dry against the skin.

dry heat—Application that provides warm temperature but is dry against the skin.

duodenum—First part of the small intestine; connects the pylorus of the stomach and the jejunum.

dyspepsia—Difficulty in digesting food; indigestion.

dysphagia—Difficulty in swallowing.

dyspnea—Difficult or labored breathing.

dystrophy—Progressive weakening (atrophy) of a body part, such as a muscle.

dysuria—Difficult or painful urination.

E

early adulthood—Period of development from 20 to 40 years of age.

early childhood—Period of development from 1 to 6 years of age.

echocardiography—A diagnostic test that uses ultra-high-frequency sound waves to evaluate the structure and function of the heart.

edema—Swelling; excess amount of fluid in the tissues.

ejaculation—Expulsion of seminal fluid from the male urethra.

ejaculatory duct—In the male, duct or tube from the seminal vesicle to the urethra.

electrocardiogram (ECG or EKG)—Graphic tracing of the electrical activity of the heart.

electroencephalogram (EEG)—Graphic recording of the brain waves or electrical activity in the brain.

emblem—A symbol; identifying badge, design, or device.

embolus—A blood clot or mass of material circulating in the blood vessels.

embryo—Unborn infant during the first 3 months of development.

emesis—Vomiting; expulsion of the contents of the stomach and/or intestine through the mouth and/or nose.

emotional—Pertaining to feelings or psychological states.

empathy—Identifying with another's feelings but being unable to change or solve the situation.

enamel—Hardest tissue in the body; covers the outside of the crown of a tooth.

endocardium—Serous membrane lining of the heart.

endocrine—Ductless gland that produces an internal secretion discharged into the blood or lymph.

endodontics—Branch of dentistry involving treatment of the pulp chamber and root canals of the teeth; root canal treatment.

endogenous—Infection or disease originating within the body.

endometrium—Mucous membrane lining of the inner surface of the uterus.

endoplasmic reticulum—Fine network of tubular structures in the cytoplasm of a cell; allows for the transport of materials in and out of the nucleus and aids in the synthesis and storage of protein.

endorsement—A written signature on the back of a check; required in order to receive payment.

endoscope—An instrument used to examine the inside of the body.

endosteum—Membrane lining the medullary canal of a bone.

enema—An injection of fluid into the large intestine through the rectum.

enthusiasm—Intense interest or excitement.

entrepreneur—Individual who organizes, manages, and assumes the risk of a business.

enunciate—To speak clearly, using correct pronunciation.

enzyme—A chemical substance that causes or increases the rate of a chemical reaction.

epidermis—The outer layer of the skin.

epididymis—Tightly coiled tube in the scrotal sac; connects the testes with the vas or ductus deferens.

epigastric—Pertaining to the area of the abdomen above the stomach.

epiglottis—Leaf-shaped structure that closes over the larynx during swallowing.

epilepsy—A chronic disease of the nervous system characterized by motor and sensory dysfunction, sometimes accompanied by convulsions and unconsciousness.

epiphysis—The end or head at the extremity of a long bone.

epistaxis—Nosebleed.

epithelial tissue—Tissue that forms the skin and parts of the secreting glands, and that lines the body cavities.

ergonomics—An applied science used to promote the safety and well-being of a person by adapting the environment and using techniques to prevent injuries.

erythema—Redness of the skin.

erythrocyte—Red blood cell (RBC).

erythrocyte count—Blood test that counts the number of red blood cells (normally 4 to 6 million per cubic millimeter of blood).

erythrocyte sedimentation rate (ESR)—Blood test that determines the rate at which red blood cells settle out of the blood.

esophagus—Tube that extends from the pharynx to the stomach.

essential nutrients—Those elements in food required by the body for proper function.

esteem—Place a high value on; respect.

ethics—Principles of right or good conduct.

ethnicity—Classification of people based on national origin and/or culture.

ethnocentric—Belief in the superiority of one's own ethnic group.

etiology—The study of the cause of a disease.

eustachian tube—Tube that connects the middle ear and the pharynx, or throat.

eversion—Turning a body part outward.

exocrine—Gland with a duct that produces a secretion.

exogenous—Infection or disease originating outside of or external to the body.

expectorate—To spit; to expel mucus, phlegm, or sputum from the throat or respiratory passages.

expiration—The expulsion of air from the lungs; breathing out air.

extension—Increasing the angle between two parts; straightening a limb.

external auditory canal—Passageway or tube extending from the auricle of the ear to the tympanic membrane.

F

facial surface—The tooth surface nearest the lips or cheek; includes the labial and buccal surfaces.

fainting—Partial or complete loss of consciousness caused by a temporary reduction in the supply of blood to the brain.

fallopian tubes—Oviducts; in the female, passageway for the ova (egg) from the ovary to uterus.

false imprisonment—Restraining an individual or restricting an individual's freedom.

fanfold—Folding in accordion pleats; done with bed linens.

fascia—Fibrous membrane covering, supporting, and separating muscles.

fasting blood sugar (FBS)—Blood test that measures blood serum levels of glucose (sugar) after a person has had nothing by mouth for a period of time.

fat—Also called a *lipid;* nutrient that provides the most concentrated form of energy; highest-calorie energy nutrient; overweight.

fat-restricted diet—Diet with limited amounts of fats, or lipids.

febrile—Pertaining to a fever, or elevated body temperature.

feces—Also called *stool;* waste material discharged from the bowel.

Federation Dentaire International System—Abbreviated means of identifying the teeth that uses a two-digit code to identify the quadrant and tooth.

femur—Thigh bone of the leg; the longest and strongest bone in the body.

fertilization—Conception; impregnation of the ovum by the sperm.

fetus—Unborn infant from the end of the third month of pregnancy until birth.

fever—Elevated body temperature, usually above 101°F, or 38.3°C, rectally.

fibula—Outer and smaller bone of the lower leg.

filing—Arranging in order.

fire extinguisher—A device that can be used to put out fires.

first aid—Immediate care given to a victim of an injury or illness to minimize the effects of the injury or illness.

fixed expenses—Those items in a budget that are set and usually do not change (e.g., rent and car payments).

flatus—Air or gas in the intestines.

flexion—Decreasing the angle between two parts; bending a limb.

fomite—Any substance or object that adheres to and transmits infectious material.

foramina—A passage or opening; a hole in a bone through which blood vessels or nerves pass.

Fowler's position—The patient lies on the back with the head elevated at one of several different angles.

fracture—A break (usually, a break in a bone or tooth).

frontal plane—Imaginary line that separates the body into a front section and a back section.

frostbite—Actual freezing of tissue fluid resulting in damage to the skin and underlying tissue.

full liquid diet—Diet consisting of liquids and foods that are liquid at body temperature.

fungi—Group of simple, plantlike animals that live on dead organic matter (e.g., yeast and molds).

G

gait—Method or manner of walking.

gallbladder—Small sac near the liver; concentrates and stores bile.

gastric—Pertaining to the stomach.

generic name—Chemical name of a drug; name not protected by a trademark.

genital—Pertaining to the organs of reproduction.

geriatrics, gerontology—The study of the aged or old age and treatment of related diseases and conditions.

gingiva—The gums (tissues surrounding the teeth).

glaucoma—Eye disease characterized by increased intraocular pressure.

glomerulus—Microscopic cluster of capillaries in Bowman's capsule of the nephron in the kidney.

glucose meter—Instrument used to measure blood-glucose (blood-sugar) level.

glucose—The most common type of sugar in the body.

glycosuria—Presence of sugar in the urine.

goal—Desired result or purpose toward which one is working.

Golgi apparatus—That structure in the cytoplasm of a cell that produces, stores, and packages secretions for discharge from the cell.

gonads—Sex glands, ovaries in the female and testes in the male.

Gram's stain—Technique of staining organisms to identify specific types of bacteria present.

graphic chart—Record used to record vital signs (e.g., temperature, pulse, and respirations) and other information.

groin—Area between the abdomen and upper inner thigh.

gross income—Amount of pay earned before deductions are taken out.

gynecology—The study of diseases of women, especially those affecting the reproductive organs.

H

halitosis—Bad breath.

hard copy—Computer term for a printed copy of information.

hard palate—Bony structure that forms the roof of the mouth.

hardware—Machine or physical components of a computer system (usually, the parts of the computer and the peripherals).

heading—That section of a letter containing the address of the person sending the letter and the date of writing.

heart attack—*See* **myocardial infarction.**

heat cramp—Muscle pain and spasm resulting from exposure to heat and inadequate fluid and salt intake.

heat exhaustion—Condition resulting from exposure to heat and excessive loss of fluid through sweating.

heat stroke—Medical emergency caused by prolonged exposure to heat, resulting in high body temperature and failure of sweat glands.

hemacytometer—Specially calibrated instrument with a measured and lined area for counting blood cells.

hematemesis—Vomiting of blood.

hematocrit—Blood test that measures the percentage of red blood cells per a given unit of blood.

hematology—The study of blood and blood diseases.

hematuria—Blood in the urine.

hemiplegia—Paralysis on one side of the body.

hemoglobin—The iron-containing protein of the red blood cells; serves to carry oxygen from the lungs to the tissues.

hemolysis—Disintegration of red blood cells, causing cells to dissolve or go into solution.

hemoptysis—Spitting up blood; blood-stained sputum.

hemorrhage—Excessive loss of blood; bleeding.

hemorrhoids—Varicose veins of the anal canal or anus.

hemostat—Instrument used to compress (clamp) blood vessels to stop bleeding.

heparin—A substance formed in the liver to prevent the clotting of blood; an anticoagulant.

hepatitis—Inflammation of the liver.

high-fiber diet—Diet containing large amounts of fiber, or indigestible food.

high-protein diet—Diet containing large amounts of protein-rich foods.

high-velocity evacuator—Dental handpiece used to remove particles and large amounts of liquid from the oral cavity.

holistic health care—Care that promotes physical, emotional, social, intellectual, and spiritual well-being.

home health care—Any type of health care provided in a patient's home environment.

homeostasis—A constant state of natural balance within the body.

honesty—Truthfulness; integrity.

horizontal recumbent position—*See* **supine position.**

hormone—Chemical substance secreted by an organ or gland.

HOSA—Health Occupations Students of America, a national organization for students enrolled in health occupations programs.

hospice—Program designed to provide care for the terminally ill while allowing them to die with dignity.

hospital—Institution that provides medical or surgical care and treatment for the sick or injured.

humerus—Long bone of the upper arm.

hydrocollator packs—Gel-filled packs that are warmed in a water bath to provide a moist heat application.

hygiene—Principles for health preservation and disease prevention.

hyperglycemia—Presence of sugar in the blood; high blood sugar.

hyperopia—Farsightedness; defect in near vision.

hypertension—High blood pressure.

hyperthermia—Condition that occurs when body temperature exceeds 104°F, or 40°C, rectally.

hypoglycemia—Low blood sugar.

hypotension—Low blood pressure.

hypothalamus—That structure in the diencephalon of the brain that regulates and controls many body functions.

hypothermia—Condition in which body temperature is below normal, usually below 95°F (35°C) and often in the range of 78° to 95°F (26° to 35°C).

hypothermia blanket—Special blanket containing coils filled with a cooling solution; used to reduce high body temperature.

hypoxia—Without oxygen.

I

ice bag/collar—Plastic or rubber device filled with ice to provide dry-cold application.

idiopathic—Without recognizable cause; self-originating.

ileostomy—A surgical opening connecting the ileum (small intestine) and the abdominal wall.

ileum—Final section of small intestine; connects the jejunum and large intestine.

immunity—Condition of being protected against a particular disease.

impaction—A large, hard mass of fecal material lodged in the intestine or rectum; a tooth that does not erupt into the mouth.

impression—Negative reproduction of a tooth or dental arch.

incisal surface—The cutting or biting surface of anterior teeth.

incision—Cut or wound of body tissue caused by a sharp object; a surgical cut.

incisors—Teeth located in the front and center of the mouth; used to cut food.

income—Total amount of money received in a given period (usually a year); salary is usually the main source.

incontinent—Unable to voluntarily control urination or defecation.

index—To put names in proper order for filing purposes.

infancy—Period of development from birth to 1 year of age.

infection—Invasion by organisms; contamination by disease-producing organisms, or pathogens.

inferior—Below; under.

inflammation—Tissue reaction to injury characterized by heat, redness, swelling, and pain.

informed consent—Permission granted voluntarily by a person who is of sound mind and aware of all factors involved.

inguinal—Pertaining to the region of the body where the thighs join the trunk; the groin.

inhalation—Breathing in.

initiative—Ability to begin or follow through with a plan or task; determination.

input—Computer term for information that is entered into a computer.

inquiry—Search for information.

insertion—End or area of a muscle that moves when the muscle contracts.

inside address—That section of a letter that contains the name and address of the person or firm to whom the letter is being sent.

inspiration—Breathing in; taking air into the lungs.

insulin shock—Condition that occurs in diabetics when there is an excess amount of insulin and a low level of glucose (sugar) in the blood.

insurance form—A form used to apply for payment by an insurance company.

intake and output (I & O)—A record that notes all fluids taken in or eliminated by a person in a given period of time.

integumentary—Pertaining to the skin or a covering.

interactive video—The color, sound, and motion of video technology integrated with computer-assisted instruction to create a new technology.

intercostal—Pertaining to the space between the ribs (costae).

interproximal space—The area between two adjoining teeth.

intestine—That portion of the alimentary canal from the stomach to the rectum and anus.

intradermal—Inserted or put into the skin.

intramuscular—Injected or put into a muscle.

intravenous—Injected or put into a vein.

intubate—To insert a tube.

invasion of privacy—Revealing personal information about an individual without his or her consent.

invasive—Pertains to a test or procedure that involves penetrating or entering the body.

inversion—Turning a body part inward.

involuntary—Independent action not controlled by choice or desire.

iris—Colored portion of the eye; composed of muscular, or contractile, tissue that regulates the size of the pupil.

ischemia—Inadequate blood flow to the body tissues caused by an obstruction in circulation.

isolation—Method or technique of caring for persons who have communicable diseases.

J

jackknife position—The patient lies on the abdomen with both the head and legs inclined downward and the rectal area elevated.

jaundice—Yellow discoloration of the skin and eyes, frequently caused by liver or gallbladder disease.

jejunum—The middle section of the small intestine; connects the duodenum and ileum.

job interview—A face-to-face meeting or conversation between an employer and an applicant for a job.

joint—An articulation, or area where two bones meet or join.

K

kcal-controlled diet—Diet containing low-calorie foods; frequently prescribed for weight loss.

kidney—Bean-shaped organ that excretes urine; located high and in back of the abdominal cavity.

kilocalorie—Unit used to measure the energy value of food.

kilojoule—Metric unit used to measure the energy value of food.

knee–chest position—The patient rests his or her body weight on the knees and chest; used for sigmoidoscopic and rectal examinations.

L

labia majora—Two large folds of adipose tissue lying on each side of the vulva in the female; hairy outer lips.

labia minora—Two folds of membrane lying inside the labia majora; hairless inner lips.

labial surface—Crown surface of the anterior teeth that lies next to the lips; facial surface of the anterior teeth.

laboratory—A room or building where scientific tests, research, experiments, or learning takes place.

laceration—Wound or injury with jagged, irregular edges.

lacrimal—Pertaining to tears; glands that secrete and expel tears.

lactation—Process of secreting milk.

lacteal—Specialized lymphatic capillary that picks up digested fats or lipids in the small intestine and transports them to the thoracic duct.

lancet—Sharp, pointed instrument used to pierce the skin to obtain blood.

laryngeal mirror—Instrument with a mirror, used to examine larynx.

larynx—Voice box, located between the pharynx and trachea.

late adulthood—Period of development beginning at 65 years of age and ending at death.

late childhood—Period of development from 6 to 12 years of age.

lateral—Pertaining to the side.

lead—An angle or view of the heart that is recorded in an electrocardiogram.

leadership—Ability to lead, guide, and direct others.

ledger card—A card or record that shows a financial account of money charged, received, or paid out.

left lateral position—*See* **Sims' position.**

legal—Authorized or based on law.

legal disability—A condition in which a person does not have legal capacity and is therefore unable to enter into a legal agreement (e.g., as is the case with a minor).

lens—Crystalline structure suspended behind the pupil of the eye; refracts or bends light rays onto the retina; also, the magnifying glass in a microscope.

lethargy—Abnormal drowsiness or sluggishness; state of indifference or stupor.

letterhead—Preprinted heading at the top of paper used for written correspondence.

leukocyte—White blood cell (WBC).

leukocyte count—Blood test that counts the total number of white blood cells (normally 5,000 to 10,000 cells per cubic millimeter of blood).

libel—False written statement that causes a person ridicule or contempt or causes damage to the person's reputation.

licensure—Process by which a government agency authorizes individuals to work in a given occupation.

life stages—Stages of growth and development experienced by an individual from birth to death.

ligament—Fibrous tissue that connects bone to bone.

light diet—Also called a *convalescent diet;* diet that contains easy-to-digest foods.

line angle—Area on crown surfaces of a tooth formed by a line drawn between two surfaces.

liner—Dental material that covers or lines exposed tooth tissue, usually in the form of a varnish.

lingual surface—The crown surface of teeth that is next to the tongue.

listen—To pay attention, make an effort to hear.

lithotomy position—The patient lies on the back with the feet in stirrups and knees flexed and separated.

liver—Largest gland in the body; located in the upper right quadrant of the abdomen; two of its main functions are excreting bile and storing glycogen.

living will—A legal document stating a person's desires on what measures should or should not be taken to prolong life when his or her condition is terminal.

low-cholesterol diet—Diet that restricts foods high in saturated fat.

low-protein diet—Diet that limits foods high in protein.

low-residue diet—Diet that limits foods containing large amounts of residue, or indigestibles.

low-speed handpiece—Slower handpiece in dental units; used to remove caries and for fine finishing work.

lung—Organ of respiration located in the thoracic cavity.

lymph—Fluid formed in body tissues and circulated in the lymphatic vessels.

lymph node—A round body of lymph tissue that filters lymph.

lymphatic duct—Short tube that drains purified lymph from the right sides of the head and neck and the right arm.

lymphatic vessels—Thin-walled vessels that carry lymph from tissues.

lysosomes—Those structures in the cytoplasm of a cell that contain digestive enzymes to digest and destroy old cells, bacteria, and foreign matter.

M

macule—A discolored but neither raised nor depressed spot or area on the skin.

magnetic resonance imaging (MRI)—Process that uses a computer and magnetic forces, instead of X-rays, to visualize internal organs.

mainframe computer—Largest type of computer; many users can access this computer at the same time.

malignant—Harmful or dangerous; likely to spread and cause destruction and death (e.g., cancer).

malnutrition—Poor nutrition; without adequate food and nutrients.

malpractice—Providing improper or unprofessional treatment or care that results in injury to another person.

mammogram—X-ray examination of the breasts.

mandible—Horseshoe-shaped bone that forms the lower jaw; only movable bone of the skull.

master's degree—Degree awarded by a college or university after completion of one or more years of prescribed study beyond a bachelor's degree.

mastication—The process of chewing with the teeth.

Material Safety Data Sheets (MSDSs)—Information sheets that must be provided by the manufacturer for all hazardous products.

matriarchal—Social organization in which the mother or oldest female is the authority figure.

maxilla—Upper jawbone; two bones fused or joined together.

meatus—External opening of a tube (e.g., the urinary meatus).

mechanical lift—Special device used to move or transfer patient.

medial—Pertaining to the middle or midline.

Medicaid—Government program that provides medical care for people whose incomes are below a certain level.

medical history—A record that shows all diseases, illness, and surgeries that a patient has had.

medical record—Also called a *patient chart;* written record of a patient's diagnosis, care, treatment, test results, and prognosis.

Medicare—Government program that provides medical care for elderly and/or disabled individuals.

medication—Drug used to treat a disease or condition.

medulla—Inner, or central, portion of an organ.

medulla oblongata—The lower part of the brain stem; controls vital processes such as respiration and heartbeat.

medullary canal—Inner, or central, portion of a long bone.

meiosis—The process of cell division that occurs in gametes, or sex cells (ovum and spermatozoa).

melanin—Brownish-black pigment found in the skin, hair, and eyes.

memorandum—A short, written statement or message.

meninges—Membranes that cover the brain and spinal cord.

menopause—Permanent cessation of menstruation.

mental—Pertaining to the mind.

mesial surface—The side surface of teeth that is toward the midline of the mouth.

metabolism—The use of food nutrients by the body to produce energy.

metacarpal—Bone of the hand between the wrist and each finger.

metastasis—The spread of tumor or cancer cells from the site of origin.

metatarsal—Bone of the foot between the instep and each toe.

microcomputer—Desktop or personal computer found in the home or office.

microorganism—Small, living plant or animal not visible to the naked eye.

microscope—Instrument used to magnify or enlarge objects for viewing.

micturate—Another word for *urinate;* to expel urine.

midbrain—That portion of the brain that connects the pons and cerebellum; relay center for impulses.

middle adulthood—Period of development from 40 to 65 years of age.

midsagittal—An imaginary line drawn down the midline of the body to divide the body into a right side and a left side.

midstream specimen—Urine specimen in which urination is begun before catching the specimen in the specimen cup.

minerals—Inorganic substances essential to life.

mitered corner—Special folding technique used to secure linen on a bed.

mitochondria—Those structures in a cell that provide energy and are involved in the metabolism of the cell.

mitosis—Process of asexual reproduction by which cells divide into two identical cells.

mitral valve—Flap or cusp between the left atrium and left ventricle in the heart.

model—Also called a *cast;* a positive reproduction of the dental arches or teeth in plaster or similar materials.

modified block—Letter-writing format in which all parts of the letter start at the left margin except the heading, complimentary close, signature, and title, which start at the center line.

moist cold—An application that provides cold temperature and is wet against the skin.

moist heat—An application that provides warm temperature and is wet against the skin.

molars—Teeth in the back of the mouth; largest and strongest teeth; used to grind food.

motivated—Stimulated into action; incentive to act.

mouth—Oral cavity; opening to the digestive tract, or alimentary canal.

muscle tissue—Body tissue composed of fibers that produce movement.

muscle tone—State of partial muscle contraction providing a state of readiness to act.

myocardial infarction—Heart attack; a reduction in the supply of blood to the heart resulting in damage to the muscle of the heart.

myocardium—Muscle layer of the heart.

myopia—Nearsightedness; defect in distant vision.

myth—A false belief; an established belief with no basis.

N

nasal cavity—Space between the cranium and the roof of the mouth.

nasal septum—Bony and cartilaginous partition that separates the nasal cavity into two sections.

nasogastric tube—A tube that is inserted through the nose and goes down the esophagus and into the stomach.

nausea—A feeling of discomfort in the region of the stomach accompanied by the tendency to vomit.

necrosis—Death of tissue.

need—Lack of something required or desired; urgent want or desire.

needle holder—Instrument used to hold or support a needle while sutures (stitches) are being inserted.

negligence—Failure to give care that is normally expected, resulting in injury to another person.

neonate—Newborn infant.

neoplasm—New growth or tumor.

nephron—Structural and functional unit of the kidney.

nerve—Group of nerve tissues that conducts impulses.

nerve tissue—Body tissue that conducts or transmits impulses throughout the body.

net income—Amount of pay received for hours worked after all deductions have been taken out; take-home pay.

neurology—The study of the nervous system.

neuron—Nerve cell.

nocturia—Excessive urination at night.

noninvasive—Pertaining to a test or procedure that does not require penetration or entrance into the body.

nonpathogen—A microorganism that is not capable of causing a disease.

nonverbal—Without words or speech.

nose—The projection in the center of the face; the organ for smelling and breathing.

nosocomial—Pertaining to or originating in a health care facility such as a hospital.

nucleolus—The spherical body in the nucleus of a cell that is important in reproduction of the cell.

nucleus—The structure in a cell that controls cell activities such as growth, metabolism, and reproduction.

nutrition—All body processes related to food; the body's use of food for growth, development, and health.

nutritional status—The state of one's nutrition.

O

observation—To look at, watch, perceive, or notice.

obstetrics—The branch of medicine dealing with pregnancy and childbirth.

occlusal surface—The chewing or biting surface of posterior teeth.

occult—Hidden, concealed, not visible (e.g., an internal [occult] hemorrhage).

occult blood—Blood that is hidden; also, a test done on stool to check for the presence of blood.

occupational therapy—Treatment directed at preparing a person requiring rehabilitation for a trade or for return to the activities of daily living.

occupied bed—A bed that is made while the patient is in bed.

odontology—Study of the anatomy, growth, and diseases of the teeth.

olfactory—Pertaining to the sense of smell.

oliguria—Decreased or less-than-normal amounts of urine secretion.

ombudsman—Specially trained individual who acts as an advocate for others to improve care or conditions.

Omnibus Budget Reconciliation Act (OBRA)—Federal law that regulates the education and testing of nursing assistants.

oncology—The branch of medicine dealing with tumors or abnormal growths (e.g., cancer).

open bed—A bed with the top sheets fanfolded to the bottom.

ophthalmologist—A medical doctor who specializes in diseases of the eye.

ophthalmology—The study of the eye and diseases and disorders affecting the eye.

ophthalmoscope—An instrument used to examine the eye.

optician—An individual who makes or sells lenses, eyeglasses, and other optical supplies.

optometrist—A licensed, nonmedical practitioner who specializes in the diagnosis and treatment of vision defects.

oral—Pertaining to the mouth.

oral cavity—The mouth.

oral hygiene—Care of the mouth and teeth.

oral-evacuation system—Special machine that uses water to form a suction or vacuum system to remove liquids and particles from the oral cavity.

organ—Body part made of tissues that have joined together to perform a special function.

organ of Corti—Structure in the cochlea of the ear; organ of hearing.

organelles—Structures in the cytoplasm of a cell, including the nucleus, mitochondria, ribosomes, lysosomes, and Golgi apparatus.

origin—End or area of a muscle that remains stationary when the muscle contracts.

originator—The person who writes a check to issue payment.

orthodontics—The branch of dentistry dealing with prevention and correction of irregularities of the alignment of teeth.

orthopedics—The branch of medicine/surgery dealing with the treatment of diseases and deformities of the bones, muscles, and joints.

orthopnea—Severe dyspnea in which breathing is very difficult in any position other than sitting erect or standing.

orthotist—An individual skilled in straightening or correcting deformities by the use of orthopedic appliances (e.g., brace or special splints).

os coxae—The hipbone; formed by the union of the ilium, ischium, and pubis.

ossicles—Small bones, especially the three bones of the middle ear that amplify and transmit sound waves.

osteopathy—A field of medicine and treatment based on manipulation, especially of the bones, to treat disease.

osteoporosis—Condition in which bones become porous and brittle because of lack or loss of calcium, phosphorus, and other minerals.

ostomy—A surgically created opening into a body part.

otoscope—An instrument used to examine the ear.

output—Computer term for processed information, or the final product obtained from the computer; also, total amount of liquid expelled from the body.

ovary—Endocrine gland or gonad that produces hormones and the female sex cell, or ovum.

P

palate—Structure that separates the oral and nasal cavities; roof of the mouth.

pallor—Paleness; lack of color.

palpation—The act of using the hands to feel body parts during an examination.

pancreas—Gland that is dorsal to the stomach and that secretes insulin and digestive juices.

panoramic—Dental X-ray that shows the entire dental arch, or all of the teeth and related structures, on one film.

Papanicolaou test—Also called a *Pap test;* a test to classify abnormal cells obtained from the vagina or cervix.

papule—Solid, elevated spot or area on the skin.

paraffin wax treatment—Heated mixture of paraffin and mineral oil; used to provide a moist heat application.

paralysis—Loss or impairment of the ability to feel or move parts of the body.

paraplegia—Paralysis of the lower half of the body.

parasite—Organism that lives on or within another living organism.

parasympathetic—A division of the autonomic nervous system.

parathyroid—One of four small glands located on the thyroid gland; regulates calcium and phosphorus metabolism.

parenteral—Other than by mouth.

partial bath—Bath in which only certain body parts are bathed or in which the health care provider bathes those parts of the body that the patient is unable to bathe.

patella—The kneecap.

pathogen—Disease-producing organisms.

pathology—The study of the cause or nature of a disease.

pathophysiology—Study of how disease occurs and the responses of living organisms to disease processes.

patience—Ability to wait, persevere; capacity for calm endurance.

patients' rights—Factors of care that all patients can expect to receive.

patriarchal—Social organization in which the father or oldest male is the authority figure.

patriotism—Love and devotion to one's country.

payee—Person receiving payment.

pediatrics—The branch of medicine dealing with care and treatment of diseases and disorders of children.

pedodontics—The branch of dentistry dealing with treatment of teeth and oral conditions of children.

pegboard system—Method of maintaining financial accounts and records in an office.

pelvic—Pertaining to the pelvis area below the abdominal region and near the sacrum and hip bones.

penis—External sex organ of the male.

percussion—Process of tapping various body parts during an examination.

percussion hammer—Instrument used to check reflexes.

periapical—Around the apex of a root of a tooth; dental X-ray that shows the entire tooth and surrounding area.

pericardium—Membrane sac that covers the outside of the heart.

perineum—Region between the vagina and anus in the female and between the scrotum and anus in the male.

periodontal ligament—Dense fibers of connective tissue that attach to the cementum of a tooth and the alveolus to support or suspend the tooth in its socket.

periodontics—The branch of dentistry dealing with the treatment of the gingiva (gum) and periodontium (supporting tissues) surrounding the teeth.

periodontium—Structures that surround and support the teeth.

periosteum—Fibrous membrane that covers the bones except at joint areas.

peripheral—That part of the nervous system apart from the brain and spinal cord; also, a device connected to a computer.

peristalsis—Rhythmic, wavelike motion of involuntary muscles.

peritoneal—Pertaining to the body cavity containing the liver, stomach, intestines, urinary bladder, and internal reproductive organs.

permanent (succedaneous) teeth—The 32 teeth that make up the second, or permanent, set of teeth.

personal hygiene—Care of the body including bathing, hair and nail care, shaving, and oral hygiene.

perspiration—The secretion of sweat.

pH—A scale of 0 to 14 used to measure the degree of acidity or alkalinity of a substance, with 7 being neutral.

phalanges—Bones of the fingers and toes.

pharmacology—The study of drugs.

pharynx—The throat.

phlebitis—Inflammation of a vein.

phlebotomist—Also called a *venipuncture technician;* individual who collects blood and prepares it for tests.

physical—Of or pertaining to the body.

physical therapy—Treatment by physical means, such as heat, cold, water, massage, or electricity.

Physicians' Desk Reference (PDR)—Reference book that contains essential information on medications.

physiological needs—Basic physical or biological needs required by every human being to sustain life.

physiology—The study of the processes or functions of living organisms.

pineal—Glandlike structure in the brain.

pinna—Also called the *auricle;* external portion of the ear.

pituitary—Small, rounded endocrine gland at the base of the brain; regulates function of other endocrine glands and body processes.

placenta—Temporary endocrine gland created during pregnancy to provide nourishment for the fetus; the afterbirth.

plane—Flat or relatively smooth surface; an imaginary line drawn through the body at various parts to separate the body into sections.

plaque—Thin, tenacious, filmlike deposit that adheres (sticks) to the teeth and can lead to decay; made of protein and microorganisms.

plasma—Liquid portion of the blood.

platelet—*See* **thrombocyte.**

pleura—A serous membrane that covers the lungs and lines the thoracic cavity.

podiatrist—An individual who specializes in the diagnosis and treatment of diseases and disorders of the feet.

point angle—Area on the crown surface of a tooth that is formed when three surfaces meet.

poisoning—Condition that occurs when contact is made with any chemical substance that causes injury, illness, or death.

polycythemia—Excess number of red blood cells.

polydipsia—Excessive thirst.

polyuria—Increased production and discharge of urine; excessive urination.

pons—That portion of the brain stem that connects the medulla oblongata and cerebellum to the upper portions of the brain.

positron emission tomography (PET)—Computerized body scanning technique in which the computer detects a radioactive substance injected into a patient.

posterior—Toward the back; behind.

posterior teeth—Teeth toward the back of the oral cavity, including the bicuspids and molars.

postmortem care—Care given to the body immediately after death.

postoperative—After surgery.

postpartum—Following delivery of a baby.

Power of Attorney (POA)—A legal document authorizing a person to act as another person's legal representative or agent.

prefix—An affix attached to the beginning of a word.

prejudice—Strong feeling or belief about a person or subject that is formed without reviewing facts or information.

preoperative—Before surgery.

pressure (decubitus) ulcer—A pressure sore; a bedsore.

primary teeth—Also called deciduous teeth; the first set of 20 teeth.

privileged communications—All personal information given to health personnel by a patient; must be kept confidential.

proctoscope—Instrument used to examine the rectum.

prognosis—Prediction regarding the probable outcome of a disease.

projection—Defense mechanism in which an individual places the blame for his or her actions on someone else or circumstances.

pronation—Turning a body part downward; turning "palm down."

prone position—The patient lies on the abdomen, with the legs together and the face turned to the side.

prophylactic—Preventive; agent that prevents disease.

prophylaxis angle—Dental handpiece attachment that holds polishing cups, disks, and brushes used to clean the teeth or polish restorations.

prostate gland—In the male, gland near the urethra; contracts during ejaculation to prevent urine from leaving the bladder.

prosthesis—An artificial part that replaces a natural part (e.g., dentures or a limb).

prosthodontics—The branch of dentistry dealing with the construction of artificial appliances for the mouth.

protective isolation—*See* **reverse isolation.**

protein—One of six essential nutrients needed for growth and repair of tissues.

protoplasm—Thick, viscous substance that is the physical basis of all living things.

protozoa—Microscopic, one-celled animals often found in decayed materials and contaminated water.

proximal—Closest to the point of attachment or area of reference.

pruritus—Itching.

psychiatry—The branch of medicine dealing with the diagnosis, treatment, and prevention of mental illness.

psychology—The study of mental processes and their effects on behavior.

psychosomatic—Pertaining to the relationship between the mind or emotions and the body.

puberty—Period of growth and development during which secondary sexual characteristics begin to develop.

pulmonary—Pertaining to the lungs.

pulmonary valve—Flap or cusp between the right ventricle of the heart and the pulmonary artery.

pulp—Soft tissue in the innermost area of a tooth and made of nerves and blood vessels held in place by connective tissue.

pulse—Pressure of the blood felt against the wall of an artery as the heart contracts or beats.

pulse deficit—The difference between the rate of an apical pulse and the rate of a radial pulse.

pulse pressure—The difference between systolic and diastolic blood pressure.

puncture wound—Injury caused by a pointed object such as a needle or nail.

pupil—Opening or hole in the center of the iris of the eye; allows light to enter the eye.

pustule—Small, elevated, pus- or lymph-filled area of the skin.

pyrexia—Fever.

pyuria—Pus in the urine.

Q

quadriplegia—Paralysis below the neck; paralysis of arms and legs.

R

race—Classification of people based on physical or biological characteristics.

radial deviation—Moving toward the thumb side of the hand.

radiograph—X-ray; an image produced by radiation.

radiology—The branch of medicine dealing with X-rays and radioactive substances.

radiolucent—Transparent to X-rays; permitting the passage of X-rays or other forms of radiation.

radiopaque—Not transparent to X-rays; not permitting the passage of X-rays or other forms of radiation.

radius—Long bone of the forearm, between the wrist and elbow.

rale—Bubbling or noisy sound caused by fluid or mucus in the air passages.

random access memory (RAM)—Form of computer memory known as read/write memory because data can be stored or retrieved from it.

range of motion (ROM)—The full range of movement of a muscle or joint; exercises designed to move each joint and muscle through its full range of movement.

rate—Number per minute, as with pulse and respiration counts.

rationalization—Defense mechanism involving the use of a reasonable or acceptable excuse as explanation for behavior.

read only memory (ROM)—Nonerasable, permanent form of computer memory built into a computer to control many of the computer's internal operations.

reagent strip—Special test strip containing chemical substances that react to the presence of certain substances in the urine or blood.

reality orientation—Activities to help promote awareness of time, place, and person.

recall—To call back; letter or notice that reminds a patient to return for periodic treatment or examination.

receipt—Written record that money or goods has been received.

rectal, rectum—Pertaining to or the lower part of the large intestine, the temporary storage area for indigestibles.

rectal tube—Tube inserted into the rectum to aid in the expulsion of flatus (gas).

red marrow—Soft tissue in the epiphyses of long bones.

reference initials—Initials placed at the bottom of a letter to indicate the writer and/or preparer.

refractometer—An instrument used to measure the specific gravity of urine.

registration—Process whereby a regulatory body in a given health care area administers exams and/or maintains a list of qualified personnel.

rehabilitation—The restoration to useful life through therapy and education.

religion—Spiritual beliefs and practices of an individual.

repression—Defense mechanism involving the transfer of painful or unacceptable ideas, feelings, or thoughts into the subconscious.

resistant—Able to oppose; organisms that remain unaffected by harmful substances in the environment.

respiration—The process of taking in oxygen (inspiration) and expelling carbon dioxide (expiration) by way of the lungs and air passages.

responsibility—Being held accountable for actions or behaviors; willing to meet obligations.

restoration—Process of replacing a diseased portion of a tooth or a lost tooth by artificial means, including filling materials, crowns, bridges, or dentures.

restraints—Protective devices that limit or restrict movement.

resumé—A summary of a person's work history and experience, submitted when applying for a job.

retina—The sensory membrane that lines the eye and is the immediate instrument of vision.

retractor—Instrument used to hold or draw back the lips or sides of a wound or incision.

reverse isolation—Technique used to provide care to patients requiring protection from organisms in the environment.

rheostat—Foot control in dental units; used to operate handpieces.

rhythm—Referring to regularity; regular or irregular.

ribs—Also called *costae;* twelve pairs of narrow, curved bones that surround the thoracic cavity.

rickettsiae—Parasitic microorganisms that live on other living organisms.

root—The anatomic portion of a tooth that is below the gingiva (gums); helps hold the tooth in the mouth.

rotation—Movement around a central axis; a turning.

rubber base—Dental impression material that is elastic and rubbery in nature.

S

safety standards—Set of rules designed to protect both the patient and the health care worker.

saliva ejector—Handpiece in dental units that provides a constant, low-volume suction to remove saliva from the mouth.

salivary glands—Glands of the mouth that produce saliva, a digestive secretion.

salutation—A greeting; the greeting in a letter (e.g., "Dear").

satisfaction—Fulfillment or gratification of a desire or need.

scalpel—Instrument with a knife blade and used to incise (cut) skin and tissue.

scapula—Shoulder blade or bone.

sclera—White outer coat of the eye.

screen—To evaluate; to determine the purpose of telephone calls so they can be referred to the correct person.

scrotum—Double pouch containing the testes and epididymis in the male.

sebaceous gland—Oil-secreting gland of the skin.

secretion—Substance produced and expelled by a gland or other body part.

self-actualization—Achieving one's full potential.

self-esteem—Satisfaction with oneself.

self-motivation—Ability to begin or to follow through with a task without the assistance of others.

semicircular canals—Structures of the inner ear that are involved in maintaining balance and equilibrium.

seminal vesicle—One of two saclike structures behind the bladder and connected to the vas deferens in the male; secretes thick, viscous fluid for semen.

senile lentigines—Dark-yellow or brown spots that develop on the skin as aging occurs.

senility—Feebleness of body or mind caused by aging.

sensitive—Susceptible to a substance; organisms that are affected by an antibiotic in a culture and sensitivity study.

sensitivity—Ability to recognize and appreciate the personal characteristics of others.

septum—Membranous wall that divides two cavities.

serrated—Notched; toothed.

sharps container—A puncture-resistant container for disposal of needles, syringes, and other sharp objects contaminated by blood or body fluids.

shock—Clinical condition characterized by various symptoms and resulting in an inadequate supply of blood and oxygen to body organs, especially the brain and heart.

sigmoidoscope—Instrument used to examine the sigmoid, or S-shaped, section of the large intestine.

sign—Objective evidence of disease; something that is seen.

signature—A person's name written by that person.

Sims' position—The patient lies on his or her left side with the right leg bent up near the abdomen.

sinus—Cavity or air space in a bone.

sitz bath—Special bath given to apply moist heat to the genital or rectal area.

skeleton—The bony structure of the body.

skill—Expertness, dexterity; an art, trade, or technique.

SkillsUSA-VICA—A student organization for students enrolled in technical and industrial vocational programs.

skin puncture—A small puncture made in the skin to obtain capillary blood.

slander—Spoken comment that causes a person ridicule or contempt or damages the person's reputation.

small intestine—That section of the intestine that is between the stomach and large intestine; site of most absorption of nutrients.

smear—Material spread thinly on a slide for microscopic examination.

Snellen charts—Special charts that use letters or symbols in calibrated heights to check for vision defects.

social—Pertaining to relationships with others.

sodium-restricted diet—Special diet containing low or limited amounts of sodium (salt).

soft diet—Special diet containing only foods that are soft in texture.

soft palate—Tissue at the back of the roof of the mouth; separates the mouth from the nasopharynx.

software—Programs or instructions that allow computer hardware to function intelligently.

specific gravity—Weight or mass of a substance compared with an equal amount of another substance that is used as a standard.

speculum—Instrument used to dilate, or enlarge, an opening or passage in the body for examination purposes.

sphygmomanometer—Instrument calibrated for measuring blood pressure in millimeters of mercury (mm Hg).

spinal—Pertaining to the vertebral column or spinal cord.

spinal cord—A column of nervous tissue extending from the medulla oblongata of the brain to the second lumbar vertebra in the vertebral column.

spirituality—Individualized and personal set of beliefs and practices that evolve and change throughout an individual's life.

spleen—Ductless gland below the diaphragm and in the upper-left quadrant of the abdomen; serves to form, store, and filter blood.

sprain—Injury to a joint accompanied by stretching or tearing of the ligaments.

sputum—Substance coughed up from the bronchi; contains saliva and mucus.

standard precautions—Recommendations that must be followed to prevent transmission of pathogenic organisms by way of blood and body fluids.

statement–receipt—Financial form that shows charges, amounts paid, and balance due.

statistical data—Record containing basic facts about a patient, such as address, place of employment, insurance, and similar items.

stereotyping—Process of assuming that everyone in a particular group is the same.

sterile—Free of all organisms, including spores and viruses.

sterile field—An area that is set up for certain procedures and is free from all organisms.

sterilization—Process that results in total destruction of all microorganisms; also, surgical procedure that prevents conception of a child.

sternum—Breastbone.

stethoscope—Instrument used for listening to internal body sounds.

stoma—The opening of an ostomy on the abdominal wall.

stomach—Enlarged section of the alimentary canal, between the esophagus and the small intestine; serves as an organ of digestion.

stool—Material evacuated from the bowels; feces.

strain—Injury caused by excessive stretching, overuse, or misuse of a muscle.

stress—Body's reaction to any stimulus that requires a person to adjust to a changing environment.

stroke—*See* **cerebrovascular accident.**

subcutaneous—Beneath the skin.

subcutaneous fascia—Layer of tissue that is under the skin and connects the skin to muscles and underlying tissues.

sublingual—Under the tongue.

succedaneous teeth—The 32 teeth that make up the second set of teeth; also called permanent or secondary teeth.

sudoriferous gland—Sweat-secreting gland of the skin.

suffix—An affix attached to the end of a word.

suicide—Killing oneself.

superior—Above, on top of, or higher than.

supination—Turning a body part upward; turning "palm up."

supine position—The patient lies flat on the back, face upward.

suppository—Solid medication that has a base of cocoa butter or glycerine and is designed to melt after insertion into a body cavity (e.g., the rectum or vagina).

suppression—Defense mechanism used by an individual who is aware of unacceptable feelings or thoughts but refuses to deal with them.

surgery—The branch of medicine dealing with operative procedures to correct deformities, repair injuries, or treat disease.

surgical hose—Elastic or support hose used to support leg veins and increase circulation.

surgical scissors—Special scissors used to cut tissue.

surgical shave—Removal of hair and cleansing of skin prior to an operation.

suture—Surgical stitch used to join the edges of an incision or wound; also, an area where bones join or fuse together.

suture-removal set—Set of instruments, including suture scissors and thumb forceps, used to remove stitches (sutures).

sympathetic—That division of the autonomic nervous system that allows the body to respond to emergencies and stress; also, to understand and attempt to solve the problems of another.

symptom—A subjective indication of disease that is felt by the patient.

syncope—Fainting; temporary period of unconsciousness.

system—A group of organs and other parts that work together to perform a certain function.

systole—Period of work, or contraction, of the heart.

systolic pressure—Measurement of blood pressure taken when the heart is contracting and forcing blood into the arteries.

T

tachycardia—Fast, or rapid, heartbeat (usually more than 100 beats per minute in an adult).

tachypnea—Respiratory rate above 25 respirations per minute.

tactful—Able to do or say the correct thing; thoughtful.

tarsal—One of seven bones that forms the instep of the foot.

tartar—*See* **calculus.**

teamwork—Cooperative effort by the members of a group to achieve a common goal.

technician—A level of proficiency usually requiring a 2-year associate's degree or 3 to 4 years of on-the-job training.

technologist—A class of expertise in a health career field, usually requiring at least 3 to 4 years of college plus work experience.

teeth—Structures in the mouth that physically break down food by chewing and grinding.

temperature—The measurement of the balance between heat lost and heat produced by the body.

temporary—Dental material used for restorative purposes for a short period of time until permanent restoration can be done.

tendon—Fibrous connective tissue that connects muscles to bones.

tension—Uncomfortable inner sensation, discomfort, strain, or stress that affects the mind.

terminal illness—An illness that will result in death.

testes—Gonads or endocrine glands that are located in the scrotum of the male and that produce sperm and male hormones.

thalamus—That structure in the diencephalon of the brain that acts as a relay center to direct sensory impulses to the cerebrum.

therapeutic diet—Diet used in the treatment of disease.

therapy—Remedial treatment of a disease or disorder.

thermometer—Instrument used to measure temperature.

thermotherapy—Use of heat applications for treatment.

thoracic—Pertaining to the chest or thorax.

thoracic duct—Main lymph duct of the body; drains lymph from the lymphatic vessels into the left subclavian vein.

thrombocyte—Also called a *platelet;* blood cell required for clotting of the blood.

thrombus—A blood clot.

thymus—Organ in the upper part of the chest, lymphatic tissue and endocrine gland that atrophies at puberty.

thyroid—Endocrine gland that is located in the neck and regulates body metabolism.

tibia—Inner and larger bone of the lower leg, between the knee and ankle.

time management—System of practical skills that allows an individual to use time in the most effective and productive way.

tissue—A group of similar cells that join together to perform a particular function.

tissue forceps—An instrument with one or more fine points (teeth) at the tips of blades; used to grasp tissue.

tongue—Muscular organ of the mouth; aids in speech, swallowing, and taste.

tonometer—An instrument used to measure intraocular (within the eye) pressure.

tonsil—Mass of lymphatic tissue found in the pharynx (throat) and mouth.

tort—A wrongful or illegal act of civil law not involving a contract.

tourniquet—Device used to compress the blood vessels.

trachea—Windpipe; air tube from the larynx to the bronchi.

transdermal—Through the skin.

transfer (gait) belt—Band of fabric or leather that is placed around a patient's waist; grasped by the health care worker during transfer or ambulation to provide additional support for the patient.

transfusion—Transfer of blood from one person to another person; injection of blood or plasma.

transverse plane—Imaginary line drawn through the body to separate the body into a top half and a bottom half.

Trendelenburg position—The patient lies on the back with the head lower than the feet, or with both the head and feet inclined downward.

triage—A method of prioritizing treatment.

tricuspid valve—Flap or cusp between the right atrium and right ventricle in the heart.

tri-flow syringe—Handpiece in dental units that provides air, water, or a combination of air and water for various dental procedures.

trifurcated—Having three roots (as do some teeth).

tuning fork—An instrument that has two prongs and is used to test hearing acuity.

24-hour urine specimen—Special urine test in which all urine produced in a 24-hour period is collected in a special container.

tympanic membrane—The eardrum.

typing and crossmatch—A determination of blood types and antigens prior to a blood transfusion.

U

ulcer—An open lesion on the skin or mucous membrane.

ulna—Long bone in the forearm, between the wrist and elbow.

ulnar deviation—Moving toward the little finger side of the hand.

ultrasonic unit—Piece of equipment that cleans with sound waves.

ultrasonography—Noninvasive, computerized scanning technique that uses high-frequency sound waves to create pictures of body parts.

ultra-speed handpiece—High-speed handpiece used in dental units to cut and prepare a tooth during a dental procedure.

umbilicus—Naval; in slang, "belly button."

Universal Numbering System—Abbreviated means of identifying the teeth.

Unopette—Disposable, self-filling, blood-diluting pipette unit used for blood cell counts.

uremia—Excessive amounts of urea (a waste product) in the blood.

ureter—Tube that carries urine from the kidney to the urinary bladder.

ureterostomy—Formation of an opening on the abdominal wall for drainage of a ureter.

urethra—Tube that carries urine from the urinary bladder to outside the body.

urinalysis—Examination of urine by way of physical, chemical, or microscopic testing.

urinary-drainage unit—Special device used to collect urine and consisting of tubing and a collection container usually connected to a urinary catheter.

urinary meatus—External opening of the urethra.

urinary sediments—Solid materials suspended in urine.

urinate—To expel urine from the bladder.

urine—The fluid excreted by the kidney.

urinometer—Calibrated device used to measure the specific gravity of urine.

urology—The branch of medicine dealing with urine and diseases of the urinary tract.

uterus—Muscular, hollow organ that serves as the organ of menstruation and the area for development of the fetus in the female.

V

vaccine—Substance given to an individual to produce immunity to a disease.

vagina—Tube from the uterus to outside the body in a female.

vaginal irrigation—Also called *douche;* injection of fluid into the vagina.

variable expense—In a budget, an expense that can change or be adjusted (e.g., expenses for clothing and entertainment).

varicose—Pertaining to distended, swollen veins.

vas deferens—Also called the *ductus deferens;* the tube that carries sperm and semen from the epididymis to the ejaculatory duct in the male.

vasoconstriction—Constriction (decrease in diameter) of the blood vessels.

vasodilation—Dilation (increase in diameter) of the blood vessels.

vein—Blood vessel that carries blood back to the heart.

venipuncture—Surgical puncture of a vein; inserting a needle into a vein.

venous—Pertaining to the veins.

ventilation—Process of breathing.

ventral—Pertaining to the front, or anterior, part of the body; in front of.

ventricle—One of two lower chambers of the heart; also, a cavity in the brain.

venule—The smallest type of vein; connect capillaries and veins.

vertebrae—Bones of the spinal column.

vertigo—Sensation of dizziness.

vesicle—Blister; a sac full of water or tissue fluid.

vestibule—Small space or cavity at the beginning of a canal.

veterinary—Pertaining to the medical treatment of animals.

villi—Tiny projections from a surface; in the small intestine, projections that aid in the absorption of nutrients.

virus—One of a large group of very small microorganisms, many of which cause disease.

visceral—Pertaining to organs.

vital signs—Determinations that provide information about body conditions; include temperature, pulse, respirations, and blood pressure.

vitamins—Organic substances necessary for body processes and life.

vitreous humor—Jellylike mass that fills the cavity of the eyeball, behind the lens.

void—To empty the bladder; urinate.

volume—The degree of strength of a pulse (e.g., strong or weak).

voluntary—Under one's control; done by one's choice or desire.

vomit—To expel material from the stomach and/or intestine through the mouth and/or nose.

vulva—External female genitalia; includes the labia majora, labia minora, and clitoris.

W

walker—A device that has a metal framework and aids in walking.

warm-water bag—Rubber or plastic device designed to hold warm water for dry-heat application.

wellness—State of being in good health; well.

wheezing—Difficult breathing with a high-pitched whistling or sighing sound during expiration.

withdrawal—Defense mechanism in which an individual either ceases to communicate or physically removes self from a situation.

word root—Main word or part of word to which prefixes and suffixes can be added.

Worker's Compensation—Payment and care provided to an individual who is injured on the job.

wound—An injury to tissues.

X

xiphoid process—The small, bony projection at the lower end of the sternum (breastbone).

Y

yellow marrow—Soft tissue in the diaphyses of long bones.

Index

A

Abbreviations
    dental, 482, 486, 488
    medical, 88–94, 632
    medical records, 854
    states, 860
    symbols, 94, 486, 488
Abdominal
    cavity, 111, 112
    injuries, 428, 431
    regions, 111, 112
    thrusts, 386, 394–397
Abrasion, 398
Absorption, of nutrients, 163–164, 258
Abuse
    chemical/drug, 10, 61, 196, 249
    child, 76
    domestic, 76
    elder, 76, 249
    facilities, 10
    patient, 76, 249
Acceptance
    of criticism, 64
    of death, 200
Accidents
    first aid, 379–382, 398–403
    preventing, 285–291
Accounting system, 868–873
Accreditation, 27
Acculturation, 217–218
Acetone, urine, 603, 604, 605
Acne Vulgaris, 116
Acquired Immune Deficiency Syndrome, 184–185, 301, 306, 568
Acromegaly, 175
Activity director, 50, 53
Acupressure, 20, 224
Acupuncture, 20, 224
Addison's disease, 176
Adenitis, 154
Adipose tissue, 107

Administrator
    health care, 40
    medical records, 38, 39
Admitting
    officers/clerks, 40, 65, 272
    patients, 672–676
Adolescence, 189, 195–196
Adrenal gland, 174, 176
Adulthood
    early, 189, 196–197
    late, 189, 198–199, 233–251
    middle, 189, 197–198
Advance directives, 81–83
Aerobic organisms, 301
Affection, 203–204
Agar, 557–558, 562–565
Agency for Health Care Policy and Research (AHCPR), 11
Agent, 77
Aging
    confusion and disorientation, 245–248
    myths, 234–236
    needs, 198–199, 248–249
    physical changes, 198, 236–242
    psychosocial changes, 198–199, 242–245
Aide. See Assistant
AIDS, 184–185, 301, 306, 568
Air compressor, 491, 496
Air-water syringe, 492, 496
Airborne precautions, 337–339
Alcohol abuse, 61, 196, 261
Alginate, 511, 513–515
Alignment, 679–684
Alimentary canal, 161–164
Allergic reactions, 404, 407–408
Alopecia, 114
Alphabetical filing, 835, 838–841
Alternative therapies, 19–21, 223–224
Alveoli, 156, 157, 159, 238
Alzheimer's disease, 198, 246
AM care, 707–728
Amalgam, 498, 501, 503, 535–539
Amblyopia, 137

Ambulating patient, 808–820
Amino acids, 255
Amputation, 399
Anaerobic organisms, 301
Analgesia, 524
Analgesics, patient controlled (PCAs), 779–780
Anatomy, 102–187, 470–473
Anemia, 149–150, 572, 575, 582, 587
Anesthesia
    dental, 524–529
    minor surgery, 645, 646
    specialty, 43
    surgery, 779
    types, 524, 779
Anesthesiologist, 43
Aneurysm, 150
Anger, death, 200
Angioplasty, 151
Animal health technician, 55
Anorexia, 196, 261
Answering services, 844–845
Antibiotic resistant, 299, 558
Antibody screen, 592
Anticoagulant, 571, 709, 719
Antioxidants, 20, 224, 255, 256
Antisepsis, 302
Aphasia, 210
Apical pulse, 350, 369–372
Aplastic anemia, 149–150
Apnea, 365
Appearance, personal, 61–63
Appendix, 162, 164
Appendicitis, 165
Application
    job, 454–456
    letter of, 448–454
Applications, heat/cold, 420, 821–832
Appointment
    letter, 856
    scheduling, 847–850
Aquamatic pad, 821–822, 827–828
Aromatherapy, 20
Arrhythmia, 144–145, 364, 383

Art therapist, 51, 53
Arterial blood, 399, 567
Arteriosclerosis, 150, 198, 245
Artery, 146, 147
Arthritis, 122, 237, 596
Asepsis, 302, 303
Aspirating syringe, 524–529
Assault and battery, 76
Assignment sheet, 466
Assimilation, cultural, 217
Assistant
   dental, 31, 32, 470
   dietetic, 48–49
   education, 29
   geriatric, 17, 46, 47, 670–671
   home health care, 17, 46, 47,
     670–671
   medical, 41, 42, 43, 617–618
   medical laboratory, 33, 34,
     551–552
   mortuary, 45
   nurse, 17, 46, 47, 670–671
   occupational therapy, 50, 51
   ophthalmic, 56, 57
   physical therapist, 50, 52
   physician, 41, 42
   recreational therapy, 50, 53
   veterinary, 55
Assisted living facilities, 9
Associate's degree, 27, 29
Asthma, 158–159
Astigmatism, 137
Atherosclerosis, 150, 245, 253
Athlete's foot, 116, 300
Athletic trainer, 51, 53
Attorney, Power of, 81, 82
Audiologist, 51, 53
Aural temperature, 351–352, 353,
   360–361
Authorization, obtaining, 83, 288,
   682, 865
Autoclave, 302, 314–320
Autocratic leader, 67
Automated routing telephone
   system, 844
Autonomic nervous system,
   129, 132
Avulsion, 398–399
Axillary temperature, 351, 359–360
Ayer blade, 635, 636
Ayurvedic practitioner, 19

B

Bachelor's degree, 27, 29
Back
   blows, 386, 397
   supports, 284
Backrub, 709, 717–719

Bacteria, 298–299, 603
Bacterial slides, 557–567
Bandages, 399, 401–402, 424,
   437–442
Bargaining, 200
Bartholin's glands, 180, 182
Basal metabolic rate, 259
Bases, dental, 529–535
Bass method, 507–509
Bath
   bed, 707–710, 723–726
   Sitz, 821–822, 830–832
   tub, 707, 727–728
   waterless, 707–708
Battery, 76
Bed bath, 707–710, 723–726
Bedclothes, changing, 709,
   721–722
Bedmaking, 698–707
   closed, 698, 699–702
   cradle, 698, 706–707
   occupied, 698, 702–704
   open, 698, 705
   postoperative, 779, 784–785
Bedpan, 737–740
Bedsores. *See* Pressure ulcer
Belt, transfer or gait, 808, 813–815
Bias, 218–219
Bicuspids, 474
Bilirubin, 603, 604
Binders, 780, 787–789
Biofeedback, 20, 224
Biohazards, 306, 308, 310–311
Biological needs, 202
Biomedical equipment
   technician, 33, 34–35
Bite-wing X-ray, 541, 546
Bladder
   training program, 241, 744
   urinary, 168, 170, 198, 240–241
Bland diet, 264
Bleeding, first aid, 398–403
Blindness, 209–210, 631
Block-style letter, 857–860
Blood, 146–149, 551–601, 603
Blood and body fluid precautions.
   See Standard precautions
Blood cells
   anatomy, 146–149
   counting, 579–585
   erythrocytes (red), 146, 149,
     570, 574, 579–585, 587,
     595–597, 598, 603, 611
   leukocytes (white), 146–147,
     149, 579–582, 585–587,
     603, 611
   platelets, 148–149, 587
   thrombocytes, 148–149, 587
Blood film, 587–591
Blood pressure, 350, 372–376
Blood smear, 587–591

Blood tests, 268, 272, 274, 551–601
   cell counts, 579–587
   computers, 268, 272, 274
   differential, 587, 591
   erythrocyte sedimentation, 552,
     595–597
   fasting blood sugar, 598
   film, 587–591
   glucose, 552, 598–601
   glucose tolerance, 598
   glycohemoglobin, 598
   hematocrit, 551, 570–574
   hemoglobin, 552, 574–579
   microhematocrit, 551, 570–574
   quick stain, 588, 590–591
   skin puncture, 567–570
   smear, 587–591
   typing, 591–595
   Wright's stain, 588, 590–591
Blood typing, 591–595
Blood vessels, 146, 147, 148,
   149, 238
Bloodborne Pathogen Standard,
   287, 306
Body
   cavities, 111, 112
   defenses, 302
   fluids, 307
   mechanics, 283–285, 679
   planes, 110–111
   structure, 103–109
   systems, 108, 109, 113–186
Body positions
   bed, 679–681, 682–688
   dental chair, 409–491, 505–507
   examination, 625–630
   shock, 403–406
Bone injuries, 122, 123, 419–425
Bones, 108, 109, 117–124, 198, 237
Bookkeeping system, 868–873
Botanical medicine, 20
Bradycardia, 364
Bradypnea, 366
Brain
   anatomy, 130–131
   injury, 426–427, 430
   syndrome, 246
Breasts
   anatomy, 183
   self examination, 183–184
Breathing, 157–158, 198, 238,
   365–367, 384
Bronchitis, 159, 238
Brushing teeth
   method, 507–509
   oral hygiene, 708, 710–714
Buccal cavity, 111, 112, 162
Budget, 462–463
Bulimarexia, 196
Bulimia, 196
Bulk purchasing, 16

Bureau of Immigration Reform Act, 459
Burns
 chemical, 407, 409
 first aid, 410–414
 types, 410–411
Burs, dental, 493–494
Bursitis, 122
Business
 letters, 856–861
 skills, 834–882

C

Calcium hydroxide, 530, 532
Calculus, renal, 171
Calorie
 controlled diet, 263–264
 definition, 259
Cancer
 breast, 183–184
 cervical, 184
 lung, 159, 160
 ovarian, 184
 skin, 116
 testicular, 180
 uterus, 184
Canes, 810–812, 818–819
Cannula, oxygen, 790
Capillaries, 146
Capillary blood, 399, 567
Carbohydrate
 digestion, 162–164, 258
 function, 254
Carbon monoxide, 407
Carboxylate, 530, 533
Cardiac
 compressions, 384–393
 computer tests, 274
Cardiopulmonary resuscitation, 382–398
Cardiovascular
 system, 108–109, 142–152, 198, 238
 technologist, 32, 33
Career passport, 452–453
Careers, health care, 25–59, 103, 113, 118, 125, 129, 135, 142, 152, 155, 161, 168, 172, 178, 470, 551–552, 617, 670–671, 800
Caries, dental, 507, 535
Carpules, anesthetic, 524–529
Cartilage, 107, 198
Cataract, 137, 138, 239
Catheter
 condom, 742
 oxygen, 790
 urinary, 742–746

urine specimen, 743–744, 753–754
Caution, explanation of, 466
Cavity
 body, 111, 112
 dental, 507, 535
CDC, 11, 307, 337, 512
Cell
 stem, 106–107
 structure, 104–107, 109
Cellular
 respiration, 158
 telephone, 845
Cellulose, 254
Celsius temperature, 350, 351, 887–888
Cements, dental, 529–535
Centers for Disease Control and Prevention, 11, 307, 337, 512
Centigrade temperature, 350, 351, 887–888
Central nervous system, 129–132
Central/sterile supply technician, 40, 41
Cerebral palsy, 133
Cerebrospinal fluid, 132, 427, 430
Cerebrovascular accident (CVA), 133, 244, 245, 432–433, 436
Certification, 27, 470, 551, 617
Cervical cancer, 184
Chain
 of command, 13–15
 of infection, 301–302, 303
Chair
 dental, 490–491, 495, 505–507
 sitz, 821–822, 830–832
 transfer to, 681–682, 690–693
CHAMPUS, 13
Characteristics, personal, 61–63, 446–447
Charge slips, 868–869, 872–873
Charting
 admission, 672–676
 errors, 78, 84, 212
 Federation Dentaire International System, 477–478, 480
 intake and output, 728–733
 medical records, 38–40, 78–79, 211–212, 850–856
 teeth conditions, 483–489
 teeth surfaces, 481–483
 temperature, pulse, respiration, 354, 367–369
 Universal Numbering System, 476–477, 479
Checkpoints, explanation of, 466
Checks, 873–874, 876–877
Chemical
 abuse, 10, 61, 196

burns, 407, 409
 disinfection, 321–323
 Material Safety Data Sheets (MSDSs), 285–287, 290
 restraints, 772
Chest
 cavity, 111, 112
 compressions, 384–393
 injuries, 427–428, 430–431
Cheyne-Stokes respirations, 366
Child
 choking, 386, 394–398
 CPR, 385–386, 392–393
 growth and development, 189, 193–195
Chinese medicine, 19
Chiropractic, 19, 41, 224
Chlamydia, 185
Choking victim, 386, 394–398, 734–735
Cholecystitis, 165
Cholesterol
 definition, 254–255
 diet, 264
Chronic obstructive pulmonary disease (COPD), 159
Cilia, 156
Circulation, checking, 425, 438, 568, 773
Circulatory system, 108–109, 142–152, 198, 238
Cirrhosis, 165
Clean catch urine specimen, 753, 757–758
Cleansing enemas, 705, 764–769
Clinical laboratory
 assistant, 33, 34
 technician, 33, 34
 technologist, 33, 34
Clinical Laboratory Improvement Amendment (CLIA), 551–552
Clinics, 9–10
Clock, 24-hour, 889
Closed
 bed, 698, 699–702
 wound, 400–401
Clothing
 health worker, 62
 patient, 709, 721–722
Clotting, blood, 148–149
Cold
 applications, 420, 821, 823–824, 828–830
 exposure, 417–419
 first aid, 417–419
Colitis, 167
Colon, 162, 164
Color blindness, 631–632
Color-coded indexing, 836–837
Colostomy, 748, 749
Coma, diabetic, 434, 437

Communication
  barriers, 209–211
  careers, 38–40
  electronic (e-mail), 272, 845
  interruptions, 208
  language differences, 208,
    210–211
  non-English speaking, 77,
    210–211
  nonverbal, 209
  privileged, 78
  services, 38–40
  skills, 206–212
  verbal, 76, 206–211
  written, 76, 211–212
Communicable diseases, 336–341
Compensation, 205
Competence, 64
Complementary therapies, 19–21,
  223–224
Complete bed bath, 707–710,
  723–726
Composite, 498, 502, 503,
  535–537, 539–541
Compress, moist, 821–822,
  828–830
Computer, 78, 267–281, 837, 848,
  865, 870–871
  applications, 268, 271–277, 337,
    848, 865, 870–871
  assisted instruction, 268,
    276–277
  back-up system, 273, 837
  components, 269–271
  confidentiality, 78, 273, 837
  history, 268–269
  Internet, 278–280
  literacy, 268
Computerized tomography (CT),
  35, 268, 274–275
Conditions, teeth, 483–489
Condom catheter, 742
Confidential information, 78, 79,
  80, 84, 273, 846, 850, 854
Confusion, 244–248
Congestive heart failure, 150
Conjunctivitis, 137
Connective tissue, 107, 109
Consent, obtaining patient, 76,
  83–84, 288–289, 381, 625
Conservation, energy, 16
Constipation, 165
Contact precautions, 339–340
Continuing education units
  (CEUs), 27–28
Contracts, 77
Contracture, 127, 679–681
Convulsions, 133, 433, 436–437
Coronary
  occlusion, 151, 432, 436
  stent, 151

Correspondence. *See* Letters
Cost containment, 15–16
Counseling centers, 10
Cover letter, 448–454
Cowper's gland, 179
CPR, 382–398
CPT codes, 864–865, 867
Cradle, bed, 698, 706–707
Cranial cavity, 111, 112
Cranium, 109
Cretinism, 175–176
Cross index/references, 836, 839
Crossmatch blood, 592
Crutches, 809–810, 815–817
CT, 35, 268, 274–275
Cultural diversity, 210–211,
  215–232, 248, 249, 261, 854
  communication barrier, 210–211
  eye contact, 211, 222
  family organization, 219–220
  gestures, 222
  health beliefs, 210, 211,
    222–225, 226–229
  language, 210–211, 220–221
  personal space, 221–222
  religion, 225–230
  respecting, 210–211, 230,
    249, 854
  touch, 211, 221–222, 248
Culture, 210–211, 216, 249, 261
  beliefs, 210–211, 249, 261
  characteristics, 216
Cultures, 557–567
  agar, 557–558, 562–565
  Gram's stain, 558–559, 565–567
  obtaining, 557, 559–560
  slides, 557–558, 561–562
  transfers, 557–558, 561–565
Curing light, 537, 540
Current Procedural Terminology
  (CPT) codes, 864–865, 867
Cushing's syndrome, 176
Cuspidor, 493
Cuspids, 474
Custom trays, 522–523
Cuvette, 574–575, 577–578,
  600–601
Cyanosis, 115, 366, 710
Cystitis, 170

D

Dance therapist, 51, 53
Dangling, 681, 689–690
Data sheet, 850–856
Databases, 272, 837
Daydreaming, 205–206
Daysheet, 868, 869, 872–873
Deafness, 139, 209, 239

Death
  cultural beliefs, 211
  post-mortem care, 794–796
  religious beliefs, 226–229
  stages, 199–200
  types, 382
Deciduous teeth, 470–471, 472,
  474–476
Decubitus ulcer, 679, 680, 710, 774
Defamation, 76–77
Defense mechanisms, 205–206
Defibrillator, 145, 383
Deficit pulse, 370
Dehydration, 107, 412, 607, 728
Dementia, 246
Democratic leader, 67
Denial
  death, 199–200
  defense mechanism, 206
Dental
  abbreviations, 482, 486, 488
  anesthesia, 524–529
  assistant, 31, 32, 470
  bases, 529–535
  brushing, 507–509
  careers, 30–32
  carts, 492–494
  cements, 529–535
  chair, 490–491, 495, 505–507
  conditions, 483–489
  custom tray, 522–523
  equipment, 489–498
  Federation Dentaire
    International System,
    477–478, 480
  flossing, 507–508, 509–510
  handpieces, 493–494, 497–498
  hygienist, 31
  impressions, 510–517
  instruments, 498–505
  laboratories, 10
  laboratory technician, 31
  light, 490, 495, 505, 506
  models, 510–512, 517–522
  offices, 9
  oral hygiene, 507–510, 708,
    710–714
  radiographs, 541–547
  restoratives, 498, 503, 535–541
  skills, 468–549
  specialties, 31
  surfaces of tooth, 481–483
  symbols, 482, 486, 488
  trays, 498, 503, 504–505
  Universal Numbering System,
    476–477, 479
  X-rays, 541–547
Dentist, 31
Denture care, 708, 712–713
Department of Health and Human
  Services (USDHHS), 11, 551

Dependability, 64
Deposit slips, 874–875, 878–879
Depression, 200
Dermatitis, 116
Developing X-rays, 541–545
Diabetes
  first aid, 433–435, 437
  insipidus, 175, 607
  mellitus, 177, 433–434, 604, 607
Diabetic
  blood tests, 598
  coma, 434, 437
  diet, 263
Diagnosis codes, 862–864, 867
Diagnostic
  careers, 32–36
  cluster standards, 28–29, 30
  computers, 268, 272, 273–276
  related groups (DRGs), 15
  services, 32–36
  vascular technologist, 33
Dialysis, 53–54, 170, 171
Dialysis technician, 51, 53–54
Diaphoresis, 403, 710
Diarrhea, 165
Diastole, 143
Diastolic pressure, 372, 376
Diet, 61, 252–266
  balanced, 61, 259–261
  bland, 264
  calorie-controlled, 263–264
  diabetic, 263
  fat-restricted, 264
  feeding patient, 734–737
  five major food groups, 61,
    259–261
  liquid, 261–263
  low-cholesterol, 264
  low-residue, 264
  personal, 61, 259–261
  protein, 264
  regular, 61, 259–261
  religious restrictions, 261, 262
  requirements, 61, 259–261
  sodium-restricted, 264
  soft, 262
  therapeutic, 261–264
Dietary services, 48–49
Dietetic
  assistant, 48–49
  technician, 48–49
Dietitian, 48–49, 273
Differential count, 587, 591
Digestion, 162–164, 258
Digestive system, 108–109,
    161–167, 240, 258
Direct smear, 557, 561–562
Directives, legal, 81–83
Disability
  legal, 77
  physical, 209–210, 211, 244–248

Discharging patients, 672–674,
    677–678
Discretion, 64
Diseases
  aging, 198, 237–242, 244–246
  circulatory, 149–152, 198, 238
  communicable, 336–341
  cultural beliefs, 210, 211,
    222–225
  digestive, 165–167, 240
  ear, 139, 239
  endocrine, 175–176, 177, 241
  eye, 137–138, 239
  heart, 149–152, 238
  integumentary, 116–117,
    236–237
  International Classification of,
    862–864, 867
  lymphatic, 154
  muscular, 127–128, 237
  nervous, 133–134, 198, 238–240
  pathophysiology, definition, 104
  reproductive, 180, 183–184,
    241–242
  respiratory, 158–160, 238
  sexually transmitted, 184–186
  skeletal, 122–124, 237
  urinary, 170–171, 240–241
Disinfection, chemical, 302,
    321–323
Disk, ruptured, 123
Dislocation, 122, 419–425
Disorientation, 244–248
Displacement, 205
Disposable
  enema, 763, 767–769
  thermometer, 353, 354
Diverticulitis, 165–166
DNR order, 81, 386
Doctor
  degree, 27, 29
  dental, 31
  eye, 43, 56
  medical, 41–43
  psychiatric, 43, 44
Dorsal
  cavity, 111, 112
  recumbent position, 627–628
Drainage
  irrigation, 730
  urinary, 742–745, 747–748
Dress code, 61–63
Dressings
  application, 334–336, 401–402,
    437–442
  bandages, 399, 401–402, 424,
    437–442
  first aid, 401–402, 424, 437–442
  sterile, 326–336
  surgical, 779
  tape application, 336

  tray, 326–328, 330–332
  types, 399, 437
DRGs, 15
Drop technique, 326, 327, 328,
    330, 331
Droplet precautions, 339
Drug
  abuse, 10, 61, 196
  administering, 660–663
  *Physicians' Desk Reference
    (PDR)*, 658–660
  resistant organisms, 299, 558
Dry heat sterilization, 314
Durable Power of Attorney, 81, 82
Durelon, 530, 533
Dwarfism, 175
Dycal, 530, 532
Dying, stages of, 199–200
Dysphagia, 240, 734
Dyspnea, 238, 365, 710

E

Ear
  anatomy, 138–139
  diseases, 139
  examination, 634, 637–638
  injuries, 426, 430
Ear, eye, nose, throat (EENT)
    examination, 634, 637–638
Early adulthood, 189, 196–197
Early childhood, 189, 193–194
Earthquake safety, 293
Eating disorders, 196
Echocardiograph, 32, 35, 274
Eczema, 116
Edema, 107, 618, 710, 728
Educational requirements, 17,
    27–28, 29
Elastic
  bandages, 438
  hose, 780, 785–787
Elderly
  care, 16–17, 233–251
  confusion and disorientation,
    245–248
  myths, 234–236
  needs, 198–199, 248–249
  physical changes, 198, 236–242
  psychosocial changes, 198–199,
    242–245
Electrocardiogram, 32, 145, 274,
    636, 647–658
Electrocardiograph technician,
    28, 32, 33
Electroencephalographic
    technologist, 28, 32–34
Electroneurodiagnostic
    technologist, 33, 34

Electronic
mail, 272, 845
thermometers, 353, 362–363
Embalmer, 45
Embolus, 150
Emergency medical
paramedic, 37, 38
services, 10, 36–38, 380–381
technician, 36–38
Emotional
development, 189, 192–199
wellness, 18
Empathy, 63
Emphysema, 159, 238
Employability skills, 445–465
Employment Eligibility
Verification Form, 459
Encephalitis, 133
Endocrine system, 108–109,
172–177, 241
Endodontics, 31
Endogenous infection, 301
Endometriosis, 184
Enema, 763–770
disposable, 763, 767–769
oil retention, 763, 769–770
soap solution, 763, 764–767
tap water, 763, 764–767
Energy conservation, 16
English measurements,
665–666, 732
Enteral feedings, 729
Enthusiasm, 64
Entrepreneur, 28
Environmental services
cluster standards, 29, 30
careers, 40, 41
Enzymes, digestive, 162–163,
165, 258
Epididymitis, 180
Epiglottis, 156, 157
Epilepsy, 133
Epistaxis, 159, 427, 430
Epithelial tissue, 107, 109
Equipment
biomedical, 33, 34–35
dental, 489–498
personal protective, 306, 308,
309–310, 312–313
physical examination, 635,
636, 640
safety, 287–288, 290–291
Ergonomics, 283–285, 287
Erikson's stages of psychosocial
development, 190, 191
Errors, 78, 84, 212
Erythema, 115, 710
Erythrocyte
anatomy, 146, 149, 587, 598
count, 579–585
microhematocrit, 551, 570–574

sedimentation rate, 552, 595–597
urine, 603, 611
Esophagus, 162, 163, 258
Esteem, 204
Ethics, 79–80
Ethnic groups, 216–217, 218,
223–224
Ethnicity, 216–217, 218
Eustachian tube, 139
Evacuator, oral, 491–493, 496–497
Evaluation sheet, 467
Examination
breast self, 183–184
ear, eye, nose, throat (EENT),
634, 637–638
dental, 498, 503
gynecological, 634, 638–640
physical, 634–637, 640–642
positions, 625–630
testicular self, 180
Excretory system, 108–109,
167–171, 240–241
Exercises
benefits, 61
range of motion, 125, 126, 237,
801–808
Exogenous infection, 301
Expiration, 157, 365
Expressed contracts, 77
Extended care facility, 8–9
External respiration, 157–158
Extinguisher, fire, 292, 293–294
Extracorporeal circulation
technologist, 51, 54
Eye
anatomy, 136–137
cavity, 111, 112
changes in aging, 198, 239
contact, 211, 222
diseases, 137–138, 239
examination, 634, 637
injuries, 412, 414, 425–426, 429
irrigation, 412, 414
protection, 308, 309–310,
312–313
vision screening, 630–633

F

Face shields, 308, 309–310, 312–313
Facilities, health care, 8–11, 40
Fahrenheit temperatures, 350,
351, 887–888
Fainting, 433, 436
Fallopian tubes, 180–182
False imprisonment, 76
Family organization, 219–220
Fascia, 125
Fasting blood sugar, 598

Fats
digestion, 162–164, 258
function, 254–255
restricted-diet, 264
tissue, 107
Fax machine, 845–846
FDA, 11
Federation Dentaire International
System, 477–478, 480
Feeding
patient, 734–737
tube, 729
Female reproductive system,
180–184
Fever, 352
Fibromyalgia, 127
Filing records, 835–841
Fillings, dental, 498, 503, 535–541
Film
blood, 587–591
X-ray, 541–542
Financial records, 272, 868–873
Finger puncture, 567–570
Fire safety, 291–295
First aid, 378–444
abdominal injury, 428, 431
bandages, 399, 401–402, 424,
437–442
bleeding, 398–403
bone injury, 122, 123, 419–425
burn, 410–414
cardiopulmonary resuscitation,
382–398
cerebrovascular accident, 133,
244, 245, 432–433, 436
chest injuries, 427–428, 430–431
choking, 386, 394–398
cold exposure, 417–419
convulsion, 433, 436–437
diabetic reactions, 433–435, 437
dressings, 399, 401–402,
437–442
ear injury, 426, 430
emergency medical services,
10, 36–38, 380–381
epistaxis, 159, 427, 430
eye injury, 412, 414, 425–426, 429
fainting, 433, 436
fracture, 122, 123, 419–425
frostbite, 417–419
genital injury, 428–429, 431
head injury, 426–427, 430
heart attack, 151, 432, 436
heat exposure, 415–417
illness, 432–437
injury, 425–431
insect bite, 407, 409–410
joint injury, 122, 419–425
moving victim, 380, 381, 404, 422
nosebleed, 159, 427, 430
obstructed airway, 386, 394–398

poisoning, 406–410
priorities of care, 379–382
shock, 403–406
snakebite, 407, 410
stroke, 133, 244, 245,
432–433, 436
tick, 407, 410
triage, 381
wounds, 398–403
First responder, 37
Flossing teeth, 507–508, 509–510,
708, 710–714
Flu, 159–160
Foley catheter, 742
Food
feeding patient, 734–737
groups, 61, 259–261
nutrition, 252–266
pyramid, 61, 259–261
religious restrictions, 261, 262
service workers, 48–49
Food and Drug Administration
(FDA), 11
Foot drop, 127, 679–681
Forceps, transfer, 326–327,
329–330, 331
Forms
admission, 672–676
financial, 868–873
job application, 454–456
insurance, 862–868
intake and output, 728–733
medical, 850–856
Fowler's position, 626, 627, 629
Fracture bedpan, 738
Fractures, 122, 123, 419–425
Frontal plane, 110–111
Frostbite, 417–419
Full mouth X-rays, 541, 546
Funeral director, 45
Fungi, 299–300

G

Gait belt, 808, 813–815
Gaits
canes, 810–812, 818–819
crutches, 809–810, 815–817
Gallbladder, 164–165, 258
Gastroenteritis, 166
Gastrostomy tube, 729
Genetic counseling, 10, 150
Genital injury, 428–429, 431
Geographic filing, 835–836, 839
Geriatric
assistant, 17, 46, 47, 670–671
care, 16–17, 233–251
confusion and disorientation,
245–248

facilities, 8–9, 234–235, 243–244
late adulthood, 189, 198–199,
233–251
myths, 234–236
needs, 198–199, 248–249
physical changes, 198, 236–242
psychosocial changes, 198–199,
242–245
Geriatrician, 43
Gerontology, 234
Gestures, 222
Giantism, 175
Gingiva, 472
Gland
Bartholin's, 181, 182
Cowper's, 179
endocrine, 172–177
lacrimal, 136
lymph, 153
prostate, 179
salivary, 162–163, 258
sebaceous, 114, 115
sudoriferous, 114, 115
Glaucoma, 137–138, 239
Glomerulonephritis, 170
Glossary, 890–910
Gloves
donning and removing, 309,
312, 332–334
infection control, 308, 309, 312
isolation, 337, 339–340, 342
sterile, 327–328, 332–334
Glucose meter, 598–601
Glucose
blood, 552, 598–601
fasting blood sugar, 598
glycohemoglobin, 598
tolerance test, 598
urine, 603, 604, 605
Glycosuria, 598
Goiter, 175
Gonorrhea, 185, 298
Government
agencies, 11, 19
hospitals, 8
Gown
changing, 709, 721–722
infection control, 308, 309, 312
isolation, 337, 340, 341–343
Gram's stain, 558–559, 565–567
Graphing
National Center for Health
Statistics, 618, 619
TPR, 367–369
Graves' disease, 175
Groin temperature, 351
Gross income, 460–462
Growth and development, 188–214
Gynecological examination, 634,
638–640
Gynecologist, 43

H

Hair
anatomy, 114
care, 708, 715–716
standards for health workers, 63
Handpieces, dental, 493–494,
497–498
Handwashing, 289, 290, 303–306,
308, 309
Head
circumference, 618, 619,
623–624
injuries, 426–427, 430
Health
department, 11
information and
communications, 38–40
insurance, 12–13, 862–868
maintenance organizations,
11, 12
occupations education (HOE),
27, 29
services manager, 40
Health care
administrator, 40
advance directives, 81–83
alternative therapies, 19–21,
223–224
careers, 25–59, 103, 113, 118,
125, 129, 135, 142, 152, 155,
161, 168, 172, 178, 470,
551–552, 617, 670–671, 800
complementary therapies,
19–21, 223–224
core standards, 28, 30
cultural beliefs, 210, 211,
222–225
facilities, 8–11
geriatric, 16–17, 233–251
history of, 3–8
holistic, 18, 219
home, 10, 16, 17
hospice, 10, 200–201
industrial, 11
insurance, 12–13, 862–868
national plan, 22
Policy and Research Agency, 11
power of attorney (POA),
81, 82
records, 38–40, 78–79, 211–212,
850–856
religious beliefs, 225–230
school, 11
skill standards, 28–29, 30
systems, 2–24
trends, 15–22
Health occupations education
(HOE), 27, 29

Health Occupations Students of America (HOSA), 883–884
Hearing
aid, 139, 209, 239
loss, 139, 198, 207, 209, 239
Heart
anatomy, 108, 109, 142–145, 647–648
attack, 151, 432, 436
changes in aging, 198, 238
congestive failure, 150
echocardiograph, 32, 35, 274
electrical pathway, 144–145, 647–648
electrocardiogram, 32, 145, 274, 647–658
sounds, 370
stress test, 32, 274
Heat
applications, 420, 821, 825–832
cramps, 415–416
exhaustion, 415–416
sterilization, 314
stroke, 415–416
Height, 618–624
Hematocrit, 551, 570–574
Hemiplegia, 134, 244
Hemoccult slide, 755, 761–762
Hemocytometer counting chamber, 579–581, 584, 585–586
Hemodialysis machine, 53–54, 170, 171
Hemoglobin, 146, 552, 574–579, 598
Hemolytic disease, 592, 604
Hemophilia, 150
Hemorrhoids, 166
Hemovac, 730
Hepatitis, 166, 300–301, 306, 339, 568, 596, 604
Herbal medicine, 20
Hernia, 166
Herpes, 185, 300, 339
High-speed handpiece, 494, 497–498
Histologic technician, 34
History
of computers, 268–269
health care, 3–8
physical forms, 850–856
HMOs, 11, 12
Hodgkin's disease, 154
HOE, 27, 29
Holistic health care, 18, 219
Holter monitoring, 32
Home health care
agencies, 10, 16
assistant, 17, 46, 47, 670–671
Homeopaths, 19, 20, 224
Homeostasis, 351

Honesty, 64
Horizontal recumbent position, 625, 628–629
Hormones, 172, 173–174, 241
HOSA, 883–884
Hose, surgical, 780, 785–787
Hospice, 10, 200–201
Hospital, 8, 13–14, 268
Household measurements, 665–666, 732
Housekeeping worker, 40
Human
anatomy and physiology, 102–187
growth and development, 188–214
needs, 201–206
Hurricane safety, 293
Hydrocephalus, 133
Hydrotherapy, 20
Hygiene
health worker, 63
oral, 708, 710–714
patient, 707–728
Hygienist, dental, 31
Hyperglycemia, 598
Hyperopia, 137, 138, 631, 632
Hyperparathyroidism, 176
Hypertension, 150–151, 253, 372
Hyperthermia, 352, 415–416
Hyperthyroidism, 175
Hypnotherapy, 20, 224
Hypnotist, 19, 224
Hypoglycemia, 434–435, 598
Hypoparathyroidism, 176
Hypotension, 372
Hypothermia, 237, 352, 417–419
Hypothyroidism, 175–176

I

I & O records, 728–733
ICD-9–CM codes, 862–864, 867
Ice bag/collar, 821–824
Identifying patient, 83–84, 288, 291
Identifying teeth, 474–489
conditions, 483–489
Federation Dentaire International System, 477–478, 480
names, 474–476
surfaces, 481–483
Universal Numbering System, 476–477, 479
Ileostomy, 748
Illness
cultural beliefs, 210, 211, 222–225
first aid, 432–437

needs, 202–203, 204, 244–245, 749–750
terminal, 199–201, 211
Illustrator, medical, 38–40
Imagery, 20, 69, 224
Impaction, 763–764
Impetigo, 116, 339
Implied contracts, 77
Impressions, dental, 510–517
alginate, 511, 513–515
polysiloxane, 511–512
polysulfide, 511, 515–517
polyvinylsiloxane, 511–512
rubber base, 511, 515–517
Imprisonment, false, 76
Incision, 398
Incisor, 474
Income, 460–462
Incontinence, 170, 241, 744
Independence, elderly, 244
Independent living facilities, 9
Industrial health care centers, 11
Infant
cardiopulmonary resuscitation, 385, 392–393
choking, 386, 396–397
growth and development, 189, 190–192
head circumference, 618, 619, 623–624
height and weight, 190, 618, 619, 623–624
Infection
chain of, 301–302, 303
control, 297–347, 489–490, 494, 698
wound, 400, 402
Infectious-waste bags, 306, 308, 310–311, 313
Influenza, 159–160, 300, 339
Information
careers, 38–40
section, 466
services cluster standards, 29, 30
systems, 38–40, 268, 271–273
Informed consent, 76
Inhalation
medication, 662
oxygen, 293, 789–793
poison, 407, 409
Injection, types, 661
Injury
first aid, 425–431
preventing, 285–291
reporting, 290, 311
Insect bites, 407, 409–410
Inspiration, 157, 365
Instruments
chemical disinfection, 321–323
dental, 498–505
minor surgery, 642–643

physical examination, 635, 636, 640
sterilization, 314–320
suture removal, 643–644, 647
wrapping for autoclave, 314, 316–319
Insulin
function, 174, 177, 433–434
shock, 434–435, 437
Insurance
forms, 862–868
health, 12–13, 22
liability, 84
State Children's Health Program, 13
Intake and output records, 728–733
Integumentary system, 108–109, 113–117, 140, 198, 236–237
Internal respiration, 158
International Classification of Diseases (ICD), 862–864, 867
Internet, 278–280
Interpreter, 77, 210–211, 220–221, 854
Interview, job, 456–460
Intestine, 162, 163–164, 258
Intravenous (IV), 661, 730, 779
Invasion of privacy, 76
Inventory
personal list, 672, 675, 676, 678
supplies, 272, 273
Ionization therapy, 20
IRM, 530, 534–535
Iron-deficiency anemia, 149
Irrigation
enema, 763–770
eye, 412, 414
nasogastric tube, 730
types, 730
Ishihara method, 631–632
Isolation, 336–346

J

Jacket restraint, 773, 775–777
Jackknife position, 628, 630
Jaundice, 115, 710
Jewelry
health worker, 63
postmortem, care of, 794, 795
surgery, care of, 778, 783
valuables, care of, 672, 675, 676, 678, 778, 783, 794, 795
Job, 445–465
application, 454–456
cover letter, 448–454
income, 460–462
interview, 456–460

keeping skills, 446–447
resumé, 448–454
Joint
anatomy, 121
injuries, 122, 419–425
movements, 125, 126, 802–803
range of motion, 801–808
types, 121

K

Ketones, urine, 603, 604, 605
Key terms
anatomy and physiology, 103, 110, 113, 117, 124, 129, 135, 141–142, 152, 155, 161, 167–168, 172, 178
business and accounting skills, 835
careers in health care, 26
computers in health care, 268
cultural diversity, 216
dental assistant skills, 469
first aid, 379
geriatric care, 234
health care systems, 3
human growth and development, 189
infection control, 298
laboratory assistant skills, 551
legal and ethical responsibilities, 75
medical assistant skills, 617
medical terminology, 88
nurse assistant skills, 670
nutrition and diets, 253
personal qualities of a health care worker, 61
physical therapy skills, 800
preparing for the world of work, 446
safety, 283
vital signs, 349
Kidney, 168–169, 198, 240–241
Kilocalorie, 259
Knee-chest position, 626, 629
Kübler-Ross, Elizabeth, 199
Kyphosis, 123, 124

L

Laboratory
careers, 33–34, 551–552
dental, 10, 31
facilities, 10, 551–552
Improvement Amendment, 551–552

medical, 10, 33–34, 551–552
ophthalmic, 56, 57
skills, 550–615
waived tests, 551–552
Labstix, 605
Laceration, 398
Lacrimal gland, 136
Laissez-faire leader, 67
Language
barriers, 210–211
differences, 77, 210–211, 220–221, 854
therapist, 51, 53
Laryngitis, 160
Larynx, 156, 157, 635, 636
Late adulthood, 189, 198–199, 233–251
Late childhood, 189, 194–195
Law
civil, 75–77
criminal, 75
Laws
Bloodborne Pathogen Standard, 287, 306
Bureau of Immigration Reform Act, 459
Clinical Laboratory Improvement Amendment, 551–552
Needlestick Safety and Prevention Act, 306–307
Occupational Exposure to Hazardous Chemicals Standard, 285–287
Older American Act, 249
Omnibus Budget Reconciliation Act, 17, 47, 772
Patient Self-Determination Act (PSDA), 81–83
Patient's Bill of Rights, 80–81
Leadership, 66–67
Leads, ECG, 649–651
Ledger
appointment, 847–850
card, 869, 870, 872–873
financial, 868–873
Left lateral position, 626, 629
Legal
directives, 81–83
disability, 77
responsibilities, 17, 19, 30, 66, 75–79, 84, 201, 249, 287, 293, 382, 459, 551, 567, 671, 679, 716, 749, 772, 789, 802, 846, 850
Letters
application, 448–454
business, 856–861
Leukemia, 151, 587, 596
Leukocyte
anatomy, 146–147

Leukocyte, *(continued)*
  count, 579–582, 585–587
  types, 146–147, 149
  urine, 603, 611
Leukocytosis, 581
Leukopenia, 581
Liability insurance, 84
Libel, 77
Librarian, medical, 38–40
Lice, 185, 300, 339
Licensed Practical Nurse (LPN), 46, 47
Licensed Vocational Nurse (LVN), 46, 47
Licensure, 27, 551, 800
Life stages, 188–201
Ligament, 121
Lift, mechanical, 681–682, 695–697
Light
  curing, 537, 540
  dental, 490, 495, 505, 506
Limb restraints, 772–775
Lines of authority, 13–15
Linen
  bed, 698–699
  infection control, 308, 311, 345, 698–699
  isolation, 345
  wrapping autoclave, 316–318
Lipids
  digestion, 162–164, 258
  function, 254–255
Liquid
  diet, 261–263
  measurements, 663–664, 665, 730–731, 887–888
Listening, 208
Lithotomy position, 626–627, 629–630
Liver, 164, 165, 258
Living will, 81, 82
Long term care
  facilities, 8–9, 234–235, 243–244
  training programs, 17, 47, 772
  workers, 17, 46, 47, 670–671
Lordosis, 123, 124
Love, 203–204
Low-calorie diet, 263–264
Low-cholesterol diet, 264
Low-residue diet, 264
Low-speed handpiece, 493–494, 497
Lung
  anatomy, 156, 157
  cancer, 159, 160
Lymphangitis, 154
Lymphatic, system, 108–109, 152–154

M

Macrobiotic diet, 21
Magnetic resonance imaging (MRI), 35, 268, 275
Makeup, health worker, 63
Male reproductive system, 178–180
Malnutrition, 253–254
Malpractice, 75
Mammogram, 183–184
Managed care, 13
Mandibular
  block, 524
  bone, 119, 121, 474
  teeth, 474–475
Mask
  high efficiency particulate air, 338–339
  infection control, 308, 309–310, 312–313
  isolation, 338–339, 340, 341, 342–343
  oxygen, 790
Maslow's hierarchy of needs, 201–204
Mass purchasing, 16
Massage
  back, 709, 717–719
  Swedish, 21
  therapeutic, 21, 224
  therapist, 50, 52
Master's degree, 27, 29
Material Safety Data Sheets (MSDSs), 285–287, 290
Math
  conversion chart, 351, 732, 887–888
  English/household measurements, 665–666, 887–888
  metric measurements, 663–665, 732, 887–888
  Roman numerals, 663
  temperature conversion, 350, 887–888
Matriarchal, 220
Maxillary
  bone, 119, 121, 474
  infiltration, 524
  teeth, 474–475
Mechanical lift, 681–682, 695–697
Medicaid, 12–13
Medical
  abbreviations, 88–94, 854
  assistant, 41, 42, 43, 617–618
  careers, 41–43, 617–618
  doctor, 41–43
  emergency services, 10, 36–38, 380–381

illustrator, 38–40
laboratories, 10, 551–552
laboratory assistant, 33, 34, 551–552
laboratory technician, 33, 34, 551–552
laboratory technologist, 33, 34, 551–552
librarian, 38–40
offices, 9
skills, 616–668
specialties, 43
symbols, 95, 854
terminology, 95–100
transcriptionist, 38, 39
Medical records
  administrator, 38, 39
  careers, 38–40
  completing, 38–40, 78–79, 211–212, 850–856
  confidentiality, 78–79, 80, 84, 273, 846, 850, 854
  errors, 78, 84, 212
  filing, 835–841
  technician, 38, 39
Medical terminology, 87–101, 208
Medicare, 12–13
Medications
  dental anesthesia, 525, 528
  disposal of, 662
  math, 663–667
  Physician's Desk Reference (PDR), 658–660
  transdermal, 115, 661–662
  types, 660–662
Meditation, 21, 69, 224
Meiosis, 106–107
Melanoma, 116
Memorandums, telephone, 843–844, 846
Meniere's disease, 139
Meninges, 132
Meningitis, 133, 298, 339
Mental health
  careers, 41–43
  development, 189, 192–198
  facilities, 10
  services, 41–43
  technician, 44
  wellness, 18
Mercury
  dental, 535–536
  disposal, 352–353
  poisoning, 352–353, 535–536
Messages
  communication, 207–208
  telephone, 843–844, 846
Metabolism, 258–259
Metric
  conversion chart, 351, 732, 887–888

measurements, 663–665, 732, 887–888
Microbiology, 34, 298–303
Microhematocrit, 551, 570–574
Microorganism, 298–303
Microscope, 553–557
Middle adulthood, 189, 197–198
Midsagittal plane, 110, 111, 477
Midstream urine specimen, 753, 757–758
Military time, 889
Minerals, 254, 255, 257
Mitered corner, 698, 699–700
Mitosis, 105–106
Mitten
  restraint, 773
  transfer technique, 326, 327, 329
Models, dental, 510–512, 517–522
Modified-block letters, 857–860
Moist compress, 821–822, 828–830
Molars, 474
Montgomery straps, 780–781
Morgue kit, 794
Mortuary
  assistant, 45
  careers, 45–46
Mounting
  electrocardiogram, 653, 657, 658
  X-rays, 543, 546–547
Mouth
  anatomy, 162–163, 258, 470–473
  care, 507–510, 708, 710–714
Mouthpieces, 308, 311, 313, 383
Moving patient
  bed, 679–688
  chair, 681–682, 690–693
  emergency care, 380, 381, 404, 422
  mechanical lift, 681–682, 695–697
  stretcher, 681–682, 693–695
  wheelchair, 681–682, 690–693
MRI, 35, 268, 275
Multicompetent or multiskilled worker, 28
Multiple sclerosis, 134
Multistix, 605
Muscle
  aging changes, 198, 237–238
  anatomy, 124–128
  contracture, 127, 679–681
  movements, 125, 126, 802–803
  range of motion, 125, 126, 237, 801–808
  skeletal, 107–108, 125–128
  spasms, 128, 415–416
  tissue, 107–108, 109
  types, 107–108, 109
  using correctly, 283–285

Muscular
  dystrophy, 127
  system, 108–109, 124–128, 237, 238
Music therapist, 51, 53
Myasthenia gravis, 127
Myocardial infarction, 151, 432, 436
Myopia, 137, 138, 631, 632
Myths, aging, 234–236
Myxedema, 175–176

N

Nails
  anatomy, 114
  care, 708, 716–717
  health worker, 63
Name badge, 62
Nasal cavity, 111, 112
Nasogastric tube, 729
National Center for Health Statistics, 618, 619
National health care plan, 22
National Health Care Skill Standards (NHCSS), 28–29, 30
National Institutes of Health (NIH), 11, 19
Naturopaths, 19, 224
Needles
  dental anesthesia, 524–529
  disposal, 306–307, 308, 310, 313, 526–527, 568
Needlestick Safety and Prevention Act, 306–307
Needs
  elderly, 198–199, 248–249
  human, 201–206
Negligence, 75–76
Nephritis, 170, 171
Nephron, 169, 240
Nerve tissue, 107, 109, 129
Nervous system, 108–109, 129–134, 238–240
Net income, 460–462
Neuralgia, 134
Neurologist, 43
Neuron, 129, 130
NIH, 11, 19
Nonpathogen, 298
Nonprofit agencies, 11–12
Nonretention enemas, 763, 764–769
Nonverbal communication, 209
Nose
  anatomy, 140, 141, 156
  cavity, 111, 112
  examination, 634, 637
  injuries, 159, 427, 430

Nosebleed, 159, 427, 430
Nosocomial infection, 301
Note, explanation of, 466
Nuclear medicine technologist, 35
Numerical filing, 835, 839–840, 841
Nurse
  anesthetist, 46–47
  assistant, 17, 46, 47, 670–671
  careers, 46–48, 670–671
  educator, 46–47
  midwife, 46–47
  practical, 46, 47
  practitioner, 46–47
  registered, 46–47
  skills, 669–798
  vocational, 46, 47
Nursing homes, 8–9, 234–235, 243–244
Nutrients, 254–259, 260
Nutrition
  careers, 48–49
  diet, 252–266
  feeding patient, 734–737
Nutritionist, 48, 49

O

OBRA, 17, 47, 772
Observations, 211–212, 379–380, 634, 682, 709–710, 738, 744, 750, 780
Obstetrician, 43
Obstructed airway, 386, 394–398, 734–735
Obstructive pulmonary disease, 159
Obtaining direct smear, 557, 559–560
Occult blood, stool, 552, 755, 761–762
Occupational Exposure to Hazardous Chemicals Standard, 285–287
Occupational health clinics, 11
Occupational Safety and Health Administration (OSHA), 11, 285, 306, 373
Occupational therapist, 49–51
Occupied bed, 698, 702–704
Odontology, 470
Office
  business and accounting skills, 834–882
  dental, 9
  medical, 9, 13–14, 616–668
Office of Alternative Medicine (OAM), 19
Oil retention enema, 763, 769–770

Older American Act, 249
Olfactory receptors, 140, 141
Ombudsman, 249
Omnibus Budget Reconciliation Act (OBRA), 17, 47, 772
Oncologist, 43
Open
　bed, 697, 705
　wound, 398–399
Operating room technician, 46, 47–48
Operative care, 777–787
Ophthalmic
　assistant, 56–57
　laboratory technician, 56–57
　medical technologist, 56
　technician, 56–57
Ophthalmologist, 43, 56
Ophthalmoscope, 632, 635, 636
Opportunistic infection, 301
Optical centers, 10
Optician, 56, 57
Optometrist, 56
Oral
　cavity, 111, 112, 162–163, 258, 470–473
　evacuator, 491–493, 496–497
　intake, 788
　hygiene, 507–510, 708, 710–714
　medication, 660–661
　surgery, 31, 498, 502–503
　temperature, 351, 353, 354, 356–357, 362
Orbital cavity, 111, 112
Orchitis, 180
Orderlies, 47, 670–671
Organ
　anatomy, 108, 109
　donation, 226–229
Organisms
　classes of, 298–301
　human, 102–186
Organizational structure, 13–15
Orthodontics, 31
Orthopedist, 43
Orthopnea, 366
OSHA, 11, 285, 306, 373
Osteomyelitis, 122
Osteopathic medicine, 41
Osteoporosis, 122, 237, 253, 802
Ostomy care, 748–752
Otitis, 139, 339
Otosclerosis, 139
Otoscope, 635, 636
Outpatient services, 10, 15–16
Output records, 728–733
Ovarian cancer, 184
Ovaries, 174, 177, 180, 181
Oximeter, pulse, 791–792
Oxygen, 293, 789–793

P

Pacemaker, cardiac, 145
Paging systems, 845
Pain, 223–224, 240, 349, 779–780
Pajamas, changing, 709, 721–722
Palliative care, 200–201
Pancreas, 165, 174, 177, 258
Pancreatitis, 166
Panoramic X-ray, 542
Papanicolaou (Pap) test, 634
Paralysis, 134, 244, 277, 422, 772
Paramedic, 37, 38
Paraplegia, 134, 277
Parasympathetic nervous system, 67, 132
Parathyroid gland, 174, 176
Parenteral medications, 661
Parkinson's disease, 134
Partial bed bath, 707
Passport, career, 452–453
Pathogens, 298–301
Pathologist, 34, 43
Pathophysiology. *See* Diseases
Patience, 64
Patient care technician, 46, 47, 65, 670–671
Patient controlled analgesics (PCAs), 779–780
Patient Self-Determination Act (PSDA), 81–83
Patient's
　rights, 19, 80–81, 224, 249
　safety, 84, 240, 246, 288–289, 291
Patriarchal, 220
PDR, 658–660
Pediatrician, 43
Pedodontics, 31
Pegboard system, 868–873
Pelvic
　cavity, 111, 112
　girdle, 120–121
　inflammatory disease (PID), 184
Peptic ulcer, 167
Perfusionist, 51, 54
Periapical X-rays, 541
Perineal care, 725–726, 738
Perineum, 182, 183
Periodontics, 31, 541
Periodontium, 472, 473
Peripheral nervous system, 129, 132
Peritonitis, 166–167
Permanent teeth, 470–471, 472, 475–476
Pernicious anemia, 150
Personal
　appearance, 61–63
　characteristics, 63–64, 446–447

　hygiene, 63
　protective equipment, 306, 308, 309–310, 312–313
　qualities, 61–64, 446–447
　safety, 202–203, 290, 291, 311
　space, 221–222
PET, 35, 268, 275
Pet therapy, 21
pH of urine, 603, 604, 605
Pharmacist, 50, 51–52, 272–273
Pharmacy technician, 50, 52
Pharynx, 156–157, 162, 163
Phlebitis, 151
Phlebotomist, 33, 34
Photometer, 574–575, 577–579
Physiatrist, 43
Physical
　abuse, 76, 249
　changes of aging, 198, 236–242
　development, 189, 190–198
　disabilities, 209–210, 211, 244–248
　examination, 634–642
　needs, 202
　records, 850–856
　restraints, 772–777
　therapist, 50, 52, 53, 800
　therapy, 52, 799–833
　wellness, 18
Physician
　assistant, 41, 42
　careers, 41–43
　specialties, 9, 43
Physicians' Current Procedural Terminology, 864–865, 867
Physicians' Desk Reference (PDR), 658–660
Physiological needs, 202
Physiology, 102–187
Phytochemicals, 21
Pick-up transfer technique, 326–327, 329–330, 331
Pigmentation of skin, 115
Pineal body, 174, 177
Pipettes, diluting, 581, 582–584, 585
Pituitary gland, 172–173
Placenta, 174, 177
Planes, body, 110–111
Plaque, 507
Plasma, 146
Plaster models, 510–512, 517–519
Platelets, 148–149, 587
Play therapy, 21
Pleurisy, 160
Pneumonia, 160, 298, 339
Podiatric medicine, 41
Poisoning, first aid, 406–410
Polycythemia, 572, 575, 582
Polysiloxane, 511–512

Polysomnographic technologist, 34
Polysulfide, 511, 515–517
Polyvinylsiloxane, 511–512
Portfolio, career, 452–453
Positron emission tomography
        (PET), 35, 268, 275
Positioning patient
    bed, 679–688
    dental chair, 490–491, 505–507
    examinations, 625–630
    shock, 403–406
Positive thought, 21, 69
Postmortem care, 794–796
Postoperative, 779–781, 784–787
Post-secondary education, 27
Posture, 61
Power of Attorney (POA), 81, 82
PPOs, 12
Practical nurse, 46, 47
Precautions, standard. *See*
        Standard precautions
Preferred Provider Organizations
        (PPOs), 12
Prefixes, 95–100
Prejudice, 210, 218–219
Premenstrual syndrome (PMS), 184
Preoperative, 777–779, 781–784
Presbyopia, 137, 138
Pressure
    bandage, 399, 401–402
    points, 399–400, 402
    ulcer, 679, 680, 710, 774
Preventive services, 16
Primary teeth, 470–471, 472,
        474–476
Privacy
    invasion of, 76
    providing, 288, 625, 738, 852–853
Privileged communications, 78
Procedure section, 466
Professional
    appearance, 61–63
    education, 27, 29
    ethics, 79–80
    negligence, 75–76
    standards, 83–85
Projection, 205
Prone position, 625–626, 629
Prostate gland, 179, 241
Prostatic hypertrophy, 180
Prosthodontics, 31
Protective
    equipment, personal, 306, 308,
        309–310, 312–313
    isolation, 340
Proteins
    diet, 264
    digestion, 162–164, 258
    function, 254, 255
    urine, 603, 604, 605
Protoplasm, 104

Protozoa, 299, 300
Psoriasis, 117
Psychiatric technician, 44
Psychiatrist, 43, 44
Psychiatry careers, 43–45
Psychological
    abuse, 76, 249
    barriers to communication,
        210, 749–750
Psychologist, 44
Psychosocial
    changes, 190, 192–199, 242–245
    development, 190, 191, 192–199
Puberty, 195
Pubic lice, 185
Pulmonary disease, 159
Pulse
    apical, 350, 369–372
    deficit, 370
    oximeter, 791–792
    pressure points, 399–400, 402
    pressure, 372
    radial, 350, 363–365
    rates, 363–364
    sites, 364
Puncture
    skin, 567–570
    wound, 398
Pyelonephritis, 171
Pyramid, food, 259–261
Pyrexia, 352

Q

Quadrants, abdominal, 111, 112
Quadriplegia, 134, 277
Quick stain, 588, 590–591

R

Race, 217
Radial pulse, 399–400, 402
Radiation therapist, 35
Radiographer, 35
Radiologist, 34, 43
Radiology
    careers, 33, 34–35
    dental, 541–547
Rales, 366
Range-of-motion (ROM) exercises,
        125, 126, 237, 801–808
Rationalization, 205
Reagent strips
    automated strip reader, 605
    blood, 598–601
    glucose, 598–601
    urine, 551, 602–607

Reality orientation, 247–248
Recap device, 526–527, 529
Receipts, 874, 879–880
Records
    admission, 672–676
    dental, 483–489
    filing, 835–841
    financial, 868–873
    insurance, 862–868
    intake and output, 728–733
    medical, 38–40, 78–79, 211–212,
        850–856
Recreational therapist, 50,
        52–53
Rectal
    enemas, 763–770
    examination, 641
    medication, 661
    temperature, 351, 353,
        358–359, 362
    tube, 764, 770–772
Rectum, 162, 164
Red blood cells. *See* Erythrocytes
Reflex actions, 190
Reflexology, 21
Refractometer, 607–610
Regions, abdominal, 111, 112
Registered nurse, 46–47
Registration, 27, 551
Regular diet, 61, 259–261
Rehabilitation
    careers, 49–55
    facilities, 11
Reiki, 20
Religion, 225–230, 249, 261, 262
Renal
    calculus, 171
    failure, 171
Reporting
    errors, 78, 84, 212
    injuries, 290, 311
    observations, 211–212
Repression, 206
Reproductive system, 108–109,
        178–186, 241–242
Research, computer, 268, 277
Resident's Bill of Rights, 80–81
Resistant, antibiotic, 299, 558
Respiration
    counting, 350, 365–366
    process, 157, 365
    stages, 157–158
Respiratory
    infection, 160
    system, 108–109, 155–160, 238
    therapist, 50, 53
    therapy technician, 50, 53
Responder, first, 37
Restorative materials
    amalgam, 498, 501, 503,
        535–539

Restorative materials, *(continued)*
  composite, 498, 502, 503, 535–537, 539–541
  instruments, 503
Restraints, 772–777
Resumé, 448–454
Resuscitation devices, 308, 311, 313, 383
Retention enemas, 763, 769–770
Retirement, 235, 242
Reverse isolation, 340
Rh factor, 591–592, 594–595
Rhinitis, 160
Ribs, 120, 121
Rickettsiae, 300
Right to die, 201
Rights, patient's, 19, 80–81, 224, 249
Ringworm, 117, 300
Roman numerals, 663
ROMs, 125, 126, 237, 801–808
Roots, word, 95–100
Rubber base impression, 511, 515–517
Ruptured disk, 123

S

Safety, 84, 202–203, 240, 246, 282–296
  environment, 240, 246, 290–291
  equipment, 287–288, 290–291
  ergonomics, 283–285, 287
  fire, 291–295
  material data sheets, 285–287, 290
  medications, 662–663
  needs, 202–203
  oxygen, 293, 791, 793
  patient, 84, 240, 246, 288–289, 291, 812, 814, 822
  personal, 202–203, 290, 291
  precautions, 84, 285–290
  solutions, 287–288, 290
Salary, 460–462
Saliva
  ejector, 492, 496
  functions, 162–163, 258
Salivary gland, 162–163, 258
Sanitary manager, 40
Satellite clinics/centers, 9–10
SCANS skills, 453
Scheduling appointments, 272, 847–850
School health services, 11
Scoliosis, 123, 124
Search engines, 278–279
Sebaceous gland, 114, 115, 236
Secondary
  education, 27

teeth, 470–471, 472, 475–476
Secretary
  skills, 834–882
  unit, 38, 39
Sedimentation
  erythrocyte, 552, 595–597
  urine, 602, 610–613
Sediments, urinary, 602, 610–613
Seizure, 133, 433, 436–437
Self-actualization, 204
Senses, special, 108–109, 135–141, 211, 379
Sensitivity
  personal, 218
  study, 558, 563
Sexual abuse, 76, 249
Sexuality, 203–204, 241–242
Sexually transmitted diseases, 184–186
Sharps, disposal of, 306–307, 308, 310, 313, 526–527
Shaving
  operative, 778, 781–782
  patient, 709, 719–720
Shingles, 134, 337
Shock
  first aid, 403–406
  insulin, 434–435, 437
  types, 404
Shoes, 63
Shower, 707, 727–728
Sickle cell anemia, 150, 587
Sigmoid colon, 162, 164
Sigmoidoscope, 635
Sim's position, 626, 629
Sinuses, 119, 156
Sinusitis, 160, 339
Sitz bath, 821–822, 830–832
Skeletal system, 108–109, 117–124, 237
Skilled care facilities, 8–9
SkillsUSA-VICA, 883–886
Skin
  aging, 198, 236–237
  anatomy, 108–109, 113–117, 140, 236–237
  burns, 410–414
  chemical injuries, 407, 409
  layers, 113–114
  preparation, surgery, 778, 781–782
  puncture, 398, 567–570
Skill Standards, National Health Care, 28–29, 30
Slander, 77
Slides
  bacterial, 557–567
  blood, 587–591
  hemoccult, 755, 761–762
  urine, 602, 610–613
Slings, 422, 424–425

Smear
  blood, 587–591
  culture, 557–567
  direct, 557, 561–562
Smell, 140, 141, 240
Snakebite, 407, 410
Snellen chart, 630–631
Soap solution enema, 763, 764–767
Social
  changes in aging, 199, 242–245
  development, 189, 192–199
  services, 43–45
  wellness, 18
  worker, 44
Sociologist, 44
Sodium-restricted diet, 264
Soft diet, 263
Solutions
  chemical, 285–287, 321
  safety, 285–288, 290
  ultrasonic, 323–326
Sonographer, 35
Space, personal, 221–222
Spasm, muscle, 128, 415–416
Specific gravity, urine, 603, 607–610
Specimens
  culture, 557–567
  stool, 755, 760–762
  urine, 602, 605, 610, 743–744, 752–760
Speculum, 635, 636
Speech impairment, 210
Speech-language therapist, 51, 53
Sphygmomanometer, 372, 373–374, 635, 636
Spinal
  anesthesia, 779
  cavity, 111, 112
  column, 119–120
  cord, 132
  curvatures, 123, 124
Spiritual
  therapies, 21, 226–229
  wellness, 18
Spirituality, 225
Spleen, 153–154
Splenomegaly, 154
Splints, 420–425
Sports medicine, 43
Sprains, 122, 420
Spreadsheets, 272
Standard precautions, 306–313, 336–337, 489–490, 494, 512, 559, 568, 602, 636–637, 644, 698–699, 710, 732, 738, 744–745, 750, 755, 764, 781, 822
Standards
  Bloodborne Pathogen, 287, 306

National Health Care Skill, 28–29, 30
Occupational Exposure to Hazardous Chemicals, 285–287
professional, 83–85
safety, 84, 285–290
State abbreviations, 860
Statement-receipt, 868, 869, 872–873
Statistical data sheet, 850–856
Stem cell, 106–107
Stent, coronary, 151
Stereotype, 210, 218–219
Sterile supply technician, 40, 41
Sterile techniques, 326–336, 642–647
  dressing change, 334–336
  dressing tray, 326–328, 330–332
  gloves, 332–334
  minor surgery, 642–646
  opening supplies, 326–330
  suture removal, 643–644, 646–647
  tray set-up, 326–328, 330–332, 642–647
Sterile urine specimen, 743–744, 753–754
Sterilization, 302, 314–320
  autoclave, 314–320
  dry heat, 315–316
  wrapping for, 314, 316–319
Sternum, 120, 121, 338
Stethoscope, 369, 370, 374, 635, 636
Stoma, 748, 750
Stomach, 162, 163, 258
Stone models, 510–512, 520
Stool specimen, 552, 755, 760–762
Strabismus, 138
Straight binder, 787–789
Strains, 128, 420
Stress
  management, 67–69
  test, 32, 274
Stretcher, 681–682, 693–695
Stroke
  cerebrovascular, 133, 244, 245, 432–433, 436
  heat, 415–416
Subject filing, 836
Sublingual medication, 662
Succedaneous teeth, 470–471, 472, 475–476
Sudoriferous gland, 114, 115, 236
Suffixes, 95–100
Sugar
  blood, 552, 598–601
  nutrient, 254
  urine, 603, 604, 605
Suicide, 196
Supine position, 625, 628–629

Suppository, 661, 764
Suppression, 206
Surfaces, teeth, 481–483
Surgeon, 43
Surgery
  careers, 43, 46, 47–48
  dental, 31, 498, 502–503
  minor, 642–646
  oral, 31, 498, 502–503
  tray, 642–646
Surgical
  care, 777–787
  clinics/centers, 10
  extraction tray, 498, 502–503
  hose, 780, 785–787
  instruments, 498, 642–643
  technologist/technician, 46, 47–48
Suture removal, 643–644, 646–647
Symbols
  dental, 482, 486, 488
  medical, 95, 854
  religious, 225–230, 249
Sympathetic nervous system, 67, 132
Syphilis, 185, 299
Syringes
  air-water, 492, 496
  aspirating, 524–529
  tri-flow, 492, 496
Systems
  body, 108–109, 113–186
  health care, 2–24
Systole, 143
Systolic pressure, 372, 375, 376

T

Tachycardia, 364
Tachypnea, 366
Tact, 64
T'ai Chi, 21, 224
Tap-water enema, 763, 764–767
Tape application, 336
Taste, 139–140, 240
Taxes, 460–462
Teamwork, 64, 65–66, 447
Technician
  animal health, 5
  biomedical equipment, 33, 35–36
  central/sterile supply, 40, 41
  dental laboratory, 31
  diagnostic vascular, 33
  dialysis, 51, 53–54
  dietetic, 48–49
  education, 29
  electrocardiograph, 28, 32, 33
  emergency medical, 36–38

  medical laboratory, 33, 34, 551–552
  medical records, 38, 39
  mental health, 44
  nurse, 46, 47
  ophthalmic, 56–57
  ophthalmic laboratory, 56, 57
  patient care, 46, 47
  pharmacy, 50, 52
  psychiatric, 44
  respiratory therapy, 50, 53
  surgical, 46, 47–48
  veterinary, 55
Technologist
  cardiovascular, 32, 33
  education, 29
  electroencephalographic, 28, 32–34
  electroneurodiagnostic, 33, 34
  extracorporeal circulation, 51, 54
  medical laboratory, 33, 34
  nuclear medicine, 35
  ophthalmic medical, 56
  polysomnographic, 34
  radiologic, 33, 34–35
  surgical, 46, 47–48
  ultrasound, 35
Teeth
  abbreviations, 482, 486, 488
  anatomy, 162, 163, 470–473
  brushing, 507–509, 708, 710–714
  conditions, 483–489
  deciduous, 470–471, 472, 474–476
  eruption, 470–471
  Federation Dentaire International System, 477–478, 480
  flossing, 507–508, 509–510
  function, 470–472, 474
  identification, 474–476
  impressions, 510–517
  models, 510–512, 517–522
  oral hygiene, 507–510, 708, 710–714
  permanent, 470–471, 472, 475–476
  primary, 470–471, 472, 474–476
  radiographs, 541–547
  restoratives, 498, 503, 535–541
  secondary, 470–471, 472, 475–476
  succedaneous, 470–471, 472, 475–476
  surfaces, 481–483, 507
  tissues, 470–473
  types, 474
  Universal Numbering System, 476–477, 479
  X-rays, 541–547

Telemedicine, 17–18
Telephone, 842–847
Temperature, 349–363
    aural, 351–352, 353, 360–361
    axillary, 351, 359–360
    charting, 354, 367–369
    converting, 350, 888
    graphing, 367–369
    groin, 351
    oral, 351, 353, 354, 356–357, 362
    rectal, 351, 353, 358–359, 362
    regulation, 114–115, 131,
        349–350, 351
    thermometers, 350, 352–353
    tympanic, 351–352, 353,
        360–361
    variations, 351–352
Tendon, 125
Tent, oxygen, 790
Terminal illness, 199–201, 211
Terminology
    medical, 95–100
    *Physician's Current Procedural
        Terminology*, 864–865, 867
Testes, 174, 177, 178, 179, 241
Testicular
    cancer, 180
    self-examination, 180
Tests, waived, 551–552
Tetanus, 400, 402
Thallium scan, 32
Therapeutic
    careers, 49–55
    cluster standards, 28–29, 30
    diets, 261–264
    massage, 21, 224
    services, 49–55
    touch, 21, 224
Therapist
    art, music, dance, 51, 53
    education, 29
    massage, 50, 52
    occupational, 49–51
    physical, 50, 52, 53
    radiation, 35
    recreational, 50, 52–53
    respiratory, 50, 53
    speech/language, 51, 53
Therapy
    alternative/complementary,
        19–21, 223–224
    pet, 21
    play, 21
    spiritual, 21, 226–229
Thermometer
    cleaning, 354–356
    clinical, 350, 352–356
    disposable, 353, 354
    electronic, 353, 362–363
    mercury disposal, 352–353
    reading, 353–354

tympanic, 351–352, 353,
    360–361
types, 350, 352–353
Thoracic
    cavity, 111, 112
    duct, 153, 154
Thought, positive, 21, 69
Thrombocyte, 148–149, 587
Thrombolytic drugs, 133, 151, 433
Thrombophlebitis, 151
Thrombus, 151, 238
Thymus, 154, 174, 177
Thyroid gland, 174, 175–176
Time, military, 889
Tissues
    body, 107–108, 109
    lymph, 152–154
    teeth, 470–473
Tobacco abuse, 61
Tongue, 139–140, 635
Tonometer, 632, 635, 636
Tonsillitis, 154
Tonsils, 153
Toothbrushes, 507–508
Toothpastes, 508
Topical anesthetic, 524
Tornado safety, 293
Torts, 75–77
Touch
    cultural differences, 211,
        221–222, 248
    healing, 20
    nonverbal communication,
        209, 248
    therapeutic, 21, 224
TPR graphs, 367–369
Trachea, 156, 157
Training, health care, 27, 29
Transcriptionist, medical, 38, 39
Transdermal medication, 115,
    661–662
Transfer
    belt, 808, 813–815
    forceps, 326–327, 329–330, 331
Transfers
    chair, 681–682, 690–693
    culture specimens, 557–565
    gait belt, 808, 813–815
    mechanical lift, 681–682,
        695–697
    room/unit, 672–674, 676–677
    sterile, 326–330, 331
    stretcher, 681–682, 693–695
    wheelchair, 681–682, 690–693
Translator, 77, 210–211, 220–221,
    854
Transmission-based isolation,
    336–346
Transient ischemic attacks (TIAs),
    245–246
Transverse plane, 110, 111, 477

Trays
    custom, 522–523
    dental, 498, 503, 504–505
    dressing, 326–328, 330–332
    minor surgery, 642–646
    sterile technique, 326–332
    suture removal, 643–644,
        646–647
Trendelenberg position,
    627–628, 630
Trends
    health care, 15–22
    historical, 3–8
Triage, 381, 842–843
TRICARE, 13
Trichomonas vaginalis, 185–186
Tri-flow syringe, 492, 496
Trimming models, 521–522
Tub bath, 707, 727–728
Tub, sitz, 821–822, 830–832
Tube
    catheter, 742–746
    drainage, 730, 742–746, 780
    feedings, 729
    gastrostomy, 729
    nasogastric, 729
    rectal, 764, 770–772
Tuberculosis, 160, 299, 337
Tuning fork, 635, 636
Turning patient, 681, 686–688
24-hour
    clock, 889
    urine specimen, 754–755,
        759–760
Tympanic
    membrane, 139
    temperature, 351–352, 353,
        360–361
Typing blood, 591–595

U

Ulcer
    digestive, 167
    pressure, 679, 680, 710, 774
    skin, 116, 679, 680, 710, 774
Ulcerative colitis, 167
Ultrasonic cleaning, 323–326
Ultrasonography, 35, 268, 275–276
Ultrasound technologist, 35
Uniforms, 62
Unit coordinator, 38, 39
Unit secretary, 38, 39
Universal Numbering System,
    476–477, 479
Universal precautions. *See*
    Standard precautions
Unopette, 581, 582–584, 585
Uremia, 171

Ureterostomy, 748
Urethritis, 171
Urinal, 737–738, 741
Urinalysis, 602–605
Urinary
    calculus, 171
    catheter care, 742–746
    conditions, 170, 241
    drainage unit, 742–745,
        747–748
    sediments, 602, 610–613
    system, 108, 109, 167–171,
        240–241
Urine
    components, 170, 603, 604, 611
    production, 169–170, 240–241
    specimens, 602, 605, 610,
        743–744, 752–760
Urine tests, 602–613
    reagent strips, 551, 602–607
    sediment, 602, 610–613
    specific gravity, 603, 607–610
    urinalysis, 602–605
Urinometer, 607, 608–609
Urobilinogen, 603, 604, 605
U.S. Department of Health and
    Human Services (USDHHS),
    11, 551
Uterus, 181, 182, 241

Venipuncture, 567
Venous blood, 399, 567
Ventilation, 157
Ventral cavity, 111, 112
Ventricles
    brain, 130, 132
    heart, 142, 143
Verbal
    abuse, 76, 249
    communication, 206–211
Verrucae, 117, 300
Vertebrae, 119–120
Veterinarian, 55
Veterinary careers, 55
VICA, 884–886
Villi, 163–164
Viruses, 300–301, 302
Vision
    aging changes, 198, 239
    careers, 56–57
    defects, 137–138, 207, 209–210,
        239, 631, 632
    screening, 630–633
    services, 10, 56–57
Vital signs, 348–377, 778, 779
Vitamins, 254, 255, 256
Voluntary agency, 11–12
Vomiting, inducing, 406–407, 409
Vulva, 182–183

Weight, 259, 618–624
Wellness, 18, 253
Wheelchair, 681–682, 690–693
White blood cell. *See* Leukocyte
Will, Living, 81, 82
Withdrawal, 206
Word
    elements, 95–100
    processing, 272
Work
    applying for, 445–465
    changes in aging, 199, 235, 242
Workers' compensation, 13
World Health Organization
    (WHO), 11
Wounds
    cleansing, 400, 402
    dressing, 334–336, 402
    first aid, 398–403
    types, 398–399
Wraps
    autoclave, 314, 316–319
    bandage, 439–442
Wright's stain, 588, 590–591
Written consent, 76

Vaccine
    hepatitis, 166, 300–301, 306
    influenza, 160
Valuables, care of, 672, 675, 676,
    678, 778, 783, 794, 795
Varicose veins, 152, 166
Varnish, dental, 529, 530–531
Vasectomy, 179
Veins
    anatomy, 146, 148, 149
    obtaining blood, 567
    varicose, 152, 166

Walker, 812, 819–820
Ward clerk, 38, 39
Warm water bag, 821–822,
    825–827
Warts, 117, 300
Washing hands, 289, 290,
    303–306, 308, 309
Waste
    disposal, 306, 308, 310–311, 313
    mercury spill, 352–353, 536
Water, 254, 255
Waterless bath, 707–708

X-rays
    careers, 33, 34–35
    dental, 541–547

Yoga, 21, 224

Z

Zinc phosphate, 530
Zinc oxide eugenol, 530, 534–535